Introduction to Epilepsy

Introduction to Epilepsy

Edited by
Gonzalo Alarcón

Antonio Valentín
Institute of Psychiatry, King's College London, London, and King's College Hospital, London, UK

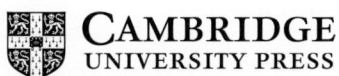

CAMBRIDGE UNIVERSITY PRESS
Cambridge, New York, Melbourne, Madrid, Cape Town,
Singapore, São Paulo, Delhi, Mexico City

Cambridge University Press
The Edinburgh Building, Cambridge CB2 8RU, UK

Published in the United States of America
by Cambridge University Press, New York

www.cambridge.org
Information on this title: www.cambridge.org/9780521691581

© Cambridge University Press 2012

This publication is in copyright. Subject to statutory exception
and to the provisions of relevant collective licensing agreements,
no reproduction of any part may take place without
the written permission of Cambridge University Press.

First published 2012

Printed in the United Kingdom at the University Press, Cambridge

A catalogue record for this publication is available from the British Library

Library of Congress Cataloging-in-Publication Data

Introduction to epilepsy / edited by Gonzalo Alarcón, Antonio Valentín.
  p. ; cm.
  ISBN 978-0-521-69158-1 (Paperback)
  I. Alarcón, Gonzalo, 1960– II. Valentín, Antonio, 1969–.
  [DNLM: 1. Epilepsy. WL 385]
  LC classification not assigned
  616.8′53–dc23
                                                                    2011030293

ISBN 978-0-521-69158-1 Paperback

Cambridge University Press has no responsibility for the persistence or
accuracy of URLs for external or third-party Internet websites referred to
in this publication, and does not guarantee that any content on such
websites is, or will remain, accurate or appropriate.

Every effort has been made in preparing this book to provide accurate
and up-to-date information which is in accord with accepted standards
and practice at the time of publication. Although case histories are
drawn from actual cases, every effort has been made to disguise the
identities of the individuals involved. Nevertheless, the authors, editors
and publishers can make no warranties that the information contained
herein is totally free from error, not least because clinical standards are
constantly changing through research and regulation. The authors,
editors and publishers therefore disclaim all liability for direct or
consequential damages resulting from the use of material contained in
this book. Readers are strongly advised to pay careful attention to
information provided by the manufacturer of any drugs or equipment
that they plan to use.

To Professors Colin D. Binnie and Charles E. Polkey, who inspired, developed and taught Epileptology at the Denmark Hill Campus, London, for over 20 years.

Contents

List of contributors xii
Foreword by Dr Edward H. Reynolds xvi
Preface xvii
Acknowledgements xviii

Section 1 Basic principles

1. **History of epilepsy** 1
   Edward H. Reynolds

2. **What is epilepsy?** 6
   Gonzalo Alarcón

3. **Functional anatomy of the central nervous system** 8
   Gonzalo Alarcón

4. **Introduction to neurochemistry and receptor pharmacology** 17
   Gonzalo Alarcón

5. **Cellular electrophysiology: membrane, synaptic and action potentials** 22
   Gonzalo Alarcón

6. **Techniques used to study epilepsy in the laboratory: experimental techniques in basic neurophysiology** 31
   Antonio Valentín

7. **Techniques used to study epilepsy in the laboratory: neuropathological methods** 35
   Nuria T. Villagra and Istvan Bodi

8. **Functional anatomy and physiology of the hippocampus** 37
   Gonzalo Alarcón

9. **Neurotransmission and biochemistry of neurotransmitters in epilepsy** 40
   Brian Meldrum

10. **Experimental models of epilepsy** 46
    John G. R. Jefferys

11. **Epileptogenesis in vitro** 52
    Antonio Valentín

12. **Epileptogenesis in vivo** 58
    Gonzalo Alarcón

13. **Neuropathology of epilepsy** 64
    Istvan Bodi and Mrinalini Honavar

14. **Introduction to the electroencephalogram (EEG)** 76
    Gonzalo Alarcón

15. **Phenomenology of normal EEG: effects of age and state of awareness** 81
    Franz Brunnhuber

16. **Pathological EEG phenomena and their significance** 96
    Lee Drummond

Section 2 Classification and diagnosis of epilepsy

17. **Electroclinical classification of seizures and syndromes** 107
    Gonzalo Alarcón

18. **Clinical use of EEG in epilepsy** 119
    Gonzalo Alarcón

19. **General overview of epileptic syndromes in childhood and adolescence** 131
    Archana Desurkar

20. **Neonatal seizures** 142
    Ronit Pressler

Contents

21 **Epileptic encephalopathies in the first year of life** 150
William Whitehouse

22 **Epileptic encephalopathies in early childhood** 153
William Whitehouse

23 **Febrile convulsions/seizures and related epileptic syndromes** 156
William Whitehouse

24 **Idiopathic focal epilepsies** 158
Colin D. Ferrie

25 **The idiopathic generalized epilepsies** 163
Colin D. Ferrie

26 **Temporal lobe epilepsy** 168
Robert D. C. Elwes

27 **Frontal lobe epilepsy** 174
Gonzalo Alarcón

28 **Parietal and occipital focal symptomatic epilepsies** 177
Gonzalo Alarcón

29 **Epilepsy and myoclonus** 181
Gonzalo Alarcón

30 **Progressive myoclonic epilepsies** 185
J. Helen Cross

31 **Acute symptomatic seizures** 189
Gonzalo Alarcón

32 **EEG in neonates and children** 191
Sushma Goyal

33 **Applications of EEG other than epilepsy** 213
Bidi Evans

34 **Evoked potentials in epilepsy** 217
Graham E. Holder

35 **Introduction to neuroimaging and relevant anatomical landmarks** 224
Gonzalo Alarcón and Jozef M. Jarosz

36 **The role of structural imaging in the assessment of epilepsy** 226
Gonzalo Alarcón, Antonio Valentín, Richard P. Selway and Jozef M. Jarosz

37 **Indications for neuroradiological investigation of epilepsy** 237
Mark P. Richardson

38 **Volumetric MRI and MRI spectroscopy** 240
Andrew Simmons

39 **Functional MRI in epilepsy** 244
Mark P. Richardson

40 **SPECT in epilepsy** 248
T. J. von Oertzen

41 **PET in epilepsy** 252
Mathias Koepp

42 **Advanced MRI sequences – diffusion tensor imaging** 259
Mathias Koepp

43 **EEG-correlated fMRI in epilepsy** 266
Louis Lemieux

44 **Source localization methods** 269
Stefano Seri and Antonella Cerquiglini

45 **Magnetoencephalography in epilepsy** 273
Stefano Seri, Jade N. Thai and Paul L. Furlong

46 **History-taking and physical examination in epilepsy** 276
Gonzalo Alarcón

47 **The role of video-EEG monitoring in epilepsy** 281
Gonzalo Alarcón

48 **Cardiovascular syndromes simulating epilepsy** 285
R. Shane Delamont

49 **Sleep disorders simulating epilepsy** 287
Bidi Evans

50 **Psychiatric disorders mistaken for epilepsy** 290
John D. C. Mellers

51 **Differential diagnosis of epilepsy: migraine and movement disorders** 293
Yvonne Hart

52 **Differential diagnosis of epilepsy in children** 296
Elaine Hughes

53 **Investigation of newly diagnosed and chronic epilepsy in adults**   299
Robert D. C. Elwes

54 **The role of investigations in the management of epilepsy in children**   304
J. Helen Cross

55 **Case scenarios in paediatric epilepsy**   308
David McCormick

56 **Psychogenic non-epileptic seizures: diagnostic approach**   313
Franz Brunnhuber

57 **Seminar: paediatric EEG reporting session**   318
Ronit Pressler

Section 3 Epidemiology

58 **Epidemiology of epilepsy**   329
Gonzalo Alarcón

59 **Prognosis of newly diagnosed and chronic epilepsy**   332
Gonzalo Alarcón

60 **Single seizures**   335
Robert D. C. Elwes

61 **Epidemiology of epilepsy in childhood**   337
Euan M. Ross

62 **Mortality in epilepsy**   340
Lina Nashef

Section 4 Genetics of epilepsy

63 **Introduction to modern molecular genetics: a genetics timeline**   345
Robert Robinson

64 **Methods of molecular genetics**   347
Robert Robinson

65 **Progress in the genetics of the epilepsies**   350
Robert Robinson

Section 5 Management of epilepsy

66 **Neurochemistry of antiepileptic drug action**   353
Brian Meldrum

67 **Antiepileptic drug pharmacokinetics and therapeutic drug monitoring**   358
Philip N. Patsalos

68 **Antiepileptic drug trials and their methodology**   367
Graeme J. Sills

69 **Treatment with traditional antiepileptic drugs**   374
Robert D. C. Elwes

70 **Treatment with 'new' antiepileptic drugs**   380
Lina Nashef

71 **Pharmacological interactions**   385
Philip N. Patsalos

72 **Monotherapy or polytherapy?**   392
Edward H. Reynolds

73 **Antiepileptic drugs currently under development**   396
Philip N. Patsalos

74 **Antiepileptic drug withdrawal**   401
R. Shane Delamont

75 **Behavioural effects of antiepileptic drugs**   403
Frank M. C. Besag

76 **Epilepsy emergency treatment**   406
Frank M. C. Besag and Gonzalo Alarcón

77 **Clinical neuropsychological evaluation**   410
Robin G. Morris

78 **Neuropsychological effects of antiepileptic drugs**   413
Laura H. Goldstein

79 **The Wada test (intra-arterial amobarbital procedure)**   415
Robin G. Morris

80 **General principles of surgical treatment**   417
Richard P. Selway

Contents

81 **Preoperative assessment** 419
Gonzalo Alarcón

82 **Surgical techniques** 431
Richard P. Selway

83 **Outcome of surgery** 434
Charles E. Polkey

84 **Epilepsy surgery in children** 438
Charles E. Polkey

85 **Vagus nerve stimulation** 441
Richard P. Selway

86 **Brain stimulation for the treatment of epilepsy** 442
Richard P. Selway

87 **Diagnosis and treatment of hypothalamic hamartomas** 444
Nandini Mullatti

88 **Intraoperative (acute) electrocorticography (ECoG)** 447
Gonzalo Alarcón

89 **Single-pulse electrical stimulation** 452
Antonio Valentín

90 **Ketogenic diet in the management of childhood epilepsy** 456
J. Helen Cross

Section 6 Epilepsy in specific circumstances

91 **Reflex epilepsies** 459
Michalis Koutroumanidis

92 **Photosensitive and language-induced seizures and epilepsies** 461
Simeran Sharma, Mark Stevenson and Michalis Koutroumanidis

93 **Audiogenic epilepsies** 464
Nicholas Moran

94 **Reading epilepsy** 466
Michalis Koutroumanidis

95 **Status epilepticus: classification and pathophysiology** 468
Matthew Walker

96 **Status epilepticus: diagnosis and management** 471
Matthew Walker

97 **Management of epilepsy in women** 474
Gonzalo Alarcón

98 **Catamenial seizures** 476
Nandini Mullatti

99 **The management of epilepsy in children** 478
David McCormick

100 **Learning and educational issues in epilepsy** 483
Corina O'Neill

101 **Epilepsy in old age** 486
Gonzalo Alarcón

102 **Epilepsy and learning** 489
Frank M. C. Besag

103 **Epilepsy in chromosomal and related disorders** 492
Elaine Hughes

104 **Epilepsy and cerebral trauma** 494
Charles E. Polkey

105 **Epilepsy after cerebral tumours, hamartomas and neurosurgery** 497
Charles E. Polkey

106 **Epilepsy and cerebrovascular disease** 501
R. Shane Delamont

107 **Abnormalities of neuronal migration** 504
R. Arunachalam

108 **Malformations of cortical development** 506
Charles E. Polkey

109 **Rasmussen's disease and epilepsia partialis continua** 510
Charles E. Polkey

110 **Behavioural treatment of epilepsy** 513
Peter Fenwick

Section 7 Psychiatric, social and legal aspects

111 **Affective disorders and epilepsy** 515
Nozomi Akanuma

112 **Anxiety disorders and epilepsy** 518
John Moriarty

113 **Personality and epilepsy** 520
Peter Fenwick

114 **The psychoses of epilepsy** 522
Brian Toone

115 **Epilepsy and aggression** 524
Peter Fenwick

116 **Epilepsy in childhood: effects on behaviour and mental health** 526
Sarah H. Bernard

117 **Psychogenic non-epileptic (dissociative) seizures: psychiatric aspects** 529
John D. C. Mellers

118 **Psychiatric effects of surgical treatment for epilepsy** 532
Richard P. Selway

119 **Use of psychotropics in people with epilepsy** 533
Nozomi Akanuma

120 **Time-limited psychodynamic counselling for people with epilepsy** 536
Shiri Spector

121 **Evaluation of quality of life in epilepsy** 538
Jennifer Nightingale

122 **Cultural aspects of epilepsy: stigma, prejudice, self-image** 543
Jennifer Nightingale

123 **Epilepsy, marriage and the family** 545
Jennifer Nightingale

124 **Epilepsy and employment** 548
Rona Eade, Sally Gomersall and Stella Pearson

125 **Drivers' and pilots' licences** 553
Peter Fenwick

126 **Treatment with limited pharmacopoeia** 555
Dominic C. Heaney

127 **The role of primary care in the management of epilepsy** 557
Greg Rogers

128 **Residential care and special centres for epilepsy** 561
Frank M. C. Besag

129 **Main UK charities supporting epilepsy** 564
Shiri Spector

130 **Public education and resources** 566
Stephen Brown

131 **Organizations and support services for people with epilepsy** 569
Stephen Brown

132 **Can a joined-up primary–secondary care approach help people with epilepsy?** 572
Leone Ridsdale

133 **Support groups and their role in care in the community** 576
Jane Juler

134 **The International League Against Epilepsy (ILAE) and the International Bureau for Epilepsy (IBE)** 578
Edward H. Reynolds

135 **Health economics and epilepsy** 581
Dominic C. Heaney

136 **Epilepsy, crime and legal responsibility** 585
Peter Fenwick

137 **The law and its consequences for people with epilepsy** 587
Peter Fenwick

138 **Epilepsy and lifestyle issues** 589
Frank M. C. Besag

139 **Bereavement, SUDEP and Epilepsy Bereaved** 592
Maureen Lahiff and Jane Hanna

Index 594
The colour plates will be found between pages 238 and 239.

Contributors

Nozomi Akanuma
Consultant Psychiatrist, South London & Maudsley NHS Foundation Trust; Visiting Senior Lecturer in Clinical Neuroscience, Institute of Psychiatry, King's College London, London, UK

Gonzalo Alarcón
Reader and Honorary Consultant in Clinical Neurophysiology, Institute of Psychiatry and Institute of Epileptology, King's College London, and at King's College Hospital, London, UK

R. Arunachalam
Consultant, Clinical Neurophysiology, Southampton University Hospitals NHS Trust, Southampton, UK

Sarah H. Bernard
Consultant Psychiatrist, Child and Adolescent Learning Disability, The Michael Rutter Centre, London, UK

Frank M. C. Besag
Consultant Neuropsychiatrist, CAMHS-LD, Mid Beds Clinic, SEPT: South Essex Partnership University NHS Foundation Trust, Bedfordshire, UK

Istvan Bodi
Consultant Neuropathologist, Visiting Senior Lecturer, Institute of Psychiatry, King's College London, London UK

Stephen Brown
Consultant Neuropsychiatrist, Honorary Professor of Developmental Neuropsychiatry, Peninsula Medical School, Exeter, UK

Franz Brunnhuber
Consultant, Department of Clinical Neurophysiology, King's College Hospital, London, UK

Antonella Cerquiglini
Department of Child Neurology and Psychiatry, University La Sapienza, Rome, Italy

J. Helen Cross
Head of Neuroscience Unit, UCL Institute of Child Health, London, UK

R. Shane Delamont
Consultant Neurologist, King's College Hospital, London, UK

Archana Desurkar
Department of Paediatric Neurology, Evelina Children's and St Thomas' Hospitals, London, UK

Lee Drummond
Senior Chief Technician, Dept Clinical Neurophysiology, King's College Hospital, London, UK

Rona Eade
Epilepsy Information Manager, Epilepsy Society, Buckinghamshire, UK

Robert D. C. Elwes
Consultant Neurologist and Clinical Neurophysiologist, King's College Hospital and Institute of Epileptology, London, UK

Bidi Evans
Department of Clinical Neurophysiology, King's College Hospital, London, UK

Peter Fenwick
Consultant Neuropsychiatrist emeritus, Epilepsy Unit, Maudsley Hospital

Colin D. Ferrie
Consultant Paediatric Neurologist, General Infirmary of Leeds, Leeds, UK

Paul L. Furlong
Wellcome Laboratory for MEG Studies, School of Life and Health Sciences, Aston University, Birmingham, UK

List of contributors

Laura H. Goldstein
Professor of Clinical Neuropsychology
Institute of Psychiatry, King's College London,
London, UK

Sally Gomersall
Epilepsy Society, Buckinghamshire, UK

Sushma Goyal
Department of Clinical Neurophysiology, King's
College Hospital, London, UK

Jane Hanna
Director, Epilepsy Bereaved, Oxon, UK

Yvonne Hart
Consultant Neurologist, Royal Victoria Infirmary,
Newcastle upon Tyne, UK

Dominic C. Heaney
Consultant Neurologist, National Hospital for
Neurology and Neurosurgery, University College
London, London, UK

Graham E. Holder
Clinical Neurophysiologist, King's College Hospital,
London, UK

Mrinalini Honavar
Department of Clinical Neuropathology, King's
College Hospital, London, UK

Elaine Hughes
Consultant Paediatric Neurologist, King's College
Hospital, London, UK

Jozef M. Jarosz
Consultant, Neuroimaging Unit, King's College
Hospital, London, UK

John G. R. Jefferys
Professor of Neuroscience, Neuronal Networks Group,
School of Clinical and Experimental Medicine,
University of Birmingham, Birmingham, UK

Jane Juler
Division of Neuroscience, Guy's, King's and
St Thomas' School of Medicine, London, UK

Mathias Koepp
Professor, Institute of Neurology, University College
London, London, UK

Michalis Koutroumanidis
Consultant Clinical Neurophysiologist and
Neurologist, Honorary Senior Lecturer, GKT School
of Medicine, King's College, London, UK

Maureen Lahiff
Academic Coordinator and Lecturer, School of Public
Health, University of California, Berkeley, Berkeley,
CA, USA

Louis Lemieux
Professor of Physics Applied to Medicine, Institute of
Neurology, University College London, London, UK

David McCormick
Clinical Director – Child Health, King's College
Hospital, London, UK

Brian Meldrum
Professor of Experimental Neurology, Centre
for Neuroscience, King's College London,
London, UK

John D. C. Mellers
Consultant Neuropsychiatrist, Maudsley Hospital,
London, UK

Nicholas Moran
Consultant, Department of Neurology, King's College
Hospital, London, UK

John Moriarty
Consultant Neuropsychiatrist, South London and
Maudsley NHS Foundation Trust, London, UK

Robin G. Morris
Professor of Neuropsychology and Head of the
Neuropsychology Department, King's College
Hospital, London, UK

Nandini Mullatti
Consultant in Clinical Neurophysiology and Epilepsy,
King's College Hospital, London, UK

Lina Nashef
Consultant Neurologist and Honorary Senior
Lecturer, King's College Hospital, London, UK

Jennifer Nightingale
Epilepsy Nurse Specialist, Barts and the London NHS
Trust, London, UK

List of contributors

T. J. von Oertzen
Consultant Neurologist/Epileptologist and Honorary Senior Lecturer Atkinson Morley Neuroscience Centre, St. George's Hospital, London, UK

Corina O'Neill
Specialist Children's Service, Wood Street Health Centre CDC, London, UK

Philip N. Patsalos
Professor of Clinical Pharmacology, Dept of Clinical and Experimental Epilepsy, Institute of Neurology, University College London, London, UK

Stella Pearson
Epilepsy Information Services, Epilepsy Society, Buckinghamshire, UK

Charles E. Polkey
Consultant Neurosurgeon, Department of Neuroscience, Institutes of Psychiatry and Epileptology King's College London, London, UK

Ronit Pressler
Department of Clinical Neurophysiology, King's College Hospital, London, UK

Edward H. Reynolds
Institute of Epileptology, King's College London, London, UK

Mark P. Richardson
Paul Getty III Professor of Epilepsy, Director, Institute of Epileptology, King's College London, London, UK

Leone Ridsdale
Professor of Neurology and General Practice, Department of Clinical Neuroscience, King's College Hospital, London, UK

Robert Robinson
Consultant Paediatric Neurologist, Great Ormond Street Hospital, London, UK

Greg Rogers
GPwSI in epilepsy, East Kent Health Authority, Kent, UK

Euan M. Ross
Emeritus Professor, King's College London, London, UK

Richard P. Selway
Consultant Neurosurgeon, King's College Hospital, London, UK

Stefano Seri
Wellcome Laboratory for MEG Studies, School of Life and Health Sciences, Aston University; Comprehensive Paediatric Epilepsy Programme, The Birmingham Children's Hospital NHS Foundation Trust, Birmingham, UK

Simeran Sharma
Clinical Physiologist, Neurophysiology and Epilepsies, Guy's and St. Thomas' NHS Foundation Trust, London, UK

Graeme J. Sills
Lecturer in Pharmacology, University of Liverpool, Liverpool, UK

Andrew Simmons
Reader in Neuroimaging/Consultant Clinical Scientist, Institute of Psychiatry, King's College London, UK

Shiri Spector
Psychotherapy Unit, King's College Hospital, London, UK

Mark Stevenson
Clinical Physiologist/Manager, Neurophysiology and Epilepsies, Guy's and St. Thomas' NHS Foundation Trust, London, UK

Jade N. Thai
Wellcome Laboratory for MEG Studies, School of Life and Health Sciences, Aston University, Birmingham, UK

Brian Toone
Department of Psychological Medicine, King's College Hospital, London, UK

Antonio Valentín
Lecturer in Epilepsy, Institute of Psychiatry and Institute of Epileptology, King's College London, London, UK

Nuria T. Villagra
Visiting SpR in Neuropathology, Department of Clinical Neuropathology, King's College Hospital, London, UK

Matthew Walker
Professor of Neurology, Institute of Neurology,
National Hospital for Neurology and Neurosurgery,
London, UK

William Whitehouse
Clinical Senior Lecturer, Faculty of Medicine &
Health Sciences, University of Nottingham,
Nottingham, UK

Foreword
by Dr Edward H. Reynolds

The Fund, the Centre and the Institute

In the summer of 1991 a group of 10 professional colleagues involved in nearly every aspect of the multi-disciplinary subject of epilepsy, and who were working in several physically related but, at that time, administratively unrelated medical institutions in South London, agreed to combine their expertise in a major initiative that had three strands. First, a charity, The Fund for Epilepsy, was registered in December 1992. Second, a new comprehensive clinical Centre for the treatment and care of children and adults with epilepsy was opened at the Maudsley Hospital in July 1994, but transferred to King's College Hospital under reorganized Neuroscience arrangements in 1995. Third, in November 1994 the world's first university-based academic Institute of Epileptology was launched at King's College London.

The clinical Centre provides epilepsy services to a population of 4 million people in South London and the South East of England.

Since 1995 the various parent institutions of the Institute of Epileptology have themselves all combined under the umbrella of King's College London. Although clinical neurosciences, including the Centre for Epilepsy, are based at King's College Hospital, the three hospitals of Guy's, King's and St. Thomas' are now incorporated into a single Medical School and the post-graduate Institute of Psychiatry and its associated Maudsley Hospital are also now a School at King's College London.

The virtual Institute of Epileptology now has over 60 personnel working in every discipline related to epilepsy, within these various institutions of King's College.

A generous private donation from Paul Getty III has enabled King's College to establish the Paul Getty III Chair in Epilepsy, to which a recent Chair of Paediatric Epilepsy has also been added. The Fund for Epilepsy has recently combined with the Epilepsy Research Fund, ERF, to establish a single national research charity, ERUK. There are plans for the research facilities of the Institute of Epileptology to be transferred to a new Neurosciences institution at the Denmark Hill Campus of King's College in the next few years.

The MSc Course in Epilepsy

From the beginning one of the main objectives of the Institute of Epileptology has been teaching, in addition to research. In 1995 it established the world's first university degree course in association with King's College. The course is open to post-graduates from varied backgrounds, e.g. neurology, neurosurgery, psychiatry, paediatrics, clinical neurophysiology, pharmacology, pharmacy, industry, psychology, nursing and social sciences. It may be undertaken on a full-time basis for one year or a part-time basis for two years. It has been one of the most successful of King's College MSc Courses with over 150 students from many countries graduating over the last 12 years and thus training a much-needed new generation of epileptologists.

This book is based on the current teaching course of the Institute of Epileptology MSc in Epilepsy at King's College. Most but not all the lectures are from members of the Institute within King's College itself but a few distinguished teachers from other institutions in the UK have kindly agreed to contribute to this MSc Course and are represented in this book.

Reference

Reynolds EH (ed.). Scientific meeting for the launch of the Institute of Epileptology, King's College University of London. *Epilepsia* 1995; Supplement 1.

Preface

'Even when they teach, men learn'.
Seneca 'The Younger', c 4 Bc–Ad 65. *Epistulae Morales*

Learning and teaching any discipline is necessarily complex. Relevant concepts and related subtle hues need to be intertwined in the appropriate order and proportion for the mix to settle solidly. Yet, time erodes it fast. Despite epilepsy being one of the most common neurological conditions, there are surprisingly few formal academic qualifications and teaching textbooks on Epileptology. The present volume compiles the essence of our 16-year experience in training epileptologists from all over the world in the Masters in Science Course in Epilepsy (MSc in Epilepsy) at King's College London. When we initially set up this course, we met a degree of scepticism suggesting that Epileptology was not a broad enough discipline to provide teaching for a full-year MSc. Needless to say that this proved not to be the case. However, students and professionals wanting to specialize in epilepsy often have difficulties in finding a textbook pitched to the appropriate level of learning, as textbooks tend to be either too elementary, or too encyclopaedic, or too specialized. We have chosen a structural approach starting with elementary fundamental concepts building up to socio-economic issues, while covering all aspects of Epileptology. Each chapter has been adapted to the specific nature of the topic. In our experience, students find most difficult the fundamental but conceptually complex concepts necessary to understand Neuroscience, Basic Epileptology and Classifications of seizures and syndromes. Consequently, those chapters have been structured as written tutorials, containing multiple tables, bullet points, clarifying text boxes and simple diagrams. For the chapters on practical issues, a down-to-earth approach has been adopted by virtue of clear hands-on advice aided by multiple bullet points, illustrations and tables. Finally, those subjects currently evolving have been critically reviewed by leading experts on the topic. The end product is a volume that would benefit a large variety of professionals seeking deep and practical knowledge and updates on epilepsy, should they be general practitioners, technicians, nurses, students, researchers, auditors, specialist registrars, consultants or patients suffering with epilepsy.

Each chapter contains a limited number of key reading references in addition to 'learning objectives'. The latter, we believe, constitute a novel approach in Epileptology, which will aid the reader in focusing their learning by identifying the key concepts, skills and knowledge required to master the subject.

Finally, we would greatly appreciate any constructive criticism, which could lead to improvements in this textbook. Please send any comments to gonzalo.alarcon@kcl.ac.uk.

Acknowledgements

The authors would like to express their most sincere gratitude to:
- All the students of the MSc in Epilepsy, who inadvertently taught us how to write this book
- The faculty of the MSc in Epilepsy, many of whom have directly contributed towards this volume
- The staff of Cambridge University Press

Section 1 Basic principles

Chapter 1

History of epilepsy

Edward H. Reynolds

Introduction

Throughout its recorded history of at least 3 to 4 millennia, epilepsy has usually been defined by its most visible and dramatic symptom, i.e. mysterious brief periodic attacks of one kind or another. Thus the ancient Sumerian term 'antasubba' and the later Babylonian and Assyrian word 'miqtu' both refer to 'the falling sickness' (Kinnier Wilson and Reynolds 1990), a term also adopted by the Greeks and Romans and employed by Temkin (1971) as the title of his classic history of epilepsy 'from the Greeks to the beginning of modern neurology', i.e. the late nineteenth century. Since the nineteenth century the paroxysms have been variously referred to as 'fits', 'convulsions', 'seizures' or 'epileptic attacks'. Currently the word 'seizure' is favoured by the International League Against Epilepsy (ILAE) in its classification of such paroxysmal episodes, but whatever word is chosen there are always similar or borderline non-epileptic attacks to confuse the physician in the differential diagnosis.

The word 'epilepsy' is of Greek origin and means to seize, to take hold of or to attack. The word 'seizure' is of Latin origin from 'sacire', i.e. to claim. These words reflect the ancient belief that the sufferer has been seized or claimed by a supernatural power, spirit or god.

Ancient descriptions and concepts

The oldest detailed description of epilepsy is in a Babylonian clay tablet in the British Museum from the second millennium BC (Kinnier Wilson and Reynolds, 1990). The tablet is one of 40 such tablets comprising a Babylonian 'textbook' of medicine and in number 26 the cuneiform text is wholly concerned with epilepsy. The Babylonians were remarkable observers of human illness and behaviour. They accurately described many of the seizure types we recognize today, which we call tonic clonic, absence, complex partial, Jacksonian or even gelastic seizures. They also documented status epilepticus, provocative and prognostic factors and inter-seizure events, including psychoses of epilepsy. However, they had no understanding of pathology or brain function and each seizure type was thought to be the result of an invasion of the body by a particular evil spirit or demon.

The first line of the text states:

> If epilepsy falls once upon a person or falls many times, it is the result of possession by a demon or a departed spirit.

The Babylonians apparently had no doubt about whether a single seizure is epilepsy. Every attack, whether single or multiple, was the result of possession. Here is a remarkable account, for example, of a left-sided focal motor attack in which the progression to loss of consciousness makes it harder to drive out the demon:

> If at the time of his possession, while he is sitting down, his left eye moves to the side, a lip puckers, saliva flows from his mouth, and his hand, leg and trunk on the left side jerk like a newly slaughtered sheep, it is miqtu. If at the time of the possession his mind is consciously aware, the demon can be driven out; if at the time of possession his mind is not so aware, the demon cannot be driven out.

By the time of the later Greco-Roman period, the responsible invading supernatural powers now included Gods. This is reflected in Hippocrates' famous fifth-century BC treatise on 'The sacred disease' in which he doubted whether the human body could be polluted by a God and for the first time suggests a natural causation mediated through disorder of brain

---

Introduction to Epilepsy ed. Gonzalo Alarcón and Antonio Valentín. Published by Cambridge University Press.
© Cambridge University Press 2012.

function: 'The brain is the seat of this disease as it is of other very violent diseases'.

Epilepsy as a brain disorder

Unfortunately this Hippocratic insight had little influence on the prevailing supernatural view of epilepsy until the seventeenth and eighteenth centuries AD, when the concept of a brain disorder began to take root in Europe. By now the focus was on motor paroxysms and the problem was how to distinguish a particular form of motor convulsion, with or without loss of consciousness, from other periodic 'convulsive diseases', such as hysteria, tetanus, tremors, rigors and other paroxysmal movement disorders. The latter were gradually separated off from epilepsy in the nineteenth century especially in the Lumleian Lectures on 'convulsive diseases' by Todd in 1849 and Jackson in 1890.

Functional localization and unilateral seizures

Also the nineteenth century saw the development of the concept of functional localization in the brain (Ferrier, 1876) and the discovery, for example, of the motor cortex (Fritsch and Hitzig, 1870). The concept of 'epileptiform', focal, or partial seizures arose as models for the study of 'generalized' seizures (Jackson, 1870 and 1890). By meticulously studying the clinical features of unilateral motor seizures arising in the motor cortex, Jackson was able to conclude, as was later confirmed experimentally, that the motor cortex was concerned with movements rather than individual muscles.

Idiopathic and symptomatic epilepsy

It was apparent to Jackson and to many others that unilateral or focal seizures were often associated with various local brain pathologies, e.g. vascular, tumour, tuberculosis, neuro-syphilis etc. There therefore began in the second half of the nineteenth century a very long-running debate, still with us today, concerning the distinction between primary idiopathic epilepsy in which the brain is macroscopically normal, and secondary symptomatic epilepsy with focal and generalized seizures, associated with various brain pathologies. Russell Reynolds (1861) and Gowers (1881) both viewed true epilepsy as the primary idiopathic variety, whereas Sieveking (1858) concluded that it was impossible to separate primary from secondary or idiopathic from symptomatic epilepsy. This debate continues in the twenty-first century and is at the heart of current controversies concerning modern ILAE classifications of seizures and epilepsy syndromes (Reynolds and Rodin, 2009).

Basic mechanisms: vascular and electromagnetic theories

As the neurological foundations of epilepsy became more firmly established, the dominant view in the nineteenth century was that it had a vascular origin, perhaps due to some temporary insufficiency of blood supply. Even the Babylonians understood that a sacrificed sheep displayed terminal convulsions associated with severe blood loss. The experimental studies by Brown-Sequard (1860), who influenced Jackson, supported this view and in his early writings in the 1860s Jackson favoured wholly vascular theories. Even when he later developed his famous hypothesis of neuronal instability and discharge in the 1870s he continued to invoke a vascular dimension.

Vascular theories were first challenged by Todd in 1849, who found them unsatisfactory. Todd was a scientific physician and Professor of Physiology and Morbid Anatomy at King's College in London, where he had a special interest in disorders of the nervous system before the discipline of neurology existed. He was greatly influenced by his contemporary in London, the famous Michael Faraday (1791–1867), at the Royal Institution, who at that time was laying the foundations of our modern understanding of electromagnetism. As a pioneering neuro-histologist Todd saw each nerve vesicle (cell) and its related fibres (neuron in later terminology) as a distinct apparatus for the development and transmission of 'nervous polarity' based on Faraday's concepts of the polar forces of electricity and magnetism. Todd applied these concepts to epilepsy in which he envisaged a periodic rise in electrical tension in grey matter, which could, at a certain threshold, result in a sudden change in polar state, leading to a seizure discharge, comparable to the spark from a battery or lightning. In his 1849 Lumleian Lectures Todd emphasized:

> These periodical evolutions of the nervous force may be compared to the electrical phenomena described by Faraday under the name of 'disruptive discharge'.

Todd supported his views by electrical experiments in the rabbit.

Although Jackson, who was more of a philosopher than a scientist, later in 1873 developed a theory of 'excessive discharge' in epilepsy, his concept was very different, based on chemistry, anabolism and catabolism. He had no understanding of physics or electromagnetism and he overlooked or ignored Todd's prior electrical theory of discharge. However, vascular theories continued to dominate late nineteenth century and early twentieth century thinking, reaching their peak with Turner in 1907.

Electromagnetic concepts of epilepsy were finally established in the middle of the twentieth century following the discovery of the human electroencephalogram (EEG) by Berger in 1929. Earlier Caton (1873) had reported electrical potentials from the cortex of various animal species, but relatively little notice was taken of this until Berger's human studies. Hans Berger was Head of the University Psychiatric Hospital in Jena, where he spent 27 years studying the electrical activity of cats, dogs and, later, human volunteers and patients. By 1933 he had described the interictal resting EEG, the EEG response to hyperventilation, the post-ictal EEG following a tonic-clonic seizure, and the ictal EEG of focal motor seizures. This led to a rapid growth in the discipline of electroencephalography in the middle of the twentieth century. Electromagnetic concepts of epilepsy were reinforced in the second half of the twentieth century by the development and application of video-telemetry.

In the meanwhile in 1906 Ramón y Cajal and Golgi received the Nobel Prize for their histological development of the 'neuron doctrine', already glimpsed more than 50 years earlier by Todd. It took another half century for the ionic basis of Todd's 'nervous polarity' or neurotransmission to be confirmed by the Nobel Prize-winning work of Hodgkin and Huxley (1953), who identified the role of sodium, potassium and chloride, elements that had first been discovered by Faraday's mentor at the Royal Institution, London, i.e. Sir Humphry Davy (1778–1829).

The psychiatry of epilepsy

Throughout most of its documented history, epilepsy has been viewed as a mental disorder, beginning with the supernatural concepts of the ancients.

Despite the neurological progress in the late nineteenth and early twentieth centuries the concept of epilepsy as a psychiatric disorder prevailed in most parts of the world until the middle of the twentieth century, especially as epilepsy has always been noted to be associated with a high incidence of psychological, behavioural and personality disorders. Indeed in the nineteenth century it was widely believed in Europe by 'alienists' in charge of mental institutions, where much epilepsy was treated, that epilepsy, like much insanity, was a hereditary degenerative disorder leading to cognitive and moral decline. Some went so far as to diagnose 'epilepsy', 'epilepsy equivalent' or 'masked epilepsy' in patients with paroxysmal disorders of mood or behaviour in the absence of any clinical seizures. It was only in the middle of the twentieth century with the widespread acceptance of electromagnetic concepts and the rapid development of the discipline of neurology that the World Health Organization (WHO) in 1960 finally separated 'epilepsy per se' from 'epilepsy with deterioration or psychosis' in their International Classification of Diseases. At the same time epidemiological studies now revealed that most patients with epilepsy were leading relatively normal lives in the community, often well controlled by the relatively new antiepileptic drugs of phenobarbitone (1912) and phenytoin (1938). Only about a third of patients had significant psychological, behavioural or personality disorders, especially in the presence of underlying brain lesions or learning disabilities (Reynolds and Trimble, 1981).

By the middle of the twentieth century clinical neurophysiology, including cortical stimulation studies (Penfield and Jasper, 1954), had refined the concepts of temporal and frontal lobe epilepsy; and neuropsychology was clarifying their behavioural and cognitive associations. The stage was now set for increasingly precise distinction between pre-ictal, ictal, post-ictal and interictal psychiatric disorders, e. g. transient ictal mood change, hallucinations or automatisms; the rare brief interictal psychoses associated with cessation of seizures and 'forced normalization' of the EEG (Landolt, 1958); or the occasional chronic interictal psychoses associated with temporal lobe epilepsy (Slater, Beard and Glithero, 1963); all of which are much less common than interictal anxiety or depressive states.

At the turn of the nineteenth century neurology and psychiatry were diverging and epilepsy remained

Section 1: Basic principles

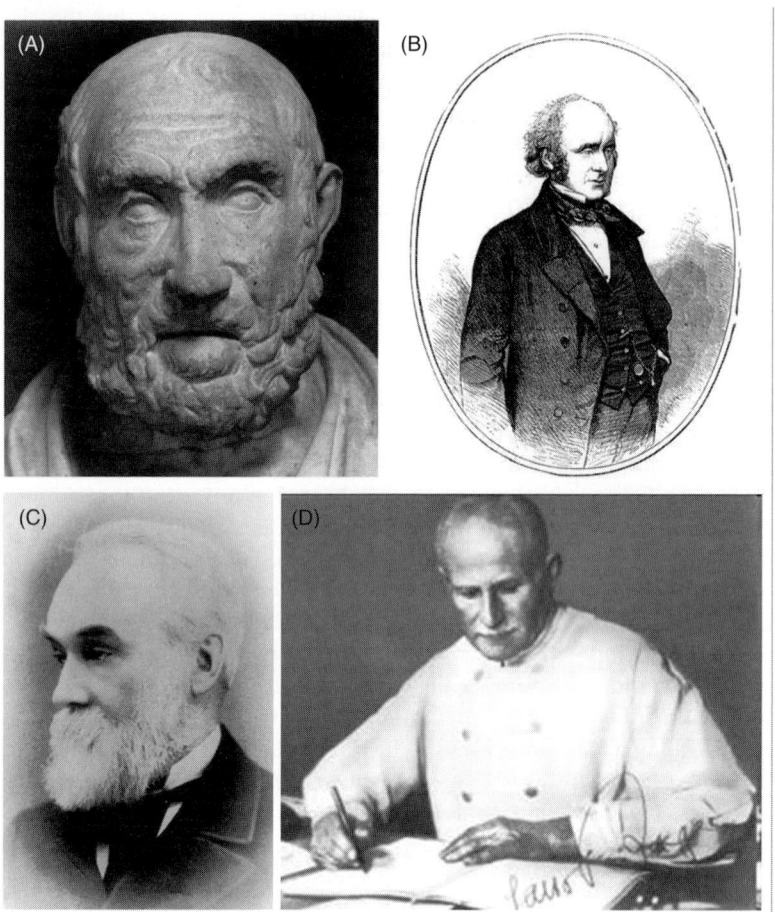

Figure 1.1. Four key people in the history of epilepsy. (A) Hippocrates (460?–377 or 359 BC); (B) Robert Bentley Todd (1809–1860); (C) John Hughlings Jackson (1835–1911); (D) Hans Berger (1873–1941).

to some extent in both camps. At the turn of the twentieth century the two disciplines have been converging again, led in many respects by epilepsy, which has provided several useful models of mental illness, a window on brain function, and a bridge between the two disciplines (Reynolds and Trimble, 1981 and 2009).

Epilepsy as a social disorder

No history of epilepsy would be complete without acknowledging the enormous social consequences of the disorder throughout the ages (Temkin, 1971). Seizures are such unusual, sudden, dramatic, frightening, potentially harmful and, until quite recently, mysterious events that they have always given rise to misunderstanding, fear, neglect, social penalties and stigma at all ages in all social classes, cultures and countries. Such misunderstanding and anxiety have profoundly affected family and other relationships, and the potential for marriage, employment and personal fulfilment. So deep is this legacy that notwithstanding greater knowledge of the disorder, negative public attitudes are still widespread, undermining fundraising, research, services and social integration. Against this background in 1997 the ILAE, IBE and WHO launched a global campaign to bring epilepsy 'out of the shadows' especially in developing countries (see Chapter 134: 'The International League Against Epilepsy (ILAE) and the International Bureau for Epilepsy (IBE)').

References

Berger H. Über das Electroenkephalogramm de Menschen. *Arch Psychiatr Nerverkr* 1929;**87**:527–70.

Ferrier D. *The Function of the Brain*. London; Smith Elder, 1876.

Gowers WR. *Epilepsy and Other Chronic Convulsive Diseases*. London: Churchill, 1881.

Jackson JH. A study of convulsions. *Trans St Andrews Med Grad Assoc* 1870;3:162–204.

Jackson JH. On convulsive seizures. *Lancet* 1890;1:685–788.

Kinnier Wilson JV, Reynolds EH. Texts and documents. Translation and analysis of a cuneiform text forming part of a Babylonian treatise on epilepsy. *Med Hist* 1990;34(2):185–98.

Reynolds EH. Milestones in epilepsy. *Epilepsia* 2009;**50**:338–42.

Reynolds EH, Rodin E. The clinical concept of epilepsy. *Epilepsia* 2009;**50**(suppl 3):2–7.

Reynolds EH, Trimble MR (eds). *Epilepsy and Psychiatry*. Edinburgh: Churchill Livingstone; 1981.

Reynolds EH, Trimble MR. Epilepsy, psychiatry, and neurology. *Epilepsia* 2009; **50**(suppl 3):50–5.

Slater E, Beard AW, Glithero E. The schizophrenia-like psychoses of epilepsy. *Br J Psychiatry* 1963; **109**:95–150.

Temkin O. *The Falling Sickness*. 2nd edn. Baltimore, MD: The Johns Hopkins University Press; 1971.

Todd RB. On the pathology and treatment of convulsive diseases. *London Medical Gazette* 1849;8:661–846.

Learning objective

(1) To be aware of the main hallmarks in the historical development of Epileptology.

Section 1 Basic principles

Chapter 2

What is epilepsy?

Gonzalo Alarcón

Epilepsy is one of the most common neurological conditions. Epilepsy is usually defined as a tendency to suffer recurrent epileptic seizures. Epileptic seizures show a variety of clinical and electroencephalographic characteristics which are described in Chapter 17: 'Electroclinical classification of seizures and syndromes'. More pragmatically, epilepsy can be defined as suffering two or more unprovoked epileptic seizures occurring within a time frame of two years. This definition implies that epilepsy is essentially a chronic condition. The term 'unprovoked' refers to the absence of underlying acute conditions that can induce seizures in subjects who would not otherwise have seizures (hypoglycemia, alcohol withdrawal, hypercalcemia, encephalitis, electroconvulsive therapy, etc.; see Chapter 31: 'Acute symptomatic seizures').

In a small proportion of patients with epilepsy, seizures can be triggered by specific stimuli that do not trigger seizures in the general population (flashing lights, visual patterns, reading, music, intellectual activity, etc.). This type of epilepsy is called reflex epilepsy (see Chapters 91 to 94).

Besides the formal definition of epilepsy, there is the more practical problem of how to identify (diagnose) the condition. Epilepsy is often misdiagnosed (Leach et al., 2005). The diagnosis of epilepsy is complicated by the fact that many key symptoms and signs of epilepsy are intermittent and brief (e.g. epileptic seizures, interictal epileptiform EEG discharges). This means that clinical and EEG examinations can appear normal, although they might have shown abnormalities had they been obtained earlier or later. This means that detailed medical history is of paramount importance for diagnosis (see Chapter 46: 'History-taking and physical examination in epilepsy'). To complicate matters further, epileptic seizures can show such a variety of clinical manifestations (see Chapter 17: 'Electroclinical classification of seizures and syndromes') that a reliable definition of epileptic seizures based on their clinical manifestations alone is impossible.

In practice, an epileptic seizure can be defined as a sensation, feeling, autonomic change, abnormal or automatic movement or alteration of consciousness associated with abnormal EEG changes. EEG changes can be detected on the scalp, unless seizures are very localized or restricted to deep brain regions (hippocampus, medial aspect of the hemispheres). In this case, EEG changes may only be detectable by intracranial electrodes.

There is a widespread misconception that the diagnosis of epilepsy is purely clinical (i.e. that it relies solely on history and clinical examination). This is not necessarily the case. Indeed, it may be more realistic to say that, in general, the diagnosis of epilepsy is electro-clinical. As in any medical condition, a good history will raise the suspicion of epilepsy as part of a differential diagnosis (a differential diagnosis is a list of conditions that can explain the symptoms). In many patients, a detailed history with a reliable witness will be sufficiently convincing to diagnose epilepsy, but in others epilepsy needs to be confirmed with the identification of EEG abnormalities consistent with the suspected epilepsy syndrome. The EEG is also instrumental in the classification of epilepsy, which can be seen as a refined diagnosis. Indeed, the diagnosis of some epilepsy syndromes cannot be made without specific EEG abnormalities (e.g. West syndrome, epilepsy with continuous spike and waves during sleep, childhood absence epilepsy, Lennox-Gastaut syndrome). What appears to be clear is that the diagnosis of epilepsy is not only electrical, i.e. finding EEG abnormalities without a compatible

---

Introduction to Epilepsy ed. Gonzalo Alarcón and Antonio Valentín. Published by Cambridge University Press.
© Cambridge University Press 2012.

history of epilepsy should not trigger the diagnosis of epilepsy.

Of course, in some patients it may not be possible to obtain sufficient clinical or EEG information to confirm the diagnosis of epilepsy, either because there are not reliable witnesses to the seizures or because EEG abnormalities are repeatedly absent, or both. In such cases, it may not be possible to confirm the diagnosis of epilepsy.

A further difficulty arises because in some syndromes, particularly in adults, a normal interictal EEG cannot rule out the diagnosis of epilepsy, as abnormalities can be intermittent. Nevertheless a repeatedly normal interictal EEG should cast a doubt on the diagnosis of epilepsy. In such cases, ictal EEG recordings or videos of seizures may be necessary (see Chapter 47: 'Role of video-EEG monitoring in epilepsy').

Reference

Leach JP, Lauder R, Nicolson A, Smith DF. Epilepsy in the UK: misdiagnosis, mistreatment, and undertreatment? The Wrexham area epilepsy project. *Seizure* 2005;**14**:514–20.

Learning objectives

(1) To be aware of the main issues and difficulties met in defining epilepsy.
(2) To understand the present definition(s) of epilepsy.
(3) To understand the principles and difficulties involved in the diagnosis of epilepsy.

Section 1 **Basic principles**

Chapter 3
Functional anatomy of the central nervous system

Gonzalo Alarcón

Cerebral hemispheres

The upper brain contains two symmetrical round structures called the cerebral hemispheres (or simply the hemispheres). A section of the hemispheres will reveal grey areas (grey matter) and white areas (white matter). Grey matter contains dendrites, neuronal bodies and axons, whereas white matter contains largely axons. There is a strip of grey matter surrounding each hemisphere, immediately under its surface, called the cerebral cortex (in plural, cortices). Each hemisphere also contains multiple internal islands of grey matter (nuclei in plural and nucleus in singular) such as the thalamus, basal ganglia and hypothalamus. The cerebral cortex surrounds both cerebral hemispheres and folds in a complicated fashion, defining depressions of the surface of the brain (the sulci, or sulcus in singular) and bulging regions (the gyri, or gyrus in singular) (Figure 3.1). In addition, there are two deep depressions called fissures: the rolandic or central fissure between frontal and parietal lobes, and the sylvian fissure between frontal and temporal lobes. We will hereafter use the term cortex to refer to the cerebral cortex since the other brain cortex, the cerebellar cortex, is not directly involved in the generation of epileptic seizures.

The sylvian fissure is particularly deep and ends in a virtual space surrounded by cortex, called the insula. The cortical regions around the sylvian fissure which cover the insula are called the operculum.

Both hemispheres communicate with each other though several structures: mainly the corpus callosum, but also the anterior and posterior commissures and the fornix (trigon). The beginning of the fornix is called fimbria, runs medial to the hippocampus on the floor of the temporal horn and contains the main output from the hippocampus.

A line defined by the imaginary plane that runs between both hemispheres is called the midline. Structures near the midline are called medial (or mesial) whereas structures furthest away from the midline are called lateral.

The hemispheres contain cavities filled with cerebrospinal liquid, called ventricles. There are two lateral ventricles, one within each hemisphere, and one medial ventricle (between both hemispheres), called the third ventricle. Each lateral ventricle has portions that extend within the frontal, temporal and occipital lobes, often referred to as horns (the frontal or anterior horn, the temporal or inferior horn and the occipital or posterior horn). Each lateral ventricle communicates with the third ventricle through the interventricular foramen or foramen of Monro (foramen is a medical term for hole, the plural is foramina). Ventricles will enlarge if there is loss of brain tissue or if there is an obstacle to the normal circulation of cerebrospinal liquid. There is a thin wall existing between both lateral ventricles outside the interventricular foramen. This wall is called the septum pellucidum. The anterior and superior region of the septum pellucidum contains islands of grey matter called the septum nuclei.

Cerebral cortex

Seizure manifestations result from dysfunction of the cerebral cortex and its interaction with subcortical structures. The cortex is the structure responsible for complex brain functions (the so-called 'higher brain functions'): perception, voluntary movement, memory, motivation, production and understanding of language. During seizures, the cortex functions abnormally. This has two consequences:

Introduction to Epilepsy ed. Gonzalo Alarcón and Antonio Valentín. Published by Cambridge University Press.
© Cambridge University Press 2012.

Chapter 3: Functional anatomy of the central nervous system

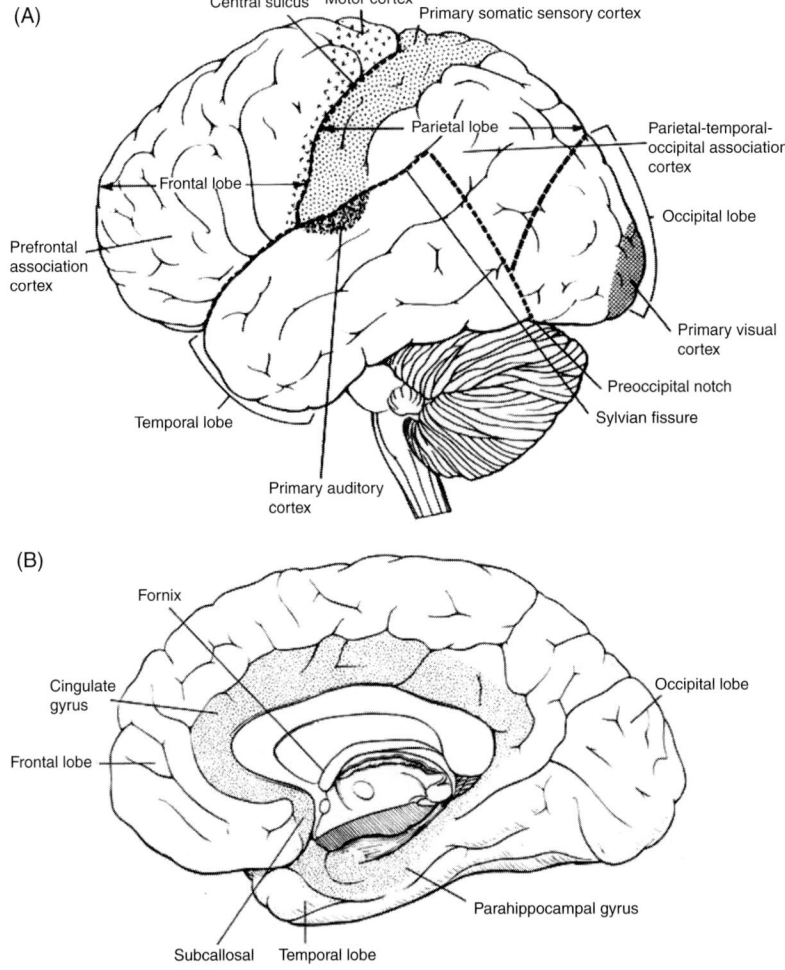

Figure 3.1. The major divisions of the human cerebral cortex. (A) Lateral view of the hemisphere. (B) Medial view of the brain showing the limbic lobe as dotted areas (reproduced with permission, *Principles of Neural Science*, second edition, edited by ER Kandel and JH Schwartz, Elsevier, New York, 1985, Figures 19–3A of page 214 and 46–1A of page 613).

- Normal functions of the cortex can be suppressed during seizures: lack of memory for the event, unresponsiveness, aphasia, behavioural arrest, etc.
- Additional abnormal behaviour and perceptions can occur during seizures: hallucinations, illusions, automatic unconscious movements, convulsions.

To a large degree, the nervous system's function is hierarchical. The cortex appears to be the most dominant structure, responsible for higher functions. The remaining brain structures (such as the thalamus, brainstem and cerebellum) are sometimes termed subcortical structures.

Regions of cortex

The cortex is divided into lobes (frontal, temporal, parietal, occipital, limbic), which are shown in Figure 3.1.

Some regions of the cortex are specialized in processing certain tasks:

- The primary motor cortex (in the posterior portion of the frontal lobes, immediately anterior to the rolandic fissure) commands voluntary movements to muscles. The primary motor cortex is sometimes called the motor strip.
- The supplementary motor cortex (in the medial aspect of the frontal lobes, anterior to the primary motor cortex) is crucial for planning movements.
- The somatosensory cortex (in the anterior region of the parietal lobes, immediately posterior to the rolandic fissure) processes information from the body (somatosensory information), i.e. information from skin, joints, muscles, tendons. It is necessary to feel sensations from skin and to be aware of our body posture in the absence of visual information.

Section 1: Basic principles

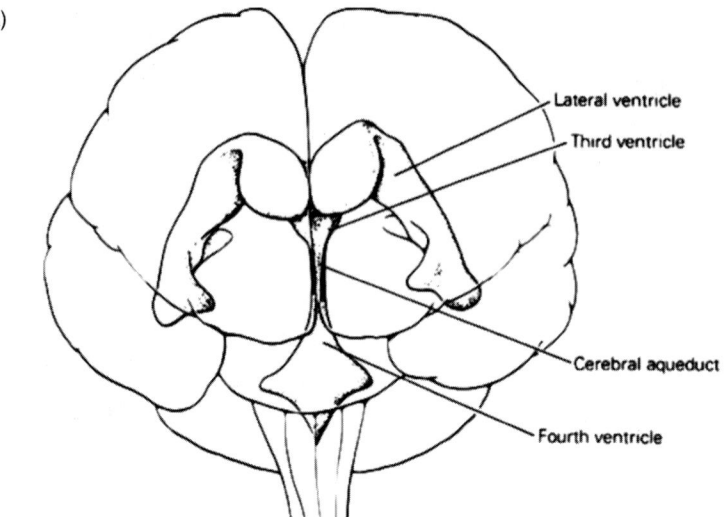

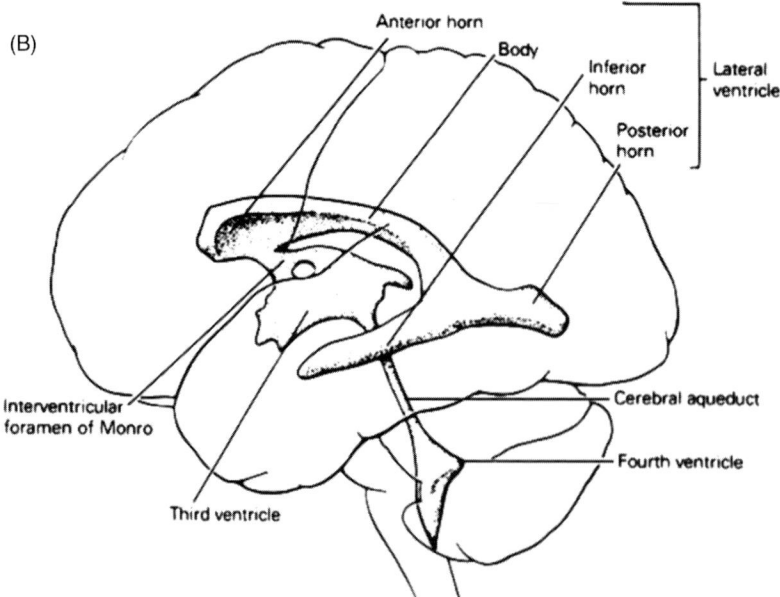

Figure 3.2. The ventricular system of the human brain. (A) Frontal view; (B) lateral view (reproduced with permission, *Principles of Neural Science*, second edition, edited by ER Kandel and JH Schwartz, Elsevier, New York, 1985, Figure 1.19–4, page 216; adapted from Noback and Demarest, 1981).

- The auditory cortex (in the lateral cortex of the temporal lobes) is involved in processing sound.
- The visual cortex (in the occipital lobes) is involved in processing visual information.
- The sensory speech area (usually in the left temporal lobe), also called Wernicke's area, is responsible for interpreting language (both spoken and written) (Figure 3.5).
- The motor speech area (also called Broca's area, located in the lateral inferior and posterior regions of the frontal lobe, usually on the left) is responsible for generating speech (Figure 3.5).
- The hippocampus is involved in processing memories and emotions.
- The limbic system is involved in processing emotions (see below).

Topographic and contralateral organization of motor and sensory cortices

Motor, somatosensory and visual cortices have a topographic organization (somatotopic representation). This means that each area of these cortices processes information from (or for) specific areas of

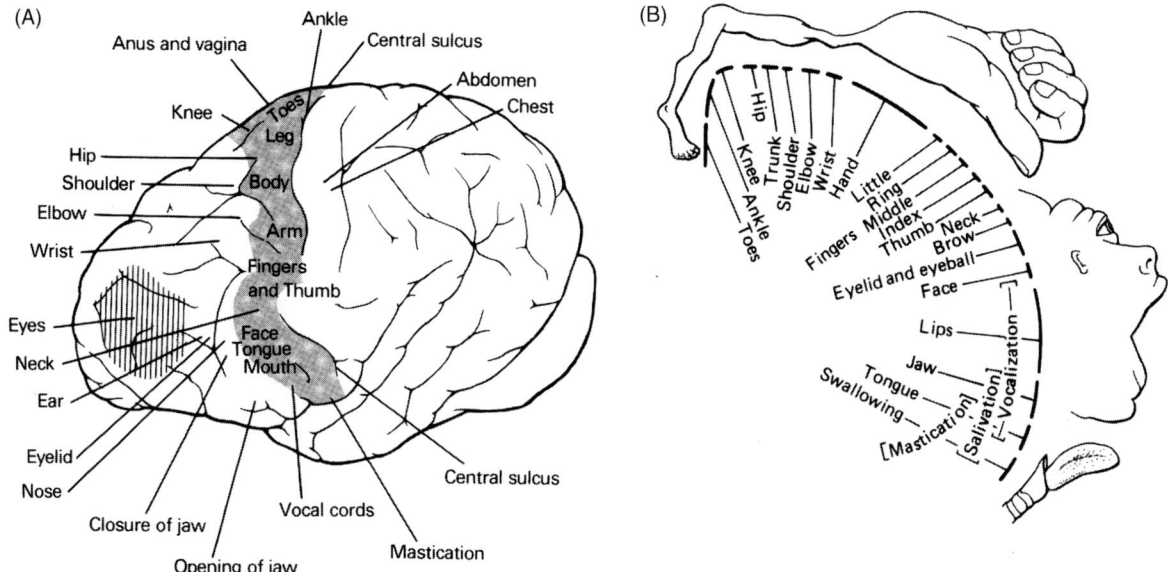

Figure 3.3. The body is somatotopically represented in the motor cortex. (A) Map of the body representation in a lateral view of the motor cortex of the chimpanzee (left side of the picture is anterior brain and right side is posteriorr). The shaded area indicates the precentral gyrus. Electrical stimulation of the region highlighted by vertical lines produces eye movements (reproduced with permission, *Principles of Neural Science*, second edition, edited by ER Kandel and JH Schwartz, Elsevier, New York, 1985, Figure 1.38–1, page 488; adapted from Sherrington, 1906). (B) Body representation in the human motor cortex and corresponding homunculus on a coronal (transversal) section of one hemisphere at the level of the precentral gyrus (reproduced with permission, *Principles of Neural Science*, second edition, edited by ER Kandel and JH Schwartz, Elsevier, New York, 1985, Figure 1.38–1, page 488; adapted from Penfield and Rasmussen, 1950).

the body or visual fields (Figure 3.3). Auditory cortex shows a tonotopic organization (i.e. certain areas process specific tones). Some parts of the body have more cortical representation than others in the somatosensory and motor cortices. In particular, hand, tongue and face appear to engage particularly large areas of cortex. It is standard practice to draw a subject next to the cortex with the size of body parts proportional to the cortical areas representing them. This creates a distorted figure called the Penfield homunculus (Figure 3.3). Motor, somatosensory and visual processing is crossed (each hemisphere moves and feels the opposite side of the body, and sees the contralateral visual field). Auditory processing is bilateral (each hemisphere receives information from both ears). Consequently, removing or damaging cortex unilaterally can generate severe contralateral motor, somatosensory or visual deficits, but not major auditory deficits.

The areas other than those mentioned above are generically designated 'association areas'. The functions of association areas are not as clear as those of the areas mentioned above. Most of what we know about the functions of association cortex derives from studying the effects of acute lesions occurring in humans (stroke, accidental injury) or induced in animals. The frontal lobe is involved in thinking, motivation, volition and making decisions. The parietal lobe (particularly on the right side) is involved in processing spatial information and body self-image. The main deficits induced by lesions in association cortex are shown in Box 3.1.

> **Box 3.1. Effects of lesions on association cortex of different brain lobes**
>
> (1) Effects of lesions in parietal association cortex:
>
> - Neglect of contralateral space (Figure 3.4)
> - Motor deficits: ataxia, poor coordination
> - Sensory deficits: stereo-agnosia (deficits in recognizing objects by touching them, without visual cues)
> - Deficits in spatial perception
> - Affective deficits: neglecting contralateral stimuli
>
> (2) Effects of lesions in temporal association cortex:
>
> - Lateral and posterior lesions are associated with deficits in discriminating complex auditory or visual stimuli, and with visual field defects
> - Memory deficits

Section 1: Basic principles

> **Box 3.1.** (cont.)
> - Short-term deficits
> - Verbal memory if left-sided
> - Prosopagnosia (deficits in recognizing faces) in bilateral occipito-temporal lesions
>
> (3) Effects of lesions in frontal association cortex
> - Behavioural and emotional changes
>   - Acute: apathy, akinesia, mutism
>   - Chronic: hyperactivity, dysinhibition, jocularity
> - Deficit in initiating/changing behaviour
> - Deficits in neuropsychological tests: card-sorting, mazes, Necker cube, visual search

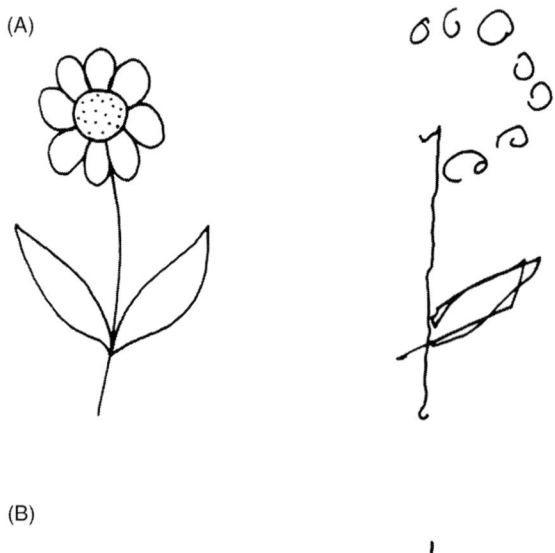

Figure 3.4. Examples of hemispatial neglect in a patient with a right parietal lobe lesion. In (A) the patient was asked to copy the flower on the left, and in (B) to bisect the line (reproduced with permission, *Textbook of Physiology*, volume 1, 21st edition, edited by HD Patton, AF Fuchs, B Hille, AM Scher, R Steiner, W.B Saunders Company, Philadelphia, 1989, Figure 1.31–2, page 666; after Hellman KM, Watson RT, Valenstein E, published in Hellman KM, Valenstein E, *Clinical Neuropsychology*, Oxford University Press, Oxford, 1985).

Connections of the cortex

The cortex receives massive input from subcortical structures, particularly from the thalamus, which is the main subcortical centre involved in processing sensory information. Thalamus and brainstem modulate cortical excitability and control sleep cycles (see below). Each cortical area receives and sends information from and to other cortical areas. The main output of the cortex is the pyramidal tract, composed of axons from the motor area, which convey motor orders to the spinal tracts. Association areas from contralateral hemispheres communicate through the corpus callosum. In man, the medial cortex of frontal lobes is particularly well connected though the corpus callosum (Lacruz *et al.*, 2007).

Functional anatomy of speech function

Speech function is one of the most complex cortical functions. In addition to the mechanical generation or perception of strings of sounds (or letters), it involves complex associations between concepts and sounds (or written words), and associations between complex concepts and symbols according to specific rules to generate or interpret sentences. Speech function is highly localized in the cortex. The posterior regions of the superior temporal gyrus are involved in understanding speech (Wernicke's area) and the inferior lateral aspect of the frontal lobe is involved in generating speech (Broca's area). Wernicke's and Broca's areas are connected by the arcuate fasciculus (see Figure 3.5).

In most subjects, speech areas are present only on the left hemisphere. The hemisphere that processes speech is called the dominant hemisphere for speech. The laterality of speech dominance depends on handedness.

- Among right-handed people, 96% of subjects have the dominant hemisphere on the left.
- Among left-handed people, 70% have the dominant hemisphere on the left, 15% on the right and 15% have speech processing on both sides (co-dominant).

Hemisphere specialization (asymmetries)

Although both hemispheres can independently process information and make decisions, there is a degree of specialization. The right hemisphere tends to be better at processing spatial information (e.g. reading maps, solving spatial puzzles) whereas the left hemisphere processes speech in most (not all) subjects. Memory tends to be processed independently by both hemispheres.

The fact that both hemispheres process information independently has been shown by a series of

Chapter 3: Functional anatomy of the central nervous system

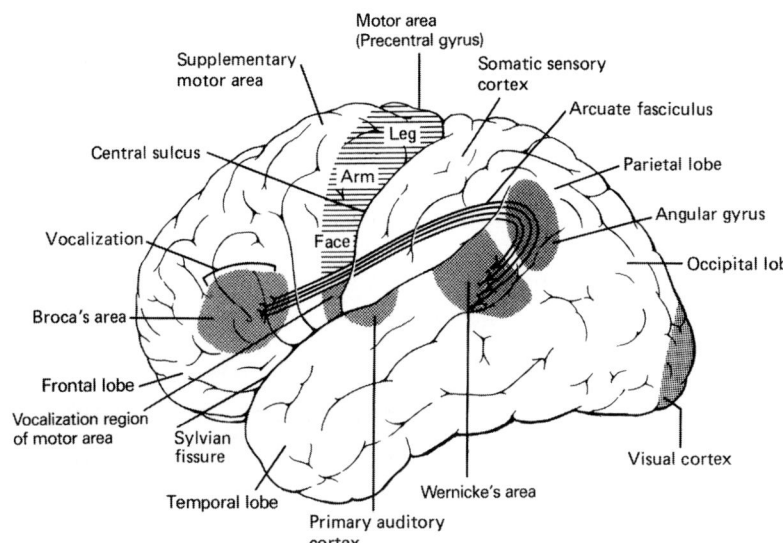

Figure 3.5. Lateral view of the human left cerebral hemisphere, highlighting the main areas involved in movement control and language. The main lobes, sulci and gyri are also shown (reproduced with permission from *Principles of Neural Science*, second edition, edited by ER Kandel and JH Schwartz, Elsevier, New York, 1985, Figure 1.1–5, page 8).

> **Box 3.2.** Useful terms to describe speech disturbances
>
> Dysarthria: abnormal pronunciation of speech.
>
> Aphasia (dysphasia): difficulty in speaking or understanding speech in the absence of dysarthria.
>
> Alexia: inability to read aloud or silent.
>
> Agraphia: inability to express speech in writing.
>
> Expressive, motor or non-fluent aphasia: speech is slow, laboured, telegraphic, or absent. Grammatical errors are common. Understanding is preserved (patient can obey commands). This aphasia can be seen in processes affecting Broca's area.
>
> Receptive, sensory or fluent aphasia: speech understanding is impaired in the absence of hearing deficits. Patient perceives speech as incomprehensible sounds. Some patients can understand slowly spoken, familiar and redundantly conveyed ideas. The patient's own speech is abnormal, rapid, often failing to use the correct word or using circumlocutory phrases (e.g. 'the thing to write' for 'pencil') or empty words (e.g., 'the other', 'that', 'thing'). This aphasia can be seen in processes affecting Wernicke's area.
>
> Conduction aphasia: patient can understand words or sentences but cannot repeat them. It can occur in processes affecting the arcuate fasciculus.
>
> Apraxia: inability to understand and execute learned motor commands in the absence of motor deficits.

elegant experiments carried out in patients who are born without corpus callosum or where the corpus callosum has been surgically severed (for instance for the treatment of seizures). In these patients, both hemispheres do not communicate significantly, so that information delivered to one hemisphere does not cross to the other hemisphere. If discordant information is shown to both visual hemifields and patients are asked to select with each hand the object shown, the right hand will tend to point at what was shown in the right hemifield and vice versa. If asked to name the object, the subject will usually name what was shown in the right hemifield, processed by the left hemisphere.

The limbic system and the physiology of emotions

The limbic system is thought to be involved in processing emotions, an important component of many epileptic seizures. Since the early twentieth century, physiologists have been puzzled by the mechanisms of normal emotions. On the one hand, emotions have much in common with sensations in that they can be triggered by external stimuli. On the other hand, they differ from usual 'sensory' experiences in that they can become independent from the external stimulus, often outlasting it by minutes or hours, or even occurring without an apparent external trigger. Moreover, emotions are often associated with an autonomic or behavioural response (restlessness, flushing, pupillar changes, aggression, sweating, pallor).

The limbic lobe was initially described by Broca (1878) on anatomical grounds, comprising the regions having a common origin along the border ('limbus') of the foramen of Monro. The limbic lobe

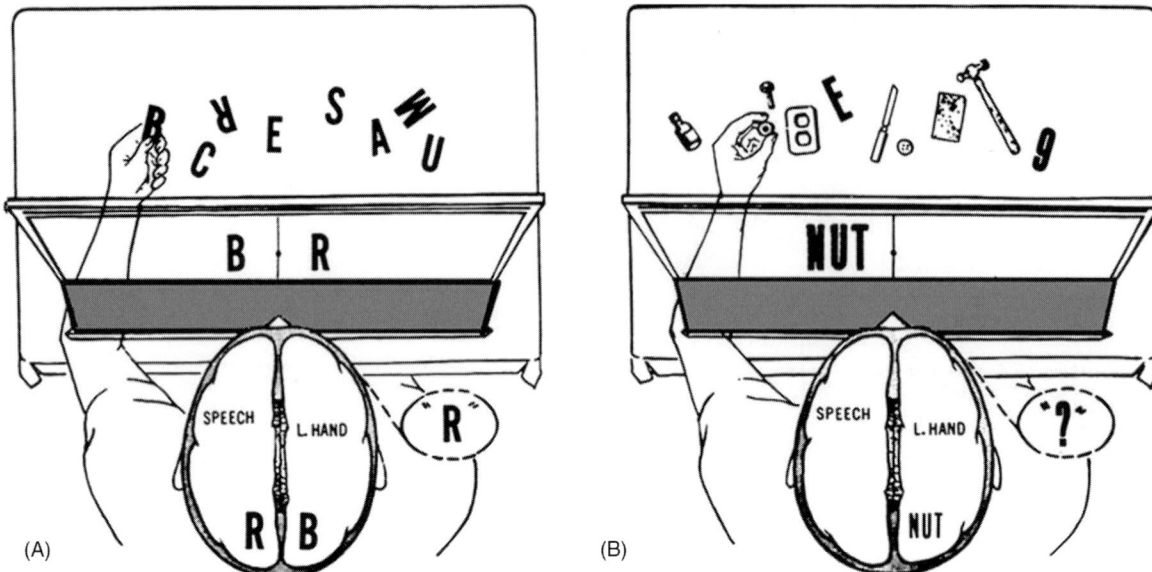

Figure 3.6. Responses of a commissurotomized patient to the tachistocopic presentation of stimuli to the left and right visual fields, which reach the right and the left hemispheres, respectively. (A) When stimuli are presented simultaneously to the right and left hemifields, the subject can name the right-field stimulus but retrieves the left-field stimulus with the left hand. (B) The subject can read and understand the names of objects presented in the left hemifield and can retrieve the appropriate items with his left hand but cannot name them (reproduced with permission, *Textbook of Physiology*, volume 1, 21st edition, edited by HD Patton, AF Fuchs, B Hille, AM Scher, R Steiner, W.B Saunders Company, Philadelphia, 1989, Figure 1.31–18 page 685; after Sperry RW, Gazzaniga MS, Bogen JE, published in Vinken PJ, Bruya GW, *Handbook of Clinical Neurology*, volume 4, pages 273–290, Elsevier Science Publishers, Biomedical Division, 1969).

included the cingulate gyrus (gyrus in the medial aspect of the hemispheres running around the corpus callosum), hippocampal formation, parahipocampal gyrus and subiculum (see Figure 3.1 and Chapter 6). Papez, in 1937, suggested that the limbic lobe in conjunction with the thalamus, hypothalamus and mammillary bodies constituted the limbic system, which was the system responsible for elaborating emotions and emotional behaviour (response). In Papez circuit, activity originating in the cortex (sensation, perception, thoughts) is relayed via the hippocampus to the hypothalamus, which is responsible for the emotional-autonomic response. The mammillary bodies, a subregion of the hypothalamus, then relay the activity to the cingulate gyrus via the anterior thalamus to generate the feelings associated with emotion. Cortical connections from the cingulate gyrus then return activity to the hippocampus, and emotional activity is sustained via reverberating activity within this circuit. The concept of the limbic system has more recently been expanded by MacLean (1952) to include cortical association areas, septum, amygdala, basal ganglia and brainstem structures (mesencephalic reticular formation and tegmentum).

Several classic experiments have gradually identified the structures involved in generating and processing emotions. Electrical stimulation of the lateral hypothalamus induces sham rage in cats (rage directed not only at other animals but also self-directed and directed at inanimate objects) and continuous self-stimulation in rats. Lesions in ventromedial hypothalamus can induce changes in food intake, suggesting that these structures are involved in controlling appetite. Electrical stimulation of the septum nuclei in primates and cats is associated with autonomic changes (decreased heart rate and respiration) and septal stimulation in rats induces septal rage (aversion to all sensory stimuli, which make animals extremely aggressive and intractable to handle) and docility later on. Several sensory modalities appear to converge in the amygdala. Electrical stimulation of the amygdala in patients being assessed for surgery can induce déjà vu, hallucinations, aggressive feelings and visceral sensations. Destruction or removal of the amygdala in animals and humans is associated with flat behaviour and a reduction in responses to environmental stimuli. The physiology of the hippocampus is summarized in Chapter 8.

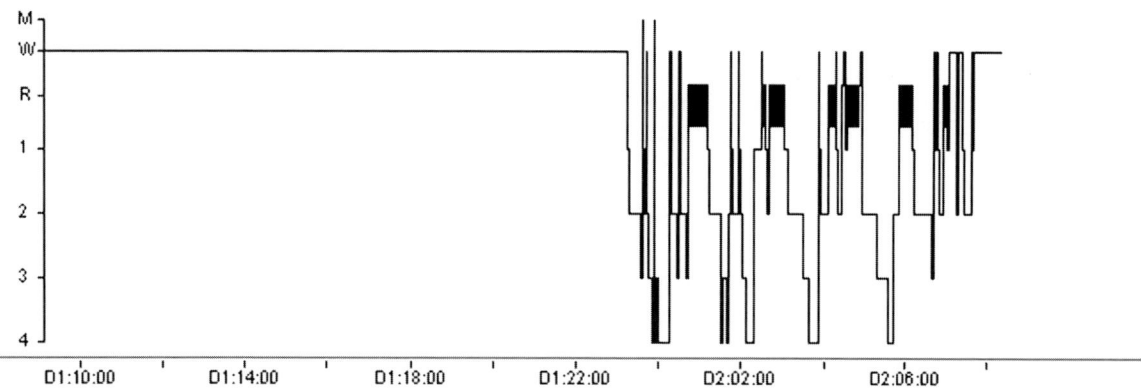

Figure 3.7. One-day sleep staging from a patient (hypnogram). The graph represents sleep stage (awake, 1, 2, 3, 4 and REM versus time of the day) during a 24-hour period, from 10 am of day 1 to 10 am of day 2. The patient remains awake until 11 pm of day 1. He then falls asleep until 8 am of day 2. Note alternating cycles between deep and lighter/REM sleep through the night. REM sleep is shown as periods of thick horizontal bars. The patient suffered from restless leg syndrome and woke up frequently in the night. Deep sleep becomes less common towards the end of sleep. M, movement; W, awake; R, REM; 1, sleep stage 1; 2, sleep stage 2; 3, sleep stage 3; 4, sleep stage 4; D1, day 1; D2, day 2.

Subcortical structures

The thalami (in singular, thalamus) and brainstem are connected to the cortex and appear to control global cortical excitability and sleep cycles. The thalami are bilateral egg-shaped sets of grey matter nuclei located in the centre of each hemisphere. Thalamic nuclei are classified into two types:

- specific nuclei, involved in processing specific afferent peripheral information (somatosensory, visual, auditory), and relaying it to the corresponding cortical areas;
- nonspecific and association nuclei, which project to widespread areas of the cortex and to other subcortical structures. They are involved in regulating global cortical excitability and are key structures involved in generating seizures in idiopathic generalized epilepsies.

Because of the intricate relations between thalamus and cortex, both structures are sometimes referred to as the thalamo-cortical system. Thalamic electrical stimulation induces cortical responses (Morison and Dempsey, *Am J Physiol* 1942;**135**:281–92): high-frequency stimulation induces spindle-like responses whereas low-frequency induces recruiting responses (diffuse but with parietal and frontal emphasis).

Sleep

In many epileptic syndromes, the incidence of interictal epileptiform discharges and seizures increase during sleep. The physiology of sleep is complex and poorly understood. Several neuronal structures appear to be involved in regulating sleep cycles: the brainstem, the hypothalamus (preoptic area and suprachiasmatic nucleus) and the thalamo-cortical system. During a night of sleep, there are changes in the depth of sleep according to how difficult it is to wake up the subject. Sleep depth in humans has been classified into stages 1 (or drowsiness, the most superficial) to 4 (the deepest), and REM sleep (REM stands for 'rapid eye movements'). Stages 1–4 are sometimes called non-REM sleep. The electroencephalogram and electromyogram are used to identify each sleep stage. REM sleep has also been called 'paradoxical sleep' because the EEG resembles an awake stage but the subject is deeply asleep. During a normal night, a subject will enter and leave each stage several times, usually showing a higher proportion of stage IV in the first half of the night, and more REM sleep in the second half of the night (see Figure 3.7).

Recommended reading

Kandel ER, Schwartz JH, Jessell TM. *Principles of Neural Science*. 4th edn. New York: McGraw-Hill; 2000.

Patton HD, Fuchs AF, Hille B, Scher AM, Steiner R. *Textbook of Physiology*, pp. 663–736. Vol 1. 21st edn. Philadelphia, PA: W.B. Saunders; 1989.

Reference

Lacruz ME, García Seoane JJ, Valentín A, Selway R, Alarcón G. Frontal and temporal functional connections of the living human brain. *Eur J Neurosci* 2007; **26**:1357–70.

Learning objectives

(1) To understand the basic anatomical concepts and anatomical terminology of the following structures:
- cerebral hemispheres
- limbic system
- cerebral cortex
- subcortical structures.

(2) To be aware of the functional roles of these structures, particularly in relation to:
- cortical motor function
- cortical sensory functions
- cortical speech function
- hemisphere specialization
- physiology of emotions
- control of cortical excitability by subcortical structures
- sleep physiology.

Section 1 Basic principles

Chapter 4
Introduction to neurochemistry and receptor pharmacology

Gonzalo Alarcón

Neurons and glia

Two main types of cells are located in the cortex: neurons, which process information mainly coded as chemical and electrical signals; and glia, whose functions are much debated, but appear to be related to appropriately maintaining the cellular environment, including immune defence.

There are several types of neurons with rather complex and variable shapes (Figure 4.1). Each neuron has very large number of connections (synapses), receiving and sending information from and to many other neurons. It is estimated that the typical human brain contains around one hundred billion neurons, each with an average of 7000 synapses.

The cell membrane of the neurons

The cell membrane separates the inside and outside of the cell. Both sides of the membrane contain mainly fluids: the intracellular and the extracellular (interstitial) fluids, with different composition. The cell membrane is constituted by a double layer of phospholipids (fat), which contains sparsely scattered proteins. The proteins can behave as receptors, or as ion channels or as both (see below, and also Chapter 5: 'Cellular electrophysiology: membrane, synaptic and action potentials').

Basic anatomy of the neuron

Most neurons have the following parts (Figure 4.1):

(A) Neuronal body (or cell body or soma, plural is somata): a round or triangular central structure containing cellular nucleus and organelles.

(B) Dendrites: ramifications arising from the neuronal body, showing complex shapes, often resembling tree branches. Dendrites are specialized in picking up mostly chemical signals from other neurons and converting them into electrical signals that travel along the dendrite. Dendrites and body are the neuronal elements responsible for processing information coming from other neurons.

(C) Axon: a single ramification, usually longer than the dendrites, with an initial wider portion called the axon hillock. Under normal conditions, the axon hillock can initiate self-propagating electrical signals, called action potentials (see Chapter 5, 'Cellular electrophysiology: membrane, synaptic and action potentials'). Action potentials

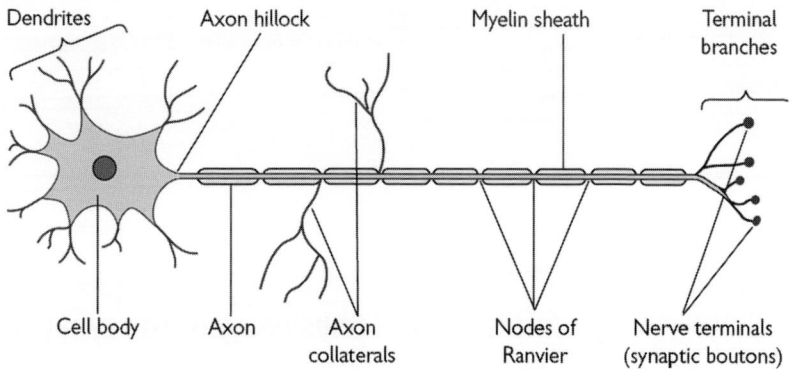

Figure 4.1. Anatomy of the neuron. Diagramatic representation of a central nervous system neuron (reproduced with permission from Pocock G and Richards CD, *Human Physiology*, 3rd edition, 2006, Oxford University Press, Oxford).

Introduction to Epilepsy ed. Gonzalo Alarcón and Antonio Valentín. Published by Cambridge University Press.
© Cambridge University Press 2012.

Section 1: Basic principles

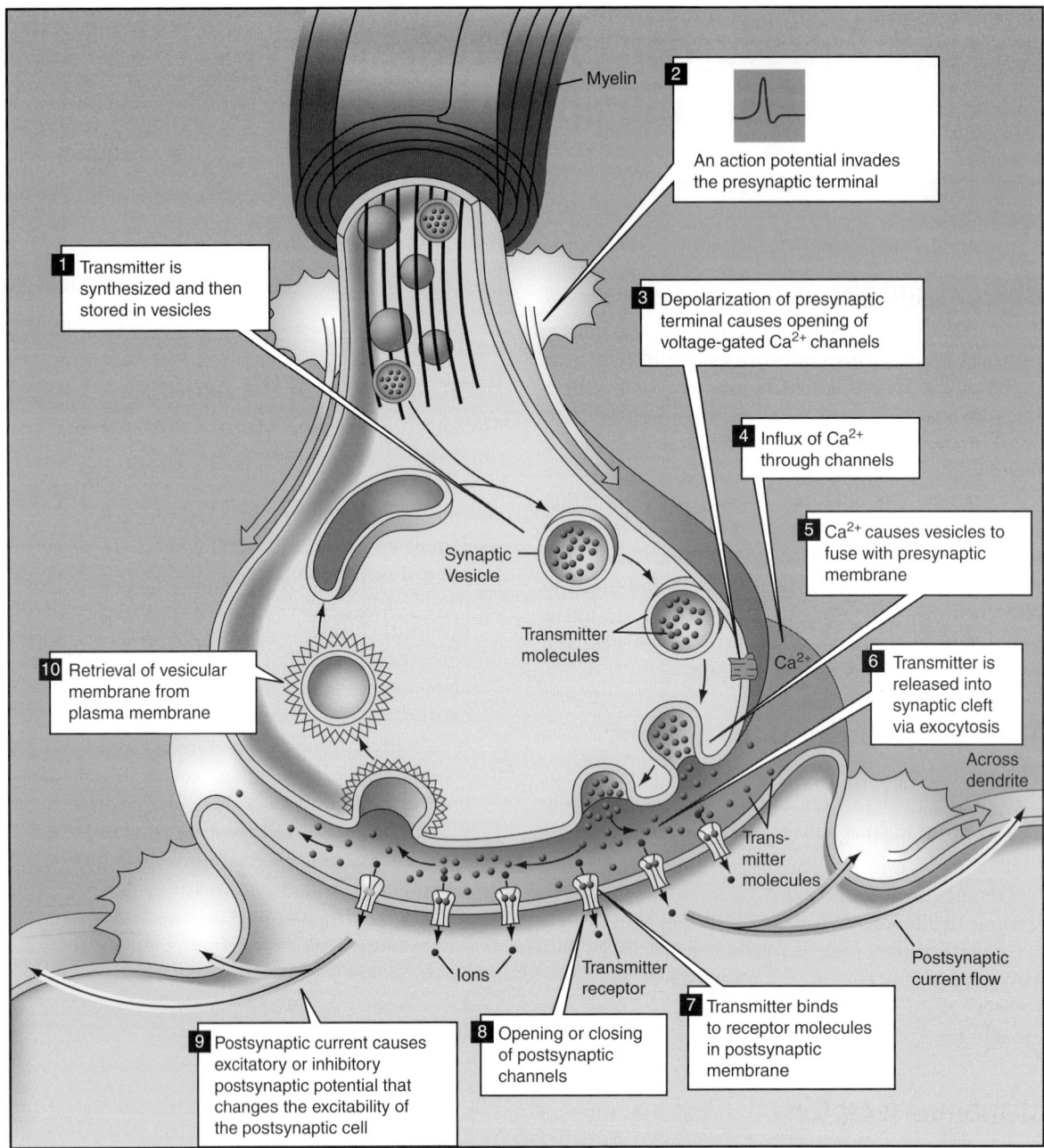

Figure 4.2. Anatomy and physiology of a chemical synapse (reproduced from scholarpedia.com).

travel along the axon and are directly responsible for releasing the chemical compounds (called neurotransmitters and neuromodulators) necessary to communicate with other neurons through a structure called a synapse.

Anatomy and physiology of the synapse

The synapse (Figure 4.2) is the region where two neurons become very close, in contact or nearly in contact with each other, and it is the neuronal structure involved in transferring information from one neuron to another. Synapses usually involve the axon of one neuron and the dendrite of another neuron. With the standard (optical) microscope, synapses look like a little pimple on the surface of the neuron (called synaptic boutons or synaptic processes; Figure 4.2). However, when seen with the electron microscope, membranes from the two communicating neurons come nearly into contact, being separated by a narrow space of around 20 nm called the synaptic cleft. The membrane from the neuron providing information is called the presynaptic membrane (usually from an axon), and the membrane from the neuron receiving information is called the postsynaptic membrane (usually from a dendrite; Figure 4.2).

When an action potential reaches the presynaptic membrane, specific chemical compounds called neurotransmitters (different types, depending on the class of neurons involved) are released into the synaptic cleft via exocytosis of presynaptic vesicles. For this process, a minimum concentration of intracellular calcium is necessary. The postsynaptic membrane has certain proteins (receptors) that can specifically couple with a neurotransmitter and bind with it (see below). When neurotransmitters bind to the specific receptors, pores for specific ions open in the postsynaptic membrane, a process that triggers changes in electrical voltage across the membrane (the postsynaptic potential; see Chapter 5: 'Cellular electrophysiology: membrane, synaptic and action potentials'). The end product is that electrical phenomena in the presynaptic membrane give rise to electrical changes in the postsynaptic membrane via a neurochemical process.

Some synapses are thought to be only electrical, having pre- and postsynaptic membranes in direct contact. In the human brain, such synapses are thought to be a minority and their role is uncertain.

Membrane receptors

A membrane receptor is a protein to which one or more specific molecules can bind. The molecule that binds to a receptor is called a ligand. In epileptology, most ligands involved are neurotransmitters or drugs. Most ligands and receptors bind through spatial coupling ('like a key in a lock'). A receptor may bind to different ligands. Ligand binding determines a specific receptor molecular shape (conformation) with no change in amino acid sequence. The conformational change may generate a biological effect (the response).

If the binding of ligand and receptor induces a response, the receptor is said to have been activated. Activation of neuronal receptors is ordinarily associated with opening of nearby ionic channels in the membrane, resulting in changes in ion permeability across the membrane (see Chapter 5: 'Cellular electrophysiology: membrane, synaptic and action potentials').

Most neurotransmitter receptors are membrane receptors (proteins embedded in the phospholipid bilayer of the cell membrane). They have been classified into:

- Ionotropic receptors or ligand-gated ion channels: the receptor contains a pore which opens when binding to the ligand;
- metabotropic receptors, which are coupled to intracellular G-proteins that indirectly affect membrane ion currents through enzymes which control ion channels.

Agonists and antagonists

Neurotransmitters are ligands to their receptor, but receptors may have other ligands which are not neurotransmitters. When bound to the receptor, not all ligands activate it. Several types of ligands have been identified:

- Agonists: ligands that activate the receptor. Two types of agonists exist:
  - full agonists: activate the receptor and result in a maximal biological response;
  - partial agonists: induce an incomplete activation of the receptor, originating responses which are smaller compared to those of full agonists.
- Antagonists: they bind to receptors but do not activate them. This blocks the receptor and reduces the binding of agonists.
- Inverse agonists: reduce the activity of receptors.

Cortical neurons

There are several types of cortical neurons, and classifications have been made based upon the size and form of neuronal bodies, the length and distribution of their dendritic trees, and the destination and degree of branching of their axons. The principal neuron types and their connections are shown in Figure 4.3. The simplest classification divides neurons into two major classes: pyramidal cells and interneuron cells.

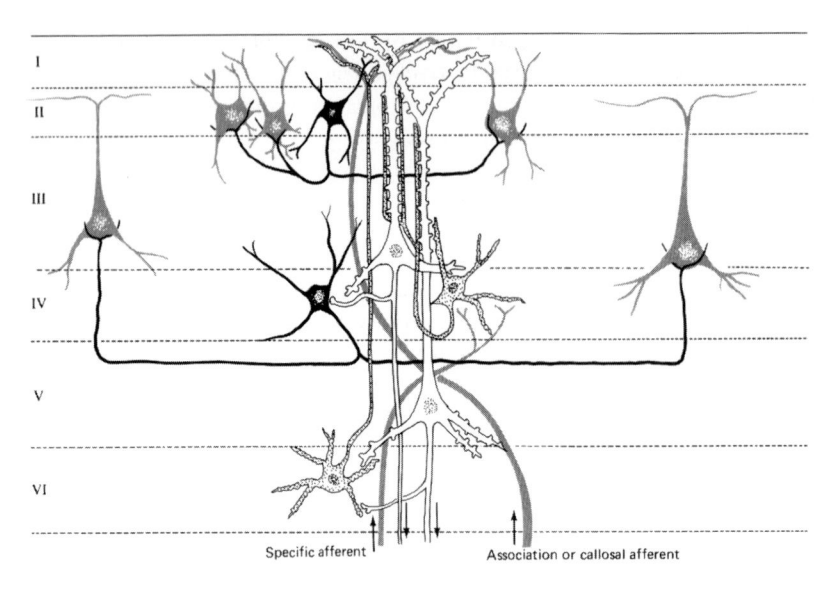

Figure 4.3. The principal neuron types and their interconnections. The two large pyramidal cells (white) in layers III and V receive multiple synaptic connections from the interneurons (stellate cells, stippled) in layer IV. Basket cell (black) inhibition is directed to the body of cortical neurons. Most input to the cortex arrives from specific thalamic nuclei (specific afferents) and is directed mostly to layer IV. Association and callosal input (association and callosal afferents) is mainly directed to more superficial layers (reproduced with permission from Kandel ER and Schwartz JH (eds.) (1985). *Principles of Neural Science*, 2nd edition. Elsevier, New York; adapted from Szentágothai (1969)).

(a) Pyramidal cells have bodies similar to small pyramids. Their axons are usually long, connecting with other areas of the cortex or brain or to the spinal cord. They are excitatory.

(b) Interneurons have a body that is round or oval. They are small neurons with dendrites that may spring in all directions (stellate cells, i.e. resembling a star). They are called interneurons because their axons typically make synapses with nearby neurons, and do not leave the cerebral cortex. Several types of interneurons have been described: stellate cells, granule cells, basket cells, chandelier (axo-axonic) cells, and doublebouquet cells. They are inhibitory neurons, with gamma-aminobutyric acid (GABA) being their main neurotransmitter.

The regions of the brain with plenty of neuronal bodies and dendrites appear grey, and therefore are called grey matter. The cerebral cortex is grey matter. The regions with few neuronal bodies tend to have plenty of axons, look whiter and are called white matter.

Layers of cortex

Cortical cells are not randomly distributed. Different types of cells and axons tend to lay across the cortex with a distribution that, in most regions, makes up six layers running parallel to the surface of the cortex:

- layer I, molecular or plexiform: with few neuronal bodies; this layer is the most external, in contact with the meninges;
- layer II or external granular layer: with small pyramidal neurons and interneurons;
- layer III or pyramidal cell layer: with small pyramidal bodies;
- layer IV or granular cell layer or internal granular layer: rich in stellate (granular) cells and axons from pyramidal cells;
- layer V or ganglion cell or giant pyramidal layer: with large bodies of pyramidal cells;
- layer VI or fusiform or multiform cell layer: with cells of different size and shape; this layer is the most internal, in contact with the white matter.

Long extracortical axons leave or enter perpendicularly to the cortex through the underlying white matter. Axons leaving the cortex are called efferent, whereas axons entering the cortex, coming from neurons in thalamus or remote cortex, are called afferent. The corpus callosum (callosal fibres) is composed of axons connecting cortex between both hemispheres.

Regions rich in pyramidal cells are predominantly output regions, whereas those rich in granular-stellate cells are mainly input regions, where afferent axons from thalamus and other structures terminate. For instance, layer IV is expanded in thickness in the primary visual cortex, whereas layer V is expanded in the primary motor cortex.

Surround inhibition

When information is processed in a cortical region, the local interneurons are activated and tend to release the inhibitory neurotransmitter GABA. This creates a small region of inhibition around an excitatory area, called surround or lateral inhibition. Such inhibition limits the extent of active cortex, often to a rather small area similar to a column of cortex. Such small columns are considered the functional units of the cortex.

Neuromodulators

Neurotransmitters are released in the synaptic cleft and then destroyed or reabsorbed by the presynaptic membrane and glia, so that their effects are localized. Neuromodulators are compounds which show more widespread activity because they are not so readily destroyed or re-absorbed.

Learning objectives

(1) To know the functions of glia and neurons.
(2) To know the basic anatomy of neurons and synapses.
(3) To understand the concepts of neurotransmitters, membrane receptors, agonists, antagonists and neuromodulators.
(4) To understand the basic histology of the cortex and understand the concept of surround inhibition.

Section 1   **Basic principles**

Chapter 5

Cellular electrophysiology: membrane, synaptic and action potentials

Gonzalo Alarcón

Some key concepts about the physiology of cell membrane

- The cell membrane separates intracellular and extracellular (interstitial) fluids.
- The cell membrane is constituted by a double layer of lipids (essentially fat), which contains sparsely scattered proteins.
- Lipids are impermeable to water or ions.
- Some proteins have pores, which can be open or closed, and allow specific charged ions to move between intracellular and extracellular fluids. Such protein pores are called ion channels (Figures 8.2 and 8.4).
- Each ion channel type is permeable to one type of ion or to a limited number of ion types.
- For each ion, the density of ion-specific channels open in the membrane defines the permeability of the membrane to that ion.
- Since ion channels determine the permeability of the membrane to specific ions, they are responsible for specific ion currents. For this reason, ion channels and currents are sometimes referred to under the same name, although they are conceptually different (for instance, some channels may be permeable to more than one ion type; and one channel might be active but blocked, resulting in no current).
- Some ion channels open or close when the voltage across the membrane reaches a certain value. This type of channel is called voltage-dependent or voltage-gated.

Behaviour of the cell membrane at rest

- Generally speaking, in every cell there is a voltage difference (potential difference; see Box 5.1)

Box 5.1. Synonyms

The following terms refer to the same concept:
  Potential difference
  Voltage difference
  Electrical field
  Electrical force
  Potential gradient
  Voltage gradient
  Electrical gradient

between intracellular and extracellular fluids (i.e. across the membrane). This is called the membrane potential.
- The voltage difference between inside and outside the neuron at rest is called the resting potential (Figure 5.1).
- In neurons at rest, the intracellular fluid is 60–70 mV more negative than the extracellular fluid. This concept is sometimes expressed with sentences such as:
  - 'At rest, the membrane is polarized at −60 mV' or
  - 'At rest, the membrane potential is −60 mV' or
  - 'The resting membrane potential is −60 mV'.
- The resting potential is commonly described as having a value of −60 to −70 mV because it is usually measured with the reference electrode (considered as having a voltage of 0) located outside the cell. Since the resting potential is generally different from 0, the membrane at rest is said to be polarized.
- In addition to voltage differences, there are also differences in ion concentrations between inside and outside the cell.

Introduction to Epilepsy ed. Gonzalo Alarcón and Antonio Valentín. Published by Cambridge University Press.
© Cambridge University Press 2012.

Chapter 5: Cellular electrophysiology: membrane, synaptic and action potentials

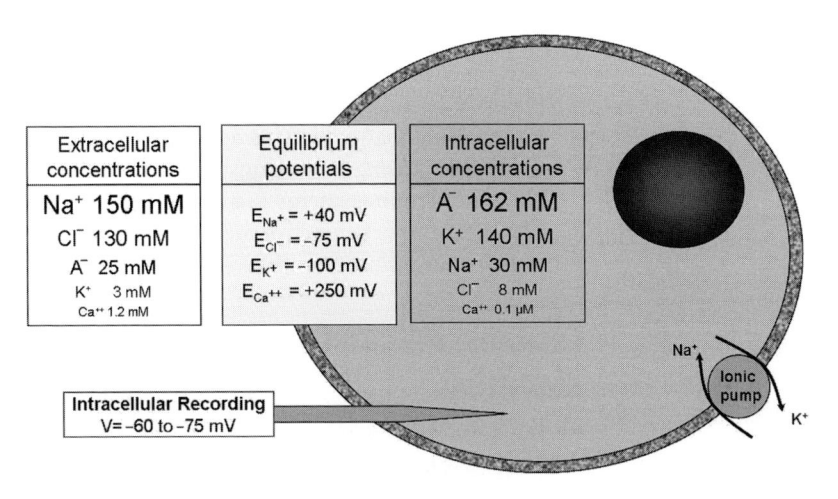

Figure 5.1. Distribution of ions across neuronal membranes (concentrations in mM) and their equilibrium potentials (expressed as mV). At rest, the cell membrane is permeable to K^+, Na^+ and Cl^-, and exhibits a voltage difference (inside versus outside) of approximately −60 to −70 mV, as seen by an intracellular recording electrode. E, equilibrium potential.

Extracellular concentrations
Na^+ 150 mM
Cl^- 130 mM
A^- 25 mM
K^+ 3 mM
Ca^{++} 1.2 mM

Equilibrium potentials
E_{Na^+} = +40 mV
E_{Cl^-} = −75 mV
E_{K^+} = −100 mV
$E_{Ca^{++}}$ = +250 mV

Intracellular concentrations
A^- 162 mM
K^+ 140 mM
Na^+ 30 mM
Cl^- 8 mM
Ca^{++} 0.1 μM

Intracellular Recording V= −60 to −75 mV

Ionic pump

- Outside, Na^+, Ca^{2+} and Cl^- exist in higher concentrations than inside. On the inside, the concentration of K^+ and non-permeable anions (mainly proteins) is higher than outside the cell (Figure 5.1).
- Differences in ion concentration, and in electrical potential, existing between inside and outside the cell are called gradients. Consequently, there are generally two gradients across the membrane (i.e. between inside and outside the cell): a voltage (electrical) gradient and a concentration (chemical) gradient.
- For each ion, the electrical and concentration gradients are forces that move ions between inside and outside the cell, depending on the ion charge and membrane permeability to that ion. According to voltage gradients, positively charged ions move towards negative regions, and negatively charged ions move towards positive regions. According to concentration gradients, ions tend to move from regions with higher concentration to regions of lower concentration.
  - For instance, at rest, Na^+ ions will tend to be pushed into the cell because of the concentration gradient (concentration higher outside) and because of the electrical gradient (inside more negative, attracts positively charged external Na^+).
  - On the other hand, K^+ ions are pushed inside by the electrical gradient (inside negativity attracts positively charged K^+) and are pushed outside by the concentration gradient (higher concentration inside than outside).
- The strength of the force is proportional to the gradient (difference) between inside and outside the cell. For instance, if the membrane potential is −100 mV, the electrical force moving sodium inside the cell would be five times stronger than if the membrane potential was −20.
- The passage of charged ions across the membrane behaves as an electrical current (ionic current). Since the electrical resistance of the membrane is high, large voltage changes can be generated by relatively small ionic currents (Ohm's law, $V = I \cdot R$). This means that ion concentrations inside and outside the cell tend to change little with voltage changes, unless massive neuronal firing occurs.

Equilibrium potential

- As mentioned above, ion concentrations inside and outside the cell change little during normal function, even while membrane potential is changing and ions are moving (i.e. too few ions move to change ion concentration). Consequently, it can be assumed that the concentration gradient for each ion is generally constant.
- For each ion, there will be a membrane potential at which the forces due to electrical and concentration gradients have similar values and push ions in opposite directions. This is the equilibrium potential.
- At the equilibrium potential there will be no net movement of ions across the membrane (since the number of ions that leave the cell due to one gradient will be equal to the number of ions that enter the cell due to the other gradient).
- For each ion type, its equilibrium potential depends on its intracellular and extracellular concentrations and its charge. For each value of

these variables, the value of the equilibrium potential is given by the Nernst equation:

$$E = (RT/FZ) \log_e [C_e/C_i]$$

where E = equilibrium potential, R = 8.31 joules per mole, T = absolute temperature, or 310 for body temperature (37°C), F = 96 500 coulombs per equivalent, Z = ion charge, C_e = extracellular concentration and C_i = intracellular concentration.

- Consequences of the Nernst equation: for positive ions (K^+, Na^+, Ca^{2+}), increasing their extracellular concentration will increase their equilibrium potential, and decreasing their extracellular concentration will decrease their equilibrium potential. Increasing their intracellular concentration will decrease their equilibrium potential and decreasing their intracellular concentration will increase their equilibrium potential. The opposite will occur for negative ions (e.g. Cl^-).
- For the normal conditions of mammalian cells, the values for equilibrium potentials are:

  for $K^+ = -100\text{mV}$
  for $Na^+ = +40\text{mV}$
  for $Cl^- = -75\text{mV}$
  for $Ca^{2+} = +250\text{mV}$

- Since the value of the equilibrium potential is different for different ions, when the membrane is permeable to more than one ion an overall equilibrium potential cannot exist, because an equilibrium potential for one ion would be a non-equilibrium potential for another ion. The membrane potential will settle closest to (but not at) the equilibrium potential of the ion of highest permeability. This is described by Goldman constant field flux and voltage equations, whose analysis is beyond the scope of this book.
- Consequently, if the cell membrane becomes largely permeable to one ion (i.e. the permeability to that ion increases), the membrane potential will move towards the equilibrium potential of that ion.
- In a living cell, the resting potential is relatively constant and different from the equilibrium potential of any individual ion. Consequently, there is permanently movement of ions due to electrical and chemical gradients (passive movement). This means that, since the resting potential is constant, there have to be other mechanisms that move ions against the gradients. Moving ions against gradients (forces) obviously requires energy (active movement). The most important active mechanism is the sodium–potassium pump.

Excitable cells and postsynaptic potentials

- For each cell, the value of the resting potential is fairly constant in time.
- In excitable cells (mainly muscle cells and neurons), the membrane potential can change due to changes in ionic permeability occurring as a response to external stimulation. Such stimulation can be the result of the application of electrical current across the membrane, or of the release of specific chemicals (e.g. neurotransmitters) into the extracellular fluid.
- In the postsynaptic membrane, changes in the membrane potential seen as a consequence of the release of neurotransmitters are called postsynaptic potentials.
- Postsynaptic potentials can be generated by changes in permeability to specific ions. This occurs due to opening of ion channels as a response to activation of specific membrane receptors by neurotransmitters.
- Neurotransmitters that increase permeability to specific ions tend to drive the membrane potential closer to the equilibrium potentials for these ions.
- Thus, neurotransmitters that increase permeability to Na^+ and/or Ca^{2+} tend to drive the membrane potential closer to the equilibrium potentials for these ions. Since their equilibrium potentials are positive, the membrane potential will become less negative than at rest (and therefore the membrane will become less polarized). This is called depolarization (Figure 5.2).
- In contrast, neurotransmitters that increase permeability to K^+ and/or Cl^- tend to make the membrane potential more negative (and therefore the membrane will become more polarized). This is called hyperpolarization (Figure 5.2).

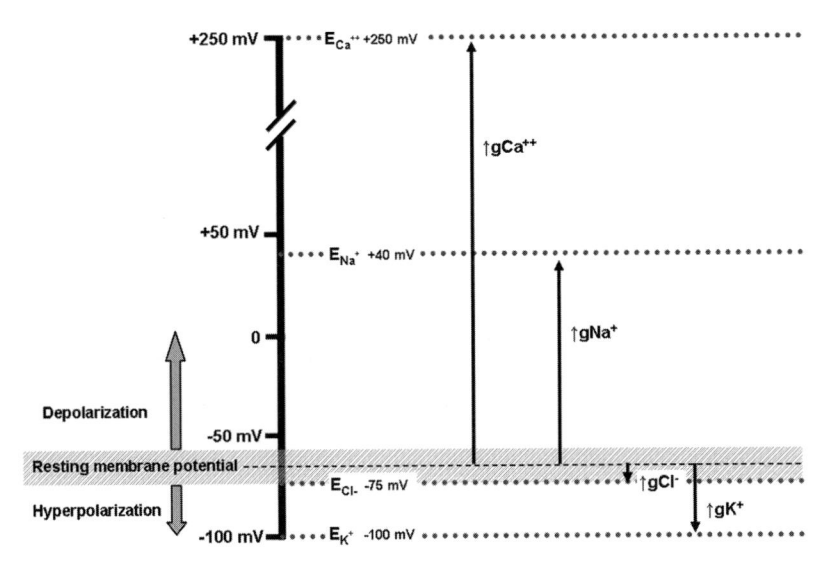

Chapter 5: Cellular electrophysiology: membrane, synaptic and action potentials

Figure 5.2. Effect of increasing membrane permeability (or conductance, symbolized as g) to Cl^-, K^+, Ca^{2+} or Na^+. Increases in gCl^- or gK^+ move the membrane potential toward more negative values (hyperpolarization), whereas increases in gNa^+ or gCa^{2+} bring the membrane potential toward more positive values (depolarization). E, equilibrium potential.

- Postsynaptic depolarization potentials drive the membrane potential closer to the threshold for action potentials (see below). Therefore, they increase the likelihood of neuronal firing and are called excitatory postsynaptic potentials (EPSPs).
- Postsynaptic potentials consisting of hyperpolarization drive the membrane potential away from the threshold for action potentials. Therefore, they decrease the likelihood of neuronal firing and are called inhibitory postsynaptic potentials (IPSPs).
- Postsynaptic potentials can add up (Figure 5.3) and travel along the membrane with progressive decrement.

Action potentials

- In neurons and muscle fibres, when the membrane is depolarized to a particular value of membrane potential (called threshold), an action potential will occur (Figure 5.4). Due to their sharp appearance, action potentials are also called spikes (this is different from the EEG spikes that can be seen in epilepsy; see Chapter 16: 'Pathological EEG phenomena and their significance').
- The value of the threshold is normally between –60 and –50 mV.

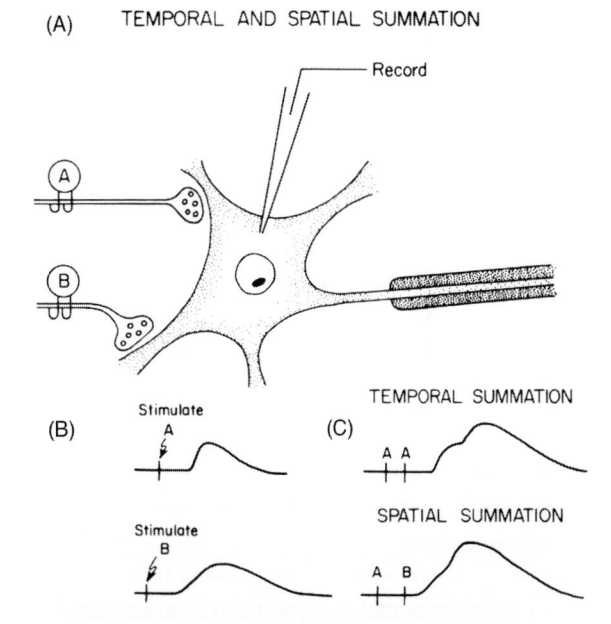

Figure 5.3. Temporal and spatial summation of synaptic inputs to a central neuron. A shows the experimental arrangement in which a neuron is impaled by an intracellular recording electrode, and stimulating electrodes. A and B activate two separate inputs that make synaptic contact near each other. (B) Stimulaton of either synaptic input alone evokes an EPSP. (C) The amplitude of the EPSP can be increased either by stimulating the same synaptic contact twice at a short interval (temporal summation) or by stimulating one contact shortly after the other (spatial summation) (reproduced with permission from Patton DH, Fuchs AF, Hille B, Scher AM, Steiner R, *Textbook of Physiology*, volume 1, 21st edition, W.B. Saunders Company, Philadelphia, 1989, Figure 1.11–8, page 242).

Section 1: Basic principles

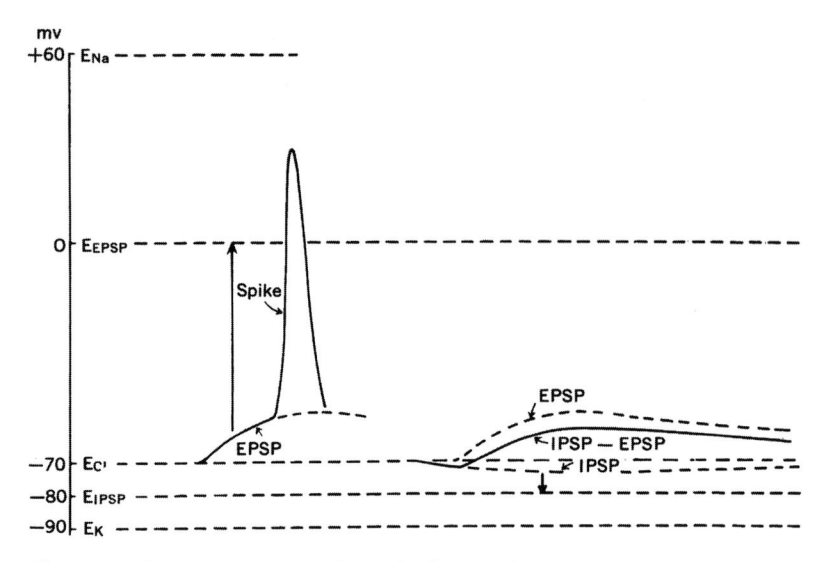

Figure 5.4. Diagram summarizing the mode of action of postsynaptic excitation and inhibition at chemically operated synapses in the central nervous system in terms of ionic hypothesis. Equilibrium potentials for Na$^+$, K$^+$ and Cl$^-$, and for EPSP and IPSP are shown as dotted lines. At left, EPSP is seen driving membrane potential in depolarizing direction, and at threshold eliciting an action potential in the cell. To right, IPSP and EPSP are shown alone (dotted lines) and when they interact (net effect, continuous line). EPSP is now so depressed by simultaneous IPSP that the membrane potential does not reach cell threshold. Interaction of synaptic influences of opposite signs is the essence of integrative action of single neurons (reproduced from Mountcastle VB, *Medical Physiology*, volume 1, 13th edition, The C.V. Mosby Company, Saint Louis, 1974, Figure 1.6–16, page 202; itself reproduced from Eccles JC, *Modes of Communications Between Nerve Cells*. Australian Academy of Science Yearbook, Sydney, 1963, Waite & Bull.)

- An action potential is a complex electrical event, which is commonly initiated by opening of voltage-gated channels, inducing a sudden increase in permeability to Na$^+$ which is followed by increases in permeability to K$^+$ (Figure 5.5).
- Action potentials generated by the same neuron are nearly identical (all-or-nothing).
- Action potentials are self-propagating (travel along the membrane with no decrement).
- During or shortly after the generation of an action potential, a second action potential cannot be induced (absolute refractory period) or, if induced, the second action potential may be smaller (relative refractory period). Following the initiation of an action potential, there is an absolute refractory period followed by relative refractory period lasting for a few milliseconds (Table 5.1).
- Action potentials are responsible for triggering the release of neurotransmitters when they reach the presynaptic terminal in the axon. Action potentials are the final electrical events that are responsible for the release of neurotransmitters and therefore for communication of information to the 'next' neuron.
- A neuron is said to 'fire' when it generates one action potential or a run of action potentials.
- If a neuron is depolarized above threshold and this level of depolarization is maintained, sustained repetitive firing usually occurs during the duration of depolarization, although a slight attenuation in the frequency of spikes may occur during the duration of depolarization.
- Some normal neurons show a marked decrease in the frequency of action potentials during sustained supra-threshold depolarization. This is called adaptation.
- The onset of adaptation associated with infusion of drugs has been used to screen for potential anticonvulsants.
- Action potentials are usually immediately followed by a relatively long period of hyperpolarization (after-hyperpolarization).

Table 5.1. Main differences between postsynaptic potentials and action potentials

Postsynaptic potentials	Action potentials
Usually initiated close to synapses	Usually initiated at axon hillock
Passive propagation with voltage decrement	Self-propagation without voltage decrement
Voltage amplitude proportional to stimulus	All-or-nothing
Temporal and spatial voltage summation	No voltage summation (refractory period)

Membrane channels and currents

Ion channels are responsible for specific ion currents, and consequently ion channels and currents are sometimes referred to under the same name. However, they are conceptually different, as some channels may be permeable to more than one ion type, or some types of channels might be active (open) but simultaneously blocked, resulting in no ions passing through and therefore no ion current generated.

Sodium channels

- Sodium channels induce depolarization by allowing sodium ion influx into the cell. In the neurons, voltage-dependent sodium channels are involved in the rising phase of action potentials. At resting potential they are mainly closed, opening quickly with depolarization and closing and inactivating during the repolarizing phase. During hyperpolarization, voltage-dependent sodium channels activate but remain closed until the threshold is reached again.

- One type of sodium channels quickly opens and closes (transient) during the initial half of action potentials, and was the first to be described. This type is blocked by tetradotoxin and its current is called I_{Na} (I stands for current intensity). Blocking this type of channel prevents the initiation and spread of action potentials. Alterations in the functional characteristics of the sodium channels are thought to be one of the main mechanisms of action of many anticonvulsant drugs (see Chapter 66: 'Neurochemistry of antiepileptic drug action').

- The duration of the inactivated state of voltage-dependent sodium channels contributes to the cell refractory period. Consequently, it is one of the parameters that determine the maximal firing rate of action potentials in the neuron. Therefore, drugs that change the functional characteristics of voltage-dependent sodium channels can block repetitive firing and decrease the occurrence of seizures.

- Conversely, late long-lasting sodium channel openings can result in prolonged neuronal depolarization, as observed during paroxysmal depolarizing shifts (see Figure 5.6).

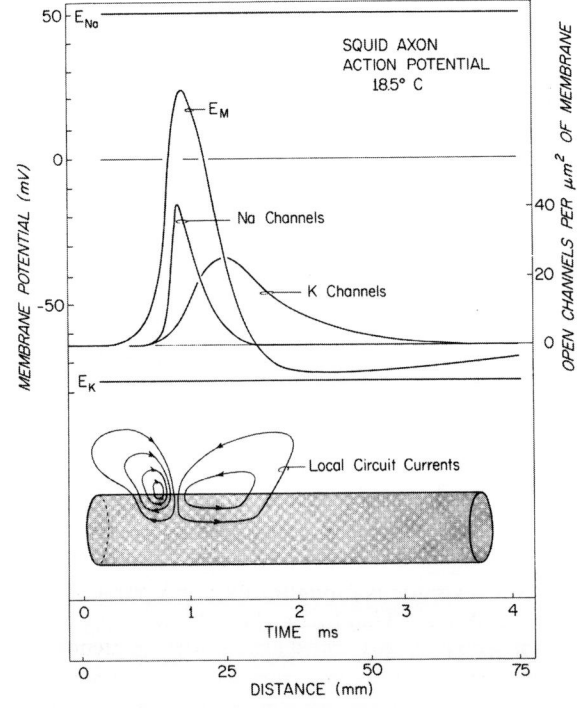

Figure 5.5. Opening and closing of Na$^+$ and K$^+$ channels during propagated action potential (E_M), calculated from the Hodgkin-Huxley model. Because the action potential is a non-decrementing wave, the diagram shows the time course of events at one point on the axon or the spatial distribution of event at one time as the action potential propagates from right to left. The absolute calibration in terms of channels per µm^2 is only approximate. The lower diagram shows the local circuit current flowing during the action potential in an axon with greatly exaggerated diameter (reproduced with permission from Patton DH, Fuchs AF, Hille B, Scher AM, Steiner R, *Textbook of Physiology*, volume 1, 21st edition, W.B. Saunders Company, Philadelphia, 1989, Figure 1.3–14, page 69; adapted after Hodgkin AL and Huxley AF, *J Physiol* (Lond), 1952;117:500–44).

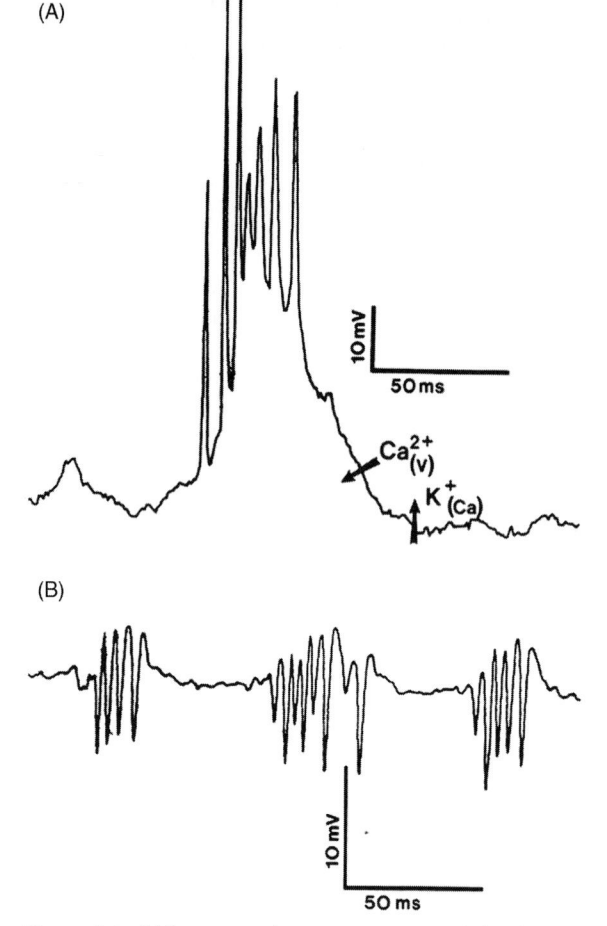

Figure 5.6. (A) Spontaneously occurring paroxysmal depolarizing shift (PDS) recorded intracellularly in a CA3 pyramidal cell. A burst of action potentials ride on a depolarization produced by an inward voltage-sensitive calcium current. Repolarization is produced by a potassium efflux triggered by incoming calcium. (B) Extracellular recording from several CA3 neurons that have been induced to fire synchronously (reproduced with permission from Patton DH, Fuchs AF, Hille B, Scher AM, Steiner R, *Textbook of Physiology*, volume 1, 21st edition, W.B. Saunders Company, Philadelphia, 1989, Figure 1.32–10, page 708).

- Other types of sodium channels remain open for much longer, resulting in non-inactivating persistent sodium currents (I_{NaP}). They are also blocked by tetradotoxin. As these channels activate at voltage levels below threshold, they probably contribute in driving the membrane towards threshold, and in initiating transient I_{Na} (and action potentials).

Calcium channels

Calcium currents induce cell depolarization. Voltage-dependent calcium channels in brain cells are subclassified into L, P/Q, N and T channels. Significant membrane depolarization is required for the activation of L, P/Q and N channels. T channels can be activated by smaller depolarizations or by hyperpolarization. The currents resulting from opening calcium channels are often called $I_{Ca(L)}$, $I_{Ca(P)}$, $I_{Ca(N)}$ or $I_{Ca(T)}$.

- L channels are located in the postsynaptic cell membrane. They are responsible for calcium influx during depolarization, and inactivate slowly. This calcium influx can be necessary for gene regulation and for long-term potentiation (see below). Blockade of L-calcium current could be considered as anticonvulsant by inhibiting synaptic potentiation, but also proconvulsant by inhibiting after-hyperpolarization.

- N and P/Q receptors are located in synaptic boutons (presynaptic cell membrane) and mediate calcium entry necessary for neurotransmitter release into the synaptic cleft. They are regulated by G-proteins, and modulated by G-protein linked receptors such as $GABA_B$. Inhibiting these calcium currents reduces synaptic release of neurotransmitter.

- T channels are activated either by hyperpolarization or by small depolarizations, and quickly inactivate. They appear to contribute to the generation of spike-and-wave discharges in absence seizures. Hyperpolarization of thalamo-cortical neurons results in activation of T calcium channels which are opened by subsequent repolarization, resulting in calcium entry, consequent depolarization, an action potential and recurrent EEG discharges. Ethosuximide is thought to act as a potent anti-absence drug by blocking T-type calcium channels.

Potassium channels

Potassium channels generally induce cell hyperpolarization. Persistent potassium currents ($I_{K,leak}$) are responsible for maintaining the membrane resting potential, and voltage-dependent potassium currents can alter neuronal excitability. Voltage-dependent potassium currents influence the resting potential (directly affecting excitability) and are involved in the repolarization after action potentials. Repolarization rate determines the duration of action potentials, and influences neurotransmitter release and the propensity for repetitive firing (refractory period).

Voltage-dependent potassium channels are subclassified into:

- A-type channels (IA): they activate by depolarization of the membrane positive to −60 mV, delaying the onset of action potentials. They have rapid activation and inactivation dynamics.
- Delayed rectifier channels (IK): they are responsible for currents that activate during the second half of action potentials. These channels open during depolarization and do not significantly inactivate.
- Muscarine-sensitive potassium currents (IM): they are activated by depolarization above −65 mV, and do not inactivate. They are blocked by stimulation of muscarinic cholinergic receptors. As they generate slow and small potassium currents, they do not appear to affect the morphology and function of the action potentials, but might contribute to the adaptation of action potential frequency.
- Inward-rectifying channels (Kir): they open at the resting potential and close during depolarization. Inward rectification is the ability of an ion channel to allow greater influx than efflux of ions. In the case of Kir channels, inward rectification is caused by cytoplasmic ions including polyamines and Mg^{2+}, which plug the conduction pathway when the neuron is depolarized and block the outward flow of K^+. Some channels are linked to G-proteins being activated by G-protein related receptors such as $GABA_B$ receptors, and other channels are activated with intracellular ATP.

The main non-voltage-dependent potassium channels are the calcium-activated potassium channels or $I_{K,Ca}$. They are activated by intracellular cyclic nucleotides, mainly in retinal photoreceptors. They are opened by intracellular calcium, and mediate after-hyperpolarization. Two calcium-activated potassium currents have been described: I_C and I_{AHP}. I_C is sensitive to intracellular calcium and is also voltage-dependent, increasing with depolarization. It regulates the frequency of action potentials by causing marked hyperpolarization after each action potential. I_{AHP} is slower and generates prolonged after-hyperpolarization. It is considered to be responsible for frequency adaptation during repetitive firing.

Sodium–potassium currents or hyperpolarizing inward rectification (I_h)

These channels are permeable to potassium and sodium, and are involved in depolarizing the membrane from a hyperpolarized potential. They activate during hyperpolarization, allowing an inward current, and they inactivate during depolarization. As they are potassium currents that depolarize the membrane potential (toward resting potential), they are also called I_Q ('queer') or I_f ('funny'). They inactivate T-type calcium currents, depolarizing thalamo-cortical neurons, and contribute to terminating thalamo-cortical oscillations responsible for spike-wave activity during absence seizures. Because I_h resists attempts to depolarize the cell, it keeps the resting membrane positive to the equilibrium potential for potassium, closer to the action potential threshold.

The paroxysmal depolarizing (or depolarization) shift (PDS)

The pyramidal cells in the CA3 region of the rat hippocampus show a combination of ionic currents that make them particularly prone to generate bursts of action potentials (burst firing). The action potentials are sodium- and/or calcium-dependent, riding on large depolarizations, which result from an intrinsic, voltage-dependent, slow calcium current (the paroxysmal depolarizing shift or PDS; Figure 5.6A). The action potential bursts are stopped by a calcium-dependent outward potassium current, which is activated by an increase in intracellular calcium. The potassium current is necessary to repolarize the neuron, because the calcium current is inactivated very slowly, if at all, and consequently tends to keep the neuron depolarized. Under normal conditions, PDSs in different CA3 neurons occur asynchronously and are not usually observed on extracellular recordings. However, if CA3 neurons are made to fire synchronously, either by electrical stimulation or by suppression of inhibition, the action potentials from neighbouring CA3 neurons can add to generate bursts of spikes that can be recorded by extracellular electrodes.

Recommended reading

Bear MF, Connors BW, Paradiso MA. *Neuroscience. Exploring the Brain.* Baltimore, MD: Williams & Wilkins; 1996.

Kandel ER, Schwartz JH, Jessell T. *Principles of Neural Science*. 4th edn. New York: Elsevier: 2000.

Shepherd GM. (2003). *The Synaptic Organization of the Brain*. 5th edn. Oxford: Oxford University Press; 2003.

Learning objectives

(1) To understand the basic structure and physiology of the cell membrane.

(2) To understand the concept behind and the mechanisms involved in the generation of:

- equilibrium potential
- resting potential
- postsynaptic potentials
- action potentials.

(3) To know the differences between:

- resting potential
- postsynaptic potentials
- action potentials.

Section 1 Basic principles

Chapter 6

Techniques used to study epilepsy in the laboratory: experimental techniques in basic neurophysiology

Antonio Valentín

The purpose of this chapter is to describe the experimental methods used in animal studies to understand the working processes of neurons, from membrane function to the neural circuits in the central nervous system (CNS).

Experimental models in vitro

Artificial membrane-channel preparations

At cellular level, the electrical activity of neurons consists of the movement of ions through neuronal membranes. Models using artificial lipid bilayer membranes have been designed to determine the functions of ion channels. Some models include insertion of natural ion channels from a variety of cell types, and to carry out neurophysiological recordings in the presence of different concentrations of ions or drugs. Other models use natural membranes with artificially inserted natural receptor-channel complexes.

Acutely isolated neuron

Isolated and relatively intact neurons are prepared using enzymes and agitation of brain tissue to separate neurons. This model provides neurons with relatively normal functions, but altered neuronal morphology.

Chronically cultured neurons

This method has been used to study the electrophysiology of synaptic connections between neurons. The model has the advantage of direct microscopic visualization and manipulation of cells.

Slice culture

Slice cultures are prepared by long-term incubation of brain slices. The slices are converted into a monolayer of neurons keeping some local connections.

Brain slices

This technique consists in preparing brain slices (usually 100–500 mm) quickly cut from a fresh brain and rapidly cooled. Slices can survive for many hours in a proper bath of cerebrospinal fluid saturated with carbogen gas (artificial cerebrospinal fluid or ACSF, 95% O_2, 5% CO_2). Neurophysiological recordings are usually performed after 1–2 hours of incubation to allow recovery from the surgery. During the recording the slice is perfused with ACSF, and drugs at known concentration could be added to this perfusion bath. With this system, electrophysiological recordings could be stable for several hours. Hippocampal slices are some of the most widely used brain slices.

Advantages of slice techniques:

- simple preparation
- control of experimental conditions
- absence of movement due to pulse or breathing
- good visualization of tissue
- easy to modify extracellular medium (to add drugs or change ionic concentrations)
- intrinsic hippocampal connections are maintained in the slice (tri-synaptic circuit).

Disadvantages of slice techniques:

- absence of normal extrinsic afferents
- absence of normal extrinsic efferents
- a degree of tissue damage is unavoidable
- neurons can lose their electrophysiological characteristics with time
- excitability can change with anoxia associated with slice manipulation.

Isolated brain

This technique consists in removing and keeping the entire brain alive in an incubation system. This method

Introduction to Epilepsy ed. Gonzalo Alarcón and Antonio Valentín. Published by Cambridge University Press.
© Cambridge University Press 2012.

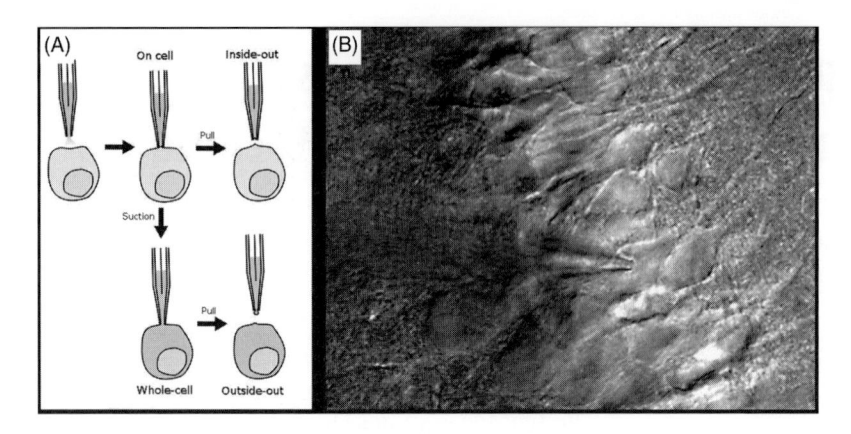

Figure 6.1. (A) Diagram showing different variations of the patch clamp; (B) whole cell recording of a hippocampal neuron. The micropipette in the photograph has been shaded with a blue hue (from Wikipedia). See colour version in plate section.

shares many advantages of brain slices in terms of recording stability and capability for intracellular recordings, but it is complicated to keep the whole brain alive *in vitro*.

Experimental techniques in vitro

Single-channel patch clamp

The 'patch clamp' method is used for recording small currents passing through single ion channels. A glass micropipette is used, allowing the creation of a very high-resistance seal between glass and the neuronal membrane (of the order of giga-ohms). Two main types of single-channel patch clamp can be performed:

- Cell-attached: recordings of single channels are made after formation of the seal without disruption of the cell membrane.
- Patch-attached: a small piece of the cell membrane is separated from the neuron and remains attached to the micropipette. There are two different types of patch-attached techniques:
  - Inside-out patch clamp: the membrane patch is directly detached from the neuron after the seal, with the extracellular side of the membrane now exposed to the micropipette solution.
  - Outside-out patch clamp: the cell is initially attached with a whole-cell patch clamp (see below) and the micropipette is slowly withdrawn, the membrane is torn and a portion of the membrane is then taken away from the cell attached to the micropipette. Coalescence of the membrane attached to the micropipette leaves the intracellular side of the membrane exposed to the micropipette solution (Figure 6.1).

Whole-cell patch clamp

Whole-cell patch clamp (Figure 6.1) allows recording of the current flowing through all channels in the entire cellular membrane. After the pipette is sealed to the neuronal membrane, a vacuum is applied to the tip, breaking the membrane within it. The solution in the pipette mixes over time with the intracellular solution. The whole cell becomes attached to the micropipette and the micropipette solution becomes the intracellular fluid.

Perforated patch clamp

Perforated patch clamp is similar to the whole-cell patch clamp, but instead of vacuum the membrane is perforated using small amounts of drugs (e.g. amphotericin-B or gramicidin) in the micropipette solution. When this technique is used, the intracellular solution remains similar to normal intracellular fluid for longer.

Intracellular recordings (sharp electrode technique)

With this technique it is possible to record the membrane potential, without significantly changing the composition of the intracellular solution. A micropipette with a very small tip (high electrical resistance) is introduced in the cell. The exchange between intracellular and micropipette fluids is not significant, leaving cell properties relatively preserved. Several types of dyes can be used to see the morphology of neurons.

Chapter 6: Techniques used to study epilepsy in the laboratory

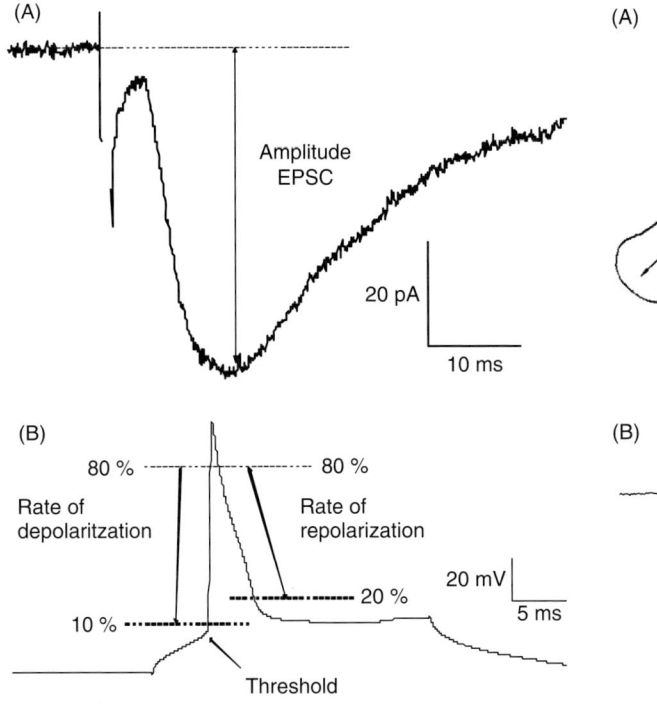

Figure 6.2. Examples of whole-cell patch clamp recordings. (A) Voltage clamp recording. Excitatory postsynaptic current (EPSC) recorded from a neuron in the region CA1 of the hippocampus. The region stimulated was CA3. (B) Current clamp recording. Typical action potential recorded from a neuron in the region CA1 of the hippocampus, after injecting a pulse of constant current. Some of the parameters of the action potential usually considered for study are identified.

Figure 6.3. Example of electrical extracellular orthodromic stimulation in a hippocampal slice. (A) Position of the stimulating electrode (in the Schaffer collateral) and the recording electrode (in the dendrites of CA1 neurons). (B) Typical extracellular recording from the CA1 region. Please note the initial fibre volley (recording of the response of the axons in the Schaffer collateral) and the excitatory postsynaptic potential (EPSP) recorded from CA1 neurons. GD = gyrus dentate.

Current and voltage clamp recordings

In the techniques described above, neuronal activity can be recorded using current or voltage clamp (Figure 6.2) techniques:

- Current clamp involves the measurement of the voltage difference across the neuronal membrane while electrical current across the cell membrane is maintained constant. With this technique it is possible to study how ion channels behave during membrane voltage changes and the mechanisms of action potentials.
- Voltage clamp involves the measurement of the current required to hold a neuronal membrane at a constant voltage and measures current across the membrane. Voltage clamp is used to study how the membrane currents behave at different voltages, to identify the equilibrium potential (and consequently the ions involved in the currents) and to establish how current behaviour can be modified by different drugs and channel blockers.

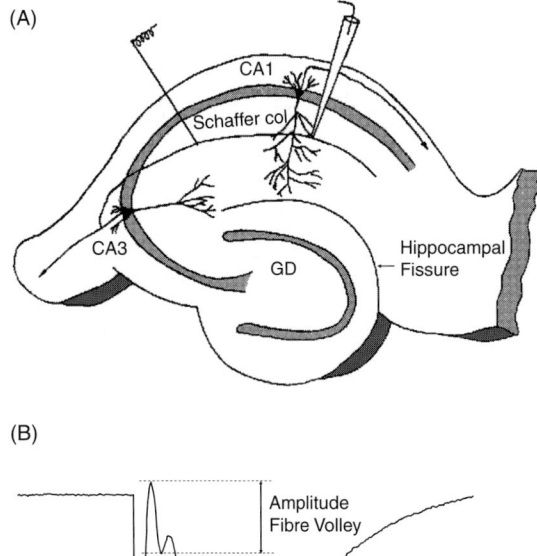

Optical recording methods

Several optical techniques have recently been developed using voltage-sensitive dyes and resins that allow tracking of membrane potential changes by eye.

Electrical extracellular stimulation

Pulses of electrical stimulation are applied to a brain region and neuronal responses recorded with intra- or extracellular recordings (Figure 6.3). This technique is used to identify synaptic connections between different regions. Since axons can conduct action potentials towards and away from the soma, two types of electrical stimulation can be considered:

- orthodromic stimulation: stimulation of the axons projecting to the neurons surrounding the recording electrode;
- antidromic stimulation: stimulation of axons from the neurons surrounding the recording electrode.

Experimental models and experimental techniques in vivo

Single-cell extracellular recordings
Microelectrodes with very thin tips can record from single neurons or from a limited number of neurons (multiunit activity). The microelectrodes are implanted in the brain using stereotaxic instruments during anaesthesia, and recordings can be performed while the subject is awake or anaesthetized. This model has been mainly used in animals, but several hospitals and clinical centres around the world are also studying single-cell recording in patients with severe intractable epilepsy. Single-neuron recordings in awake patients provide an extraordinary opportunity to directly study the neural correlates of human brain function.

Intracranial EEG recordings
Intracranial EEG electrodes can be implanted in the brain to study brain activity, connectivity between different areas, and functional activity related to physiological conditions in animals and in humans.

Local drug application
These methods study the effects of application of drugs by iontophoresis or local micropressure application in the intact brain.

Microdialysis
A tiny tube made of a semi-permeable membrane is inserted in the brain to determine the chemical components of the extracellular fluid. The semi-permeable membrane has micro-pores through which small molecules can pass. It can be used to estimate the concentration of drugs and neurotransmitters in the extracellular fluid.

Lesional models
Deficits associated with focal lesions of brain structures have been used to estimate the function of severed areas and their connected regions.

Learning objective

(1) To understand the basic principles and usefulness of the techniques used in basic neurophysiology, both in vivo and in vitro.

Section 1 Basic principles

Chapter 7

Techniques used to study epilepsy in the laboratory: neuropathological methods

Nuria T. Villagra and Istvan Bodi

In many cases, epilepsy is due to structural disorders of the central nervous system (symptomatic epilepsies). The structural abnormalities responsible for epilepsy can be demonstrated by neuropathological techniques applied to tissue samples obtained after biopsy, after surgical resections for the treatment of epilepsy or after post-mortem examination. Histological stains, immunohistochemistry, confocal microscopy, electron microscopy and posttranscriptional and molecular genetics studies might be used during routine neuropathological investigations and in experimental epileptology. Neuropathology plays an important role in the diagnosis of the causes of epilepsy and in the classification of epilepsy.

Handling of epilepsy surgical specimens

The epileptic surgery specimens are usually received in 10% neutral buffered formalin in the neuropathology laboratory. The tissue is routinely fixed for at least 24–48 hours. The specimen should be oriented, measured and weighed. The larger specimens are cut in the coronal plane into 5-mm-thick slices using metal grids, numbered with ink and embedded in separate blocks. Detailed description of whole specimen is mandatory, including surface and gyral abnormalities, grey and white matter demarcation, presence of heterotopic grey matter and focal lesions. The extent of the abnormalities should be noted according to individual slices. Surgical haemorrhages and electrode tracks may be encountered. Presence of identifiable anatomical structures, such as hippocampus and amygdala, should be recorded. The intact tissue and the posterior surface of each slice are photographed. Close-up photographs are to be taken of any specific findings.

Histochemistry

Paraffin embedded, hematoxylin and eosin (H&E; Figures 13.2, 13.3, 13.5) stained 7-µm tissue sections are used for routine histological examination. The features of the Nissl substance in the neurons can be seen by the classic Nissl stain. Myelination and the grey-white matter demarcation are best assessed by myelin stain, such as luxol fast blue/Nissl (LFB/N; Figure 13.7). The latter stain also helps assess the cortical architecture and distribution of neurons, any reduction in number of neurons (e.g. mesial temporal sclerosis), disruption of normal cortical lamination, dysmorphic or ectopic neurons seen in cortical dysplasia, heterotopic neuronal nodules and the nodularity of certain tumours. Bielschowsky or Glees silver stains highlight dendritic arborization of the dysmorphic neurons in cortical dysplasia (Figures 13.7F and 13.8D).

PAS and Lugol's iodine stain the cytoplasmic inclusions of polyglycosan bodies in neurons, astrocytes and also in apocrine sweat glands where presence of inclusions contributes to the diagnosis of Lafora's disease (Figure 13.13). Specific techniques to stain collagen components, such as elastic Van Gieson (EVG), are useful to study vascular malformations.

Immunohistochemistry

Immunohistochemistry against specific neuron proteins is very useful. NeuN, expressed in the neuronal nucleus and cytoplasm, is the most specific nuclear neuronal marker and is used to estimate neuronal density and distribution. Synaptophysin highlights the neuropil and the synaptic connections around neurons and labels most neurons. Chromogranin is concentrated in the neuroendocrine synaptic vesicles and usually expressed in abnormal ganglion cells in gangliogliomas. The recently introduced nestin and

---

Introduction to Epilepsy ed. Gonzalo Alarcón and Antonio Valentín. Published by Cambridge University Press.
© Cambridge University Press 2012.

doublecortin may help identify neurons in early developmental stages.

The classic phosphotungstic acid hematoxylin (PTAH) stain for the glial fibrils has been replaced by immunohistochemistry against GFAP (glial fibrillary acidic protein) to study reactive astrocytes and glial tumours. Reactive changes in primary or secondary lesions in epilepsy are frequently accompanied by microglial activation. H&E only displays the rod nuclear morphology that appears in the activated microglia. However, HLA-DR immunostain is the most sensitive and specific marker for recognizing early steps of microglial activation. The other frequently used microglial and macrophage marker is CD68. CD34 is frequently expressed in focal cortical dysplasia type IIB and certain glioneuronal tumours (ganglioglioma and some dysembryoplastic neuroepithelial tumours), although the expression profile of the immunoreactive cells is yet to be clarified.

Oligodendroglial cells have small round nuclei with delicate chromatin and lack of specific markers. The Del Río Hortega silver carbonate impregnation technique and carbonic anhydrase II immunohistochemistry may be applied, but these techniques are not routinely used in the diagnosis. Sometimes the interpretation of the oligodendroglial component is difficult in gliomas or dysembryoplastic neuroepithelial tumours. MIB1 or Ki67 markers are used to assess the proliferation activity of these tumours.

There are some cases where inflammatory components seen by H&E have to be characterized. Specific inflammatory markers for T (CD3) and B (CD20) lymphocytes, plasma cells or macrophages are useful in conditions such as in idiopathic, infectious or vasculitic encephalitis. Microbiological infection has to be ruled out by special techniques such as Gram, Grocott or Ziehl-Neelsen, useful to detect bacteria, fungi or acid-alcohol resistant bacteria respectively.

Electron microscopy

Special fixation by glutaraldehyde and specific resin embedding are necessary to prepare the tissue for electronic microscopy (EM). The classic transmission EM is not really helpful in epilepsy diagnosis, but might be useful in research and in experimental models of epilepsy. Application of immuno-gold EM may help locate expressed surface markers and subcellular molecular components.

Molecular and genetic techniques for diagnosis and research of epilepsy diagnosis

Freshly frozen tissue is necessary to carry out most molecular studies at the protein level. In epilepsy research, Western blotting, electrophoresis, proteomics, cell sub-fractionation, protein aggregates, protein–protein interactions, immunoprecipitation, enzymatic activities, etc. could give a molecular neurobiological approach to the mainly obscure pathogenesis of epilepsy.

DNA studies might be carried out in frozen tissue, blood or the proper deparaffinized tissue. From a diagnostic point of view, DNA is useful to determinate genetic mutations in already known hereditary conditions by means of *in situ* hybridization, FRLP, direct sequencing, etc. PCR to detect fragments of microbiological DNA sequences, such as herpes virus, JC virus, mycobacterium, *Tropheryma whipplei*, etc., can be helpful.

Recommended reading

Honavar M, Meldrum BS. Epilepsy. In *Greenfield's Neuropathology*, pp. 931–71. 6th edn. London: Arnold; 1997.

Thom M. Recent advances in the neuropathology of focal lesions in epilepsy. *Expert Rev Neurother* 2004;4(6):973–84.

Learning objective

(1) To understand the basic principles and indications of neuropathological techniques.

Section 1 Basic principles

Chapter 8
Functional anatomy and physiology of the hippocampus

Gonzalo Alarcón

The hippocampus is a long structure that runs from anterior to posterior along the medial portion of each temporal lobe (Figure 8.1). The main functions of the hippocampus are processing of emotions, short-term memory and spatial information. These functions have been identified in animal experiments showing that

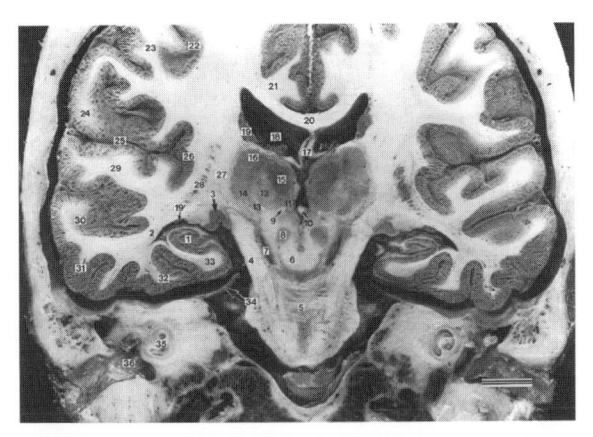

Figure 8.1. Coronal section of the human brain. (1) Hippocampal bodi; (2) temporal stem; (3) lateral geniculate bodi; (4) crus cerebri; (5) pons, ventral part; (6) brachium conjunctivum; (7) substantia nigra; (8) red nucleus; (9) habenulopeduncular tract; (10) posterior commissure; (11) parafascicular nucleus; (12) centromedian thalamic nucleus; (13) ventral posteromedial thalamic nucleus; (14) ventral posterolateral thalamic nucleus; (15) dorsomedial thalamic nucleus; (16) lateral thalamic nucleus; (17) fornix; (18) body of lateral ventricle; (19) body of caudate nucleus; (19) tail of caudate nucleus; (20) corpus callosum; (21) cingulate gyrus; (22) central sulcus; (23) postcentral gyrus; (24) inferior parietal gyrus; (25) lateral (sylvian) sulcus; (26) insula; (27) posterior limb of internal capsule; (28) cellular bridges joining caudate nucleus and putamen (pontes grisei caudatolenticulares); (29) superior temporal gyrus; (30) middle temporal gyrus; (31) inferior temporal gyrus; (32) gyrus fusiformis; (33) parahippocampal gyrus; (34) tentorium cerebelli; (35) internal ear; (36) middle ear. (reproduced with permission from Figure 1.42, page 66, *The Human Hippocampus. An Atlas of Applied Anatomy.* By Henri M. Duvernoy. J.F. Bergmann Verlag, Munchen, 1988).

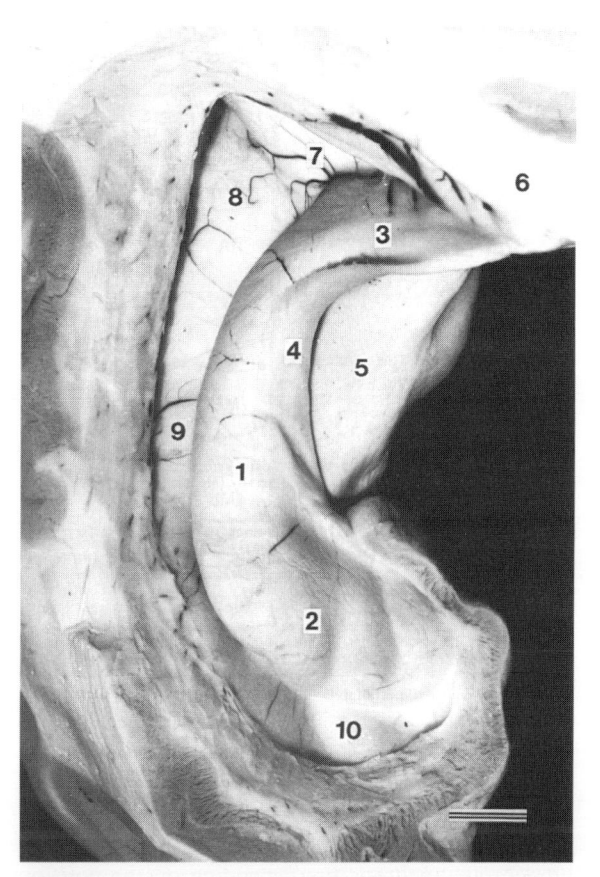

Figure 8.2. Intraventricular aspect of the hippocampus. The temporal horn has been opened and the choroids plexuses removed. Bar: 6.5 mm. (1) Hippocampal body; (2) head and digitations hippocampi or internal digitations; (3) hippocampal tail; (4) fimbria; (5) subiculum (parahippocampal gyrus); (6) splenium of the corpus callosum; (7) calcar avis; (8) collateral trigone; (9) collateral eminence; (10) uncal recess of the temporal horn (reproduced with permission from Figure 1.2, page 15, *The Human Hippocampus. An Atlas of Applied Anatomy.* By Henri M. Duvernoy. J.F. Bergmann Verlag, Munchen, 1988).

Introduction to Epilepsy ed. Gonzalo Alarcón and Antonio Valentín. Published by Cambridge University Press.
© Cambridge University Press 2012.

Section 1: Basic principles

Situation of CA1 and CA3 in rats and humans

Small arrows show the hippocampal sulcus.
ca1 Regio superior
ca3 Regio inferior
Th Thalamus
The large arrow indicates the inversion of arrangements in the hippocampus in these two species.

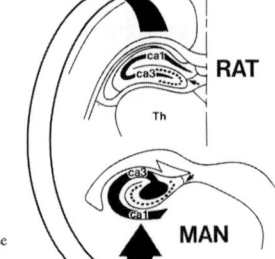

Figure 8.3. Transversal sections of the hippocampal formation showing its connections and anatomical inversion between rat and man (reproduced with permission from Figure 1.9, page 23, *The Human Hippocampus. An Atlas of Applied Anatomy*. By Henri M. Duvernoy. J.F. Bergmann Verlag Munchen, 1988).

Connexions of the hippocampus

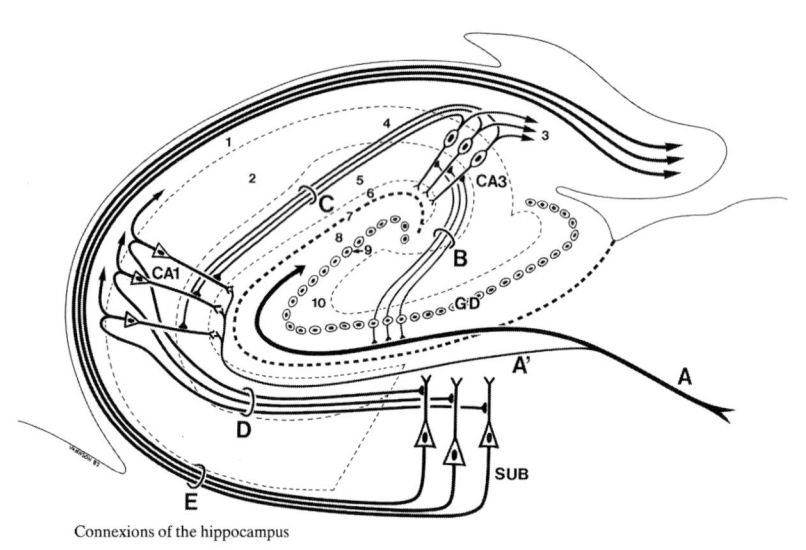

Diagram of principal pathways. A B C D E are parts of neuronal chains forming the principal pathways. A': These perforant fibres join the apical dendrites of the pyramidal neurons directly.

Cornu ammonis:
1 Alveus
2 Stratum pyramidale
3 Axon of pyramidal neurons
4 Schaffer collateral
5 Stratum radiatum and lacunosum
6 Stratum moleculare
7 Hippocampal sulcus

Gyrus dentatus:
8 Stratum moleculare
9 Stratum granulosum
10 Polymorphic layer

GD Gyrus dentatus
CA3, CA1 Fields of the cornu ammonis
SUB Subiculum

hippocampal neurons fire depending on the position of the animal within its environment, and in human experiments showing that hippocampal neurons fired to particular pictures and faces. Bilateral ablation or inactivation of the human hippocampus is associated with profound memory deficits. The hippocampus is particularly important in epileptology because it is the source of a high proportion of focal seizures and the most common source of temporal lobe epilepsy. In addition, it has a relatively simple anatomy and internal synaptic connections, which makes it ideal to study the basic mechanisms of synaptic transmission, the mechanisms of epileptogenesis and the mechanisms of memory.

Seen from above (from within the temporal horn of the lateral ventricle), the hippocampus resembles a sea horse (which is the origin of its name) having a head (anterior), feet (pes hippocampi), fingers (digitations hippocampi), body and tail (posterior) (Figure 8.2). A transversal section of the hippocampus reveals two sheets of grey matter coiled together. The external coil resembles a ram's horn and is called cornu ammonis (CA) or Ammon's horn or hippocampus proper. The internal coil is called gyrus dentatus, because it looks like teeth when seen from the lateral ventricle after lifting the hippocampus proper. The hippocampus proper plus the gyrus dentatus are sometimes generically called the hippocampal formation, or simply the hippocampus. The cornu ammonis has traditionally been subdivided into four regions or fields: CA1 (most lateral in man, also called Sommer sector), CA2, CA3 (most medial in man) and CA4 (or hillum, between gyrus dentatus and CA3). The cortical gyrus running immediately inferior and parallel to the hippocampus in the medial aspect of the temporal lobe is called the parahippocampal gyrus. The upper surface of the parahippocampal gyrus, where the hippocampus lies, is called the subiculum.

The basic circuitry of this region is shown in Figure 8.3, on a transversal section of the hippocampal formation. The main input comes from the entorhinal cortex, which itself receives information from widespread association cortical areas and subcortical structures (thalamus and amygdala). The main output is to the hypothalamus via the fimbria and fornix (trigon).

Most of the input from the entorhinal cortex (A) is excitatory (glutaminergic) and reaches the hippocampal formation through the perforant path, which perforates the subiculum to reach hippocampal structures. Most of the input reaches the granular neurons in the gyrus dentatus, which project to dendrites of pyramidal neurons in CA3 through axons called mossy fibres, running across CA4. Axons from CA3 divide, one branch joining the fornix and the other branch (Schaffer collateral) going along the cornu ammonis to CA1. Axons from neurons in CA1 project to the hypothalamus via the fimbria and to the subiculum. A small proportion of entorhinal fibres separate from the main branch and synapse directly with dendrites of neurons in CA1. Most of the output of the hippocampus is composed of axons from neurons in CA1, which run along the alveus to join the fimbria and fornix. These axons also produce collaterals that project to the subiculum.

Recommended reading

Duvernoy HM. *The Human Hippocampus. An Atlas of Applied Anatomy*. Munich: JF Bergmann; 1988.

Lacruz ME, Valentín A, Garcia Seoane JJ, *et al*. Single pulse electrical stimulation of the hippocampus is sufficient to impair human episodic memory. *Neuroscience* 2010;**170**:623–32.

Quiroga RQ, Reddy L, Kreiman G, Koch C, Fried I. Invariant visual representation by single neurons in the human brain. *Nature* 2005;**435**:1102–7.

Scoville WB, Milner B. Loss of recent memory after bilateral hippocampal lesions. *J Neurol Neurosurg Psychiatry* 1957;**20**:11–21.

Shepherd GM. *The Synaptic Organization of the Brain*. 5th edn. Oxford: Oxford University Press; 2004.

Learning objectives

(1) To become familiar with the macroscopic and microscopic anatomy of the hippocampus and related structures, and their terminology.

(2) To understand the basic input, output and internal neuronal circuitry of the hippocampal formation.

(3) To be aware of the functional relevance of the hippocampal formation, and to understand the relevance and usefulness of hippocampal studies.

Section 1 **Basic principles**

Chapter 9

Neurotransmission and biochemistry of neurotransmitters in epilepsy

Brian Meldrum

Glutamate and excitatory neurotransmission

Glutamate and aspartate are dicarboxylic amino acids that are universal constituents of living organisms. They are among the most bountiful amino acids found in animal proteins. They are found free in neurons at high concentration (glutamate 10 mM, aspartate 4 mM). Glutamate is the principal excitatory neurotransmitter in the mammalian brain. Glutamate binds to ionotropic receptor molecules in nerve cell membranes to produce the opening of cation-selective ion channels, permitting the inward movement of Na^+ and sometimes Ca^{2+}, and the outward movement of K^+. The net effect, given the very severe inward gradient for $[Na^+]$ and $[Ca^{2+}]$, is depolarization of the resting membrane potential. Glutamate also binds to metabotropic receptors located pre- and post-synaptically on neurons and astrocytes.

- Glutamate is transported into synaptic vesicles by three transporters (VGLUT-1–3) that have distinctive distributions in the brain and are highly selective for glutamate (unlike the plasma membrane glutamate transporters, they do not bind D- and L-aspartate). Glutamate is present at 100 mM in synaptic vesicles.
- Glutamate is transported from the synaptic cleft by plasma membrane transporters in astrocytes (GLAST and GLT-1) and neurons (EAAC1).
- Glutamate and glutamine are interconverted (by glutamine synthetase and glutaminase) in astrocytes and neurons. Glutamate can be decarboxylated to form GABA by glutamate decarboxylase. It can also participate in a variety of transaminase reactions (Figure 9.1).

Table 9.1. Ionotropic and metabotropic glutamate receptors and their subunits

Ionotropic (tetrameric)			Metabotropic (dimeric)		
AMPA	Kainate	NMDA	Group I	Group II	Group III
GluR1(A)	GluR5	NMDAR1	mGluR1	mGluR2	mGluR4
GluR2(B)	GluR6	NR2A	mGluR5	mGluR3	mGluR7
GluR3(C)	GluR7	NR2B			mGluR8
GluR4(D)	KA1	NR2C			
	KA2	NR2D			
		NR3A			
		NR3B			

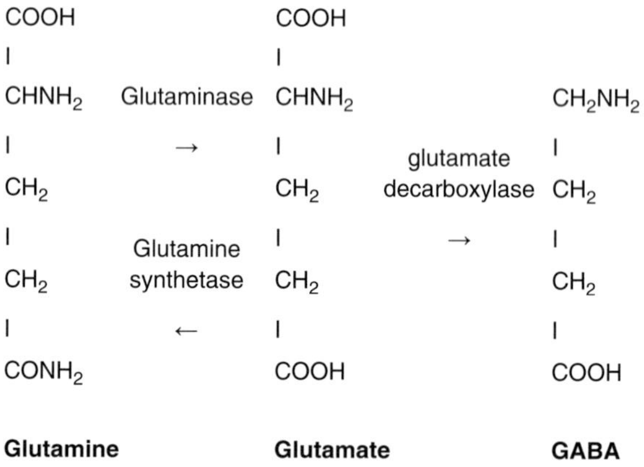

Figure 9.1. Glutamate metabolism.

AMPA and NMDA receptors

The AMPA and NMDA receptors (Figure 9.2) are tetrameric, i.e composed of four subunits. When one

Introduction to Epilepsy ed. Gonzalo Alarcón and Antonio Valentín. Published by Cambridge University Press.
© Cambridge University Press 2012.

of the four units in an AMPA receptor is a GluR2, then the open channel is permeable to Na$^+$ but impermeable to Ca^{2+}. The AMPA receptors are the principal post-synaptic glutamate receptors and they generate the fast excitatory (depolarizing) potentials. Trafficking of AMPA receptors provides an important mechanism of synaptic plasticity and is an important component of long-term potentiation (LTP) and learning.

NMDA receptors have two agonist sites: one recognizes glutamate and aspartate, the other recognizes glycine and D-serine. Glycine and D-serine are not released synaptically in the cortex. Their extracellular concentration is dependent on transporter activity; e.g. glycine-transporter 1 in astrocytic membranes. The NMDA receptor channel has a high Ca^{2+} permeability. The NMDA ion channel shows a voltage-dependent Mg^{2+} block, such that the channel when opened by agonist binding tends to be blocked by Mg^{2+} ions moving into it unless concurrent AMPA-receptor activation produces a membrane depolarization (which relieves the block by allowing the Mg^{2+} to move away).

Kainate receptors

Kainate receptors are sensitive to glutamate, kainate and the related compound, domoate (found in algae and blue mussels). Kainate receptors have a very limited expression in the mammalian brain but are particularly prominent in the hippocampus. Kainate or domoate induce limbic seizures when given systemically to rodents or humans.

All types of glutamate ionotropic receptor antagonists have been shown to possess some anticonvulsant properties in animal models of epilepsy. NMDA receptor antagonists are particularly effective against reflexly induced seizures in rodents and baboons. They are relatively ineffective and toxic against kindled seizures in rats. AMPA receptor antagonists are effective anticonvulsants in a wide range of models, including kindled seizures. Preliminary clinical trials have been negative in the case of NMDA antagonists (e.g. D-CPPene) but positive in the case of AMPA antagonists (e.g. talampanel).

Table 9.2. Glutamate ionotropic receptor antagonists

	AMPA	Kainate	NMDA
Competitive with glutamate	NBQX YM900 LY293,558	NBQX NS102 LY293,558	AP7 CPPene CGS 19355 selfotel
Competitive with glycine			ACEA10211 licostinel GV150526A
Allosteric	GYKI52466 Talampanel		
Open channel blockers			MK801 dizocilpine CNS1102 cerestat
Polyamine site			Eliprodil RO25,6981

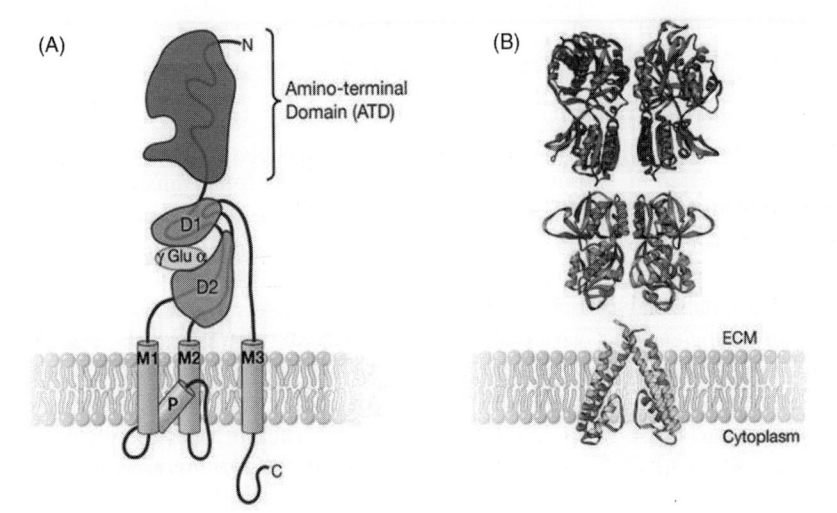

Figure 9.2. Molecular morphology of AMPA and NMDA glutamate receptors. (A) Showing the extracellular amino-terminal domain, the 'venus fly trap' (that binds glutamate) composed of two extracellular loops, the three transmembrane segments, the intramembrane segment forming the ion-selective pore and the intracellular carboxyterminal. (B) Showing the dimeric functional unit. In the NMDA receptor one dimer is composed of NR1 subunits and binds glycine or D-serine, and the other dimer is composed of NR2A-D subunits and binds glutamate. Binding of 2 glutamate and 2 glycine/D-serine is required for channel opening (from Meldrum and Rogawski, Parts A and B of Figure 1.5, *Neurotherapeutics*, vol. 4, January 2007, with permission).

Glutamate metabotropic receptors

These receptors are directly coupled to certain enzymes and through G-protein fragments modulate some voltage-gated ion channels in neuronal membranes. Group I of the glutamate metabotropic receptors (mGluR1, mGluR5) are principally post-synaptic. They activate phospholipase C, leading to the formation of diacylglycerol and IP3, which in turn activate protein kinase C and release Ca^{2+} from internal stores. Group II (mGluR2, mGluR3) and Group III (mgluR4, mGluR7, mGluR8) receptors inhibit adenylate cyclase, thus reducing the availability of cAMP for various phosphorylations. They also, through a G-protein-linked mechanism, reduce Ca^{2+} entry through voltage-gated channels in synaptic terminals, thereby reducing neurotransmitter release.

Antagonists acting on Group I receptors show anticonvulsant action in some animal models of epilepsy. This includes competitive antagonists acting on both mGluR1 and mGluR5 (such as AIDA and LY367385), but also non-competitive antagonists acting on mGluR5 (such as MPEP). A lack of activity in kindled seizures has been reported. Agonists acting at presynaptic group II receptors such as LY 354740 and 2R,4R APDC are anxiolytic and anticonvulsant in rodents. Some agonists at Group III receptors, such as ACPT-1 and (R,S) PPG, are anticonvulsant in animal models.

GABA and inhibitory neurotransmission

GABA (γ-aminobutyric acid) is the principal inhibitory neurotransmitter in the mammalian brain.

GABA, as its name indicates, is an omega-amino acid (i.e. the amino group is attached to the carbon atom chain at the opposite end to the carboxyl group). Unlike the alpha-amino acids, GABA does not participate in the formation of protein molecules. It is synthesized in nerve cells by the enzymic decarboxylation of glutamic acid (Figure 9.3). The enzyme glutamic acid decarboxylase is selectively expressed in GABA-ergic neurons and its staining with antibodies is used as a histological marker for GABA-ergic neurons. The enzymatic reaction is dependent on pyridoxal phosphate and is impaired in animals and children with pyridoxine (vitamin B6) deficiency. Pyridoxal phosphate antagonists, such as isoniazid and 6-deoxypyridoxine, are convulsant.

GABA is transported into synaptic vesicles by vesicular transporters (that are selective for GABA and glycine). Following membrane depolarization

```
COOH
|
CHNH₂                    CH₂NH₂              CHO
|         glutamate      |          GABA     |
CH₂       decarboxylase  CH₂      transaminase CH₂
|                        |                    |
CH₂                      CH₂                  CH₂
|                        |                    |
COOH                     COOH                 COOH

Glutamate                GABA                 Succinic
                                              semialdehyde
```

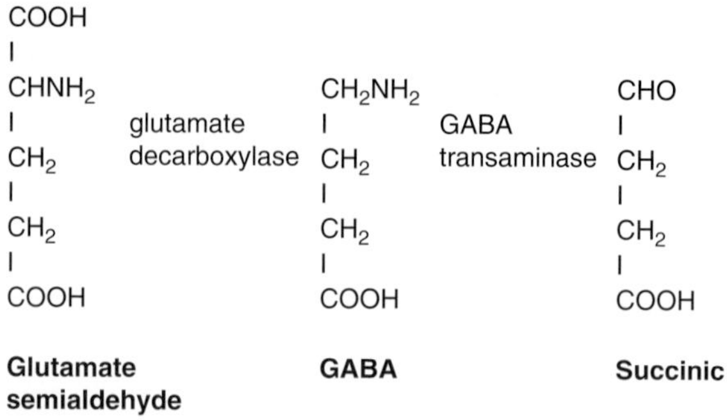

Figure 9.3. Metabolism of GABA.

and the entry of Ca^{2+} into the nerve terminal, vesicles release GABA into the synaptic cleft, where it binds to $GABA_A$ (ionotropic) and $GABA_B$ (metabotropic) receptors. The effect of GABA on $GABA_A$ receptors is to increase Cl^- conductance and thereby increase the resting negative intracellular potential (hyperpolarize the neuron) and decrease the probability of the cell firing. Its effects on $GABA_B$ receptors include a G-protein-mediated enhancement of K^+ conductance that also has the effect of increasing the negative intracellular potential.

GABA transporters

There are four GABA transporters in neuronal membranes, referred to (in man and rat) as GAT-1, GAT-2, GAT-3 and BGT-1. GAT-1 is found around nerve terminals in the forebrain and helps to shape phasic inhibition (see below). GAT-3 is prominent in astrocytes and helps to control tonic inhibition (see below). Many compounds that inhibit GABA transporters show some selectivity between the different transporters. Tiagabine selectively inhibits GAT-1.

$GABA_A$ receptors

$GABA_A$ receptors are pentameric structures composed of subunits (each with four trans-membrane helical segments) selected from various families (Figure 9.4). These include six α subunits (α1–6), three β subunits (β1–3), three γ subunits (γ1–3), one δ and one ϵ subunit. The subunit composition varies according to the brain region and the type of neuron. It determines whether the channel provides phasic inhibition (commonly with a γ subunit) or tonic inhibition (with a δ subunit) and the pharmacological responsiveness of the receptor, especially the nature of the response to benzodiazepines such as

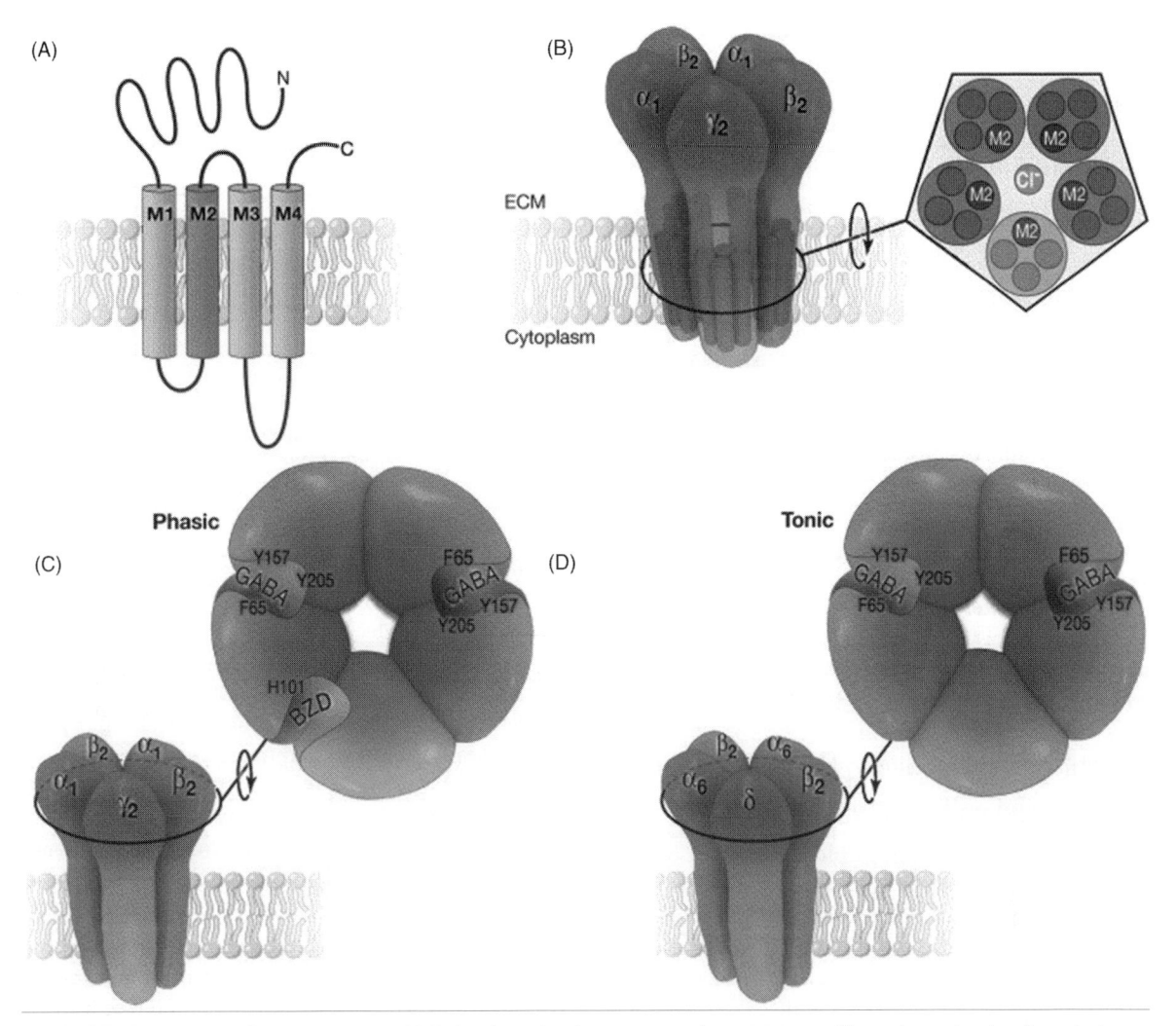

Chapter 9: Neurotransmission and biochemistry of neurotransmitters in epilepsy

Figure 9.4. Morphology of GABA$_A$ receptors. (A) Each subunit has four trans-membrane segments. The amino and carboxyl terminals are extracellular. (B) Five subunits comprise the receptor. The second TM segment (M2) lines the ion channel. (C) A 'phasic' receptor contains a γ subunit. The two GABA binding sites involve three amino acids at the α-β junction. The single benzodiazepine binding site is at the α-γ junction. (D) A 'tonic' receptor contains a δ subunit (from Meldrum and Rogawski, Figure 1.4, *Neurotherapeutics*, vol. 4, January 2007, with permission).

diazepam. Benzodiazepines potentiate the effect of GABA (by increasing the frequency of channel opening in response to a given GABA concentration) when the receptor contains an α1, α2, α3 or α5 subunit, but not when it contains an α4 or α6 subunit. The expression of the α subunits varies according to the brain region, and particular neurological side effects of benzodiazepines are dependent on receptors containing particular α subunits. The GABA binding site involves α and β subunits; the benzodiazepine binding site involves α and γ subunits.

In benzodiazepine-insensitive receptors, enflurane and ethanol act at an allosteric site (involving α and β subunits) prolonging channel openings.

GABA$_A$ receptor antagonists are powerful convulsants producing focal epileptic activity if locally applied to the cortex or generalized motor seizures if given systemically. They can act either by competition at the GABA recognition site, e.g. bicuculline, or by action on the channel, e.g. picrotoxinin. Allosteric antagonists, e.g. ethyl β-carboline-3-carboxylate (β-CCE) and 6,7-dimethoxy-4-ethyl-β-carboline-3-carboxylate

(DMCM), acting as an inverse agonist at the benzodiazepine site, i.e. decreasing the effect of GABA at the receptor, are also convulsants.

Phasic inhibition and tonic inhibition

$GABA_A$ receptors provide two inhibitory functional systems, phasic and tonic inhibition. Phasic inhibition is the fast inhibitory response, with a rise time of 1 ms and a decay time of 10–200 ms, which is the immediate product of the synaptic release of GABA. It is produced by $GABA_A$ receptors, usually containing γ subunits and showing benzodiazepine responsiveness, located in the post-synaptic membrane. Tonic inhibition is produced by $GABA_A$ receptors located extrasynaptically and involves a sustained Cl^- current. The $GABA_A$ receptors involved contain α4, α5 or α6 and δ subunits and are not responsive to benzodiazepines, but do respond to neurosteroids such as progesterone metabolites and ganaxolone. They show a low EC_{50} for GABA and slow desensitization. Tonic inhibition is enhanced by tiagabine and vigabatrin.

Genetic defects involving the $GABA_A$ receptor and epileptic syndromes

A remarkable range of idiopathic generalized seizures has been linked to mutations involving subunits of the $GABA_A$ receptor. These are sometimes phenotypically very similar to syndromes associated with mutations in subunits of voltage-gated ion channels. A mutation affecting the α1 subunit has been found in a family with juvenile myoclonic epilepsy (JME). Mutations in γ2 and in δ subunits have been found in families with GEFS+. These mutations either reduce the inward current induced by GABA or reduce the surface expression of the $GABA_A$ receptor.

A deletion involving the β3 subunit is commonly found in Angelman syndrome. Seizures and a cleft palate are produced in mice with a β3 subunit knockout. Mutations involving the δ subunit have been described in some families with GEFS+.

$GABA_B$ receptors

$GABA_B$ receptors are heterodimeric – that is, they are composed of one B1 and one B2 subunit, each of which has seven transmembrane elements. They are G-protein-coupled to K^+ channels, whose activation enhances the resting negative membrane potential,

Table 9.3. Drugs acting on GABA receptors

	Agonists	Antagonists
$GABA_A$		
GABA site	Muscimol	Bicuculline
Ion channel		Picrotoxin
Benzodiazepine site	Diazepam	β-CCE
	Clobazam	DMCM
	Clonazapam	
Neurosteroid site	Ganaxolone	
Other sites	Chlormethiazole	
	Topiramate	
	Felbamate	
	Loreclezole	
$GABA_B$	Baclofen	Phaclofen

and to Ca^{2+} channels, whose activation decreases channel opening thus decreasing presynaptic release of neurotransmitter. They are negatively coupled to adenylyl cyclase, decreasing cAMP synthesis.

Baclofen (p-chlorophenyl GABA) is a specific agonist at $GABA_B$ receptors. Baclofen is an antispasticity agent but it also induces or enhances spike-and-wave discharges in the cortex and thalamus similar to those recorded in absence epilepsy attacks. Antagonists at $GABA_B$ receptors such as phaclofen suppress spike-and-wave discharges in animal models of absence epilepsy.

GABA-transaminase and the further metabolism of GABA

After re-uptake into neurons and astrocytes, GABA is further metabolized by the mitochondrial enzyme GABA-transaminase (4-aminobutyrate:2-oxoglutarate aminotransferase). This enzyme converts GABA to succinic semialdehyde by transferring the amino group to α-ketoglutarate, thereby forming glutamic acid. Succinic semialdehyde is converted to succinic acid by a dehydrogenase enzyme and re-enters the tricarboxylic acid cycle.

GABA-ergic circuitry is the basis of recurrent inhibition and surround inhibition

There are many morphologically distinct forms of GABA-ergic interneurons (more than 16 have been described in the hippocampus). The most consistent pattern is that the interneurons provide multiple synapses either on the soma of principal neurons or around the axon initial segment. In the cortex, hippocampus and thalamus GABA-ergic interneurons provide recurrent inhibitory feedback to principal neurons, which has the effect of limiting the intensity and duration of any excitatory output. The lateral spread of the output of the interneurons is usually greater than the extent of the excitatory input to the interneurons. This gives rise to the phenomenon of inhibitory surround that prevents the lateral spread of excitation in the cortex and other structures.

References

Conn PJ. Physiological roles and therapeutic potential of metabotropic glutamate receptors. *Ann NY Acad Sci* 2003;**1003**:12–21.

Dingledine R, Borges K, Bowie D, Traynelis SF. The glutamate receptor ion channels. *Pharmacol Rev* 1999; **51**:7–61.

Farrant M, Nusser Z. Variations on an inhibitory theme: phasic and tonic activation of $GABA_A$. *Nat Rev Neurosci* 2005;**6**:215–29.

Macdonald RL, Gallagher MJ, Feng HJ, Kong J. $GABA_A$ receptor epilepsy mutations. *Biochem Pharmacol* 2004; **68**:1497–506.

Mayer ML, Armstrong N. Structure and function of glutamate receptor channels. *Annu Rev Physiol* 2004; **66**:161–81.

Meldrum BS, Rogawski MA. Molecular targets for antiepileptic drug development. *Neurotherapeutics* 2007; 4:18–61.

Moldrich RX, Chapman AG, De Sarro G, Meldrum BS. Glutamate metabotropic receptors as targets for drug therapy in epilepsy. *Eur J Pharmacol* 2003;**476**:3–16.

Rudolph U, Möhler H. GABA-based therapeutic approaches: $GABA_A$ receptor subtype functions. *Curr Opin Pharmacol* 2006;**6**:18–23.

Somogyi P, Klausberger T. Defined types of cortical interneurone structure space and spike timing in the hippocampus. *J Physiol* 2005;**562**:9–26.

Watkins JC, Evans DE. The glutamate story. *Br J Pharmacol* 2006;**147**:S100–8.

Learning objectives

(1) To understand the basics of glutamate and GABA metabolisms.
(2) To know the different types of glutamate and GABA receptors and their properties:
- their structure
- the membrane currents induced by their activation and their postsynaptic effects
- their agonists and antagonists.

Section 1 **Basic principles**

Chapter 10

Experimental models of epilepsy

John G. R. Jefferys

There are two broad reasons for using experimental models of epilepsies. The first is to develop new treatments, and in particular to screen compounds as potential antiepileptic drugs (AEDs). The second is to discover the complex pathophysiological mechanisms responsible for epileptic seizures. The requirements for these two uses are rather different so I will consider them in turn, after first introducing another fundamental division within the experimental models of epilepsy: acute versus chronic.

Acute experimental models of epilepsy use some treatment to trigger epileptic activity in normal brain tissue. Usually the trigger is a convulsant drug or other chemical, but can be electrical stimulation. In reality these are models of symptomatic seizures rather than epilepsy. Chronic experimental models of epilepsy use some intervention that reduces seizure thresholds permanently, or at least for long periods, and usually leads to spontaneous epileptic seizures.

Drug screening

The requirements to screen compounds for their potential use as antiepileptic drugs are that they need (1) to predict antiepileptic activity in humans with epilepsy, and (2) to allow high throughput, which in general means the tests need to be quick and cheap. Most of this work is performed within pharmaceutical companies, but a small number of centres funded by national agencies or academic bodies are also involved in screening AEDs.

Perhaps the highest-throughput screens are those that assume a specific molecular target, for the AEDs usually the voltage-gated sodium channel or the GABA-gated chloride channel. They may be 'in silico', that is, computer modelling of the molecular interactions between real or prospective chemical compounds and specific binding sites on the molecular target. Often closely allied with this approach is the in vitro high-throughput patch clamp where cells that express the relevant molecular target are introduced to a machine that automatically sucks them onto fluid-filled microscopic holes that provide electrophysiological recordings while compounds are perfused onto the outside of the cells. These highly targeted approaches can work well, but they do miss the opportunity to identify AEDs with novel mechanisms, and they ignore the considerable complexity of the pathophysiology of epilepsy.

For many years the mainstays of drug screening were based on convulsant treatments applied to normal mice or rats in vivo. The most common versions used either electroshock or a chemical convulsant, usually intravenous or subcutaneous Metrazol (pentylenetetrazol or PTZ). These methods were validated by their sensitivity to existing AEDs. Broadly electroshock is sensitive to drugs that work best on tonic-clonic epilepsy, and PTZ to drugs that work best on absence epilepsy. These tests have identified new compounds, usually with mechanisms broadly similar to the drugs originally used for validation.

These traditional screens used normal, not epileptic, brains; that is to say the experimental models are acute rather than chronic. They also omit two important classes of epilepsy: partial epilepsies, including temporal lobe epilepsy, and the broad class of drug-resistant epilepsies. To help address these omissions, kindling (a chronic model discussed below) and 6 Hz corneal stimulation (an acute model) were introduced. Both models have been used to address the problem of drug resistance, in the case of kindling by selecting individual rats by their resistance to phenytoin.

Introduction to Epilepsy ed. Gonzalo Alarcón and Antonio Valentín. Published by Cambridge University Press.
© Cambridge University Press 2012.

Chapter 10: Experimental models of epilepsy

These kinds of investigation have to be complemented by a range of tests designed to look for adverse reactions, such as sedation, impaired motor control and so on. This allows estimation of the therapeutic index. Successful drugs then enter the clinical trials' pipeline.

Basic mechanisms

The other major use of experimental models of epilepsy is in understanding the basic mechanisms, especially the pathophysiology, of epilepsy.

Acute models have played a major role in developing modern concepts of epilepsy, especially the partial or focal epilepsies. The first of these kinds of studies used injections of convulsant compounds into the brains of experimental animals in vivo, while systemic injections of certain convulsants produce models of primary generalized epilepsies. A large and influential body of work is based on an in vitro preparation, the brain slice.

Brain slices are prepared from brains removed from humanely killed animals (or occasionally from humans undergoing neurosurgery). They are cut thin enough to allow adequate diffusion of oxygen and other compounds to keep the cells alive, while being thick enough to preserve enough of the neurons and neuronal circuitry to sustain the functions under investigation, in this case epileptic activity. One of the most commonly used types of slice is the rodent hippocampal slice (Figure 10.1).

Acute convulsant treatments used to model focal epilepsies in brain slices, and in some cases in vivo, include several distinct groups.

(1) Impaired synaptic inhibition mediated through $GABA_A$ receptors can be produced by several acute treatments, including penicillin, bicuculline, picrotoxin, and replacing Cl^- with anions that will not pass through the $GABA_A$ receptor. It can also be induced by withdrawal of $GABA_A$ activating or amplifying treatments, such as repeated doses of GABA, benzodiazepines or barbiturates, which progressively weaken $GABA_A$-receptor mediated IPSPs.

(2) Increased excitability: increasing the K^+ in the bathing medium, from 3 to ~8 mM, induces epileptic activity partly due to the depolarization of neuronal membranes, and partly to an indirect weakening of IPSPs (the smaller gradient of K^+ reduces the effectiveness of the chloride transporter known as KCC2, reducing intracellular Cl^- which in turn makes IPSPs less hyperpolarizing and less effective).

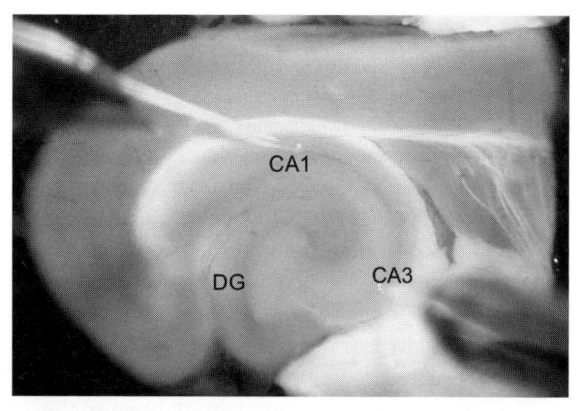

Figure 10.1. Hippocampal slice in vitro (unstained, 0.4 mm thick) from a rat photographed during an electrophysiological recording session. Glass micropipettes can be seen descending from top left and bottom right, respectively into the pyramidal layers of the CA1 and CA3 of the hippocampus. DG is the dentate gyrus. The white band above CA1 is known as the alveus. The blood vessels to the left and above 'DG' are in the hippocampal fissure. The hippocampus is about 3–4 mm along the longest axis shown.

(3) Strengthened synaptic excitation: the best-characterized example uses reductions in the extracellular concentrations of Mg^{2+}. The main mechanism is the strengthening of excitatory glutamate NMDA receptors. These have the curious property of being blocked with an Mg^{2+} ion at resting membrane potentials. The block is relieved when the membrane is depolarized, and this complicated physiology is thought to play critical roles in synaptic plasticity and in learning and memory. If Mg^{2+} ions are depleted then the EPSPs are considerably stronger than those normally produced by the non-NMDA receptors and this leads to epileptic activity.

(4) Weakened voltage-gated K^+ membrane currents, for instance with application of 4-aminopyridine, dendrotoxin or Mast Cell Degranulating peptide. Voltage-gated K^+ currents are perhaps most widely known in the context of the repolarization of the action potential, but there are many different sorts of K^+ current which are beyond the scope of this chapter. Blocking them tends to increase neuronal excitability. In the case of convulsants such as 4-aminopyridine, the major effect is increasing the release of neurotransmitters from presynaptic terminals. Both inhibitory and excitatory terminals are affected in the

same way, providing one illustration of why the idea of epilepsy being due to an imbalance of excitation over inhibition is an oversimplification.

(5) Non-synaptic mechanisms: decreasing the concentration of Ca^{2+} in the medium bathing hippocampal slices to below 0.2 mM leads to a dramatic epileptic activity in the hippocampal region called CA1. The epileptic bursts can last tens of seconds, which is very long for the small volume of tissue in a brain slice preparation. Such a low level of Ca^{2+} stops synaptic transmission. It also increases neuronal excitability because the positively charged layer of Ca^{2+} ions around the outer surface of sodium channels is depleted. While the low-Ca^{2+} condition is not obviously physiological, similar mechanisms may be engaged in models where synapses are not blocked, notably in the increased-K^+ model, and in vivo Ca^{2+} can drop during seizures to levels required for the non-synaptic seizure-like events in the in vitro model.

Acute models of this kind have led to a well-documented working model of the generation of brief epileptic discharges in the hippocampus and other cortical structures, which resemble interictal spikes on the EEG. Essentially they show that focal epileptic discharges are a kind of chain reaction of excitatory pyramidal cells. In the case of the hippocampus it is the CA3 region that is most susceptible, probably because the connections between the pyramidal cells are particularly strong.

The requirements for this chain reaction are:

(1) Excitatory connections between pyramidal cells in the region must diverge – i.e. each must excite more than one other neuron on average. In practice the connectivity is much higher.
(2) The connections between pyramidal cells must be strong. EPSPs between pyramidal cells in CA3 are about 1 mV in amplitude, which is stronger than in most other cortical areas. It is not only the strength of the synapses that matter: it turns out that CA3 pyramidal cells are prone to discharge bursts of action potentials because they express a voltage-gated calcium current which, when activated, triggers several action potentials mediated by the faster voltage-gated sodium current. (These 'intrinsic bursts' depend on a slow depolarization, which in other cells, including CA1 pyramidal cells, can be due to a slow form of sodium current.)
(3) The population of neurons must be larger than some minimum aggregate (or critical mass, to make an analogy with nuclear fission). This is necessary if excitation is not to die out before most or all the neurons can be recruited.

The connections between pyramidal cells in normal brain do not exist to cause epilepsy. They are part of the circuitry necessary for normal function: perceiving the outside world, laying down memories and so on. Normally this circuitry is held in check by inhibitory interneurons. These neurons form a minority in hippocampus and neocortex, perhaps around 10–20% of the total number of neurons. But they play a crucial role in preventing excitation spreading through the majority excitatory neuron population, as evidenced by drugs and toxins that are convulsants because they block the inhibitory $GABA_A$ receptor (penicillin, picrotoxin and quinolones, and, rather less selectively, cocaine). Seizures on withdrawal of benzodiazepine, barbiturates and perhaps alcohol also appear to be due to impaired functioning of $GABA_A$ receptors.

Acute models of idiopathic generalized epilepsies are much more limited. The best understood use systemic administration of penicillin, or some other $GABA_A$ receptor antagonists, to produce widely generalized spike-and-wave discharges similar to those seen in clinical absence epilepsy. These kinds of model led to the understanding that absence seizures are due to the interplay between the neocortex and the thalamus (the relay for much of the sensory input into the cortex). It is thought that rhythmic inhibitory activity generated within the thalamus paces the spike-and-wave discharges recorded from the neocortex (see Chapter 12). The pathological rhythmic interplay of synaptic excitation, and their interaction with the intrinsic properties of the neurons involved, is quite distinct from the runaway spread of excitation and recruitment of neurons characteristic of focal seizures. This fundamental difference may be a factor in the distinctive pharmacological profiles of these clinical conditions.

It has been difficult to model absence seizures in slices in vitro, because of the importance of long-range connections between thalamus and neocortex, which are extremely difficult to preserve in slices that are not so thick that they suffer from anoxia in their centres. One way round this has been to prepare thalamic slices and use a computer simulation in place of the real cortex (an innovation pioneered by the groups of McCormick and Destexhe in 2000). Essentially, if thalamic activity triggers an input to the 'electronic cortex' that results in a single stimulus to the descending output from cortex to thalamus, the thalamus produces a strengthened 6–10 Hz physiological spindle oscillation. If the electronic cortex is modified to produce a burst of stimuli (or descending action potentials), the thalamic oscillation converts to a slower and more synchronous 3 Hz similar to absence epilepsy. This approach shows that the way that the neocortex transforms input from the thalamus into output back to it plays a critical role in transforming physiological spindle oscillations into the rhythmic pathophysiology of the absence seizure.

Chronic models – focal epilepsy

As is made clear in Chapter 1, epilepsy is by definition chronic. Diagnosis generally requires more than one seizure without an obvious cause such as intoxication, or metabolic or cardiovascular problem. Essentially the functional organization of the epileptic brain is such that it will generate seizures under conditions that would normally be innocuous. 'Functional organization' here means some combination of the wiring of the neuronal circuitry and the properties of the neurons themselves.

Chronic models of temporal lobe epilepsy in general depend on some initial 'precipitating event' which leads to the induction of epileptic foci. These models are more difficult and labour-intensive than acute models, but do mimic epilepsy as distinct from symptomatic seizures. The means of induction is normally targeted at a particular structure (typically the hippocampus for temporal lobe epilepsy), although in some cases systemic administration of drugs or toxins can be used, albeit often with more widespread abnormalities. These kinds of model fall into three broad categories (Figure 10.2).

(1) Models induced by an episode of status epilepticus (Figure 10.2A). This is triggered by one of the following: injection of kainic acid into the hippocampus, systemic injection of pilocarpine or kainic acid, or repetitive intracranial electrical stimulation until self-sustaining status epilepticus is achieved. Status is normally terminated by a suitable drug after 1–2 hours, which is long enough to induce the focus. After a week or two the animals (rats or mice) start to have spontaneous seizures which will recur for the rest of their lives. The status epilepticus produces a focal loss of neurons in the hippocampus, which is similar, but not identical, to hippocampal sclerosis in humans.

(2) Kindling involves the repeated stimulation of certain brain regions, such as the amygdala, every day (or in some cases several times a day or every several days; Figure 10.2B). Kindling does not induce status epilepticus, nor does it result in hippocampal sclerosis; it usually does not produce spontaneous seizures either. The lack of spontaneous seizures is something of a drawback as a realistic model of temporal lobe epilepsy, but the need to evoke seizures by stimulation does have the advantage of predictability when it comes to testing drug efficacy. (In contrast, spontaneous seizures are by definition unpredictable, and care is needed to ensure that any change in seizure frequency when a drug administered is not just a chance variation.) Kindling has proved valuable; for instance it played a key role in recognizing the potential of levetiracetam as an AED. The enduring change induced by kindling is a reduction in seizure threshold, so that initially innocuous stimulations result in secondarily generalized seizures once kindling has been established.

(3) Tetanus toxin injected into the rat hippocampus (Figure 10.2C) has no immediate clinical effects: there is no early status epilepticus, and no hippocampal sclerosis. Approximately 1 week later the animals start to experience spontaneous seizures, which recur intermittently for 6–8 weeks before most of the animals gain seizure remission. The remission appears to be an active process because some animals do not gain remission, and those with neocortical foci never gain remission. All animals with hippocampal foci show cognitive impairments, especially in learning and memory. The lack of hippocampal sclerosis means that intrahippocampal tetanus toxin models non-lesional temporal lobe epilepsy, which is a significant clinical problem. A small proportion of these animals go on to develop hippocampal sclerosis, showing that this pathology can result from repeated brief (<2 min) seizures.

Many different kinds of cellular pathology and pathophysiology can be identified in chronic models of

Section 1: Basic principles

(A)
Status epilepticus ← pilocarpine (ip)/kainic acid (ip or intracranial)/repetitive stimulation
Silent or "latent" period of up to 2 weeks.
Spontaneous seizures
0 2 4 6 8   26   weeks

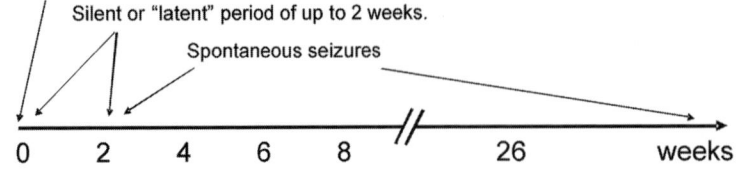

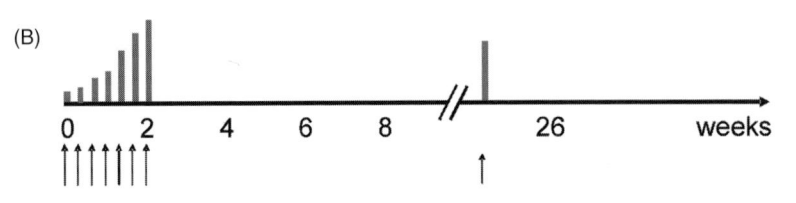

(B)
0 2 4 6 8   26   weeks

(C) Inject ng dose of tetanus toxin into hippocampus or other brain region
Seizures start after 1–2 weeks and recur intermittently for many weeks
Seizures normally remit after 6–8 weeks
Behavioural changes persist; seizures may recur
0 2 4 6 8   26   weeks

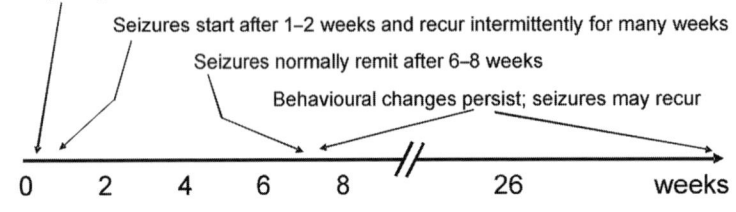

Figure 10.2. Time lines for three major classes of chronic experimental temporal lobe epilepsy. (A) Status epilepticus can be induced by several treatments, and is allowed to continue for at least 40 minutes, and more typically 90 min to several hours. After a latent period of 1–2 weeks spontaneous seizures occur and continue for the rest of the animal's life. (B) Kindling is induced by repetitive stimulation (stimuli shown by arrows). Repetition increases the strength of the response, which is indicated by the height of the vertical lines in this panel. (C) Injection of a small dose of tetanus toxin does not cause status epilepticus or other obvious response. Spontaneous seizures start after a latent period of 1–2 weeks, usually with seizure remission after 6–8 weeks, but with permanent changes in behaviour.

focal epilepsy. This complicates research, but perhaps matches the complexity of clinical epileptic foci. The challenge for future research on basic mechanisms is to characterize these changes, and determine which are pro-epileptic, which are antiepileptic and which are neutral epiphenomena. A complete list of chronic changes is beyond the scope of this chapter, but some recurring themes include changes in intrinsic neuronal properties (voltage-gated ion channels of several kinds), altered synaptic transmission, selective losses of neurons, and 'sprouting' of new connections.

Patients with epilepsy have not usually received intracranial injections of toxins or repeated electric shocks or doses of convulsant drugs, so the chronic models outlined above cannot be completely faithful reproductions of specific clinical conditions. One or two models exist that do attempt just that. For instance, there are simulated forms of head injury (such as fluid percussion through a burr hole in the skull), and advances in the genetics of epilepsy are starting to lead to genetically modified mice that express such mutations, and in some cases appear to have epileptic symptoms.

Secondarily generalized seizures

Brain slices can sustain seizure-like activity, in the sense that they can discharge for tens of seconds. Examples of seizure-like events are found in the low-Ca^{2+}, high-K^+, low-Mg^{2+} and 4-AP models in hippocampal slices. Often these prolonged discharges are generated by different networks from those responsible for brief interictal discharges. The prolonged discharges are typically associated with increases in extracellular potassium ion levels, which result in a negative DC shift of the extracellular potential. Interestingly, DC recordings from human epileptic cortex have also revealed negative shifts during seizures (most clinical recordings are AC and automatically filter out these negative shifts).

Models in vivo, both acute and chronic, show that secondarily generalized seizures recruit multiple brain regions, and suggest that the interplay between these regions may be crucially important in seizure generation. In most cases there are no consistent delays between different regions, arguing against excitation cycling around a series of connected structures, and for coupled or mutually interconnected oscillators.

Chronic models – idiopathic generalized epilepsies

Myoclonic and/or tonic-clonic seizures can be induced by sensory stimulation in photosensitive baboons,

Mongolian gerbils and several lines of rats and mice. The latter include the Genetically Epilepsy Prone Rat (GEPR), which responds to auditory stimulation with tonic-clonic seizures, which do respond to at least some of the appropriate AEDs. However, the cellular mechanisms of this model are not well understood.

Several kinds of rodents spontaneously develop absence epilepsy and have been bred to optimize this trait. Notable examples amongst mice include tottering, lethargic and stargazer, all of which have generalized spike-and-wave epilepsy and have been the subject of intensive molecular investigations. Amongst the rat models, WAG/Rij and GAERS (the Genetic Absence Epilepsy Rat of Strasbourg) have provided significant advances in our understanding of the dynamics of spike-and-wave discharges. Both played roles in the fundamental advance of recognizing that absence seizures depend on a focal cortical pathophysiology, blurring the distinction between focal/partial and idiopathic generalized epilepsies (see also the outline above of experiments on thalamic slices connected to an electronic cortex).

Conclusions

Experimental models have told us much about the physiological dynamics and molecular pathology of epilepsies. Perhaps most notable is the chain reaction of excitation in the focal epilepsies and the rhythmic interplay of excitation and inhibition in the absence epilepsies. Drug discovery has relied on experimental models to screen putative compounds and several useful compounds have resulted from this process. However, it may be that really novel antiepileptic drugs need to use more realistic, but often more labour-intensive, models, such as kindling and other chronic models.

Recommended reading

Huguenaerd J. Thalamocortical circuits and excitability. *Epilepsy Currents* 2001;**1**:13. http://www.pubmedcentral.nih.gov/articlerender.fcgi?artid=320682.

Jefferys JGR. Epilepsy in vitro: electrophysiology and computer modeling. In Engel J, *et al.*, eds. *Epilepsy: A Comprehensive Texbook*. Philadelphia: Lippincott, Willams & Wilkins; 2007.

Pitkänen A, Schwartzkroin PA, Moshé SL (eds). *Models of Seizures and Epilepsy*. Amsterdam: Elsevier; 2006.

Learning objectives

(1) To understand the relevance and usefulness of the study of animal models of epilepsy.
(2) To understand the strengths and weaknesses of animal models of epilepsy.
(3) To know the existing types of animal models of epilepsy and, for each model, the:

- animal species used
- principles behind
- time-course
- type of epilepsy modelled
- role in testing potential new anticonvulsants.

Section 1 Basic principles

Chapter 11

Epileptogenesis in vitro

Antonio Valentín

Introduction

Since the nineteenth century, the pathophysiology of seizures has been explained as alterations in neuronal activity. Different lines of evidence suggest that neuronal activity during epileptic seizures becomes hypersynchronous, excessive, autonomous and disordered. The process by which a normal area of the brain acquires a long-lasting propensity to generate spontaneous epileptic seizures is called epileptogenesis. In vitro studies have been used to identify mechanisms of epileptogenesis that could occur in vivo (in the living complete animal). Epileptic seizures are defined in terms of behavioural changes in the complete animal, a feature that is absent in vitro. As behavioural changes are absent in vitro, it is difficult to identify changes in neuronal activity equivalent responsible for epileptic seizures in vivo. Two types of electrical neuronal activity are often studied in vitro (Figure 11.1):

- Paroxysmal depolarizing shift (PDS) appears on intracellular recordings as a burst of action potentials riding on a sustained depolarization, lasting for 0.05 to 0.2 seconds (see detailed description below). This phenomenon is usually interpreted as a model of in vivo interictal epileptiform discharges.
- Electrographic seizures: consisting of repeated bursts of action potentials occurring at regular intervals and lasting for 3–200 seconds. They often resemble runs of several PDS occurring regularly. They are usually interpreted as a model of in vivo epileptic seizures.

Slice models are usually models of focal seizures, as the amount of brain studied is necessarily limited. Nevertheless, some slice preparations including cortex and thalamus have been used as models of absence seizures.

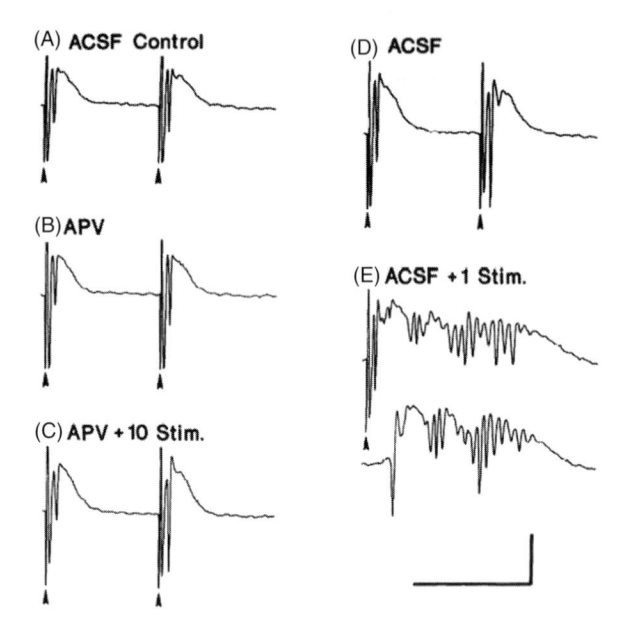

Figure 11.1. DL-2-amino-5-phosphonovaleric acid (APV) blocked burst induction by trains of electrical stimuli. (A) triggered twin excitatory potentials (EPSPs) in artificial cerebrospinal fluid (ACSF) control. (B) 10 min in 200 microM APV. (C) Absence of bursting after 10 stimulus trains (2 s, 60/s, one every 5 min). (D) 25 min in ACSF wash. (E) Triggered and spontaneous (bottom) bursting after one stimulus train in ACSF. Calibrations vertical 2mV; horizontal, 50 ms (reproduced with permission from William W. Anderson, H. Scott Swartzwelder and Wilkie A. Wilson. The NMDA receptor antagonist 2-amino & phosphonovalerate blocks stimulus train-induced epileptogenesis but not epileptiform bursting in the rat hippocampal slice. *J Neurophysiol* 1987;57(1)).

Types of epileptogenesis

To describe epileptogenesis it is necessary to understand the mechanisms, stages, experimental models and seizure types necessary for the brain to become epileptic.

Introduction to Epilepsy ed. Gonzalo Alarcón and Antonio Valentín. Published by Cambridge University Press.
© Cambridge University Press 2012.

Mechanisms of epileptogenesis

The mechanisms of epileptogenesis may be classified as genetic or acquired:

- Genetic: genetic mechanisms are responsible for some types of generalized and focal epilepsies. New genetic abnormalities related to epilepsy are described on a day-to-day basis.
- Acquired: epileptogenesis could result from any neuronal insults, including hypoxia, trauma, sclerosis, infection, tumours, stroke, neuronal degeneration, developmental abnormalities, and toxic and metabolic conditions.

Stages of epileptogenesis

During development of epileptogenesis, three different stages can be seen:

- rapid phase: occurring during the first minutes to hours following an insult to the brain, mainly at the cellular and molecular level;
- intermediate phase: occurring during days, at the level of cellular connections and networks;
- long-lasting phase: lasting for weeks to months, creating a brain prone to generate seizures.

Seizure types

Experimental models are necessary to study the mechanisms and stages of epileptogenesis, and they can be studied acutely or chronically in animals in vivo or in vitro. The type of seizures generated with the different models could be classified as:

- reactive (induced): if seizures occur in normal tissue while applying an epileptogenic condition (drug, electrical stimulation, changes in perfusion medium, etc.);
- epileptic (spontaneous): if seizures arise spontaneously in an area of the brain that has been altered either genetically or inducing long-lasting tissue changes or damage.

Reactive seizures and epileptogenesis

PDS and electrographic seizures can be induced in normal tissue by applying drugs or by manipulations in extracellular ionic concentrations. These studies provide models for acute symptomatic seizures (see Chapter 31) and for some of the mechanisms contributing to seizure generation. For instance:

- When artificial cerebrospinal fluid in brain slices contains very low calcium concentration, synaptic transmission is lost. Nevertheless, electrographic seizures can still occur, suggesting that non-synaptic mechanisms such as gap junctions may contribute to seizure generation. Low calcium concentration may occur in vivo after repetitive firing, perhaps contributing to prolongation and propagation of seizures.
- Changes in other extracellular ion concentrations: high synaptic activity is associated with an efflux of potassium and increase in extracellular potassium concentration. This may lead to depolarization (bringing the membrane potential closer to threshold) and to a reduction in the driving force of potassium-mediated inhibition. Low extracellular magnesium levels increase excitability by removing the normal voltage-dependent physiological block of NMDA glutamate receptors. Low extracellular calcium also increases excitability (see Chapter 10). Increases in extracellular potassium and reductions in extracellular calcium and magnesium can occur during repetitive firing and seizures, leading to increased neuronal excitability.

Epileptogenesis at molecular level

Epileptogenesis at molecular level involves changes in the molecular components synthesized by neurons. These include synaptic neurotransmitter and neuromodulator systems (see also Chapter 3):

(a) Excitatory neurotransmitter systems:

- NMDA receptors generate an increase in the calcium influx inside the neuron:

    - increasing in NMDA and AMPA synaptic transmission
    - acutely decreasing GABAergic inhibition
    - changing other regulatory systems (protein kinase systems, metabolic glutamate receptors, tyrosine kinase, gene expressions, changes in mRNA of neurotransmitters, etc.).
    - Acute epileptogenesis is blocked by NMDA antagonists (Figure 11.1)
    - However, once bursting activity is induced, NMDA antagonists have an attenuated effect or no effect at all.

- Non-NMDA receptors (AMPA and kainate) can be also involved in the epileptogenesis although their role is currently unclear.
  - AMPA and kainate receptors are involved in spontaneous recurrent seizure activity.
  - Blockade of AMPA or kainate receptors is one of the most effective research techniques to reduce epileptiform activity.
  - AMPA and kainate receptors are increased in epileptic brain tissue in humans and animals.
- Pharmacological manipulation of metabotropic glutamate receptors can increase neuronal excitability.

(b) Inhibitory neurotransmitter systems:
- GABA has been considered as one of the most important neurotransmitters involved in epileptogenesis.
- Defects of the GABA system have been implicated in epileptogenesis since the 1970s, when loss of GABA neurons was considered responsible for seizures (absence of inhibition).
- However, some physiological studies in animal models of epilepsy did not find a reduction in GABAergic inhibition.

(c) Neuromodulators, neuropeptides, neurotrophines, growth factors and cytokines:
- These peptides and small proteins were not previously recognized as having a clear relevance to epilepsy, but some studies are starting to demonstrate that they may influence neuronal neurotransmission.
- However, their role in epileptogenesis is still unknown.

Epileptogenesis at cellular level

Epileptogenesis at cellular level can involve changes in cellular morphology and function, developmental defects, acute neurotoxicity or intrinsic electrophysiological properties of some neuronal types. Proposed cellular mechanisms of epileptogenesis include:

- presence of ectopic neurons or groups of neurons with morphological changes, including aberrant and displaced synaptic connections, inadequate sprouting or pruning of axons, or abnormal dendrites;
- increments in excitatory synaptic connections due to changes in dendrite morphology and function (e.g. increments in AMPA receptors, sprouting);
- altered glial function inducing changes in neurotransmitter uptake or in extracellular ion concentrations;
- cellular swelling and associated contraction of extracellular space, which can enhance ephaptic coupling between cells (depolarization due to electrical fields associated to firing of nearby neurons);
- acute neurotoxicity provoking cell damage and cell loss; some cellular types, mainly interneurons, are severely affected, modifying the neuronal network excitability;
- passive membrane properties: induction and propagation of action potentials depend on input resistance, membrane time constant and resting membrane potential, which are largely determined by cellular geometry and resistivity; not all studies have confirmed changes in these variables in epileptic tissue;
- gap junctions: electrical synapses may play a role in seizure initiation and propagation in the postnatal period or in areas where they are more common (e.g. the hippocampus);
- alterations in the intrinsic electrophysiological properties of neuronal membrane ion channels:
  - Blocking or slowing recovery of voltage-sensitive sodium channels can prevent high-frequency firing and is thought to be the mechanism of action of several anticonvulsant drugs.
  - There are many types of potassium channels. In general, their activation may prevent burst firing by hyperpolarizing the cell, although the IQ current depolarizes the cell under some circumstances (see below)
  - Voltage-dependent calcium channels are responsible for a depolarizing after-potential in some thalamic neurons and have been implicated in absence seizures (see below).

Two examples of neuronal electrophysiological properties that could be the basis of epileptogenesis are oscillating currents in thalamic neurons, and paroxysmal depolarizing shifts (PDS) in the hippocampus:

- Oscillating currents in thalamic relay neurons are involved in the pathophysiology of generalized epilepsies (see Chapter 10). Thalamic relay neurons have peculiar ion currents (Figure 11.2). Two ion currents appear to be responsible for such an oscillating process (Figure 11.2B).

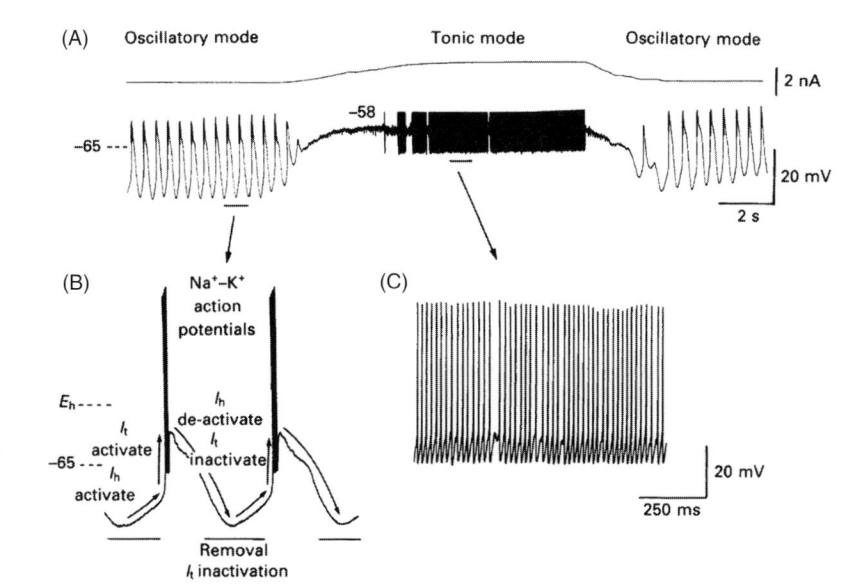

Figure 11.2. Examples of the two different firing modes of thalamic relay neurons. (A) Rhythmic burst firing at a rate of about 2 Hz in a thalamic cell in a cat. Depolarization of the cell to −58 mV with the intracellular injection of current (top trace) halted the rhythmic activity and switched the neuron to the tonic mode of action potential generation. Removal of the depolarization reinstated the oscillatory activity. (B) Expanded trace of oscillatory activity with the proposed currents, which largely mediate it. (C) Expanded trace of tonic activity (reproduced with permission from McCormick DA. and Pape HC. Properties of a hyperpolarization-activated cation current and its role in rhythmic oscillation in thalamic relay neurones. *J Physiol* 1990;431:291–318).

- Calcium IT current: this current triggers low-threshold calcium spikes (calcium action potentials occurring when the neuron is only slightly depolarized). After an action potential, this current is inactivated and is re-activated by hyperpolarization.
- Potassium IH (IQ) current: this is a potassium current which is paradoxically activated by hyperpolarization and results in a slight depolarization of the membrane.
- When a thalamic cell is hyperpolarized, IH potassium current induces membrane depolarization which is followed by calcium IT currents resulting in action potentials. The subsequent post-spike hyperpolarization re-activates IH and IT currents, re-starting the cycle again. This phenomenon explains the repetitive firing nature of thalamic neurons.
- When a thalamic cell is maintained depolarized above threshold, calcium IT and potassium IH currents are inactivated, and their associated rhythmic activity ceases. Under such conditions, the thalamic cell fires at high frequency (tonic mode; Figure 11.2.C).
- The paroxysmal depolarizing shifts (PDS; Figure 11.3) are considered the cellular correlate of the interictal EEG spikes and may be the physiological basis for some types of focal epilepsies:
  - PDS are large depolarizations of the neuronal membrane (20–40 mV), lasting for 50–200 ms, similar to a giant EPSP. Indeed, voltage clamping experiments have shown that PDS and EPSP reverse at the same potential, suggesting that PDS are a type of EPSP.
  - PDS can be evoked by repetitive electrical stimulation or by altering physiological conditions (e.g. drugs such as 4-AP, bicuculline or kainate, changes in ionic concentration, particularly an increase in extracellular potassium).
  - PDS drive the membrane potential above threshold, making the neurons fire rapid bursts of action potentials.
  - PDS are followed by a period of hyperpolarization lasting for 200–500 ms.
  - PDS depend on glutamate acting through voltage-sensitive calcium and sodium channels.
  - PDS occur only in large populations of highly connected neurons ('minimum aggregate', around 1000 in animal models). This suggests that PDS arise from the properties of the neuronal networks rather than being an intrinsic property of the neurons.

Epileptogenesis at the network level (slices)

In experimental models studying epileptogenesis in tissue slices, the most important condition to generate epileptic seizures appears to be an imbalance between

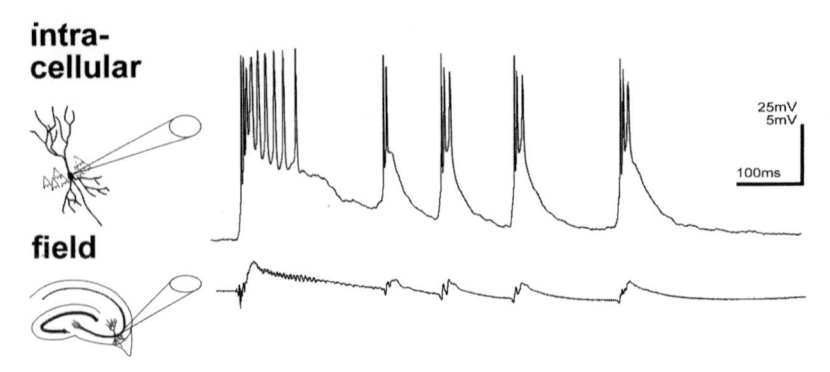

Figure 11.3. Electrophysiology of epileptic discharges and paroxysmal depolarizing shifts. Simultaneous intracellular (IC) and field potential recordings were made from the CA3 region of a hippocampal slice. The first 200 ms correspond to an interictal spike (modified with permission from Figure 1.1, page 49, chapter 2, Pathophysiology of experimental epilepsies, by JGR Jefferys and RD Traub, published in *Neuropathology of Epilepsy*, edited by F. Scaravilli, 1998, World Scientific, Singapore, ISBN 9810231709).

excitation and inhibition, resulting in excessive and hypersynchronous neuronal activity. Acute experimental models of epileptogenesis usually modify the relation between excitation and inhibition by blocking inhibitory synapses, by strengthening excitatory synapses or by increasing neuronal excitability.

A particular problem in interpreting results from tissue slices is that it is rather difficult to know what behaviour of neurons corresponds to seizures or interictal discharges in the whole brain. Runs of fast activity and repetitive spikes or spike-wave in the slices are commonly considered as correlates of proper seizures in the whole brain.

Epileptogenesis in tissue slices has the following features:

- Epileptogenesis can be induced by convulsant drugs, altered ion concentrations, or repeated stimulus trains.
- Time course ranges from minutes to hours (they are 'acute' models).
- Some mechanisms are different from those underlying chronic epileptogenesis.
- Epileptogenesis may be reversible.
- Mechanisms can become long-lasting, sometimes continuing after withdrawal of the epileptogenic agent or stimulus.
- Epileptogenesis may or may not involve acute cell loss.
- Epileptiform activity may induce cell damage.

The role of synchronization

In addition to increased excitability resulting from the mechanisms mentioned above, synchronized firing from many neurons is thought to be necessary to generate interictal epileptiform discharges or seizures in vivo. Several mechanisms may be involved in neuronal synchronization, including increments in the number of excitatory synapses, gap junctions, ephaptic effects and changes in extracellular ionic concentration.

The epileptic hippocampus

The hippocampal slices are one of the most commonly used models for epileptogenesis in tissue slices. Several theories have been developed to understand the acquisition of epileptogenesis in the hippocampus:

- Inhibitory loss and axonal sprouting
  - Destruction of inhibitory cells.
  - Deafferentation of inhibitory cells (e.g. because of destruction of the hillum).
  - Sprouting of mossy fibres.
  - Axonal sprouts from relatively mature neurons tend to synapse very locally rather than travelling long distances.
  - New synapses, most of which are excitatory, occur locally and produce increased positive feedback networks.
  - Some axons synapse onto inhibitory interneurons, resulting in a net strengthening of recurrent inhibition.
- Excess in hypersynchrony:
  - Under normal conditions, brain slices do not show spontaneous field potentials in the hippocampus.
  - If inhibition is blocked, spontaneous multipeaked field potentials can be seen in CA1, CA2 and CA3.
  - CA3 and CA2 show 'bursting activity' even when isolated whereas CA1 requires input from CA3 and/or CA2.
  - If inhibition is intact, CA3 can not drive spontaneous activity in CA1.

- Changes in extracellular ionic concentrations: increases in extracellular potassium concentration after prolonged cellular discharges can induce further hyperexcitability and changes in the extracellular volume.
- Changes in the balance between excitation and inhibition: increase in excitation and/or decrease in inhibition; both possibilities have been considered as possible mechanisms for epileptogenesis.
  - A relative increase in excitation would create a hyperexcitable cortex.
  - A relative increase in inhibition would contribute to an excess in neuronal hypersynchrony.

Conclusion

The main objective of this chapter was to show how epilepsy research studies can increase our knowledge of the mechanisms involved in acute epileptogenesis. Understanding epileptogenesis can generate new diagnostic and treatment options in the future, eventually helping prevent seizures in patients with predisposition to epilepsy.

Recommended reading

Delgado-Escueta AV, Wilson WA, Olsen RW, Porter RJ. *Jasper's Basic Mechanisms of the Epilepsies.* 3rd edn. *Advances in Neurology*, vol. 79. Philadelphia, PA: Lippincott Williams and Wilkins; 1999.

Jefferys JGR, Traub RD. Pathophysiology of experimental epilepsies. In Scaravilli F, ed. *Neuropathology of Epilepsy*, pp. 45–76. Singapore: World Scientific; 1998.

Schwartzkroin PA. *Epilepsy: Models, Mechanisms and Concepts.* Cambridge: Cambridge University Press; 1993.

Wyllie E. *The Treatment of Epilepsy. Principles and Practice.* 2nd edn. *Part 1 (Basic Mechanisms of Epileptogenesis)*, pp. 9–150. Baltimore, MD: Williams & Wilkins; 1997.

Learning objective

(1) To understand the preparations used to study epileptogenesis in vitro:
- methodology
- time course (e.g. acute/chronic)
- how epileptogenesis manifests itself
- interpretation of how epileptogenesis arises
- usefulness.

Section 1 **Basic principles**

Chapter 12

Epileptogenesis in vivo

Gonzalo Alarcón

In vivo animal models of epilepsy

The mechanisms of epileptogenesis in vivo have been extensively studied in animal models, including the mechanisms of initiation and propagation of seizures. Kindling and local cortical application of convulsant agents have been used as models of focal epilepsy. Intravenous injections of convulsant agents have been used as models of idiopathic generalized epilepsies. Genetic models have been developed by breeding epileptic animals to model idiopathic epilepsies. The methodology and results of animal models are discussed in Chapter 9. In essence, multiples lines of evidence suggest that an imbalance between excitation and inhibition is the most important condition to generate epileptic seizures in animals. Such imbalance results in excessive, rapid and hypersynchronous neuronal activity. A number of specific mechanisms have been identified in vivo:

- Proliferation of excitatory neurons or axons (sprouting): kindling, pilocarpine model, kainate lesions, tetanus toxin model.
- Loss of inhibitory interneurons: in the pilocarpine model there is selective loss of GAD-positive neurons.
- Disconnection of excitatory input to inhibitory interneurons ('dormant cells'; see below): sustained electrical stimulation of the dentate gyrus.
- Increase in excitation: low magnesium model, kindling, kainate lesions.
- Decrease in presynaptic GABA release: tetanus toxin model, kainate lesions.
- Changes in post-synaptic receptors or in the properties of ionic currents.

The dormant cell hypothesis to explain temporal lobe epilepsy postulates that epilepsy is caused by hilar cell loss resulting in the interruption of an inhibitory circuit which includes dentate granule cells, hilar mossy cells and inhibitory interneurons. Loss of hilar mossy cells reduces excitatory input to the inhibitory interneurons which then become 'dormant' and no longer inhibit granule cells. Later mossy cell sprouting results in excitatory direct synapses between mossy cells and granule cells.

In Wyler's hypothesis of focal epileptogenesis, neurons at the centre of the epileptic focus ('Type I') are de-afferented. Hence the lack of control by input permits disordered and autonomous, notably oscillatory, neuronal activity in the centre of the focus. Dysfunctional Type I neurons recruit surrounding normal Type II neurons into hypersynchronous firing, inducing propagation of discharges from abnormal to normal regions (Wyler and Ward, 1986).

Sustained electrical activity such as that seen in status epilepticus can kill neurons, probably due to abnormally high activation of NMDA glutamate receptors which is associated with excessive cellular entry of calcium (Meldrum, 1993)

Mechanisms of focal seizures in man

As the basic histology of the human brain and that of other mammals is essentially similar, the human cortex is vulnerable to the same pro-convulsant conditions and agents mentioned above. Nevertheless, the pathophysiology of spontaneous focal seizures in man is puzzling, and largely derives from the study of spontaneous seizures with intracranial electrodes during presurgical assessment. It might initially be expected that focal EEG changes, particularly spike-and-wave activity, will be the first electrical change seen in partial seizures. However, the onset of focal seizures often shows a number of subtle focal as well

---

Introduction to Epilepsy ed. Gonzalo Alarcón and Antonio Valentín. Published by Cambridge University Press.
© Cambridge University Press 2012.

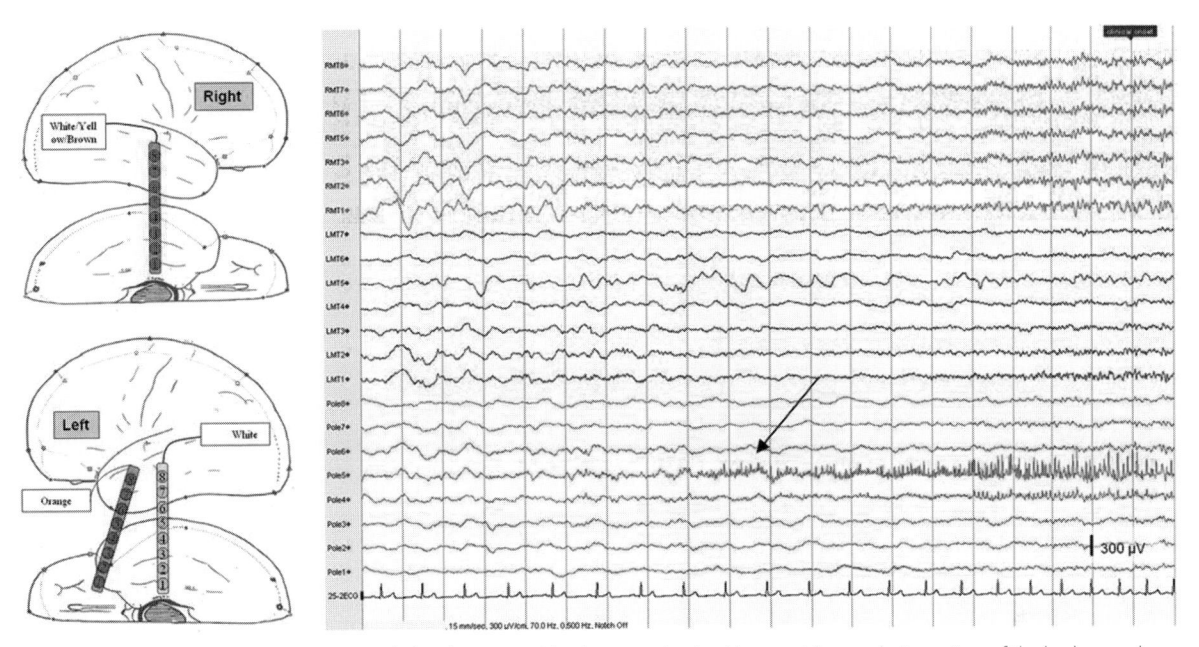

Figure 12.1. Onset of a focal seizure recorded with intracranial subtemporal strips. Note a widespread attenuation of the background activity occurring as rhythmic sharp spike activity occurs at contact 5 of the polar strip. See colour version in plate section.

as widespread electrical changes (Alarcón et al., 1995). These include focal or generalized attenuation in the amplitude of the ongoing EEG (electrodecremental event), focal or diffuse low-amplitude high-frequency activity, focal rhythmic theta or delta activities, and focal rhythmic spikes or spike-wave activity. Of these, sharply localized high-frequency activity at or above 20 Hz appears to be the most likely marker of the seizure onset site. It appears that only 7–14% of neurons contribute at any one time to the EEG discharge at seizure onset in man (Babb et al., 1987). Indeed, very high-frequency focal oscillations (termed fast ripples) at frequencies over 200 Hz appear to have the highest pathological significance and coincide with the epileptogenic zone (for review, see Engel et al., 2009). After a few seconds or minutes, focal discharges increase in rhythmicity and amplitude as they decrease in frequency and spread to neighbouring regions (rhythmic ictal transformation; Geiger and Harner, 1978), gradually giving way to more widespread spike-and-wave or sharpened slow activity in the course of several seconds or minutes. The relationship between these electrical phenomena and clinical symptoms is variable and depends on their duration, their extent and functional relevance of the area involved. Discharges restricted to one gyrus can induce focal convulsions or a perception of elementary sensations if located in primary motor or sensory areas but produce minimal or no symptoms if restricted to association areas. Often discharges propagate to neighbouring cortical regions or to widespread areas of the cortex. If there is extensive bilateral spread of discharges, a complex partial or secondarily generalized tonic-clonic seizure may result.

About a third of focal seizures are preceded by a generalized or focal electrodecremental event, a brief attenuation of the ongoing activity lasting for several seconds. When generalized it does not preclude a favourable outcome (Alarcón et al., 1995). The occurrence of an event that could be generalized as the first electrical manifestation of a focal seizure is perplexing. The absence of particularly poor outcome associated with such diffuse ictal changes at seizure onset may reflect generalized cerebral changes that allow particularly susceptible regions to develop paroxysmal discharges. In particular, electrodecremental events tend to be associated with increased neuronal firing, suggesting that they are due to neuronal desynchronization rather than deactivation (Figure 12.2). In any case, the phenomenon suggests a deficiency in our understanding of the underlying pathophysiology of focal seizures and questions current criteria for the distinction between focal and generalized seizures.

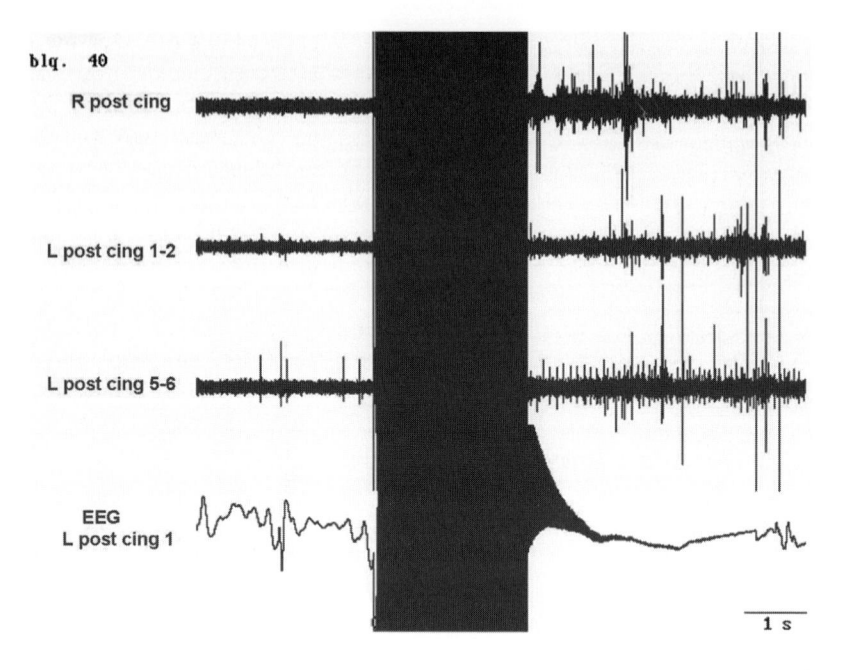

Figure 12.2. Neuronal firing during an electrodecremental event in a human seizure. Habitual seizure induced by electrical stimulation at 50 Hz during 2 s. Note increment in firing rated during attenuation of background activity. R = right; L = left; post = posterior.

The significance of interictal epileptiform discharges is no less puzzling. In patients with unilateral focal seizures, focal interictal discharges can occur independently in several regions, often in separate hemispheres, suggesting that interictal discharges can occur in areas that do not originate seizures (Alarcón et al., 1994, 1997). Nevertheless, seizures tend to arise from areas with the highest incidence of interictal discharges. Single-pulse electrical stimulation is a new tool to map cortical excitability and identify areas originating seizures (see Chapter 89: 'Single-pulse electrical stimulation'). Interestingly, simultaneous EEG and single-neuron recordings have shown striking similarities in neuronal firing patterns during interictal discharges and during responses to single-pulse electrical stimulation. Around 32% of cells do not show changes in firing rate whereas the remaining show a brief burst of action potentials, lasting for less than 100 ms, or a period of inhibition lasting for around 200–600 ms or both (Alarcón et al., 2008).

Mechanisms of generalized seizures in man

The mechanisms responsible for the sudden onset of simultaneous bilateral electrical EEG changes during generalized seizures, particularly bilaterally synchronous discharges during absence seizures, have been a puzzle for epileptologists for many decades. The finding that large bilateral areas of the cortex can suddenly synchronize suggests that the phenomenon may be driven by a subcortical structure. Partially inspired by current sleep research, which had shown that cortical excitability was largely influenced by midbrain structures in the cat, Penfield and Jasper (1954) postulated that a deep midbrain pacemaker was responsible for triggering and maintaining synchrony of bilateral discharges (the centrencephalic hypothesis). This hypothesis was supported by the fact that brainstem structures and thalamic nuclei (nonspecific thalamic nuclei, intralaminar nuclei) project to many cortical regions. The observation that generalized seizures in animals can be induced by various manipulations of subcortical structures (Shouse and Ryan, 1984; Gale, 1985; Burnham, 1987; Garrant and Gale, 1987; Browning, 1994) provides further evidence in favour of the centrencephalic hypothesis. Further support was provided by the finding that unilateral thalamic stimulation can induce bilateral cortical responses (Dempsey and Morison, 1942; Morison and Dempsey, 1942), and that absence-like seizures at 3 Hz can be induced by electrical stimulation of intralaminar thalamic nuclei (Jasper and Droogleever-Fortuyn, 1947). Moreover, simultaneous thalamic and cortical recordings during absence seizures in humans showed thalamus leading the cortex by 1–2 s (Williams, 1953), and the centrencephalic hypothesis gradually transformed into a 'thalamic theory'.

Nevertheless, the centrencephalic model has been questioned by the following experimental and clinical evidence:

- Both intravenous administration and unilateral local cortical application of penicillin (a weak GABA$_A$ antagonist) in cats are associated with generalized discharges (Gloor, 1968).
- Generalized spike-wave activity could also be induced by direct bilateral application of penicillin to the cortex but not to the thalamus (Marcus and Watson, 1966; Gloor et al., 1979; Gloor and Fariello, 1988).
- Generalized discharges induced by local application of penicillin are rendered unilateral, confined to the side of application, by section of the corpus callosum in the presence of normal thalamic structures (Marcus et al., 1968).
- Some localized medial frontal cortical lesions in humans can be associated with generalized seizures with bilaterally symmetrical spike-wave discharges arising from the vicinity of the frontal lesion (Pruvot et al., 1972). These discharges can be clinically and electroencephalographically indistinguishable from primarily generalized absence seizures unless invasive intracerebral recordings are performed.
- 'Absence'-like attacks can be induced by electrical stimulation of the frontal lobe in man (Bancaud et al., 1974). In addition, callosotomy can be used to ameliorate the degree of generalization of such seizures (Huck et al., 1980), suggesting that direct interhemispheric pathways are at least partially involved in generalization of seizures.

The sodium amytal test (Wada test, amobarbital procedure), used in the evaluation of epilepsy surgery, has provided further insights into the pathogenesis of seizures (Bennett, 1953; Gloor, 1968). The test involves injecting sodium amytal into the internal carotid artery, which supplies most of ipsilateral neocortex (see Chapter 79: 'The Wada test', and Chapter 81: 'Preoperative assessment'). Since amytal is anticonvulsant and anaesthetic, intracarotid injection is usually associated with the interruption of discharges arising from the ipsilateral neocortex, and with the abolition of cognitive function in the ipsilateral hemisphere, thus allowing an estimation of potential neuropsychological deficits resulting from removal of cortical structures of that hemisphere. In the initial protocol, a pro-convulsant agent such as pentylenetetrazol was also injected after the effects of amytal had worn off in order to localize the site of seizure onset. Occasionally, injections were inadvertently made into the vertebrobasilar system, which supplies blood to the thalamus and hippocampus. Unilateral injections of amytal into the internal carotid artery, supplying the cortex, suppressed generalized spike-and-wave activity bilaterally whereas injection of convulsant (pentylenetetrazol) induced generalized spike-wave discharges. However, injections in the vertebrobasilar system, supplying the thalamus, had little effect.

These findings led Gloor (1968) to postulate the model of generalized corticoreticular epilepsies, which assumes that the principal functional abnormality in the generation of generalized seizures is that of widespread cortical excitability, resulting in generalized spike-and-wave discharges as a response to essentially normal physiological afferent activity arriving from the thalamus and reticular activating system. The thalamus becomes secondarily involved in widespread synchronous discharges via reverberating cortico-thalamic pathways. Once oscillatory burst firing in the cortex and thalamus is established, the electrical activity of either structure may lead the other, but neither can be regarded as the initial pacemaker as both are necessary to maintain the periodic discharges (Avoli and Kostopoulos, 1982). This model is supported by findings from the feline model of generalized epilepsy induced by intramuscular injection of penicillin, which shows a gradual dose-dependent transformation of spindle responses into generalized spike-wave discharges (Prince and Farrell, 1969). The corticoreticular model postulates that there is a diffuse increase in cortical excitability, resulting in the cortex responding to afferent thalamo-cortical volleys by generating spike-and-wave rather than spindles.

Within the corticoreticular model, an initially localized discharge arising from a focal cortical pacemaker may quickly spread to originate apparently generalized discharges in conditions with widespread cortical hyperexcitability ('secondary bilateral synchrony'; Gloor 1968). This is seen in Landau-Kleffner syndrome during slow-wave sleep (Martín Miguel et al., 2011) and in the cat after focal application of penicillin. It may perhaps be argued that simultaneous activation of the entire cortex is implausible and that the distinction between partial and generalized seizures, fundamental to the international classifications of both epileptic seizures and syndromes, is only a matter of the rate and extent of spread of an initially focal physiological disturbance.

> **Box 12.1. Thalamic hypothesis revisited**
>
> There has recently been a renewal of interest in the centrencephalic hypothesis after evidence from neuroimaging and genetic models.
>
> - Genetic models of generalized epilepsies in the rat (Genetic Absence Epilepsy Rats from Strasbourg or GAERS; Wistar Albino Glaxo/Rijswijk or WAG/Rij rats; Fischer344) suggest a lateral thalamic origin for spike-wave activity:
>   - *The thalamic clock theory*: thalamic neurons fire phase locked with spike-wave discharges, and thalamic microinjection of NMDA blockers (ketamine or AP5) slows or abolishes discharges (Buzsáki, 1991).
>   - Lesions to the reticular thalamic nucleus abolish spike-wave activity, and the firing of thalamic neurons time-locked with spike-and-wave discharges precedes cortical neuronal firing (for review, see Meeren *et al.*, 2005).
>   - Normal cortical (sensori-motor) excitability (Tolmacheva *et al.*, 2004).
>   - Nevertheless, the perioral sensory cortex appears to be initiating area for generalized spike-and-wave discharges (for review, see van Luijtelaar and Sitnikova, 2006).
> - Neuroimaging has shown thalamic changes in idiopathic generalized epilepsy:
>   - PET (Prevett *et al.*, 1995).
>   - fMRI (Salek-Haddadi *et al.*, 2003).

Cellular and synaptic mechanisms of generalized spike-wave

- $GABA_A$- and $GABA_B$-mediated intra-cortical inhibition appears to be preserved in the penicillin model (Giaretta *et al.*, 1985).
- Properties of thalamic cells: as explained in the previous chapter, the interaction between potassium I_H currents and calcium I_T currents has been suggested as an explanation of the tendency to repetitive firing of thalamic neurons, which could explain the recurrent spike-wave EEG discharges seen during absence seizures. Ethosuximide is thought to act as a potent anti-absence drug by blocking T-type calcium channels.

Recommended reading

DeFelipe J. Cortical interneurons: from Cajal to 2001. *Prog Brain Res* 2002;**136**:215–38.

Delgado-Escueta AV, Wilson WA, Olsen RW, Porter RJ. *Jasper's Basic Mechanisms of the Epilepsies*. 3rd edn. *Advances in Neurology*, vol. 79. Philadelphia, PA: Lippincott Williams and Wilkins; 1999.

Meeren H, van Luijtelaar G, Lopes da Silva F, Coenen A. Evolving concepts on the pathophysiology of absence seizures. the cortical focus theory. *Arch Neurol* 2005;**62**:371–6.

Schwartzkroin PA. *Epilepsy: Models, Mechanisms and Concepts*. Cambridge: Cambridge University Press; 1993.

References

Alarcón G, Binnie CD, Elwes RDC, Polkey CE. Power spectrum and intracranial EEG patterns at seizure onset in partial epilepsy. *Electroencephalogr Clin Neurophysiol* 1995;**94**:326–37.

Alarcón G, Garcia Seoane JJ, Binnie CD, *et al.* Origin and propagation of discharges in the acute electrocorticogram: implications for physiopathology and surgical treatment of temporal lobe epilepsy. *Brain* 1997;**120**:2259–82.

Alarcón G, Guy CN, Binnie CD, *et al.* Intracerebral propagation of interictal activity in partial epilepsy: implications for source localisation. *J Neurol Neurosur Ps* 1994;**57**:435–49.

Alarcón G, Valentin A, Lacruz E, *et al.* Single cell electrical activity during human spontaneous interictal epileptiform discharges and responses to single pulse electrical stimulation (SPES). *Eur J Neurol* 2008;**15**(suppl 3):304.

Avoli M, Kostopoulos G. Participation of corticothalamic cells in penicillin-induced generalized spike and wave discharges. *Brain Res* 1982;**247**(1):159–63.

Babb TL, Wilson CL, Isokawa-Akesson M. Firing patterns of human limbic neurons during stereoencephalography (SEEG) and clinical temporal lobe seizures. *Electroencephalogr Clin Neurophysiol* 1987;**66**:467–82.

Bancaud J, Talairach J, Morel P, *et al.* 'Generalized' epileptic seizures elicited by electrical stimulation of the frontal lobe in man. *Electroenceph Clin Neurophysiol* 1974;**37**:275–82.

Bennett FE. Intracarotid and intravertebral metrazol in petit mal epilepsy. *Neurology* 1953;**3**:668–73.

Browning RA. Anatomy of generalized convulsive seizures. In Malafosse A *et al.*, eds. *Idiopathic Generalized Epilepsies: Clinical, Experimental and Genetic Aspects*, pp. 399–413. London: John Libbey; 1994.

Burnham WM. Electrical stimulation studies: generalized convulsions triggered from the brain-stem. In Fromm GH, *et al.*, eds. *Epilepsy and the Reticular Formation: the Role of the Reticular Core in Convulsive Seizures*, pp. 25–38. New York: Alan Liss; 1987.

Buzsáki G. The thalamic clock: emergent network properties. *Neuroscience* 1991;**41**:351–64.

Dempsey EW, Morison RS, The production of rhythmically recurrent cortical potentials after localized thalamic stimulation. *Am J Physiol* 1942;**135**:293–300.

Engel J Jr, Bragin A, Staba R, Mody I. High-frequency oscillations: what is normal and what is not? *Epilepsia* 2009;**50**:598–604.

Gale K. Mechanisms of seizure control mediated by gamma-aminobutyric acid: role of the substantia nigra. *Fed Proc* 1985;**44**:2414–24.

Garrant DS, Gale K. Substantia nigra-mediated anticonvulsant actions: role of nigral output pathways. *Exp Neurol* 1987;**97**:143–59.

Geiger LR, Harner RN. EEG patterns at the time of focal seizure onset. *Arch Neurol* 1978;**35**:276–86.

Giaretta D, Kostopoulos G, Gloor P, Avoli M. Intracortical inhibitory mechanisms are preserved in feline generalized penicillin epilepsy. *Neurosci Lett* 1985;**59**:203–8.

Gloor P. Generalized cortico-reticular epilepsies. Some considerations on the pathophysiology of generalized bilaterally synchronous spike and wave discharge. *Epilepsia* 1968;**9**:249–63.

Gloor P, Fariello RG. Generalized epilepsy: some of its cellular mechanisms differ from those of focal epilepsy. *Trends Neurosci* 1988;**11**:63–8.

Gloor P, Pellegrini A, Kostopoulos GK. Effects of changes in cortical excitability upon the epileptic bursts in generalized penicillin epilepsy of the cat. *Electroenceph Clin Neurophysiol* 1979;**46**:274–89.

Huck FR, Radvany J, Avila JO. Anterior callosotomy in epileptics with multiform seizures and bilateral synchronous spike and wave EEG pattern. *Acta Neurochirurg (Wien)* 1980;**30**(Suppl):127–35.

Jasper HH, Droogleever-Fortuyn J. Experimental studies on the functional anatomy of petit mal epilepsy. *Res Publ Assoc Res N* 1947;**26**:272–98.

Marcus EM, Watson CW. Bilateral synchronous spike wave electrographic patterns in the cat. Interaction of bilateral cortical foci in the intact, the bilateral cortical-callosal, and adiencephalic preparation. *Arch Neurol* 1966;**14**:601.

Marcus EM, Watson CW, Simon SA. An experimental model of some varieties of petit mal epilepsy: Electrical-behavioral correlations of acute bilateral epileptogenic foci in cerebral cortex. *Epilepsia* 1968;**9**:233–48.

Martín Miguel MC, García Seoane JJ, Valentín A, et al. EEG latency analysis for hemispheric lateralisation in Landau-Kleffner syndrome. *Clin Neurophysiol* 2011;**122**:244–52.

Meldrum BS. Excitotoxicity and selective neuronal loss in epilepsy. *Brain Pathol* 1993;**3**:405–12.

Meeren H, van Luijtelaar G, Lopes da Silva F, Coenen A. Evolving concepts on the pathophysiology of absence seizures: the cortical focus theory. *Arch Neurol* 2005; **62**:371–6.

Morison RS, Dempsey EW. A study of thalamo-cortical relations. *Am J Physiol* 1942;**135**:281–92.

Penfield W, Jasper H. *Epilepsy and the Functional Anatomy of the Human Brain*, pp. 27–9. Boston, MA: Little, Brown & Co; 1954.

Prevett MC, Duncan JS, Jones T, Fish DR, Brooks DJ. Demonstration of thalamic activation during typical absence seizures using H2(15)O and PET. *Neurology* 1995;**45**:1396–402.

Prince DA, Farrell D. 'Centrencephalic' spike and wave discharges following parenteral penicillin injection in the cat. *Neurology* 1969;**19**:309–10.

Pruvot P, Bancaud J, Delandsheer JM, Bordas-Ferrer M, Talairach J. Generalized epileptic crises and focal cortical lesion. (A propos of a post-traumatic frontal epilepsy). *Rev Electroencephalogr Neurophysiol Clin* 1972;**2**(2):165–70.

Salek-Haddadi A, Lemieux L, Merschhemke M, et al. Functional magnetic resonance imaging of human absence seizures. *Ann Neurol* 2003;**53**:663–7.

Shouse MN, Ryan W. Thalamic kindling: electrical stimulation of the lateral geniculate nucleus produces photosensitive grand mal seizures. *Exp Neurol* 1984;**86**:18–32.

Tolmacheva EA, van Luijtelaar G, Chepurnov SA, Kaminskij Y, Mares P. Cortical and limbic excitability in rats with absence epilepsy. *Epilepsy Res* 2004;**62**:189–98.

van Luijtelaar G, Sitnikova E. Global and focal aspects of absence epilepsy: the contribution of genetic models. *Neurosci Biobehav Rev* 2006;**30**:983–1003.

Williams D. A study of thalamic and cortical rhythms in petit mal. *Brain* 1953;**76**:50–69.

Wyler AR, Ward AA Jr. Neuronal firing patterns from epileptogenic foci of monkey and human. *Adv Neurol* 1986;**44**:967–89.

Learning objectives

(1) To understand the principles behind in vivo animal models of epilepsy and the mechanisms by which epilepsy arises in each model.
(2) To be aware of the EEG features seen in focal seizures in man when recorded with intracranial electrodes and their significance.
(3) To be aware of the relation between focal seizures and focal interictal epileptiform discharges in man and its significance.
(4) To understand the different theories to explain generalized seizures in man and how they were generated.

Section 1 **Basic principles**

Chapter 13

Neuropathology of epilepsy

Istvan Bodi and Mrinalini Honavar

Introduction

Epilepsy is not a single disease. It may be the consequence of a very wide range of conditions that affect the brain and hence the neuropathology of the condition is extremely varied. Chronic seizures may themselves induce damage in the brain, as may therapeutic endeavours, medical and surgical. Abnormalities detected in the brain in individuals with epilepsy are not always responsible for the disorder, and thus may be divided into those causing the seizures and those resulting from the epilepsy. In a good proportion of cases no morphological changes may be observed.

Changes secondary to epilepsy

Regardless of aetiology of epilepsy, secondary neuropathological changes may occur, such as:
- acute neuronal damage due to status epilepticus
- chronic seizures result in neuronal loss and chronic gliosis
- traumatic brain injury due to falls
- possibility of iatrogenic damage related to surgery or drugs.

Status epilepticus

Status epilepticus is defined as continuous seizure activity for 5 minutes, or two or more seizures with incomplete recovery of consciousness (60 minutes for adults and 30 minutes for children). The prognosis is poor, with high morbidity and mortality even with treatment. It may occur in both previously seizure-free and known epileptic patients. In the latter group the most common cause is non-compliance with anti-epileptic treatment.

Post-mortem examination in patients dying in status epilepticus reveals extensive but selective neuronal damage mainly affecting:
- pyramidal neurons in the hippocampus
- purkinje cells in the cerebellar cortex
- pyramidal neurons in laminae II and III in the neocortex.

Acute nerve cell loss or alterations similar to ischaemic ('red') neurons are noted, sometimes with an acute astrocytic reaction, and are similar to those of diffuse hypoxic injury. The mechanism of acute neuronal cell damage is linked to excitotoxicity. Continuous activation of excitatory NMDA (glutamate) receptors during seizures leads to sodium and particularly calcium entry into neurons, which in turn activates cytotoxic enzymes. The most vulnerable areas probably contain the most NMDA receptors. In prolonged survival, extensive neuronal loss and gliosis are detected in the affected areas. A frequent finding is laminar necrosis in the neocortex, particularly in the watershed areas.

In patients without a history of epilepsy, status epilepticus may be associated with:
- cerebrovascular disease
- drug overdose
- tumour
- trauma
- cardiac arrest
- alcohol withdrawal
- hyperpyrexia.

Chronic epileptic brain damage

The neuropathological changes most frequently found in the brains of chronic epileptics consist of neuronal loss and subsequent astrocytic gliosis in a

---

Introduction to Epilepsy ed. Gonzalo Alarcón and Antonio Valentín. Published by Cambridge University Press.
© Cambridge University Press 2012.

distribution that is similar to that seen in status epilepticus, although they may not be as severe. It raises the question as to whether the neuronal loss results from an early severe seizure or the cumulative effect of repeated minor damage, or both.

Mesial temporal sclerosis (MTS)

The presence of atrophy and sclerosis of the medial temporal lobe, particularly the hippocampus, has been noted in the brains of epileptic subjects from early in the nineteenth century. Over the next 150 years, the discussion has been centred on whether the changes seen are the effect of chronic epilepsy or the cause. The causative association of MTS with temporal lobe epilepsy received strong support from the demonstration of the lesion in a large proportion of specimens from patients undergoing surgery for this type of epilepsy, and their subsequent clinical improvement.

Also referred to as medial temporal sclerosis, Ammon's horn sclerosis or hippocampal sclerosis, MTS is present in 20–80% of autopsies on individuals with epilepsy and is predominantly unilateral (up to 40% bilateral) (Figure 13.1). MTS is found in up to 75% of temporal lobectomy specimens.

The possible aetiology of MTS includes prolonged and repeated febrile convulsions in childhood, birth trauma and childhood CNS infections. Early insult is thought to induce changes in areas of the brain vulnerable to damage, which over time may become spontaneous epileptic foci.

In classic hippocampal sclerosis, the most severe neuronal loss is seen in the CA1 segment (also called Sommer sector), then the CA3–4 segment, while the CA2 segment is relatively preserved (Figure 13.2). The dentate fascia may also show neuronal loss and/or dispersion. The neuronal cell loss is accompanied by astrocytic gliosis. Similar changes are usually detected in the amygdala and the surrounding medial temporal neocortical areas, accounting for the term mesial or medial.

There have been attempts to grade mesial temporal damage based on the distribution and severity of neuronal loss and gliosis, although whether the grades have a clinical correlation remains to be verified.

Dual pathology may exist, in which MTS may be associated with other pathology such as a cortical malformation or tumour in the temporal lobe or elsewhere in the brain

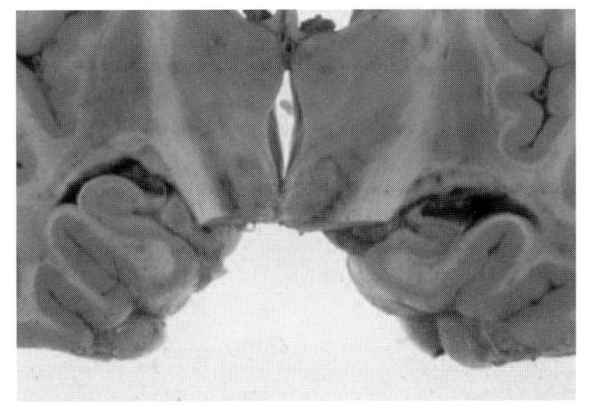

Figure 13.1. Unilateral (right) hippocampal atrophy.

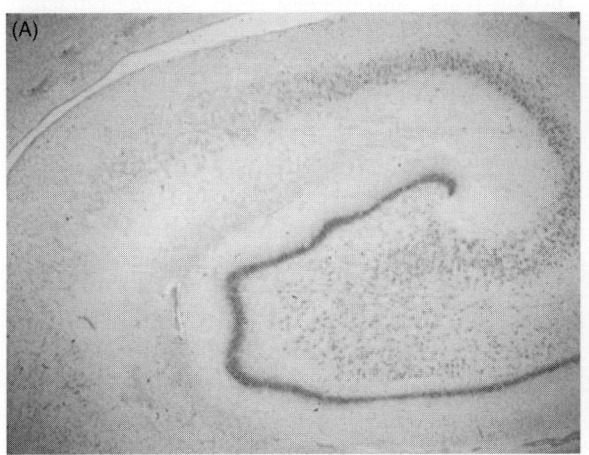

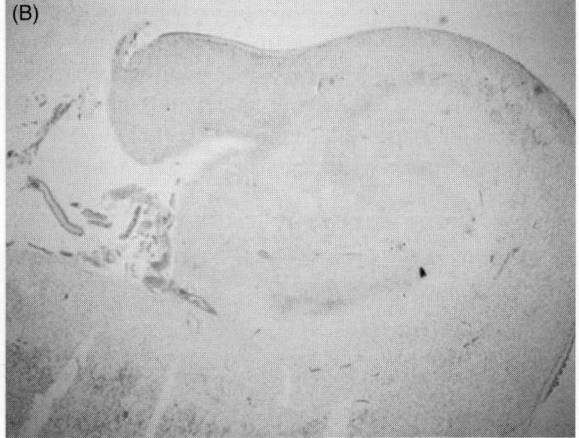

Figure 13.2. Normal hippocampus (A) and severe hippocampal sclerosis (B). See colour version in plate section.

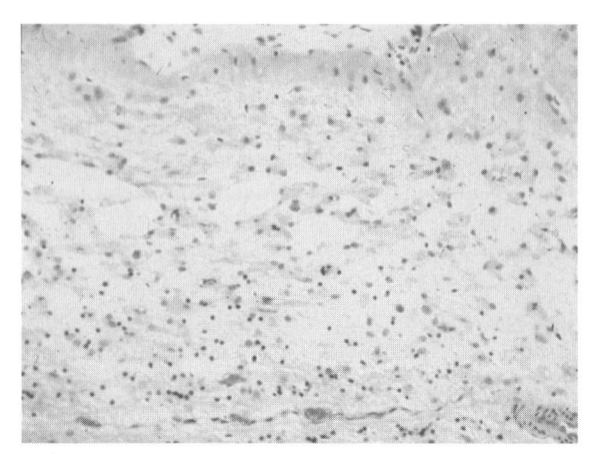

Figure 13.3. Severe laminar necrosis. The tissue is vacuolated due to loss of neurons. See colour version in plate section.

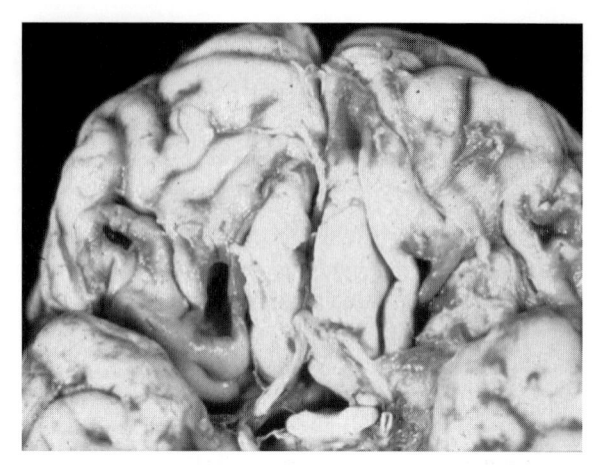

Figure 13.4. Old contusions in the frontobasal brain. The lesions are cavitated and show brownish decolourization.

Regardless of primary cause of MTS, the secondary changes (gliosis) may lead to development of additional seizure activity within the hippocampus, making the epilepsy more severe. In such cases surgical treatment, temporal lobectomy, may be beneficial in controlling further seizures.

Cerebellar atrophy

Loss of Purkinje cells with associated Bergmann's gliosis in the molecular layer is a common finding in epilepsy as the Purkinje cells are sensitive to excitotoxic injury.

Diffuse neocortical atrophy

Selective neuronal loss and astrocytic gliosis in laminar distribution may be seen in the neocortex (laminar necrosis) (Figure 13.3). The lamina III appears to be the most vulnerable, followed by lamina II, while the laminae V and VI are often preserved. Neuronal loss in the basal ganglia, particularly in the thalamus, is also described. Another frequent but nonspecific finding is the presence of subpial (Chaslin's) gliosis in the cortex. These changes are patchy and variable in intensity.

Traumatic injuries due to epileptic falls

Among various traumatic injuries, head injury is a common complication and may even be fatal. Contusions have been reported in 11–36% of autopsies in chronic epileptics, typically located in the basal frontal and temporal lobes or temporal and frontal poles (Figure 13.4). Multiple contusions of different chronology may be found.

Possible iatrogenic damage

Phenytoin was suspected to cause cerebellar atrophy, although it is more likely that the atrophy related to chronic epileptic neuronal damage. Epileptic drugs are known to be teratogenic in pregnancy.

Sudden unexpected death in epileptics (SUDEP)

Epileptic patients have increased risk of premature death, due to accidents, traumatic injuries, drowning and aspiration during seizures. The incidence of SUDEP in patients with chronic epilepsy is 1–2/1000 person-years, and highest with severe, refractory seizures, 3–9/1000. This includes witnessed or non-witnessed, non-traumatic and non-drowning death, with or without evidence of seizures at the time of death. However, evidence of status epilepticus and toxicological or anatomical causes, including non-neurological causes of death, must be excluded by post-mortem examination, which in the UK must be carried out under the auspices of the Coroner.

Neuropathological findings at autopsy have been sparse and nonspecific, suggestive of hypoxia. It has been postulated that death results from cardiac arrhythmia or respiratory failure during or immediately after seizure, or some form of autonomic dysfunction. Most patients die during sleep. The risk of SUDEP is higher in young patients, males, and those

Chapter 13: Neuropathology of epilepsy

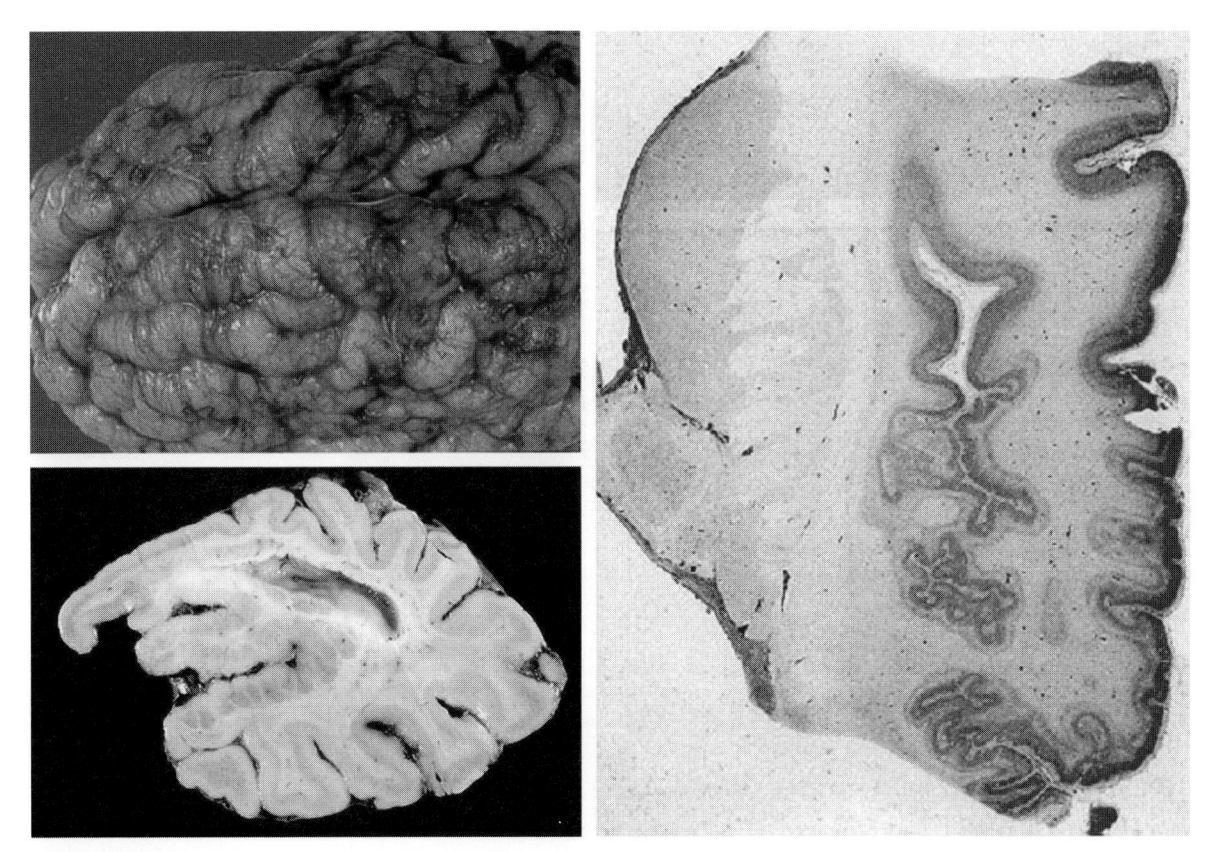

Figure 13.5. Polymicrogyria. The surface shows cobblestone appearances due to abnormal gyri. Cross sections reveal fused gyri in the affected area (unlayered polymicrogyria).

with symptomatic epilepsy, head injury and poor compliance with medication.

Symptomatic epilepsy

Although in a large proportion of patients the cause of epilepsy remains unknown, a number of neuropathological lesions are associated with epilepsy. Early-onset epilepsy is most commonly linked to cerebral malformations or intrauterine damage or associated with birth trauma. Recurrent childhood febrile illness may lead to epilepsy in a small proportion of cases. Any glial scar secondary to a variety of causes may result in epilepsy. Epileptogenic lesions:

- cerebral malformations
- perinatal vascular or hypoxic brain injury
- emerging from childhood febrile illness
- inflammatory lesions and sequelae
- post-traumatic scars
- vascular lesions
- neoplasms

Cerebral malformations

Numerous developmental disorders are associated with chronic seizures. They may be seen in various disturbances of cerebral growth or agenesis of certain structures or characterized by disordered architecture and aberrant neuronal arrangement. Some conditions are related to neuronal migrational defects and may be focal. The spectrum of changes is determined by the timing of disruption of neuronal migration. Early migrational disruption results in focal cortical dysplasia, damage in the intermediate period (10–24 weeks of gestation) leads to polymicrogyria or neuronal heterotopia, while late events may cause only microdysgenesis or mild malformation of cortical development. Most of these malformations may be associated with learning difficulties and motor dysfunction.

- Microcephaly
- Macrocephaly
- Megalencephaly, hemimegalencephaly
- Corpus callosum agenesia (partial or complete)
- Tuberous sclerosis

Section 1: Basic principles

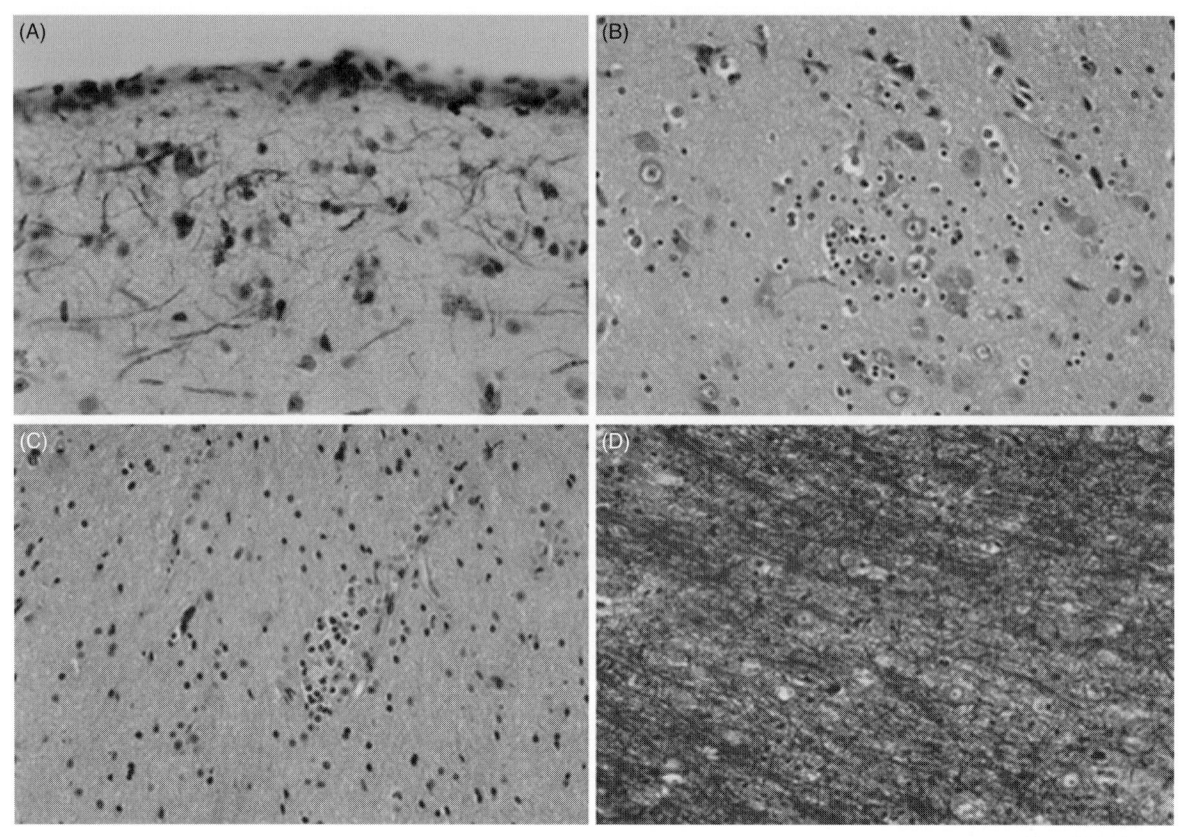

Figure 13.6. MCD. (A) Ectopic neurons and myelinated subpial axons. (B, C) Clusters of immature neurons in the cortex and white matter. (D) Heterotopic neurons in white matter. See colour version in plate section.

- Lissencephaly, pachygyria
- Polymicrogyria (Figure 13.5)
- Schizencephaly
- Laminar or nodular heterotopia
- Cortical dysplasia

Cortical dysplasia

Cortical dysplasia describes malformative lesions predominantly affecting cerebral neocortex, resulting in disorganized brain architecture. The normal cortical lamination is disturbed and neurons are abnormally located. The adjacent white matter is frequently involved. Cortical dysplasia forms a spectrum from minor microscopical abnormalities to focal lesions often detectable by MRI or macroscopic examination. The cortical dysplasias have been recently re-classified and divided into mild malformation of cortical development (mild MCD) and focal cortical dysplasia (FCD) (Palmini *et al.*, 2004).

Mild malformation of cortical development (MCD)
- Type I: ectopic neurons in layer I.
- Type II: microscopic neuronal heterotopia outside layer I (cluster of misplaced neurons).

Mild MCD is characterized by minor microscopical abnormalities and is divided into type I if only ectopic neurons are detected in layer I, and type II in cases of microscopic neuronal heterotopia in other layers of the neocortex. The latter include indistinct cortical lamination, small grey-matter heterotopia, increased neuronal satelitosis, rows of perivascular glia, dispersed granular cell layer in dentate fascia, microdysgenetic nodules or glioneuronal hamartia (Figure 13.6). It is debated whether all these changes are truly of developmental origin or secondary to seizures. Some mild MCD changes are also found in normal brain, raising the question of their relationship to the pathogenesis of epilepsy.

Chapter 13: Neuropathology of epilepsy

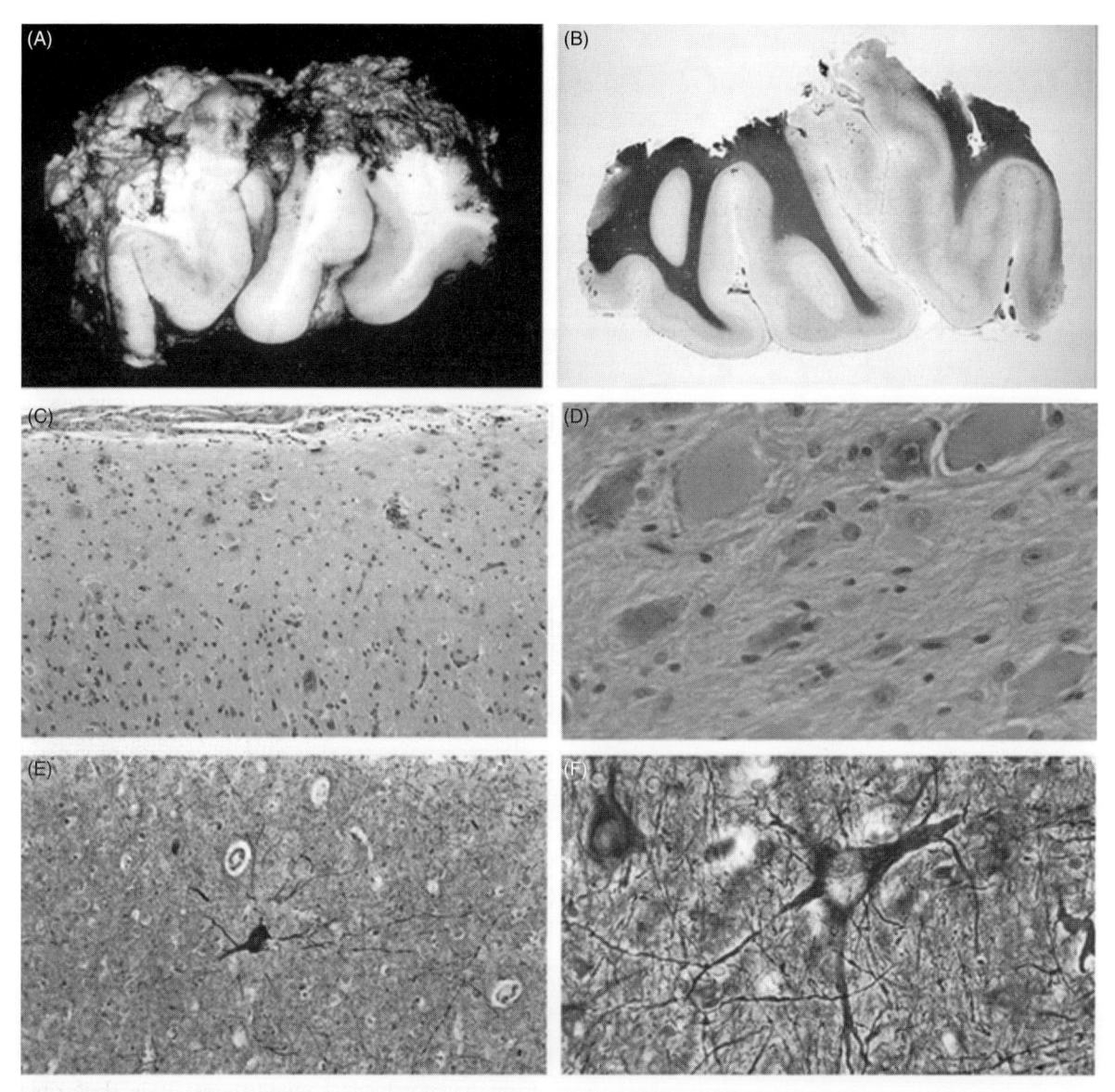

Figure 13.7. FCD type IIB. (A, B) Blurred grey–white matter border in temporal lobectomy specimen (B: LFB/Nissl). (C, D) Abnormal lamination with dysmorphic neurons and balloon cells. Neurofilament (E) and silver stain (F) highlights abnormally oriented neurites in the dysmorphic neurons. See colour version in plate section.

Focal cortical dysplasia (FCD)

- Type IA: dyslamination only
- Type IB: dyslamination + giant or immature neurons
- Type IIA: dyslamination + dysmorphic neurons with no balloon cells
- Type IIB: dyslamination + dysmorphic neurons and balloon cells

This is a morphologically distinct form seen mainly in patients with medically intractable partial epilepsy. The lesion might be visualized by MRI, making localization and surgical excision possible. Macroscopically widened gyri and blurred grey–white matter boundary are seen. Histologically, abnormal cortical lamination and organization are evident. Giant and bizarre, dysmorphic neurons with prominent dendritic arborization and abnormal orientation are demonstrated by silver impregnation or neurofilament immunostain (Figure 13.7). Heterotopic neurons may be seen in the underlying white matter,

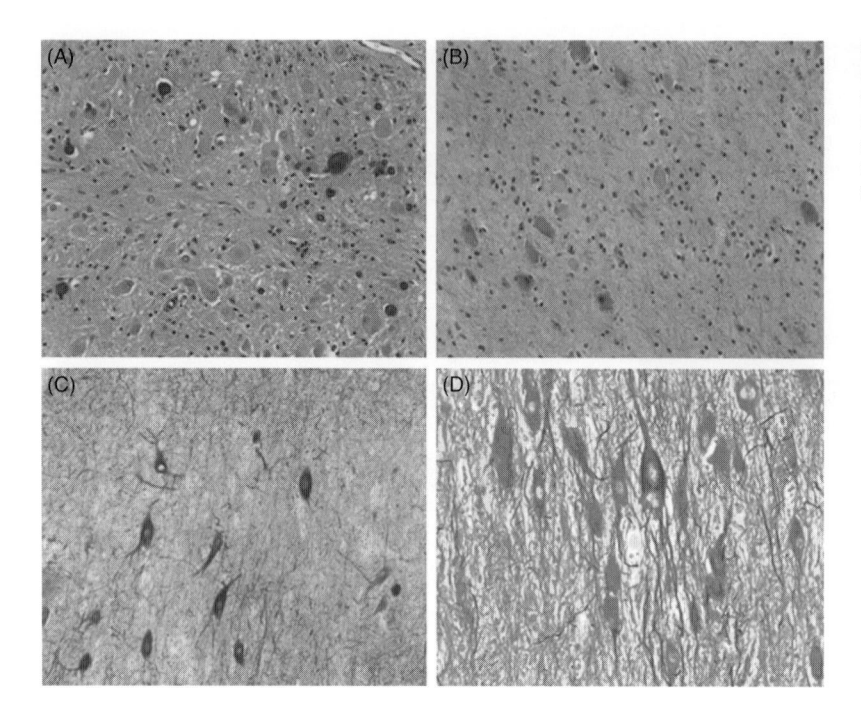

Figure 13.8. Cortical tuber. (A, B) Giant dysmorphic neurons and balloon cells similar to FCD type IIB. Calcification is also noted (A). Neurofilament (C) and silver stain (D) highlights abnormally oriented neurites in the giant neurons. See colour version in plate section.

sometimes also showing gliosis and atrophy. Large balloon cells with glassy cytoplasm and pleomorphic nuclei are detected in type IIB, which may show immunoreactivity with both astrocytic and neuronal markers. Most cases of FCD type IIB also show scattered nestin and CD34-positive cells, particularly in the deep cortex and subcortical white matter. FCD associated with other pathology is classified FCD type III: e.g., with hippocampal sclerosis IIIa, epilepsy-associated tumor IIIb, vascular malformations IIIc, epileptogenic lesions acquired in early life IIId. Good seizure control may be achieved by complete surgical excision, if possible.

Tuberous sclerosis

The tuberous sclerosis complex is an autosomal dominant disorder caused by a mutation on either the *TSC1* or *TSC2* genes on 9q and 16p, respectively, characterized by hamartomas and benign tumours in the CNS, eyes, skin, heart and kidneys. The CNS lesions present with epilepsy and often mental retardation from childhood:

- Cortical tuber: firm nodules projecting from the surface (Figure 13.8), a hamartoma composed of giant bizarre neurons and astrocytes dispersed in disorganized and very gliotic cortex.
- Subependymal nodule: a hamartoma protruding into the ventricles, composed of atypical large glial cells and often calcified.
- Subependymal giant cell astrocytoma: a low-grade glioma (WHO grade I) arising from the subependymal nodules.

Perinatal brain damage

Epilepsy is a frequent complication of birth asphyxia, perinatal brain damage and hydrocephalus. Premature babies are prone to develop intraventricular haemorrhage and periventricular leukomalacia. The risk of developing epilepsy is particularly increased from haemorrhagic complications. It is postulated that the iron liberated from haemoglobin and transferrin may be important to epileptogenesis via free radical formation.

Vascular malformations

Epilepsy is a common and sometimes the sole clinical manifestation of vascular malformations. Arteriovenous malformation (AVM) and cavernous angioma (cavernoma) are frequently associated with seizures (Figure 13.9). Mass effect, haemorrhage and ischemia causing gliosis and neuronal loss are implicated in the seizure production. Haemorrhage, leading to haemosiderin deposition and subsequent iron-induced free

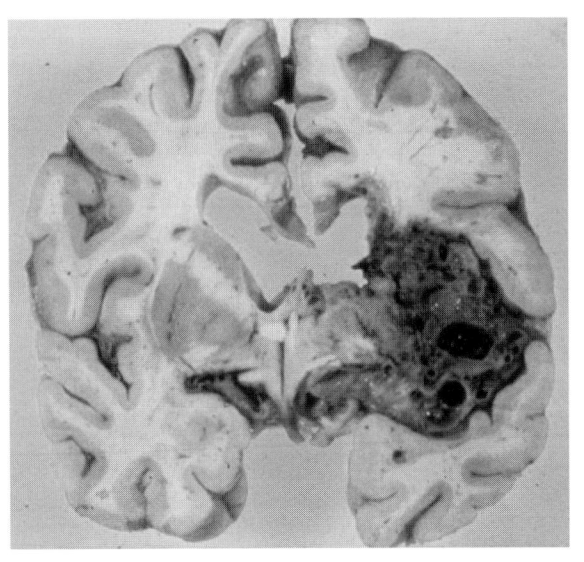

Figure 13.9. AVM showing tortuous and dilated vascular channels.

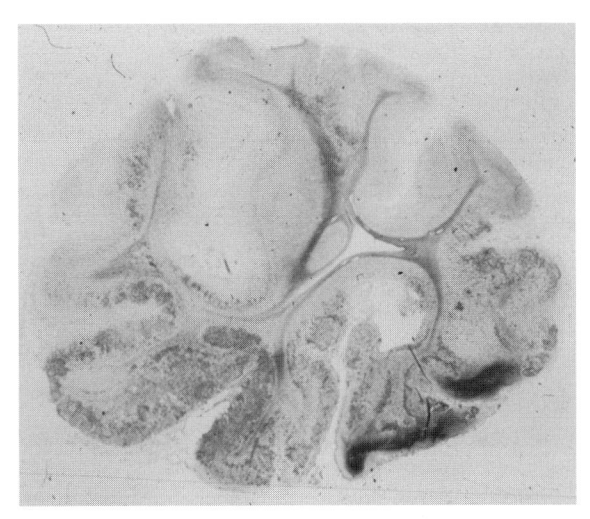

Figure 13.10. Sturge-Weber syndrome. Extensive calcified leptomeningeal deposits. See colour version in plate section.

radical generation, appears to be the most important. Although small venous and capillary teleangiectasia are more common than AVM and cavernoma, they are usually not associated with seizures.

Sturge-Weber syndrome is a rare congenital malformation characterized by unilateral facial angiomatous nevus and ipsilateral parieto-occipital teleangiectatic venous angioma of the leptomeninges (Figure 13.10), with seizures starting early in childhood. Calcified deposits within the lesion in the leptomeninges and the underlying parenchyma may be detected by skull X-ray.

Infections

Seizures may occur during or as a sequel to any inflammatory intracranial process in the acute stage and the resultant scarring. Seizure risk is significantly increased if glial scarring occurs in the chronic stage. Some patients may develop mesial temporal sclerosis, resulting in new seizure activity.

Seizure frequency appears to increase from bacterial meningitis and viral encephalitis to chronic cerebral abscess up to 25%. Epilepsy is a well-recognized complication of HIV-related disease, cerebral tuberculosis and parasitic infections, such as malaria, neurocysticercosis, toxoplasmosis, African trypanosomiasis and hydatid disease; all of which explain the high prevalence of epilepsy in the developing world.

Rasmussen's encephalitis

It is characterized by chronic intractable unilateral seizures with progressive neurological deficit. Seizures begin abruptly, usually in childhood, with onset of focal motor, complex partial and generalized seizures, followed by hemiplegia, hemianopsia and intellectual deterioration. The condition progresses to cerebral hemiatrophy, which might be partly localized or may involve the whole hemisphere. Histology reveals chronic perivascular lymphocytic inflammation, neuronophagia and microglial nodules within the active lesions in the affected hemisphere (Figure 13.11). These features are similar to those seen in viral encephalitis, but no viral particles have been identified. The aetiology is unknown, but an autoimmune process against the neurotransmitter receptor GluR3 is suspected. Early hemispherectomy may result in a better prognosis.

Febrile convulsions

Two to three per cent of children between 6 months and 6 years of age have generalized seizures associated with fever. About one-third of affected children will have subsequent febrile convulsions, and approximately 5% develop complex partial seizures, probably due to mesial temporal sclerosis. The risk of developing epilepsy is increased if the febrile convulsions are prolonged (>20 minutes), contain focal features, post-ictal hemiparesis develops, there is a family

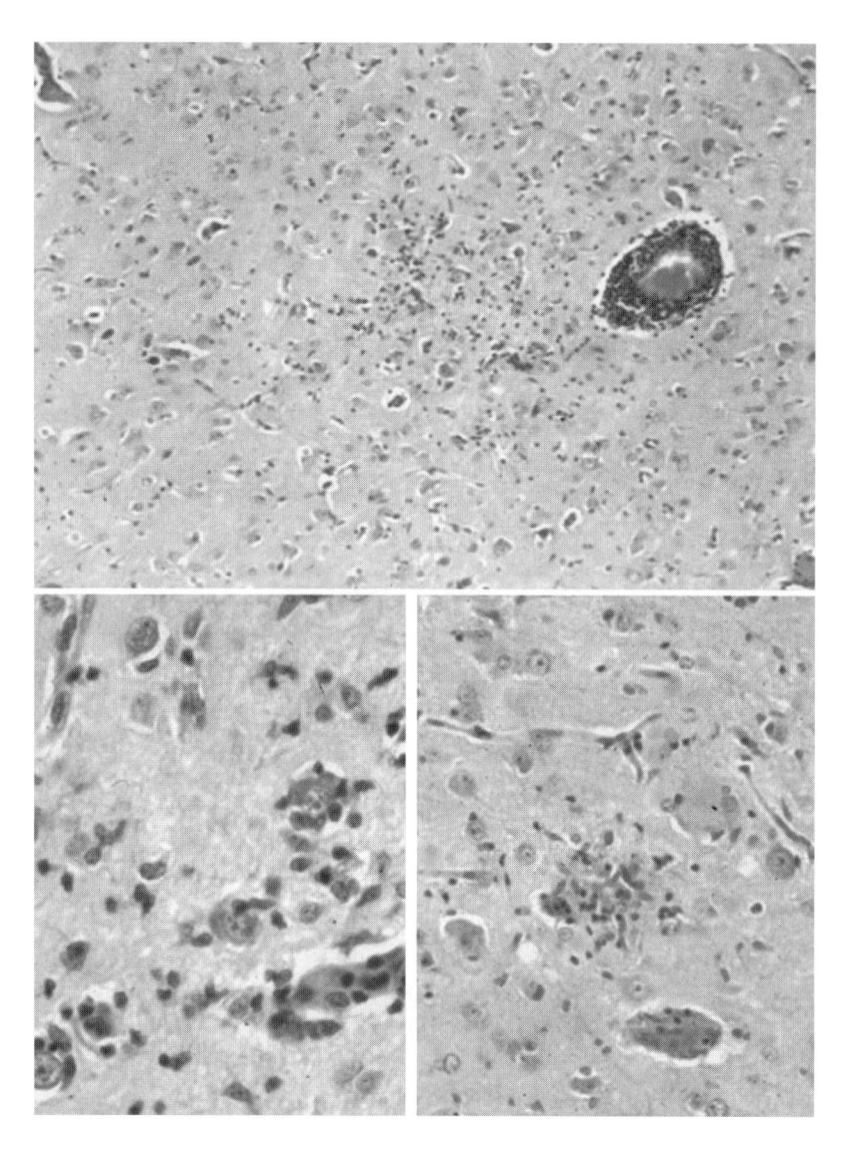

Figure 13.11. Rasmussen's encephalitis showing perivascular lymphocytic inflammation, neuronophagia and microglial nodules. See colour version in plate section.

history of epilepsy or prior abnormal neurological development. The increased risk may reflect common genetic and acquired underlying factors.

Trauma

Epilepsy may be the late consequence of head injury. Risk of developing post-traumatic epilepsy is related to the severity and type of trauma. Depressed skull fractures, dural penetration, loss of brain tissue, intracerebral haemorrhage and retained foreign material increase the risk. This is related to glial scarring. Haemorrhage, via free radicals from iron deposition, also appears to be a significant risk factor.

Tumours

Seizures are common (35%) and frequently the first symptom in intracranial tumours. The incidence of epilepsy appears to correlate conversely with the rate of tumour growth. Low-grade gliomas are twice as frequently associated with seizures as glioblastoma. Seizures are seen in decreasing frequency in oligodendroglioma (70%), low-grade astrocytoma (58%), meningioma (36%) and glioblastoma (28%). There is significant reduction of seizure activity after surgical removal.

A group of unusual, mixed glio-neuronal tumours deserve attention, as they present almost invariably

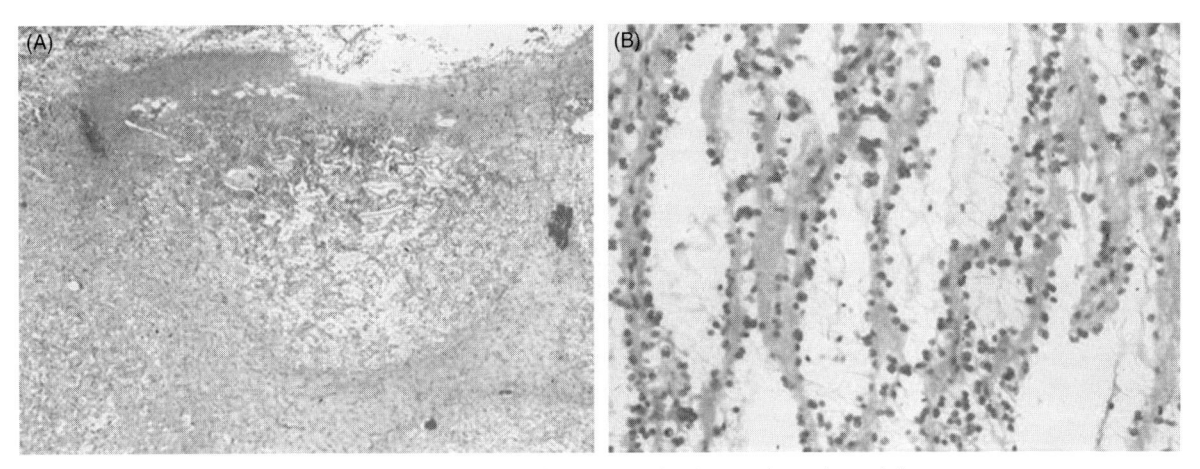

Figure 13.12. DNT. (A) Multinodular intracortical tumour nodules. (B) Specific glio-neural complex with floating neurons. See colour version in plate section.

with chronic seizures: ganglioglioma, dysembryoplastic neuroepithelial tumour (DNT) and the recently described angiocentric glioma.

Ganglioglioma

A low-grade (WHO grade I) tumour presenting most often in children and young adults, ganglioglioma is one of the most commonly seen tumours in surgical specimens from patients with epilepsy. It consists of neuronal and glial cells, the former showing nuclear abnormalities and the glial component resembling an astrocytoma. The tumour has a good prognosis. In the very rare anaplastic ganglioglioma (WHO grade III) the malignant features are usually in the astrocytic component.

Dysembryoplastic neuroepithelial tumour (DNT)

These patients have a history of long-standing intractable epilepsy which is usually present in childhood or early adulthood. MRI reveals a predominantly intracortical lesion, most frequently occurring in the temporal lobe. The lesions are intracortical or subcortical, more likely to be multinodular but solitary nodules are also seen. Histology shows oligodendroglial-like cells with perinuclear halo, astrocytes and neurons that appear to float in a myxoid matrix, together referred to as the specific glio-neuronal element, although proportions of the cells may vary (Figure 13.12). A diffuse form of DNT without nodularity is also described which may also show transition to classical DNT and/or ganglioglioma. DNT (WHO grade I) is usually recurrence-free and characterized by good seizure control after even incomplete surgical resection.

Myoclonic epilepsy

Myoclonus is defined by sudden, brief, shock-like involuntary movements caused by muscle contractions or muscle inhibitions arising from the CNS. It may affect single muscles or groups of muscles, and the jerks may be single or repetitive.

Myoclonic seizures may occur in childhood epilepsies, such as Lennox-Gastaut syndrome. However, they usually present in two broad types of progressive neurological diseases. Myoclonus may be noted in the late stage of progressive encephalopathy, or myoclonic epilepsy might be the presenting and major symptom, leading to progressive neurological deterioration later.

A. Progressive encephalopathy accompanied by myoclonic jerks

- Prion diseases
- Alzheimer's disease
- Dementia with Lewy bodies
- Inborn metabolic errors (e.g., gangliosidoses, Krabbe disease, Nieman-Pick diseases, neuronal ceroid lipofuschinosis)
- Subacute sclerosing panencephalitis

B. Myoclonus is a presenting symptom leading to progressive neurological deterioration

Lafora body disease (see also Chapter 30: 'Progressive myoclonic epilepsies')

This is an autosomal recessive condition due to EPM2A gene mutation coding laforin. Laforin is involved in glycogen metabolism, regulation of ion

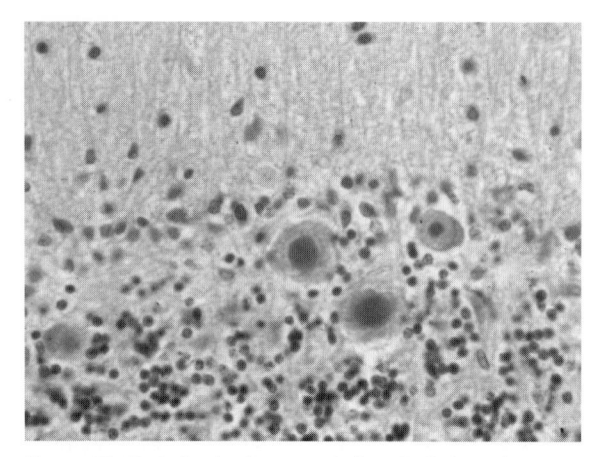

Figure 13.13. Lafora bodies in cerebellum (PAS). See colour version in plate section.

channels and synaptic transmission, but it is unknown how the laforin deficit leads to epilepsy. The disease presents in young adults with generalized seizures followed by myoclonus. The brain reveals mild diffuse atrophy. The histological hallmark is the presence of Lafora (polyglycosan) bodies in neurons and astrocytes in the CNS, and also in extracranial sites; e.g. sweat glands and liver (Figure 13.13). Diagnosis can be readily achieved by axillary skin biopsy.

Unverricht-Lundborg disease (Baltic myoclonus epilepsy)

It presents in childhood with myoclonus provoked by light, touch and other stimuli, followed by other neurological abnormalities late in the course. Phenytoin has an adverse effect and is associated with rapid progression of the disease. The most conspicuous finding is severe loss of Purkinje cells in the cerebellum, which might be related to the effect of phenytoin. This is an autosomal recessive condition due to mutation in cystatin B gene.

Mitochondrial myopathy with ragged red fibres (MERRF)

The symptoms begin in the second decade with myoclonus and ataxia. Other features include hearing loss, peripheral neuropathy and optic atrophy. Although the muscle weakness is mild or absent, muscle biopsy reveals ragged red fibres due to mitochondrial accumulation. Point mutation of mitochondrial DNA is found in most cases.

Ramsay Hunt syndrome

The combination of progressive cerebellar atrophy and myoclonus is referred to as Ramsay Hunt syndrome. Most cases of this clinical syndrome are examples of mitochondrial encephalopathy and Unverricht-Lundborg disease.

Neurosurgery and neurosurgical pathology of epilepsy

Neurosurgery may be an effective treatment in chronic drug-resistant epilepsies. Two categories of procedures are carried out, functional and resective surgery.

Functional surgery is performed for control of seizures rather than cure. The success of surgery depends more on the extent rather than on the pathology of the underlying lesion.

- Corpus callosum resection is performed to prevent propagation of seizures to the contralateral hemisphere. Generalized seizures with falls abate but the partial seizures persist.
- Subpial resections are done to control partial seizures in unresectable areas (motor, sensory or speech areas). Interruption of horizontal intracortical superficial fibres of the molecular layer may limit the spread of epileptic activity without causing major cortical damage.
- Temporal lobotomy is transection of the white matter connection of temporal lobe for the treatment of complex partial seizures.
- Stereotactic lesions can be made to ablate deep epileptic foci or control seizures if they are multiple.

Resective surgery is aimed to remove the epileptic focus and may also disconnect the rest of the brain from seizure focus if resection is incomplete. The epileptic focus is to be localized by EEG and sometimes by MRI before surgery.

- Temporal lobectomy is carried out for drug-resistant temporal lobe epilepsy. Mesial temporal sclerosis is the most commonly found lesion, in which marked seizure reduction or complete seizure control can be achieved. Double pathology may be present with mesial temporal sclerosis. Other frequent lesions include malformations, cortical dysplasias, vascular malformations, glial scars and neoplasms, such as ganglioglioma, DNT and low-grade gliomas.

Chapter 13: Neuropathology of epilepsy

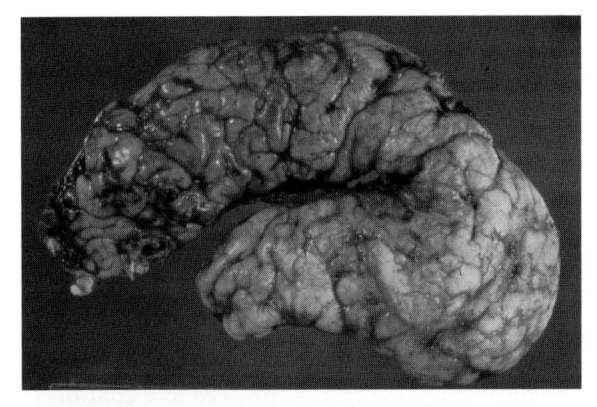

Figure 13.14. Hemispherectomy specimen with polymicrogyria affecting the posterior lobes.

- Cortical resection is performed for focal cortical abnormalities, most frequently for focal cortical dysplasia, located in the non-functionally eloquent areas.
- Hemispherectomy is surgical removal of cortex and underlying white matter, while the basal ganglia are usually spared (total hemispherectomy). Functional hemispherectomy means that portions of cerebral tissue are removed, functionally disconnecting the remainder. Hemispherectomy is performed for intractable chronic unilateral seizures (usually with hemiplegia) or multiple epileptogenic foci in one hemisphere. The most frequently found abnormalities are perinatal anoxic-ischaemic damage, hemimegalencephaly, Rasmussen's encephalitis and Sturge-Weber syndrome (Figure 13.14).

Genetics of epilepsy

There have been great advances in the understanding of genetic background in epileptic conditions. Idiopathic generalized forms of epilepsy have a genetic basis, such as demonstrable Mendelian inheritance, chromosomal deletions or are assumed to be polygenic. Mutations have been identified in genes for ion receptors, neurotransmitter receptors, neuromodulators and protein kinases, predisposing to neuronal hyperexcitability.

A number of mutations are associated with cerebral malformations and migrational disorders leading to epilepsy; e.g. Angelman syndrome, Aicardi's syndrome, tuberous sclerosis, lissencephaly types I and II. Mutations in certain diseases with myoclonic epilepsy, such as Lafora body disease and Unverricht-Lundborg disease, have been recently identified. Genetic abnormalities in mitochondrial disorders presenting with seizures are divided into two groups. Mutations in regulating proteins of mitochondrial function coded in nuclear DNA follow Mendelian inheritance. Mitochondrial genome deletions and duplications may be sporadic (e.g. Kearns-Sayres syndrome) and point mutations of mitochondrial DNA follow maternal inheritance (MELAS, MERRF and MILS).

Recommended reading

Blumcke *et al.* The clinicopathologic spectrum of focal cortical dysplasias: a consensus classification proposed by an ad hoc Task Force of the ILAE Diagnostic Methods Commission. *Epilepsia* 2011;52:158–174.

Bodi *et al.* Diffuse form of dysembryoplastic neuroepithelial tumour: the histological and immunohistochemical features of a distinct entity showing transition to dysembryoplastic neuroepithelial tumour and ganglioglioma. *Neuropathol Appl Neurobiol* 2011. doi: 10.1111/j.1365-2990.2011.01225.x

Honavar M, Meldrum BS. Epilepsy. In *Greenfield's Neuropathology*, pp. 931–71. 6th edn. London: Arnold; 1997.

Scaravilli F. *Neuropathology of Epilepsy*. Singapore: World Scientific; 1998.

Thom M. Recent advances in the neuropathology of focal lesions in epilepsy. *Expert Rev Neurother* 2004;4(6):973–84.

Learning objective

(1) To know the histopathological features of lesions causing seizures in different epilepsy syndromes and, if possible, their significance to the pathophysiology of epilepsy.

Section 1 Basic principles

Chapter 14

Introduction to the electroencephalogram (EEG)

Gonzalo Alarcón

The electroencephalogram (EEG)

- The EEG is a record of variations in electrical activity recorded from different regions on the head.
- The EEG represents the compound electrical field generated by neuronal function, mainly originating from postsynaptic potentials in the cerebral cortex.
- The most commonly used EEG recordings in humans are obtained with electrodes on the scalp (the scalp EEG). More rarely, intracranial electrodes can be used for presurgical assessment of epilepsy (see Chapter 81: 'Preoperative assessment').
- Because electrical fields quickly attenuate with distance, electrical activity from deep brain structures (basal ganglia, hippocampus, amygdala) is hardly detectable on the scalp.
- The scalp EEG is most sensitive to radial electrical currents (perpendicular to the scalp surface) and very insensitive to tangential currents (parallel to the surface of the scalp).
- It is commonly assumed that the scalp EEG records mainly activity from the cortical gyri for two reasons:
  - the cortex in gyri is closer to the scalp than cortex in sulci;
  - assuming that most of the currents generated during cortical function are perpendicular to the cortical surface, currents in the gyri would be radial whereas those of the sulci would be tangential.

How is an EEG recorded?

- EEGs are most commonly recorded with silver electrodes on the scalp.

- The EEG is displayed as simultaneous graphs of electrical activity versus time (see Figures 14.1 and 14.2).
- Nowadays, most EEG recordings are digital, which allows reformatting, unlike previous paper recordings.
- Each graph (channel) represents changes over time in electrical activity in a region(s).
- The standard EEGs used to study epilepsy show 10 s of recording at a time (10 s per page or screen).
- Electrical activity is measured as the voltage difference between two electrodes, showing negative polarity upwards (the opposite to the standard convention in physics and mathematics).
- A typical EEG will record the electrical activity generated by the patient's brain for around 30 min if it is not intended to include a sleep period (the so-called awake or routine EEG), or for 60–90 min

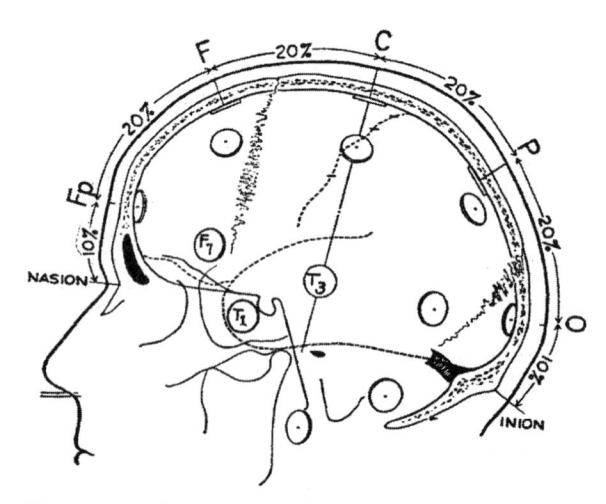

Figure 14.1. The 10–20 electrode positioning system for scalp electrodes.

Introduction to Epilepsy ed. Gonzalo Alarcón and Antonio Valentín. Published by Cambridge University Press.
© Cambridge University Press 2012.

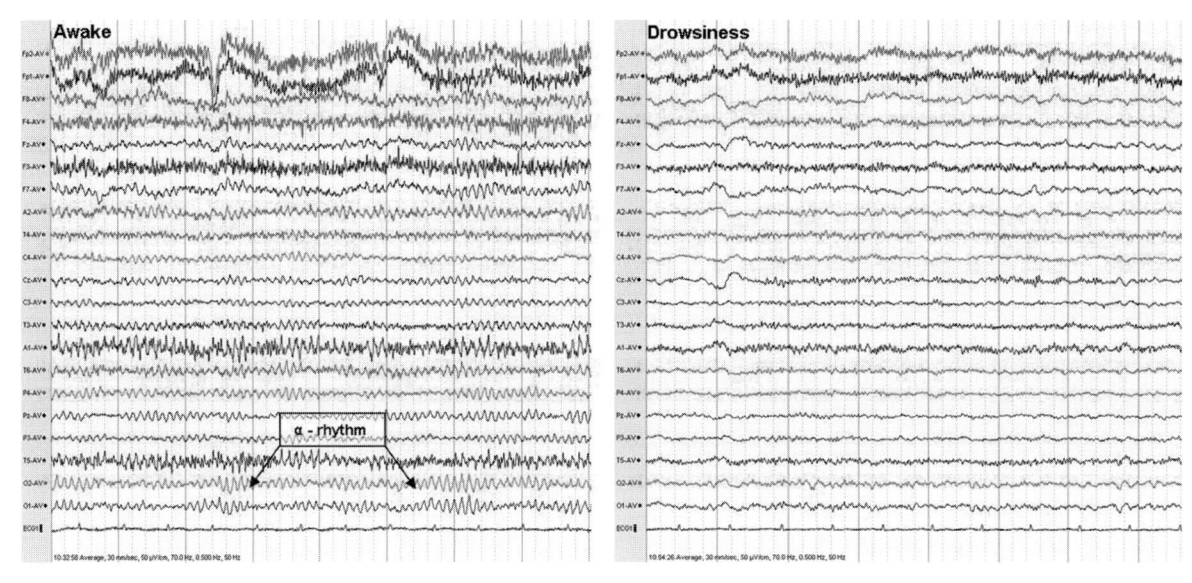

Figure 14.2. Several EEG normal activities.

or more if it is intended to include a period of sleep (a sleep EEG). The latter can be obtained after sleep deprivation or with drug-induced sleep, using an agent that does not significantly affect the EEG (for instance, quinalbarbitone).

- Most EEGs include a period of overbreathing (hyperventilation) and some stimulation with flashing lights (photic stimulation).
- Hyperventilation is achieved by asking the patient to breathe as quickly and deeply as possible for 3 min. A toy windmill can be helpful to encourage children to hyperventilate. Hyperventilation should be avoided in patients above 50 because it is associated with cerebral vasoconstriction and a small increase in the risk of stroke.
- Photic stimulation is carried out by asking patients to look into a light that repeatedly flashes, located around 30 cm away from the face.
- The frequency of the flashing light is measured in Hz (number of flashes delivered during 1 s). For each frequency tested, the patient is exposed to the flashing light for around 10 s. Several frequencies between 2 and 60 Hz are used on each patient.
- There are reservations about performing photic stimulation on adult patients holding a driving licence, since there is a small risk of inducing a seizure in susceptible individuals, and consequently having the driving licence withdrawn. There is no need to carry out photic stimulation when epilepsy is not under consideration (e.g. hepatic encephalopathy) or is very unlikely (e.g. atypical psychosis). Some individuals find photic stimulation uncomfortable even if no photoparoxysmal discharges are recorded.

Recording and reviewing principles

The electric field (voltage difference) can only be recorded between two sites. Like distance, the electric field cannot be measured at a point, only between two points. This means that each EEG channel necessarily represents voltage difference between two sites. Each site can be in the head, on the scalp, outside the head or it may even be a calculated voltage (e.g. the average of all the electrodes). In clinical practice, to record the scalp EEG, a number of electrodes are applied covering most of the scalp according to standard systems to position EEG electrodes. One of the most popular is the 10–20 System (Jasper, 1958) (Figure 14.1). Although almost universally accepted, this system does not provide appropriate cover of inferior and anterior temporal regions, and consequently might not be entirely satisfactory for the study of temporal lobe epilepsy and during pre-surgical assessment. Additional electrodes have been used to overcome this difficulty (e.g. the anterior temporal Silverman electrode, the percutaneous sphenoidal electrode). The Maudsley System (Margerison et al., 1970, based on modifications of the system by Pampiglione, 1956) superficially resembles the 10–20 and uses the same number of electrodes, allowing for the use of similar conventions and headboxes. Nevertheless, some electrodes are applied over lower regions, providing more adequate cover of the temporal lobe. For instance, the anterior temporal electrodes of the Maudsley System are as effective as sphenoidal electrodes to detect temporal epileptiform discharges and seizures (Fernández Torre et al., 1999; Kissani et al., 2001).

The table that allocates pairs of measuring sites to each EEG channel is called montage. There are two basic designs for designing a montage:

- bipolar or differential montage: each channel measures the voltage difference between two nearby electrodes;
- common reference montage: one of the measuring voltages for each channel is common to all channels. This common electrode or voltage is called reference. In common reference montage, each channel measures voltage difference between a specific electrode and the reference. Consequently, channels are sometimes labelled with the name of the electrode that is specific to the channel.

Modern digital recording systems allow changing filter settings and montages after recording (during reviewing). Sometimes this can be invaluable because, for the characterization of some phenomena, it may be necessary to change filters or to review it on different montages (see Box 14.1)

> **Box 14.1. References and montages**
>
> A lot of electroencephalographers' time and effort has been devoted to the search for a generic reference with zero voltage (an 'indifferent reference'). This is a chimerical enterprise. Because voltage difference can only be recorded between two points, the reference could only have zero voltage when compared to a second point having the same voltage, which will not generally be the case. Pragmatically, it is best to choose a reference located as far as possible from the process to be studied or a common average reference (the average of all recording electrodes), which will be largely inert to signals recorded in a localized region. Even better, always review your EEGs with a variety of montages including bipolar and common reference montages.

How to interpret an EEG

As cortical electrical activity changes with time, so does the EEG. EEG traces are always changing and these time variations appear as waves of different frequencies on the EEG record. EEG waves have traditionally been classified into frequency bands according to the Greek alphabet:

- δ (read as delta): waves of frequency below 4 Hz
- θ (read as theta): waves of frequency between 4 and 8 Hz
- α (read as alpha): waves of frequency between 8 and 14 Hz
- ς (read as sigma): waves of frequency largely restricted to 14 Hz
- β (read as beta): waves of frequency above 14 Hz, also called fast activity or fast rhythms
- γ (read as gamma): waves of very high frequency (20 Hz or above).

The ongoing electrical activity on the EEG is called the background activity. The α rhythm is an important part of the background activity in awake subjects. It is a sinusoidal rhythm that waxes and wanes, is blocked by eye opening, shows maximal amplitude over posterior regions of the head, and is fairly symmetrical, although often slightly larger on the nondominant hemisphere (usually the right). The frequency composition of the background activity changes with age, level of consciousness, and disease. Background activity that contains mainly activity in δ and θ ranges is called slow activity. Normal children and teenagers tend to show more slow activity than normal adults, particularly posteriorly. Slow activity increases during normal sleep, confusional states or coma, and in the presence of brain damage or structural abnormalities.

In addition to the ongoing background activity, the EEG can show brief waveforms that occur occasionally. These are called paroxysmal events, and are thought to result from sudden synchronization of neuronal activity. Some paroxysmal events are normal (e.g. vertex sharp waves and K-complexes often seen in sleep; see Chapter 15: 'Phenomenology of normal EEG: effects of age and state of awareness'). Other paroxysmal events are abnormal (e.g. epileptiform discharges, as described in Chapter 16: 'Pathological EEG phenomena and their significance', and in Chapter 18: 'Clinical use of EEG in epilepsy').

Chapter 14: Introduction to the electroencephalogram (EEG)

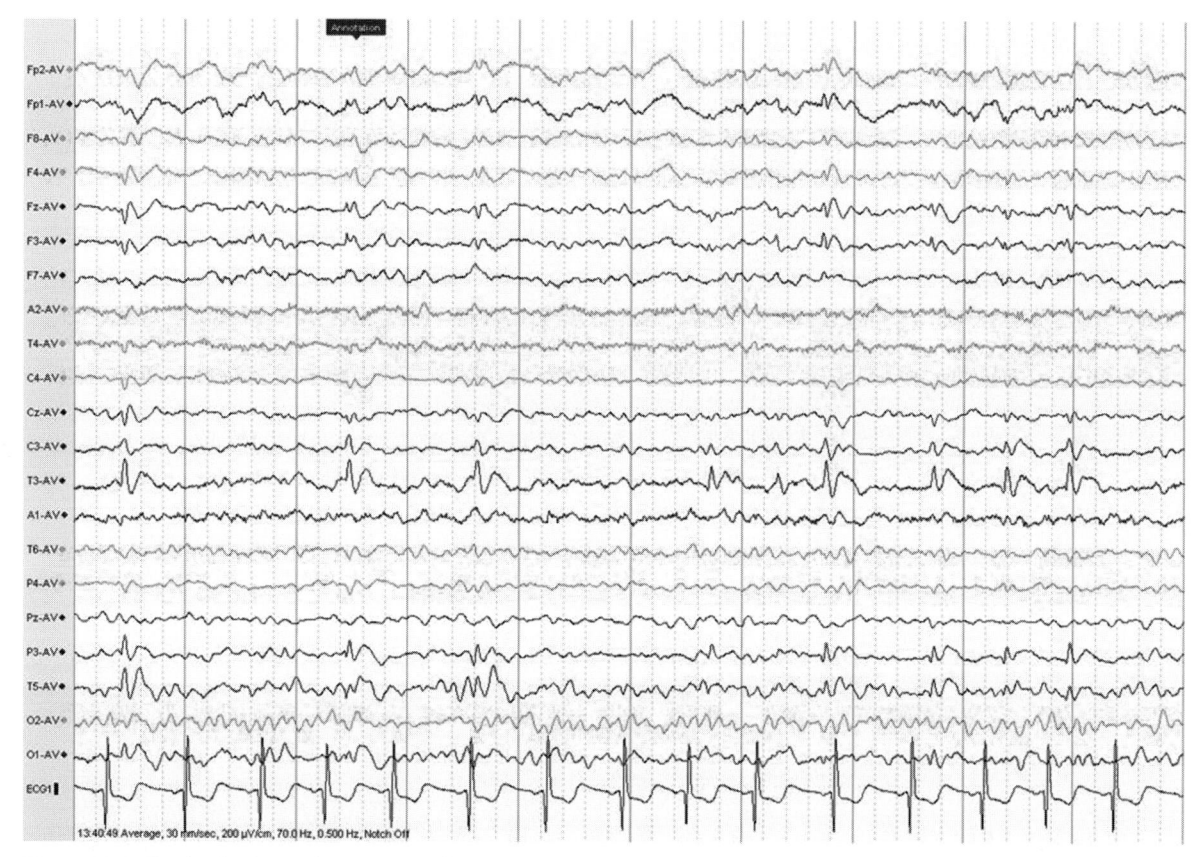

Figure 14.3. Dipolar distribution between T3 and Fz in common reference montage in a patient with benign childhood epilepsy with centro-temporal spikes.

Useful EEG terminology

- Background activity: activity occurring continuously or during most of the time under specific conditions.
- Paroxysmal activity: appearing suddenly and persisting for a short period (usually for shorter than a second or two).
- Focal: phenomena which are unilateral and restricted to a localized area of the scalp.
- Diffuse or generalized: phenomena which can be recorded all over the scalp.
- Multifocal abnormalities: focal abnormalities seen over different regions at different times. Multifocal abnormalities restricted to one side or seen mainly on one side are said to be lateralized.
- Regular or rhythmic: the terms regular or rhythmic are often used to describe waveforms of similar shape occurring repeatedly, usually for several seconds.
- EEG artefacts: in the context of epileptology, an artefact is an electrical signal that did not originate in the brain. EEG artefacts can have a variety of shapes and mechanisms. The most common artefacts are due to muscle activity (electromyogram), artefacts generated by movement of cables, eye movement, chewing and the electrocardiogram.
- Ictal: occurring during a seizure.
- interictal: occurring in the period between seizures.
- Isoelectric trace: a flat trace or channel (containing no changes in time or space).
- Complex: a set of waveforms with complex morphology (for instance spike-and-wave complexes, or K-complexes).
- Dipole (Figure 14.3): this term can be applied to a localized intracranial current or to the scalp electric field generated by such current.

References

Fernández Torre JL, Alarcón G, Binnie CD, Polkey CE. Comparison of sphenoidal, foramen ovale and anterior temporal placements for detecting interictal epileptiform discharges in presurgical assessment for temporal lobe surgery. *Clin Neurophysiol* 1999;**110**:895–904.

Jasper HH. Report of the committee on methods of clinical examination in electroencephalography. *Electroencephalogr Clin Neurophysiol* 1958; **10**:370–5.

Kissani N, Alarcón G, Dad M, Binnie CD, Polkey CE. Sensitivity of recordings at sphenoidal electrode site for detecting seizure onset: evidence from scalp, superficial and deep foramen ovale recordings. *Clinical Neurophysiol* 2001;**112**:232–40.

Margerison JH, Binnie CD, McCaul IR. Electroencephalographic signs employed in the location of ruptured intracranial arterial aneurysms. *Electroencephalogr Clin Neurophysiol* 1970;**28**:296–306.

Pampiglione G. Some anatomical considerations upon electrode placement in routine EEG. *Proc Electrophysiol Technol Assoc* 1956;**7**:20–30.

Learning objectives

(1) To understand the concept of the electroencephalogram (EEG) and what it records.
(2) To understand how EEGs are recorded.
(3) To understand how EEGs are reviewed.
(4) To become familiar with the waveforms seen in a normal EEG.
(5) To understand the basic principles of EEG interpretation.
(6) To become familiar with common EEG terminology.

Section 1 Basic principles

Chapter 15
Phenomenology of normal EEG: effects of age and state of awareness

Franz Brunnhuber

Introduction

With illustrations and examples, this chapter attempts to be a pragmatic approach to the visual, phenomenological, non-quantitative, recognition of normal EEG patterns and transients.

The phenomena described here include the age groups from infancy to adulthood. EEGs in preterm babies, neonates and the first 12 months of age are covered in Chapter 32. The range of normal responses to photic stimulation is not covered.

This chapter stresses the importance of recognizing normality, its range and benign variants to avoid over-interpretation of the EEG, which could lead to over-diagnosing pathology, notably epilepsy.

To understand normality it is often helpful to study distinctly abnormal phenomena, or pathology. This applies as much to the assessment of the EEG as it applies to medicine as a whole. Therefore chapters dealing with the abnormal EEG, epileptiform activity and the EEG in epilepsy are complementary to this text.

That the EEG can be falsely negative or, in other words, that some patients with epilepsy can have 'normal' EEGs, or falsely positive, that normal subjects can have abnormal EEGs, can be understood by applying the principles of sensitivity and specificity for this test (Table 15.1 and Chapter 18: 'Clinical use of EEG in epilepsy').

Normal background

From a phenomenological point of view the background or ongoing EEG activity can be distinguished from transients which are short-lasting EEG changes. This dichotomy can be summarized in the algorithm of EEG examination shown in Figures 15.1 and 15.2.

Table 15.1. Approximate sensitivity and specificity of the interictal EEG in epilepsy (various sources)

Epileptiform activity	Subjects with epilepsy	Normal subjects
First interictal awake EEG		
Present	40% (true positives)	0.5–4% (false positives)
Absent	60% (false negatives)	>96% (true negatives)
Second interictal sleep EEG		
Present	80–90% (true positives)	0.5–4%[a] (false positives)
Absent	10–20% (false negatives)	<96%[b] (true negatives)

[a] 0.5–1% in the adult population, 3.6% in paediatric population.
[b] interictal epileptiform discharges can be seen in normal subjects and in a variety of conditions.

Considering the wake EEG the following normal background activities are seen. The effects of age and state of awareness are summarized below.

- Alpha: (>86% as the dominant rhythm, Figure 15.3) 8–13 Hz, during wakefulness, over the posterior region of the brain, maximum amplitudes over occipital area: amplitudes below 50 μV. Best seen with eyes closed and during physical relaxation and relative mental inactivity. Blocked on eye opening.
- Beta: (>7% as the dominant rhythm) 13–35 Hz over fronto- central region, wakefulness amplitude below 30 μV, a normal phenomenon, or fast alpha variant (see drugs).
- Theta: (>5% as the dominant rhythm) 4–7 Hz, irregular theta is a usual feature of the normal adult EEG in the awake state and is of greatest amplitude in the posterior temporal region.

Introduction to Epilepsy ed. Gonzalo Alarcón and Antonio Valentín. Published by Cambridge University Press.
© Cambridge University Press 2012.

Section 1: Basic principles

Figure 15.1. Algorithm for EEG assessment (Reproduced with permission from Drury *et al.*, Pitfalls of EEG Interpretation in Epilepsy, Neurologic Clinics, November 1993 11:4).

Algorithm of EEG assessment

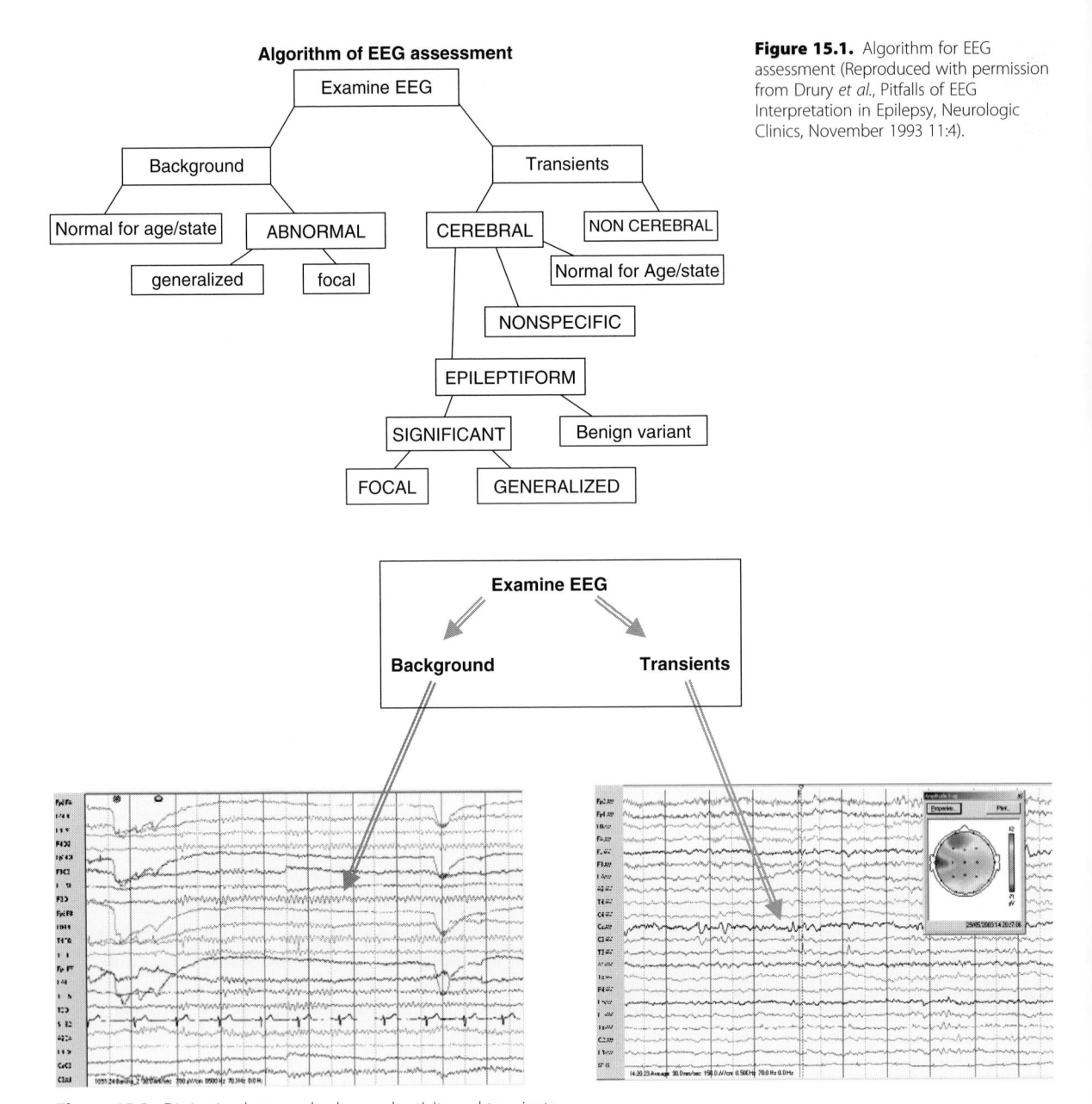

- Examine EEG
  - Background
    - Normal for age/state
    - ABNORMAL
      - generalized
      - focal
  - Transients
    - CEREBRAL
      - Normal for Age/state
      - NONSPECIFIC
      - EPILEPTIFORM
        - SIGNIFICANT
          - FOCAL
          - GENERALIZED
        - Benign variant
    - NON CEREBRAL

Figure 15.2. Distinction between background activity and transients.

- Delta: 0.5–4 Hz. Normal in the first year of life. Also occurs in adults during sleep, but rhythmic delta is usually abnormal in adults.
- The low 'voltage' EEG: a low amplitude is often a normal EEG. Reactivity to eye opening may, however, be difficult or impossible to assess.
- Slow alpha variants: in some subjects slow rhythms often in the theta range can be seen along with faster rhythms (Figure 15.4). These components are reactive to eye opening and disappear in sleep. Despite their apparent abnormality, they are a background variation of no clinical significance and can easily lead to over-interpretation (suggesting that it is an abnormal finding when it is not).

Artefacts

One of the biggest challenges for the recording and interpreting of the EEG are the 'non-cerebral

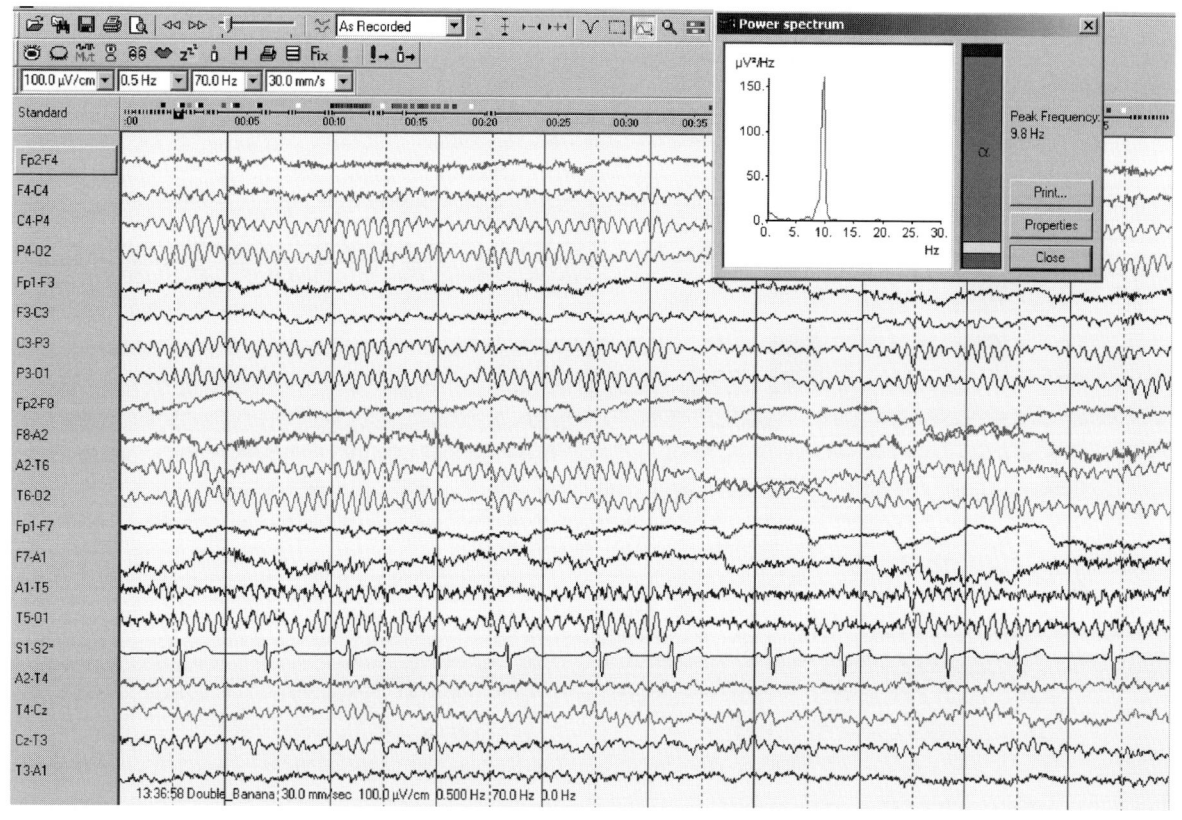

Figure 15.3. Alpha activity over posterior regions with peak frequency at 9.8 Hz.

transients' or artefacts. EEG technicians are often able to eliminate them or at least identify them. The electroencephalographer needs to be aware of the ubiquity and abundance of artefacts as a potential source of misinterpretation.

Normal transients and benign variants

Short-lasting deflections, so-called cerebral transients, represent either normal physiological phenomena or variants, which are not known to be clinically significant. Benign variants either occur as transients or patterns.

Lambda waves (Figure 15.6) are isolated electropositive sharp waves of up to 30 μV in amplitude and 200 ms in duration. They are seen over the occipital region extending to the parietal region. Lambda waves are elicited by scanning a patterned visual field.

Mu rhythm ('comb' (Figure 15.7)) is a rhythm at 7–11 Hz composed of arch-shaped waves occurring over the centro-parietal regions with amplitudes below 50 μV. It is blocked or attenuated by contra-lateral hand movements, the anticipation of a movement or the readiness to move or by tactile stimulation.

Posterior temporal slow waves (Figures 15.8 and 15.9) are isolated delta waves in children and young adults. They are regarded as a reflection of the immaturity of the brain and taken to be normal up to the twenties. With some non-10–20 electrode placement systems, such as the modified Maudsley system, these transients were seen also in the early thirties.

Vertex sharp waves (V wave, vertex sharp transient, Figure 15.10) are most prominent during stage I of sleep. They have moderate high voltage (100–250 μV), and a negative polarity which can be followed by a positive element. They occur as isolated transients or in runs, with maximum over Cz (vertex electrode).

Positive occipital sharp transient of sleep (POST, Figure 15.11): triangular, monophasic positive transient of 200–300 ms duration with maximal amplitude over the occipital electrode. They are usually seen during sleep stage I. The old term for this phenomenon, 'lambdoid' waves, is now considered obsolete.

Section 1: Basic principles

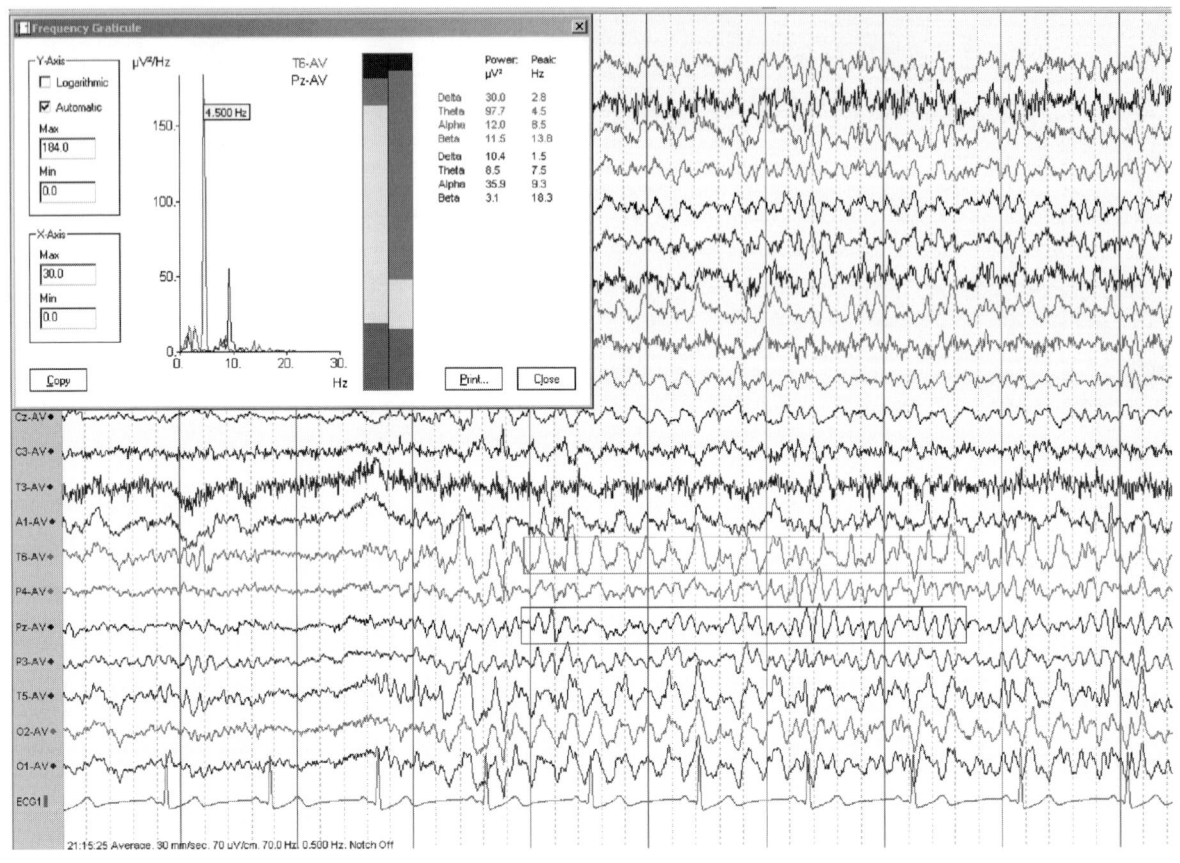

Figure 15.4. Slow alpha variant with widespread bilateral distribution, but clearest at T6 and O2. Note its reactivity to eye closure.

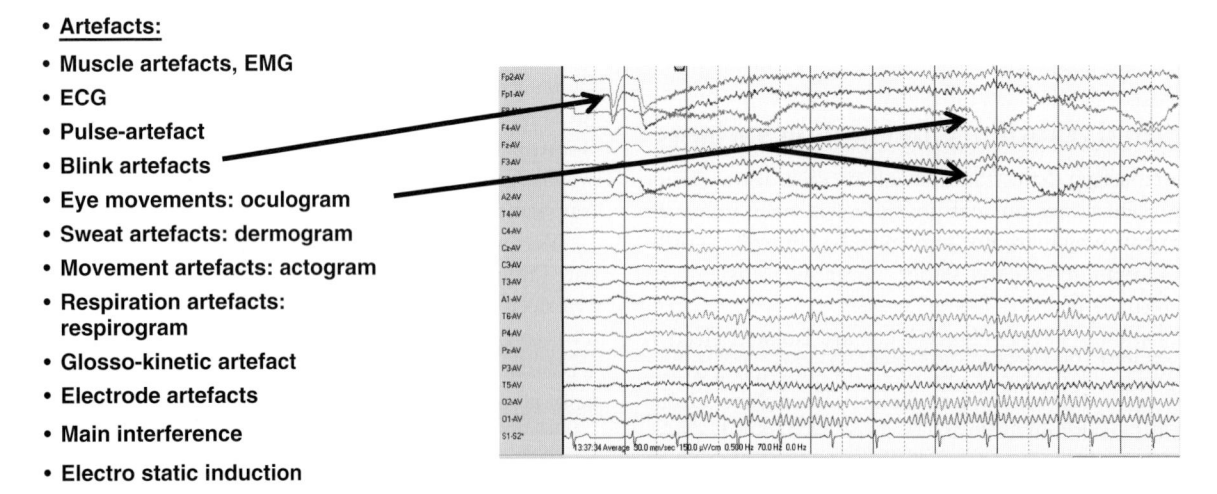

- **Artefacts:**
- Muscle artefacts, EMG
- ECG
- Pulse-artefact
- Blink artefacts
- Eye movements: oculogram
- Sweat artefacts: dermogram
- Movement artefacts: actogram
- Respiration artefacts: respirogram
- Glosso-kinetic artefact
- Electrode artefacts
- Main interference
- Electro static induction

Figure 15.5. Common non-cerebral transients often seen on EEG recordings.

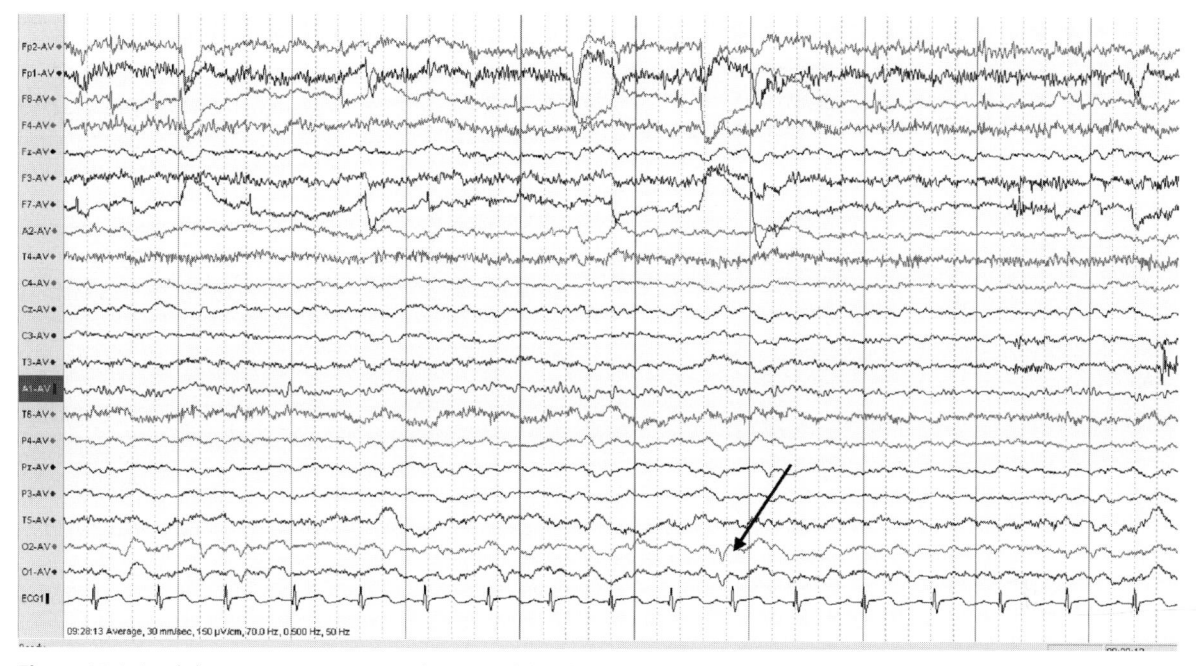

Chapter 15: Phenomenology of normal EEG: effects of age and state of awareness

Figure 15.6. Lambda waves seen over occipital regions while subject is awake.

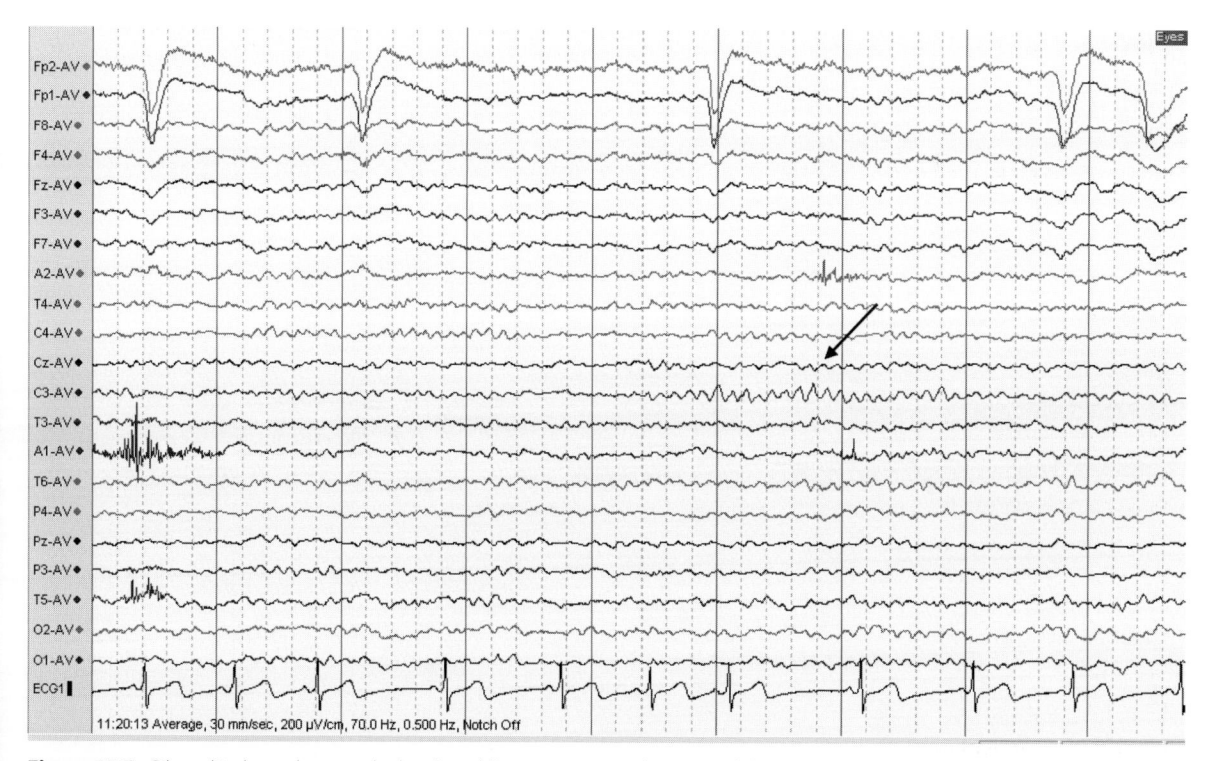

Figure 15.7. Bilateral independent mu-rhythm ('comb') seen over central regions while patient is awake.

Section 1: Basic principles

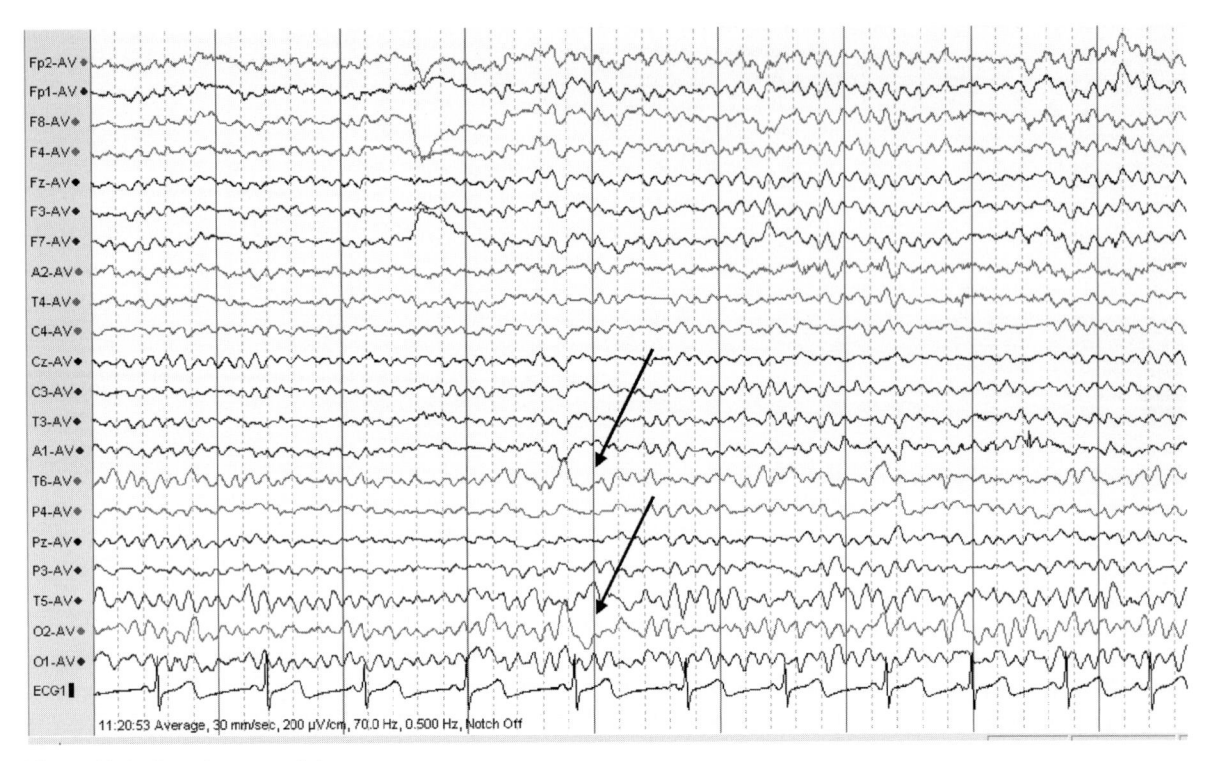

Figure 15.8. Posterior temporal slow waves.

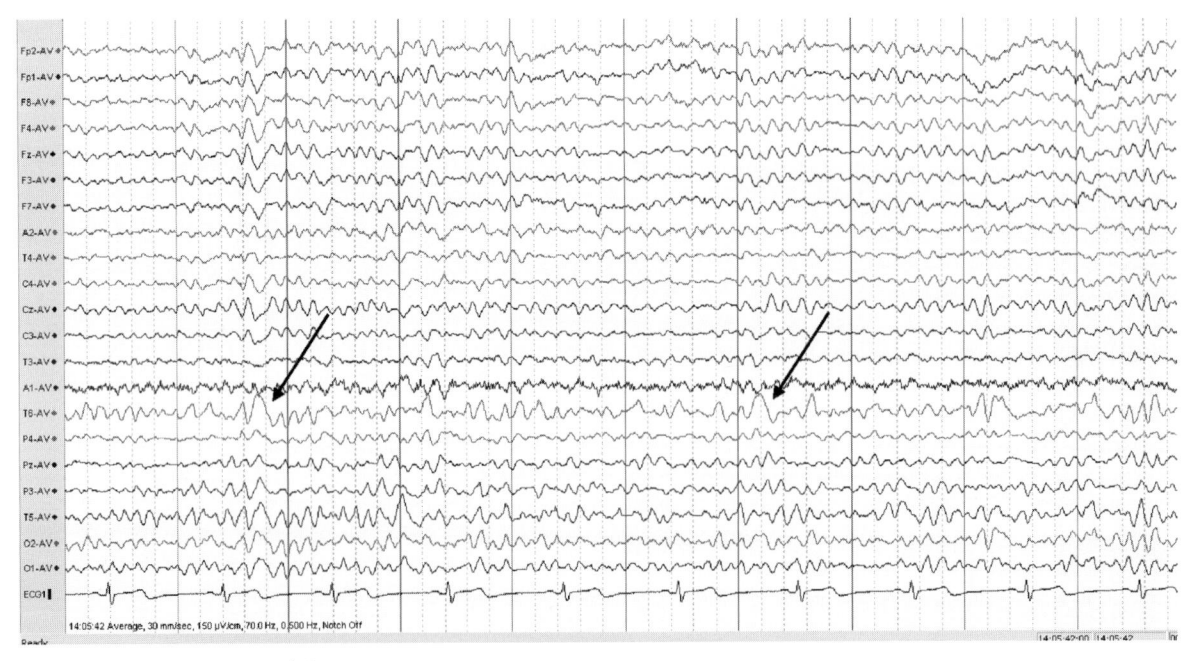

Figure 15.9. Posterior temporal slow waves.

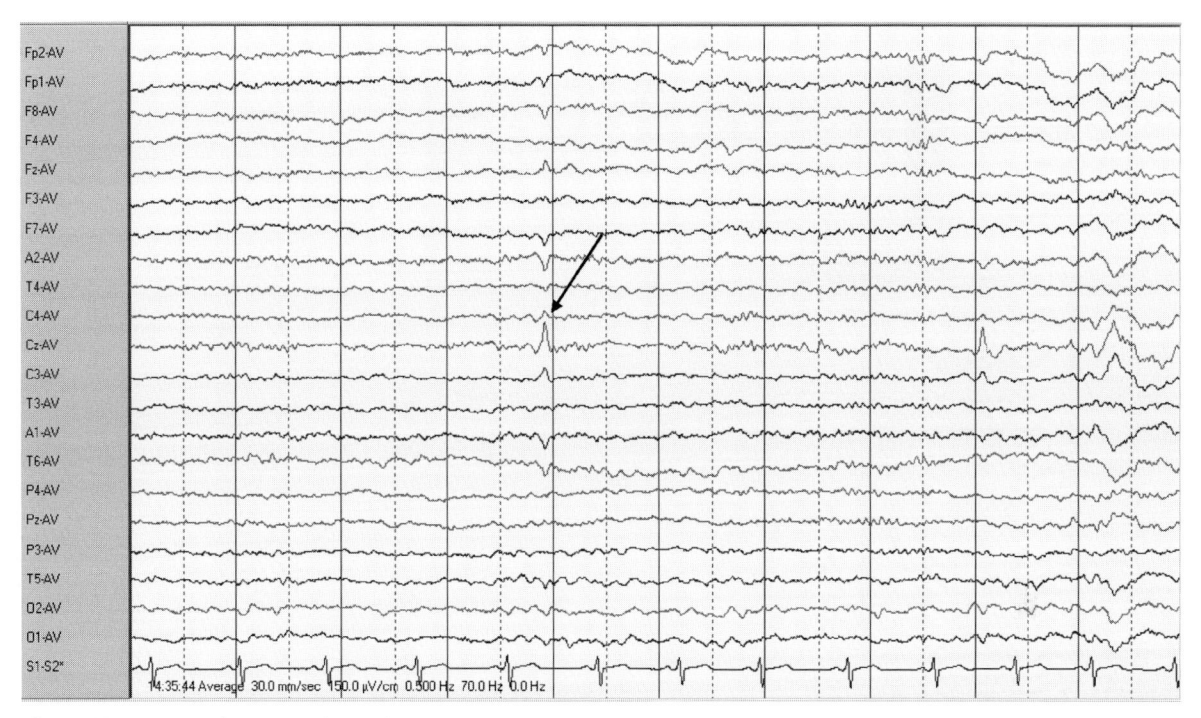

Figure 15.10. Vertex sharp wave during sleep.

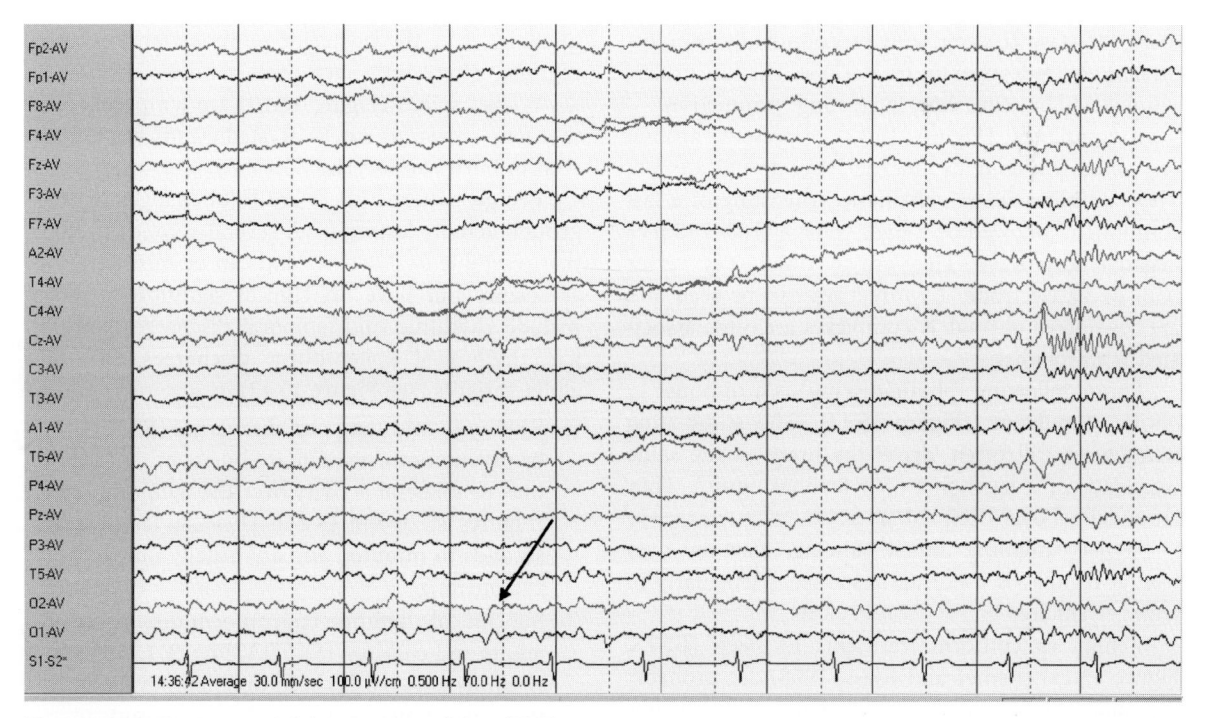

Figure 15.11. Positive occipital sharp transient of sleep (POST).

Section 1: Basic principles

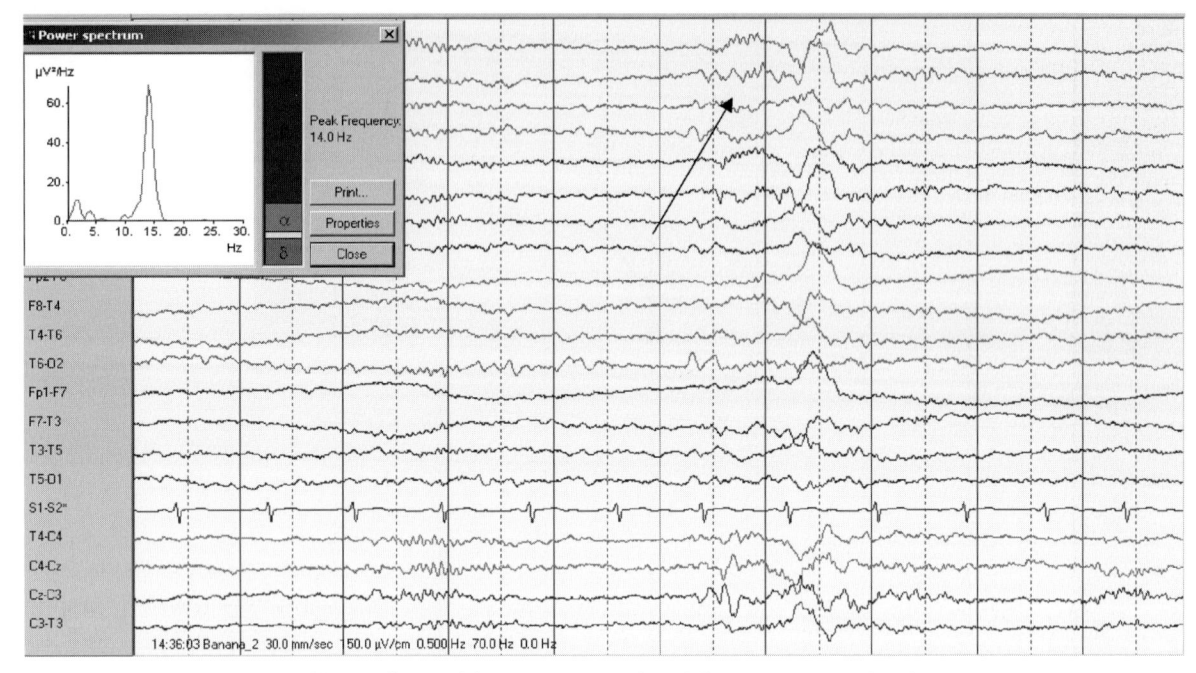

Figure 15.12. Sleep spindle. Brief bursts of sinusoidal activity (arrow) with peak frequency at 14 Hz (inset).

Sleep spindles (sigma activity, Figure 15.12): bursts of 0.5–2 s duration, usually at 14 Hz, they are the hallmark for stage II sleep, seen predominantly over the midline electrodes over the frontal lobe. They are usually symmetrical but may show fluctuating asymmetries.

K-complexes (Figure 15.13) represent arousal responses triggered by internal or external stimuli. They are biphasic, or polyphasic, consisting of a fast component followed by a high voltage (100–250 μV) negative slow wave. They are maximal over vertex (Cz) or Fz electrode. Asymmetries can be seen and are considered normal. K-complexes are often associated with spindles.

Photic following (photic driving) is a response to photic stimulation (Figure 15.14). The stimulating frequencies will often 'drive' the brain at the same frequency or a harmonic of it (subharmonic). They are maximal over occipital areas.

Hyperventilation: diffuse slowing, maximal over frontal regions, is a normal response, particularly in younger children.

Benign epileptiform transients of sleep (BETS, Figure 15.15) (Reiher and Klass, 1968) are probably the same phenomenon as small sharp spikes (Gibbs and Gibbs, 1963). They have very short duration and low amplitude, occurring in the temporal region(s) during drowsiness and light sleep.

6–14 Hz positive spike waves (Figures 15.16, 15.17 and 15.18) are runs of spikes at these frequencies over the posterior temporal and occipital regions, where the sharp peak is positive.

Wicket spikes (Figure 15.19) are temporal spikes that may appear as single isolated events but are also seen in bursts at 5–7 Hz.

Benign patterns: there are focal changes in background activity lasting from several seconds to hours that resemble ictal activity and can be misinterpreted as seizure but have no clinical significance. These include rhythmic mid-temporal discharges, subclinical rhythmical epileptiform discharges and slow alpha variants (see Figure 15.12).

(a) Rhythmic mid-temporal discharges (RMTD) or psychomotor variant are bursts of 6–7 Hz uni- or bilateral activity over the temporal region (Figures 15.20 and 15.21). They can last several seconds to minutes, and are usually unreactive to eye opening.

(b) Subclinical rhythmic epileptiform discharges of adults and children (SREDA, Figure 15.22) are rhythms at 0.5–6 Hz seen over temporal and parietal regions, occurring during seconds to minutes, usually unreactive to eye opening. Their significance is uncertain but they are not clearly associated with epilepsy.

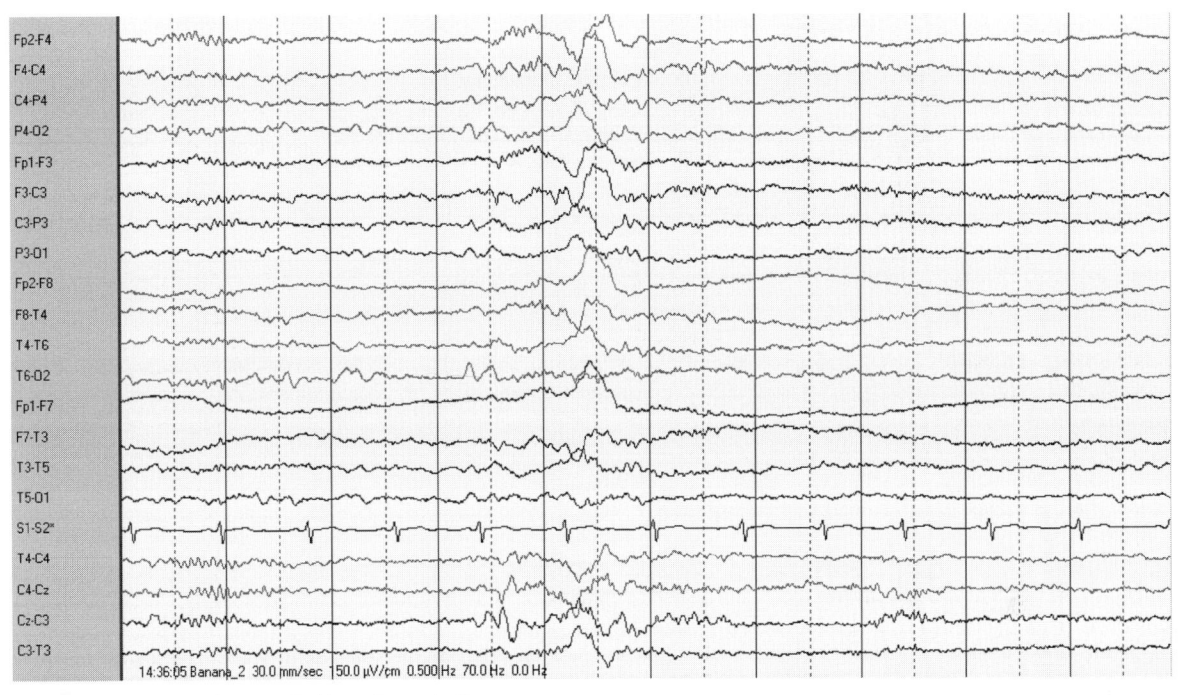

Chapter 15: Phenomenology of normal EEG: effects of age and state of awareness

Figure 15.13. K-complex preceded by a sleep spindle.

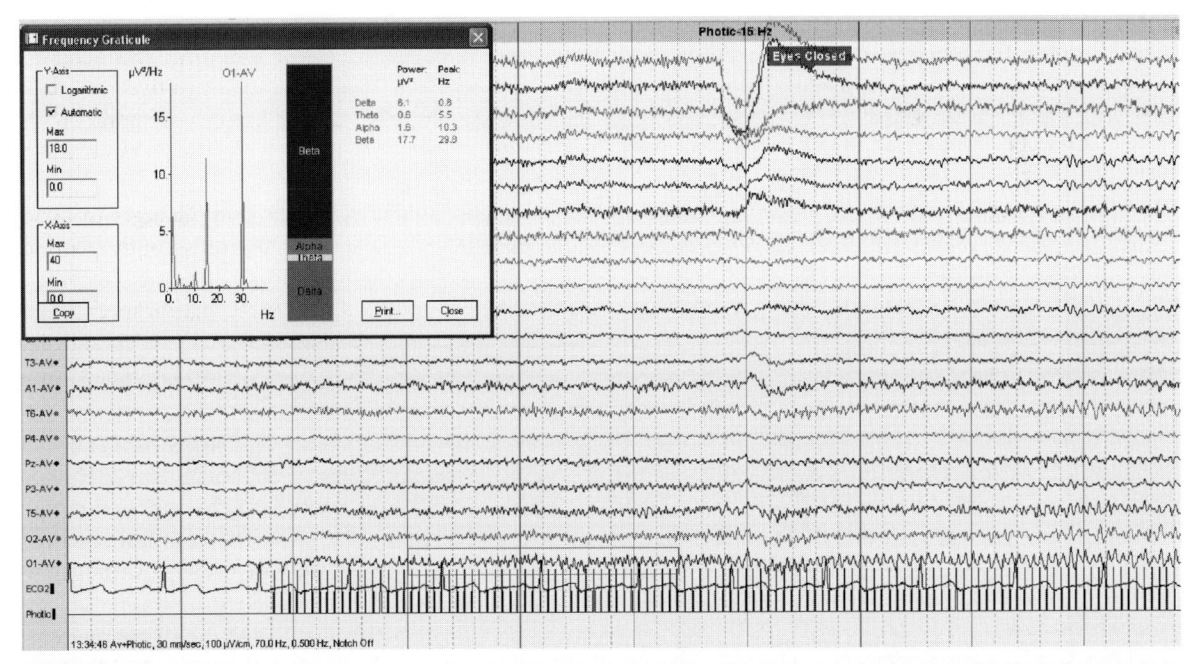

Figure 15.14. Photic following responses at 15 Hz and its 30 Hz harmonic. Note small deflections over posterior regions locked with the light flashes (black bottom trace).

Section 1: Basic principles

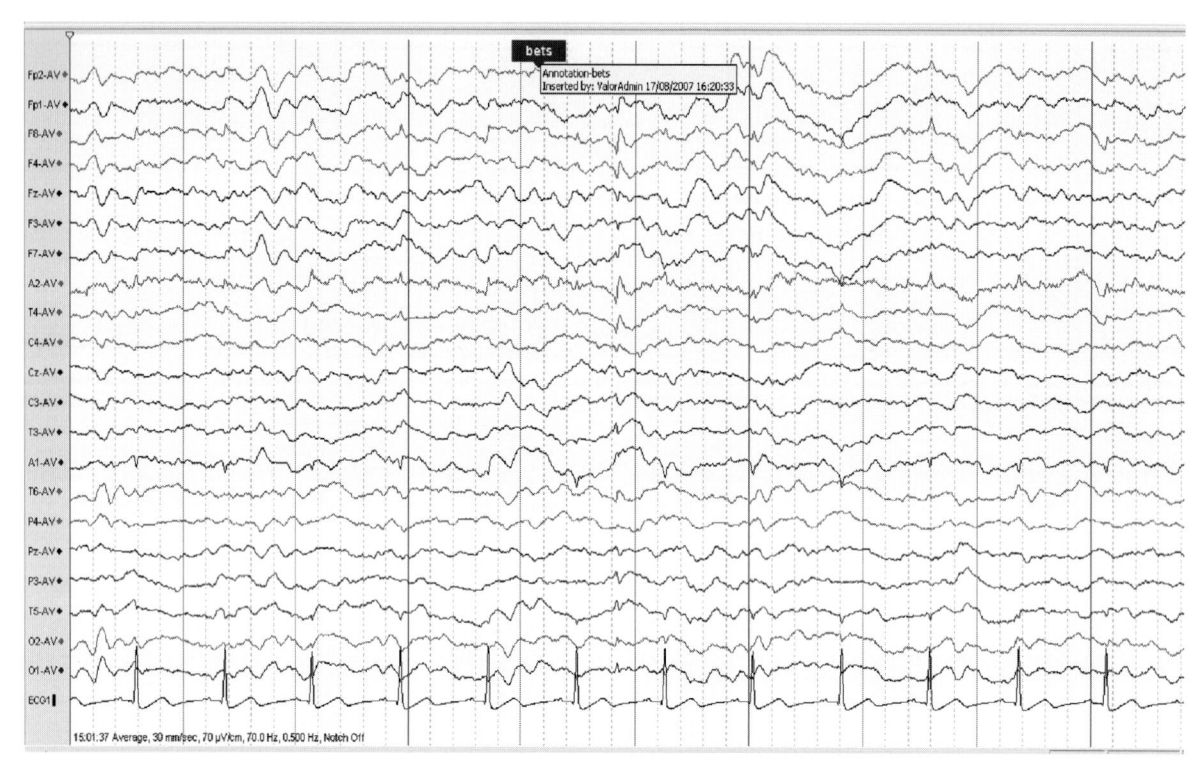

Figure 15.15. A single BETS seen at F8, F4, A2 and T4.

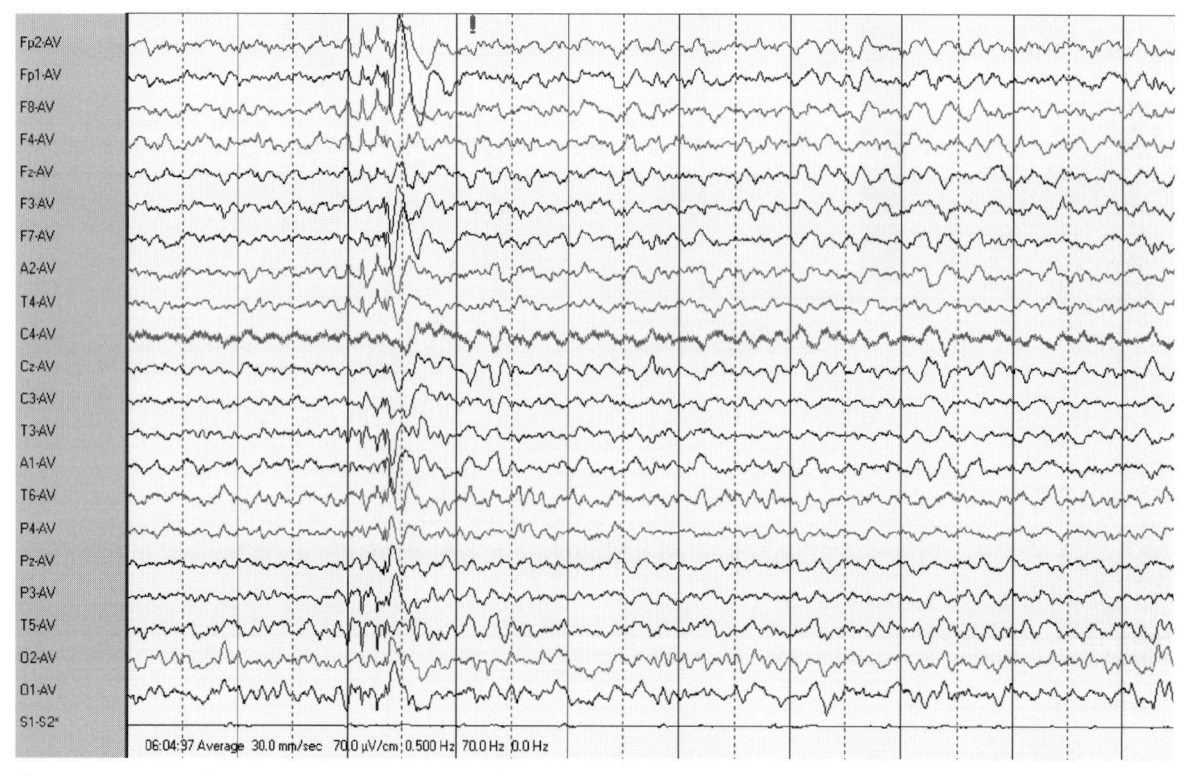

Figure 15.16. Run of 6–14 Hz positive spikes with peak frequency at 6 Hz.

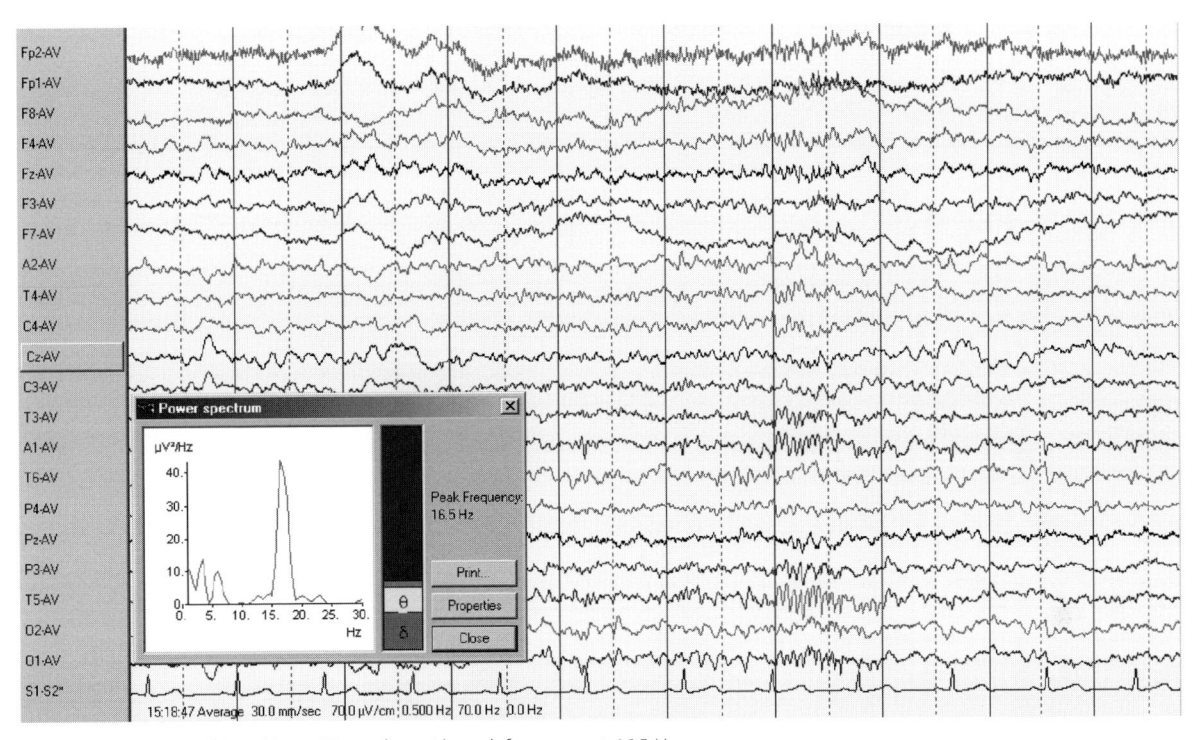

Chapter 15: Phenomenology of normal EEG: effects of age and state of awareness

Figure 15.17. Run of 6–14 Hz positive spikes with peak frequency at 16.5 Hz.

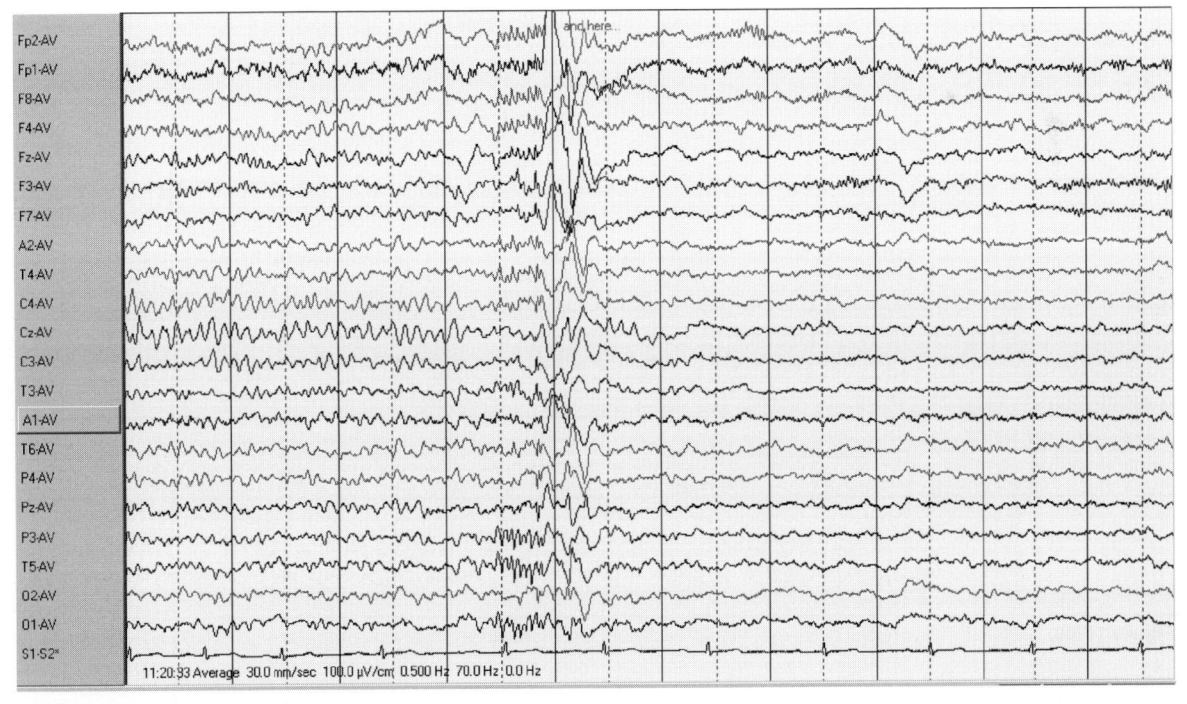

Figure 15.18. Run of 6–14 Hz positive spikes.

Section 1: Basic principles

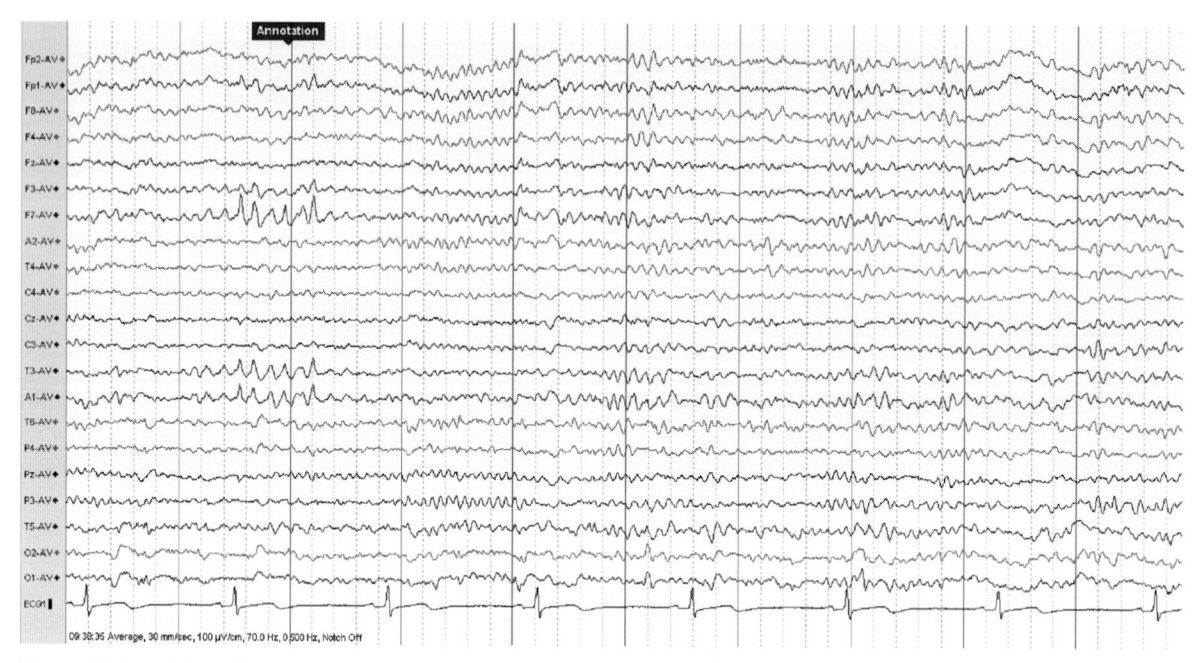

Figure 15.19. Wicket spikes seen clearest over left anterior temporal regions (at F7).

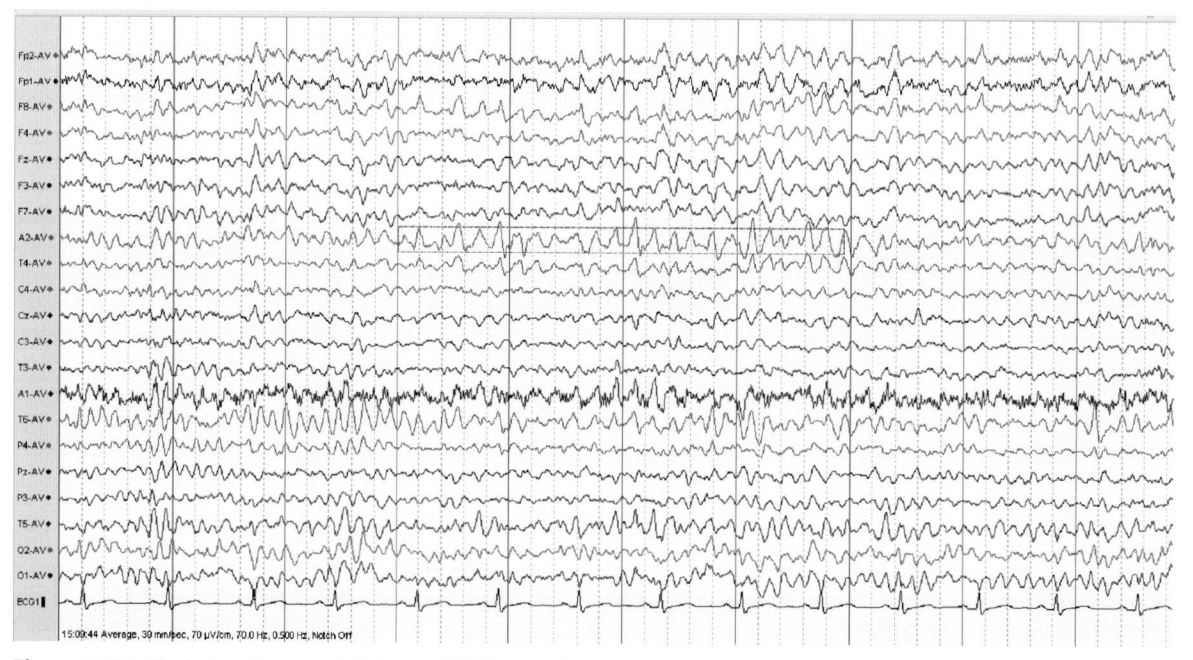

Figure 15.20. Rhythmic mid-temporal discharges (RMTD) or psychomotor variant seen over right temporal regions (mainly at A2 and F8).

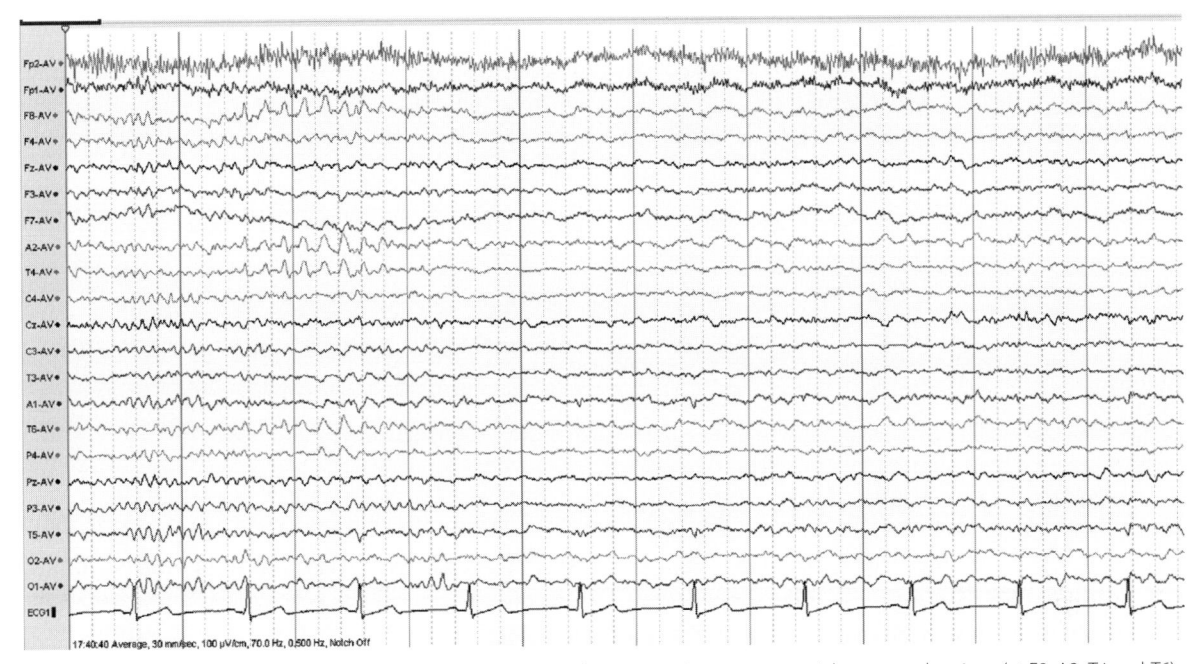

Chapter 15: Phenomenology of normal EEG: effects of age and state of awareness

Figure 15.21. Rhythmic mid-temporal discharges (RMTD) or psychomotor variant seen over right temporal regions (at F8, A2, T4 and T6).

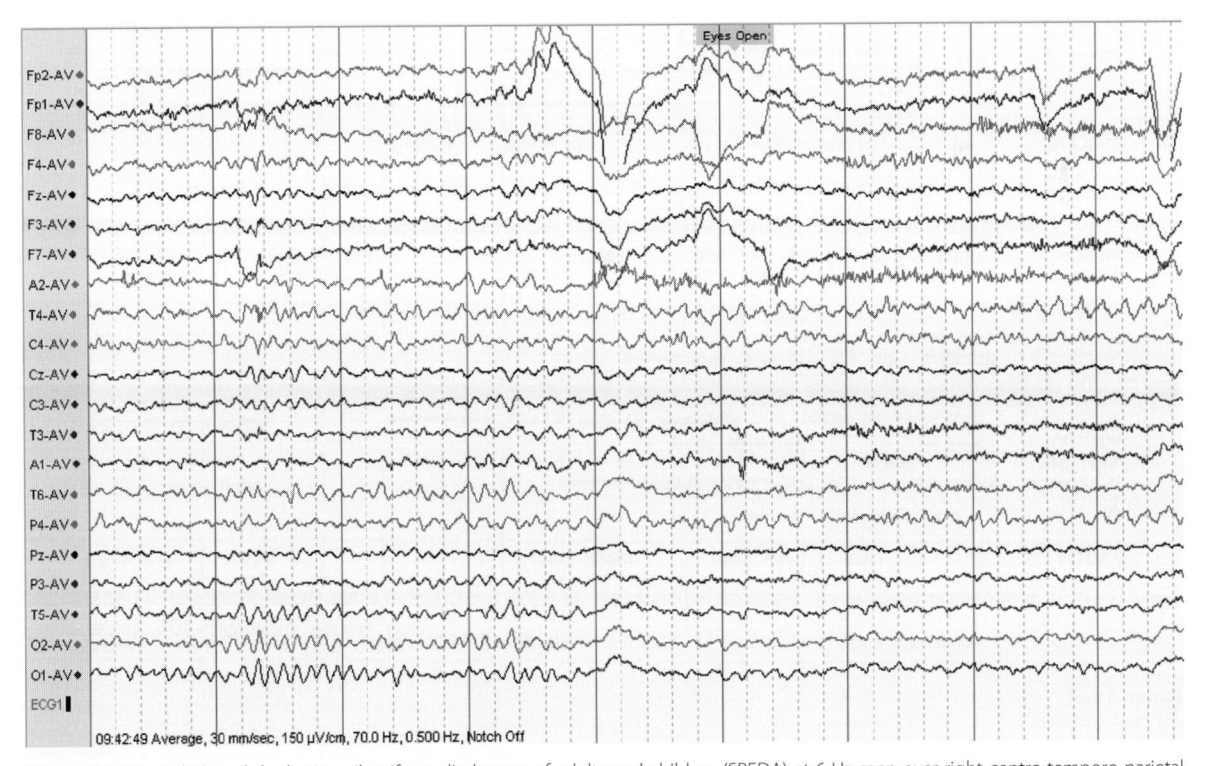

Figure 15.22. Subclinical rhythmic epileptiform discharges of adults and children (SREDA) at 6 Hz seen over right centro-temporo-parietal regions (at C4, T4, T6 and P4).

Table 15.2. Normal sleep EEG stages (Rechtschaffen and Kales, 1968)

Awake	More than 50% of 10 s epochs show alpha
Very light sleep (stage I)	Alpha is disintegrating, increase of theta, SEM (slow lateral eye movements), vertex sharp waves, paradoxical alpha activity
Light sleep (stage II)	Sleep spindles and K-complexes. Delta not more than 20% (50% of sleep)
Deeper sleep (stage III)	Slow-wave sleep: there are some sleep spindles and K-complexes, but delta activity dominates during 20–50% of the time
Deep sleep (stage IV)	Slow-wave sleep: delta activity dominates during more than 50% of the time
REM stage	Rapid eye movements (REM), theta or delta, reduced muscle tone. Usually around six cycles per night; one cycle is about 95 minutes

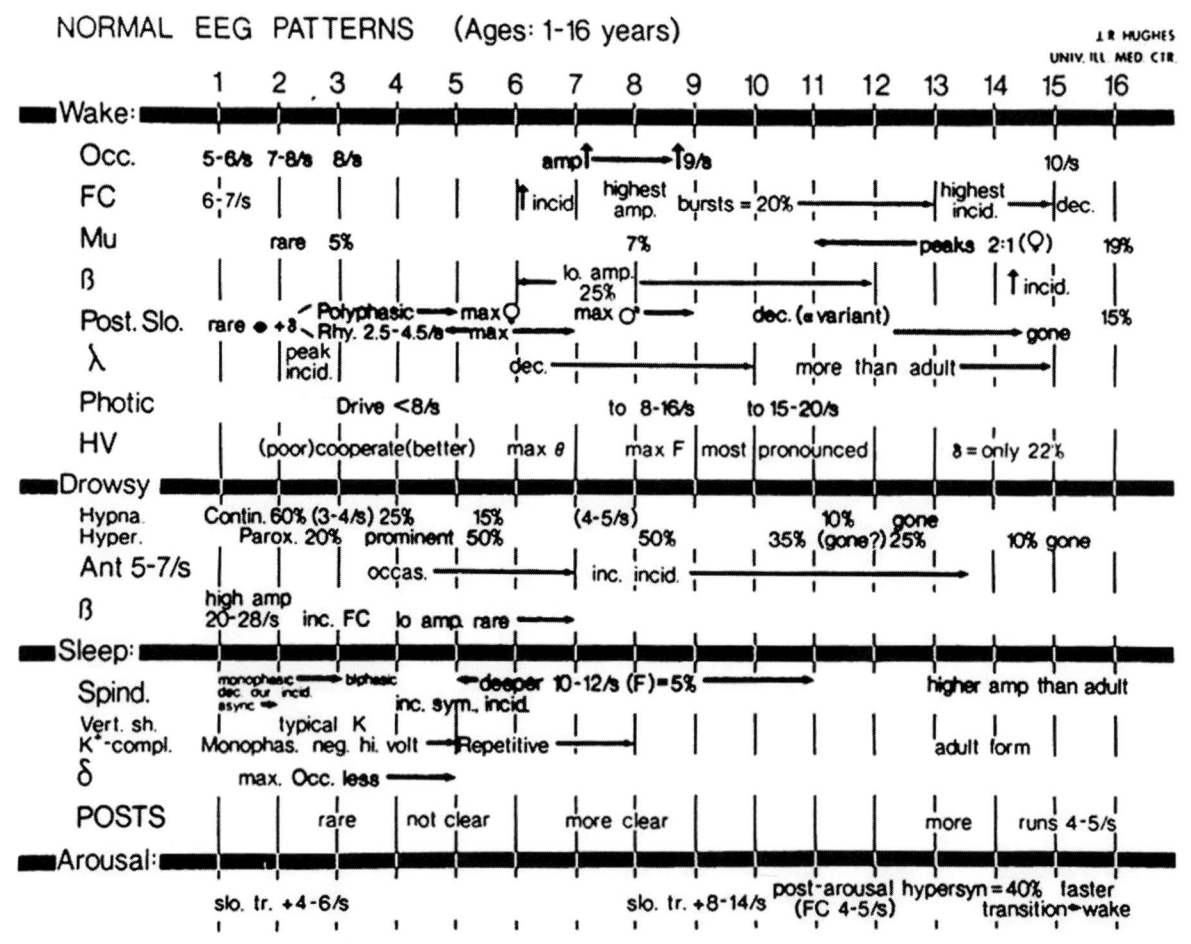

Figure 15.23. Summary of normal patterns during awake, drowsy and arousal stages for ages between 1 and 16 years. Occ, background occipital rhythms; FC, fronto-central theta rhythms; Mu, μ(mu)-rhythm; β, β-rhythms; Post. Slo., posterior slow waves; λ, lambda-waves; Photic, photic following responses; HV, response to hyperventilation; Hypna. Hyper., hypnagogic hypersynchrony at 3–5 Hz; Ant 5-7/s, anterior theta activity at 5–7 Hz; Spind, sleep spindles; Vert. sh, vertex sharp waves; K-compl., K-complexes; δ, delta-activity; POSTS, positive occipital sharp transients of sleep; amp, amplitude; incid, incidence; max, maximal amplitude; lo, low; Monophas., monophasic; neg, negative; hi, high; hypersyn, hypersynchrony; slo., slow; tr., transients (reproduced with permission from Figure 1.5.35, page 101, *EEG in Clinical Practice*, second edition, edited by John R Hughes, published by Butterworth-Heinemann, Boston, 1994, ISBN 0–7506–9511–0).

Effects of state and age

The EEG is very sensitive to changes in the state of awareness and/or alertness and reflects the development, maturing and ageing of the brain. It is an ideal tool for sleep staging (Table 15.2). Figure 15.23 captures the dynamic changes through various age groups.

Recommended reading

Rechtschaffen A, Kales A. *A Manual of Standardized Terminology, Techniques and Scoring System of Sleep Stages in Human Subjects*. Los Angeles: Brain Information Service/Brain Research Institute, University of California; 1968.

Hughes JR (ed). *EEG in Clinical Practice*. 2nd edn. Boston, MA: Butterworth-Heinemann; 1994.

Binnie CD, van Emde Boas, Prior PF, Shaw JC. EEG phenomenology. In Binnie C, et al., eds.*Clinical Neurophysiology*, vol. 2. Amsterdam: Elsevier; 2003.

Binnie CD. Activation procedures. In Binnie C, et al., eds. *Clinical Neurophysiology*, vol. 2. Amsterdam: Elsevier; 2003.

References

Binnie CD, Cooper R, Mauguiere F, *et al. Clinical Neurophysiology*, vol. 2. Amsterdam: Elsevier; 2003.

Chiofalo N, Fuentes A, Gálvez S. Serial EEG findings in 27 cases of Creutzfeldt-Jakob disease. *Arch Neurol* 1980;**37**(3):143–5.

Connolly JH, Allen IV, Hurwitz LJ, Millar JH. Measles-virus antibody and antigen in subacute sclerosing panencephalitis. *Lancet* 1967;**1**(7489):542–4.

Dawson JR. Cellular inclusions in cerebral lesions of lethargic encephalitis. *Am J Pathol* 1933;**9**(1): 7–16.3.

Drury I *et al.* Pitfalls of EEG interpretation in epilepsy. *Neurol Clin* 1993;**11**:4.

Gibbs FA, Gibbs EL. Age factor in epilepsy: a summary and synthesis. *N Engl J Med* 1963;**269**:1230–6.

Hughes JR. *EEG in Clinical Practice*. 2nd edn. Boston, MA: Butterworth-Heinemann; 1994.

Rechtschaffen A, Kales A. *A Manual of Standardized Terminology, Techniques and Scoring System of Sleep Stages in Human Subjects*. Los Angeles: Brain Information Service/Brain Research Institute, University of California; 1968.

Reiher J, Klass DW. Two common EEG patterns of doubtful clinical significance. *Med Clin North Am* 1968;**52**:933–40.

Zschocke S.*Klinische Elektroenzephalographie*. 2nd edn. Berlin: Springer; 2002.

Learning objectives

(1) To become familiar with:

- normal EEG waveforms according to patient's age and state of awareness
- common artefacts
- normal variants.

(2) To be able to correctly interpret normal EEG phenomena that can resemble epileptiform activity.

Section 1 Basic principles

Chapter 16

Pathological EEG phenomena and their significance

Lee Drummond

The EEG is often fundamental to the management of epilepsy and other conditions. In the present section, we briefly discuss the significance and provide examples of abnormal EEG findings in epilepsy and in other conditions where the EEG can show waveforms resembling those seen in epilepsy. These include brain tumours, cerebrovascular disease, anoxic brain damage, encephalitis, encephalopathy, status epilepticus and cardiac arrhythmia. The EEG can help in the diagnosis of these conditions and their differential diagnosis with epilepsy. The latter is complicated by the fact that many of these conditions can lead to symptomatic epilepsy or to acute symptomatic seizures (see Chapter 31: 'Acute symptomatic seizures').

Epilepsy

A number of EEG abnormalities can be seen in patients with epilepsy: slowing of the background activity, sharp wave, spikes, polyspikes, spike-and-wave activity. Some abnormalities such as background slowing or sharp waves can be secondary to the underlying lesions causing seizures. They are not specific and can be seen in patients with lesions with or without seizures. Other abnormalities are more specific and tend to be seen in patients having seizures. When interpreting the EEG in patients with epilepsy, the following questions should be considered:

(1) What does the wave look like?
(2) Where do they appear to come from?
(3) Age of the patient?
(4) State of awareness of the patient?
(5) Is this an artefact?
(6) Could this be another physiological potential?

Spikes (Figure 16.1) are paroxysmal abnormalities with a pointed peak at conventional recording speeds (10 s/screen) and duration of 20–70 ms. The first large peak is generally negative and the amplitude is variable. Positive spikes are rarely seen in the scalp recordings but may be evident in intracranial recordings.

A sharp wave (Figure 16.2) can be distinguished from the background with a more blunted peak of 70–200 ms duration. Sharp waves are generally negative.

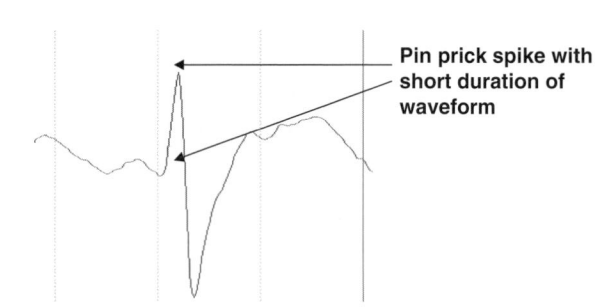

Figure 16.1. Spike. 200 ms per division.

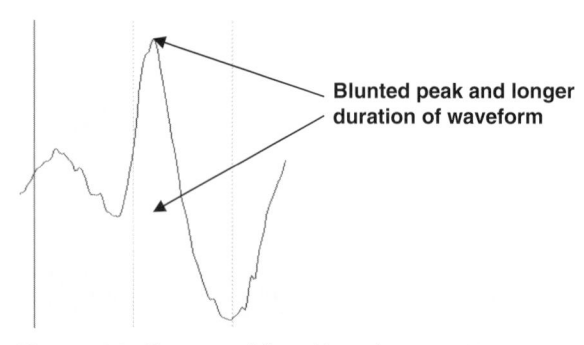

Figure 16.2. Sharp wave followed by a slow wave. 200 ms per division.

Introduction to Epilepsy ed. Gonzalo Alarcón and Antonio Valentín. Published by Cambridge University Press.
© Cambridge University Press 2012.

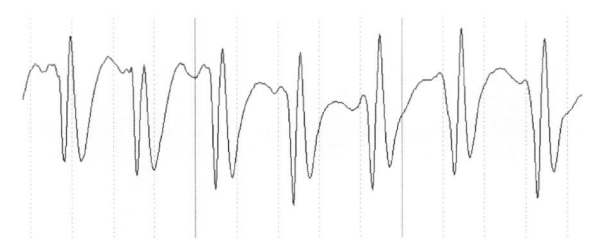

Figure 16.3. Spike-wave activity. 200 ms per division, 1 s between solid vertical lines.

Spike-wave complex (Figure 16.3) is a repetitive pattern consisting of a spike followed by a slow wave. The classic variety occurring three times per second (at 3 Hz) is the hallmark of childhood absence seizures.

Brain tumours

At present the EEG is seldom necessary for the initial diagnosis of intracranial tumours due to modern neuroimaging techniques. However, because tumours can be associated with seizures, the EEG can be useful in their management, either to confirm symptomatic epilepsy or during presurgical assessment.

EEG findings in intracranial tumours

- Focal theta activity
- Focal delta activity (often high voltage; polymorphic and/or monomorphic)
- Regional decrease in voltage and loss of organization of normal frequencies and/or background activity (alpha and beta)
- Focal sharp waves and/or spikes. Focal spike activity is seen in 20–30% of patients with hemispheric tumours
- Asymmetries of the sleep architecture (sleep spindles, K-complexes and vertex sharp waves) may also be seen, but may be difficult to evaluate as such phenomena can be asymmetrical in normal subjects

Cerebrovascular disorders

The normal functions of the brain depend on oxygen carried in the blood via the cerebral circulation. If depleted of oxygen for more than 5 minutes, neurons can die, causing cerebral infarction.

Interference with the cerebral circulation may be caused by a sudden reduction in blood pressure or by:

- reduction of blood flow due to occlusion of a blood vessel (ischaemic stroke)
- rupture of a blood vessel (haemorrhagic stroke).

EEG findings in cerebrovascular disorders

In the case of a cerebrovascular accident the EEG may be the first test following a stroke that becomes positive. An important initial feature to diagnose and localize the process is the asymmetry in background activity and/or in sleep patterns. Polymorphic delta is seen in the area near an infarction. Fast activity may be lost due to cortical damage.

If the cerebrovascular accident involves the brainstem, generalized slow waves can be seen. These are usually bilateral but may be attenuated on the side of the infarction. The characteristic EEG features are of high-voltage unilateral epileptiform activity which is periodic or quasiperiodic with a tri- or biphasic morphology. These are decribed as periodic lateralized epileptiform discharges (PLEDs; Figure 16.4), which may be associated with contralateral seizures. PLEDs are most readily seen in cerebrovascular disease but not exclusively. They may also be seen in neoplasmic and inflammatory brain disorders.

Hypoxic brain damage

A number of EEG patterns are associated with ischaemic-hypoxic states. The clinical presentation of hypoxia is typically metabolic in character with progressive confusion, stupor and coma, often with seizures and focal features.

The EEG displays an array of unique appearances and a number of EEG patterns can be described associated with hypoxic states. A simple grading system can be employed to classify the EEG:

Grade 1 – dominant alpha rhythm with some theta activity; reactive

Grade 2 – dominant theta, rare alpha; or dominant delta with other activity; reactive

Grade 3 – continuous delta with little other activity; or continuous spike activity; or episodic low-voltage or isoelectric periods of less than 1 second; poorly or non-reactive (Figure 16.5)

Grade 4 – isoelectric periods greater than 1 second (burst-suppression); low-voltage diffuse delta or low-amplitude/power EEG; un-reactive

Grade 5 – isoelectric EEG.

Section 1: Basic principles

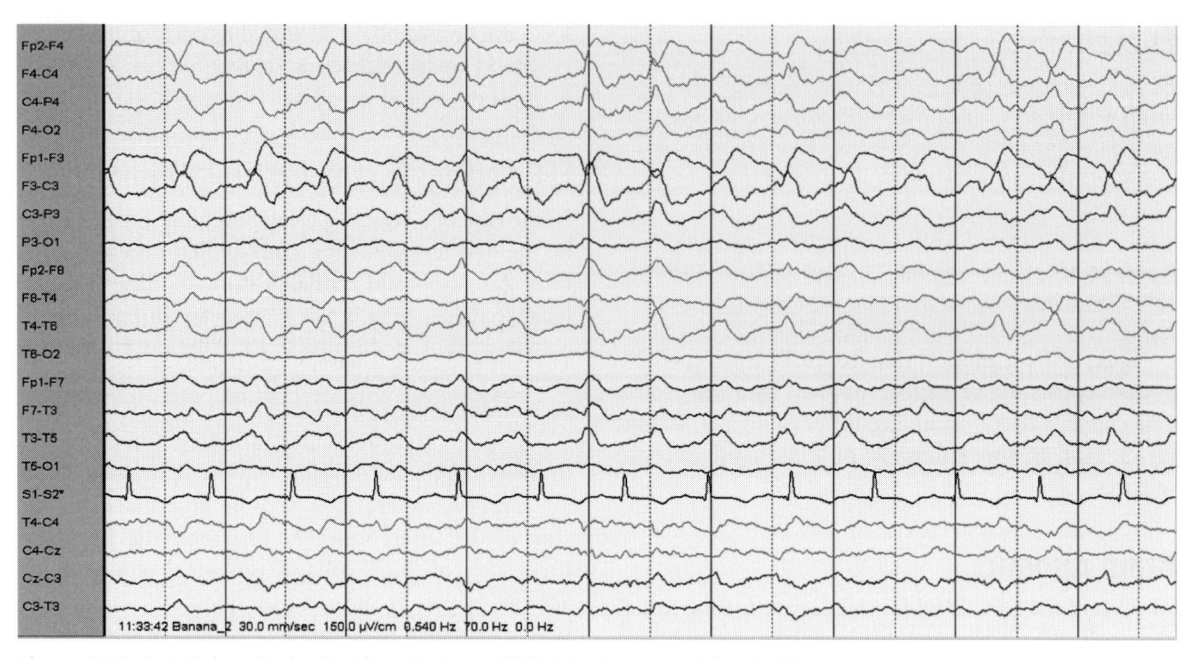

Figure 16.4. Periodic lateralized epileptiform discharges (PLEDs). 1 s between solid vertical lines.

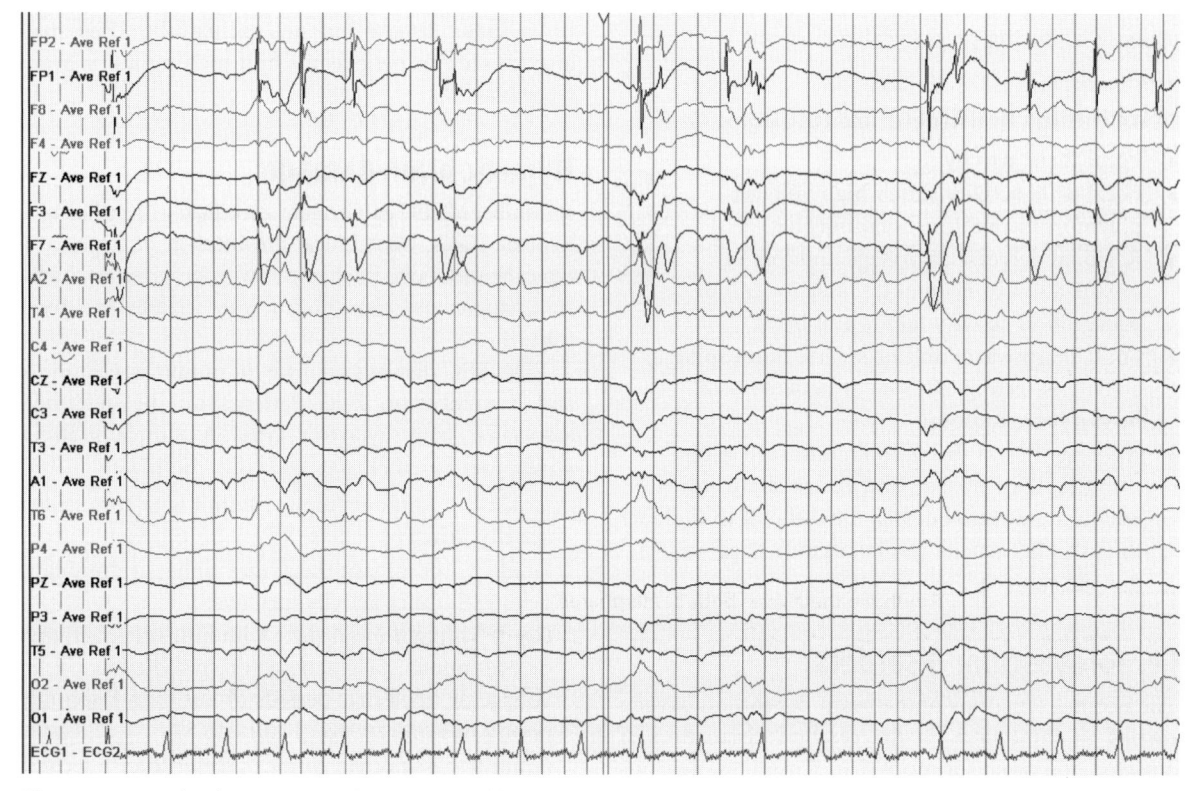

Figure 16.5. Grade 3 hypoxia. 100 ms between vertical lines.

98

Encephalitis

Encephalitis and meningitis can be caused by bacterial, viral or fungal infections. EEG findings in encephalitis are similar to those in meningitis, but tend to appear more severe, which can aid in the differential diagnosis. The EEG is abnormal in the acute phase. The different types of encephalitis tend not to generate specific EEG patterns. EEG abnormalities are usually expressed as diffuse or focal slowing (Figure 16.6), the extent of which is dependent on the amount of parenchymal involvement. When the white matter is involved, slow activity tends to be polymorphic and arrhythmic. When the grey matter is involved, slow activity tends to be bilateral synchronous and paroxysmal. The degree of slowing depends on the severity of the infection, the amount of cerebral involvement and the level of consciousness.

Nevertheless, there are a few encephalitic illnesses which do produce stereotyped EEG characteristics which aid in the differential diagnosis and classification of the disease.

Herpes simplex encephalitis

This is usually due to the herpes simplex virus type I, which is also responsible for oral herpes ('coldsores'). Herpes simplex encephalitis is an acute necrotizing illness, which preferentially affects the temporal lobes. The evolution can be rapid, leading to coma, hyperpyrexia and convulsions, and often hemipareisis. The EEG can be useful in the early diagnosis of the illness, especially with serial recordings. Several stages can be identified:

- Initially the EEG shows a disorganized background, with polymorphic delta, focally or lateralized with a temporal emphasis.
- As the disease progresses over the next 1–2 days, lateralized or focal sharp or slow wave complexes with maximal emphasis over the temporal regions appear.
- In the chronic phase, stereotyped, periodic discharges (complexes) recurring every 1–3 seconds, present after 2–5 days of the illness. If there is bilateral involvement of the brain, complexes tend to be bilateral, independent and synchronous, often with a time-locked relationship. Focal electrographic seizures with repetitive sharp or slow waves, spikes or polyspikes are seen over the involved hemisphere (Figure 16.7). The periodic complexes disappear during this time (NB – this phase is rarely seen these days as the patient has usually been treated with Acyclovir prior to the EEG being requested and recorded).
- Seizure discharges occur together with the periodic complexes which remain unaltered. The periodic complexes now appear broad in morphology.
- In the final stages of the evolution of the disease the EEG is almost isoelectric (flat).

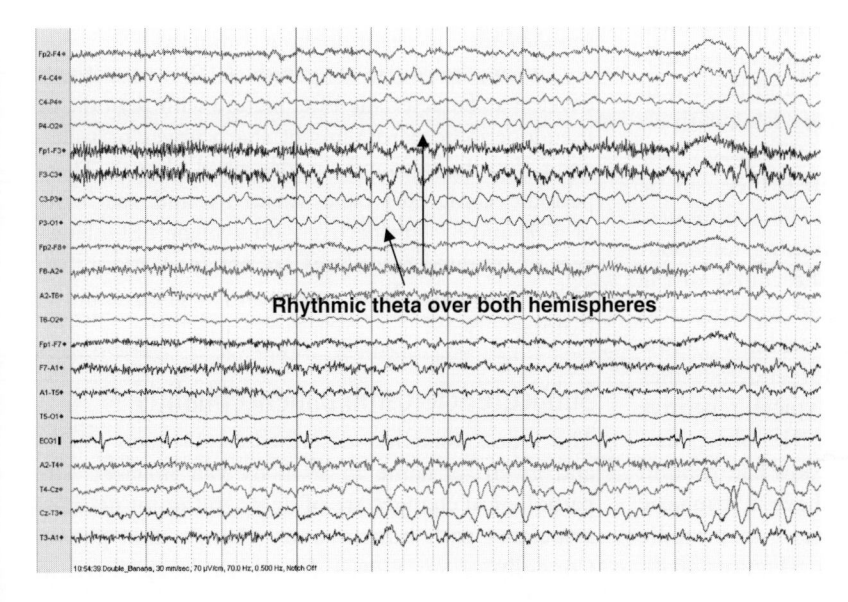

Figure 16.6. Encephalitis showing bilateral rhythmic theta activity. 1 s between solid vertical lines.

Section 1: Basic principles

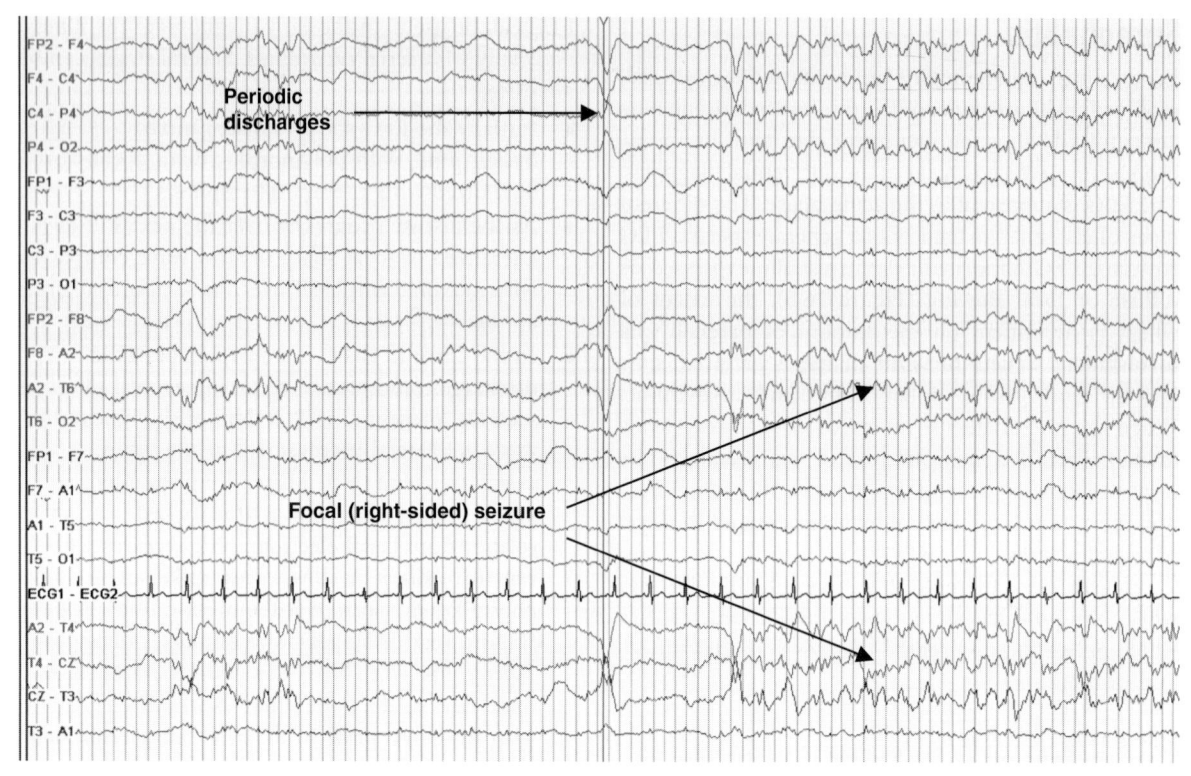

Figure 16.7. Herpes simplex encephalitis showing periodic discharges; a right-sided focal seizure. 100 ms between vertical lines.

Creutzfeldt–Jakob disease (CJD)

Prion diseases are a large group of related neurodegenerative conditions, affecting both animals and humans. They include CJD and Gerstmann-Straussler-Scheinker (GSS) in humans, bovine spongiform encephalopathy (BSE) in cattle, chronic wasting disease (CWD) in mule, deer and elk, and scrapie in sheep. Currently all prion diseases are fatal, with no effective curative treatment. Prion diseases are unique in that they can be inherited, they can be sporadic or they can be infectious. The commonest human prion disease is CJD, accounting for about 85% of all human prion disease. The course of the illness once symptoms begin is rapid with progressive dementia, dysarthria, spastic weakness of the limbs, parkinsonian rigidity, tremor and muscular wasting. The EEG shows fairly typical repetitive patterns of high-voltage slow (1–2 Hz) sharp and wave complexes on an increasingly slow background (Figure 16.8). These waves may have a triphasic appearance, but are generally seen as periodic sharpened slow wave complexes (Figure 16.8), separated by 1–1.5 seconds. They are present while awake and disappear during sleep.

Sporadic CJD is characterized by a rapidly progressive multifocal neurological dysfunction, myoclonic jerks, a terminal state of global severe cognitive impairment and death in about 8 months.

During the course of sporadic CJD, most patients develop a characteristic EEG picture with periodic or pseudoperiodic paroxysms of sharp waves or spikes on a slow background (as described above). These periodic complexes have sensitivity and specificity of 67% and 87% respectively on a single EEG. However, if repeated recordings are obtained, more than 90% of patients show periodic EEG abnormalitites (Chofalo, 1980).

Subacute sclerosing panencephalitis

The illness was first described by Dawson (1933) and given its name in 1945 by van Bogaert. The pathological changes are of degeneration of neurons associated with inflammatory changes and gliosis. Connolly *et al.* (1967) found antibody titres to

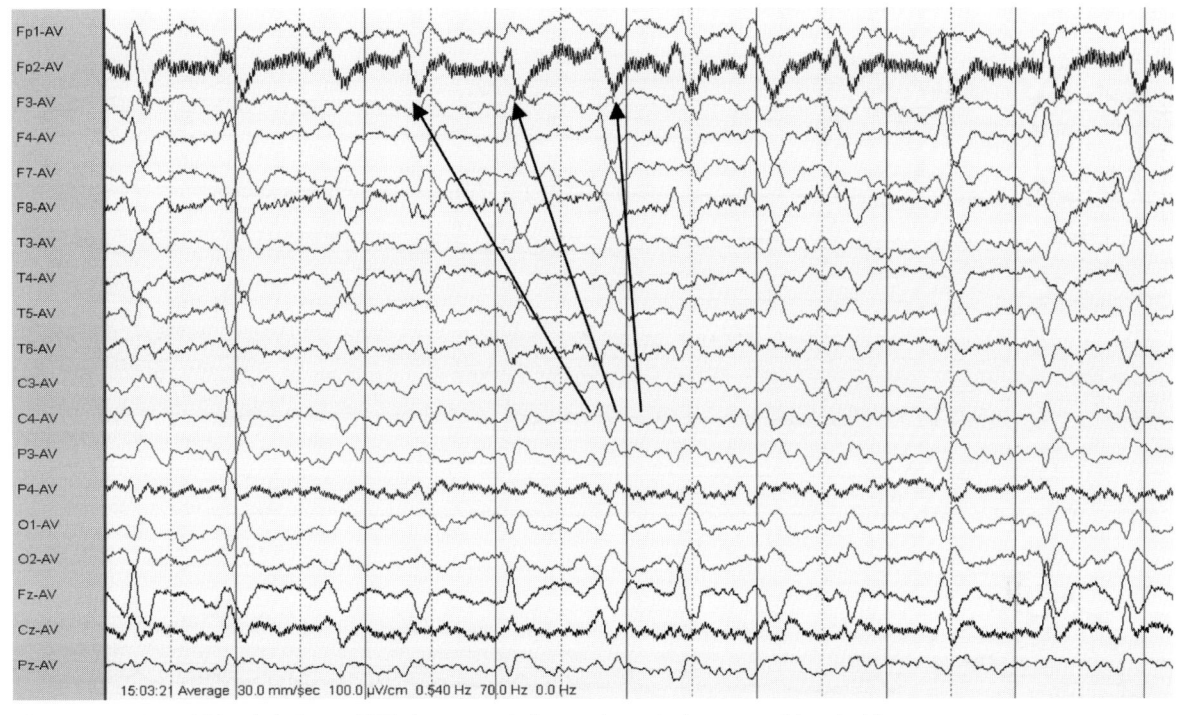

Figure 16.8. Creutzfeldt–Jakob disease (CJD) showing periodic complexes. 1 s between solid vertical lines.

measles virus rose in the serum during the illness. The condition is due to a persistence of the measles virus in the brain after suffering measles. The incidence of this condition has dramatically decreased after modern vaccination policies were implemented. The disease is slow from 2–18 months with three recognizable stages: (a) mood changes with intellectual deterioration, accompanied by epileptic changes and myoclonic jerks; (b) progressive dementia and akinetic mutism with involuntary movements; (c) decortication. The characteristic EEG changes were first described by Radermecker (1949) and Cobb and Hill (1950), consisting of high-voltage (300–1500 μV) repetitive polyphasic and sharp and slow wave complexes lasting up to 2 seconds and recurring every 4 to 15 seconds (Figure 16.9). The period between discharges shows relative electrical silence. The complexes are usually bi-synchronous and generalized, but may be asynchronous and show a time lag from one side to the next or from front to back. Initially the complexes show an irregular periodicity, which becomes more stereotypically periodic as the disease progresses. Afferent stimuli do not alter the discharges. A prominent feature of SSPE is the stereotyped jerk or spasm, which is related to the periodic complexes. At times instead of a jerk with loss of motion, there is a cessation of motion from reduced muscle tone. The motor movements often disappear during sleep. Sleep stages become less recognizable as the disease progresses. In the final stages of the disease the EEG may become almost isoelectric, although the alpha can remain until death.

Hepatic encephalopathy

Hepatic encephalopathy can be the consequence of viral or toxic hepatitis (acute) or chronic liver disease (cirrhosis). The illness causes personality changes, confusion and encephalopathy (diffuse disturbance of the brain). The EEG is sensitive to the appearance of the encephalopathy, and changes are seen prior to biochemical parameters changing. In the early stages of the illness, there is a change of personality, with confusion and cognitive decline. The EEG shows alpha at the lower end of the frequency spectrum, then theta and delta activities progressively appear in larger amounts, and sleep phenomena become disrupted. In the mid stages, when the patient becomes stuporose, the EEG is

Section 1: Basic principles

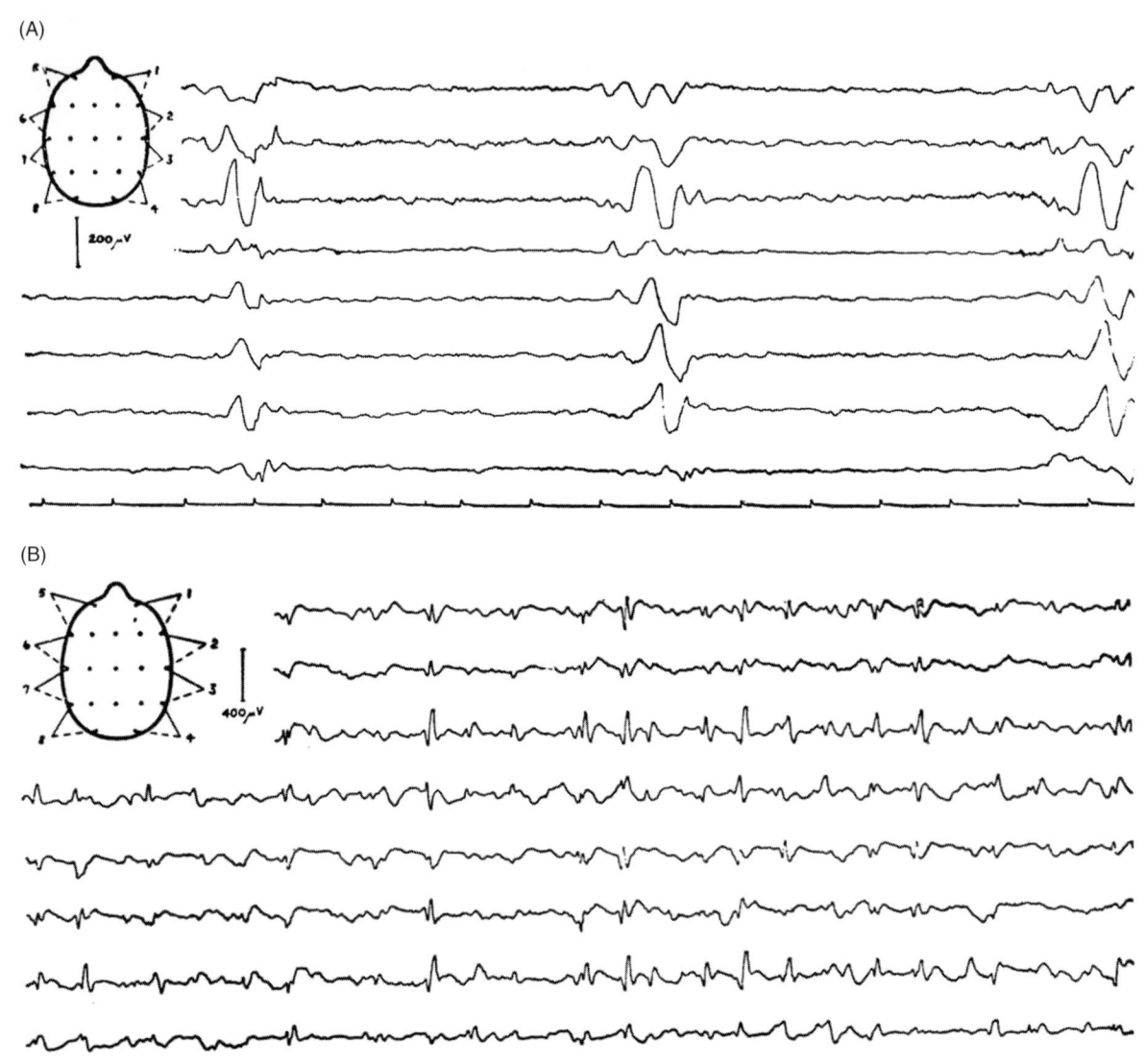

Figure 16.9. Two examples from different patients with subacute sclerosing panencephalitis showing stereotyped repetitive sharp wave complexes often associated with jerking of the limbs. (A) Girl aged 7 years, progressive organic deterioration, dyspraxia and dysphasia with generalized myoclonus for 4.5 months, died 5 months later. (B) Woman aged 70 years, onset of illness 3 weeks previously, progressive rigidity and dementia, frequent myoclonus of the upper limbs and face, died 5 weeks later (reproduced with permission from Kiloh LG, McComas AJ, Osselton JW, *Clinical Electroencephalography*, 3rd edn, Butterworths, London, 1977, Figures 8.6, page 144, and 8.7 page 145).

slow diffusely with the presence of triphasic sharp waves or sharpened slow waves. These have an initial low-voltage negative phase with a prominent positive component again followed by a broad negative wave. They occur at 2–4 Hz with an anterior emphasis and anterior-posterior time lag. Triphasic waves may also be seen in renal failure, hypercalcaemia, hyponatraemia, hypoglycaemia and lithium intoxication.

Status epilepticus (SE)

This is a common life-threatening neurological disorder. It is a prolonged epileptic seizure or a cluster of seizures without proper recovery between them. It has been defined as more than 30 minutes of continuous seizure activity or two or more sequential seizures without full recovery of consciousness between seizures (Dodson et al., 1993).

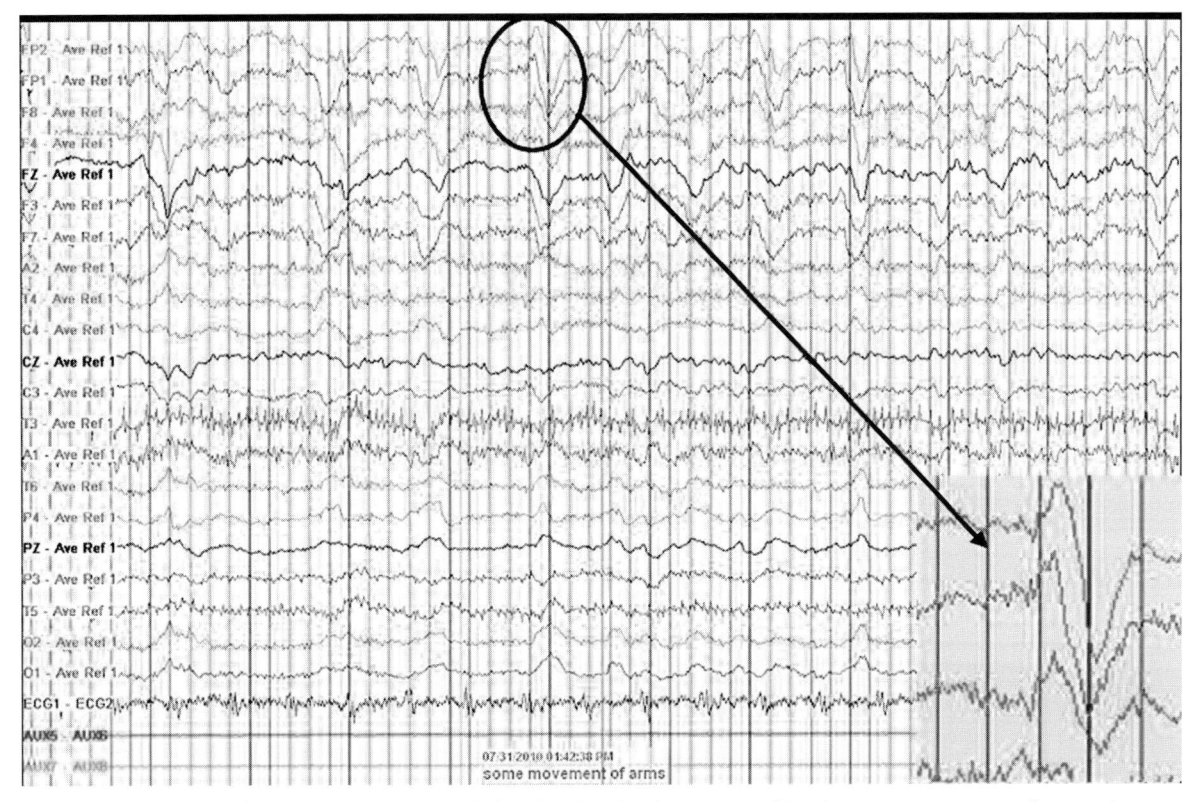

Figure 16.10. Triphasic slow waves in hepatic encephalopathy. Note the three phases of the sharp wave components: first negative (upwards), then positive (long downward arm) and then negative again.

Many patients who present with SE do not have prior history of seizures. Causes include head trauma, stroke, cardiac arrest and CNS infection. In children younger than 16 years, the commonest cause is fever/infection (36%). The most common precipitant in adults is cerebrovascular disease (25%).

Early diagnosis of status epilepticus is a priority because treatment with a sedative or anaesthetic agent is required to prevent prolonged seizures, brain damage and death. Diagnosis of convulsive status epilepticus is usually straightforward. However, nonconvulsive status epilepticus can show more subtle nonspecific signs such as confusion, slow thinking or poor memory. An early EEG is crucial to confirm the diagnosis (Figure 16.11).

If the diagnosis of status epilepticus is confirmed, antiepileptic drugs can be titrated under EEG monitoring. In severe cases, sedation may be necessary to reduce cortical activity to a burst-suppression pattern: bursts of background activity separated by periods of relative EEG flattening (Figure 16.12). This activity can then be monitored on a daily basis with the aid of a cerebral function monitor, which will display a compressed time graph of cortical activity as well as provide a spectral analysis of the frequencies contained in the EEG signal (Figure 16.13).

Cardiac arrhythmia

It is standard practice to record one electrocardiographic (ECG) lead during EEG recordings and to simultanously display EEG and ECG channels. Cardiac arrhythmias can be identified and are occasionally the cause of the patient's symptoms, most frequently faints or blackouts. The most common cardiac arrhythmias seen during EEG recordings are ectopics (Figure 16.14), which are asymptomatic in most patients.

Section 1: Basic principles

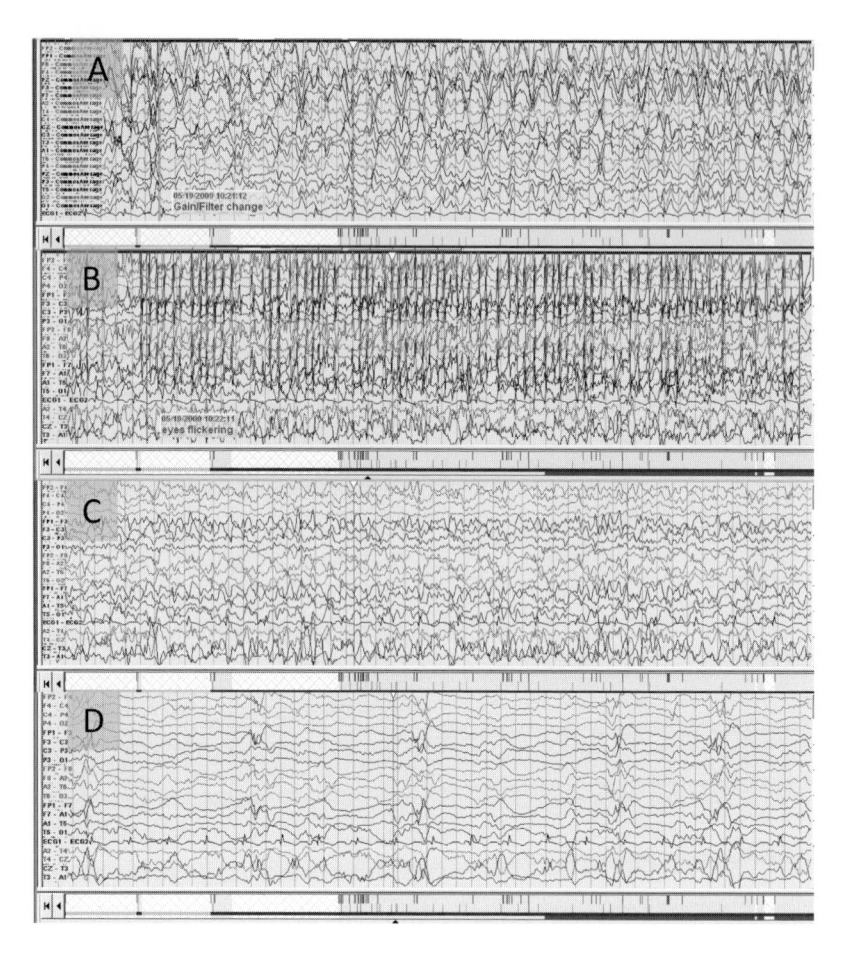

Figure 16.11. Examples of status epilepticus. (A) Build up of seizure associated with focal twitching of the face and hand. (B) Spread of discharges becoming generalized and involving both hemispheres. (C) Bilateral jerking. (D) Discharges subside and clinical features abate. 1 s between solid vertical lines.

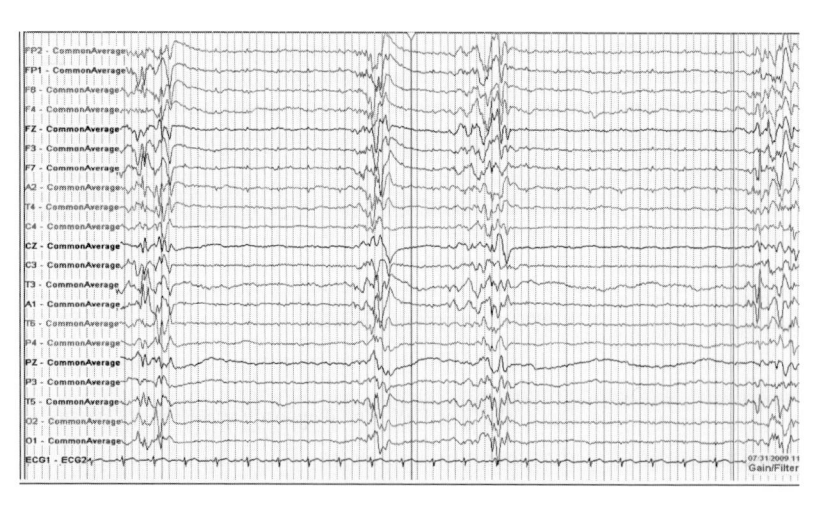

Figure 16.12. Burst suppression following administration of sedation (propofol). Time-base has been reduced to 15 mm/s to show the period of the suppressions between the bursts of complex activity. 100 ms between vertical lines.

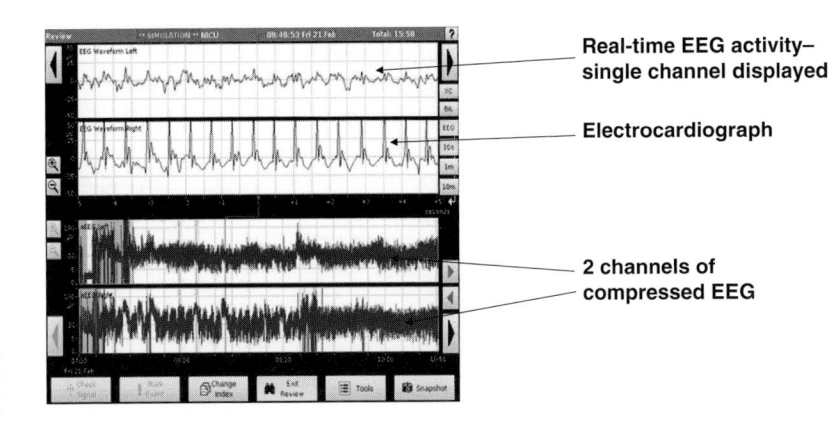

Chapter 16: Pathological EEG phenomena and their significance

Figure 16.13. Cerebral Function Analysing Monitor with single channel ECG and on-line EEG. 1 s between solid vertical lines.

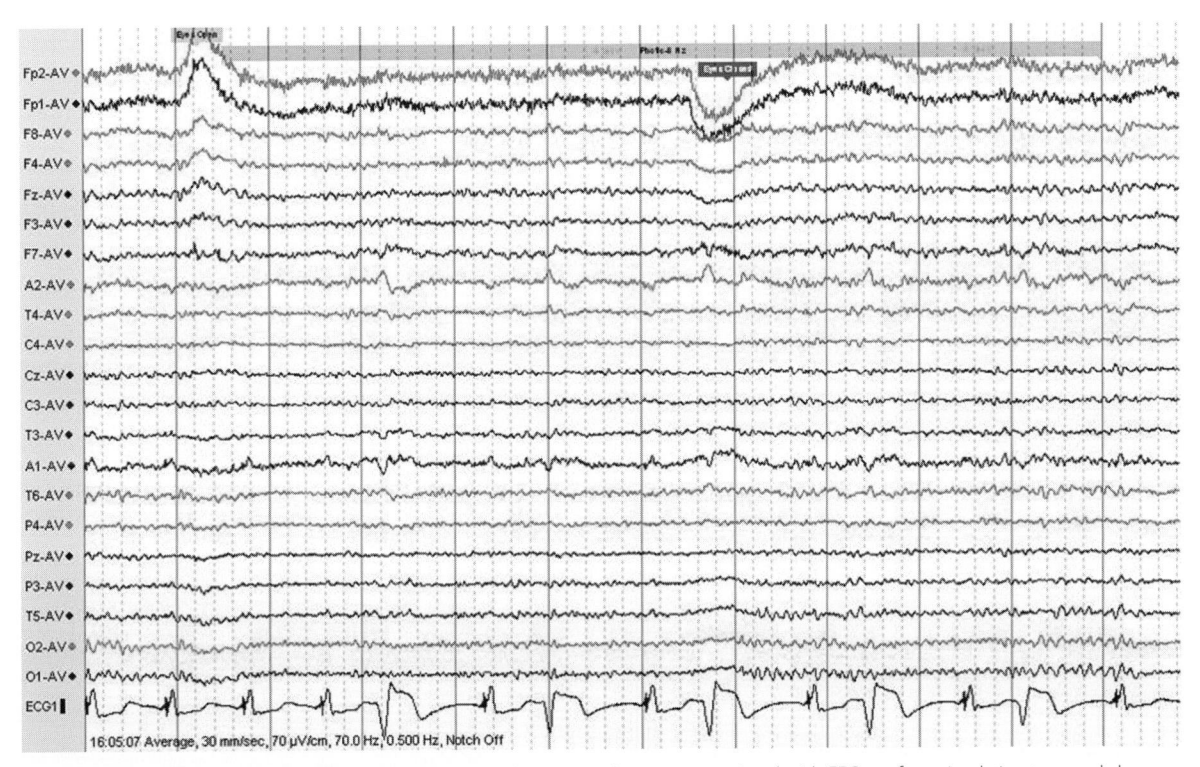

Figure 16.14. Frequent ectopic beats on the ECG. Note that ectopic beats are associated with EEG artefacts simulating temporal sharp waves. 1 s between solid vertical lines.

References

Binnie C, Cooper R, Mauguiere F, Osselton JW. *Clinical Neurophysiology*, vol. 2. Amsterdam: Elsevier; 2003.

Cobb W, Hill D. EEG in subacute progressive encephalitis. *Brain* 1950;73:392–404.

Dawson JR. Cellular inclusions in cerebral lesions of lethargic encephalitis. *Am J Pathol* 1983;9:7–16.

Fisch BJ, Klass DW. The diagnostic specificity of triphasic wave patterns. *Electroencephalogr Clin Neurophysiol* 1988;**70**(1):1–8.

Fisch BJ, Spehlman R. *EEG Primer: Basic Principles of Digital and Analogue EEG*. 2nd edn. Amsterdam: Elsevier; 1999.

Neidemeyer E, Lopes Silva FH. *Electroencephalography – Basic Principles, Clinical Applications and Related Fields*. Philadelphia, PA: Lippincott, William & Wilkins; 2005.

Rennie J, Chorley G, Pressler R, Nguyen Y, Hooper R. Non-expert use of cerebral function monitor for neonatal seizure detection. *Arch. Dis Child Fetal Neonatal Ed* 2004;**89**(1):37–40.

Scheld WM, Whitley RJ, Mama CM. *Infections of the Central Nervous System*. 3rd edn. Philadelphia, PA: Lippincott, Williams & Wilkins; 2004.

Learning objectives

(1) To be able to identify EEG waveforms commonly associated with epilepsy.
(2) To become familiar with EEG abnormalities commonly seen in conditions other than epilepsy and their significance.

Section 2: Classification and diagnosis of epilepsy

Chapter 17: Electroclinical classification of seizures and syndromes

Gonzalo Alarcón

International classifications

Anyone involved in the study of epilepsy will be confronted with two complementary classifications, which are often used in the diagnosis, management and study of epilepsy:

- the classification of epileptic seizures
- the classification of the epilepsy (epilepsy syndromes).

Epileptic seizures are specific, relatively brief, events, which are symptoms of the underlying epilepsy disorder. Each seizure is characterized by its duration and manifestations (the specific feelings, perceptions or actions that the patient has or performs during the seizure) resulting from abnormal neuronal activity. In contrast, the term epilepsy (or epileptic syndrome or epilepsy syndrome) refers to a disease characterized by a chronic propensity to suffer epileptic seizures. Like most chronic conditions, each epilepsy syndrome is characterized by an age of onset, a constellation of symptoms and signs, a prognosis (natural evolution of the disease, response to treatment), presence or absence of genetic predisposition, and specific cause or causes. Seizures are only one element among the constellation of symptoms and signs that characterize each epilepsy syndrome.

Both seizure and epilepsy classifications are necessary. There is not a one-to-one correspondence between seizure type and epilepsy syndrome. Generally, a subject will have one epilepsy syndrome but may show more than one seizure types, and a particular seizure type can be seen in several epileptsy syndromes. Nevertheless, the spectrum of seizure types seen in each epilepsy syndrome is a key element for syndrome classification.

Many classifications of seizures and epilepsies have been developed. Currently the most widely used classifications are those periodically proposed by the International League Against Epilepsy (ILAE).

Classification of seizures

Seizures have traditionally been classified considering clinical and electroencephalographic manifestations into two main groups:

- Focal seizures: focal seizures are those starting in a localized region of the cerebral cortex of one hemisphere (i.e. they arise from a cortical focus). Focal seizures have also been named partial or local seizures.
- Generalized seizures: these arise simultaneously from both cerebral hemispheres, usually involving most cerebral cortex at once.

> **Box 17.1.**
> The term 'partial seizure' can be misleading because it has sometimes been misunderstood as not referring to genuine seizures (only partially being a seizure). Nevertheless, 'partial seizures' are true epileptic seizures (focal seizures).

Focal seizures

The manifestations of focal seizures depend on the area where they originate and on how they spread to other cortical regions.

Focal seizures have been classified according to a number of criteria:

- According to severity: whether consciousness is lost or whether they lead to convulsions
- According to the site of initiation: in the four main lobes (temporal, frontal, parietal or occipital lobe seizures) or in more specific structures (limbic seizures, medial temporal seizures, medial frontal seizures, insular seizures, etc.).

Introduction to Epilepsy ed. Gonzalo Alarcón and Antonio Valentín. Published by CAMBRIDGE UNIVERSITY PRESS.
© Cambridge University Press 2012.

In clinical practice, consciousness is regarded as the ability to appropriately respond to questions or requests, and to remember events happening during the seizure. Impairment of consciousness has traditionally been considered an important feature to classify focal seizures, and was considered a cardinal classification criterion for the 1981 ILAE seizure classification, although its role has been re-assessed in more recent classifications.

Nevertheless, impairment of consciousness is an important feature to evaluate seizure severity for the following reasons:

- Since each hemisphere is able to maintain consciousness independently, impairment of consciousness means that the seizure has spread to both hemispheres.
- Seizures with impairment of consciousness can be considered more severe because patients are more prone to accidents, which can be serious or fatal.
- Loss of consciousness may be associated with severe convulsions that may lead to falls, carpet burns, bruises, fractures, respiratory arrest and convulsive status epilepticus.

Box 17.2. Useful terms to describe seizures and their features

In relation to seizure onset
Pre-ictal: occuring immediately before a seizure.
Ictal: occurring during a seizure.
Post-ictal: occurring shortly after a seizure (within minutes or sometimes hours), while the patient is not fully recovered from a seizure.
Peri-ictal: happening around the time when seizures occur.
Interictal: occurring in the periods without seizures (between seizures).
Catamenial seizures: seizures occurring in relation to menstruation.

To describe convulsive movements
Clonus or clonic movements or clonic convulsions: repetitive and rhythmic brisk contractions of muscle groups which generate fast movement of one or several parts of the body in one direction, usually followed by more gradual muscle relaxation that brings the body parts involved back to the original position before the next brisk contractions occur. Contractions usually occur at around 3 Hz. They can be focal (involving one limb or body parts on one side of the body) or generalized (involving all limbs or limbs on both sides).

Rhythmic: a movement or EEG waveform that repeats at regular intervals.
Dystonia or tonic or dystonic posture: sustained contraction of muscles for seconds, resulting in slow movement of body parts that end up rigid in a sustained posture, usually rather unnatural. Dystonia can be focal or generalized.
Fencing posture: bilateral symmetrical dystonic posture where one arm is extended and the other one is flexed. Often seen in seizures involving the supplementary motor cortex.
Head version: rotation of the head.
Forced head version: slow gradual head rotation where the head ends up in an extreme unnatural position looking to one side over the shoulder. It is due to a tonic contraction of neck muscles. Sometimes there are superimposed small head clonic movements. Forced version has lateralizing value (usually the face looks away from the side of the seizure focus).
Aversive head version: head rotation where the face looks away from the side of the seizure focus.
Myoclonus, myoclonia or myoclonic jerk: isolated sudden jerk of a body part due to a brisk contraction of a number of muscles lasting for <200 ms.

To describe speech disturbance
Aphasia: inability to speak or understand speech because of speech cortex dysfunction.
Dysphasia: impaired communication, involving language without dysfunction of the relevant primary motor or sensory pathways, manifested by impaired comprehension, anomia or difficulty in naming, paraphasic errors or a combination of these.
Post-ictal dysphasia: dysphasia occurring immediately after a seizure. It has lateralizing power, being more common in seizures arising from the dominant hemisphere for speech.
Speech arrest: sudden and temporary cessation of ongoing speech.

To describe other features
Dialeptic seizures: seizures where the predominant ictal features are alteration of consciousness, staring and no or minimal motor activity.
Hypermotor seizures: seizures dominated by bizarre, frenetic, frantic, agitated and dramatic automatisms (violent thrashing and kicking).
For a more detailed description of terms see the ILAE Commission report (Berg et al., 2010).

Depending on the functional relevance of the cortex initiating the seizure and its degree of spread, during focal seizures consciousness can be either preserved throughout the seizure, impaired from the start or initially preserved and then lost.

Focal seizures with preserved consciousness ('simple partial seizures' according to the 1981 ILAE seizure classification)

Focal seizures with preserved consciousness are seizures that remain localized and involve functionally relevant areas (visual, olfactory, auditory, somatosensory, primary motor or speech areas, hippocampus, amygdala). They can show the following manifestations, depending on the areas involved:

Motor signs

Abnormal movements can be seen depending on the motor areas involved:

- Primary motor cortex: unilateral clonic movements or tonic posturing, most commonly affecting one hand or one side of the face, since these are the body parts with largest cortical representation. Occasionally, motor seizures may propagate to neighbouring cortical areas, sequentially affecting neighbouring body parts (for instance, starting in the hand, then involving the forearm, arm, same side of the face). This phenomenon is called a 'Jacksonian march' (after Hughlings Jackson, who first described it).
- Prefrontal cortex: aversive head turning (towards the side opposite the hemisphere originating the seizure), fencing posture.
- Speech areas: aphasia, dysphasia.

Sensory symptoms

Simple sensations depend on the sensory areas involved:

- Somatosensory cortex: tingling, numbness, less frequently pain or burning sensation. These sensations most commonly affect one hand or one side of the face, since these are the body parts with the largest cortical representation.
- Visual cortex: flashing lights, simple geometrical figures such as circles, ovals or spots, and sometimes more complex figures are reported. They are seen in the visual field contralateral to the hemisphere affected.
- Auditory cortex: hearing sounds, melodies or sentences.
- Olfactory or gustatory cortex: perceiving smells (often putrid or burnt) or taste (often metallic). Sometimes, ictal smell or taste is indescribable.
- Insula and parietal lobe: vertiginous sensation.

Autonomic symptoms and signs

- Epigastric sensation: the commonest epileptic aura
- Pallor
- Flushing
- Sweating
- Pupillary dilatation
- Piloerection
- Changes in heart rate: tachycardia, bradycardia and asystole
- Changes in respiratory rate
- Erection
- Urination
- Defecation

Psychic symptoms

- Memory disturbances: flashbacks, déjà vu (sensation as if a new experience has been experienced before), jamais vu (sense of a familiar experience seeming novel or unfamiliar), panoramic vision (rapid recollection of episodes from the patient's past experience).
- Affective symptoms: fear, terror, anger, rage, depression, extreme pleasure or displeasure.
- Cognitive disturbances: forced thinking, dreamy states, distortion of time, sensations of unreality, detachment and depersonalization.
- Illusions: this term refers to an alteration of an actual perception. Illusions in seizures include distortions of object size (micropsia, macropsia), distortions of distance, distortions of sounds (microacusia, macroacusia) and altered perception of size or weight of a limb.
- Structured hallucinations: this term refers to the experience of perceptions not corresponding to external stimuli. Hallucinations seen during seizures include hearing music or seeing scenes which are not real.

> The terms aura or warning are often used to describe the subjective experience preceding loss of consciousness, or sometimes occurring on their own. Auras and warnings are very localized focal seizures that have not spread far enough to affect consciousness.

Focal seizures with impairment of consciousness

If focal seizures propagate to both hemispheres, consciousness will be impaired or lost. The patient will be unresponsive or only partially responsive and have no recollection of what is happening. After the seizure, some patients might not even be aware that they had a seizure.

In focal seizures, impairment of consciousness can be the first clinical symptom (if it arises from a cortical area that is not very functionally relevant, and symptoms only occur after spreading to both hemispheres) or consciousness may initially be preserved (showing the symptoms and signs described in the previous section) to be impaired when the seizure becomes bilateral.

Manifestations of seizures with impaired consciousness

- Patient might stare and appear distant.
- Patient might appear distant and carry out normal but apparently purposeless movements called 'automatisms', which are classified into two categories:
  - De novo automatisms: actions that appear with the seizure. They can be spontaneous (such as chewing, swallowing, lip smacking, walking, running, saying stereotyped sentences, looking around, fidgeting, fiddling or fumbling with things, clapping, carrying out bicycling movements in the air, taking clothes off), or they may be actions carried out as a response to an external stimulus occurring during the seizure (reactive mechanisms, such as pushing off an approaching observer, drinking from a nearby cup, withdrawing a limb held by an observer, etc.).
  - Perseverative automatisms: continuation of any complex activity initiated prior to loss of consciousness such as to continue eating with a spoon, chewing, carry on walking, carry on sewing or passing pages, etc.
- Patient might suffer convulsions: these seizures are often called 'tonic-clonic' seizures, secondarily generalized seizures or 'grand mal' seizures. Convulsions usually start with some or all limbs and head becoming rigid for a few seconds (tonic phase) often associated with uttering grunting noises or a scream ('the epileptic cry'). This is usually followed by repetitive contractions of all limbs and head (clonic phase) at about 3 Hz, where the body parts jerk fast and more slowly recover the initial position before jerking again. Convulsions can be preceded by forced head version. Convulsive movements can start earlier or be more pronounced on the body side contralateral to seizure focus. Convulsive seizures can be followed by paralysis or paresis (weakness) contralateral to the seizure focus (Todd's paralysis). The patient might be incontinent or bite his/her tongue (particularly the side of the tongue) or the internal wall of the cheek during convulsive seizures.

According to the 1981 ILAE Classification, the first two groups (patient staring and/or showing automatisms) are considered as 'complex partial' seizures, and the third group as 'secondarily generalized' seizures. Brief complex partial seizures can resemble absence seizures (see Box 17.5).

> **Box 17.3. Cautionary note!**
> The terms complex partial seizures, temporal lobe seizures and psychomotor seizures are often used as synonyms. This is not correct. Although the most frequent source of complex partial seizures is the temporal lobe, it is not the only one, as complex partial seizures can arise from any lobe. The term psychomotor seizure is now obsolete.

Other focal seizures

Gelastic seizures: gelastic seizures are those that include laughter as one of their clinical manifestations. Laughter is usually a short manifestation (<30 s). Laughter can be a manifestation of several seizure types such as partial seizures with motor symptoms, myoclonic seizures, axial tonic seizures, spasms, generalized convulsive seizures and petit mal absences. Gelastic seizures have been observed mainly in association with hypothalamic hamartomas, but also in temporal and frontal lobe lesions as well as in metabolic conditions (Niemann-Pick disease type C).

Focal myoclonias: they consist of an isolated, sudden, fast, brief (<200 ms) contraction affecting one muscle group.

Hemiclonic seizures: consisting of clonic movements restricted to most of one side (right or left).

Classification of focal seizures according to the site of origin

Focal seizures can be classified according to the site of initiation. The site of onset can be ascertained in many focal seizures with preserved consciousness by the motor manifestations or other symptoms experienced by the patient (see above 'Focal seizures with preserved consciousness'). Focal seizures from any location can lead to impairment of consciousness and/or convulsions.

Temporal lobe seizures tend to be associated with an epigastric sensation, memory disturbances (most commonly déjà vu), staring, oroalimentary automatisms (manual automatisms, fidgeting, fumbling with objects) unilateral dystonia and sometimes convulsions. If unilateral, automatisms tend to be ipsilateral to seizure onset and dystonia contralateral. They last for about 1 minute, ending with post-ictal confusion and gradual recovery.

Frontal lobe seizures are usually brief, with prominent bizarre motor or gestural automatisms (limb thrashing, kicking, grimacing), sometimes asymmetrical tonic postures, often occurring in clusters during sleep and with little post-ictal confusion unless they become secondarily generalized.

Insular seizures: tend to be associated with visceral sensations, retching, belching or vomiting, and cardiac arrhythmias.

Parietal seizures: tend to show contralateral somatosensory auras (tingling, numbness, pain, burning or cold sensations), distortions of body image.

Occipital lobe seizures tend to start with blinking and/or visual symptoms (flashing lights, shades, circles, lines) seen on the hemifield contralateral to the side of seizure onset.

Generalized seizures

Generalized seizures are those arising simultaneously from both cerebral hemispheres, usually from most of the cerebral cortex at once. Consequently, generalized seizures have the following characteristics:

- Consciousness is lost from the outset.
- There is no early stage where consciousness is preserved: there is no specific aura or warning to the seizures.
- There are no consistent focal features either clinically or on the ictal EEG: convulsions and muscle contractions do not consistently start on one side, there are no warnings, there is no consistent head rotation to the same side, and there are not consistent earlier EEG changes on one hemisphere compared to the other.

There are several types of generalized seizures.

Generalized tonic-clonic seizures: tonic-clonic seizures similar to those described above under focal seizures with impairment of consciousness but with no consistent focal components (movements are symmetrical from the start and if there is head rotation, it does not occur consistently to the same side).

Clonic seizures: they are similar to tonic-clonic seizures but without an initial tonic phase. There are no focal features.

Tonic seizures: the patient's limbs and neck suddenly go rigid for a few seconds and, if standing, the patient might fall backwards or forwards.

Atonic seizures: brief attacks consisting of a sudden loss of muscle tone causing the patient to suddenly nod the head or fall to the floor. Atonic seizures have previously been named 'akinetic' or 'astatic' seizures.

> **Box 17.4. Drop attacks**
>
> The term 'drop attack' is applied to seizures where patients suddenly fall to the ground and frequently injure themselves. If epileptic, they are usually tonic or atonic seizures. Patients are often at risk from injury, especially to head and face, and may require protective helmets to be worn permanently while standing or sitting.

Spasms: these consist of brief massive contractions of axial muscles that can provoke flexion or extension of the trunk. Each spasm lasts for a fraction of a second, but can occur in clusters of 5–50, several clusters each day, often on awakening. They may be symmetrical or asymmetrical, with lateral deviation of the eyes or head, or involving only one side of the body. Children often cry after each spasm. Spasms tend to occur between the age of 3 and 12 months, and are associated with learning difficulties, developmental delay and hypsarrhythmia on the EEG (West syndrome). Spasms have been sub-classified into flexor spasms, extensor spasms or flexor-extensor spasms (neck and arms flex, but legs extend). Flexor spasms have also been called 'salaam convulsions' or 'salaam attacks'.

Absence (petit mal) seizures: characterized by a period of unresponsiveness lasting for several seconds. Absences can be associated with a variety of clinical phenomena – staring, cessation of ongoing activities and speech, eyelid flutter, mild automatisms, mild clonic movements, decreased postural tone without fall (mild atonic components), mild tonic components, mild autonomic components (incontinence, pupil dilatation, pallor, flushing, tachycardia, blood pressure changes). Automatisms are mild, usually consisting of small peri-oral movements or finger fiddling and are more likely in prolonged episodes. Simple absences are those showing only impairment of consciousness. With regard to EEG features, absence seizures have been sub-classified into typical and atypical:

- Typical absences: show generalized spike-and-wave activity at 2.5–3.5 Hz. Spikes are rather sharp.
- Atypical absences: show generalized spike-and-wave activity at <2.5 Hz. Spikes are usually blunter than in typical absences.

Myoclonic absence seizures: consisting of bilateral rhythmic clonic jerks or brief tonic contractions. Jerks mainly involve muscles of the shoulders, arms and legs. Facial muscles are less commonly involved. When facial myoclonias occur, they are more evident around the chin and mouth, whereas eyelid twitching is typically absent or rare. The jerks and tonic contractions may be symmetrical or predominant on one side, causing turning of the head and body.

Eyelid myoclonia with absences: brief episodes of marked jerking of the eyelids with upwards deviation of the eyes, associated with a generalized discharge of spike-wave occurring on eye closure. All patients are photosensitive. Absence seizures are induced by changes in light associated with eyelid jerking or closure, which can be voluntary, involuntary or reflex. The majority of the seizures are induced immediately after closure of the eyes in the presence of light. Eye closure in total darkness is ineffective to induce seizures. Intermittent photic stimulation potentiates the effect of eye closure and is capable of inducing seizures when eyes are open or closed. Eyelid myclonia without prominent absences may occur particularly in adult patients.

> **Box 17.5. Cautionary note!**
> Because staring and automatisms can be seen in absence and complex partial seizures, it can be difficult to distinguish between them on clinical grounds (the ictal EEG is distinctly different):
>
> - Absence seizures are brief, usually lasting for less than 10 s and rarely for longer than 45 s, whereas complex partial seizure often last for longer than 1 min.
> - Absence seizures have a sudden onset, without warning, whereas complex partial seizures may have a warning.
> - In absence seizures, recovery of consciousness is also sudden, without post-ictal confusion, whereas complex partial seizures are often followed by a variable period of confusion sometimes lasting for several minutes.

Generalized myoclonic seizures (jerks) or generalized myoclonias (see also Chapter 29: 'Epilepsy and myoclonus'): generalized myoclonic seizures consist of an isolated, sudden, fast, brief (<200 ms) and symmetrical muscle contraction, usually involving the arms and neck. Hands and arms suddenly flex upwards while head and neck usually flex down. Sometimes there are two or three superimposed contractions within a few hundreds of milliseconds. Myoclonias are essentially isolated events, and repetitive rhythmic contractions, usually several per second, lasting for several seconds, can be considered 'clonus' or 'clonic convulsions' (see generalized tonic-clonic seizures).

Negative myoclonus: sudden and abrupt interruption of muscular activity. The EMG shows a brief (< 500 ms) silent period, not preceded by enhancement of EMG activity (i.e. not preceded by a myoclonia). Epileptic negative myoclonus is time-locked to a spike on the EEG, without evidence of a previous myoclonia. Clinically, negative myoclonus appears as a shock-like involuntary jerky movement due to a sudden brief interruption of muscular activity and can resemble real (positive) myoclonus.

Reflex seizures: reflex seizures are those triggered by specific stimuli. Stimuli that can trigger seizures include visual stimuli (flashing lights, particularly at around 18–20 Hz; and geometrical patterns, particularly stripes), thinking, music, eating, praxis, somatosensory stimulation, propioceptive stimuli, reading, hot water and startle.

> **Box 17.6. Variations of myoclonic seizures**
>
> - Myoclonic seizures may not always be truly generalized. Sometimes they are bilateral and symmetrical but do not affect all muscles. For instance, they may affect only both shoulders. Such symmetrical but not generalized myoclonic jerks are sometimes called segmental myoclonus.
> - Some patients have multiple, nearly continuous, small myoclonic jerks, affecting only a few muscles at a time, often unilaterally, involving different muscles one after another. Eventually most muscles will jerk, but not simultaneously. This is sometimes called migratory myoclonus, multifocal myoclonus, fragmentary myoclonus or polymyoclonus.
> - Myoclonic jerks can occur immediately preceding, during or at the end of an atonic seizure (myoclonic-astatic seizures).
> - Myoclonic jerks may occur in conditions other than epilepsy. They can arise from the brainstem (subcortical myoclonus) or from the spinal cord (spinal myoclonus).
> - Myoclonic seizures should be distinguished from spasms and tonic seizures (Figure 17.1)
> - Normal myoclonus occurs in sleep (Chapter 49: 'Sleep disorders simulating epilepsy.

EEG manifestations of seizures

EEG changes occurring during seizures can be very important to establish whether seizures are focal or generalized, as well as to identify certain seizure types, since EEG characteristics during seizures can be specific. The EEG changes that can be seen during different seizure types are described in Chapter 18.

Evolution of ILAE classifications of seizures

The ILAE has periodically published recommendations on seizure classifications since 1960. Table 17.1 broadly compares the most commonly used classifications from 1981 and 2001 classifications. A new very recent classification is now under evaluation (Berg *et al.*, 2010).

The classification of generalized seizures has essentially changed little, apart from the addition of spasms and reflex seizures.

However, the classification of focal seizures has changed more substantially. The 2001 proposal re-coined the term 'focal' to replace 'partial'. In addition, whereas in 1981 non-convulsive focal seizures were classified into simple (with preservation of consciousness) and complex (with impairment of consciousness), in the 2001 classification they were largely grouped according to whether symptoms were motor or sensory.

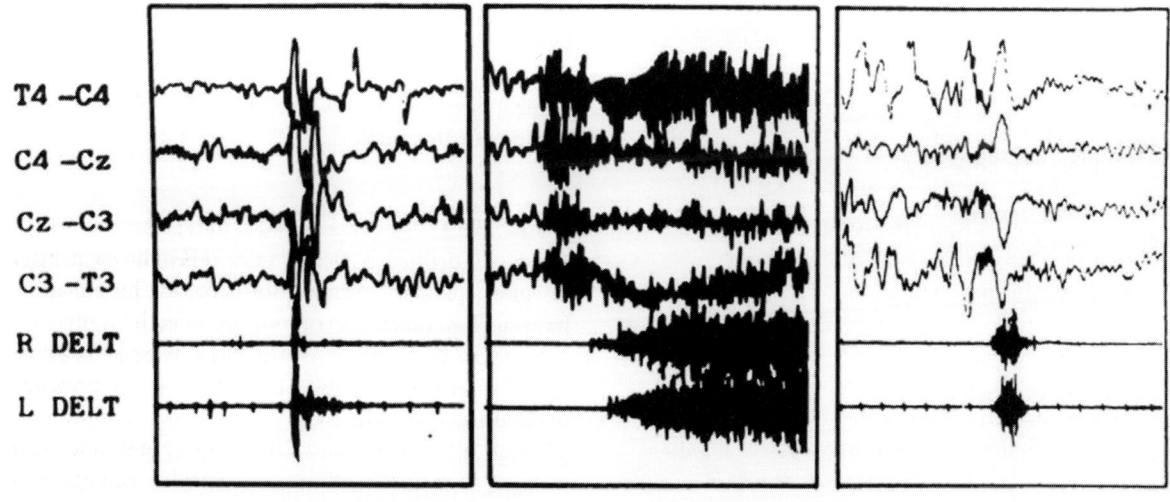

Figure 17.1. Polygraphic recording of a myoclonic seizure, a tonic seizure and a spasm. The top four channels correspond to EEG recordings and the bottom two channels correspond to right and left deltoid muscle activity (electromyogram or EMG). Note that the myoclonic jerk (left) consists of a brief burst of muscle activity lasting for less than 200 ms followed by a tail of less intense activity, whereas the spasm (right) has a more gradual build up and decay of EMG activity lasting for 1–2 s and showing a characteristic rhomboidal morphology. The tonic seizure (centre) shows more sustained EMG activity lasting for several seconds (reproduced with permission from Vigevano *et al.*, Neurophysiology of spasms. *Brain Dev* 2001;23:467–72, Figure 2.3).

Section 2: Classification and diagnosis of epilepsy

Table 17.1. Approximate equivalence of the self-limited seizure types described in the two most recent ILAE seizure classifications

ILAE Classification (1981)	ILAE Classification (2001)
Generalized seizures	
Absence seizures: • With impairment of consciousness only • With mild clonic components • With atonic components • With tonic components • With automatisms	Typical absence seizures Atypical absence seizures Myoclonic absence seizures
Atonic seizures	Atonic seizures
Tonic seizures	Tonic seizures
Tonic-clonic seizures	Tonic-clonic seizures
Clonic seizures	Clonic seizures: • With tonic features • Without tonic features
Myoclonic seizures	Myoclonic seizures Myoclonic atonic seizures Negative myoclonus
Not defined	Spasms
Not defined	Eyelid myoclonia: • With absences • Without absences
Not defined	Reflex seizures in generalized epilepsy syndromes
Focal (partial, local) seizures	
Simple partial seizures (with no impairment of consciousness)	Focal sensory seizures: • With elementary sensory symptoms • With experiential sensory symptoms • Focal motor seizures • With elementary clonic motor signs • With asymmetrical tonic motor seizures (e.g. supplementary motor seizures) • With typical (temporal lobe) automatisms (e.g., mesial temporal lobe seizures) • With hyperkinetic automatisms • With focal negative myoclonus • With inhibitory motor seizures • Gelastic seizures • Hemiclonic seizures
Secondarily generalized seizures	Secondarily generalized seizures
Not defined	Reflex seizures in focal epilepsy seizures

With the 2001 classification, the meaning of some terms has changed. For instance, the term 'focal motor seizure' traditionally referred to seizures consisting of focal convulsions thought to arise from selective involvement of the primary motor cortex, usually showing clonic convulsions involving hand or face. In the 2001 classification, the term 'focal motor seizure' has a wider meaning, referring to focal seizures with any movement, including automatisms. The 1981 classification did not really attempt to classify reflex seizures or status epilepticus (apart from epilepsia partialis continua). In contrast, the 2001 classification includes a detailed classification of reflex seizures and status epilepticus (the so-called 'continuous seizure types').

The 1981 classification is still routinely used in clinical practice, and will be used throughout some sections of this book.

Classification of the epilepsies

Epilepsy is defined as a long-lasting (chronic) propensity to suffer epileptic seizures. Normally, the patient must have suffered more than one seizure to establish that he/she suffers from epilepsy. The susceptibility to suffer epileptic seizures (epilepsy) can be caused by a variety of circumstances, which can be grouped into two:

- Brain lesions. Nearly any type of brain lesions can cause epilepsy, including stroke, scarring after head injury, brain tumours, anoxia, metabolic disorders, brain infections, etc. The epilepsies

Chapter 17: Electroclinical classification of seizures and syndromes

Table 17.2. General features of idiopathic and symptomatic epilepsies

	Idiopathic	Symptomatic
Development	Normal	Normal or abnormal
Age of onset	Infancy, childhood, early adulthood	Any time, depending on onset of brain insult
Intelligence and memory	Normal	Learning difficulties or subtle deficits (e.g., low verbal IQ) or normal, depending on extent and location of underlying brain damage
EEG background activity	Normal	Abnormal or normal
Structural neuroimaging	Normal	Abnormal or normal
Family history	Frequent	Weak or none

caused by such lesions are called 'symptomatic' epilepsies, as they are a symptom of the underlying lesion. Previously, such epilepsies were called 'secondary' epilepsies as they were secondary to brain lesions.

- Genetic predisposition with no evidence of brain damage or lesions. It appears that some families or individuals can have a particularly low threshold to suffer epileptic seizures without having any underlying brain lesion. Such epilepsies occurring without evidence of brain damage are called 'idiopathic' epilepsies (previously called 'primary'). The cause of idiopathic epilepsies is supposed to be genetic, but too subtle to show brain damage. Consequently patients with idiopathic epilepsies tend to have normal development, normal intelligence, normal memory, normal neurological function, normal imaging and normal EEG background activity. Nevertheless, if the epilepsy is severe or has early onset, it can have an adverse impact on development or function.

There is often difficulty in classifying patients where there is no direct evidence of structural brain abnormalities. A common example is patients with delayed milestones, learning difficulties and diffusely slowed EEG background, with normal neuroimaging and no clear history of a brain injury. Nevertheless, the presence of developmental delay, learning difficulties and diffusely slowed EEG background strongly suggests that these patients have suffered some form of diffuse brain damage. Thus, these patients cannot be classified as idiopathic, or as symptomatic (there is no clear underlying lesion of which epilepsy could be a symptom). The ILAE recommends the term 'presumed symptomatic' for these patients (previously called cryptogenic). Conceptually and for management purposes, presumed symptomatic epilepsies are identical to symptomatic epilepsies. Presumed symptomatic epilepsies are probably symptomatic epilepsies where our present diagnostic methods are not sensitive enough to find a specific cause.

If brain lesions in symptomatic epilepsies are localized, their impact on brain function might be undetectable, subtle, or might only become evident on performance of neuropsychological tests. For instance, a right-handed patient with left mesial temporal sclerosis might show normal speech during everyday activities or perhaps complain of difficulties in remembering some names. However, on formal neuropsychological testing, his verbal memory or IQ might be much lower than his non-verbal memory or performance IQ. In contrast, early massive diffuse brain damage (for instance, after perinatal hypoxia) usually manifests as developmental delay and learning difficulties.

In addition to establishing whether epilepsy is idiopathic or symptomatic, it is important to determine whether the seizures are focal or generalized. Epilepsies with focal seizures are called focal epilepsies and result from a focal abnormality. In contrast, epilepsies presenting generalized seizures are called generalized epilepsies and usually result from an abnormality affecting most cortex on both hemispheres. Generalized seizures occur either because there is diffuse brain damage (symptomatic generalized epilepsies), or because there is a generalized increase in cortical excitability due to abnormal interactions between cortex and thalamus (idiopathic generalized epilepsies).

Focal epilepsies have also been called local, partial, and localization-related epilepsies.

Section 2: Classification and diagnosis of epilepsy

Following the concepts above, the epilepsies can be classified into four types, according to whether they are symptomatic, idiopathic, focal, or generalized:
- idiopathic focal epilepsies,
- idiopathic generalized epilepsies,
- symptomatic focal epilepsies
- symptomatic generalized epilepsies.

Specific syndromes have been defined within each group (see Chapter 18). Table 17.3 summarizes the main characteristics and examples of each group.

Practical examples for epilepsy classification

- A patient having seizures caused by left mesial temporal sclerosis: symptomatic focal epilepsy.
- A patient having seizures caused by a stroke: symptomatic focal epilepsy.
- Patients with multiple seizure types and learning difficulties as a result of a metabolic brain disease with an autosomal recessive inheritance: probably symptomatic generalized epilepsy.
- A patient having multiple angiomas on both hemispheres with seizures arising only from an angioma located on the right frontal lobe: symptomatic focal epilepsy.
- A patient with focal cortical dysplasia on MRI who has never had a seizure: not epilepsy of any type.
- Patients with generalized and focal seizures and learning difficulties: probably symptomatic generalized epilepsy.
- Patients with infrequent focal seizures of early onset, normal development and positive family history: probably idiopathic focal epilepsy.
- Patients with generalized seizures, generalized discharges on the EEG, normal development and normal MRI: probably idiopathic generalized epilepsy.

Table 17.3. The epilepsies at a glance

2001	Idiopathic		(Presumed) symptomatic
1989	Idiopathic		Cryptogenic/Symptomatic
1970	Primary		Secondary
	Aetiology unknown or genetic		Presumed or known pathology
Generalized	Name: idiopathic generalized Pathophysiology: susceptibility to generalized seizures without brain damage or lesions EEG findings: • Generalized spike-wave • Normal background Syndrome examples: • childhood/juvenile absence • juvenile myoclonic • TC on awakening		Name: (presumed) symptomatic generalized Pathophysiology: susceptibility to generalized seizures caused by diffuse (generalized) brain damage EEG findings: • Generalized or multifocal discharges • Diffusely abnormal background Syndrome examples: • West syndrome • Lennox-Gastaut syndrome
Partial	Name: idiopathic focal Pathophysiology: susceptibility to focal seizures without brain damage or lesions EEG findings: • Focal spike-and-wave • Normal background Syndrome examples: • Benign epilepsy of childhood: rolandic, occipital, etc. • Primary reading epilepsy • Autosomal dominant nocturnal frontal lobe epilepsy		Name: focal epilepsy Pathophysiology: susceptibility to focal seizures caused by focal brain damage or lesions EEG findings: • Focal spike-and-wave • Focal background abnormality Syndrome examples: • Temporal, frontal, occipital lobe epilepsies

Relevance of epilepsy classification

Although a patient might have several seizure types, he/she will generally have only one type of epilepsy.

It is important to establish the type of epilepsy that a patient has because different types of epilepsies have different prognoses in terms of patient development, natural evolution of the seizures, treatment choices, seizure response to treatment, patient integration in society and genetic counselling.

Idiopathic epilepsies tend to have good prognosis, with no developmental delay. There is often good response to medical treatment, and seizures in some syndromes may disappear with age. Resective surgical treatment is not indicated, since there is no underlying structural abnormality to remove and patients may grow out of their seizures.

Symptomatic generalized epilepsies have poor prognosis: seizures tend to continue throughout life, with poor response to treatment, and resective surgery is not indicated since most of the brain might be structurally abnormal.

Symptomatic focal epilepsies may or may not respond to medical treatment and, if not, they may benefit from resective surgery.

Within the four broad groups of epilepsies already described, there are several subtypes of epilepsies – the so-called epileptic (epilepsy) syndromes. It is important to identify the epilepsy syndrome because different syndromes have different prognoses and response to treatment. Like any medical syndrome, epilepsy syndromes are characterized by a constellation of symptoms and signs that tend to occur together.

The criteria used to characterize epileptic syndromes are the following:

- presence of family history of epilepsy
- patient development (milestones)
- age of onset of seizures
- seizure type(s)
- patient intelligence and memory function
- interictal EEG:
  - EEG background abnormalities
  - EEG paroxysmal abnormalities (interictal epileptiform discharges)
- ictal EEG (not always available)
- neuroimaging
- aetiology.

Detailed descriptions and summaries of the specific epileptic syndromes can be found in the chapters below and in the following textbooks: Alarcón *et al.*, 2009; Panayiotopoulos, 2007.

Future perspectives

The available classifications of epilepsy rely on a few cornerstone concepts (loss vs preservation of consciousness, idiopathic vs symptomatic, focal vs generalized). Terminology is regularly revised, which often confuses the non-epileptologist physician. Although the classifications are described as 'electroclinical' the role of the EEG requires further clarification in many syndromes. The basic concepts need revision in the light of recent advances in genetics and neuroimaging which have questioned the distinction between idiopathic and symptomatic, and between focal and generalized. The role of genetic findings in classification needs to be established.

The 1981 and 1989 ILAE classifications rely heavily on distinction between generalized, focal and secondarily generalized epileptogenesis. More recently, the ILAE has effectively recommended abandoning attempts at such rigorous classification (Berg *et al.*, 2010). Some credit may be claimed from evidence of some focal features in epileptogenesis seen in idiopathic generalized epilepsies, such as the following:

- Cortical dysgenesis and local abnormalities on functional imaging in patients diagnosed with idiopathic generalized epilepsy (Meencke and Janz, 1984),
- The postulated diffuse cortical hyperexcitability in IGE is not necessarily uniform.
- Spontaneous epileptogenesis:
  - EEG and seizure semiology indicate asymmetric or focal cortical activation.
  - Focal interictal discharges in idiopathic generalized epilepsy, e.g. 34% in juvenile myoclonic epilepsy (Obeid and Panayiotopoulos, 1988).
  - High prevalence (30–40%) of focal spikes and regional accentuation of generalized spike-and-wave in idiopathic generalized epilepsy (Koutroumanidis and Smith, 2005).
- Reflex epileptogenesis is common:
  - Specific activities, sensory, motor or cognitive, can selectively activate specific cortical regions. Such activation can produce focal discharges or partial seizures, which may generalize.

- Seizure semiology indicating asymmetric or focal cortical activation.
  - Versive or rotary seizures are seen in juvenile myoclonic epilepsy.
  - Versive movements and focal clonic activity in absences (So *et al.*, 1984).
  - Cranio-caudal march in absences (Stefan, 1983).
  - Seizure activation by moving a specific body part in juvenile myoclonic epilepsy.

Other classifications

Since 1989, there have been a number of proposed classifications and diagnostic schemes (Engel, 2001; Berg *et al.*, 2010). They have emphasized the shortcomings in the physiological distinction between simple and complex, and between partial and generalized seizures. Recently, prognosis has been suggested as the main criterion to distinguish between idiopathic and symptomatic epilepsies. Recent proposals have highlighted the rich semiological variability of seizures and epilepsies, essentially approaching classification as an evolving database. Nevertheless, the main taxonomical categories have changed little.

A particularly novel approach was suggested by The Task Force of the ILAE as a diagnostic scheme intended to provide the basis for a standardized description of individual patients according to five levels, or axes (Engel, 2001). The axes are organized to facilitate a logical approach to determine diagnostic studies and therapeutic strategies to be undertaken:

- Axis 1 consists of a description of the ictal semiology, using a standardized Glossary of Descriptive Terminology.
- Axis 2 is the epileptic seizure type, or types, experienced by the patient, derived from a list of accepted seizure types which represent diagnostic entities with etiological, therapeutic and/or prognostic implications.
- Axis 3 is the syndromic diagnosis derived from a list of accepted epilepsy syndromes, although it is understood that a syndromic diagnosis may not always be possible.
- Axis 4 will specify etiology when this is known.
- Axis 5 is an optional designation of the degree of impairment caused by the epileptic condition.

References

Alarcón G, Nashef L, Cross H, Nightingale J, Richardson S Epilepsy. In *Oxford Specialist Handbooks in Neurology*, pp. 62–130. Oxford: Oxford University Press; 2009.

Berg AT, Berkovic SF, Brodie MJ, *et al*. Revised terminology and concepts for organization of seizures and epilepsies: report of the ILAE Commission on Classification and Terminology, 2005–2009. *Epilepsia* 2010;**51**:676–85.

Commission on Classification and Terminology on the International League Against Epilepsy. Proposal for Revised Clinical and Electroencephalographic Classification of Epileptic Seizures. *Epilepsia* 1981;**22**:489–501.

Engel J Jr. ILAE Commission Report. A proposed diagnostic scheme for people with epileptic seizures and with epilepsy: Report of the ILAE Task Force on Classification and Terminology. *Epilepsia* 2001;**42**;796–803.

Koutroumanidis M, Smith S. Use and abuse of EEG in the diagnosis of idiopathic generalized epilepsies. *Epilepsia* 2005;**46**(Suppl. 9):96–107.

Lüders HO, Noachtar S (eds). *Epileptic Seizures. Pathophysiology and Clinical Semiology*. New York: Churchill Livingstone; 2000.

Meencke HJ, Janz D. Neuropathological findings in primary generalized epilepsy: a study of eight cases. *Epilepsia* 1984;**25**:8–21.

Obeid T, Panayiotopoulos CP. Juvenile myoclonic epilepsy: a study in Saudi Arabia. *Epilepsia* 1988;**29**(3):280–2.

Panayiotopoulos CP. *A Clinical Guide to Epileptic Syndromes and their Treatment*. 2nd edn. London: Springer; 2007.

So EL, King DW, Murvin AJ. Misdiagnosis of complex absence seizures. *Arch Neurol* 1984;**41**:640–1.

Stefan H. Epileptic absences. Studies on the structure, pathophysiology and clinical course of the seizure. *Fortschr Med* 1983;**101**(21):996–8.

Learning objectives

(1) To understand the purpose and advantages of having classifications in medicine.
(2) To understand the underlying principles of the different classifications.
(3) To be aware of the terms and categories of the different classifications.
(4) To understand and be able to discuss the advantages, disadvantages and strong and weak points of the different classifications.

Section 2 Classification and diagnosis of epilepsy

Chapter 18

Clinical use of EEG in epilepsy

Gonzalo Alarcón

At present, the most widespread method to confirm the diagnosis of epilepsy is the electroencephalogram (EEG) recorded on the scalp. Characteristic ictal activity shown in the EEG can be considered as the pathognomonic diagnostic feature of epilepsy. However, as seizures are relatively infrequent, the diagnosis of epilepsy on most outpatient EEG recordings is based on interictal activity.

The value of interictal EEG in epilepsy
Background activity

- Patients with idiopathic epilepsy have normal background activity (apart from medication-induced changes; see below) as there is no underlying structural abnormality.
- Focal slowing of the background activity is often seen in focal epilepsy, suggesting a structural abnormality.
- Diffuse slowing is characteristic of symptomatic generalized epilepsy due to an underlying organic pathology.
- Diffuse slowing of the background activity can be induced by metabolic abnormalities and medication, including antiepileptic drugs (AEDs). Changes induced by AEDs are dose-related and are generally mild if no clinical signs of toxicity are present. AED doses should be considered during the interpretation of the EEG, as diffuse slowing of the EEG background can wrongly suggest symptomatic generalized epilepsy.
- An increase in fast rhythms (beta activity) may also be seen with some AEDs, particularly barbiturates and benzodiazepines.
- Examples of focal and generalized slowing of the background activity can be seen in Figures 18.1 to 18.8.

Paroxysmal abnormalities in epilepsy

Paroxysmal abnormalities during the interictal period are generated by sudden synchronicity of neurons occurring for periods of 50–500 ms. They are classified as:

- **S**harp waves: triangular waves with a duration longer than 70 ms.
- Spikes: sharper triangular waves shorter than 70 ms.
- Polyspikes: runs of spikes lasting for several hundreds of milliseconds, sometimes followed by a slow wave (polyspike-and-wave).
- Spike-and-wave discharges: spikes or sharp waves followed by a slow wave of opposite polarity lasting for longer than 300 ms.

Spikes, polyspikes and spike-and-wave discharges are generically called epileptiform discharges because they tend to occur (although not exclusively) in patients with epilepsy.

Sharp waves can often be seen in conditions other than epilepsy (old age, haemorrhage, infarcts, tumours, encephalitis, etc.). Examples of focal and generalized epileptiform discharges can be seen in Figures 18.2 to 18.8.

Sensitivity of the EEG: epileptiform discharges are the most reliable EEG abnormality for the diagnoses of epilepsy. In general,

- 55% of patients with epilepsy will show epileptiform discharges in a standard awake interictal EEG.

> **Box 18.1.** First commandment in EEG interpretation
>
> 'The EEG should always be interpreted in the context of a detailed clinical history and knowledge of concomitant medication, patient's age and state of awareness.'

Introduction to Epilepsy ed. Gonzalo Alarcón and Antonio Valentín. Published by CAMBRIDGE UNIVERSITY PRESS.
© CAMBRIDGE UNIVERSITY PRESS 2012.

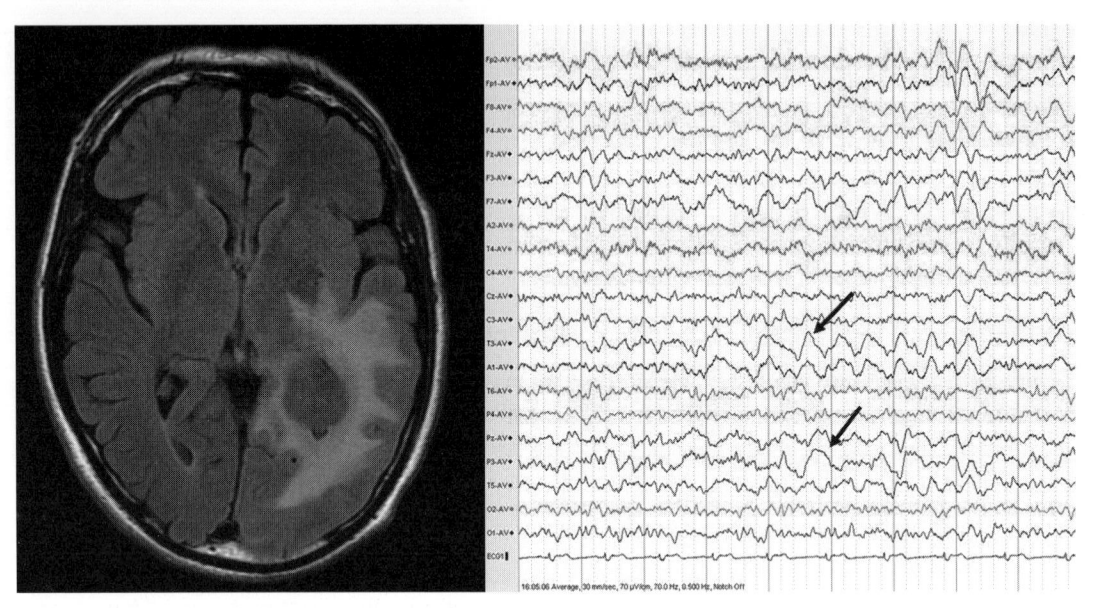

Section 2: Classification and diagnosis of epilepsy

Figure 18.1. B-cell lymphoma involving the left posterior temporo-occipital region with associated slowing of the background activity (a type of focal symptomatic epilepsy).

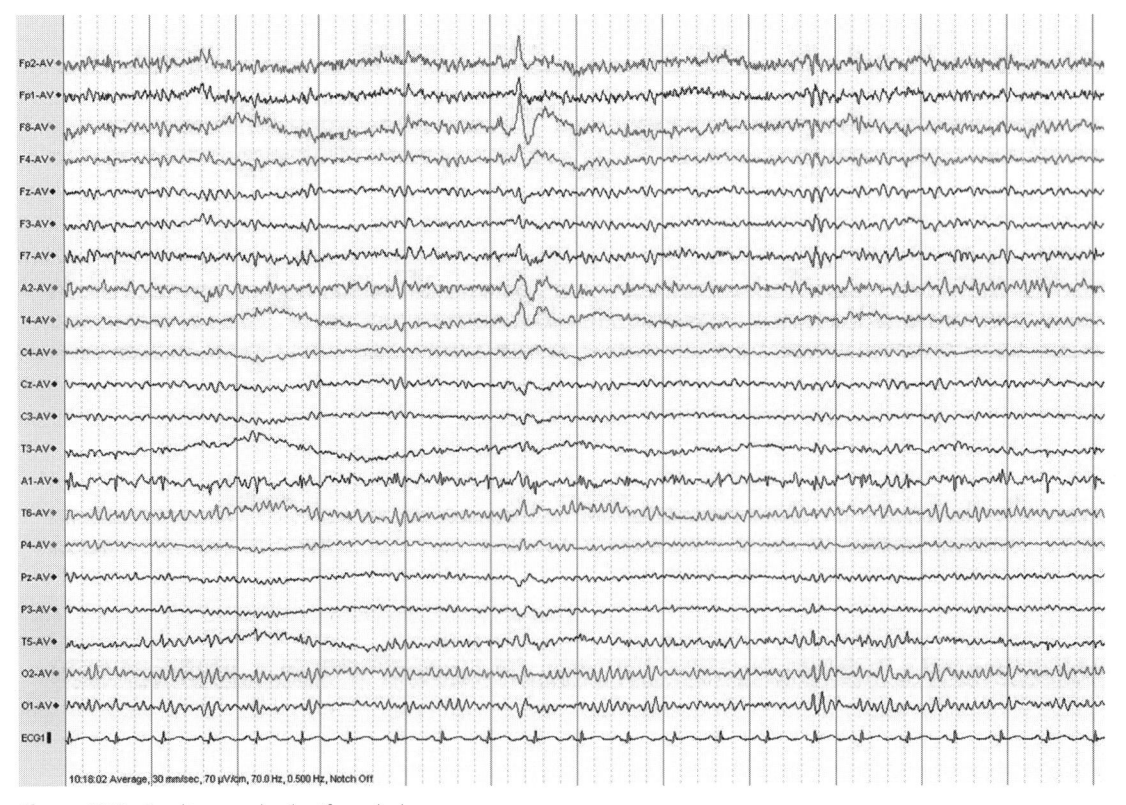

Figure 18.2. Focal temporal epileptiform discharges.

Chapter 18: Clinical use of EEG in epilepsy

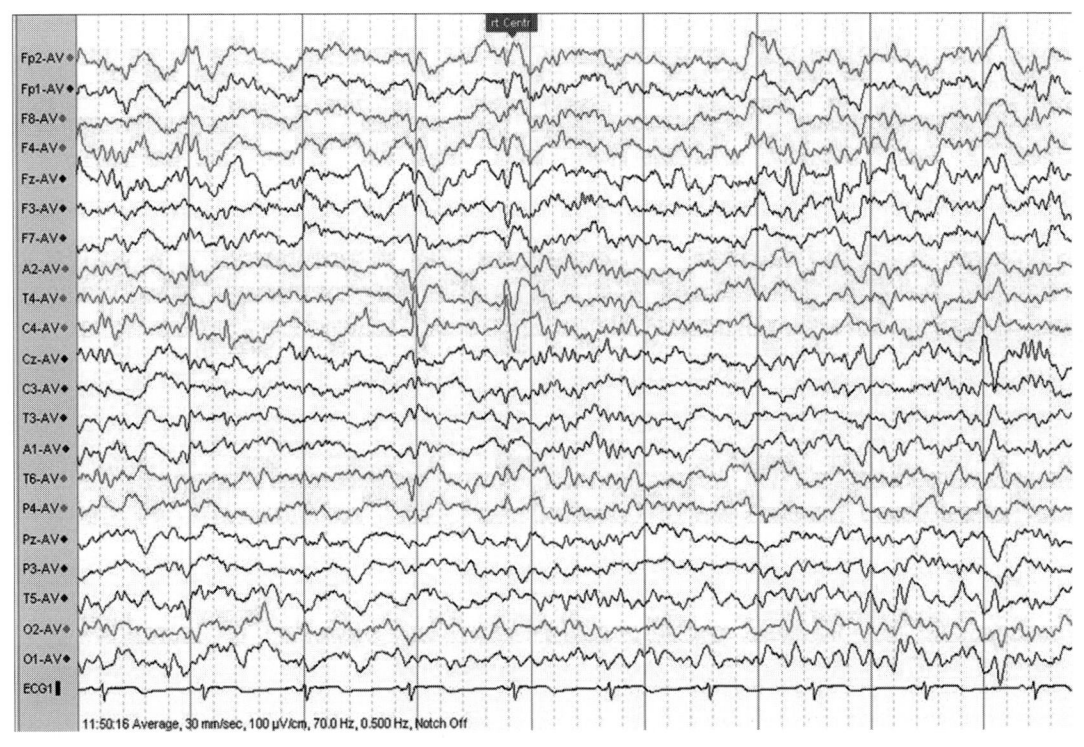

Figure 18.3. Right central epileptiform discharges (maximal at C4) in a patient who has previously suffered two secondarily generalized seizures.

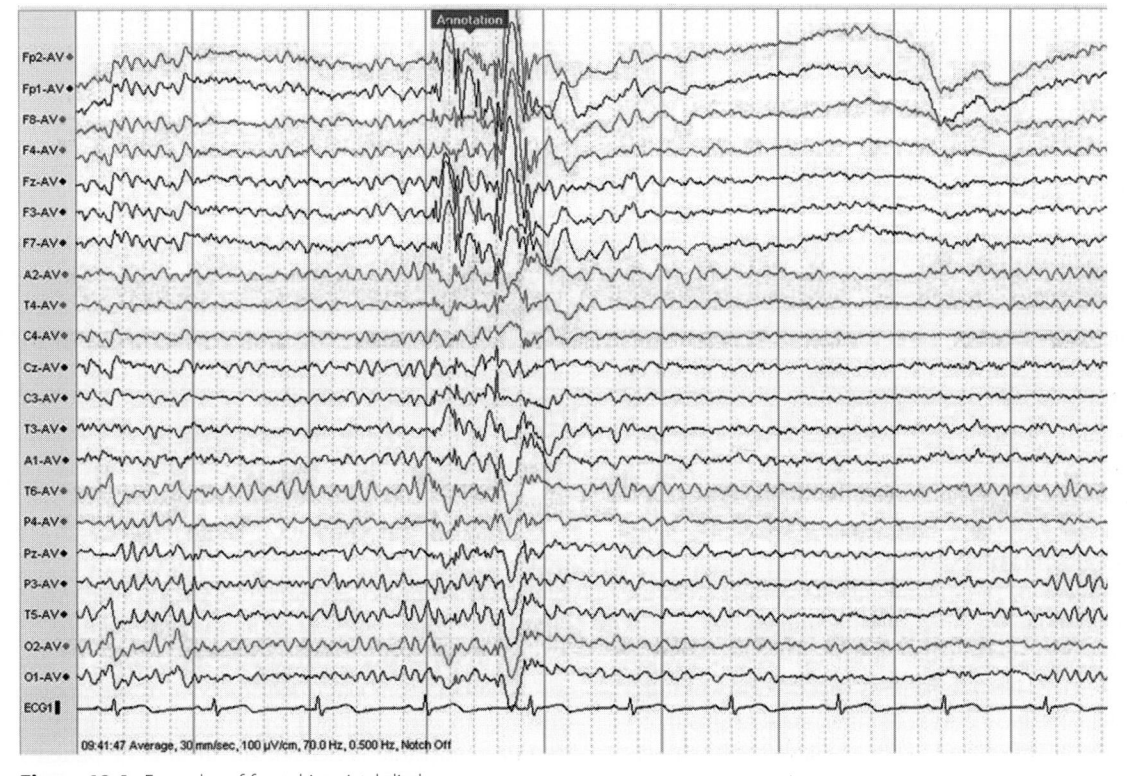

Figure 18.4. Examples of frontal interictal discharges.

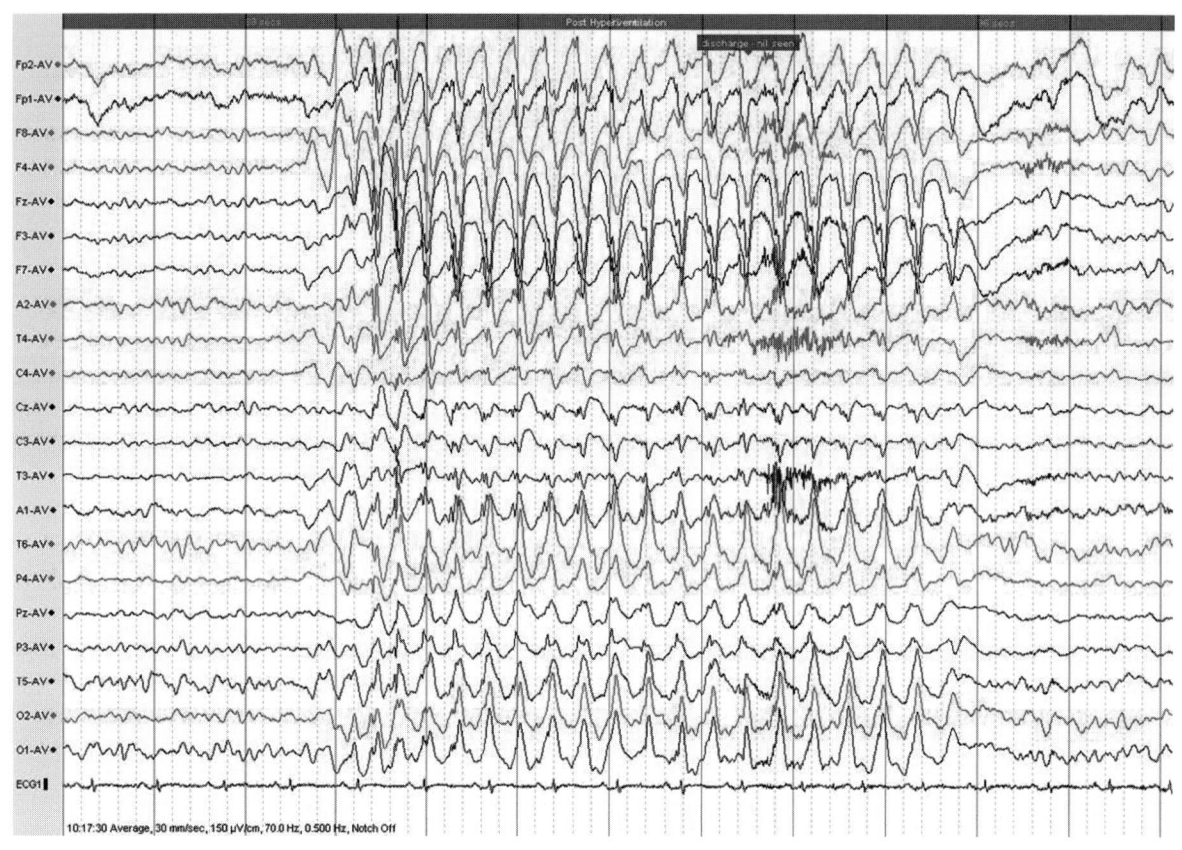

Figure 18.5. Absence seizure with associated generalized 3 per second spike and wave discharge in a patient with juvenile absence epilepsy (a type of idiopathic generalized epilepsy). Note a normal background activity. Arrows point at beginning and end of seizure.

- 80% of patients will show epileptiform discharges in a single sleep EEG.
- 92% of patients will show epileptiform discharges when at least two sleep EEGs are obtained.

Therefore, when requesting an EEG for the diagnosis of epilepsy a sleep EEG is more likely to show epileptiform discharges if the patient suffers from epilepsy. The likelihood of recording epileptiform discharges is increased if the EEG is performed relatively soon after an attack. A repeatedly normal sleep EEG should question the diagnosis of epilepsy. Epileptiform discharges associated with idiopathic epilepsy may remit beyond childhood/adolescence.

Specificity of the EEG: epileptiform discharges are very uncommon in normal healthy subjects (0.2–0.3%). However, epileptiform discharges can be more commonly seen (5–20%) in patients with a history of intracranial neurological disease or intracranial neurosurgery in the absence of epilepsy. Thus, epileptiform discharges should be interpreted with caution in these patients.

Photoparoxysmal responses

Some patients with epilepsy, and sometimes their relatives too, show spike-and-wave discharges when exposed to flashing lights (see Figure 92.1). This is more likely to occur when the frequency of the flashing light is 18–20 Hz. Spike-and-waves induced by flashing lights are called photoparoxysmal (or photoconvulsive) responses (PPRs).

PPRs can be more or less restricted to the posterior regions of the head (grades I–III), or can be generalized (grade IV). When they are generalized, they have a strong association with epilepsy and are useful in the diagnosis of epilepsy. Grade IV PPRs are commonly recorded in patients with photosensitive epilepsy and often in their asymptomatic siblings.

Patients showing generalized PPR (grade IV) are said to suffer from photosensitivity or to be photosensitive. In some epilepsy syndromes (for instance, juvenile myoclonic epilepsy), up to 40% of patients are photosensitive. In these syndromes, the presence

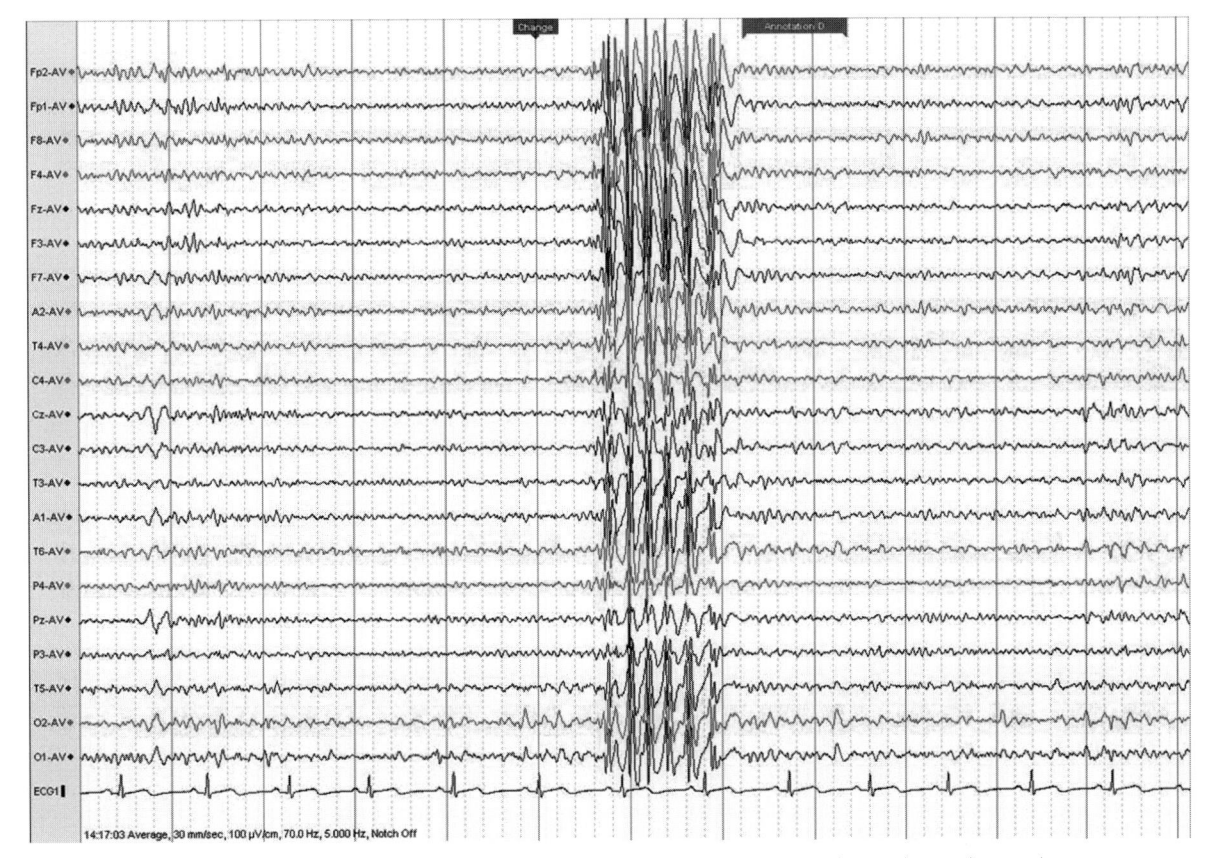

Figure 18.6. Generalized polyspike discharges with normal background activity in a patient with juvenile myoclonic epilepsy (a type of idiopathic generalized epilepsy).

of photosensitivity is a powerful diagnostic tool. PPR are more likely to occur, but not exclusively so, in generalized epilepsy syndromes.

Effects of hyperventilation

- In normal subjects, hyperventilation can be associated with bilateral slowing of the EEG background activity, particulary over frontal regions (Figure 18.9). This effect is more marked in children and young adults. It is probably due to a decrease in carbon dioxide blood levels, inducing cerebral vasoconstriction.
- To confirm the diagnosis of epilepsy, only clear epileptiform discharges should be considered, as different forms of delta waves and sharpened slow activity can be a normal response to hyperventilation.
- In patients with childhood absence epilepsy, hyperventilation nearly invariably induces absence seizures. Consequently, if no absence attacks are recorded during or shortly after well-performed hyperventilation, this type of epilepsy has to be reconsidered.
- In other syndromes, hyperventilation can less consistently activate epileptiform discharges and seizures (Figure 27.1.).

Summary on interpretation of the interictal EEG in epilepsy

The following general rules can be considered in the interpretation of the interictal EEG in epilepsy:

- Generalized epileptiform discharges without slowing of the background activity suggest that the patient has idiopathic generalized epilepsy. Photosensitivity reinforces this diagnosis.
- Focal epileptiform discharges suggest focal epilepsy arising from the area that shows discharges.
- Focal slowing of the background activity suggests symptomatic (or presumed symptomatic) focal

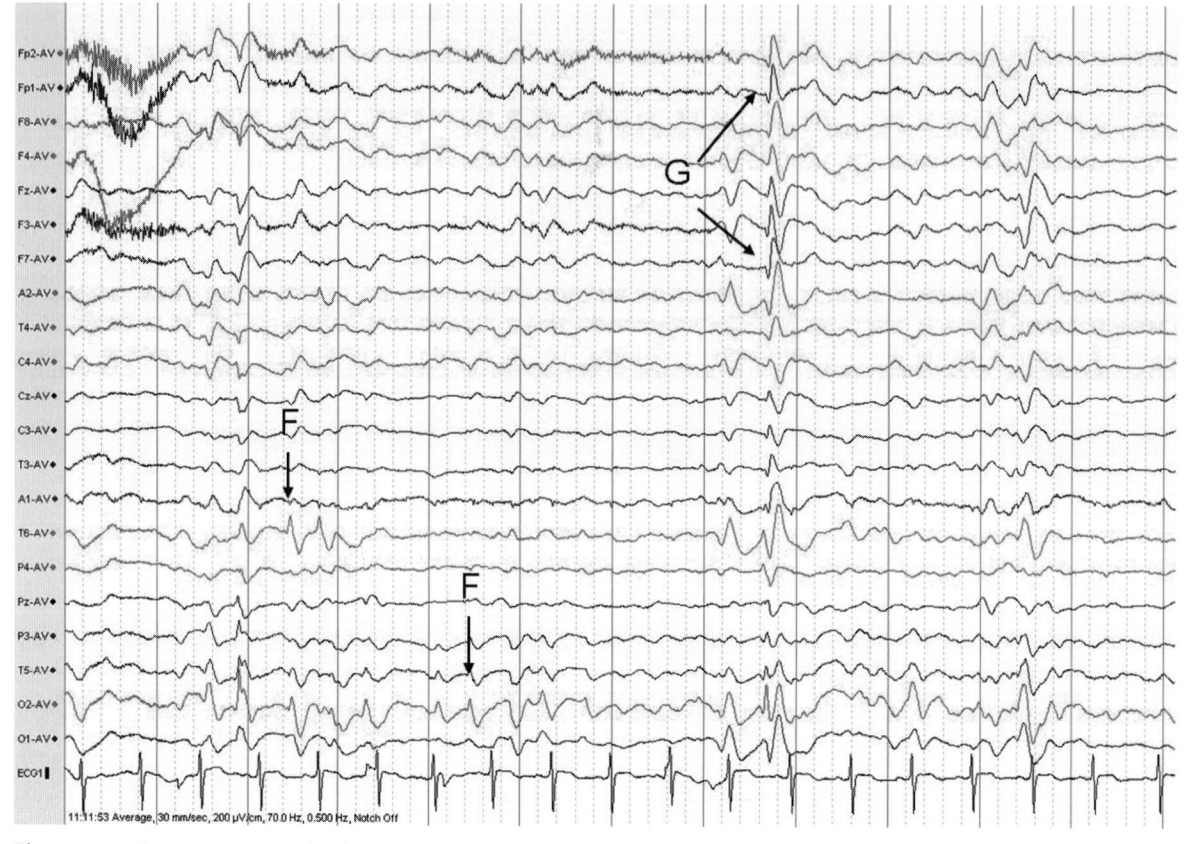

Section 2: Classification and diagnosis of epilepsy

Figure 18.7. Symptomatic generalized epilepsy in a 42-year-old patient: diffusely slow background activity with frequent superimposed focal (F) and generalized (G) discharges.

epilepsy arising from the area that shows abnormalitites. Good-quality neuroradiology is advised.
- Focal epileptiform discharges of appropriate topography and in the right age group, in the absence of slowing, can suggest idiopathic focal epilepsy.
- Focal, multifocal or generalized epileptiform discharges with diffuse background slowing suggest symptomatic (or presumed symptomatic) generalized epilepsy.
- Mild slowing of the background activity, particularly in the theta range, is often seen with antiepileptic medication.
- EEG abnormalities should be interpreted with caution in patients with a history of intracranial neurological disease or neurosurgery.
- The diagnosis of childhood absence epilepsy should be reconsidered if no absence attacks are recorded after vigorous hyperventilation.
- Finally, remember that not all patients with epilepsy will show EEG abnormalities. However, repeatedly normal EEGs should question the diagnosis of epilepsy.

Ictal EEG recordings

Ictal EEG recordings (EEG recorded during seizures) are more reliable than interictal recordings to confirm the diagnosis of epilepsy. However, they are more difficult and expensive to record, and may not be obtainable in patients with infrequent seizures.

Ictal EEG recordings can be seen if a seizure occurs during recording of a standard awake or sleep EEG. This is common in syndromes with frequent seizures, such as absence epilepsies or symptomatic generalized epilepsies, and relatively uncommon in other syndromes.

If seizures are relatively frequent or sensitive to reduction in medication or other situations (sleep deprivation), prolonged EEG recordings could be useful, usually in conjunction with simultaneous video recording

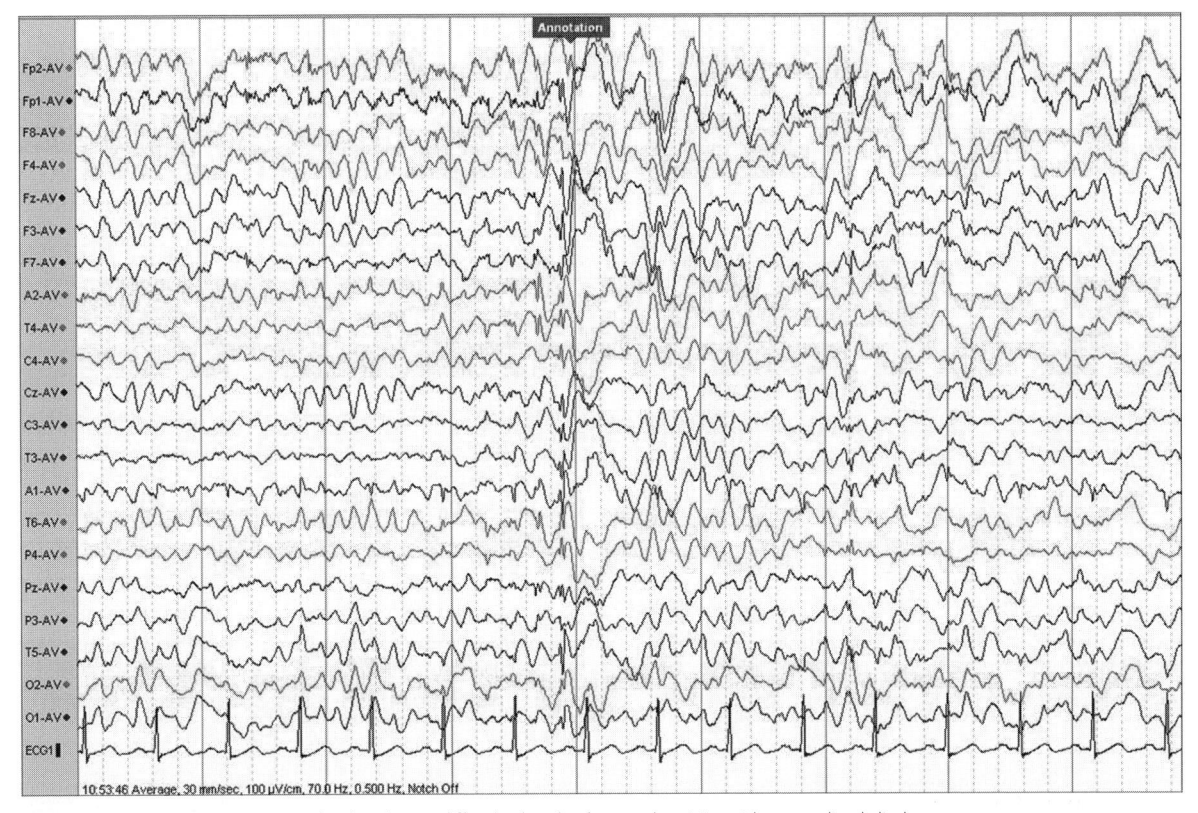

Figure 18.8. Symptomatic generalized epilepsy: diffusely slow background activity with generalized discharges.

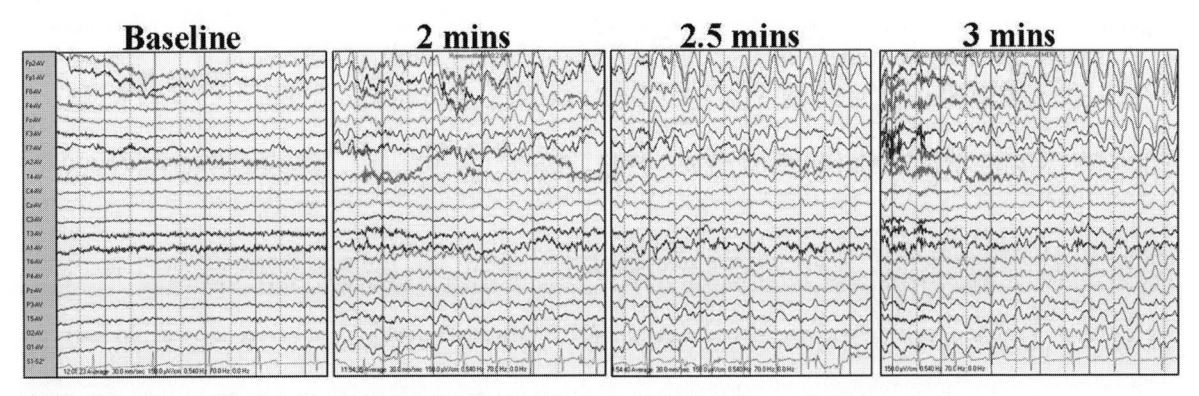

Figure 18.9. A normal finding: frontal slowing associated with hyperventilation in a 9-year-old child.

(telemetry or video-EEG monitoring, see Chapter 47: 'The role of video-EEG monitoring in epilepsy').

Indications of ictal recordings

Ictal recordings might be necessary in the following cases:

- to confirm the diagnosis of epilepsy in patients with normal EEGs, and relatively frequent seizures;
- to confirm the diagnosis of epilepsy in patients with abnormal EEG findings;
- to distinguish between epileptic and non-epileptic seizures.
- to classify seizure types;
- to establish the frequency of seizures; for instance, to monitor the effects of AED therapy, or in patients with epileptic and non-epileptic events, to establish how many events are epileptic;

- to assess surgery for the treatment of epilepsy, in order to:
  - establish beyond doubt that the patient has epilepsy;
  - determine seizure type, which is required to decide whether surgery is needed, and to choose the surgical procedure;
  - identify the location and lateralization of seizure onset.

EEG findings during ictal recordings

EEG findings seen during seizures depend on the seizure type. Ictal EEG abnormalities can consist of:

- rhythmic sharp waves;
- rhythmic spikes;
- slowing of the EEG in the θ or δ ranges;
- flattening of the EEG (electrodecremental event);
- low-amplitude fast activity with frequency above 15 Hz (high-frequency or multiunit activity) (Figure 18.14);
- a combination of the above patterns;
- changes observed during a focal seizure usually evolve and change depending on seizure spread.

Some EEG findings are characteristic of certain seizure types:

- typical absence seizures (Figure 18.10): generalized spike-and-wave activity at 2.5–3.5 Hz;
- atypical absence seizures: generalized spike-and-wave at frequency below 2.5 Hz;
- generalized myoclonic jerks (Figure 18.11): a generalized (poly-) spike-and-wave, usually intermixed with muscle artefacts;
- infantile spasms (Figure 18.12): burst of fast activity associated with rhomboid muscle artefact and followed by EEG flattening;
- focal myoclonic jerks: focal contralateral (poly-) spike-and-wave, usually over frontocentral regions; sometimes, no EEG changes are seen unless back-averaging is performed;
- focal motor (clonic) seizures: often show focal contralateral spike-and-wave synchronized with

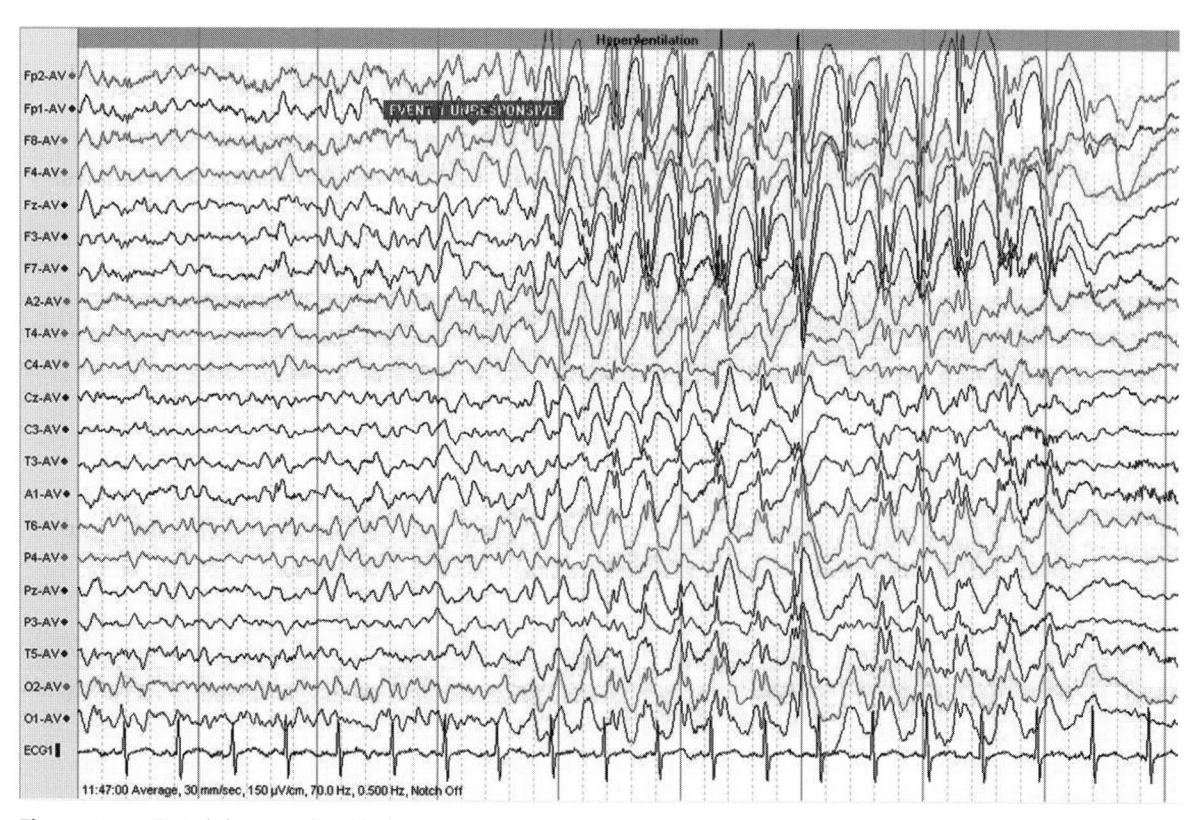

Figure 18.10. Typical absence induced by hyperventilation.

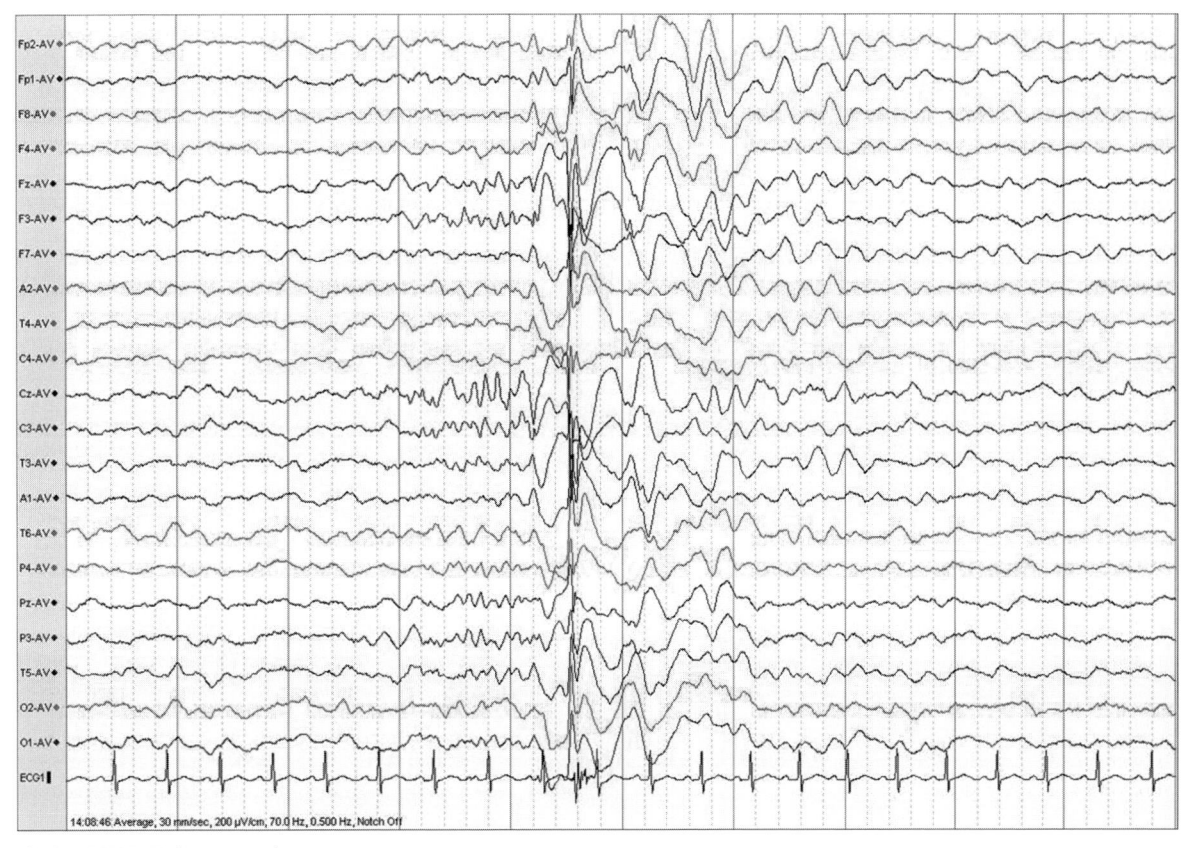

Figure 18.11. Epileptic myoclonic seizures.

the jerks, usually over frontocentral regions; sometimes no EEG changes;
- tonic and atonic seizures: flattening of the EEG, usually diffuse, and often associated with diffuse fast activity;
- simple partial seizures: EEG changes may be absent or are focal (rhythmic sharp waves, rhythmic spikes or focal slowing);
- complex partial seizures (Figures 18.13 and 18.14): slowing of the background activity usually intermixed with sharp waves or epileptiform discharges. Although these seizures are focal in origin, the scalp EEG will show a clear focal onset only in around 30% of complex partial seizures, because substantial amounts of cortex might have been recruited bilaterally by the time EEG changes are seen on the scalp (see Alarcón et al., 2001, for temporal lobe epilepsy). Therefore, a diffuse or bilateral EEG onset on the scalp does not exclude a focal seizure onset. Some complex partial seizures of frontal origin may not show EEG changes, or these may be buried among muscle and movement artefacts;
- generalized and secondarily generalized convulsive (tonic-clonic) seizures: generalized spike-and-wave activity at around 3 Hz obscured by or superimposed upon by rhythmic muscle and movement artefacts;
- post-ictal changes: complex partial, generalized and secondarily generalized convulsive seizures are often followed by a period of confusion called post-ictal confusion. During this period, the EEG often shows focal or diffuse slowing in the δ and θ ranges, with superimposed focal or multifocal sharp waves and epileptiform discharges, sometimes with intermittent periods of EEG flattening.

How to interpret ictal recordings

EEG changes occurring during a seizure will confirm that the seizure is epileptic. Conversely, most epileptic

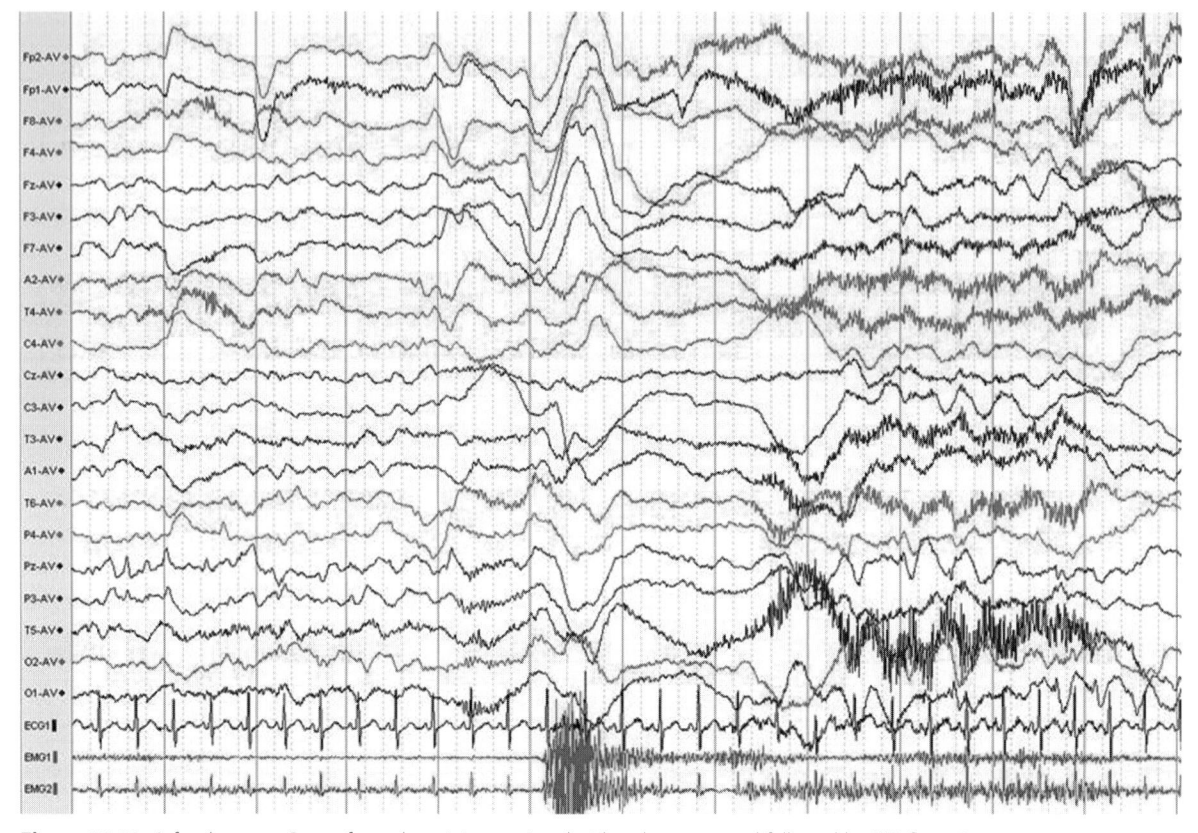

Section 2: Classification and diagnosis of epilepsy

Figure 18.12. Infantile spasm. Burst of muscle activity associated with a slow wave and followed by EEG flattening.

seizures will show EEG changes but there are a few exceptions:

- Simple partial seizures may or may not show EEG changes, as the area of cortex involved in these seizures can be rather small and sometimes deep (hippocampus–amygdala complex). Therefore, a normal EEG during a simple partial seizure cannot rule out epilepsy.
- Focal myoclonic seizures may or may not show changes on the ongoing EEG for the same reason. If jerks are relatively frequent, EEG back-averaging might show small brief EEG deflections preceding the jerks by a few milliseconds.
- Some frontal complex partial seizures may not show EEG changes, or these may be impossible to identify among muscle and movement artefacts.

If the EEG is normal while the patient appears unresponsive or while showing generalized convulsions, it is assumed that the event is not an epileptic seizure. The reason for this assumption is that in order to lose consciousness (unresponsiveness) or to suffer generalized convulsions, a substantial amount of cortex needs to be recruited bilaterally, invariably generating EEG changes.

Box 18.2. EEG phenomena resembling epileptiform discharges but not, or only weakly, associated with epilepsy (see Chapter 14)

- 6 and 14/s positive spikes
- 6/s 'spike-wave phantom'
- Rhythmic mid-temporal discharge
- Subclinical rhythmic epileptiform discharge of adults
- Mid-line spikes (some)
- Benign epileptiform transients of sleep
- 'Epileptic K-complexes'
- Frontal delta on hyperventilation
- Photoparoxysmal responses grades 1 to 3
- Posterior slow waves of youth and unusual alpha variants

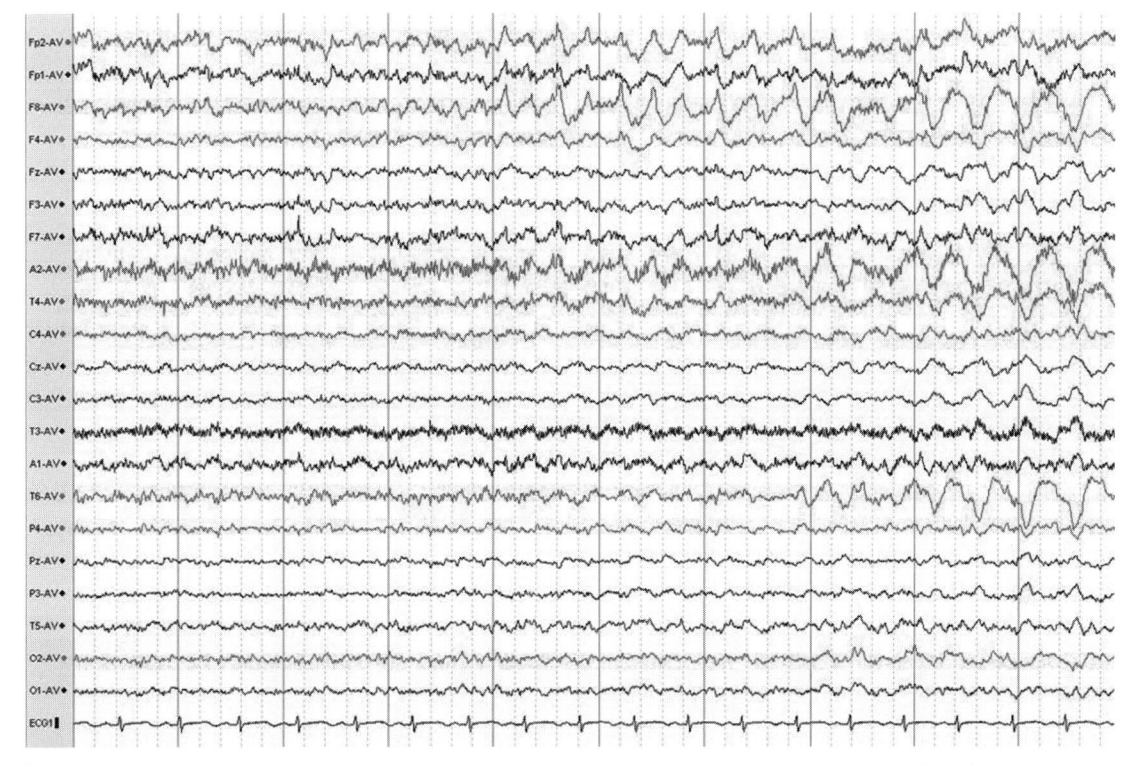

Figure 18.13. Onset of a focal temporal seizure on the scalp EEG. Note rhythmic sharp waves starting at the right anterior temporal (F8) and prefrontal electrodes (Fp2).

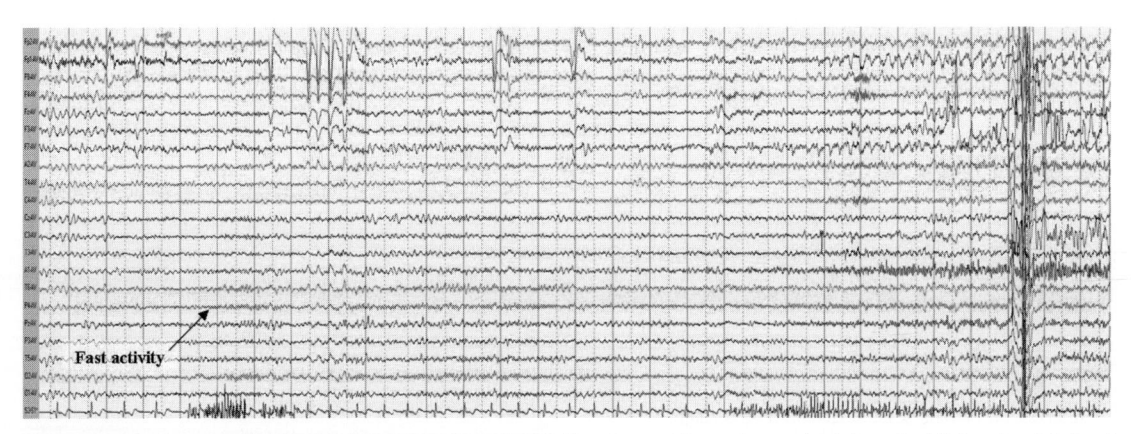

Figure 18.14. Onset of a focal parietal seizure on the scalp EEG. Note fast activity starting at the right parietal (P4) and occipital regions (O2) which later spreads to the left anterior electrodes (F7, Fp1).

Common misconceptions about the EEG in epilepsy

Further to the above, it is not in general true that:
- the interictal EEG can:
  - prove without any doubt the diagnosis of epilepsy
  - exclude epilepsy;
- an ictal EEG always shows ictal EEG changes;
- a particular interictal EEG abnormality reflects seizure severity, seizure frequency, prognosis or therapeutic response.

It is, however, true that:
- the interictal EEG can:
  - strongly support the diagnosis of epilepsy
  - exclude specific epilepsy syndromes;
- an ictal EEG in certain seizure types always shows ictal EEG changes;
- the EEG is important to identify the epilepsy syndrome, which determines seizure frequency, therapeutic response and prognosis;
- control or follow-up EEGs with no clear indication are of minimal value.

Reference

Alarcón G, Kissani N, Dad M, *et al.* Lateralizing and localizing values of ictal onset recorded on the scalp: evidence from simultaneous recordings with intracranial foramen ovale electrodes. *Epilepsia* 2001; **42**:1426–37.

Learning objectives

(1) To know and be able to recognize interictal EEG abnormalities associated with epilepsy.
(2) To quantify the sensitivity and specificity of the interictal EEG in epilepsy.
(3) To understand the significance of EEG responses to activation procedures.
(4) To know the indications and value of ictal recordings.
(5) To be able to recognize ictal changes in an EEG and be aware of their clinical interpretation.
(6) To be aware of the common misconceptions about the interpretation of the EEG in epilepsy.

Section 2 **Classification and diagnosis of epilepsy**

Chapter 19

General overview of epileptic syndromes in childhood and adolescence

Archana Desurkar

The term epilepsy is applied to a host of conditions characterized by a propensity to have recurrent paroxysmal clinical events called epileptic seizures. However, no single term can adequately describe this extremely broad spectrum of clinical manifestations and possible seizure patterns encountered in clinical practice, especially in children.

An epilepsy syndrome is defined as a cluster of signs and symptoms that include characteristic seizure types, modes of recurrence, typical neurological and other findings of special investigations, response to treatment and prognosis customarily occurring together.

Characteristics of epilepsy syndromes

- Many are age-related
- Characteristic seizure(s) – may evolve over time
- May have a typical EEG but may not be specific
- May have associated cognitive phenotype
- Outcome may be known and treatment response predictable
- An epilepsy syndrome may have more than one cause and different outcomes
- Unfortunately many children (and even more adults) don't fit into an epilepsy syndrome

Epilepsy syndromes in childhood and adolescence can be considered according to the basic classification of epilepsies as focal, generalized and undetermined with further subdivision into idiopathic, symptomatic and presumed symptomatic groups.

A proposed classification of epilepsy syndromes applicable to childhood and adolescence is shown in Box 19.1. The main features of the common syndromes are discussed below.

More recently, following the classification proposed by the ILAE commission on classification and

Box 19.1. Classification of epilepsy syndromes starting in childhood and adolescence: ILAE Task Force Report (2006)

I. **Focal epilepsy syndromes**
   Idiopathic:
   - Benign epilepsy of childhood with centrotemporal spikes (BECTS)
   - Early-onset benign childhood occipital epilepsy (Panayiotopoulos syndrome)
   - Late-onset childhood occipital epilepsy (Gastaut type)
   - Idiopathic photosensitive occipital epilepsy

   Symptomatic:
   - Chronic progressive epilepsia partialis continua of childhood (Kojewnikow syndrome)

   Presumed symptomatic (cryptogenic)

II. **Generalized epilepsy syndromes**
    Idiopathic:
    - Childhood absence epilepsy
    - Juvenile absence epilepsy
    - Juvenile myoclonic epilepsy.
    - Epilepsy with grand mal seizures on awakening
    - Reflex epilepsies

    Symptomatic or presumed symptomatic (cryptogenic)
    - Lennox-Gastaut syndrome
    - Myoclonic-astatic epilepsy
    - Myoclonic absences

III. **Undetermined whether focal or generalized**
     - Continuous spike-waves during slow-wave sleep (CSWS).
     - Acquired epileptic aphasia (Landau-Kleffner syndrome).

Introduction to Epilepsy ed. Gonzalo Alarcón and Antonio Valentín. Published by Cambridge University Press.
© Cambridge University Press 2012.

> **Box 19.2.** Epilepsy syndromes according to age of onset of syndromes
>
> **Epilepsy syndromes starting in childhood:**
> - Febrile seizures plus (FS+) (can start in infancy)
> - Early-onset benign childhood occipital epilepsy (Panayiotopoulos type)
> - Epilepsy with myoclonic atonic (previously astatic) seizures
> - Benign epilepsy with centrotemporal spikes (BECTS)
> - Autosomal-dominant nocturnal frontal lobe epilepsy (ADNFLE)
> - Late-onset childhood occipital epilepsy (Gastaut type)
> - Epilepsy with myoclonic absences
> - Lennox-Gastaut syndrome
> - Epileptic encephalopathy with continuous spike-and-wave during sleep (CSWS)
> - including: Landau-Kleffner syndrome (LKS)
> - Childhood absence epilepsy (CAE)
>
> **Epilepsy syndromes starting in adolescence and adulthood:**
> - Juvenile absence epilepsy (JAE)
> - Juvenile myoclonic epilepsy (JME)
> - Epilepsy with generalized tonic-clonic seizures alone· Progressive myoclonus epilepsies (PME)
> - Autosomal-dominant partial epilepsy with auditory features (ADPEAF)
> - Other familial temporal lobe epilepsies

terminology (Berg *et al.*, 2010) where the dichotomy of terms 'focal' and 'generalized' for syndromes is abandoned, epilepsy syndromes can be referred according to aetiology.

Benign epilepsy of childhood with centrotemporal spikes (BECTS)

This is also called rolandic or Sylvian epilepsy or lingual syndrome. It is the most common idiopathic focal epilepsy of childhood, constituting about 16% of the epilepsies seen in patients under 16 years of age.

Age of onset: usually between 3 and 10 years.

Aetiology: genetic factors play an important role as indicated by several members of the same pedigree being affected. Similar EEG abnormalities can also be found in a third of first-degree relatives. There may be a dominant inheritance with age-dependent susceptibility.

Seizure types

Partial seizures constitute 70–80% of fits; usually motor and sensory phenomena can occur. Typically seizures arise from sleep, with sensory phenomena (numbness, heaviness) involving the corner of the mouth, tongue and gums. Guttural sounds from the throat, choking and profuse salivation occur (rolandic area involved). Motor manifestations may involve facial contortion and jerking of one side of the face and eyelids. Speech arrest with retained comprehension can occur.

Secondarily generalized seizures may occur in 24–80% of patients.

Usually seizures are brief in children older than 5 years while they can be less localized and longer in younger children.

In over 50% of patients, seizures are purely nocturnal, though in 5–25% attacks occur exclusively in wakefulness.

The frequency of attacks is low and about 50% of children have fewer than five seizures altogether. If attacks occur frequently, they may cluster, separated by long intervals of several months. The duration of active epilepsy is less than 5 years in 60% of children.

Interictal EEG findings

The EEG is characteristic and interictal abnormalities are an essential part of the syndrome. The background activity is normal. The abnormalities consist of high-amplitude negative sharp waves with a blunted peak followed by a prominent positive wave mainly localized to the centrotemporal region of the side contralateral to ictal manifestations (Figure 19.1). They can be seen more posteriorly. In a third of patients, discharges can be bilateral, synchronous or independent. Sleep characteristically activates the discharges (Figure 19.2).

Course and prognosis

BECTS consistently remits at around 16 years of age, mostly between 9 and 12 years of age. Remission occurs regardless of initial treatment resistance or status epilepticus. The EEG usually normalizes after clinical remission. Most patients will not need treatment, as seizures are infrequent, nocturnal and hence minimally intrusive to normal activities. For those needing treatment, carbamazepine is a preferred choice and over-treatment should be avoided. There are controversies regarding the impact of interictal discharges on cognition.

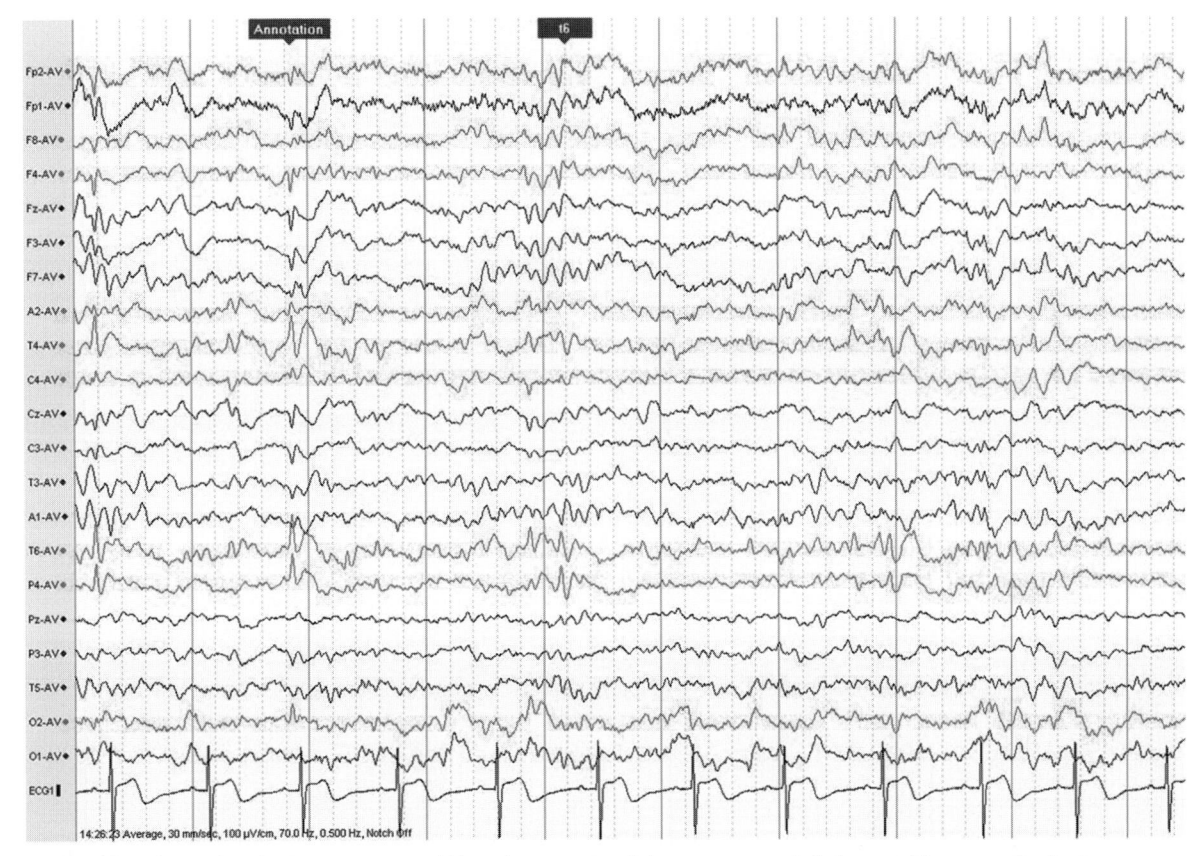

Figure 19.1. Interictal awake EEG in an 8-year-old boy demonstrating right centrotemporal discharges with accentuation in sleep.

Early-onset benign occipital epilepsy (Panayiotopoulos syndrome)

This is a common but perhaps an under-recognized epilepsy syndrome with susceptibility to autonomic seizures.

Age of onset: 1–14 years, usually 4–5 years.

Seizure types

Seizures are usually nocturnal, with ictal vomiting, slow eye deviation that evolves into a variable degree of impairment of consciousness or obtundation. Unilateral prolonged clonic jerking may occur. There is a predominance of autonomic symptoms with pallor, flushing, tachycardia and thermoregulatory alterations that occur concurrently or later in the seizure. In 10%, only autonomic seizures occur.

The attacks are infrequent and 30% of children have a single attack only.

EEG findings

The EEG is typically characterized by normal background rhythms and occipital spike complexes similar in morphology to centrotemporal spikes. They often are multifocal and high amplitude. They can be prolonged during eye closure and are abolished by eye opening (fixation-off sensitivity). They increase in sleep.

Course and prognosis

The outcome is usually favourable. About 25% may have frequent seizures within the first 2 years of onset while 75% have either a single seizure or up to five seizures.

Late-onset occipital epilepsy (Gastaut type)

This replaces the previous term 'childhood epilepsy with occipital paroxysms'. It is a rare benign epilepsy syndrome.

Age of onset: mean 6 years.

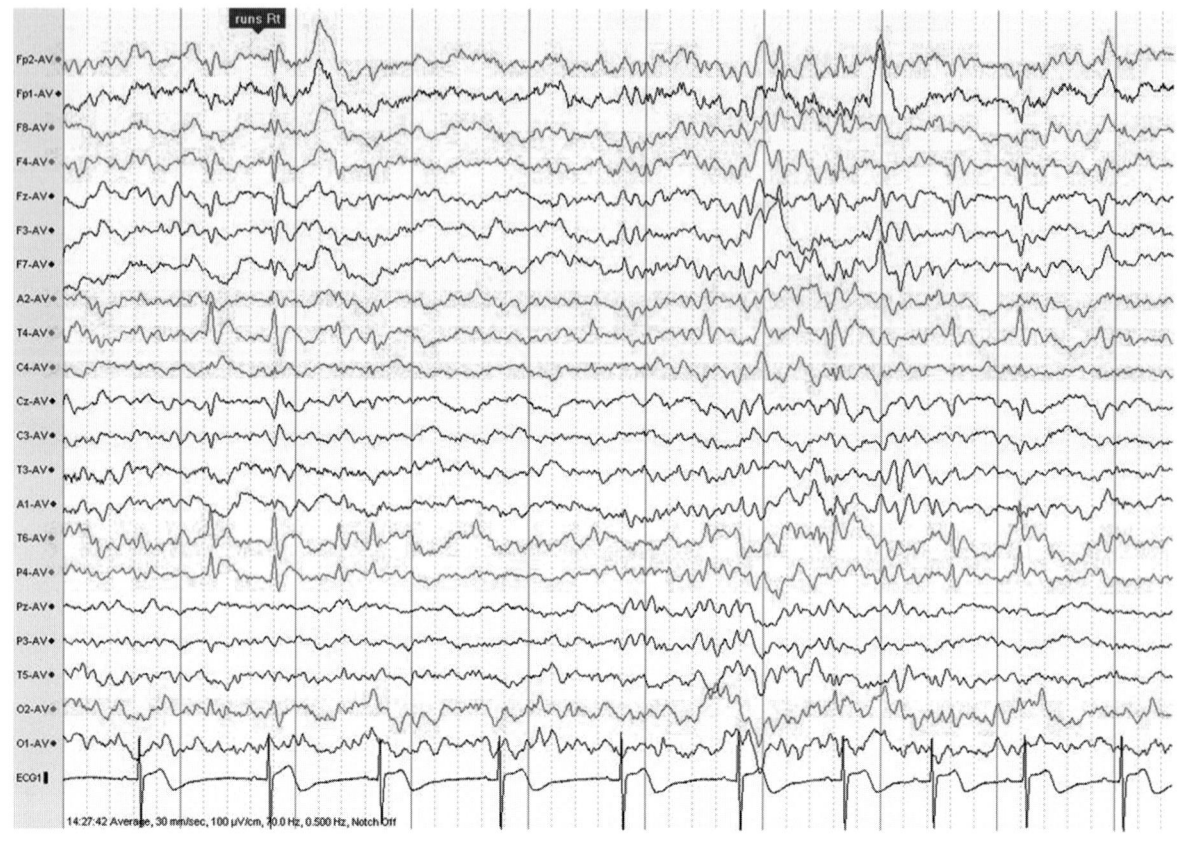

Figure 19.2. Interictal sleep record showing more frequent discharges than while awake often occurring in bursts.

Types of seizures

Seizures begin with visual symptoms such as transient amaurosis (blindness) or elementary visual hallucinations (coloured discs, formed hallucinations). Deviation of the eyes is common. Hemiclonic, complex partial or secondarily generalized seizures may occur. Post-ictal severe headache sometimes with nausea and vomiting with migrainous features is common.

Seizures are brief but frequent, often daily.

EEG findings

The EEG shows localized occipital spikes against a normal background. These occur either synchronously or independently and symmetrically or asymmetrically with fixation-off phenomenon.

Course and prognosis

Usually a benign course is anticipated, with eventual remission of seizures in 60% of patients. When treatment is required, the preferred drug is carbamazepine.

Idiopathic photosensitive occipital epilepsy

This uncommon syndrome is characterized by focal occipital seizures precipitated by photic stimulation, usually television or video games. Visual hallucinations of bright colour occur; blindness may lead to convulsive seizure and post-ictal severe headache is characteristic.

Prognosis is usually good and avoidance of triggering factors may be all that is required.

Chronic progressive epilepsia partialis continua of childhood (Kojewnikow syndrome) and Rasmussen's syndrome

Epilepsia partialis continua is defined by continuous myoclonias limited to one side of the body. The jerks are usually brief, persist in sleep and continue relentlessly. The hand, foot and/or face are the body parts most often affected.

In cases due to non-progressive cortical circumscribed lesions, epilepsia partialis continua may persist for hours, weeks or months and may suddenly stop.

Rasmussen's syndrome is a severe progressive syndrome characterized by intractable focal motor seizures, progressive hemispheric atrophy and progressive neuropsychological deterioration with hemiparesis and cognitive and language impairment. Age of onset is typically 18 months to 14 years. It evolves in phases before developing intractable epilepsy and hemiparesis. The first stage is characterized by focal motor or somatosensory seizures of increasing frequency over weeks to months. The second stage is associated with progressive neurological impairment of unilateral hemispheric involvement with worsening seizures. In the final stage epilepsy tends to subside but residual neurological deficits remain. The stages are of variable duration but early diagnosis is important though may be challenging.

Lateralized chronic inflammatory pathology is thought to be underlying aetiology.

Immunomodulatory treatment (with steroids and steroid-sparing immunosuppressant drugs, immunoglobulins) may be beneficial but eventually hemispherectomy may be required.

> **Box 19.2.** Descriptive terms for absence seizures
>
> Typical absences: they have an abrupt onset and offset, and are associated with symmetric synchronous spike-wave discharges at 2.5-3.5 Hz. No post-ictal confusion or fatigue is the essential clue. They can be:
>
> - simple typical absences: impaired consciousness with simple or limited motor activity such as eyelid fluttering or elevation of eyeballs;
> - complex typical absences: impaired consciousness associated with automatisms or prominent motor components (myoclonic, tonic or atonic movements).
>
> Atypical absence: these have progressive onset and offset and irregular generalized spike-wave bursts on the EEG at <2.5 Hz. These seizures are usually associated with symptomatic or cryptogenic epilepsies.

Childhood absence epilepsy

This is the most common absence epilepsy, constituting between 2 and 10% of childhood epilepsy.

Age of onset: 4–8 years, peak 6–7 years.

Seizure types

Typical absences (simple and/or complex) occur very frequently (dozens a day) and mostly last 10–15 s. Eyes open in the first 2–3 s. A stop-stare-start sequence is typical where the child may lose the thread of conversation or stop the activity and become unresponsive before resuming normal behaviour. Hyperventilation almost always precipitates absence seizures. If no absence is elicited with hyperventilation in an untreated child, this virtually excludes the diagnosis.

EEG findings

A normal background activity is characteristic. During absence seizures there is an abrupt onset of bilaterally synchronous and symmetrical 3 Hz spike-wave discharge, irrespective of whether typical absences are simple or complex. This EEG activity lasts for the duration of clinical absence. Often, progressive slowing to 2.5 Hz may be seen throughout the course of the absence seizure. Neither polyspikes nor photosensitivity are observed in childhood absence epilepsy compared with juvenile absence epilepsy, where photosensitivity is seen in over 50% of patients.

Course and prognosis

The outlook is usually favourable. Absence seizures disappear by adolescence in 80% of patients. Generalized tonic-clonic seizures (GTCS) may develop, occasionally several years later. The medication of choice is sodium valproate, ethosuximide or lamotrigine. Carbamazepine and vigabatrin may worsen absence seizures.

Juvenile absence epilepsy

This differs from childhood absence epilepsy in the clinical and EEG features in later age of onset, higher frequency of GTCS and myoclonic jerks.

Age of onset: 4–30 years, average 13 years.

Seizure types

Typical absences that occur less frequently than in childhood absence epilepsy, usually 1–10 a day, characterize this epilepsy. The duration of absences is 4–30 s. Impairment of consciousness can be less profound than in childhood absence epilepsy. Eye opening is not

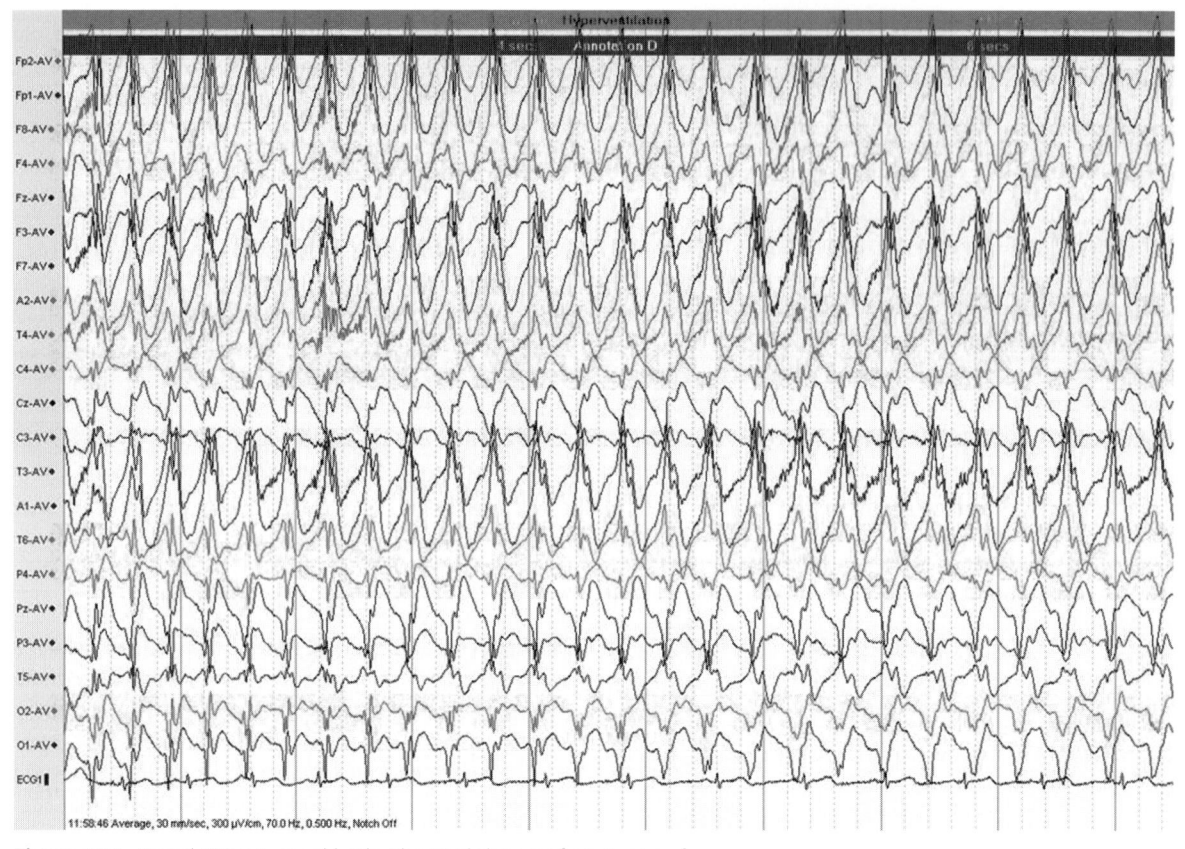

Figure 19.3. Typical EEG: a 7-year-old girl with typical absences from 6 years of age.

constant and may appear later than in childhood absence epilepsy. Automatisms are frequent. Random myoclonic jerks occur in up to 20% of patients.

EEG findings

Absence seizures show bilateral synchronous anteriorly dominant 2–5–4 Hz spike-wave discharges. Focal abnormalities as well as bursts of spikes and polyspikes are common. Twenty per cent of patients demonstrate photosensitivity. Photic stimulation may elicit an absence.

Course and prognosis

Prognosis is less favourable than in childhood absence epilepsy. In 70–80% of patients, absences are controlled. Around 80% of patients may have generalized tonic-clonic seizures following absences. Tonic-clonic seizures may persist after remission of absences, but are infrequent and often triggered by precipitating factors such as fatigue, sleep deprivation and alcohol consumption.

Juvenile myoclonic epilepsy (Janz syndrome)

This is one of the best-characterized epilepsy syndromes. Overall, it constitutes 20–27% of idiopathic generalized epilepsy and 3.1% of the overall population with epilepsy. This is a genetically determined epilepsy syndrome. Typical seizures may evolve over a period of time.

Age of onset: 6–22 years, mostly 12–18 years, with female preponderance.

Seizure types

- Absence seizures may be the first manifestation, showing an onset similar to childhood absence epilepsy. Later, absence seizures may continue, but are brief and may be unrecognized. They often occur on awakening.
- Myoclonus starts around 12–16 years of age, typically demonstrating an early morning propensity (20–30 min after awakening).

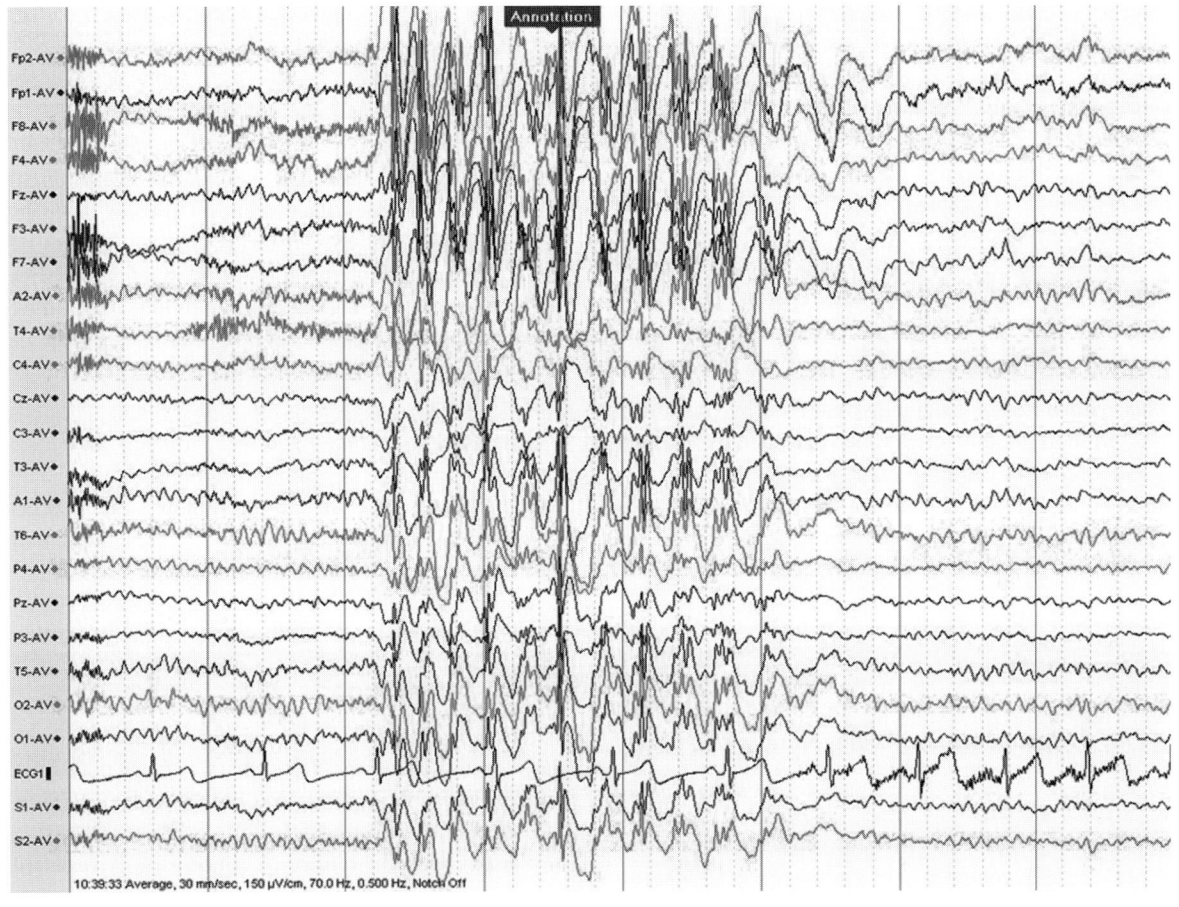

Figure 19.4. EEG: frontally dominant rather ragged polyspike wave discharge at 3–4 Hz.

Myoclonias are sudden, lightning-like, usually symmetrical, involving axial muscles (shoulders, arms) and occasionally the legs. They may be violent enough to cause a fall. They may occur singly or in clusters, which may lead to generalized tonic-clonic seizures. Sleep deprivation typically triggers myoclonus or GTCS.
- GTCS occur in 85% of patients, are infrequent, often triggered by sleep deprivation, stress, alcohol or mental activity involving planning or decision-making.
- Fifty per cent of patients are photosensitive and may show convulsive seizures triggered by flashing strobe lights, light reflected on shiny roads or the sea, etc.

EEG findings

The EEG typically shows normal background and can demonstrate classic 3 Hz spike-wave complexes as well as fast 4–6 Hz (poly)spike-wave complexes.

Myoclonus is characterized by generalized, symmetric, high-frequency clusters of spikes or polyspikes followed by slow waves. Onset and maximal voltage are in frontocentral areas.

Focal abnormalities like focal slow waves or asymmetric interictal discharges can occur in up to 55% of patients.

Photoparoxysmal responses are seen in 50% of patients.

Course and prognosis

JME is probably a life-long condition though it improves after the fourth decade.

Sodium valproate is the most effective medication (effective in 85% of patients). Addition of benzodiazepines may be required. Lamotrigine may worsen myoclonus. Carbamazepine and phenobarbitone may aggravate seizures and precipitate myoclonic status.

Response to treatment is usually excellent (80–90% achieve complete control). However, relapse with discontinuation of AED is common even after years of seizure freedom and hence long-term or life-long treatment may be required. Choice of medication, especially in adolescent females with childbearing potential, is crucial and a detailed discussion is of paramount importance. Fifteen per cent of patients are resistant to treatment, especially those showing all seizure types.

Advice about lifestyles, especially avoidance of precipitating factors, is important.

Lennox-Gastaut syndrome

This syndrome was originally described by Gastaut in 1966 though intial features were described by William Lennox in 1930, and it constitutes 1–10% of childhood epilepsies. This is one of the most misdiagnosed electro-clinical epilepsy syndromes.

Age of onset: 1–7 years, peak 3–5 years age with male preponderance.

Seizure types

Lennox-Gastaut syndrome is an epileptic encephalopathy characterized by having multiple types of seizures:

- atypical absences;
- atonic seizures: often myoatonic (with or preceded by a brief myoclonic jerk) causing drop attacks; on the EEG, rhythmic activity at around 10 Hz is seen diffusely;
- tonic seizures: are the most characteristic, usually occur in non-REM sleep; these are often associated with autonomic phenomena;
- myoclonic seizures are less common;
- status epilepticus: frequent bouts of non-convulsive status epilepticus occur in 50–75% of children, often on awakening, showing variable duration, sometimes even for days.

The presence of atypical absences, atonic seizures and tonic seizures with characteristic EEG findings of diffuse slow spike (<2.5 Hz) wave is required for the diagnosis. Some authorities also consider the presence of fast 10 Hz activity with tonic seizures in non-REM sleep as an additional necessary criterion.

Mental retardation is an important component of classic Lennox-Gastaut syndrome, and many patients are developmentally delayed at the onset of the syndrome. Lennox-Gastaut syndrome is often preceded by other forms of seizures such as infantile spasms, unilateral seizures, generalized tonic-clonic seizures and episodes of convulsive status epilepticus.

Causes

In 25–33% of patients, Lennox-Gastaut syndrome occurs without a pre-existing neurodevelopmental abnormality or imaging evidence of brain damage. In 66–75% of patients, Lennox-Gastaut syndrome has a developmental origin and is associated with malformations of cortical development, including heterotopias, focal dysplasia, polymicrogyria, etc.

EEG findings

- The EEG is characteristic with diffusely slow background activity and frequent bursts of generalized spike-wave patterns at less than 2.5 Hz (petit mal variant pattern).
- Fast 10 Hz rhythms occur during tonic seizures in non-REM sleep and this is an additional necessary criterion for diagnosis according to some authorities.

Course and prognosis

Outcome is generally unfavourable and is often associated with severe mental deficits (which may be a combination of frequent seizures, episodes of status and treatment with multiple anticonvulsant drugs).

Lennox-Gastaut syndrome is notoriously resistant to treatment and often requires multiple drug combinations, which need to be used cautiously.

Generally the following can be recommended:

- Sodium valproate and benzodiazepines are considered first-line therapy.
- Vigabatrin, steroids, intravenous immunoglobulins, felbamate, topiramate lamotrigine and leveteracetam can be used as second-line treatment.
- Rufinamide, which has marketing authorization for LGS as an orphan drug, is particularly useful for tonic and generalized tonic-clonic seizures.
- Ethosuximide may be useful for absence, atonic and myoclonic seizures. A ketogenic diet and vagus nerve stimulation can be used as non-pharmacological treatments.

Myoclonic-astatic epilepsy (MAE) (Doose syndrome)

This was initially proposed as a primary generalized epilepsy syndrome characterized by myoclonic and

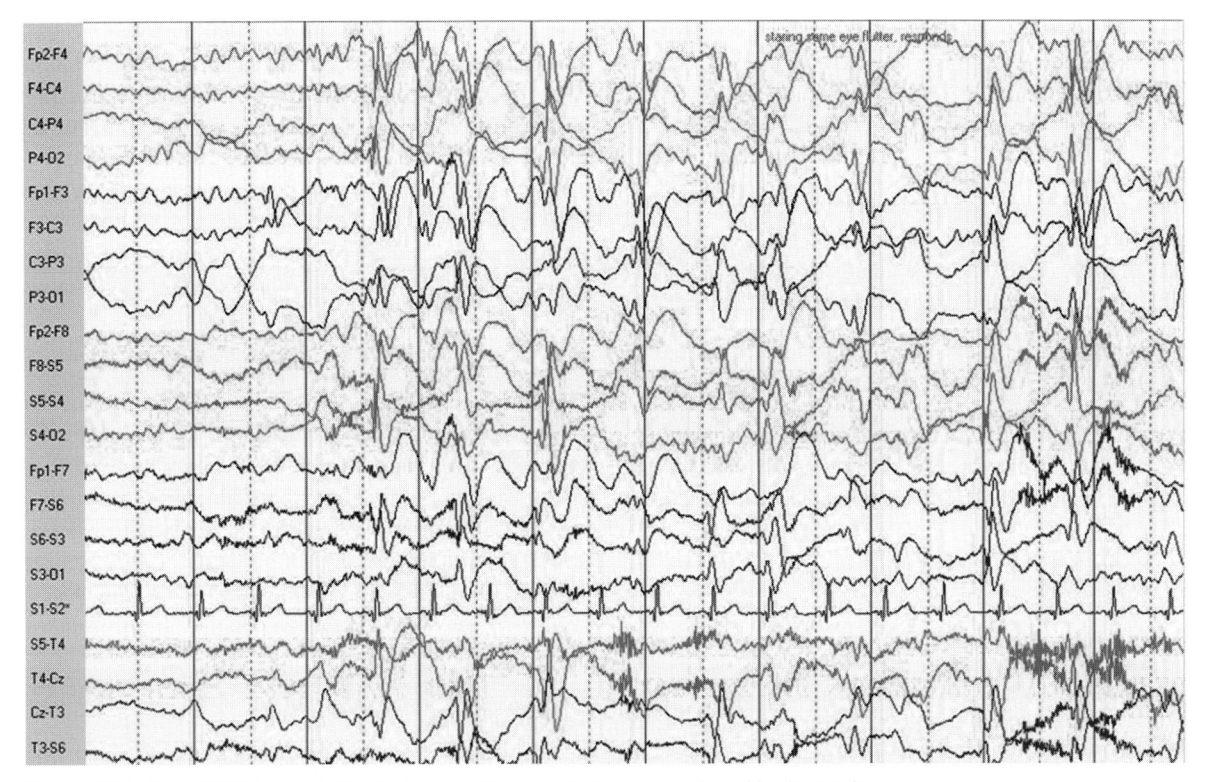

Figure 19.5. Typical EEG demonstrating 2 Hz slow spike wave discharge on a slowed background.

astatic, particularly atonic, seizures of idiopathic origin. However, in 1989 the ILAE classified this syndrome as a symptomatic/cryptogenic epilepsy. It is a relatively uncommon epilepsy syndrome. Genetic predisposition is common in a third of patients. It sits between childhood absence epilepsy and Lennox-Gastaut syndrome in terms of effects on cognition and development, difficulty to treat, and frequency of the generalized spike-and-wave on the EEG. Childhood absence epilepsy can appear as a Doose phenotype by using the wrong anticonvulsant drugs, e.g. using carbamazepine.

Age of onset: onset between 7 months and 8 years, peak at 2–6 years, and occurs usually in a previously normal child. Male preponderance is observed (3:1).

Seizure types

The first seizure is often a generalized tonic-clonic seizure, though rarely it can be a myoclonic or astatic seizure. Children typically have febrile seizures preceding afebrile seizures.

Generalized jerks or astatic falls occur several dozen times per day. Drop attacks are due to myoclonic-atonia (more common), massive myoclonus or myoatonia (loss of muscle tone). They cause frequent facial injuries.

Myoclonic seizures usually involve axial symmetrical jerks of limbs. They can be massive and violent, causing a fall, or rather subtle, resulting in brief head nods or abduction of the arms.

Atypical absences and non-convulsive status are common. Non-convulsive status presents with altered mentation, apathy, somnolence or drooling, often with erratic myoclonic jerks. They can last from minutes to weeks with fluctuations.

Tonic seizures are less common and may indicate transition to Lennox-Gastaut syndrome.

EEG findings

- The EEG initially shows a normal background.
- Three-per-second (2.5–3 Hz) spike-wave bursts without clear clinical correlate can be seen, often activated by sleep. The most suggestive findings are 4–7 Hz biparietal theta activity and occipital 4 Hz rhythms blocked by eye-opening.
- Photosensitivity may be observed.
- Myoclonic atonic seizures have associated bursts of spike-wave or polyspike-wave 2–4 Hz complexes.

Course and prognosis

The prognosis of MAE is variable. Despite recurrent falls, seizures may eventually abate, with a mean duration of active epilepsy of 3 years with satisfactory neuro-behavioural outcome in 50–89% of cases. In the remainder, epilepsy remains intractable, with variable degree of mental retardation and behavioural impairment (epileptic encephalopathy). It is not possible to predict at the onset or during the first year of the disorder, though presence of tonic seizures may indicate an adverse prognosis

- Treatment is primarily with sodium valproate, ethosuximide and benzodiazepines. Lamotrigine may be effective in controlling generalized tonic-clonic seizures rather than myoclonic seizures.
- It is important to avoid carbamazepine and vigabatrin (as it is generally in myoclonic epilepsies)
- Ketogenic diet may be particularly effective in this epilepsy syndrome.

Other myoclonic epilepsies

Myoclonic absence epilepsy occurs over a wide age range (1–12 years) with male preponderance (unlike other absence types). Absences with myoclonus are an integral part of the syndrome. Cognitive impairment may already be present at the onset and prognosis is less favourable. This syndrome can be relatively resistant to treatment with evolution to GTCS.

Eyelid myoclonia with absences (Jeavons' syndrome) is characterized by prominent jerking of the eyelids (much more intense than eyelid flutter seen with typical absences) with upward deviation of the eyes with typical absences. These can be very brief, making ascertainment of an absence difficult. There is a marked photosensitivity. In some patients, fixation-off sensitivity may be present, i.e absence of foveal fixation triggers an attack. Eyelid myoclonia with absences is usually associated with GTCS. Treatment may be difficult and require a combination of drugs (usually sodium valproate, ethosuximide and Clobazam). The attacks persist in adulthood.

Landau-Kleffner syndrome (acquired epileptic aphasia)

Landau-Kleffner syndrome (LKS) is a rare syndrome with bitemporal paroxysmal EEG abnormalities, first described in 1957. LKS is associated with ESES (electrical status epilepticus during sleep). ESES is defined as diffuse, continuous 1–3 Hz spike-waves appearing at the onset of sleep, and occupying more than 85% of slow-wave sleep.

Age of onset: the peak age of onset is 4–7 years, with male preponderance.

Seizure types

Typically, children are developmentally normal before the onset of the syndrome, showing normal language development. Regression of language occurs over a variable period, starting with auditory agnosia (inability to respond to familiar sounds, appearing deaf) leading to loss of acquired language. Nonverbal skills are relatively preserved. Clinical seizures occur in 75–85% of patients and in 60% are the first clinical manifestation (partial, complex partial or generalized motor). Behavioural disturbances may be prominent with this syndrome.

This syndrome can be regarded as epileptic encephalopathy.

EEG findings

The EEG is characteristic with high-amplitude bilateral generalized spike-wave complexes, mostly in bitemporal and parietal empahsis. These features vary in time and intensity. They augment in slow-wave sleep, leading to generalized spike-wave activity with loss of sleep architecture (ESES). This may continue in REM sleep too. However, the relationship between the language disturbance and the ESES is variable in each case.

Course, prognosis and treatment

Treatment remains difficult but sodium valproate, benzodiazepines and ethosuximide may be beneficial. Steroids and surgical procedures such as multiple subpial transactions may be useful. The prognosis is rather unpredictable but may be related to age of onset and the active period of ESES. Residual language and behavioural problems are common though EEG abnormalities tend to subside with increasing age.

Continuous spike-waves during slow-wave sleep (CSWS) syndrome

Like LKS, CSWS syndrome is also associated with ESES.

The syndrome of CSWS occurs in clinically diverse settings, in previously normal or developmentally delayed children. Approximately 20–30% of children may have identifiable brain pathology (while LKS, by definition, has no evidence of structural brain pathology). The regression is global rather than specific language impairment.

Age of onset: typical age of onset is 3–5 years, with seizures, usually nocturnal focal motor seizures, preceding the onset of CSWS.

Seizure types

CSWS may develop over months or years after the first seizures. Most have frequent nocturnal or diurnal seizures. Atonic seizures are highly suggestive (while they are not a feature of LKS), causing several falls a day. Tonic seizures are not a feature differentiating from Lennox-Gastaut syndrome where nocturnal tonic seizures are frequent. Absences are also common.

Mental and behavioural deterioration is present to a variable degree in almost all patients. Expressive aphasia rather than receptive aphasia is seen (whilst in LKS receptive aphasia occurs early, leading to expressive aphasia).

EEG findings

The EEG shows 1.5–2.5 Hz continuous diffuse spike-wave discharges at the onset of sleep, persisting throughout slow-wave sleep. Absence of this in REM sleep differentiates this from Landau-Kleffner syndrome. The initial features may appear similar to rolandic epilepsy with frequent multifocal spikes.

The long-term outlook of epilepsy is always favourable even with lesional cases. However, a variable level of mental impairment persists. Duration of CSWS longer than 2 years is a likely factor for a poor cognitive outcome.

Conclusion

Epilepsy syndromes in childhood and adolescence are phenotypically diverse. Accurate identification of these is mandatory for appropriate management and prognostication.

Recommended reading

Alarcón G, Nashef L, Cross H, Nightingale J and Richardson S. *Epilepsy. Oxford Specialist Handbooks in Neurology*. Oxford: Oxford University Press; 2009.

Berg AT, Berkovic SF, Brodie MJ, *et al*. Revised terminology and concepts for organization of seizures and epilepsies: report of the ILAE Commission on Classification and Terminology, 2005–2009. *Epilepsia* 2010;**51**:676–85.

Panayiotopoulos CP. *A Clinical Guide to Epileptic Syndromes and their Treatment*. 2nd edn. London: Springer; 2007.

Learning objective

(1) To know the following features of the main paediatric epilepsy syndromes:

- age of onset
- clinical manifestations and seizure types
- EEG manifestations
- treatment
- prognosis
- nosology.

Section 2 Classification and diagnosis of epilepsy

Chapter 20

Neonatal seizures

Ronit Pressler

Neonatal seizures are different from seizures in older children and adults in many respects such as aetiology, semiology, EEG characteristics and response to medication. The neonatal period is defined as the first 28 days of life. Seizures are more common in this time than during any other period throughout life. The incidence of clinical seizures in infants born at term (born between 37 and 42 weeks' gestational age) is 1.5–3.5 per 1000 live births (Ronen *et al.*, 1999; Saliba *et al.*, 1999). The incidence may be even higher in preterm infants (born before 37 weeks' gestational age), ranging from 1 to 13% of very-low-birthweight infants (Ronen *et al.* 1999). However, the incidence of electrographic seizures is unclear. Onset is usually within the first few days and over 60% of all cases eventually recognized have been diagnosed by the third day (Ronen *et al.*, 1999; Saliba *et al.*, 1999).

Aetiology

It is important to remember that most neonatal seizures are acute seizures, rather than symptoms of an epilepsy syndrome. This has implication for both investigations and treatment. Many causes can give rise to neonatal seizures (Table 20.1), although only a few of these conditions account for most seizures (Levene and Trounce, 1986; Mizrahi and Kellaway, 1998; Volpe, 2008). Few seizures are idiopathic (Tharp, 2002). Epileptic syndromes only rarely start in the neonatal period, but may show characteristic EEG features (Figure 20.1). At term, hypoxic ischaemic encephalopathy is the most common aetiology, typically with onset in the first 24 hours of life. In preterm infants, intracranial haemorrhage is the most common cause. Meningitis, focal cerebral infarction, metabolic disorders and congenital abnormalities of the brain can cause seizures at any gestation.

Clinical manifestation and classification

As aetiology and presentation of neonatal seizures are different from those of seizures in older children and adults, they do not easily fit into the 1981 ILAE classification of epileptic seizure types or the 1989 ILAE classification of epilepsy syndromes and epilepsies. Several classifications have been proposed, of which the classifications by Volpe (2008) and by Mizrahi and Kellaway (1987, 1998) are more widely used (Table 20.2).

Generalized tonic-clonic seizures are rare in the first month of life and are not seen in the preterm infant. Neonatal seizures are usually focal, often short-lasting. The development within the limbic system with connections to midbrain and brainstem is more advanced than the cerebral cortical organization, leading to a higher frequency of mouthing, eye deviation and apnoea in neonates than seizures in adults.

Mizrahi's classification has the advantage that it takes the origin of events into account and includes clinically silent electrographic seizures. According to Volpe's classification subtle seizures are the most common seizure type in both preterm and term babies. Manifestations include ocular, oral and autonomic phenomena as well as fragmentary body movements. Similar phenomena and motor behaviour may be seen in babies, especially in premature infants and encephalopathic infants. Although they are often less stereotyped and may be suppressed by restraints or triggered by stimulation, these are clinically very difficult to distinguish from seizures of epileptic origin (Mizrahi and Kellaway, 1998; Murray *et al.*, 2008). Prolonged video-EEG has clearly shown that the majority of infants with subtle seizures will exhibit ictal rhythmic epileptiform activity. The absence of ictal EEG discharges makes an epileptic origin of

---

Introduction to Epilepsy ed. Gonzalo Alarcón and Antonio Valentín. Published by Cambridge University Press.
© Cambridge University Press 2012.

Table 20.1. Causes of neonatal seizures

Cause	Frequency
Hypoxic-ischaemic encephalopathy	30–53%
Intracranial haemorrhage	7–17%
Cerebral infarction	6–17%
Cerebral malformations	3–17%
Meningitis/septicaemia	2–14%
Congenital infections	rare
Metabolic	
Hypoglycaemia	0.1–5%
Hypocalcaemia, hypomagnesaemia	4–22%
Hypo-/hypernatraemia	
Inborn errors of metabolism	3–4%
Glycine encephalopathy (neonatal non-ketotic hyperglycinaemia)	
Glucose transporter type 1 syndrome	
Pyridoxine/pyridoxal-5-phosphate dependent seizure	
Folinic acid responsive seizures	
Propionic aciduria	
Kernicterus	1%
Maternal drug withdrawal	4%
Idiopathic	2%
Neonatal epileptic syndromes	
Benign idiopathic neonatal convulsions (fifth-day fits)	
Benign familiar neonatal convulsions	
Early myoclonic encephalopathy	
Early infantile epileptic encephalopathy with burst-suppression pattern (Ohtahara syndrome)	

these movements less likely. This issue has been addressed in Mizrahi's classification: motor automatisms without clonic or tonic components and without EEG correlate are not considered to be of epileptic origin.

Although still considered in Volpe's seizure classification, generalized tonic posturing is unlikely to be epileptic seizures, but rather represents transient decerebrate or decorticate posturing, which can be triggered by stimulation and show no ictal EEG correlates. The EEG background activity is severely abnormal in these babies and outcome is poor. This seizure type is not classified to be of epileptic origin in Mizrahi's classification.

Diagnosis

The clinical diagnosis of neonatal seizures is recognized to be difficult, because clinical manifestations are often subtle and may be clinically silent (i.e. showing only electrographic changes). As a result the extent of the seizure burden may be greatly underestimated (Figure 20.2). This phenomenon is called electroclinical dissociation, i.e. seizures can be electroclinical, electrographic (subclinical) or clinical only (Weiner et al., 1991). However, clinical-only seizures may not be of epileptic origin, such as paroxysmal motor behaviour or tonic posturing (see above). Although there is some evidence from animal experiments suggesting that some seizures may arise in deep brainstem structures and never propagate to the surface (McCown and Breese, 1992), this is probably rare in human babies (Biagioni et al., 1998).

The large differential diagnosis following a neonatal seizure demands that the initial investigations should concentrate on the common aetiologies requiring prompt specific treatment. Certain clues to the aetiology may be present, such as a history of perinatal asphyxia or maternal narcotic abuse, but other causes such as hypoglycaemia, hypocalcaemia and CNS infection may co-exist and need excluding. Investigations should include:

- Laboratory: glucose, baseline biochemistry, magnesium, liver function, full blood count, clotting, blood gas. Also consider, ammoniac, metabolic screening, intrauterine infections (TORCH: Toxoplasmosis, Other – such as hepatitis B, syphilis, varicella-zoster virus, HIV, and parvovirus B19 – Rubella, Cytomegalovirus, Herpes simplex virus), screening for drug abuse.
- Septic screen including blood cultures and lumbar puncture (cell count, protein, glucose, lactate, pyruvate).
- Cranial ultrasound scanning, also consider MRI.
- EEG

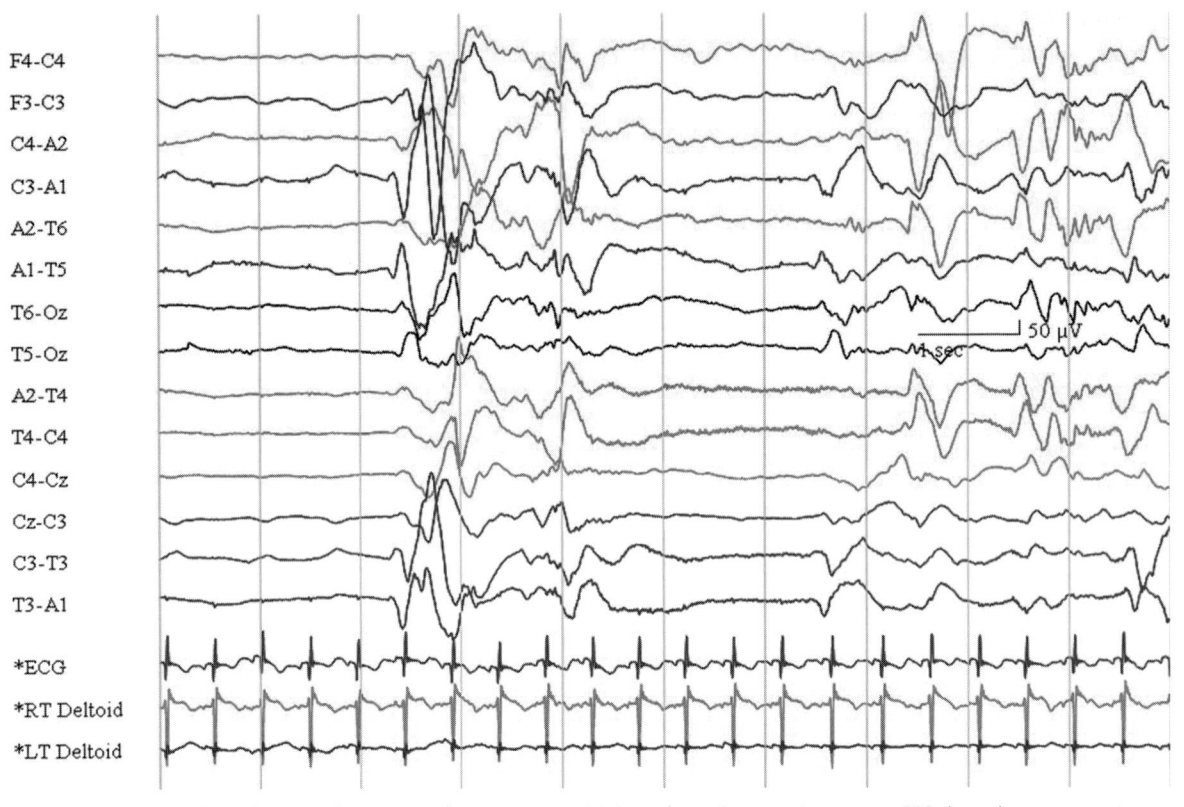

Figure 20.1. Term baby with onset of erratic myoclonic seizures at 16 days of age. Consanguine parents. EEG shows burst-suppression pattern: early myoclonic encephalopathy.

- Consider therapeutic trial of pyridoxine and pyridoxal 5-phosphate.
- In cases of unexplained/persistent hypoglycaemia investigate accordingly (lactate, ammonia, amino acids, urine organic acids, urine ketones, insulin, cortisol, free fatty acids, B-hydroxybutyrate).

EEG definitions for seizures vary, but rhythmic activity lasting more than 10 seconds is suspicious (Clancy and Ledigo, 1987). There is usually evolution of frequency, amplitude and morphology over time, typically with an increase in amplitude and a decrease of frequency (Figure 20.3). Table 20.3 summarizes EEG patterns seen during neonatal seizures. Most neonatal seizures have a focal origin but may spread to involve wider areas or even both hemispheres. The most common site of seizure onset is the temporal lobe (Figure 20.2). Neonatal seizures are usually brief, with 50% less than a minute, and tend to be shorter in preterm babies. Neonatal status is defined as a total seizure time occupying 50% of a 30 minute recording.

Discharges of less than 10 s duration have been termed BIRDs (brief interictal rhythmic discharges or brief ictal rhythmic discharges) and are of uncertain significance. However, BIRDs have been associated with seizures in the same or subsequent EEG and with poor neuro developmental outcome (Oliveira et al., 2000). Abnormal background activity is associated with an increased risk of subsequent seizures (Laroia et al., 1998) and poor neurodevelopmental outcome (Pezzani et al., 1986; Khan et al., 2008).

The amplitude integrated EEG (aEEG) has the advantage that it is widely available, and interpretation using pattern recognition can easily be learned (Hellstrom-Westas, 1992). However, short seizures (<30 s) cannot be detected, low-amplitude or focal seizures are easily missed (Figure 19.4) and movement artefacts are difficult to exclude and may look like seizures. Thus, in neonates aEEG is prone to false-negative and false-positive errors. Non-experts are prone to false-negative errors and the inter-observer agreement is low (Rennie et al., 2004).

Table 20.2. Classification of neonatal seizures

Adapted from Volpe (2008)		
Type	Characterization	Ictal EEG abnormalities
Subtle	Ocular, oral-buccal-lingual, autonomic, apnoea, limb posturing and movements.	Variable
Clonic	Repetitive jerking, distinct from jittering. Unifocal or multifocal.	Common
Myoclonic	Rapid isolated jerks. Focal, multifocal or generalized.	Common if generalized, uncommon if focal
Tonic	Stiffening. Decerebrate posturing. Focal or generalized.	Common if focal, uncommon if generalized

Adapted from Mizrahi and Kellaway (1987, 1998)		
Type	Characterization	Epileptic origin
Focal clonic	Rhythmic muscle contractions, unifocal or multifocal, synchronous or asynchronous. Not suppressed by restrain.	✓
Focal tonic	Sustained posturing of limb, trunk or neck. Also tonic eye deviation. Not provoked by external stimuli and not suppressed by restrain.	✓
Myoclonic	Random, single, rapid contractions of muscle groups. Usually not repetitive. May be generalized, focal or fragmentary. May be provoked by external stimuli.	✓/–
Spasms	Flexor or extensor. May occur in clusters. Not provoked by external stimuli and not suppressed by restrain.	✓
Electrographic	By definition none.	✓
Generalized tonic	Sustained symmetric posturing.	–
Motor automatism	Ocular, oral-buccal-lingual, progression movements of limbs or complex purposeless movements. May be provoked or intensified by external stimuli and suppressed by restrain.	–

Treatment

A recent Cochrane report has reviewed the treatment of neonatal seizures (Booth and Evans, 2004). Only two randomized controlled studies were identified using adequate methodology (Painter et al., 1999; Boylan et al., 2002), both indicating that current first-line treatment with phenobarbitone was only effective in about 40–50% of babies. Furthermore, phenobarbitone and phenytoin can increase electroclinical dissociation: clinical seizure manifestations may be suppressed but electrographic seizure activity will often persist (electroclinical dissociation or uncoupling) (Boylan et al., 2002; Scher et al., 2003) illustrating the need for EEG monitoring during treatment of neonatal seizures. A trial of pyridoxine, pyridoxal-5-phosphate and folinic acid should be considered. For a recent review on AED treatment of neonatal seizures, see Riviello 2004a and 2004b.

Table 20.4 summarizes antiepileptic drug treatment of neonatal seizures.

Prognosis

The prognosis is mainly determined by the aetiology and is overall better for term than for preterm babies (Ronen et al., 2007). In hypoxic-ischaemic encephalopathy, the prognosis depends very much on the grade (overall 30–50% normal), while CNS malformations are generally associated with poor outcome. Both animal and clinical studies suggest that neonatal seizures have an adverse effect on neurodevelopmental outcome, and predispose to cognitive, behavioural or epileptic complications in

Section 2: Classification and diagnosis of epilepsy

Table 20.3. EEG features of neonatal seizures

Rhythmic sharp waves or spikes	Common
Monomorphous delta or theta waves	Common
Sequence of alpha or beta frequencies	Relatively common
Electrodecremental event	Uncommon
PLEDs	Rare
Burst-suppression pattern	Rare
Simultaneous independent seizures	May be associated with poorer prognosis

later life (Ben Ari and Holmes, 2006; Cornejo et al., 2007). There is evidence that electrographic seizures have an impact on long-term outcome similar to electro-clinical seizures (McBride et al., 2000).

However, there is also increasing concern about the potentially adverse effects of antiepileptic drugs on the developing nervous system. In animal models, phenobarbitone has been shown to cause additional brain damage by increasing neuronal death (apoptosis) (Bittigau et al., 2002; Kim et al., 2007). Treatment improvements for neonatal seizures have been identified as a high research priority by several international expert groups with emphasis on new innovative strategies targeted specifically at the needs of babies with the ultimate aim of improving long-term outcome (Chiron et al., 2008; Silverstein et al., 2008).

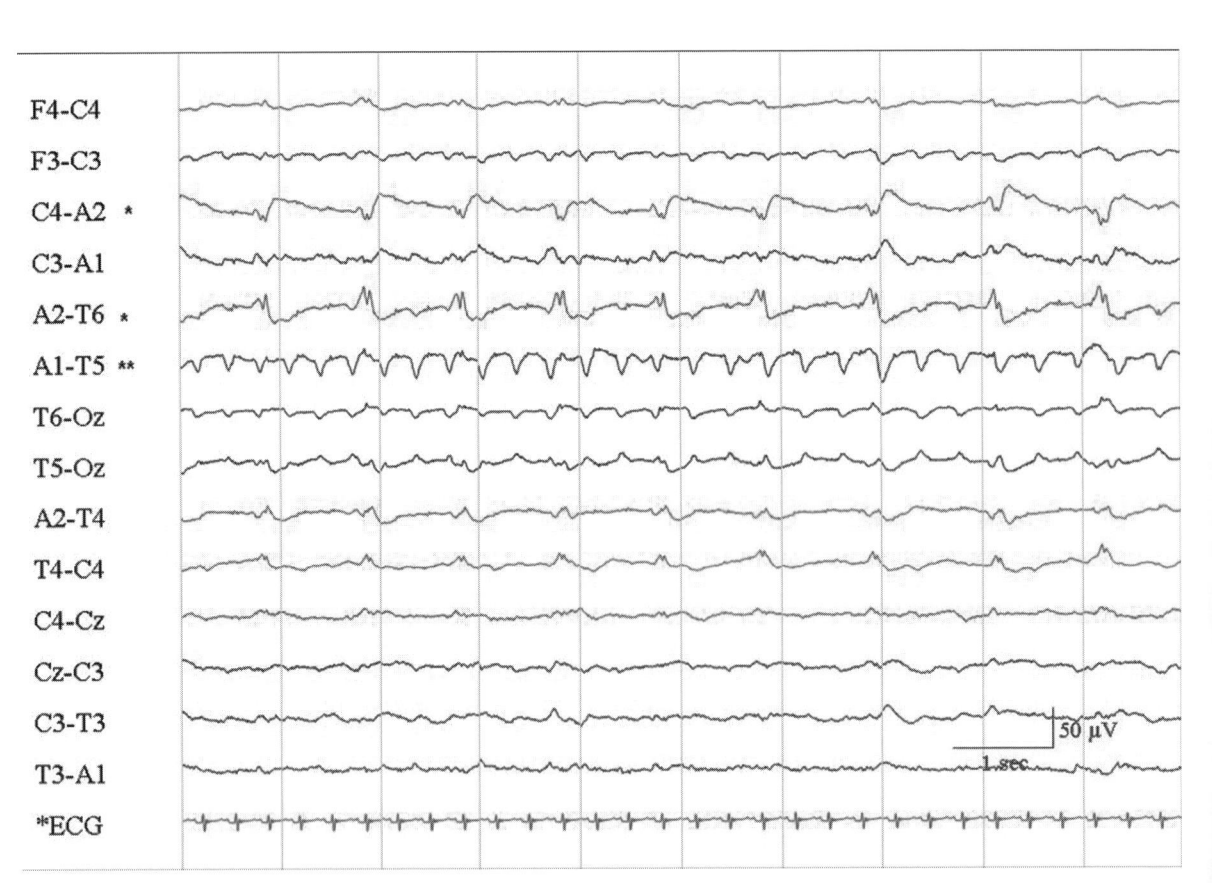

Figure 20.2. Newborn with early-onset Group B streptococcus meningitis and electrographic seizures on EEG. Characteristic features of neonatal seizures: two simultaneous, but quite different seizure pattern discharges over the two hemispheres (*right temporal and **left posterior) with independent on- and off-set. There were no obvious clinical manifestations (electro-clinical dissociation).

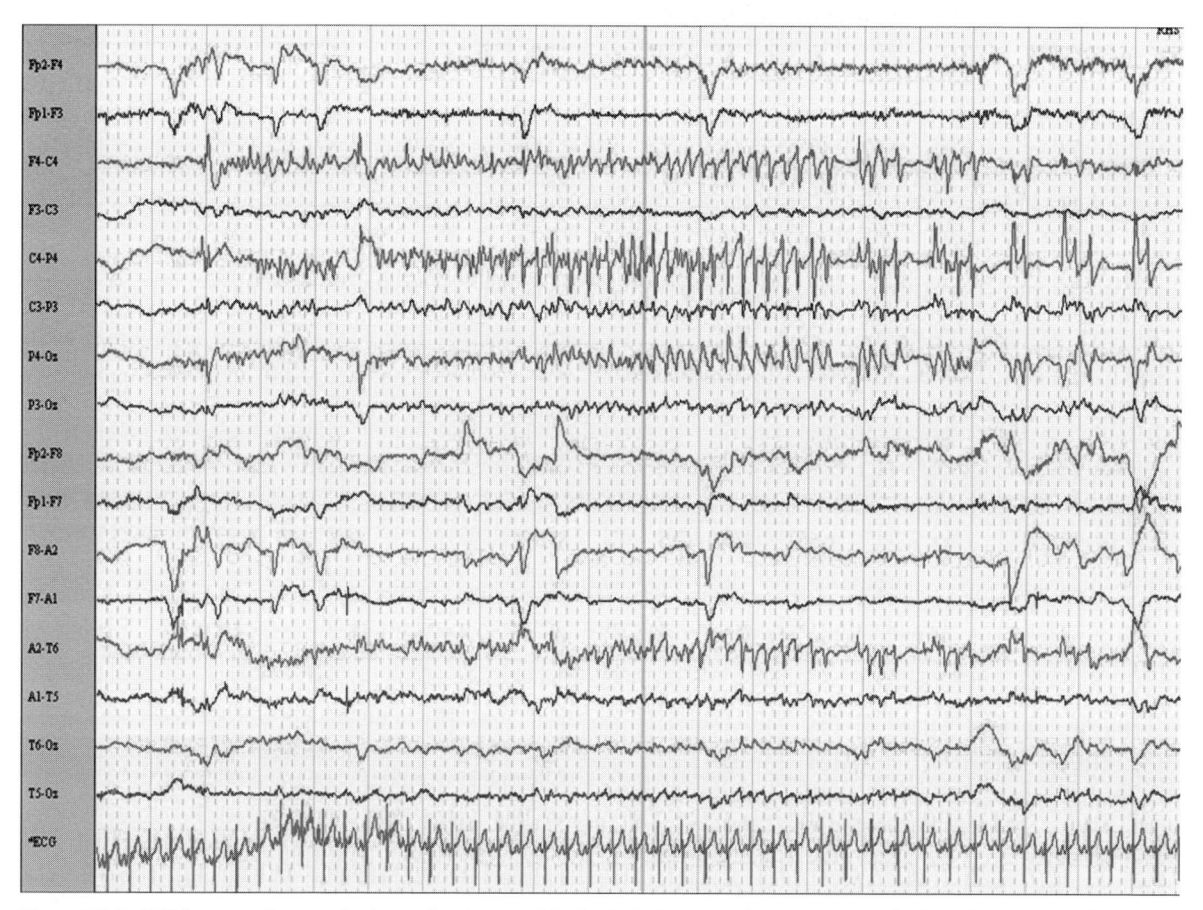

Figure 20.3. EEG features of neonatal seizures: focal onset of rhythmic discharges with increase in amplitude and a decrease of frequency, usually poorly sustained. Note different time scale.

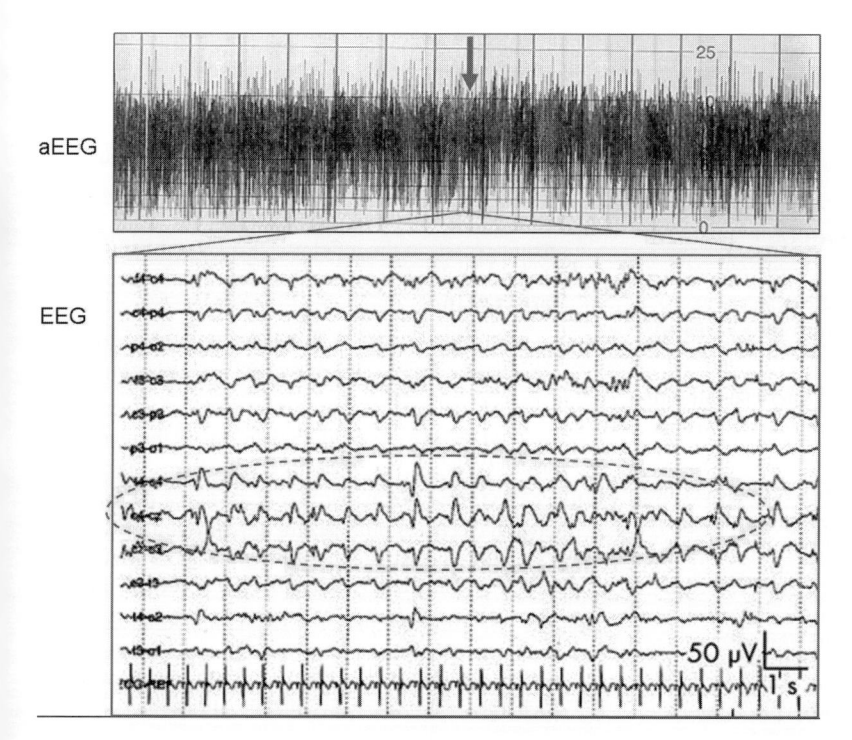

Figure 20.4. Term infant with moderate hypoxic ischaemic encephalopathy. Amplitude integrated EEG (aEEG) on day 2 shows a moderately abnormal background activity (amplitude between < 5 μV to > 10 μV), but no seizures. An EEG at point marked by arrow reveals low amplitude electrographic seizure (dotted line) lasting 30 s, which correlated to subtle eye deviation on video.

Table 20.4. Antiepileptic drug dose in the newborn

Drug	Initial dose	Route	Maintenance	Route	Therapeutic level
Phenobarbital	20–40 mg/kg	iv	3–5 mg/kg	iv/o	90–180 µmol/l
Phenytoin	15–20 mg/kg	iv/20 min	3–5 mg/kg	iv/o	40–80 µmol/l
Lorazepam	0.05–0.1 mg/kg	iv	every 8–12 h	iv	
Diazepam	0.2–0.5 mg/kg	iv	every 6–8 h	iv	
Clonazepam	0.1 mg/kg	iv/30 min			30–100 mg/l
Midazolam	0.1–0.2 mg/kg	iv	0.1–0.3 mg/kg/h	iv	
Lignocaine	2 mg/kg	iv	1–6 mg/kg/h	iv	3–6 mg/l
Valproate	10–20 mg/kg	iv/o	20 mg/kg	o	275–350 µmol/l
Paraldehyde	0.1–0.2 ml/kg	pr			
Pyridoxine (B6)	50–100 mg	iv	100 mg every 10 min (up to 500 mg)		

Please note: drug doses vary between countries and between hospitals. Local protocols and guidelines have to be considered.

References

Ben Ari Y, Holmes GL. Effects of seizures on developmental processes in the immature brain. *Lancet Neurol* 2006;**5**:1055–63.

Biagioni E, Ferrari F, Boldrini A, Roversi MF, Cioni G. Electroclinical correlation in neonatal seizures. *Eur J Paediatr Neurol*. 1998;**2**:117–25.

Bittigau P, Sifringer M, Genz K, et al. Antiepileptic drugs and apoptotic neurodegeneration in the developing brain, *Proc Natl Acad Sci USA* 2002;**99**(23):15 089–94.

Booth D, Evans DJ. Anticonvulsants for neonates with seizures. *Cochrane Database Syst Rev* 2004;**18**;(4): CD004218.

Boylan GB, Rennie JM, Pressler RM, et al. Phenobarbitone, neonatal seizures and video-EEG. *Arch Dis Child* 2002;**86**:F165–70.

Chiron C, Dulac O, Pons G. Antiepileptic drug development in children: considerations for a revisited strategy. *Drugs* 2008;**68**:17–25.

Clancy RR, Ledigo A. The exact ictal and interictal duration of electroencephalographic neonatal seizures. *Epilepsia* 1987;**28**:537–41.

Cornejo BJ, Mesches MH, Coultrap S, et al. A single episode of neonatal seizures permanently alters glutamatergic synapses. *Ann Neurol* 2007;**61**(5):411–26.

Hellstrom-Westas L. Comparison between tape recorded and amplitude integrated EEG monitoring in sick newborn infants. *Acta Paediatr* 1992;**81**:812–19.

Khan RL, Nunes ML, Garcias da Silva LF, da Costa JC. Predictive value of sequential electroencephalogram (EEG) in neonates with seizures and its relation to neurological outcome. *J Child Neurol* 2008;**23**:144–50.

Kim JS, Kondratyev A, Tomita Y, Gale K. Neurodevelopmental impact of antiepileptic drugs and seizures in the immature brain. *Epilepsia* 2007; **48**(Suppl 5):19–26.

Laroia N, Guillet R, Burchfield J, et al. EEG Background as predictor of electrographic seizures in high-risk neonates. *Epilepsia* 1998;**39**:545–51.

Levene MI, Trounce JQ. Causes of neonatal convulsions. *Arch Dis Child* 1986;**61**:78–9.

McBride MC, Laroia N, Guillet R. Electrographic seizures in neonates correlate with poor neurodevelopmental outcome. *Neurology* 2000;**55**:506–13.

McCown TJ, Breese GR. The developmental profile of seizure genesis in the inferior collicular cortex of the rat: relevance to human neonatal seizures. *Epilepsia* 1992;**33**:2–10.

Mizrahi EM, Kellaway P. Characterization and classification of neonatal seizures. *Neurology* 1987;**37**:1837–44.

Mizrahi EM, Kellaway P. *Diagnosis and Management of Neonatal Seizures*. 1st edn. Philadelphia: Lippincott-Raven; 1998.

Murray DM, Boylan GB, Ali I, et al. Defining the gap between electrographic seizure burden, clinical expression and staff recognition of neonatal seizures. *Arch Dis Child Fetal Neonatal Ed* 2008;**93**:F187–F191.

Oliveira AJ, Nunes ML, Haertel LM, et al. Duration of rhythmic EEG pattern in neonates: new evidence for clinical and prognostic significance of brief rhythmic discharges. *Clin Neurophysiol* 2000;**111**:1646–53.

Painter MJ, Scher MS, Stein AD, *et al*. Phenobarbital compared with phenytoin for the treatment of neonatal seizures. *N Eng J Med* 1999;**341**:485–9.

Pezzani C, Radvani-Bouvet MF, Relier JP, Monod N. Neonatal electroencephalography during the first 24 hours of life in full term newborn infants. *Neuropaediatrics* 1986;**17**:11–18.

Rennie JM, Chorley G, Boylan G, *et al*. Non-expert use of the cerebral function monitor for neonatal seizure detection. *Arch Dis Child* 2004;**89**:F37–F40.

Riviello JJ. Drug therapy for neonatal seizures: part 1. *NeoReviews* 2004a;**5**:215–20.

Riviello JJ. Drug therapy for neonatal seizures: part 2. *NeoReviews* 2004b;**5**:262–8.

Ronen GM, Buckley D, Penney S, Streiner DL. Long-term prognosis in children with neonatal seizures: a population-based study. *Neurology* 2007;**69**:1816–22.

Ronen GM, Penney S, Andrews W. The epidemiology of clinical neonatal seizures in Newfoundland: a population-based study. *J Pediatr* 1999;**134**:71–5.

Saliba RM, Annegers JF, Waller DK, Tyson JE, Mizrahi EM. Incidence of neonatal seizures in Harris County, Texas, 1992–1994. *Am J Epidemiol* 1999;**150**:763–9.

Scher M, Alvin J, Gaus L, *et al*. Uncoupling of EEG-clinical neonatal seizures after antiepileptic drug use. *Pediatr Neurol* 2003;**28**:277–80.

Silverstein FS, Jensen FE, Inder T, *et al*. Improving the treatment of neonatal seizures: National Institute of Neurological Disorders and Stroke workshop report. *J Pediatr* 2008;**153**(1):12–5. No abstract available.

Tharp BR. Neonatal seizures and syndromes. *Epilepsia* 2002;**43**(Suppl 3):2–10.

Volpe JJ. Neonatal seizures. In Volpe JJ, ed. *Neurology of the Newborn*, pp. 203–244. 5th edn. Philadelphia: WB Saunders; 2008.

Weiner SP, Painter MJ, Geva D, *et al*. Neonatal seizures: electroclinical dissociation. *Pediatr Neurol* 1991;**7**:363–8.

Learning objectives

(1) To know the main aetiologies of neonatal seizures.
(2) To understand the classification of neonatal seizures.
(3) To know the main criteria to diagnosis and treat neonatal seizures.
(4) To understand the prognosis of neonatal seizures.

Section 2 Classification and diagnosis of epilepsy

Chapter 21
Epileptic encephalopathies in the first year of life

William Whitehouse

Introduction

The term epileptic encephalopathy is not a disease or syndrome designation, but can be useful when used judiciously. Here it refers to diverse disorders of the brain manifest as the combination of an epilepsy (typically one that is difficult to treat) and developmental delay, arrest or regression (especially affecting cognition and learning and behaviour). Such an operational definition captures the clinical situations where an underlying disease produces both a severe intractable epilepsy and developmental/cognitive impairment in parallel, and the situation where the epileptic activity so disrupts brain function as to cause the developmental/cognitive impairment. Commonly the cognitive impairment will vary with the severity of the epilepsy, implying that at least some of the impairment is caused by the ongoing epilepsy process. The development is particularly susceptible in infancy and early childhood because of the phenomenon of 'windows for development' which once missed will never be adequately made-up for. For example, the ability to learn a language is superb in the first 2 years of life; it then declines, and if learned after about 11 years of age language abilities will probably not achieve the same level. So, even if the cognitive impairment were wholly caused by epileptic activity in a particular child, catching up after epilepsy subsides may not be possible, or only partly possible.

The archetypal epileptic encephalopathy of the first year of life is West syndrome or infantile spasms (IS). Early infantile epileptic encephalopathy or Ohtahara syndrome (OS) and early myoclonic encephalopathy (EME), and borderline or overlap cases, are neonatal or early infantile (within the first 3 months) versions of IS. Catastrophic epilepsy in infancy, of any cause, but particularly not complying with the syndromes above, covers diverse infantile epilepsies with severe and frequent epileptic seizures (many every day), typically impairing development and also often affecting cardiorespiratory function, and ability to feed, requiring extensive medical support.

West syndrome or infantile spasms

The terminology can be confusing but the terms West syndrome and infantile spasms can be considered equivalent (Lux and Osborne 2004). First described in his own son by Dr West (1841), this syndrome comprises epileptic infantile spasms, developmental arrest or regression and a particular interictal EEG appearance: 'hypsarrhythmia' or modified hypsarrhythmia. Onset ocurs from 3 to 13 months of age and the incidence is 2–4/10 000 live births.

The epileptic seizures comprise salvos of flexor and/or extensor axial epileptic spasms ('myoclonic-tonic' seizures), occurring typically close to sleep or on waking up. They may be subtle or sparse initially but generally cluster several times a day.

Developmental arrest or regression may suggest an acquired visual impairment, with loss of fixation and social regard, and smiling. The infant may appear passive and apathetic, but can be annoyed by the spasms, or less often an infant may smile after a cluster.

Hypsarrhythmia is difficult to define operationally but essentially comprises a very abnormal EEG background pattern or rhythm which is chaotic in amplitude and frequency, with diffuse, irregular, disorganized, sometimes asymmetrical, high-voltage slow waves with sharp waves and spikes mixed in (Figure 21.1). Early on in the first week or so it may not be evident in the awake record, so a sleep EEG may be needed. Ictally there is classically an abrupt lowering of the EEG amplitude

---

Introduction to Epilepsy ed. Gonzalo Alarcón and Antonio Valentín. Published by CAMBRIDGE UNIVERSITY PRESS.
© Cambridge University Press 2012.

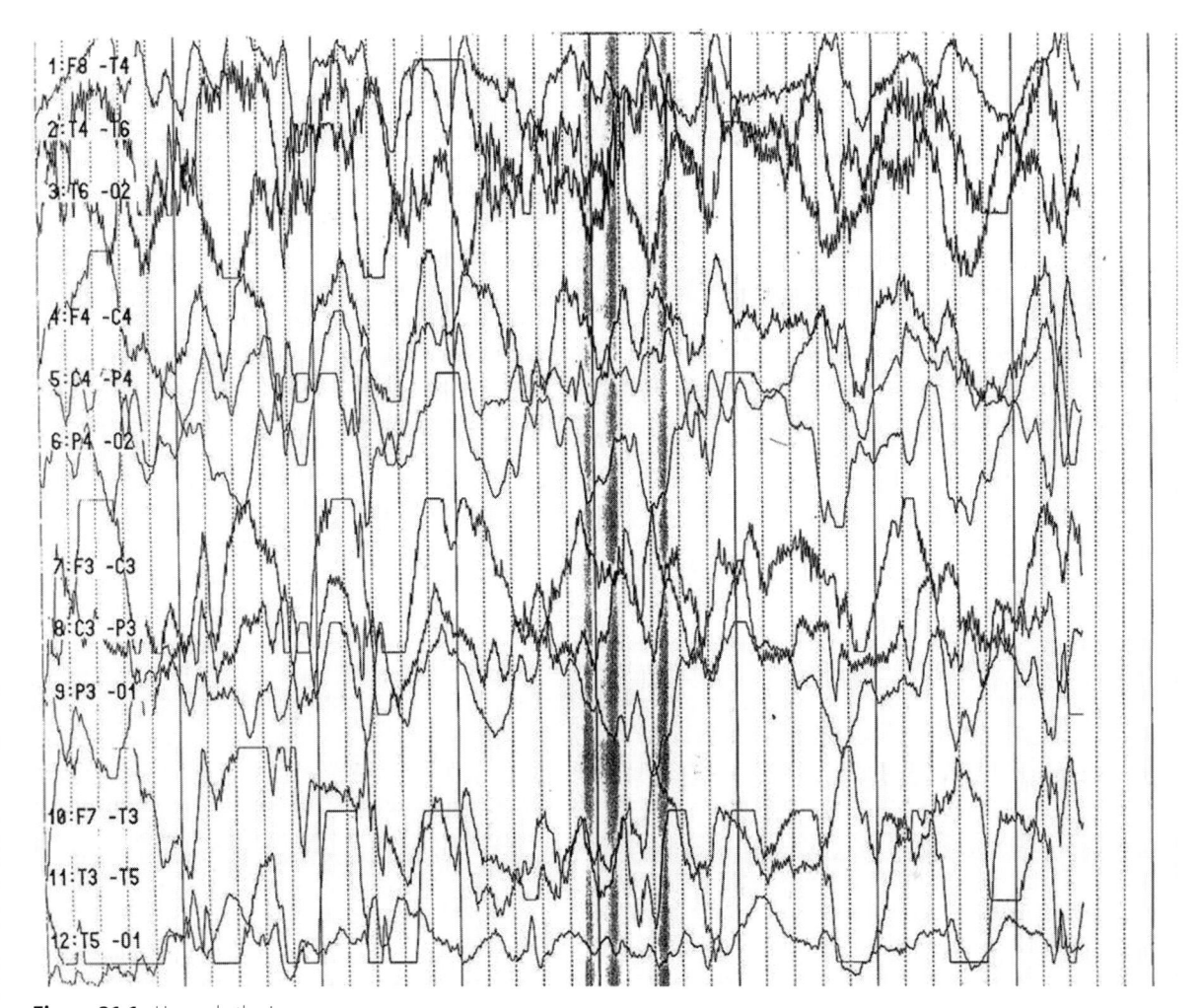

Figure 21.1. Hypsarrhythmia.

(attenuation or electrodecrement), but there may also be more spikes or focal discharges. Modified hypsarrhythmia has a periodicity, i.e. some synchronicity, to the chaotic pattern.

Many different diseases and causes can produce IS, but often the underlying cause cannot be identified. A few children (10%) can be considered to have idiopathic IS: those with previously normal development, classic EEG abnormalities and no cause found after exhaustive investigation. They have a relatively good prognosis. Cryptogenic IS refers to cases where an underlying cause seems probable, but is so far unknown. Symptomatic IS is used when the cause has been identified (50–70%). Underlying causes found include specific syndromes such as tuberous sclerosis (autosomal dominant with variable expression, found in 25% of IS), progressive encephalopathy with hypsarrhythmia and optic atrophy (autosomal recessive), Sturge-Weber syndrome (sporadic), Aicardi syndrome (X-linked dominant, seen in females), cortical dysplasias and brain malformations, metabolic diseases (e.g. pyridoxine dependency, phenylketonuria, non-ketotic hyperglycinaemia), hypoxic-ischaemic and hypoglycaemic brain injury, brain haemorrhage or trauma, cerebral infection (congenital infection, meningitis, encephalitis, brain abscess) and other causes of brain injury or dysfunction in this age group.

The EEG will exclude the most important differential diagnoses, and should be undertaken urgently (i.e. within a day or two of the diagnosis being considered). Benign myoclonic epilepsy of infancy, and non-epileptic conditions, e.g. benign myoclonus of early infancy, benign infantile sleep myoclonus, hyperekplexia, are important to consider.

First-line treatment should be started within a few days of the diagnosis being considered, but only in confirmed cases. High-dose steroids, e.g. prednisolone 10 mg four times a day increasing to 20 mg three times a day for 2 weeks followed by a tapering dose over 2–4 weeks, is popular and likely to be effective in the short term in 70%; tetracosactide 0.5 mg (40 IU) im on alternate days for 2 weeks followed by prednisolone taper (effective in 76%) or vigabatrin (effective in 54%), 50–200 mg/kg/day for up to 6 months if effective (Lux et al., 2004). If these fail consider pyridoxime, valproate, nitrazepam, topiramate and epilepsy surgery.

Prognosis is guarded, with overall 10–25% having normal or near-normal developmental outcomes, rising to 40–45% in idiopathic and cryptogenic cases. Consequently, 75–90% will have severe or profound developmental delay or mental retardation, with 25% having an autism spectrum disorder, and 50–60% developing other epilepsies as they get older, e.g. Lennox-Gastaut syndrome.

Early epileptic encephalopathies with suppression-burst EEG

Early (neonatal) myoclonic encephalopathy (EME) comprises onset under 3 months of age, fragmentary myoclonus with or without tonic/spasms, focal motor seizures and massive myoclonus, suppression-burst EEG, especially in sleep, with or without spells of hypsarrhythmia or atypical hypsarrhythmia. It overlaps with IS and OS. Some cases are autosomal recessive, including those with identified metabolic diseases e.g. non-ketotic hyperglycineaemia, proprionic acidaemia, D-glycine acidaemia. Many remain cryptogenic. The MRI is initially normal but later demonstrates acquired cerebral atrophy.

Early infantile epileptic encephalopathy or Ohtahara syndrome (OS) comprises onset under 3 months with tonic spasms, often in salvos, especially in sleep, with or without focal motor seizures, with or without alternating hemiconvulsions, or generalized tonic-clonic seizures, without clear myoclonus. There is suppression-burst on the EEG, stable in wake and sleep, evolving to West syndrome with hypsarrhythmia over time. It overlaps with IS and EME. In contrast to EME, the MRI is usually abnormal (e.g. porencephaly, cortical dysplasia, malformations, Aicardi syndrome, hypoxic-ischaemic injury). Less often, a metabolic cause is found, e.g. cytochrome oxidase deficiency. Some remain cryptogenic.

Borderline and overlap cases are relatively common.

All are generally refractory to antiepileptic drugs, steroids or pyridoxine, so care not to cause more harm than good is needed with medical treatment. Care is supportive and palliative. In the past, they have proved intractable with profound developmental delay and significant mortality, e.g. up to half by 2 years for EME. Mortality seems to have decreased with proper care and avoiding excessive drugs, using gastrostomies and with supporting families in the community.

References

Lux AL, Osborne JP. A proposal for case definitions and outcome measures in studies of Infantile Spasms and West syndrome: consensus statement of west Delphi group. *Epilepsia* 2004;**45**:1416–28.

Lux AL, Edwards SW, Hancock E, *et al*. The UK Infantile Spasms study comparing Vigabatrin with Prednisolone or tetracosactide at 14 days: a multicentre, randomised controlled trial. *Lancet* 2004;**364**:1773–8.

West JW. On a peculiar form of infantile convulsions. *Lancet* **1841**;i:724–5.

Learning objectives

(1) To understand the concept of epileptic encephalopathy.
(2) To be able to diagnose and treat infantile spasms.
(3) To recognize the spectrum of early epileptic encephalopathies with suppression-burst.

Section 2

Classification and diagnosis of epilepsy

Chapter 22

Epileptic encephalopathies in early childhood

William Whitehouse

Introduction

The term epileptic encephalopathy has already been discussed in the previous chapter on the epileptic encephalopathies of the first year of life. This chapter will focus on atypical absence seizures, Lennox-Gastaut syndrome, myoclonic-astatic epilepsy (MAE) and atypical benign partial epilepsy (ABPE). Severe myoclonic epilepsy of infancy or Dravet syndrome (DS) will be discussed in the following chapter on febrile convulsions and febrile seizures.

Atypical absence seizures are the clinical hallmark of Lennox-Gastaut syndrome. They have a less abrupt onset and termination than typical absence seizures (e.g. those seen in childhood absence epilepsy) and slower spike-wave activity, at 1.5–2.5 cycles per second (see Figure 22.1). They may be associated with hypotonia, hypertonia, erratic/fragmentary myoclonus, salivation, and are prone to absence status. The term should not be used for any kind of uncharacteristic absence seizure but specifically and only when these criteria are met.

Lennox-Gastaut syndrome (LGS)

This syndrome was originally described as an epileptic 'encephalopathy in childhood with slow spike waves'. Definitions vary.

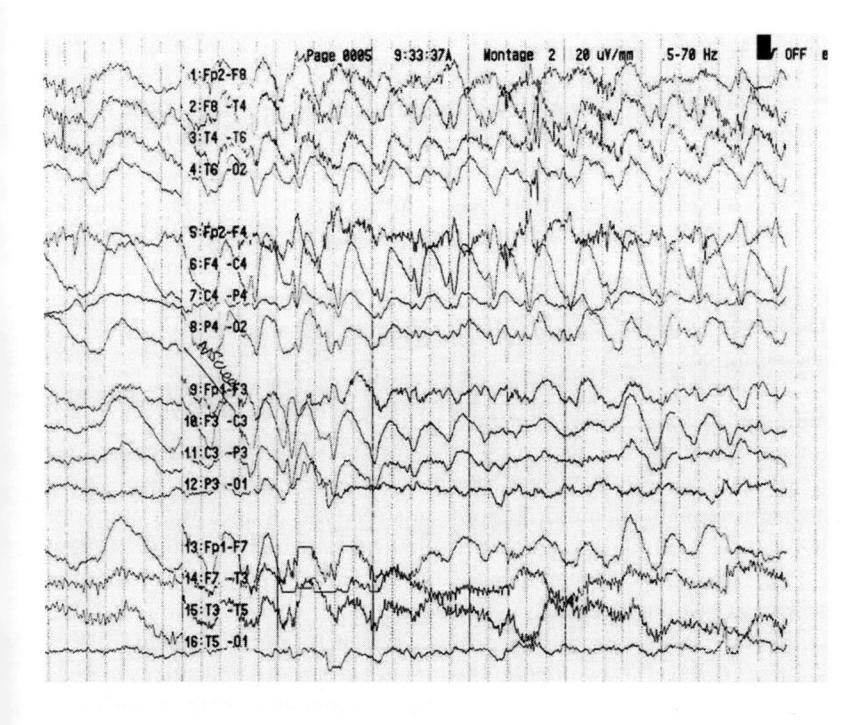

Figure 22.1. EEG demonstrating slow spike and wave of an atypical absence seizure in Lennox-Gastaut syndrome.

Introduction to Epilepsy ed. Gonzalo Alarcón and Antonio Valentín. Published by Cambridge University Press.
© Cambridge University Press 2012.

A strict (European) definition requires

- the following seizures: axial tonic seizures (typically in sleep), and atonic seizures, and atypical absence seizures (see above);
- and on EEG, diffuse slow spike wave 2–2.5 cycles per second (c/s) while awake, and fast rhythm bursts ~10 c/s while asleep;
- and developmental delay;
- and onset from age 1–8 years.

In addition there may be myoclonic seizures, absence status, GTCS or focal motor seizures. Typically there are many seizures each day, and associated head and face injuries from atonic seizures.

A loose (North American) definition: any seizures and slow spike wave 1.5–2.5 c/s.

Twenty to 40% of children with LGS have had previous West syndrome/infantile spasms (IS). Seventy to 75% have had previous developmental delay or brain lesions or significantly abnormal brain MRI, or previous epilepsy. It is essential not to think of LGS as a specific disease; remember it is an epilepsy syndrome and try to identify the underlying cause whenever possible. The list of possible causes is as for IS. The differential diagnosis includes the other epileptic encephalopathies discussed below and also, importantly, overtreatment and/or mistreatment of idiopathic generalized epilepsy with inappropriate anticonvulsants, e.g. treating childhood absence epilepsy with carbamazepine can provoke atonic and myoclonic seizures, worsen absence seizures and cause cognitive impairment, resembling LGS.

Treatment is often only partially successful and overly aggressive treatment can cause worse problems. LGS has an intractable and fluctuating course in childhood, with seizures becoming less of a problem in the teenage years, when learning and behavioural problems, often with an autism spectrum disorder, are the main issues. Valproate, clobazam, ethosuximide, lamotrigine, topiramate, levetiracetam, felbamate, stiripentiol and rufinamide can be tried, but beware of polypharmacy adverse effects on alertness, learning and quality of life. Steroids can help in short courses during exacerbations, and always consider possible referral for epilepsy surgery. Cortical resection or a palliative anterior corpus callosotomy (for atonic seizures) may be indicated. Also the ketogenic diet and vagus nerve stimulation can be very effective. Although carbamazepine or phenytoin can help prevent generalized tonic-clonic seizures, they can sometimes worsen the minor seizures.

Myoclonic-astatic epilepsy

Myoclonic-astatic epilepsy is a loosely and variably defined childhood epilepsy comprising the following seizure types: myoclonic-atonic/astatic seizures, with or without other seizures seen in idiopathic generalized epilepsies (typical absence seizures, atypical absence seizures, generalized tonic-clonic seizures), with or without myoclonic seizures, atonic seizures or absence status; an EEG with generalized spike-wave or polyspike-wave at 2.5–3.5 Hz, with or without background occipital/parietal theta rhythms at 4–7 Hz; with age of onset 1–5 years, in a previously intact child. Classically no underlying cause will be found; however, pathogenic mutations, e.g. in sodium channel SCN1A, have been found in some cases. It is a severe idiopathic generalized epilepsy and overlaps with the more idiopathic Lennox-Gastaut syndrome (so it is often classified with the 'symptomatic generalized epilepsies'). During worsening phases, cognition, learning and behaviour are impaired. Nevertheless, the prognosis is not so poor as in Lennox-Gastaut syndrome, and there is often remission or evolution to a milder epilepsy syndrome occurs (e.g. to early-onset childhood absence epilepsy). Treatment with valproate, ethosuximide or clobazam (or all three, at high dose) can help. Also consider acetazolamide, sulthiame, lamotrigine, topiramate, levetiracetam and steroids. Avoid or withdraw carbamazepine, phenytoin, vigabatrin and tiagabine. The relapse rate appears high on antiepileptic drug withdrawal.

Atypical benign partial epilepsy

This is an uncommon differential diagnosis for Lennox-Gastaut syndrome. Children have focal motor seizures in sleep, and periods with atonic or focal atonic or astatic frequent falls, with or without other seizure types. The EEG is very helpful in excluding Lennox-Gastaut syndrome by showing focal sharp waves, which are more frequent in sleep with periods with electrical status epilepticus in sleep (ESES), and irregular generalized spike wave/single spike wave while awake (Figure 22.2). The onset is from age 1–8 years. The children are generally previously intact. It can be seen in a significant minority of

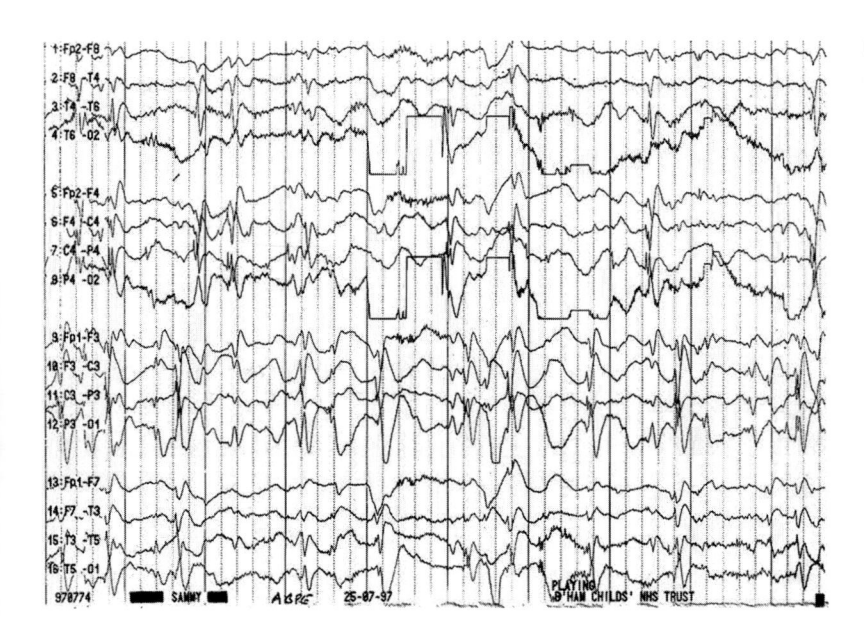

Figure 22.2. EEG in atypical benign partial epilepsy.

children treated for benign rolandic epilepsy with centrotemporal spikes and Panayiotopoulos syndrome with carbamazepine, oxcarbazepine or lamotrigine. Atypical benign partial epilepsy is part of a spectrum of idiopathic focal epilepsies in childhood including benign epilepsy of chilhood with centrotemporal spikes, benign partial epilepsy with affective symptoms, epilepsy with status epilepticus during sleep, continuous spike and wave during slow-wave sleep and Landau-Kleffner syndrome (Doose and Baier, 1989). Valproate, clobazam, sulthiame, acetazolamide and steroids can help. Seizure and developmental outcome is often good.

Reference

Doose H, Baier WK. Benign partial epilepsy and related conditions:multifactorial pathogenesis with hereditary impairment of brain maturation. *Eur J Pediatr* 1989;**149**:152–8.

Learning objectives

(1) To understand, recognize and use the term 'atypical absence seizure' correctly.
(2) To understand and use the strict definition of LGS.
(3) To be able to recognize LGS and similar but distinct epilepsies.

Section 2: Classification and diagnosis of epilepsy

Chapter 23: Febrile convulsions/seizures and related epileptic syndromes

William Whitehouse

Introduction

This chapter will focus on febrile convulsions (FCs) and febrile seizures (FSs), severe myoclonic epilepsy of infancy or Dravet syndrome (DS) and generalized epilepsy with febrile seizures plus (GEFS+). Mesial temporal lobe epilepsy (MTLE) with hippocampal sclerosis will be discussed in more detail elsewhere.

Febrile seizures

'Febrile seizures' is often used synonymously with FCs, although it is sometimes also used to cover acute symptomatic epileptic seizures accompanied by fever in addition to FCs. In its broadest sense FSs include epileptic seizures precipitated by fever: acute symptomatic epileptic seizures, exacerbations of epilepsies with fever, febrile convulsions and non-epileptic seizures such as syncopal (or 'anoxic') seizures/convulsions with fever and hypotonic-unresponsive episodes (of undetermined nature) in infants. In practice both terms are sometimes misused for any convulsions or episodes of non-convulsive transient loss of consciousness, in infants, not otherwise specified, even without fever. These could more accurately be referred to as 'infantile convulsions'.

Febrile convulsions

Febrile convulsions can be defined as occasional epileptic convulsive seizures induced by fever, onset aged 3 months–5 years, excluding those in children with previous afebrile seizures, intracranial infection or other acute symptomatic seizures, or those not associated with fever, but including prolonged convulsions and convulsive status epilepticus.

The cumulative incidence to age 5 years for FCs is 2–5%. The peak age for a first FC is 18 months. They typically occur at the start of fever, and so there may be no warning that the child is ill or has a febrile illness.

There is often a family history: the relative risk (RR) of FC occurring in a sibling is 2.5, and the risk of any first-degree relative having an FC is 10–30%. The chance of a monozygotic twin having an FC is 33% compared to a risk of 11% in a dizygotic twin. In some families FCs follow an autosomal dominant mode of inheritance.

The recurrence risk after a first FC is 25–33%, and 15% will have three or more FCs. Later epilepsy is rare, seen in only 2–7% (RR 2–10), but is higher in those with complex FCs, who can develop focal epilepsies, and those with a high number of FCs or an atypical age of first FC, who can develop idiopathic generalized epilepsies (IGEs).

Eighty to 90% of children have simple FCs: brief clonic or tonic-clonic seizures lasting less than 15 minutes. Ten to 20% have complex FCs: lasting 15 minutes or more and/or with focal semiology or a transient post-ictal (Todd's) paresis and/or repeated in the same febrile episode or within a 24-hour period. Such complex FCs carry a 10–20% chance of later MTLE. In contrast, repeated simple FCs or those with onset under 6 months or over 6 years carry a greater risk of developing later idiopathic generalized epilepsy.

The prognosis is generally good in 95%. In the past, hemiconvulsion-hemiplegia-epilepsy was a rare complication of febrile convulsive status epilepticus continuing for hours or days. Benign rolandic epilepsy (BRE) is a rare sequela, as is MTLE, idiopathic generalized epilepsy and DS. Some families will have GEFS+ and its diverse epilepsies in different individuals.

Treatment is focused on reassurance and explanation and first aid. If a convulsion is continuing on arrival in the emergency department, or lasts more

Introduction to Epilepsy ed. Gonzalo Alarcón and Antonio Valentín. Published by Cambridge University Press.
© Cambridge University Press 2012.

than 5–10 minutes, emergency rescue treatment with Buccal midazolam (McIntyre et al., 2005) or i.v. lorazepam is indicated. Phenobarbitone or valproate will reduce the recurrence risk to 20–50%. However, since there is a relatively high risk of adverse effects, such prophylactic treatment is not generally recommended for FCs and is only rarely appropriate.

Dravet syndrome or severe myoclonic epilepsy of infancy (DS)

Dravet syndrome (severe myoclonic epilepsy of infancy) presents in a previously intact child with a first convulsion between 2 and 12 months of age, e.g. a prolonged focal motor or generalized tonic-clonic seizure (often an FC). Then after a variable interval of a few weeks or months, recurrent afebrile focal motor or generalized tonic-clonic seizures ensue. From about 2 years of age, other seizures develop: e.g. myoclonic, and/or atonic/astatic, and/or absence, and/or complex partial, and/or convulsive status epilepticus, and/or convulsions in sleep. Tonic seizures are not seen.

The EEG is initially normal. Then from age 1–2 years, runs of generalized spike-waves and or polyspikes develop with a normal background activity. From 2 years the background rhythm slows and some develop photosensitivity with photoparoxysmal responses at this unusually young age. Then generalized spike-wave with focal and multifocal sharp waves develops, with the child's clinical state and EEG looking increasingly like an epileptic encephalopathy. Significant, often severe developmental delay/learning difficulties become evident at pre-school age, with an associated mild ataxia or characteristic 'diplegic-like' gait disorder, with or without upper motor neuron signs.

The epilepsy becomes intractable, although minor seizures can improve in later childhood. Valproate, clobazam and stiripentol (in combination) are often used, and ethosuximide, piracitam, other benzodiazepines, topiramate, levetiracetam, phenobarbitone and even phenytoin are worth considering (even though phenytoin often produces a choreaform movement disorder). Carbamazepine and lamotrigine should be avoided. Consider investigating for an underlying progressive myoclonus epilepsy. However, an underlying clinical cause is rarely, if ever, found, apart from a gene mutation. Mutations in *SCN* and *GABA* subunit genes have been found and it is reassuring to both the family and the physicians to find the cause is a known gene mutation in a specific case, e.g. that the child has a de novo SCN1A mutation.

Generalized epilepsy with febrile seizures plus (GEFS+)

Generalized epilepsy with febrile seizures plus (GEFS+) is a family diagnosis (Scheffer and Berkovic, 1997). The pedigree will demonstrate an autosomal dominant segregation of various epilepsy syndromes, especially FCs, but also idiopathic generalized epilepsies (such as myoclonic astatic epilepsy, childhood absence epilepsy, generalized tonic-clonic seizures and DS) and even frontal or temporal lobe focal seizures. Mutations in the sodium channel gene subunits *SCN1B*, *SCN1A*, *SCN2B* as well as in the $GABA_A$ $\gamma 2$ subunit gene *GABRG2* have been found in several families. This illustrates the pivotal role for sodium channels and $GABA_A$ receptors in the control of neuronal synchrony.

References

McIntyre J, Robertson S, Norris E, *et al*. Safety and efficacy of buccal midazolam versus rectal diazepam for emergency treatment of seizures in children: a randomised controlled trial. *Lancet* 2005;**366**:204–10.

Scheffer IE, Berkovic SF. Generalised epilepsy with febrile seizures plus. A genetic disorder with heterogenous clinical phenotypes. *Brain* 1997;**120**:479–90.

Learning objectives

(1) To understand the different definitions of febrile convulsions and febrile seizures in use.
(2) To understand the epileptic basis of febrile convulsions.
(3) To know that some sodium channel mutations can cause paroxysmal temperature-sensitive epileptic seizures.
(4) To be able to diagnose and treat Dravet syndrome.
(5) To understand the concept of GEFS+ applied to families.

Idiopathic focal epilepsies

Colin D. Ferrie

Introduction

A benign epilepsy is characterized by seizures that are easily treated or require no treatment, and remit without sequel. It is rare for an epilepsy to have no lasting effects. Nevertheless, provided the term is not taken to mean inconsequential, it is useful. The conditions considered here are all idiopathic – 'syndromes which are only epilepsy, with no underlying structural brain lesion or other neurologic signs or symptoms ...'. They occur in children who are otherwise normal. Not all idiopathic epilepsies are benign and some symptomatic ones are.

Of the syndromes currently recognized by the ILAE, the following can reasonably be considered benign: benign familial and non-familial neonatal seizures, benign familial and non-familial infantile seizures, benign childhood epilepsy with centrotemporal spikes (here called rolandic epilepsy), and early-onset benign childhood occipital epilepsy (Panayiotopoulos type) (here called Panayiotopoulos syndrome). If a less rigorous definition of 'benign' is used, other syndromes can be added: benign myoclonic epilepsy in infancy, childhood absence epilepsy, late-onset childhood occipital epilepsy (Gastaut type) (here called idiopathic childhood occipital epilepsy), and idiopathic photosensitive occipital lobe epilepsy. The neonatal and infantile syndromes are considered in Chapters 20 to 23 and the generalized syndromes are considered in Chapter 25 (The idiopathic generalized epilepsies). This leaves the following:

- rolandic epilepsy (RE)
- Panayiotopoulos syndrome (PS)
- idiopathic childhood occipital epilepsy (COE)
- idiopathic photosensitive occipital lobe epilepsy (IPOE).

These syndromes share many clinical and EEG characteristics, and 'overlap cases' are not infrequent. For example, a child with PS may develop rolandic seizures or a child with predominantly rolandic seizures may have an autonomic seizure typical of PS or a visual seizure typical of COE. Given the similarities of COE and IPOE, they will be considered together as the idiopathic occipital lobe epilepsies (IOE).

Rolandic epilepsy

Seizures in rolandic epilepsy (see also Table 24.1) have their onset in the lower part of the pre- and post-central gyri (i.e. around the lower part of the rolandic sulcus). Seizures often begin in clear consciousness (simple focal seizures) with unilateral sensory and motor symptoms affecting structures inside and around the mouth (tongue, inner cheeks, teeth and gums), pharynx and larynx. Sensory symptoms include numbness, tingling and other sensations. Motor manifestations include gurgling, grunting and guttural noises and clonic jerking around the mouth, often with ipsilateral tonic deviation of the mouth. Speech arrest is common. Seizures may remain localized. Indeed those occurring whilst awake nearly always do. However, many spread with impairment of consciousness (complex focal seizures) and/or to hemi- or generalized tonic-clonic seizures. Generalization is particularly likely to occur during seizures in sleep and RE is a common cause for school-age children having nocturnal generalized tonic-clonic seizures.

The EEG hallmark of RE is centrotemporal (or rolandic) spikes (Figure 24.1). These consist of

---

Introduction to Epilepsy ed. Gonzalo Alarcón and Antonio Valentín. Published by Cambridge University Press.
© Cambridge University Press 2012.

Chapter 24: Idiopathic focal epilepsies

Table 24.1. Clinical and EEG features of idiopathic focal epilepsies of childhood

	Rolandic epilepsy	Panayiotopoulos syndrome	Idiopathic occipital lobe epilepsies
Epidemiology	Common (15% of children with seizures aged 1–15 years)	Common (1 child with PS to every 4 with RE)	Uncommon
Sex	Boys affected slightly more than girls	Sexes affected equally	COE: sexes equally affected IPOE: females slightly more than males
Age at onset	Usually 7–10 years but occasionally from 1 year or as late as 15 years	Usually 4–5 years but occasionally from 1 year or as late as 15 years	COE: 3–15 years (peak 8 years) IPOE: 2 years – early adult life (peak 12 years)
Characteristic seizure types	Sensorimotor seizures with hemifacial and oropharyngolaryngeal symptoms	Autonomic seizures	Elementary visual seizures
Timing of seizures	70% nocturnal (usually shortly after going to sleep or shortly before rising)	70% nocturnal	Diurnal
Seizure frequency	Usually low; single seizures common. A few have frequent seizures, particularly at onset	Usually low; one-third have single seizure. A few have frequent seizures	Usually frequent, often multiple daily. In IPOE seizure frequency depends on degree of photosensitivity and level of photic exposure
Status epilepticus	Focal and convulsive status epilepticus described but exceptional	One or more episodes of autonomic status epilepticus in 40% of patients. Convulsive status exceptional	Focal and convulsive status epilepticus described but exceptional
Principal EEG features	Normal EEG background with rolandic spikes	Normal EEG background with multifocal, usually posteriorly predominant sharp- and slow-wave complexes	Normal EEG background with occipital paroxysms. Photosensitivity present in IPOE
Prognosis	Excellent: remission usually occurs within 1–2 years of onset and certainly before the age of 16 years	Excellent: remission usually occurs within 1–2 years of onset	COE: good –remission during childhood in 70% cases. IPOE: variable – for those highly photosensitive continuation into adult life very likely

high-amplitude sharp- and slow-wave complexes and localize to the central (C3/C4) electrodes or between the central and temporal (C5/C6) electrodes. They may be unilateral or bilateral, synchronous or asynchronous. Some children show similar EEG abnormalities in other brain regions. Rarely generalized discharges occur.

A minority of children with rolandic epilepsy develop mild, but not insignificant, speech, reading and behavioural problems. In part this may relate to the phenomenon of transient cognitive impairment induced by interictal discharges. Occasionally more severe cognitive impairment can occur as a consequence of the development of continuous spike-wave in slow sleep (CSWS).

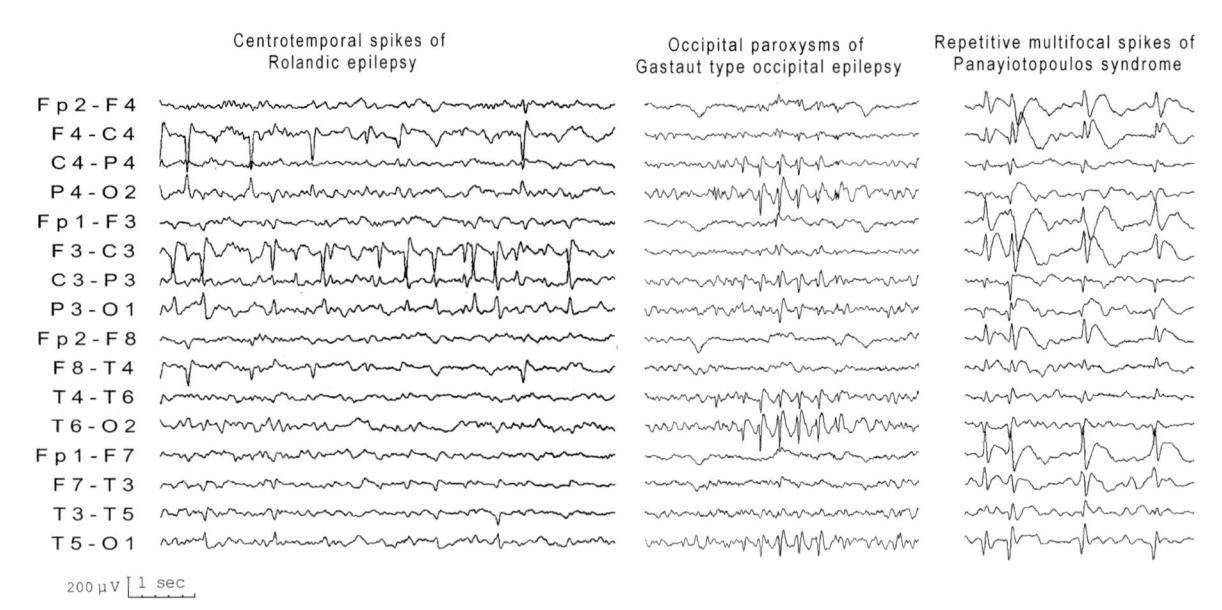

Figure 24.1. The EEG in idiopathic focal epilepsies of childhood.

Panayiotopoulos syndrome

Autonomic seizures and autonomic status epilepticus are the principal clinical manifestations of PS (see also Table 24.1). Consciousness is initially retained and the child usually complains of feeling unwell. Nausea, retching and vomiting are very common, often accompanied by behavioural changes such as agitation. Other autonomic symptoms include pallor, cyanosis or flushing, pupillary abnormalities, urinary and occasionally fecal incontinence, raised temperature and heart rate and breathing irregularities. As the seizure progresses, there is usually impairment of consciousness and, with this, deviation of the eyes and head is common. Loss of postural tone may cause syncopal-like episodes. Seizures are usually long (minutes) and autonomic status epilepticus is common. Many seizures terminate with a hemiconvulsion or generalized tonic-clonic seizure.

The characteristic interictal EEG features of PS are sharp- and slow-wave complexes similar to rolandic spikes but most commonly located posteriorly where they often occur in long runs (occipital paroxysms) and show attenuation with visual fixation caused, for example by eye-opening (fixation-off sensitivity) (Figure 24.1). However, sharp- and slow-wave abnormalities are often seen in other brain regions, including centrotemporal, frontal and midline locations. Indeed the EEG in PS is often multifocal. Generalized discharges may also occur. When first described PS was thought to be an occipital epilepsy because of the posterior predominance of interictal EEG abnormalities. However, ictal recordings have shown onset from frontal as well as posterior brain regions. It is likely that seizures in Panayiotopoulos syndrome can be triggered by discharges in various cortical areas, with initial ictal manifestations being a consequence of spread to autonomic centres.

Seizures in Panayiotopoulos syndrome are often misdiagnosed as non-epileptic events, such as syncopal attacks, migraine, gastroenteritis and cyclical vomiting. Many children with autonomic status epilepticus are intubated and ventilated, with the clinician fearing a grave cerebral insult.

The idiopathic occipital lobe epilepsies

In idiopathic occipital lobe epilepsies (see also Table 24.1), seizures arise in the occipital lobes and are mainly manifested by elementary visual seizures and ictal blindness occurring in clear consciousness. The visual seizures usually comprise hallucinations of coloured balls or similar which may move over the visual field. They are different from the black and white scintillations and fortification spectra of migraine. Formed hallucinations and visual illusions (such as distortions of form, size or distance) occur more rarely. Headache, ictal or post-ictal, is common and often migrainous in type. Seizures are short (seconds to a minute or so) although those with ictal blindness may last longer. Occasional seizures may spread, sometimes leading to generalized tonic-clonic seizures. In IPOE seizures are precipitated by photic factors, such as video-games, TV or sunlight.

The characteristic interictal EEG feature of COE is occipital paroxysms, often showing fixation-off sensitivity, as described for PS (their EEGs may be identical) (Figure 24.1). In IPOE there is, in addition, photosensitivity, which can be generalized or have a more localized distribution in the posterior regions.

Investigations

The EEG is very helpful in establishing the syndromic diagnosis. If the awake record is normal, a sleep recording should be obtained as the paroxysmal abnormalities are usually highly activated by sleep. However, repeatedly normal EEGs are compatible with diagnosis of these conditions, except IPOE, in which photosensitivity is required. Most authorities do not recommend neuroimaging in RE, provided the clinical and EEG features are typical and the expected clinical course is followed. Imaging, preferably MRI, is recommended for the other conditions.

Management

Appropriate education concerning the benign nature of these conditions, particularly RE and PS, is of great importance. Given the generally low frequency of seizures in RE and PS, antiepileptic drug treatment (AED) is often not required, especially if seizures are nocturnal and/or do not secondarily generalize. Rescue medication should be considered for PS if seizures are prolonged. Regular treatment is recommended for idiopathic childhood occipital epilepsy, given the generally high seizure frequency. Carbamazepine is probably most widely used, except for IPOE. However, it has been implicated in atypical evolutions of the idiopathic focal epilepsies of childhood, particularly if there is development of continuous spike-wave of slow sleep (CSWS). For this reason some authorities avoid its use. The drug of choice for IPOCE is unclear. However, most would choose drugs, such as sodium valproate, effective against photosensitivity.

When regular antiepileptic drugs are given, it is appropriate to attempt discontinuation after 1–2 seizure-free years. The EEG is unhelpful in helping to decide when to stop antiepileptic drugs, as EEG abnormalities may persist long after clinical seizures have remitted. The exception may be IPOE, as persistent photosensitivity is likely to be associated with a high relapse rate.

Other proposed benign focal epilepsies of childhood

Other benign focal epilepsies of childhood have been proposed and more or less well characterized. They include benign childhood seizures with affective symptoms, benign childhood epilepsy with parietal spikes and frequent giant somatosensory evoked potentials, benign childhood focal seizures associated with frontal or midline spikes, benign focal epilepsy in infants with central and vertex spikes and waves during sleep, and benign focal seizures of adolescence.

Learning objectives

(1) To be able to explain the concept of 'benign' as applied to the idiopathic focal epilepsies of childhood.
(2) To be able to list the idiopathic focal epilepsies of childhood.
(3) To be able to describe the key clinical and EEG features of the idiopathic focal epilepsies of childhood.
(4) To be able to explain the likely prognosis for children with these epilepsies.
(5) To be able to formulate a differential diagnosis for the idiopathic focal epilepsies of childhood.
(6) To be able to manage children with the idiopathic focal epilepsies of childhood appropriately.

Questions

(1) The idiopathic focal epilepsies of childhood show a strong age-dependency. Can you think of mechanisms (e.g. genetic) which might explain this?
(2) There is an ongoing and at times acrimonious debate in epileptology between those who advocate separation of epilepsy into further syndromes ('splitters') and those who prefer to classify patients into relatively broad diagnostic

groups ('lumpers'). Both approaches can be useful. What are the advantages and disadvantages of separation of the conditions considered in this chapter into individual syndromes compared with keeping them as a single entity – 'the idiopathic focal epilepsies of childhood'?

(3) A feature of these epilepsies is that in any given patient the characteristic interictal focal epileptiform abnormalities are not stable in their location. In successive EEG recordings spike foci may be located unilaterally (left or right) or bilaterally (synchronous or asynchronous) and may vary from posterior, central, midline or frontal locations or may even be generalized. Is this compatible with the concept of focal epilepsy?

(4) Do you think that the risk of SUDEP argues in favour of treating children with these epilepsies with regular antiepileptic drug medication?

Section 2 Classification and diagnosis of epilepsy

Chapter 25: The idiopathic generalized epilepsies

Colin D. Ferrie

The idiopathic generalized epilepsies (IGE) are an important group of epilepsies which occur from infancy to adult life, but which are particularly common in childhood and adolescence. As their name implies, they are without known cause, although it is widely considered that they are genetic in origin. However, with few exceptions their genetic basis is unknown. They occur in subjects who, prior to onset of seizures, have no evidence of neurological dysfunction. Significant cognitive, intellectual and behavioural problems are not expected, response to treatment is usually good and some subjects eventually become seizure-free on medication. However, there are many exceptions to these generalizations.

Seizure types

Combinations of three generalized seizure types characterize the IGE:

- typical absence seizures (TA)
- myoclonic seizures or jerks (MS)
- generalized tonic-clonic seizures (GTCS).

Typical absence seizures

TA are manifested by a relatively brief impairment of consciousness during which the subject usually stares blankly. They begin and end abruptly (like a light being switched off and then back on again). In some (simple TA) nothing else is observed. More usually there are other features (complex TA). These include automatisms, tonic (often causing retropulsion of the head), atonic (which may cause the head to slump), clonic or myoclonic features (causing, for example, jerking of the eyelids or mouth). The likelihood of automatisms is related to the severity and duration of the impairment of consciousness. They are usually simple, for example lip-smacking or fumbling with the hands. Occasionally, they can be more complicated – some children walk around in circles. TAs usually last anything from a couple of seconds up to about 20–30 seconds. Longer absences do occur, but are exceptional. TA are characteristically provoked by hyperventilation, which can be a useful diagnostic test. TA are the only seizure type which is partly defined on the basis of its EEG features. They are accompanied by a generalized 3 Hz spike-wave discharge (Figure 25.1).

TA are very strongly associated with IGE – only very rarely do they occur in other types of epilepsy. They should be distinguished from atypical absences. These may be very similar clinically, although the onset and termination are often less abrupt and atonic components with drooling are often prominent. The accompanying EEG discharge is usually a generalized spike-wave discharge but at <2.5 Hz (slow spike-wave discharge). Atypical absences are not a feature of IGE but occur in children with other neurological impairments, such as cerebral palsy and learning difficulties.

Myoclonic seizures (myoclonic jerks)

These are brief shock-like contractions of a muscle or a group of muscles and can be single or repetitive. If the latter, they can be rhythmic or arrhythmic. They can be massive, affecting the whole of the body, affect the proximal parts of limbs or else be distal and fragmentary. They can cause the subject to fall. Myoclonus occurs in a number of different types of epilepsy as well as in IGE. They can also be non-epileptic in origin.

Generalized tonic-clonic seizures (GTCS)

These comprise an initial tonic phase in which there is generalized body stiffening accompanied by loss of

Introduction to Epilepsy ed. Gonzalo Alarcón and Antonio Valentín. Published by Cambridge University Press.
© Cambridge University Press 2012.

Figure 25.1. The EEG in CAE and JME.

consciousness. This causes the subject to fall, often accompanied by a cry. There then follows rhythmical jerking of all four limbs (the clonic phase). GTCS occur in most forms of epilepsy.

Syndromes of IGE

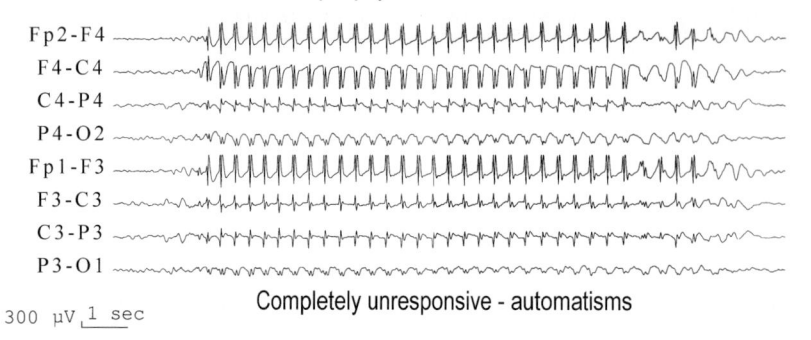

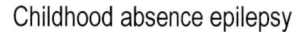

Benign myoclonic epilepsy of infancy

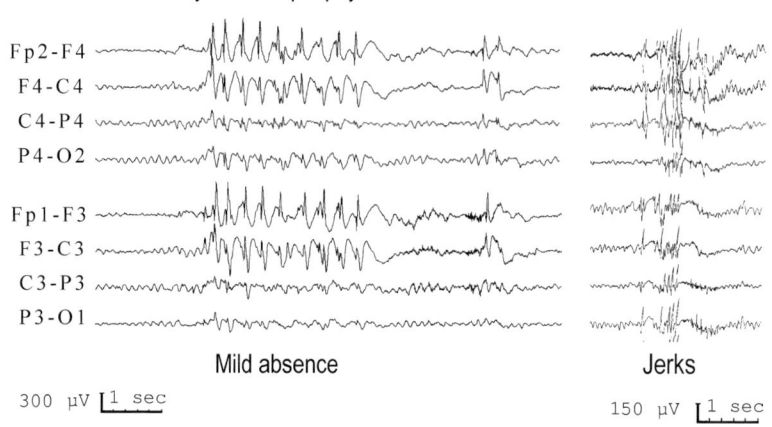

This is a rare epilepsy syndrome usually starting between 6 months and 3 years of age. The predominant, often sole, seizure type is myoclonic seizures occurring singly or in clusters. They may arise spontaneously or be provoked by noise or tactile stimuli. Remission commonly occurs between 6 months and 5 years of onset. A minority of children develop other seizure types and have educational problems.

Childhood absence epilepsy (CAE)

This is the commonest absence epilepsy (see also Table 25.1). It is characterized by frequent TA, usually many, sometimes hundreds per day – (pyknolepsy). The absences are usually relatively long with severe impairment of consciousness so that automatisms are common. There is disagreement about the prognosis of CAE. This is mainly because of differing diagnostic criteria. If broad criteria are used then the prognosis is uncertain, with many developing GTCS. However, stricter diagnostic criteria have been defined, excluding children with any seizures (other than febrile seizures) prior to the onset of TA, children with brief and/or mild impairment of consciousness during TA, children with marked myoclonic features during TA, and those who are photosensitive. If these are used, fewer children can be included but the prognosis is better.

Juvenile absence epilepsy (JAE)

This much rarer absence syndrome is characterized by absences similar in character to CAE but which occur less frequently – usually a few times per week, maximum once or twice daily (see also Table 25.1). Rare MS may occur and most patients develop GTCS. JAE usually continues into adult life when GTCS may be more troublesome.

Table 25.1. The clinical and EEG features of four IGEs

	CAE	JAE	JME	EMAb
Age of onset	2–10 years (peak 5–7)	5–20 years (peak 9–13)	From childhood to adult life	2–14 years (peak 6–8 years)
Sex	Two-thirds are girls	Sexes equally affected	Sexes equally affected	Affects many more females than males
Seizure types	TAS	TAS Infrequent MS (1/5 of patients) GTCS (nearly all)	TAS (1/3 of patients) MS (all patients) GTCS (nearly all patients)	Eyelid myoclonia with and without TAS (all patients) GTCS (nearly all patients)
EEG	Normal background sometimes with rhythmic posterior delta activity. Regular 3 Hz GSWD	Normal background. Regular 3 Hz GSWD. Focal epileptiform abnormalities may be seen. Photosensitivity in some patients	Irregular 3–6 Hz GSWD. Focal EEG abnormalities (including slow waves) common. Photosensitivity in 1/3 patients	Irregular brief 3–6 Hz GSWD occurring spontaneously, on eye-closure or during photic stimulation
Prognosis	Good: if strict diagnostic criteria used probably 90% become seizure-free	Life-long disorder in most subjects	Life-long disorder in all or nearly all patients	Life-long disorder in all or nearly all patients

CAE, childhood absence epilepsy; JAE, juvenile absence epilepsy; JME, juvenile myoclonic epilepsy; EMAb, eyelid myoclonia with absences; TAS, typical absence seizures; GTCS, generalized tonic-clonic seizures; EEG, electroencephalogram; GSWD, generalized spike-wave discharges.

Juvenile myoclonic epilepsy (JME)

This is a common epilepsy syndrome (see also Table 25.1 and Figure 25.1) which features TA, MS and GTCS. TA (if they occur – see Table 25.1) occur first, usually in mid-late childhood, with MS usually starting in early-mid adolescence and GTCS a few years later, usually in mid adolescence – early adult life. The TA, except when of early onset, are usually short with mild impairment of consciousness and are easily missed or dismissed as day-dreaming. They may be frequent or rare. MS are frequent, often daily. They usually show a diurnal pattern with a peak in the 1–2 hours following wakening and a smaller peak in the evening before bed. Many patients are so used to the jerks that they consider them normal and do not seek medical help. Specific enquiry with demonstration may be required to diagnose them. GTCS may show a similar circadian distribution, although nocturnal seizures also occur. GTCS are often preceded by showers of MS or less commonly TA. Both may lead to misdiagnosis of secondarily generalized seizures.

Seizures in IGE, particularly JME, are often precipitated by lifestyle factors. Many patients find they are more likely if they are fatigued, tired, stressed and/or hungry. Alcohol is also an important precipitant. More than 30% of patients are photosensitive.

Epilepsy with GTCS only

This is a controversial syndrome. Those authorities who recognize it consider it an IGE in which GTCS is the only seizure type. These tend to cluster within 1–2 hours of wakening. It has common features with what was previously known as epilepsy with grand mal on awakening. Onset is usually in older children, adolescence and young adults.

Epilepsy with myoclonic absences (EMyA)

This is a rare childhood epilepsy syndrome in which the characteristic seizure type is the so-called myoclonic absence seizure. This comprises a TA accompanied by rhythmic myoclonic jerks of the shoulders, arms and legs. The EEG is similar to that in CAE. Although EMyA is classified by the ILAE as an IGE, myoclonic absences also occur in children with symptomatic epilepsies. Seizures often respond poorly to medication, and cognitive and behavioural problems are common.

Eyelid myoclonia with absences (EMAb)

This syndrome is not fully recognized by the ILAE but is highly characteristic (see also Table 25.1). It comprises the triad of eyelid myoclonia occurring with and without TA (which are usually brief and inconspicuous), provocation of these seizures by eye-closure, and photosensitivity (all patients). As well as the seizures being provoked by eye-closure, so too are the characteristic EEG discharges of polyspikes or polyspikes and wave often seen with eyelid myoclonia. Induction of discharges and seizures by eye-closure is abolished in total darkness. There is controversy as to the role of self-induction of the seizures by the so-called 'slow eye-closure manoeuvre' in patients who are photosensitive. Other seizures types, notably GTCS, develop in most patients and resistance to antiepileptic drugs is the rule.

Other syndromes and possible syndromes of IGE

Many patients with IGE do not fit within the well-recognized syndromes. Proposed syndromes include IGE with absences of early childhood, perioral myoclonia with absences and IGE with phantom absences.

Absence status occurs in IGE but is exceptional in CAE.

Investigations

The EEG is very useful in the diagnosis of IGE both because they are associated with characteristic interictal features and because ictal recordings are commonly obtained during routine EEG. Epileptiform discharges are usually activated by hyperventilation, sleep and on awakening from sleep. Many patients, depending on the syndrome, are photosensitive.

The interictal hallmark of the IGE is the generalized 3 Hz spike-wave discharge (GSWD). This, if short, can be interictal but is often accompanied by a clinical TA. GSWD are provoked by hyperventilation. If the patient counts his breath during hyperventilation, errors are often seen during discharges which would otherwise be considered interictal. In CAE and JAE, GSWD are regular, with a gradual and smooth decline in frequency from the initial to the terminal phase and with well-formed spikes which retain a constant relation to the slow waves. In contrast, in JME the GSWD are usually faster (often 3.5–6 Hz), multiple spike are common, and the discharges are often irregular with the relationship between spikes and the aftercoming slow waves being inconstant and abrupt changes in frequency during discharges and fragmentations of the discharges occurring (Figure 25.1).

In IGE featuring myoclonic seizures, polyspike and/or polyspike-and-wave discharges are seen and can be interictal or ictal.

Neuroimaging is expected to be normal in IGE. Most authorities do not recommend scanning patients who have typical clinical and electrical features. However, MRI should be obtained if the clinical or EEG features are atypical and in those who do not respond to antiepileptic drugs as expected.

Treatment

Treatment with antiepileptic drugs is recommended for all the IGE. Sodium valproate has been the treatment of first choice for many years, but there are concerns about its teratogenicity. An alternative in CAE is ethosuximide. Other antiepileptic drugs active in IGE include lamotrigine, topiramate and levetiracetam. Benzodiazepines, such as clobazam and clonazepam, can be useful for myoclonic jerks. Lamotrigine may exacerbate myoclonic seizures. A minority of patients require combinations of drugs to achieve full seizure control. Sodium valproate and levetiracetam are effective for photosensitive seizures.

Many drugs, including carbamazepine, oxcarbazepine, phenytoin, gabapentin, pregabalin, tiagabine and vigabatrin, can exacerbate IGE and should be avoided.

Duration of treatment depends on the syndrome prognosis (Table 25.1). Drug withdrawal after 1–3 years is appropriate in CAE. If antiepileptic drugs are withdrawn in JME, relapse is almost certain. The EEG may be useful in that for those on medication who are seizure-free, the likelihood of relapse is higher if epileptiform abnormalities, in particular photosensitivity, persist.

Learning objectives

(1) To be able to list the main idiopathic generalized epilepsy syndromes.
(2) To be able to describe the key clinical and EEG features of the idiopathic generalized epilepsies.
(3) To be able to explain the likely prognosis for patients with these epilepsies.
(4) To be able to formulate a differential diagnosis for the idiopathic generalized epilepsies.
(5) To be able to manage patients with the idiopathic generalized epilepsies.

Questions

(1) Included within this group of epilepsies are toddlers who have frequent myoclonic seizures (only) and young adults who have occasional generalized tonic-clonic seizures (only). How valid do you think the concept of the idiopathic generalized epilepsies is?
(2) 'Lifestyle factors' (e.g. sleep deprivation, hunger, alcohol consumption) are particularly important in some patients with idiopathic generalized epilepsies in terms of precipitating seizures. Why might this be? To what extent are patients with idiopathic generalized epilepsies to blame for their epilepsy?
(3) Certain drugs, such as carbamazepine, may exacerbate the idiopathic generalized epilepsies. Can you speculate on mechanisms that might be responsible for this?
(4) Focal EEG abnormalities are common in patients with idiopathic generalized epilepsies. Are seizures in these epilepsies really generalized?

Section 2
Classification and diagnosis of epilepsy

Chapter 26

Temporal lobe epilepsy

Robert D. C. Elwes

Hughlings Jackson in 1898 gave the first complete description of temporal lobe seizures, calling them dreamy states. The patient, a physician, developed brief episodes of staring and confusion associated with chewing movements. The attacks were preceded by an epigastric sensation and an intellectual aura including a sensation of déjà vu. At autopsy, softening of the uncinate area of the temporal lobe was found. Following the discovery of the EEG by Berger, Gibbs et al. (1948) described the anterior temporal focus in people with so-called psychomotor seizures. On the basis of these findings, Pervcival Bailey carried out resective temporal lobe surgery with good results. Around the same time, electrocorticography in people undergoing temporal surgery, especially at the Montreal Neurological Institute, showed that the principal EEG abnormality was in the basal part of the temporal lobe. In the early 1950s, two important advances occurred in London and Paris. Falconer (1955) at the Maudsley Hospital developed the en bloc temporal lobectomy, which allowed detailed pathological examination. This group showed that hippocampal sclerosis and indolent glioneuronal tumours, now called DNTs, were the commonest cause of temporal lobe epilepsy (TLE) in young adults. Using the same material, focal cortical dysplasia was subsequently described. Talairach developed the stereotactic brain atlas and, with Bancaud, implanted depth electrodes chronically into the brains of people with temporal lobe seizures, recording the EEG in three dimensions, the so-called stereo EEG. Crandall in Los Angeles used technology developed in the space programme to carry out long-term telemetry EEG recordings with hippocampal depth electrodes and showed that most temporal lobe seizures did indeed start in the medial temporal areas, in keeping with the pathological findings reported by Falconer. The Commission on Classification of Epilepsy introduced the term complex partial seizures in order to emphasize that what appear to be psychomotor or temporal lobe seizures may arise at another site and spread to the amygdala and hippocampus, which seems to act as an amplifier for ictal EEG changes.

Epidemiology and etiology

Temporal lobe epilepsy is the commonest focal seizure disorder in adults. If it arises de novo in older people, a malignant tumour or cerebrovascular disease is the commonest cause. Our understanding of the aetiology in young adults is based heavily on resected temporal specimens from surgical series (Box 26.1).

Mesial temporal sclerosis is the commonest cause. About one-half give a history of a brain insult occurring in early childhood such as meningitis, trauma or, most commonly, prolonged or focal febrile convulsions. The febrile convulsions may be followed acutely by a resolving hemiparesis contralateral to the subsequent hippocampal atrophy. This disorder may be part of the spectrum of hemiconvulsions, hemiparesis and epilepsy described by

Box 26.1. Commonest aetiologies of temporal lobe epilepsy in young adults

- Mesial temporal sclerosis
- Indolent glioneuronal tumours
  - Dysembryoplastic neuroepithelial tumours (DNT)
  - Ganglioglioma
  - Oligodendroglioma
- Cavernous haemangiomas
- Arteriovenous malformations
- Cortical dysplasia
- Previous brain infections
- Meningioma

Introduction to Epilepsy ed. Gonzalo Alarcón and Antonio Valentín. Published by Cambridge University Press.
© Cambridge University Press 2012.

Gastaut. After a latent period, complex partial seizures develop, usually in the first or second decade, and continue as a lifelong disorder. Indolent glioneuronal tumours are the second commonest cause in surgical series. Trauma more frequently produces generalized or extratemporal epilepsy. Familial cases are seen, and in about two-thirds of cases no aetiology is established.

Medial/mesial temporal lobe epilepsy

Many anatomical subdivisions of temporal lobe epilepsy have been proposed. Medial temporal epilepsy appears to be by far the commonest. Distinguishing this from lateral temporal epilepsy can be difficult as seizures spread rapidly.

Semiology of seizures (Box 26.2 and Table 26.1)

The seizure may stop at the aura with the person remaining fully conscious (simple partial seizures), or may progress to loss of consciousness (complex partial seizures). Observers will notice a motionless stare. Automatisms are typical in which the person will carry out what appear to be purposeful actions over which they have no conscious control or subsequent memory. These are usually simple actions such as fiddling with clothes, perseveration of ongoing activity or reacting to nearby objects or people. Chewing movements are very characteristic and strongly associated with the presence of an epigastric aura. Sometimes the person will get up or walk around. Directed violence is very unusual although aggressive behaviour can occur if inappropriately restrained while confused. Following the active part of the seizure there is a period of post-ictal confusion. In temporal lobe seizures arising from the dominant hemisphere, post-ictal dysphasia can occur. If the seizures are brief, bland and occur with no aura, the patient may miss them or experience only a brief lapse in memory or time.

> **Box 26.2. Common leading symptoms in TLE**
> - Autonomic: rising epigastric, flushing, pallor, palpitations
> - Affective: fear, feeling of doom or dread, rarely elation or pleasure
> - Special sensory: olefactory, burning or chemical; auditory, unformed buzzing, whirring
> - Dysmnesic: déjà vu, prescience, hallucinations
> - Language: dysphasia

Table 26.1. Lateralizing features in temporal lobe seizures

Sign	Hemisphere of seizure origin
Unilateral dystonia or paralysis of limb	Contralateral
Automatisms (in non-paralysed limb)	Ipsilateral
Rhythmic ictal non-clonic hand (RINCH) motions	Contralateral
Ictal speech	Non-dominant
Post-ictal dysphasia	Dominant
Coughing, spitting, drinking	Non-dominant
Post-ictal nose-wiping with one hand	Ipsilateral
Direction of early non-forced head turning	Ipsilateral
Direction of late forced head turning	Contralateral
Relative preservation of consciousness	Non-dominant

Patients often have simple partial seizures, complex partial seizures and less frequently secondarily generalized seizures, with the latter often occurring in sleep. Seizures frequently occur in clusters within 1–2 weeks with no seizures in between. They often maintain a stable pattern over years or decades, making sufferers suitable candidates for drug trials. Seizures with a temporal semiology can occur due to spread from another site, either frontal or occipital. Interictally, cognition may be mildly impaired in temporal lobe epilepsy and memory deficits are particularly prominent, reflecting the involvement of the hippocampus in seizures, interictal discharges and pathology. Slight contralateral hemiatrophy and dystonic posturing of the hand on walking can be seen in mesial temporal sclerosis.

In assessing people with presumed TLE a number of atypical features may be obtained from the history or on telemetry suggesting extratemporal involvement:

- unformed visual symptoms (occipital)
- early lateralized motor or sensory symptoms (suprasylvian)
- mouth twitches, throat sensation, salivation (opercular/insular)
- absence of motionless stare (often frontal)
- early, abrupt onset, or hypermotor automatisms (frontal).

Lateral temporal epilepsy

Lateral temporal seizures arising from the temporal neocortex or perisylvian area (so-called insular or opercular seizures) are less common. Often there is prominent and rapid spread to the medial temporal structures producing a seizure with medial semiology. Involvement of the lateral temporal neocortex can produce unformed auditory sensations such as whirring or buzzing noises, or an early and prominent disturbance of speech. In medial temporal epilepsy speech disturbance is often a post-ictal phenomenon. Involvement of the insula produces epigastric sensations or prominent autonomic changes such as bradycardia or excessive salivation. The seizure may spread above the sylvian fissure to produce twitching in the mouth or a feeling of discomfort in the throat. Lateralized sensory symptoms due to involvement of the second sensory area also occur (the second sensory area in the superior border of the sylvian sulcus, as distinct from the primary sensory area).

Neuropsychiatric complications are particularly common in TLE, reflecting the involvement of the limbic system in this disorder, and possibly also that it is overwhelmingly the commonest focal chronic epilepsy. The following neuropsychiatric conditions can be found:

- anxiety and reactive depression
- memory deficits, not progressive
- 'temporal lobe personality'
- post-ictal psychosis
- interictal schizophreniform psychosis
- de novo post temporal lobectomy psychosis.

Investigations
EEG (Boxes 26.3 and 26.4)

The electrical field is often wide and changes may therefore be clearer with referential recording (Figure 18.13). The focus may be below the site of electrodes on the 10–20 system (a so-called basal focus), and many EEG departments use superficial or deep sphenoidal recording electrodes or lower electrodes as in the Maudsley electrode placement. The foramen ovale electrode samples the same site semi-invasively and enters the middle cranial fossa to lie near the parahippocampal gyrus.

MRI

A major advance in recent years has been the ability to use high-resolution MRI to diagnose hippocampal sclerosis and indolent glioneuronal tumours. Thin T2 cuts along

> **Box 26.3. Interictal EEG findings in TLE**
> - Focal temporal polymorphic slow activity.
> - Focal sharps or spikes, often activated in light sleep, over:
>   - anterior or mid temporal maximum, typical in medial TLE
>   - mid/posterior maximum, typical in lateral TLE
> - Bilateral independent discharges seen in 30% of subjects

> **Box 26.4. Ictal EEG findings in TLE**
> - Seizures may start with generalized decrement of EEG activity
> - Some degree of early non-localized slow (frontal not uncommon)
> - Rhythmic theta (maximal anterior temporal), usually within about 30 seconds, reflects hippocampal involvement
> - Initial scalp EEG changes may be bilateral (in up to 60%) or incorrectly lateralized (in around 10%, especially if burned out hippocampus) (Alarcón et al., 2001)
> - Usually spreads posteriorly
> - Bilateral independent onset of seizures is less common
> - Fast activity at onset suggests lateral TLE
> - On intracranial EEG, low-voltage fast activity is seen in the hippocampus and amygdala

the axis of the hippocampus are needed, and loss of the internal structure and flattening of the pes hippocampi is an early sign of sclerosis. T2 signal may be increased, which is better seen on FLAIR. Volumetric acquisition of T1 signals allows detailed assessment of hippocampal volumes, which is enhanced by quantitative measurements. Atrophy of the thalamus, fornix and mamilliary body may be seen. The presence of another lesion such as scarring or a tumour in addition to hippocampal sclerosis is referred to as dual pathology and occurs in 10% of cases in surgical series. Glioneuronal tumours are also easily identified. Cortical dysplasia, however, can be much more subtle and may be missed in about 50% of cases.

Functional investigations in TLE are of considerable use in lateralizing the disorder. A typical feature is that, although the pathology (most commonly mesial temporal sclerosis) is localized, the functional deficits may quite widespread, including:

Chapter 26: Temporal lobe epilepsy

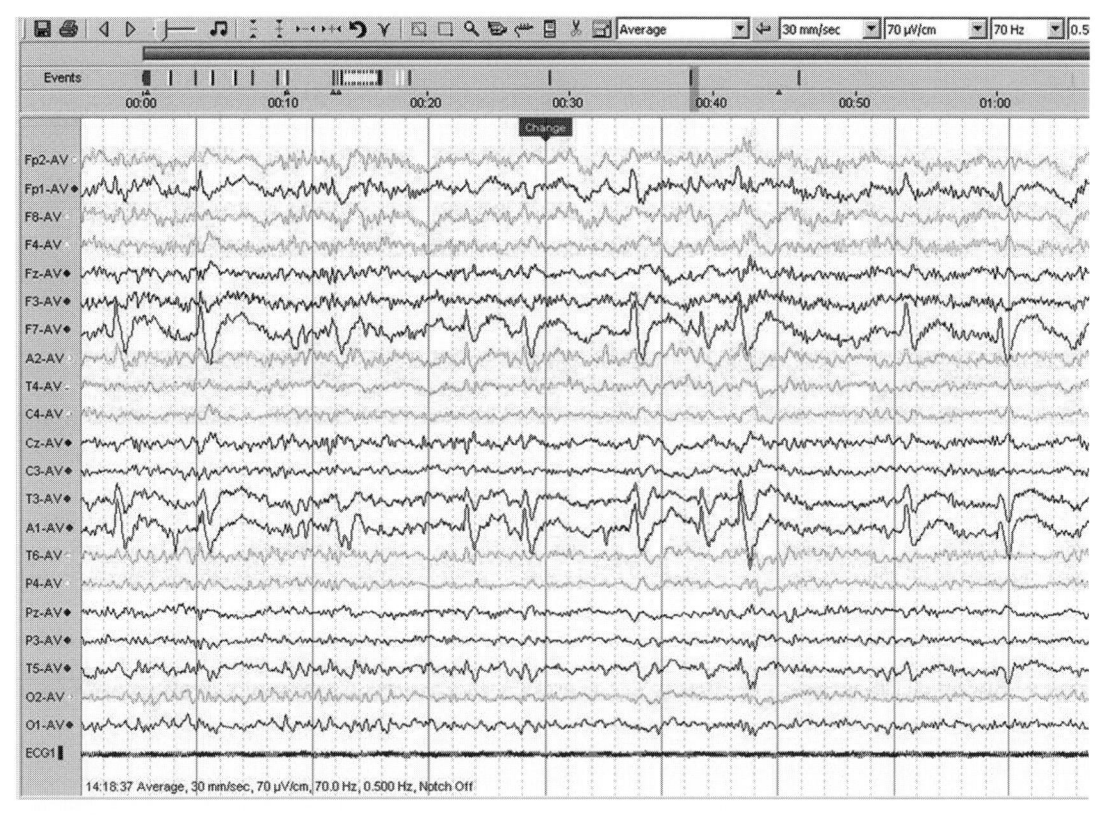

Figure 26.1. Interictal EEG in medial temporal epilepsy. Note wide field with spike maximal at F7 but spreading to A1, T3 and T5. Spikes biggest at a higher electrode, e.g. F3 or T3 suggests an extratemporal focus, frontal or sylvian.

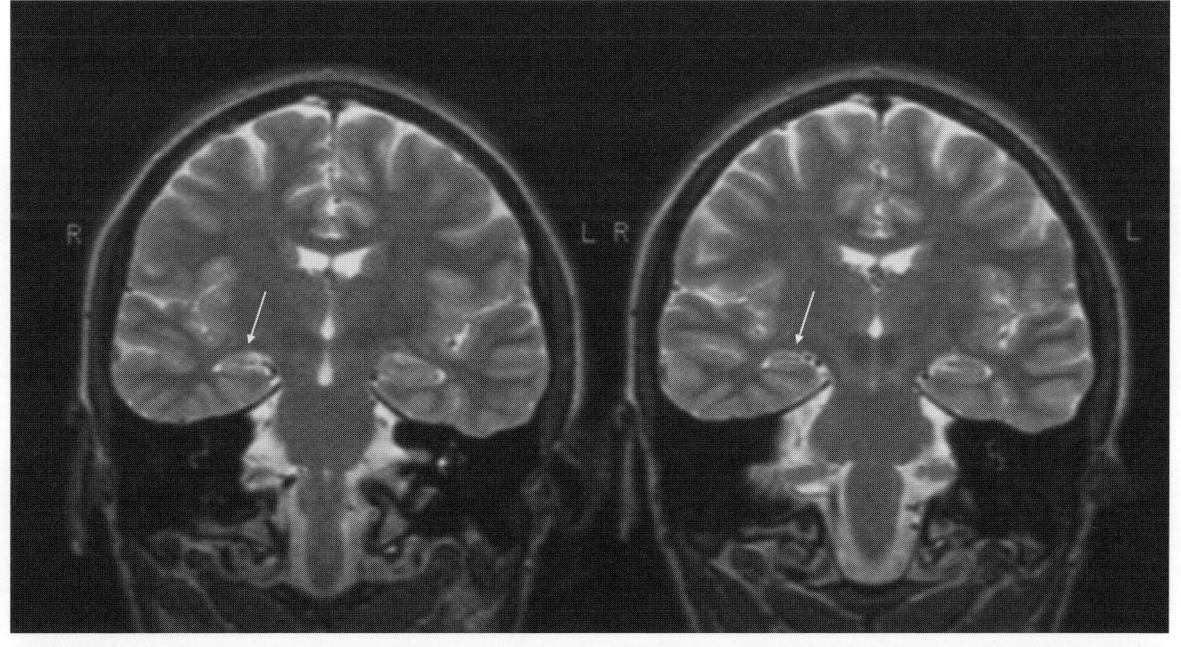

Figure 26.2. Coronal T2 MRI, 3.5 mm slices, 0.5 mm gap showing right mesial temporal sclerosis. Small right temporal lobe, atropy and increased signal in the right medial temporal area.

- ipsilateral loss of drug-induced fast activity on EEG;
- material-specific memory deficits;
- ipsilateral memory loss on carotid amytal testing;
- ipsilateral decrease in glucose uptake (often extensive) on FDG-PET, which may be extensive, usually including most of the ipsilateral temporal cortex;
- multifocal ipsilateral temporal epileptiform discharges independently arising from hippocampus, subtemporal and lateral temporal cortices on electrocorticograpy (Alarcón et al., 1997).

> **Box 26.5.** Common indications for surgical assessment in TLE include
>
> - Duration of epilepsy for 2 or years of longer
> - Full therapeutic trial of first-line and two or three second-line drugs, especially levetiracetam and topiramate
> - Seizures on a monthly basis
> - No recent prolonged remissions (e.g. 1 or more years)
> - Absence of severe learning difficulties
> - Complex partial seizures of presumed TL origin

Treatment
Medication

Drugs that act on the fast sodium channel appear particularly useful as first-line treatments in TLE. These include carbamazepine, lamotrigine, oxcarbazepine and phenytoin. Phenobarbitone is also effective but is more sedative and toxic, especially in children. Valproate may be less efficacious but may be a useful second-line medication. These drugs produce a full remission of seizures in about two-thirds of new-onset cases. If there is an idiosyncratic or adverse reaction to one first-line drug, another is usually tried. If these drugs fail, then most patients are retained on a first-line drug and rotate through second-line medications as an add-on treatment. Clinical trial evidence suggests that levetiracetam, topiramate and pregabalin are effective and this is broadly in keeping with clinical experience. The newer drugs are more expensive, have a higher incidence of neuropsychiatric side effects, may promote polytherapy and need to be administered under specialist care. With careful adjustment tailored to the individual needs of the patient, about 30 to 40% of people get an important and sustained benefit from one of these newer second-line drugs. A trial of clobazam may be helpful and some use it intermittently if there are prominent and predictable seizure clusters.

Surgery

Resective temporal lobe surgery is the commonest procedure in most epilepsy surgery programmes, accounting for about 80% of operations. It brings about complete seizure control in 60 to 80% of cases, with 2% incidence of serious morbidity. Surgical treatment should be contemplated in all patients with TLE where medication is not effective (see Box 26.5).

People with normal MRI and those with bitemporal spikes may be considered (Alarcón et al., 2006). Those with severe learning difficulties, multiple seizure types and multifocal or generalized discharges on the EEG are not as good candidates, as this may indicate more extensive disease. A fixed interictal schizophreniform psychosis is generally held to be a contraindication. Co-existent non-epileptic seizures should be identified and treated independently.

Recommended reading

Bancaud J, Angelergues R, Bernouilli C, et al. Functional stereotaxic exploration (SEEG) of epilepsy. *Electroencephalogr Clin Neurophysiol* 1970;**28**:85–6.

Berkovic SF, Andermann F, Olivier A, et al. Hippocampal sclerosis in temporal lobe epilepsy demonstrated by magnetic resonance imaging. *Ann Neurol* 1991; **29**(2):175–82.

Binnie CD, Elwes RD, Polkey CE, Volans A. Utility of stereoelectroencephalography in preoperative assessment of temporal lobe epilepsy. *J Neurol Neurosurg Psychiatry* 1994;**57**:58–65.

Currie S, Heathfield KW, Henson RA, Scott DF. Clinical course and prognosis of temporal lobe epilepsy. A survey of 666 patients. *Brain* 1971;**94**(1):173–90.

Engel J Jr, Kuhl DE, Phelps ME, Crandall PH. Comparative localization of epileptic foci in partial epilepsy by PET and EEG. *Ann Neurol* 1982;**12**:529–37.

Kotagal P, Lüders H, Morris HH, et al. Dystonic posturing in complex partial seizures of temporal lobe onset: a new lateralizing sign. *Neurology* 1989;**39**:196–201.

Wieser HG. Ictal manifestations of temporal lobe seizures. *Adv Neurol* 1991;**55**:301–15.

References

Alarcón G, Garcia Seoane JJ, Binnie CD, et al. Origin and propagation of discharges in the acute electrocorticogram: implications for physiopathology and surgical treatment of temporal lobe epilepsy. *Brain* 1997;**120**:2259–82.

Alarcón G, Kissani N, Dad M, *et al.* Lateralizing and localizing values of ictal onset recorded on the scalp: evidence from simultaneous recordings with intracranial foramen ovale electrodes. *Epilepsia* 2001;**42**:1426–37.

Alarcón G, Valentín A, Watt C, *et al.* Is it worth pursuing surgery for epilepsy in patients with normal neuroimaging? *J Neurol Neurosurg Psychiatry* 2006;**77**:474–80.

Falconer MA, Meyer A, Hill D, Mitchell W, Pond DA. Treatment of temporal-lobe epilepsy by temporal lobectomy; a survey of findings and results. *Lancet.* 1955;**268**:827–35.

Gibbs EL, Gibbs FA, Fuster B. Psychomotor epilepsy. *Arch Neurol Psychiatry* 1948;**60**(4):331–9.

Jackson H. Epilepsy with tasting movements and dreamy states. *Brain* 1898;**21**:580–90.

Learning objectives

(1) To be aware of the existing hypothesis regarding the pathophysiology of temporal lobe epilepsy.
(2) To understand the epidemiology, etiology, classification, diagnosis, treatment and prognosis of temporal lobe epilepsy.

Section 2 Classification and diagnosis of epilepsy

Chapter 27 Frontal lobe epilepsy

Gonzalo Alarcón

Epidemiology and etiology

Unless otherwise stated, the term frontal lobe epilepsy will refer to symptomatic focal frontal lobe epilepsy throughout this section. Frontal lobe epilepsy is the second most common focal epilepsy in adults. In about 50%, no clear cause is found. When a cause is found, the most common abnormalities causing frontal lobe epilepsy are: previous brain trauma (often with frontopolar scars), neoplasms (particularly low-grade astrocytomas and oligodendrogliomas), vascular malformations (arteriovenous malformations and cavernous angiomas) and developmental lesions (particularly focal cortical dysplasia, which has a predilection for pericentral regions, and hamartomas).

Manifestations

The frontal lobe extends from the rolandic (central) fissure to the frontal pole. It is the largest lobe, accounting for nearly half of each hemisphere's cortex. Consequently, frontal lobe functions are varied and complex, and manifestations of frontal lobe seizures are manifold. Nevertheless, the following features are suggestive of frontal lobe seizures: simple partial motor seizures, frequent seizures (often in clusters), nocturnal predominance (occurring during sleep), dystonic posture from onset, forced eye deviation from onset (usually contralateral to the side of seizure onset), consciousness preserved during convulsions (although usually is not), propensity to status epilepticus.

Complex partial seizures of frontal origin are often brief (<1 min), show little post-ictal confusion, and are associated with sudden, bizarre, frenetic, frantic, agitated and dramatic automatisms (violent thrashing and kicking, often called hypermotor seizures) or with bimanual and bipedal components (clapping, bicycling). Such frontal complex-partial seizures are often called hyperkinetic seizures. Vocalization is common (humming or shouting obscenities). If there are auras, they tend to be nonspecific, but forced thinking or complex visual hallucinations can be seen (e.g. scenes or panoramic travelling). Frontal complex partial seizures can arise from medial as well as dorsolateral regions of the frontal lobe.

Some manifestations of frontal seizures depend on the region from where they arise:

Primary motor (pre-central) seizures (18–25% of frontal lobe epilepsy): focal motor seizures (clonic, tonic-clonic, myoclonic convulsions involving mainly the hand and face, particularly the corner of the mouth). The seizures are often simple partial, rarely with a Jacksonian march, and they show rolandic spikes on the EEG.

Seizures from supplementary motor area: clusters of brief, unilateral or bilateral, symmetrical or asymmetrical tonic convulsions. Typically they show contralateral extension and abduction of one arm with rotation of head to the same side and flexion of the other arm (fencing posture), sometimes with preserved consciousness. Somatosensory auras are present in 45%. There may be associated frontal automatisms. The interictal EEG may show brief, frequent bursts of fast activity/spikes with largest amplitude over the midline, or generalized discharges.

Dorsolateral frontal seizures: forced thinking, complex visual illusions (abstract, intellectual), cephalic aura in 38%, loss of consciousness, tonic eye and head deviation (contralateral to the side of seizure onset), tonic posture (often bilateral and asymmetrical), automatisms (bipedal, clapping, vocalization, laughter), superior frontal or bifrontal EEG abnormalities.

Introduction to Epilepsy ed. Gonzalo Alarcón and Antonio Valentín. Published by Cambridge University Press.
© Cambridge University Press 2012.

Chapter 27: Frontal lobe epilepsy

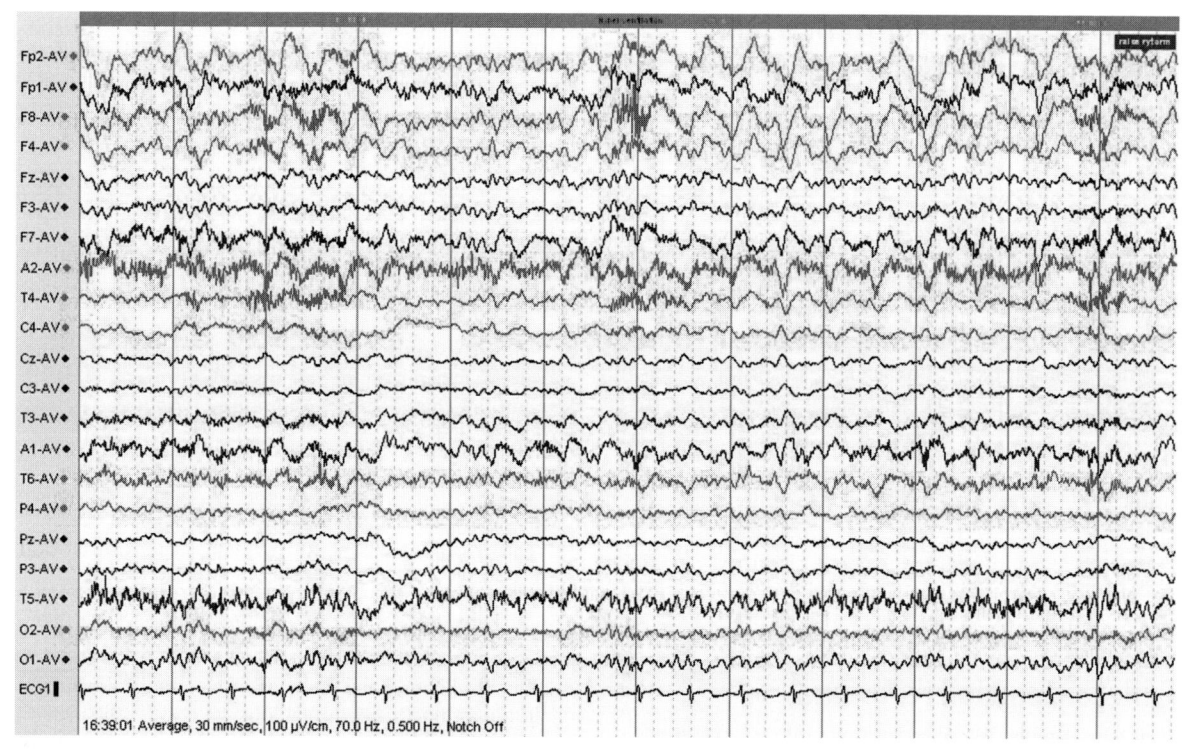

Figure 27.1. Onset of frontal seizure induced by hyperventilaton. Note maximal amplitude of slow activity at Fp2 and F8.

Fronto-polar seizures: most often due to trauma, loss of contact, fixed gaze, loss of tone and fall, followed by tonic-clonic convulsions.

Orbital frontal seizures: olfactory hallucinations, associated with loss of consciousness and automatisms. Orbital seizures may resemble temporal lobe seizures, but lack early oroalimentary automatisms. Automatisms are often brief and repetitive, often gestural or involving violent movements of limbs, such as kicking or thrashing, or involve sexual behaviour or vocalization. Sometimes an aura of fear or epigastric sensations are reported.

Interictal EEG (Figure 18.4): the EEG can be normal. Otherwise, focal epileptiform discharges and/or slowing can be seen depending on the site of origin: at Fz/Cz in medial frontal epilepsy, at F3/F4 in lateral frontal epilepsy, at F8/F7 and Fp1/2 in orbital frontal epilepsy. Secondarily generalized or bilateral discharges have been reported in up to 55% of patients, particularly in epilepsies arising from medial frontal cortex, probably due to the profuse bilateral inter-frontal connections existing through the corpus callosum (Lacruz et al., 2007). Bursts of generalized discharges may last for a few seconds and may be associated with blank spells ('frontal absences').

Ictal EEG (Figure 27.1): consisting of unilateral or bifrontal slowing (need to be differentiated from eye-movement artefacts), rhythmic discharges, or fast activity of topography according to location of underlying lesion. The EEG during seizures can be unrevealing (as often as in 58% of cases), as it is often dominated by profuse movement and muscle artefacts.

Management

Medical treatment is the first choice and includes anticonvulsant drugs effective in focal epilepsies, generally following protocols similar to those described for temporal lobe epilepsy (Chapter 26). However, response to treatment is usually worse than in temporal lobe epilepsy. Resective surgery is a possibility, particularly in patients with demonstrable lesions outside primary motor cortex or speech areas. Functional mapping with intracranial electrodes may be necessary to identify these areas. In patients with normal neuroimaging, intracranial electrodes may be necessary to identify seizure onset (Alarcón et al., 2006). Results after resective surgery are slightly worse than in temporal lobe epilepsy, with only around 55% of patients with good post-surgical outcome (Ferrier et al., 1999).

Autosomal dominant frontal lobe epilepsy (ADFLE)

This syndrome was initially seen in five families, with 45 members affected, linked to chromosome 20q (Scheffer *et al.*, 1995). Epilepsy can start at any age, but mostly in childhood. Patients present with clusters of nocturnal brief motor seizures: tonic stiffening, clonic jerking, vocalization, thrashing, consciousness often retained. There are auras in 70% of patients (somatosensory, fear, déjà vu, autonomic sensations). Physical examination and imaging are normal. The interictal EEG shows discharges only in 16% (bilateral discharges). The ictal EEG is normal or shows bifrontal discharges. It was initially thought to represent a movement disorder and has previously been named nocturnal paroxysmal dystonia. However, it is now classified as idiopathic focal frontal lobe epilepsy. The treatment of choice is carbamazepine.

Epilepsia partialis continua

This was initially described by Kojevnikov in 1895 as an epidemic, spring–summer, tic-borne epilepsy occurring several months after a febrile illness. It essentially consists of focal clonic motor status epilepticus, involving mainly face or hand. Other causes include encephalitis (particularly Rasmussen's disease), neoplasms, cortical dysplasia (particularly hemimegalencephaly), infections, vascular lesions (stroke, haemorrhage, malformations), trauma, hemiconvulsion-hemiplegia epilepsy syndrome, metabolic and mitochondrial disorders, iatrogenia (penicillin). The EEG shows focal central or fronto-central spikes, not always clearly correlated with jerks (EEG back-averaging may be needed to establish such correlation). It is often pharmacoresistant. Surgery has been used in selected cases.

References

Alarcón G, Valentín A, Watt C, *et al.* Is it worth pursuing surgery for epilepsy in patients with normal neuroimaging? *J Neurol Neurosurg Psychiatry* 2006;**77**:474–80.

Ferrier CH, Engelsman J, Alarcón G, Binnie CD, Polkey CE. Prognostic factors in presurgical assessment of frontal lobe epilepsy. *J Neurol Neurosurg Psychiatry* 1999;**66**:350–6.

Lacruz ME, García Seoane JJ, Valentín A, Selway R, Alarcón G. Frontal and temporal functional connections of the living human brain. *Eur J Neurosci* 2007;**6**:1357–70.

Scheffer IE, Bhatia KP, Lopes-Cendes I, *et al.* Autosomal dominant nocturnal frontal lobe epilepsy. A distinctive clinical disorder. *Brain* 1995;**118**:1–73.

Learning objective

(1) To understand the epidemiology, etiology, classification, diagnosis, treatment and prognosis of frontal lobe epilepsy.

Section 2   Classification and diagnosis of epilepsy

Chapter 28
Parietal and occipital focal symptomatic epilepsies

Gonzalo Alarcón

Parietal lobe epilepsy

Epidemiology and aetiology: parietal lobe epilepsy is an uncommon type of symptomatic focal epilepsy (less than 5% of patients in most surgical series). Neoplasms are the most common cause, but other causes include vascular malformations, hamartomas, cortical dysplasia (postcentral), granulomas, porencephalic cysts and old cerebral infarcts.

Manifestations: auras occur in around 94% of patients. The clinical symptoms during the auras are mainly somatosensory (numbness, tingling), but can also consist of pain (burning, abdominal and headache), disturbance of body image, sexual sensations, visual illusions, vertigo (temporo-parietal junction), aphasia, gustatory hallucinations (operculum) and retching (insula). Less common sensory symptoms include elementary visual illusions, auditory hallucinations, cephalic sensations and conscious confusion. Ictal motor phenomena can also occur such as focal motor clonus (57%), head and eye deviation (41%) and tonic posturing (28%). Less common motor symptoms include oral and gestural automatisms (17%), complex automatisms (4%), post-ictal dysphasia (7%) and Todd's paralysis (22%). Symptoms often reflect spreading to other lobes.

Occipital lobe epilepsy

Epidemiology and aetiology: symptomatic occipital lobe epilepsy is also rare (8% of some surgical series). The underlying lesion of occipital epilepsy is not found in around 25% of patients. When found, the most common causes include tumours, head injury, vascular lesions, birth injury with anoxia, focal cortical dysplasia, Sturge–Weber syndrome, coeliac disease with occipital calcifications, meningitis, encephalitis, porencephalic lesions and mitochondrial encephalomyopathy with lactic acidosis and stroke-like episodes (MELAS).

Manifestations: visual positive signs are seen in 47–73% of patients. They include simple hallucinations (contralateral spots, geometrical forms, black or coloured) or complex hallucinations (seen in 14–20%, possibly suggesting limbic involvement). Negative visual signs occur in 40%, including unilateral (contralateral) or bilateral ictal blindness (amaurosis), which can lead to status epilepticus amauroticus or permanent blindness. Forced blinking or eyelid flutter occurs in 17%. Nystagmus and tonic-clonic eye deviation (usually contralateral but sometimes ipsilateral) suggest medial occipital involvement. Seizure spread to extraoccipital regions can be associated with temporal lobe automatisms (29–88%) and focal motor symptoms (38–47%).

Investigations

Neuroimaging often shows an underlying lesion. The EEG often shows focal slowing or epileptiform discharges with distribution according to lesion location (Figures 18.14, 28.1, 28.2).

Management

Medical treatment with antiepileptic drugs effective in focal epilepsies, as described for temporal lobe epilepsy (Chapter 26), is recommended. If medical treatment is ineffective, resective surgery is possible, particularly in patients with a lesion outside

---

Introduction to Epilepsy ed. Gonzalo Alarcón and Antonio Valentín. Published by Cambridge University Press.
© Cambridge University Press 2012.

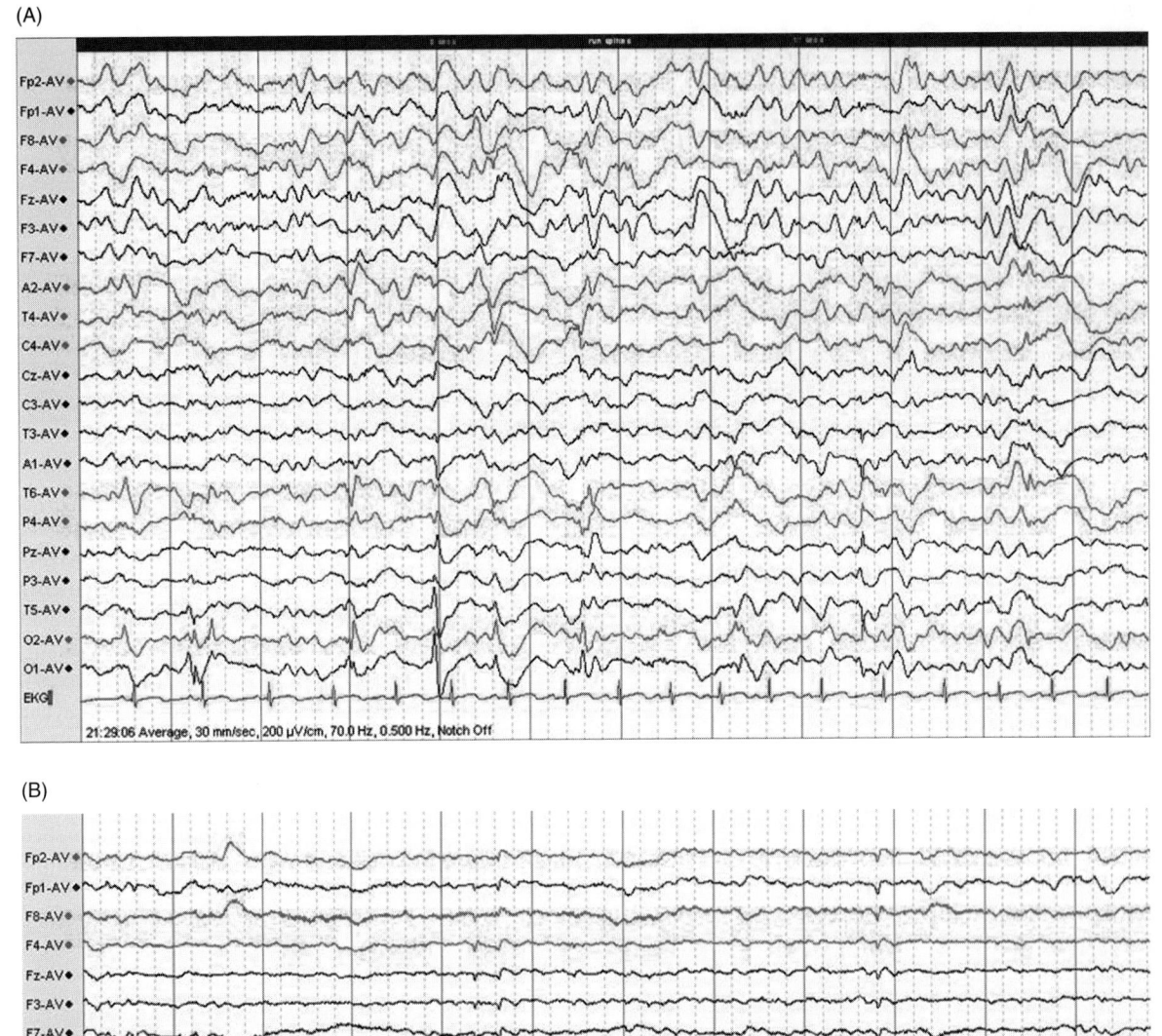

Section 2: Classification and diagnosis of epilepsy

Figure 28.1. Two examples of interictal occipital abnormalities in two different patients.

Chapter 28: Parietal and occipital focal symptomatic epilepsies

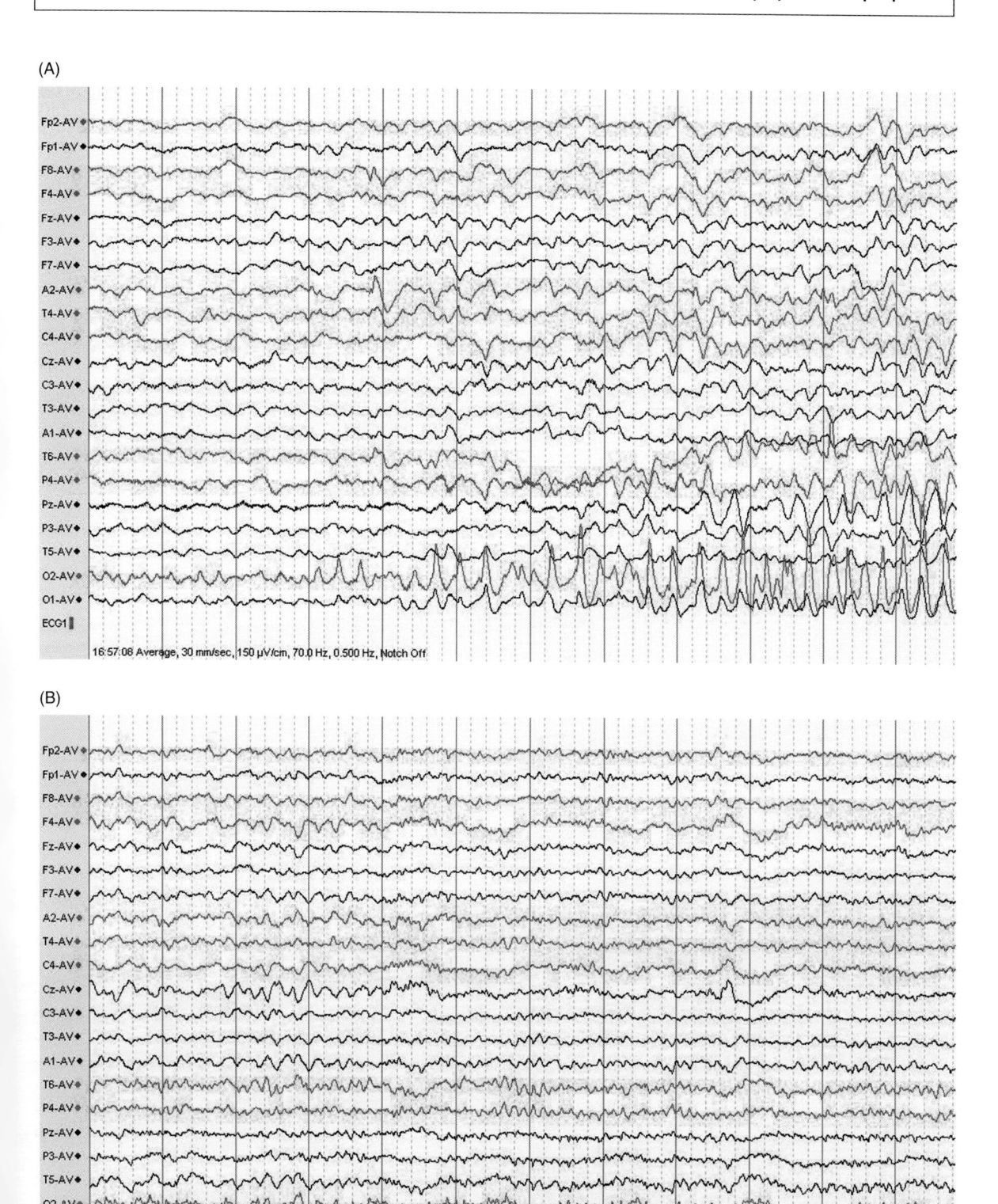

Figure 28.2. Two examples of occipital seizure onset in two different patients.

functionally relevant areas. Functional mapping with intracranial electrodes may be necessary to identify somatosensory or sensory speech areas. In patients with normal neuroimaging, intracranial electrodes may be necessary to identify seizure onset.

Learning objective

(1) To understand the epidemiology, etiology, classification, diagnosis, treatment and prognosis of parietal and occipital lobe epilepsies.

Section 2
Classification and diagnosis of epilepsy

Chapter 29

Epilepsy and myoclonus

Gonzalo Alarcón

General characteristics of myoclonus

Myoclonus (myoclonias) is isolated and involuntary brief jerky movements, frequently involving antagonist muscles (Figure 17.1). It has a heterogeneous etiology. It can be seen in normal subjects, in epilepsy (myoclonic seizures) and in chronic conditions involving brainstem and spinal cord. Myoclonus may originate from sudden muscle contraction (positive myoclonus, associated with brief EMG bursts in affected muscles) or from a sudden muscle relaxation and ensuing drop of limbs or head (negative myoclonus, associated with interruption of ongoing EMG activity in affected muscles). Because they are so brief, myoclonic seizures are often difficult to identify as seizures by patients and physicians (described by earlier physicians as 'fragment of epilepsy'). Consequently, it is unlikely that myoclonic seizures are identified unless specific questions about sudden brief jerks are made during history-taking (e.g. early morning myoclonic jerks may be interpreted by patient and relatives as clumsiness).

Physiological characteristics of epileptic myoclonus

Myoclonic seizures consist of brief sudden jerks, which are associated with synchronous electromyographic (EMG) changes in affected muscles. During positive myoclonus there are EMG bursts lasting for 10–100 ms. During negative myoclonus there is an EMG flattening lasting for 50–400 ms. The EEG changes associated with myoclonus may be detectable on the scalp EEG or after EEG averaging time-locked to EMG changes (back-averaging).

Rhythmic myoclonus

Repetitive, rhythmic myoclonic jerks can be seen in the following conditions:

- Epilepsia partialis continua: 1–2 per second focal myoclonic jerks of cortical origin usually involving face or hand unilaterally, often lasting for days or weeks. See Chapter 109.
- Angelman syndrome: myoclonus is bilateral, rhythmic, virtually continuous or occurring in fast bursts. Each jerk is preceded by a cortical EEG transient by 20–30 ms. Jerks might start focally and become generalized within milliseconds, suggesting motor cortex recruitment.
- Down syndrome: as a response to tapping on the forehead or to acoustic stimuli.
- Tuberous sclerosis: more rarely.
- Autosomal dominant cortical reflex myoclonus and epilepsy: this is a rare condition described in several Japanese families with dominant trait, cortical tremor, myoclonic jerks and tonic-clonic seizures.

Negative myoclonus

Epileptic negative myoclonus consist of a 50–400 ms period of muscle relaxation, multifocal or bilateral, time-locked to scalp sharp waves or spikes on contralateral central regions. It can be clinically difficult to distinguish from positive myoclonus.

Asterixis consists of frequent 50–200 ms periods of muscle relaxation associated with silent EMG activity, appearing as a 'flapping' tremor. Bilateral or multifocal asterixis can be seen in metabolic encephalopathies, particularly in hepatic failure. It can be observed by asking the patient to extend the arms, spread the fingers, dorsiflex the wrist and look for a 'flapping' tremor at the wrist. Unilateral asterixis can be seen in focal lesions of sensorimotor cortex, medial frontal cortex, internal capsule, midbrain or ventrolateral thalamus.

Introduction to Epilepsy ed. Gonzalo Alarcón and Antonio Valentín. Published by Cambridge University Press.
© Cambridge University Press 2012.

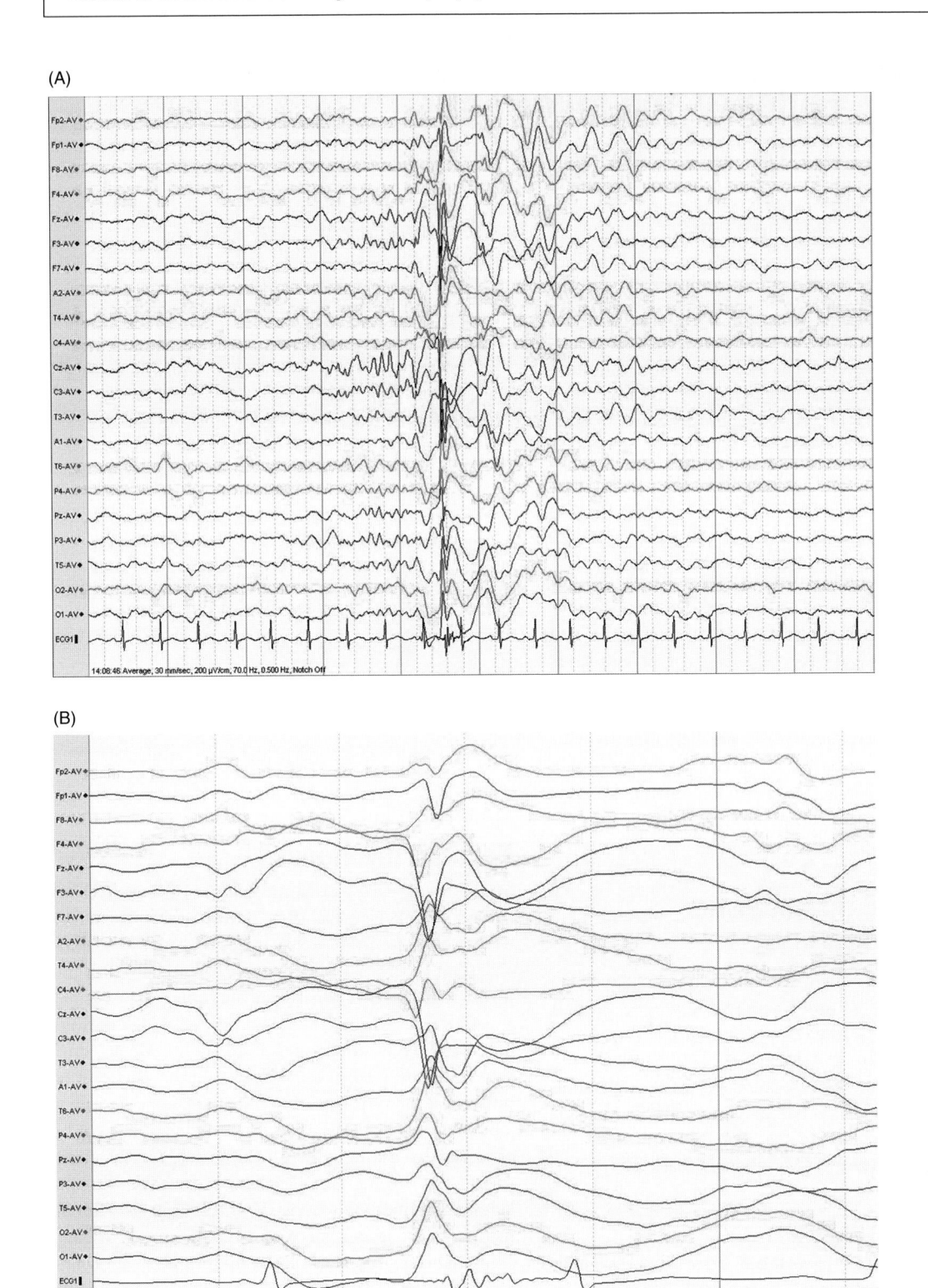

Section 2: Classification and diagnosis of epilepsy

Figure 29.1. Epileptic generalized myoclonic jerk with associated movement and muscle artefacts and spike-and-waves activity on the EEG. (A) At standard time-scale. (B) At expanded time-scale.

Chapter 29: Epilepsy and myoclonus

Box 29.1. Classifications of myoclonus

Etiological classification (Marsden et al., 1982; Fahn et al., 1986)

- Physiological myoclonus: hypnagogic jerks, hiccup, myoclonus induced by anxiety or exercise
- Essential myoclonus: no other neurological signs, often with family history of jerky movements
- Epileptic myoclonus: as part of epilepsy syndromes
- Symptomatic non-epileptic myoclonus: due to encephalopathy
- Subcortical myoclonus: driven by brainstem or spinal cord

Physiological classification

- Cortical myoclonus: with EEG changes
  - Epileptiform discharges and/or polyspikes
  - Sometimes back-averaging necessary
- Subcortical myoclonus:
  - Brainstem (reticular myoclonus): EEG changes not exactly time-locked with EMG burst, sometimes lagging behind, exaggerated startle reflex or reflex myoclonus
  - Spinal: no EEG changes.

Clinical classification

- Focal: restricted to a muscle group, usually distal
- Multifocal: if asynchronous jerks involve different musle groups. Polymyoclonus (small focal jerks, predominantly distal, leading to individual tiny finger movements) typically seen in secondarily generalized epilepsies
- Generalized: jerks involve most body segments apparently synchronously
- Spontaneous or action-induced
- Reflex: induced by peripheral stimuli
- Rhythmic
- Arrhythmic

Cortical action-reflex myoclonus

Action and reflex myoclonus can be seen in the following conditions.

- Postanoxic encephalopathy: dysarthria, ataxia, pyramidal signs, rigidity, epileptic seizures, myoclonus (spontaneous and action, multifocal and generalized, disabling, usually cortical but sometimes brainstem).

- Progressive myoclonus epilepsies: progresive myoclonus (usually head, arms and shoulders), tonic-clonic seizures, progressive neurological deterioration. It is seen in many metabolic conditions. The most common causes are Unverricht-Lundborg disease and Lafora disease. Rarer conditions include neuronal cerolipofuscinosis, type III Gaucher disease, gangliosidosis, mitochondrial disease, sialidosis. Myoclonus is cortical, often reflex or action-induced, but can be spontaneous. There may be giant somatosensory evoked potentials (Lafora's disease) and C-reflex at rest.
- Corticobasal degeneration: progressive disorder in the elderly, limb apraxia, alien limb phenomenon, slowness rigidity, cortical sensory deficits, dysarthria, aphasia, hand dystonia, stimulus-sensory myoclonus. Slowly progressive.
- Alzheimer's disease: spontaneous or action myoclonus can be seen in addition to small irregular twitching of the hands. Myoclonus is usually a late manifestation seen in 10%. Seizures are also seen in 10% of patients.
- Huntington's disease: action myoclonus (rare).

Myoclonus in symptomatic generalized epileptic syndromes

- Severe myoclonic epilepsy in infancy: onset < 3 years, febrile convulsions, massive generalized myoclonus, focal seizures and atypical absences. Generalized discharges and multifocal abnormalities in EEG. Photosensitivity in some. Distal multifocal myoclonus (polymyoclonus) can also be seen.
- Lennox-Gastaut syndrome: tonic, atonic seizures and atypical absences. Less commonly myoclonus, partial, tonic-clonic seizures and polymyoclonus.

Myoclonus in idiopathic generalized epilepsy syndromes

Myoclonus is generalized, spontaneous, arrhythmic and of axial predominance. It can be seen in:

- Benign myoclonic epilepsy of infancy: onset age <5.
- Reflex form of benign myoclonic epilepsy of infancy: photic-induced jerks, and sometimes by sounds or tactile stimulation.

- Juvenile myoclonic epilepsy: onset at around 14, myoclonus is the initial symptom in 54% of patients, often interpreted as morning clumsiness.
- Myoclonic-astatic epilepsy: learning disabilities in as many as 25% (symptomatic?). Onset between 7 months and 6 years. Seizure types include myoclonic-astatic, astatic, tonic-clonic and absence seizures. Non-convulsive status epilepticus is common. Presence of tonic seizures is an exclusion criterion. Carbamazepine may induce status.

Epileptic syndromes with myoclonus of unclear neurophysiological characteristics

- Early myoclonic encephalopathy: symptomatic or presumed symptomatic generalized epilepsy of perinatal origin (often due to inborn errors of metabolism). Multifocal severe myoclonus is seen.
- Myoclonic status in encephalopathies: myoclonus synchronized with EEG spikes is often rhythmic and bilateral.
- Epilepsy with myoclonic absences: generalized and rhythmic myoclonus can be seen synchronously with 3 Hz spike-wave.

Reticular reflex myoclonus

Reticular myoclonus is generalized, mainly involving proximal and flexor muscles, spontaneous or reflex (induced by movement, somatosensory, auditory or visual stimuli). It is believed to originate in the brainstem reticular formation because of sequential activation of muscles innervated by cranial nerves: trapezius (XI nerve) followed by sternocleidomastoid (XI nerve) followed by orbicularis oris (VII nerve) followed by masseter (V nerve). EEG activity is not well time-locked or may lag myoclonic jerks. Reticular myoclonus can be seen in postanoxic encephalopathy, myoclonic epilepsy with ragged red fibres (MERRF), Unverricht-Lundborg disease, often co-existing with cortical myoclonus.

Treatment of epileptic myoclonus

Medical treatment should be started as part of the management of the underlying epilepsy syndromes. Some drugs are particularly effective in specifically treating myoclonic seizures. Pirazetam is well tolerated and can be considered first choice for myoclonus, although clonazepam is generally more effective. Sodium valproate and lamotrigine are also used. Among the new anticonvulsants, levetiracetam appears to be particularly effective to treat myoclonus. Nevertheless, keep in mind that antiepileptic drugs can worsen myoclonus, particularly if used in combination.

Recommended reading

Guerrini R, Bonanni P, Rothwell J, Hallett M. Myoclonus and epilepsy. In Guerrini R, Aicardi J, Andermann F, Hallett M, eds. *Epilepsy and Movement Disorders*, pp. 165–210. Cambridge: Cambridge University Press; 2002.

References

Fahn S, Marsden CD, Van Woert MH. Definition and classification of myoclonus. *Adv Neurol* 1986;**43**:1–5.

Marsden CD, Hallet M, Fahn S. The nosology and pathophysiology of myoclonus. In Marsden CD, Fahn S, eds. *Movement Disorders*, pp. 196–249. London: Butterworths Scientific; 1982.

Learning objectives

(1) To know the characteristics of myoclonus and its classification.
(2) To know the conditions associated with myoclonus, with particular emphasis on epileptic syndromes associated with myoclonic seizures, and their prognosis.
(3) To understand the principles involved in treating myoclonus.

Section 2 Classification and diagnosis of epilepsy

Chapter 30

Progressive myoclonic epilepsies

J. Helen Cross

The progressive myoclonic epilepsies (PME) are a group of disorders that affect previously normal individuals, most of which have a genetic aetiology and poor outcome. The hallmark is myoclonus as a prominent part of their clinical presentation (Table 30.1). Myoclonus manifests as stimulus-sensitive segmental, arrhythmic and asynchronous, lightning jerks of muscles that may affect any muscle group of the body. Individuals also have epilepsy that usually is also stimulus-sensitive, with predominantly generalized tonic-clonic seizures and absence seizures. There is evidence of progressive neurological deterioration to a variable degree dependent on the underlying cause. Some may present in teenage years and may mimic idiopathic generalized epilepsy in the early stages. However, there may be atypical features at the presentation which guide towards further investigation.

Lafora body disease

This disease is characterized by epilepsy, myoclonus, dementia and Lafora bodies, the latter being periodic acid Schiff-positive intracellular polyglucosan inclusion bodies found in neurons, heart, skeletal muscle, liver and sweat gland duct cells. The usual presentation is in the teenage years with myoclonus and possible episodes of generalized status epilepticus. However, they may present at an earlier age with occipital seizures. Cognitive decline, dysarthria and ataxia appear early, and may progess rapidly once recognized. Most die within 10 years of onset. Diagnosis is most conveniently made by histological examination of eccrine ducts of the sweat glands from skin biopsy, usually taken from the axilla.

Lafora body disease is an autosomal recessive disorder. Up to 80% are caused by mutations in the EPM2A gene at 6q24, which encodes the laforin, a dual-specificity protein tyrosine phosphatase, primarily associated with ribosomes. This enzyme plays a role in each step of growth, development and survival of neurons, dendrites and synapses. Dysfunction leads to excessive glycogen with fewer branching points and excessively long peripheral chains, which can be seen as the Lafora inclusion bodies in the cytoplasm. There is no known treatment of the disease itself at present. Treatment is symptomatic, as will be discussed below.

Unverricht-Lundborg disease

This was first described in 1891 by Unverricht, and also by Lundborg in 1903. This may have a relatively early onset in pre-teenage years but it is more typical to mimic idiopathic generalized epilepsy (IGE) at its presentation. The first symptom is myoclonus in at least half of the individuals but they also may present with other seizure types. Patients later develop ataxia, intention tremor and dysarthria. Dementia itself may be extremely slow and difficult to detect, survival therefore highly variable. Clinically myoclonus is seen precipitated by tendon tapping, passive joint movements and auditory and light stimuli. Seizures are more typically seen on awaking and hence the mimic of juvenile myoclonic epilepsy (JME) early in the disease. The background EEG may be normal in the early stages, and with demonstrable photosensitivity may also aid the misdiagnosis of IGE, but later becomes highly abnormal and disorganized, alerting the physician to an alternative diagnosis. A useful screening test, which may be used within the neurophysiology department, is somato-sensory evoked potentials, which are highly enlarged in this group of patients.

Introduction to Epilepsy ed. Gonzalo Alarcón and Antonio Valentín. Published by Cambridge University Press.
© Cambridge University Press 2012.

Section 2: Classification and diagnosis of epilepsy

Table 30.1. Key characteristics of the progressive myoclonic epilepsies

Diagnosis	Age of onset	Presenting features	Diagnostic test	Genetics
Lafora body	Teenage	Epilepsy, myoclonus, ataxia, dementia	Axillary skin biopsy	EPM2A at 6q24
Unverricht-Lundborg	Pre-teenage	Myoclonus +/− ataxia, intention tremor	SSEP, genetics	CSTB on 21q22.3
DRPLA	6 years – adult	Myoclonus, dementia, ataxia +/− chorea	Genetics	CAG expansion at 12p13.31
Sialidosis Type 1	8–25 years	Intention + action myoclonus	Neuraminidase activity in leukocytes	NEU1-MHC locus 6p21.3 Chromosome 20
Type II	10–20 years	Myoclonus with corneal clouding, hepatomegaly, learning disability		
MERRF	Child to adult	Myoclonus, ataxia, hearing loss	Muscle biopsy for ragged red fibres, and respiratory chain enzyme activity	Adenosine to guanine substitution at nucleotide pair 8344 in the tRNA gene (MTTK) of mitochondrial DNA
Late infantile NCL	2–4 years	GTC seizures, cognitive slowing	TPP1 activity in leukocytes	CLN2 mutation
Juvenile Gaucher's	5–15 years	General/focal seizures, photomyoclonic response	Gaucher cells, glucocerebrosidase in leukocytes	
PNDC	0–10 years (can be later)	Epilepsy including EPC, cognitive slowing +/− liver dysfunction	Liver biopsy	eg POLG

The condition is caused by a mutation in the CSTB (formerly known as EPM 1) gene 21q 22.3, which encodes cystatin B, a cysteine protease inhibitor. This inhibits the papain family of cysteine proteases involved in the initiation of apoptosis. The exact pathophysiology of the disease, however, remains unknown.

Dentato-rubro-pallido-luysian atrophy (DRPLA)

This is an autosomal recessive condition due to unstable expansion of the CAG repeats of a gene at 12p13.31. Most reports of this condition come from Japan. There are three forms: ataxiachoreoathetoid, pseudo-huntingdon and the progressive myoclonic epilepsy form. Onset may be from 6 years to adult, with myoclonic epilepsy and associated dementia, ataxia and variable chorea. Progression is variable and therefore survival subsequently variable. Diagnosis is made on assessing for the trinucleotide repeat of the DRPLA gene.

Sialidosis

Two forms of sialidosis can cause a PME, both autosomal recessive in inheritance. Sialidosis type I (cherry red spot myoclonus syndrome) is caused by deficiency of α-neuraminidase. It has an onset aged 8–25 years with myoclonic and more generalized seizures. Neurological evaluation reveals ataxia and pure intention and action myoclonus. There is a slow progression with absence of cognitive deterioration. There is late onset of blindness with the characteristic cherry red spot at the macula. Sialidosis type II (also called galactosialidosis) is caused by a deficiency of both *N*-acetyl neuraminidase and β-galactosialidase. Onset varies from the neonatal period to the second decade of life. In addition to the myoclonus, clinical features include coarse facies, corneal clouding, hepatomegaly, skeletal dysplasia and learning disability. A useful screening test is urinary sialic acid, with a definitive diagnosis made by looking for lysosomal enzyme activity in white cells or cultured fibroblasts. The human sialidase gene NEU1 is located inside the locus of the MHC on chromosome 6p21.3, whereas the gene responsible for galatosialidoses is located on chromosome 20.

Mitochondrial disease (myoclonic epilepsy with ragged red fibres syndrome or MERRF)

This has onset in childhood to adulthood. It may be sporadic or familial. Clinical features involve myoclonus, ataxia and hearing loss associated with variable features of dementia, dysarthria, short stature, optic atrophy, neuropathy, myopathy, lactic acidosis and migraine. There is an overlap with the syndrome of Myoclonic epilepsy, lactic acidosis and stroke-like episodes (MELAS) but MERRF usually has a longer course and is associated with milder cognitive and behavioural deficits. As a mitochondrial disease, lactate is raised in CSF and blood. Muscle biopsy will be required to confirm the diagnosis, by the demonstration on staining of typical ragged red fibres (subsarcomlemnal aggregates of mitochondria) as well as decreased activity of respiratory chain enzymes. In more than 90% of patients the molecular defect is an adenosine to guanine substitution at nucleotide pair 8344 in the tRNA gene (MTTK) of mitochondrial DNA.

MELAS usually has an earlier onset and again presents with myoclonic epilepsy but with recurrent hemi-cranial headaches and recurrent stroke-like episodes with occipital predominance. The latter may be silent and only be demonstrated on MRI scan of the brain.

Late infantile NCL

Late infantile neuronal ceroid lipofuscinosis is one of the few neurodegenerative conditions with epilepsy as an initial manifestation, presenting between 2 and 5 years of age. The individual may present with generalized seizures and subsequently develop myoclonus, presenting with a pseudo ataxia, the result of the myoclonus. Cognitive slowing may also be quite subtle in the first instance prior to any definitive developmental regression. Other neurological findings and blindness are a late feature of this form of the disease. Neurophysiology may provide a useful screening test with characteristic abnormalities seen on EEG with prominent flash activation as well as a diminution of the electroretinogram and heightened visual evoked potential. Diagnosis is now made by screening on white cell tripeptidyl peptidase 1 (TTP1) activity, with mutations ultimately reviewed in the CLN2 gene.

Juvenile Gaucher disease

This has an age of onset between 5 and 15 years with initially generalized or partial seizures but a definitive photomyoclonic response. They may also ultimately present with eye movement abnormalities and ataxia early in the course. Diagnosis of this disease is made by looking for Gaucher cells and excessive glucocerebroside in lymphocytes, bone marrow or rectal biopsy but ultimately glucocerebrosidase activity in leukocytes or fibroblasts.

Progressive neuronal degeneration of childhood with liver disease (Alpers disease)

This has an onset usually in the first 2 years of life but actually can present at any time in childhood. Onset may be insidious with epilepsy and developmental stagnation, with the situation initially unclear as to whether it is due to a progressive disease. However, there is a high rate of status epilepticus including epilepsia partialis continua. Liver failure may be relatively late, liver involvement in some only being detected on liver biopsy. Many are thought to be due to a mitochondrial cytopathy and a proportion have been found to be the result of a mutation in polymerase gamma (POLG), the only DNA polymerase in human mitochondria, essential for mitochondrial replication and repair. However, diagnosis may still be required through liver and muscle biopsy.

Treatment of PME

Treatment of the PMEs remains largely symptomatic rather than curative. There is no question in the majority of individuals with progressive myoclonic epilepsy that myoclonus may be difficult to eradicate with treatment. The most important aspect of treatment is the avoidance of medication that may aggravate myoclonus rather than that trying to determine what may be effective, so using antiepileptic medication with a broad-spectrum action. Sodium valproate will have been used in almost all as a first-line medication but, of course, may be contraindicated in such diseases as Alpers disease. Benzodiazepines such as clobazam and clonazepam may also be useful. Piracetam has been shown to be of later benefit with regard to myoclonus itself. However, there is also evidence that the use of some of the newer medications, namely levetiracetam and zonisamide, may be useful, with anecdotal case reports suggesting they may be more effective in reduction of myoclonus and improved functioning. Certainly more research needs to be continued in this area.

Recommended reading

Ramachandran N, Girard JM, Turnbull J, Minassian BA. The autosomal recessively inherited progressive myoclonic epilepsies and their genes. *Epilepsia* 2009;**50**(s5): 29–36.

Shahwan A, Farrell M, Delanty N. Progressive myoclonic epilepsies: a review of genetic and therapeutic aspects. *Lancet Neurol* 2005;4:239–48.

Wolf NI, Rahman S, Schmitt B, *et al.* Status epilepticus in children with Alpers disease caused by POLG1 mutations: EEG and MRI features. *Epilepsia* 2009;**50**:1596–607.

Learning objectives

(1) To know the general characteristics and prognosis of progressive myoclonic epilepsies.
(2) To know the specific conditions associated with progressive myoclonic epilepsies, their prognosis, similarities and differences.
(3) To understand the principles involved in the management of progressive myoclonic epilepsies.

Section 2: Classification and diagnosis of epilepsy

Chapter 31: Acute symptomatic seizures

Gonzalo Alarcón

Epileptic seizures without epilepsy

There are a number of acute conditions (intoxication, encephalitis, metabolic problems, etc.) with seizures as part of their symptoms. In most cases, seizures disappear with remission of the underlying condition. This is not considered epilepsy, since the presence of such seizures does not necessarily imply a significantly increased tendency to suffer seizures once the underlying acute condition has resolved. Nevertheless, although this situation is not epilepsy, seizures are identical to those seen in epilepsy, and they are called 'epileptic' seizures.

> **Box 31.1. Synonyms**
> The following terms are equivalent
> Acute symptomatic seizures
> Reactive seizures
> Provoked seizures
> Situation-related seizures
> 'Gelegenheitsanfälle'

Characteristics of acute symptomatic seizures

Acute symptomatic seizures are epileptic seizures induced by an acute temporary situation. They look like epileptic seizures although they are not part of an epilepsy syndrome. They should not be considered as epilepsy but they are often wrongly considered as epilepsy in epidemiological studies. They may be treated as epilepsy in the short term, but do not usually require long-term treatment because seizures tend to remit when the underlying acute situation ceases. Where the acute situation causes brain damage, epilepsy may later occur.

The overall prognosis depends on the underlying condition. For instance:

- poor prognosis and raised mortality if associated with encephalitis;
- good prognosis if associated with drug withdrawal.

Acute symptomatic seizures are very common, representing perhaps 20–40% of newly occurring seizures. They may not be seen by neurologists, and EEG investigations may not be obtained.

Causes of acute symptomatic seizures

The most common causes of acute symptomatic seizures are febrile seizures (age-specific), traumatic brain injury, cerebrovascular disease, drug withdrawal, and infections of the central nervous system.

Incidence of acute symptomatic seizures

- 39/100 000 person/year – Rochester study (Annegers *et al.*, 1995).
- 29/100 000 person/year – French study (Loiseau *et al.*, 1990).
- 21% of newly occurring seizures – British study (Sander *et al.*, 1990).
- Approximately 40% of afebrile seizures.
- Higher risk in men than in women.
- Highest risk during first year of life – metabolic, infectious and encephalopathic causes.
- Incidence increases progressively with age after 35 years.
- Cerebrovascular disease is the cause in 50% of patients >65 years.

Introduction to Epilepsy ed. Gonzalo Alarcón and Antonio Valentín. Published by Cambridge University Press.
© Cambridge University Press 2012.

Cumulative incidence of acute symptomatic seizures

There is a 3.6% risk of having acute symptomatic seizures during an 80-year lifespan. This is higher for men (5%) than for women (2.5%).

Prognosis of acute symptomatic seizures

The prognosis of acute symptomatic seizures depends on the underlying condition. Because some conditions are serious, there is a relatively high mortality rate. There is a slightly increased risk of later developing epilepsy, compared with patients who do not suffer seizures under similar conditions.

References

Annegers JF, Hauser WA, Lee JR, *et al.* Acute symptomatic seizures in Rochester, Minnesota, 1935–1984. *Epilepsia* 1995;**36**:327–33.

Loiseau J, Loiseau P, Guyot M, *et al.* Survey of seizure disorders in the French southwest. 1. Incidence of epileptic syndromes. *Epilepsia* 1990;**31**:391–6.

Sander JWAS, Hart YM, Johnson AL, *et al.* National general practice study of epilepsy: newly diagnosed epileptic seizures in a general population. *Lancet* 1990;**336**:1267–71.

Learning objectives

(1) To understand the concept and epidemiology of acute symptomatic seizures.
(2) To be aware of the terminology used to designate acute symptomatic seizures.
(3) To know the conditions associated with acute symptomatic seizures.
(4) To understand the prognostic significance of acute symptomatic seizures.

Section 2

Classification and diagnosis of epilepsy

Chapter 32

EEG in neonates and children

Sushma Goyal

Definitions

GA = gestational age, the number of completed weeks and days from the date of the first day of the last menstrual period.

CGA = corrected gestational age, GA + number of weeks post-partum.

Term = neonate born between 37 to 42 weeks GA.

Preterm = GA less than 37 weeks.

Discontinuity = periods of hypoactivity (<10 μV) of variable duration. This is normal for preterm EEGs and abnormal in term EEGs.

Inter-burst interval = length of period of hypoactivity. Normal for preterm. Abnormal for term.

HIE = hypoxic ischaemic encephalopathy. Failure to initiate and sustain breathing immediately after delivery. This is associated with hypoxic ischaemic injury to the central nervous system, the clinical manifestations of which are termed HIE. As per the AAP (American Academy of Pediatrics) and ACOG (American College of Obstetrics and Gynecology), all the following must be present:

(1) Profound metabolic or mixed acidosis (pH < 7.00) in cord.
(2) Persistence of Apgar scores 0–3 for longer than 5 min.
(3) Neonatal neurological sequelae (e.g. seizures, coma, hypotonia).
(4) Multiple organ involvement.

Normal neonatal EEG

The neonatal EEG is in the process of maturation, thereby evolving from week to week. The terminology used to describe the neonatal EEG is largely based on the work of the Baudeloque team and retains the use of French terminology to describe the developmental features of EEG in pre-mature and full-term infants.

Box 32.1. Factors affecting the neonatal EEG
- Corrected gestational age CGA
- State
  - Awake
  - Sleep (AS – active sleep, or QS – quiet sleep)
- Medication
- Environment

Montages: Term baby/normal size for the age - full montage
Small baby for the age or pre-term –
F4-C4; C4-P4; P4-O2; F3-C3; C3-P3; P3-O1
T4-C4; C4-Cz; Cz-C3; C3-T3
see diagram neonatal montage

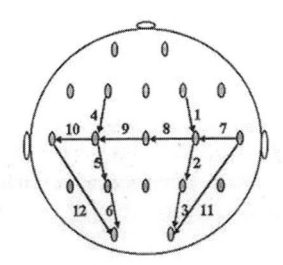

Figure 32.1. Normal neonatal montage.

Technique

Recording the neonatal EEG is challenging because the environment tends to be prone to generating artefacts and because of the size of the baby's head, which allow only a limited number of electrodes (Figure 32.1)

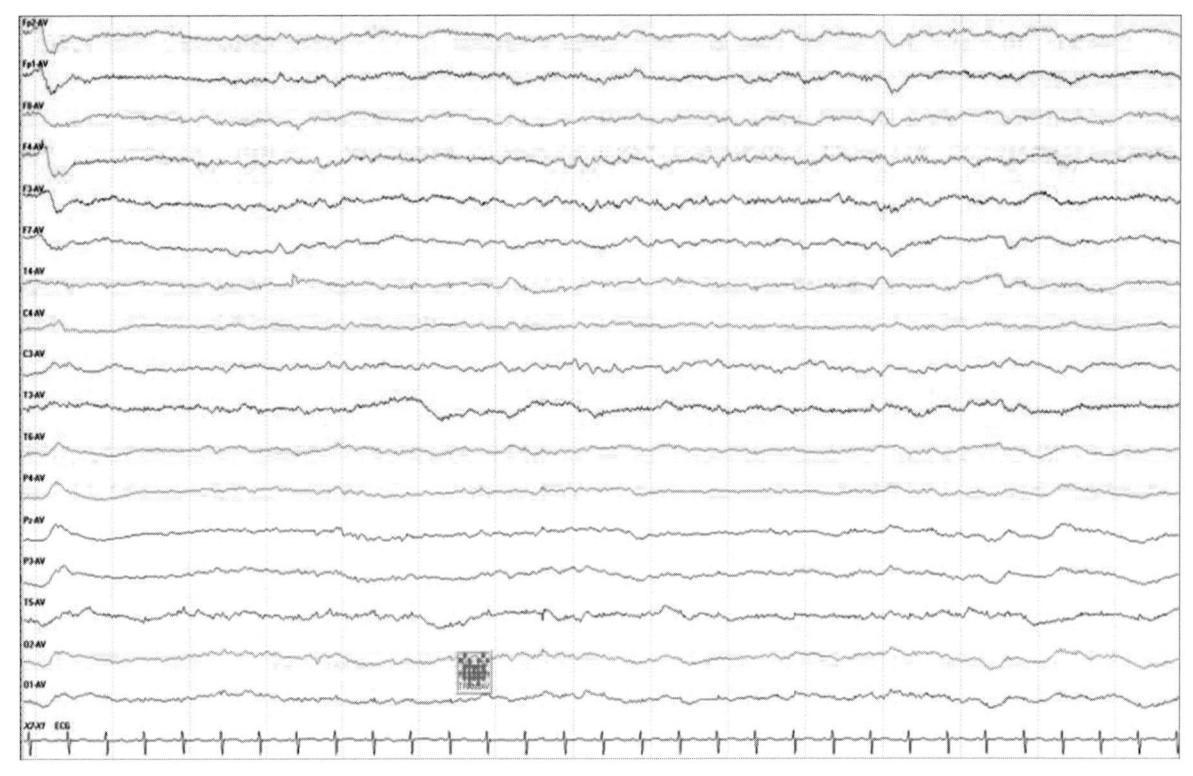

Figure 32.2. Activité moyenne.

Normal neonatal EEG

Full term

(1) Awake – Activité moyenne (Figure 32.2)

- Continuous, irregular, diffuse activity with a rolandic predominance, mainly in the theta band (4–7 Hz), with a voltage of 25–50 μV, lower occipital delta waves of similar voltage.

(2) Quiet sleep (QS)

  (a) Slow continuous tracing or high-voltage pattern:

   - Continuous delta-wave activity (1–3 Hz) with occipital predominance and variable voltage (50–150 μV).

  (b) Tracé alternant pattern: bilateral bursts of delta waves occurring on the background of continuous theta activity (4–7 Hz and 25–50 μV) (Figure 32.3). This pattern is characterized by:

   - bursts (1–3 Hz, 50–150 μV) vary from 3 to 8 seconds;
   - intervening periods of low-voltage activity (4–7 Hz, 25–50 μV) of similar duration;
   - appears between 37 and 44 weeks;
   - only in QS.

Pre-term EEG

Tracé discontinue: bursts of activity interspersed with periods of hypoactivity (<10 μV) of variable duration according to GA (Figure 32.4).

Features developing in a pre-term EEG

- Continuity: the duration of hypoactivity (inter-burst intervals or IBI) decreases with gestational age. The background becomes continuous in wakefulness from 32 weeks. In sleep at 32 weeks, IBI are equal or shorter than 15 seconds, whereas at 34 weeks IBI are equal or shorter than 10 seconds (Figure 32.5). The background becomes continuous in sleep from 37 weeks though Tracé alternant may be seen in QS until 44 weeks.
- Synchronicity: physiological patterns may occur at different times in the two hemispheres (Figure 32.6).

Chapter 32: EEG in neonates and children

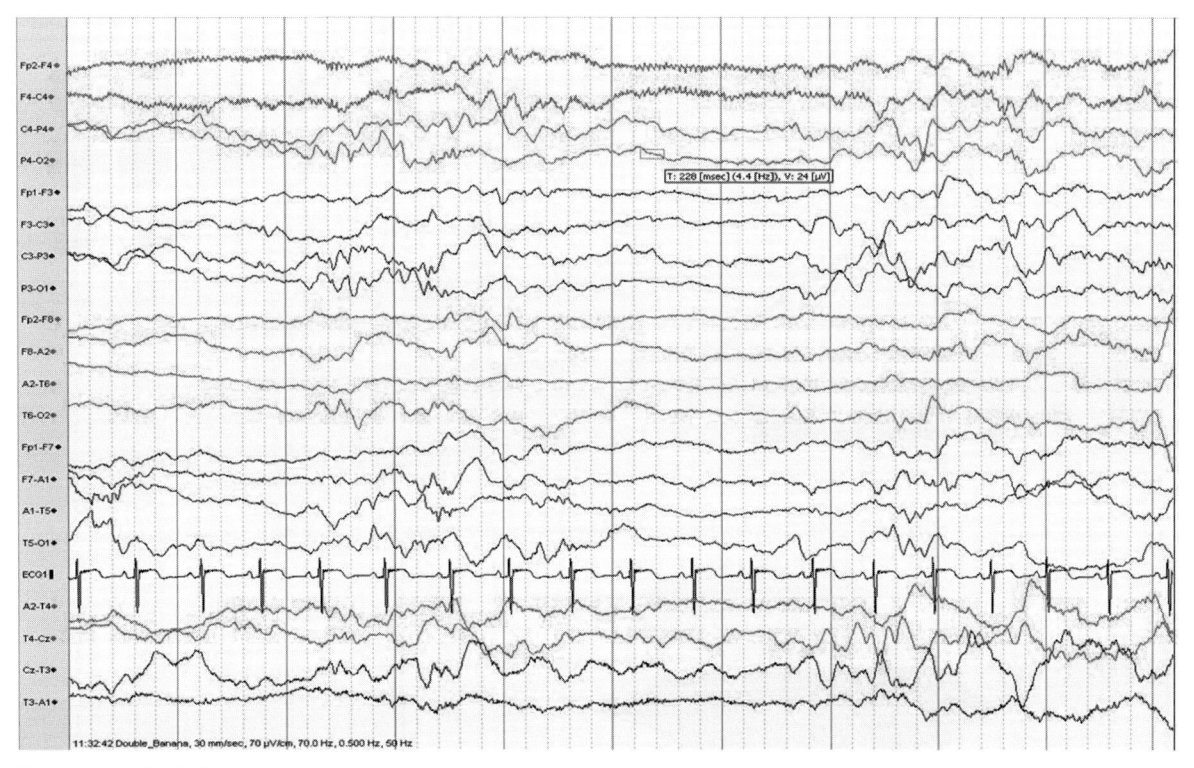

Figure 32.3. Tracé alternant in a term neonate.

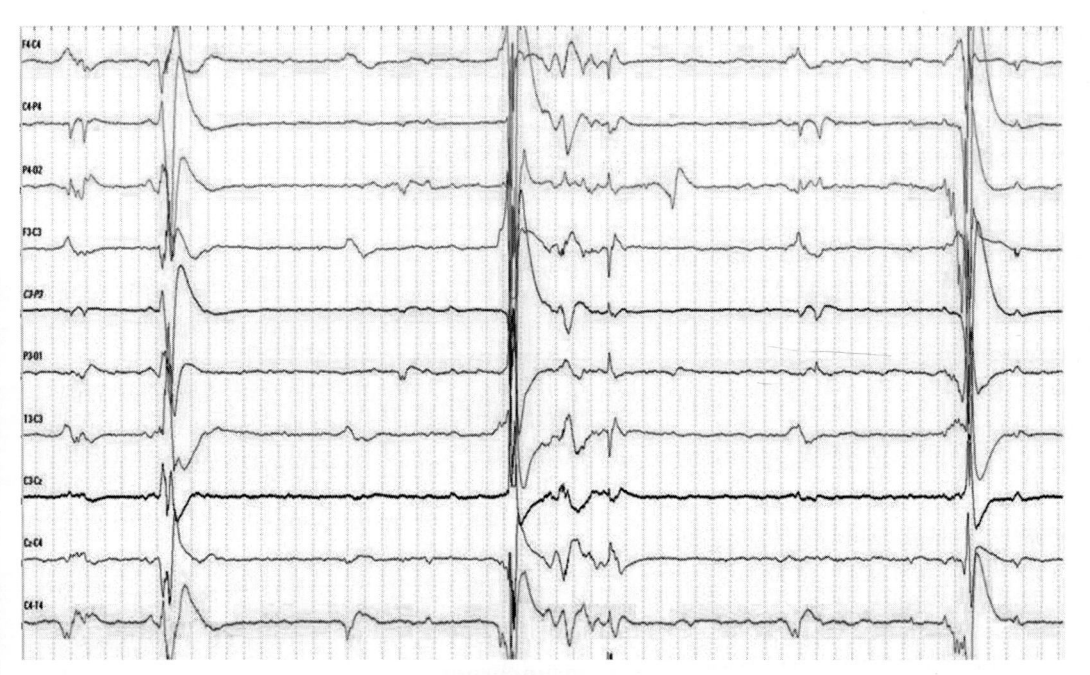

Figure 32.4. Tracé discontinue in 27 week baby with IBI 20 s during wakefulness.

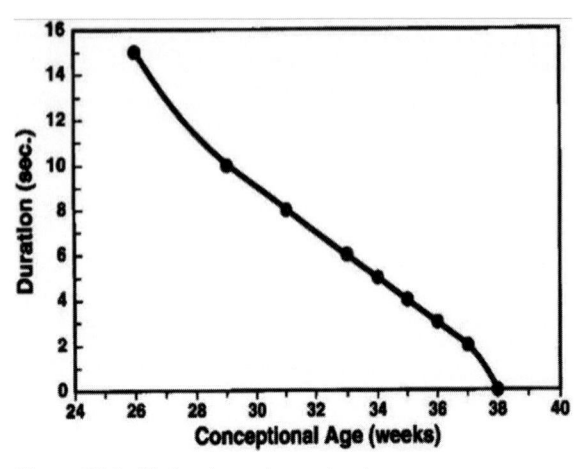

Section 2: Classification and diagnosis of epilepsy

Figure 32.5. IBI duration and gestational age.

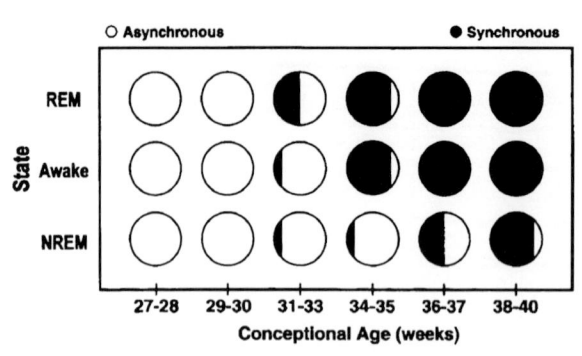

Figure 32.6. Appearance of synchronicity of activity with gestational age.

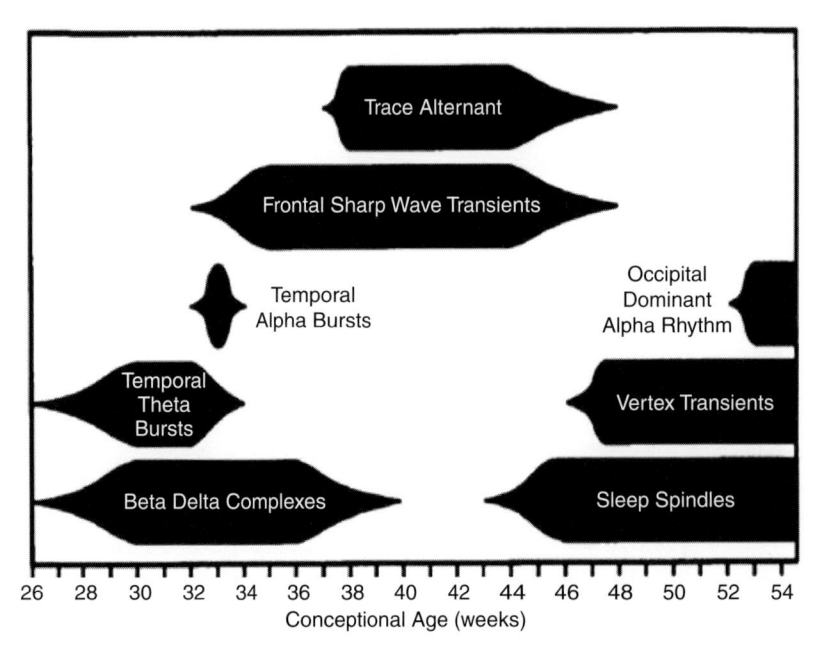

Figure 32.7. Appearance of normal transients.

- Temporal organization: organization of behavioural states:
  - active and quiet wakefulness
  - active sleep (AS1, AS2: REM sleep)
  - quiet sleep (QS: non-REM sleep)
- Spatial organization: type and location of EEG patterns specific to GA.
- Normal transients (Figure 32.7).
- Reactivity: the EEG shows a response to sensory stimulation from about 33 weeks, which becomes clear and reproducible by 35 weeks.

Abnormal neonatal EEG
Dysmaturity
This term is used when the observed maturational features are not appropriate for the CGA. The established limit for considering an EEG dysmature is a difference of > 2 weeks.

Subtle background changes asymmetry/asynchrony
See Figure 32.8.

194

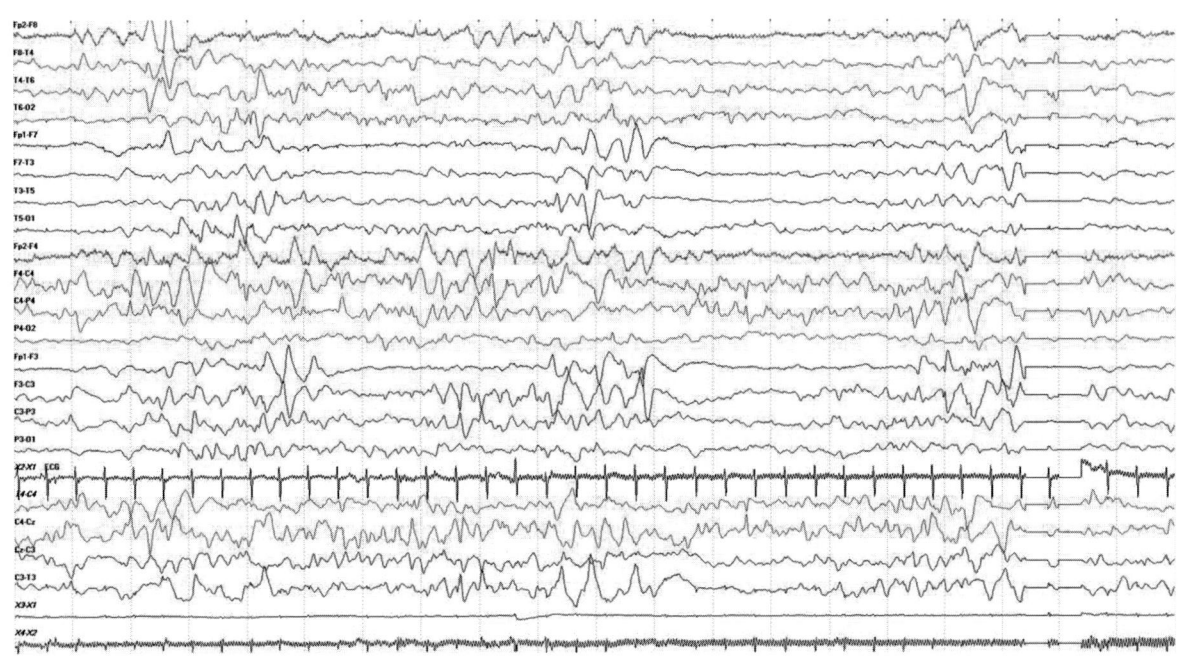

Figure 32.8. Note asynchrony between activities over the hemispheres.

Discontinuous EEG (periods of suppression < 20 μV, bursts >150 μV)

This term is used in HIE, in which this is usually a transient feature. The following factors are to be considered when reporting an EEG to evaluate prognosis in a term neonate with HIE:

(1) Clinical details of severity of HIE.
(2) Timing of EEG: early serial EEGs done in the study by Pressler (2001) showed that early EEG is an excellent prognostic indicator for a favourable outcome if normal within 8 hours of life. If the EEG remains inactive or grossly abnormal beyond 12 hours, it is indicative of a poor outcome. However, an inactive EEG within the first 8 hours could recover by 12 hours and have a good outcome. Conversely, if an EEG is done too late, then a normal background could lead to a falsely optimistic prognosis. The ideal timing to do the EEG is at the peak of the symptomatic neurological impairment, which is 12–72 hours of age.
(3) Inter-burst interval: any period of discontinuity in the background of a term neonate is abnormal (Figure 32.9). The prognostic value of the continuity of the background is well established. However, there is no consensus on the classification and grading of the background abnormalities. A simple measure proposed by Menache (2002) is the measurement of the predominant IBI (defined as the duration of more that 50% of all IBIs). A predominant IBI longer than 30 seconds in their study was associated with a 100% probability of severe neurological disabilities and 86% chance of developing subsequent epilepsy. The other parameter, that is more user-friendly, is the maximum IBI, which, if longer than 40 seconds, is associated with an 89% probability of an unfavourable outcome ($P = 0.046$).

Continuous low-voltage inactive EEG (CLV)

The amplitude of the background activity should be constantly lower than 20 μV (Figure 32.10). If it persists for more than 12 hours of age it is associated with an unfavourable outcome.

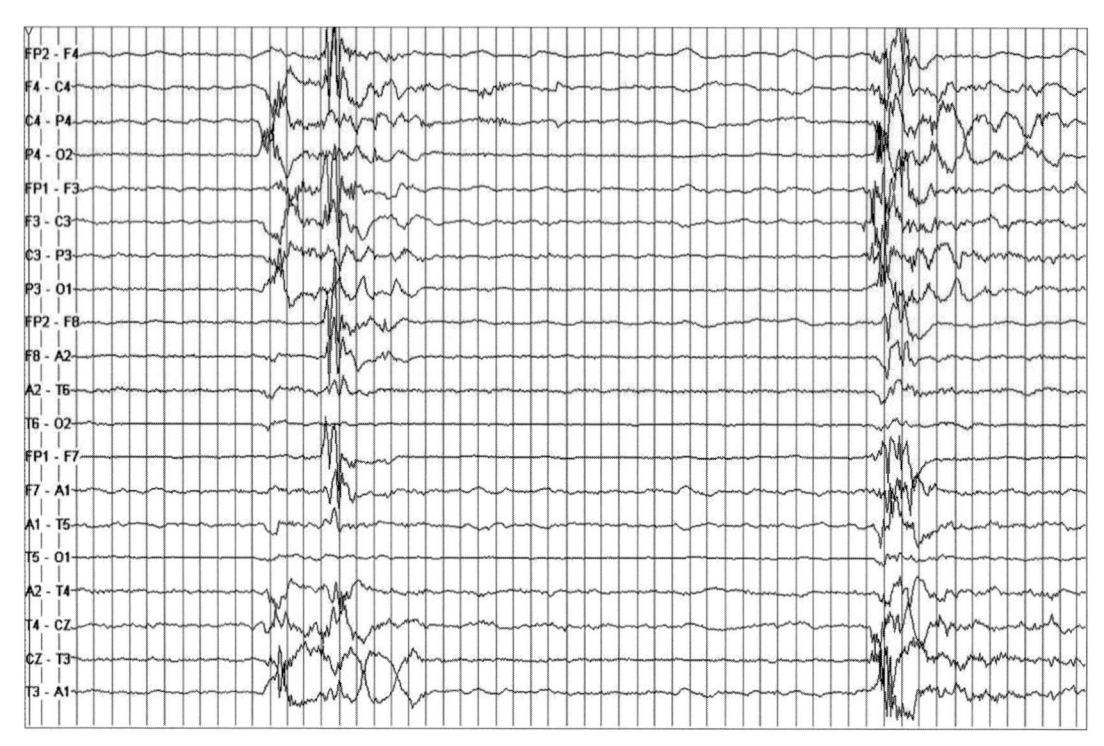

Section 2: Classification and diagnosis of epilepsy

Figure 32.9. Full-term neonate recorded day 2 with IBI = 35 s.

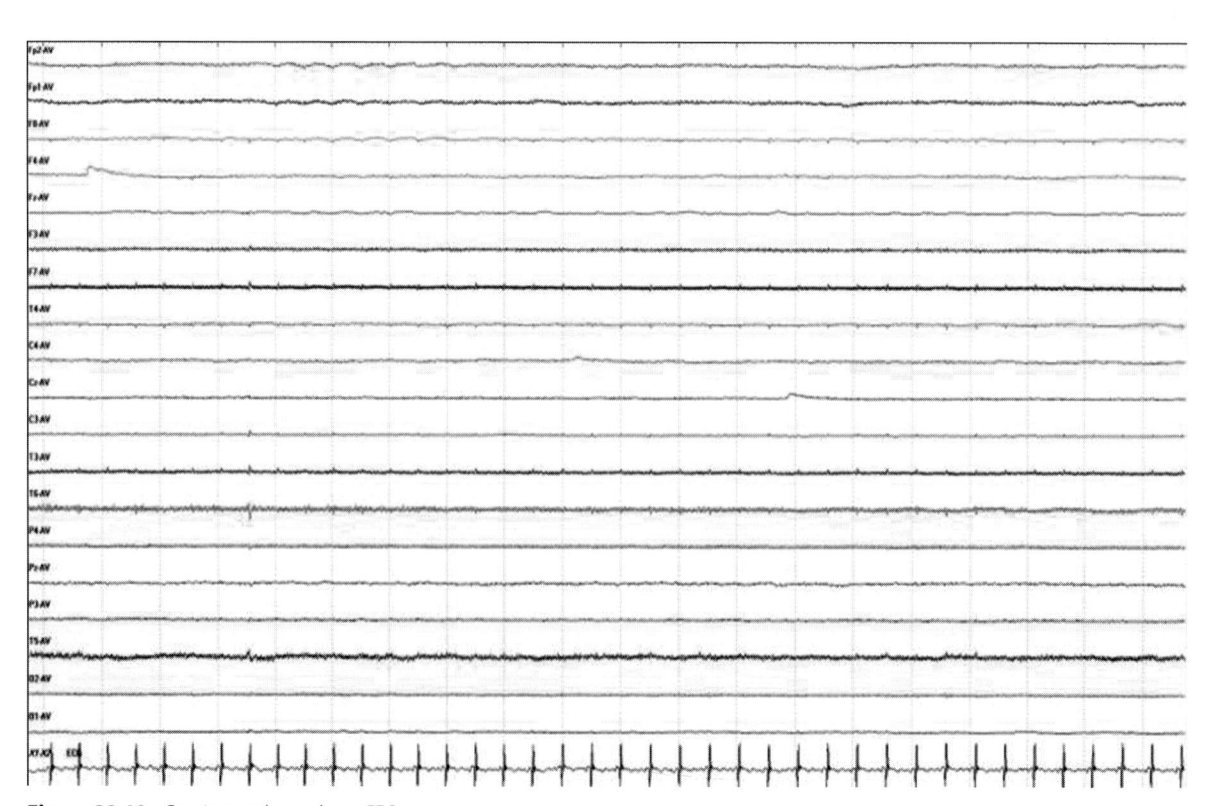

Figure 32.10. Continuous low-voltage EEG.

Burst-suppression pattern – stable or invariant for 2 weeks

Early infantile epileptic encephalopathy (EIEE or Ohtahara's syndrome)

- Early-onset tonic spasms and partial seizures; rarely massive myoclonia.
- Mostly associated with structural brain damage, especially brain malformations.
- EEG shows burst-suppression during both awake and asleep. Bursts are longer with short periods of suppression (Figure 32.11).

Early (neonatal) myoclonic encephalopathy (EME)

- Very early-onset erratic myoclonus, massive myoclonus. Tonic spasms late.
- Likely aetiology is metabolic disorders, especially non-ketotic hypoglycinaemia.
- The EEG shows burst-suppression patterns which are enhanced in sleep; shorter bursts with longer periods of suppression (Figure 32.12).

Neonatal seizures

The incidence of seizures in the neonatal period is considerably higher than at any other time (see Table 32.1). The risk of seizure recurrence in later life is 8–20%. There is also evidence from animal studies to suggest that recurrent neonatal seizures can lead to long-term morphological and behavioural changes.

Electrographic seizures are paroxysmal rhythmic activity of at least 10 s duration, not associated with clinical manifestations.

Table 32.1. Classification of neonatal seizures based on electro-clinical findings

EEG change present	No EEG change present	EEG change only
Focal clonic	Myoclonic	Sub-clinical/electrographic
Focal tonic	Generalized tonic	
Myoclonic	Motor automatisms	
Subtle		

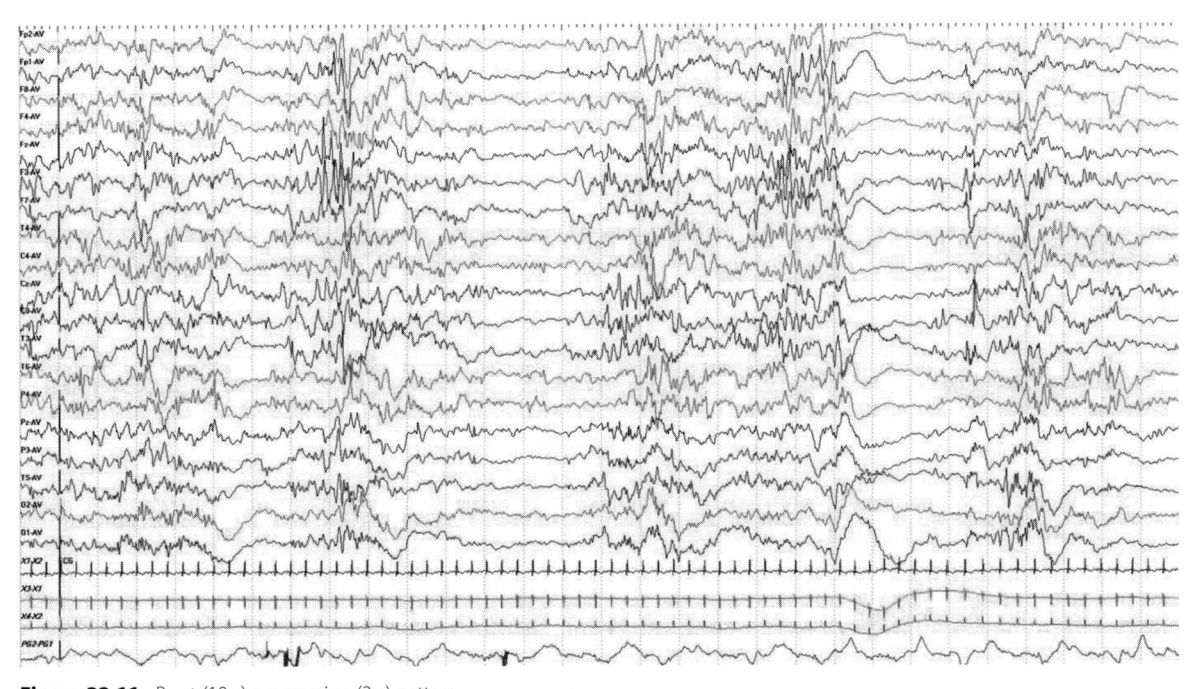

Figure 32.11. Burst (10 s)-suppression (3 s) pattern.

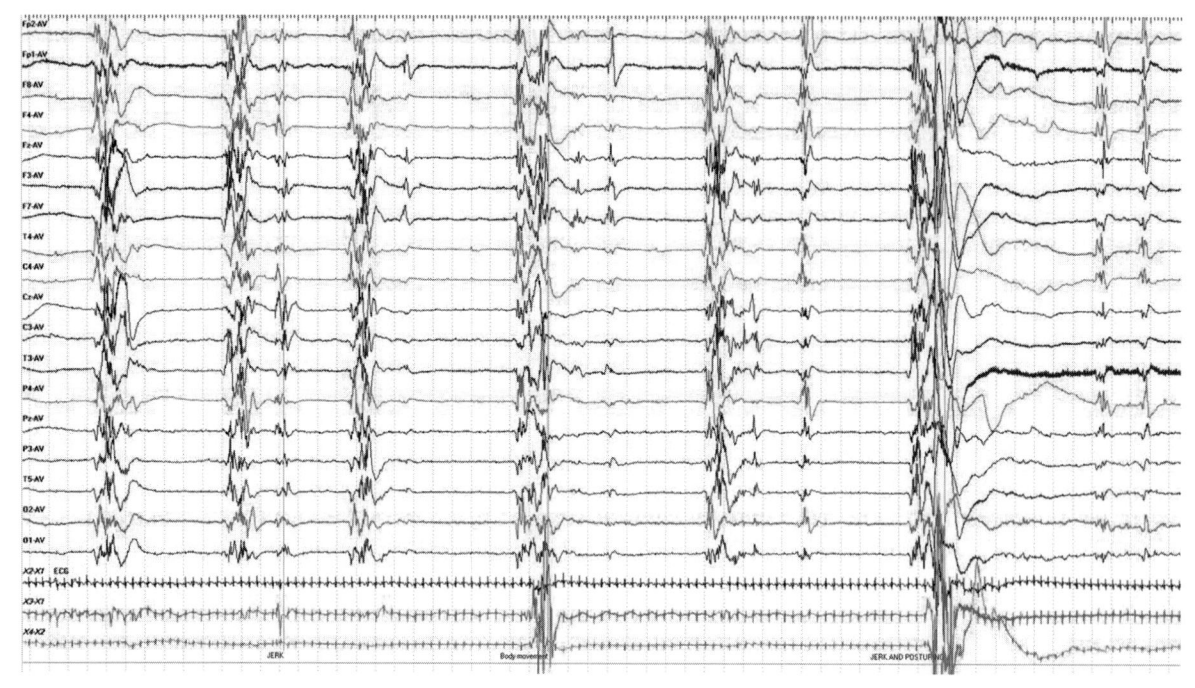

Section 2: Classification and diagnosis of epilepsy

Figure 32.12. Burst (1–2 s)-suppression (10 s) pattern. Myoclonus seen in association with the bursts.

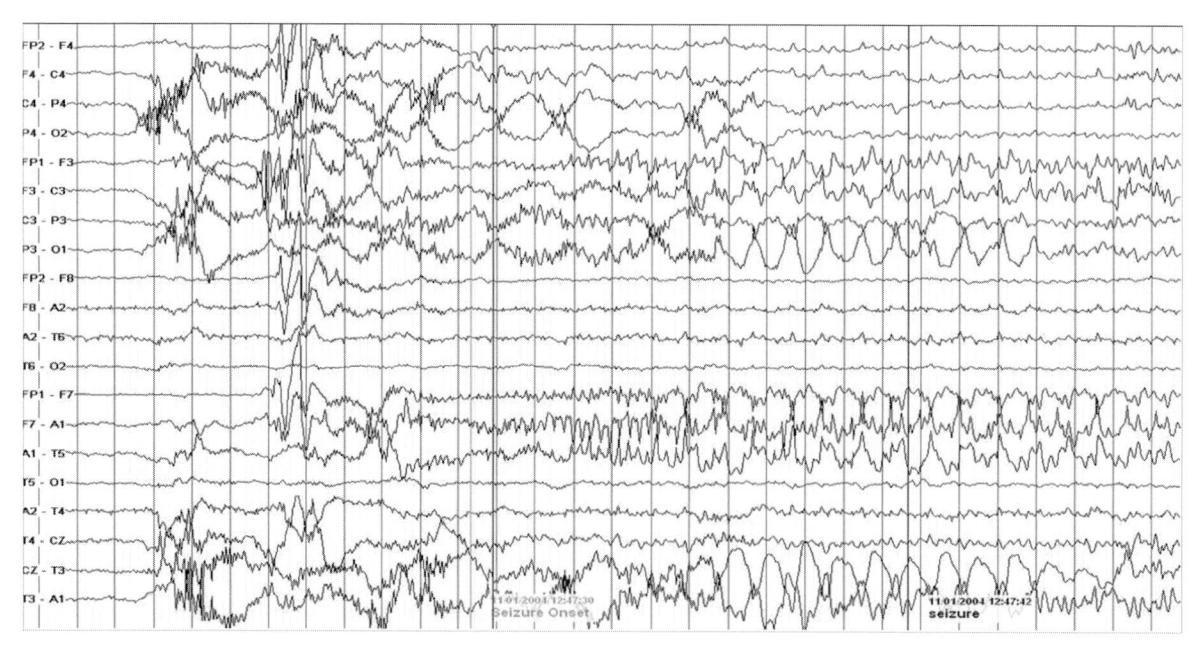

Figure 32.13. Focal electrographic seizure pattern.

The EEG in childhood

The normal EEG in childhood

Background activity: appearance of posterior dominant delta activity (50–100 μV) at around 2 months. This increases to about 7 Hz by the age of 1 year and is responsive to eye-opening. The age at which alpha appears as the dominant rhythm varies from 2 to 7 years, although 4 years is considered characteristic. Features of an adult EEG start appearing by the age of 8. Of note is

Chapter 32: EEG in neonates and children

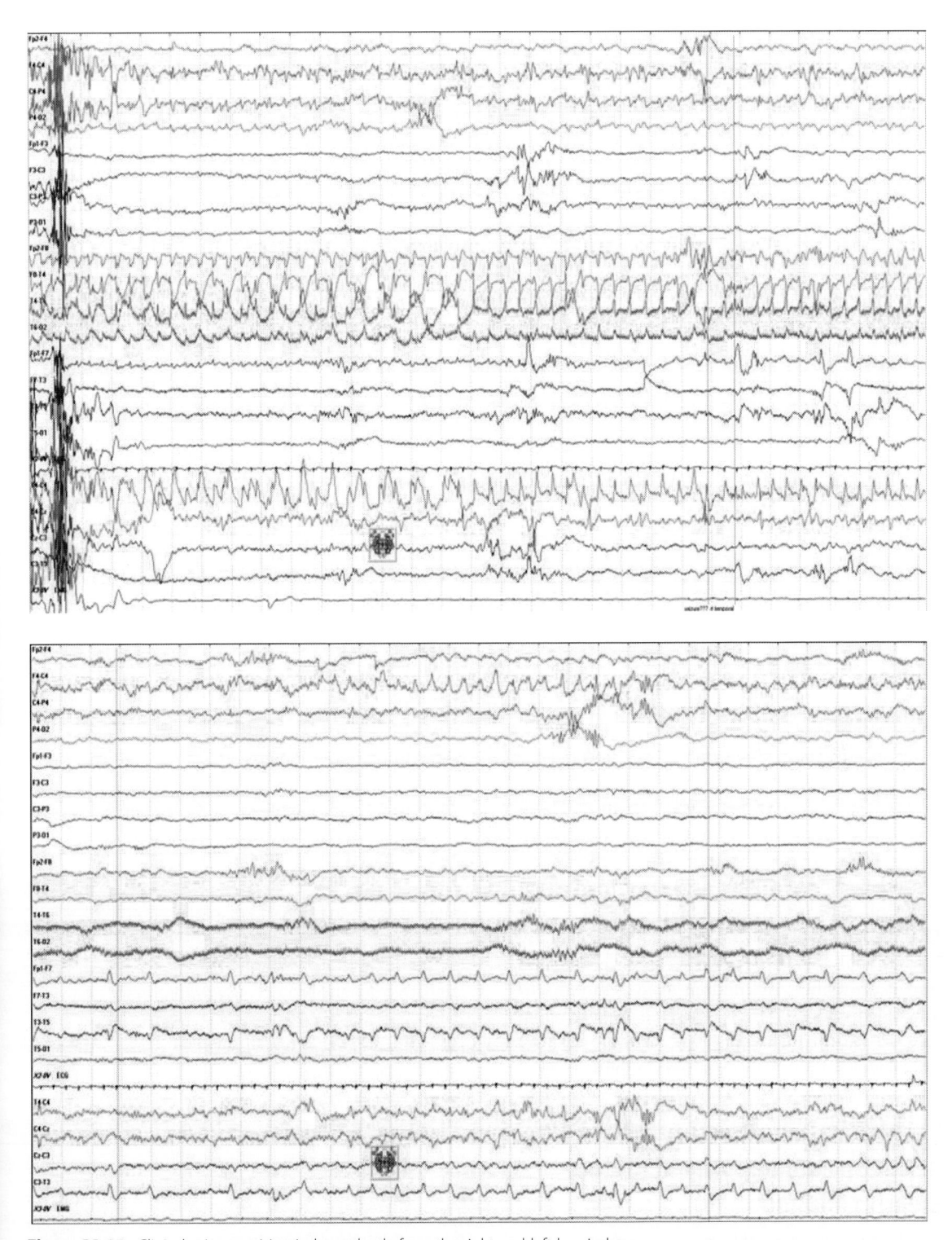

Figure 32.14. Clinical seizures arising independently from the right and left hemispheres.

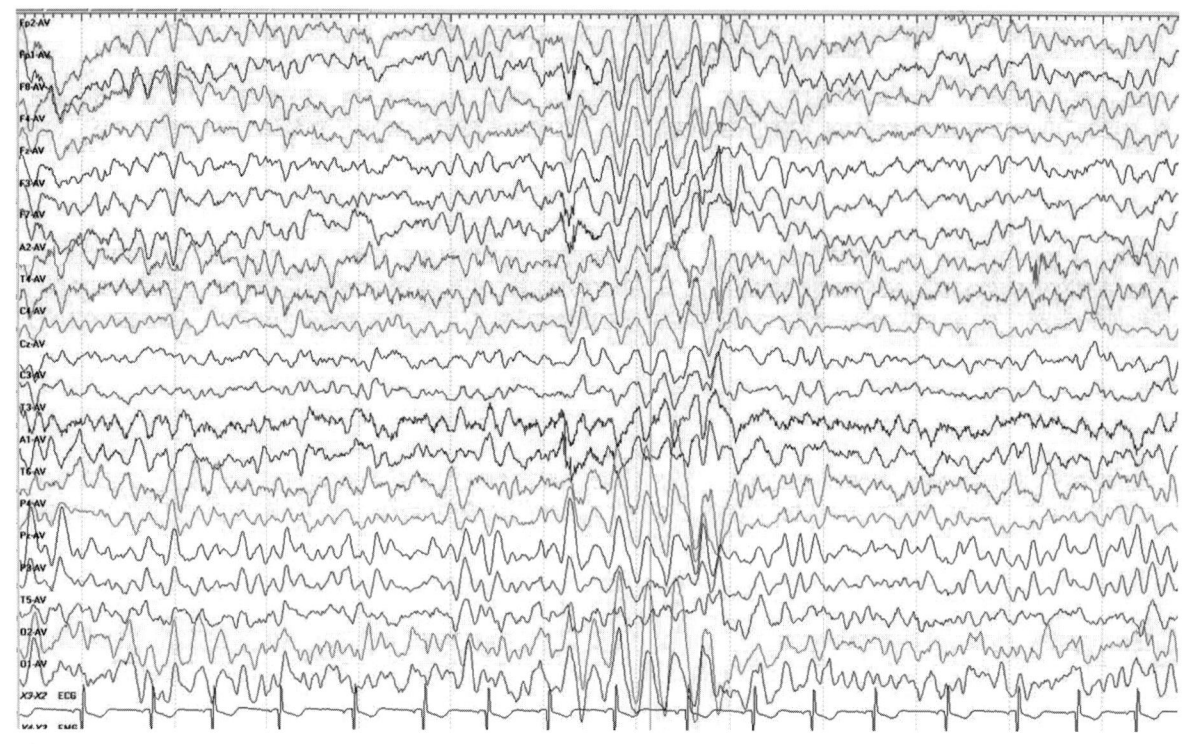

Figure 32.15. Four-year-old sleep EEG shows a burst of hypnogogic hypersynchrony during drowsiness.

the appearance of posterior slow waves of youth and slow alpha variants seen typically at around 12 years of age.

Sleep: characteristic sleep spindles are seen by 6 weeks. Spindles may have a frequency up to 14 Hz in the first year of life and occur in long trains. Vertex sharp transients and K-complexes appear by 3–5 months of age. Maturation of slow-wave sleep (non-REM sleep) into the four stages occurs by 8 months.

Hypnogogic hypersynchrony (first described by Gibbs and Gibbs, 1950) is a well-recognized normal variant of drowsiness in children aged 3 months to 13 years (Figure 32.15). This is described as paroxysmal bursts (3–5 Hz) of high-voltage (as high as 350 µV) sinusoidal waves, maximally expressed in the prefrontal to central areas, that occur as the background activity drops during drowsiness.

Epileptic encephalopathy in infancy and early childhood
Infantile spasms and West syndrome
Interictal EEG features: hypsarrhythmia is characterized by disorganized and chaotic high-voltage

---

Box 32.2. Childhood epilepsy syndromes with characteristic EEG findings

Epilepsy syndromes presenting as epileptic encephalopathy in infancy and early childhood
(1) Infantile spasms and West syndrome
(2) Severe myoclonic epilepsy in infancy (Dravet syndrome)
(3) Malignant migrating partial seizures in infancy
(4) Lennox-Gastaut syndrome

Idiopathic generalized epilepsy syndromes
(1) Benign myoclonic epilepsy in infancy
(2) Childhood absence epilepsy
(3) Juvenile myoclonic epilepsy
(4) Myoclonic-astatic epilepsy
(5) Juvenile absence epilepsy

Idiopathic focal epilepsy syndromes
(1) Benign childhood epilepsy with centrotemporal spikes
(2) Panayiotopoulos syndrome
(3) Idiopathic childhood occipital epilepsy of Gastaut

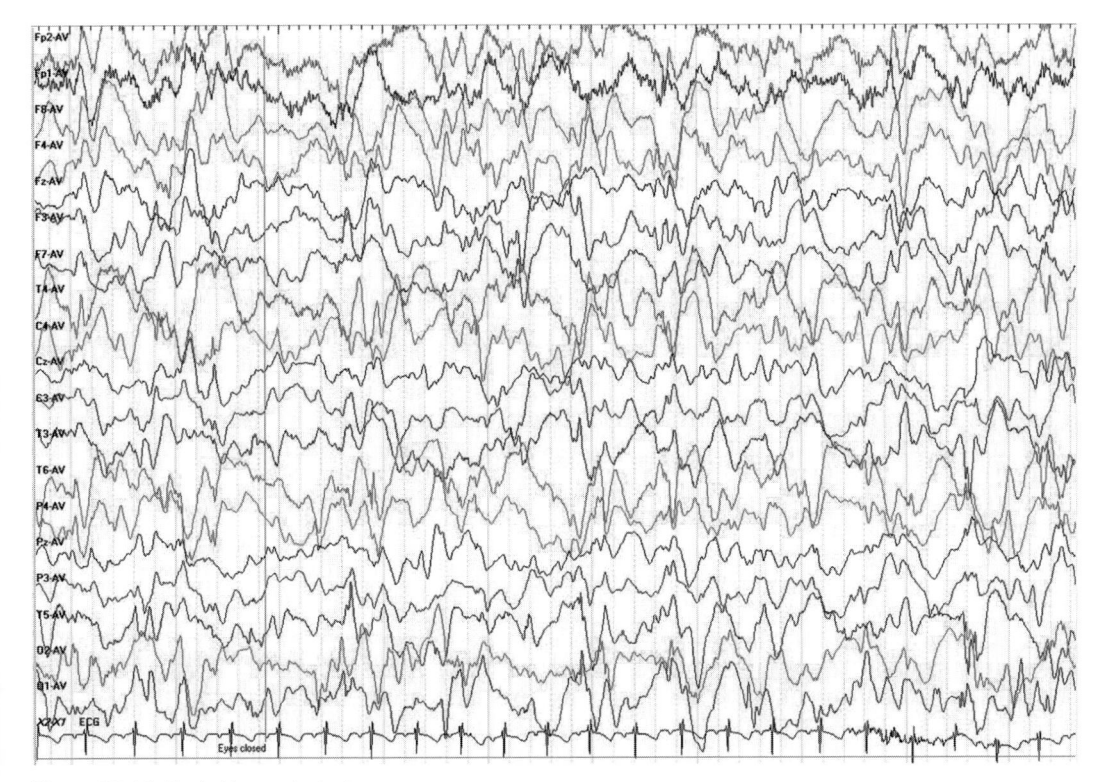

Figure 32.16. Typical hypsarrhythmia.

(>300 μV) random irregular slow waves interspersed with multiregional spikes and sharp waves over both hemispheres (Figures 32.16–32.19). During sleep, there is an increase in spikes and polyspikes, with discharges appearing more synchronous. Atypical hypsarrhythmia occurs when the discharges are more synchronous. Unilateral or asymmetric hypsarrhythmia are seen in symptomatic cases such as hemimegancephaly. About 33% of patients with infantile spasms do not have hypsarrhythmia (Jeavons and Bower, 1974).

EEG during spasms: spasms are brief axial contractions of the head, trunk and limbs lasting 0.2–2 s. They can be flexor, extensor or mixed. Subtle spasms with eye deviation are seen occasionally. Spasms usually occur in clusters with spasm occurring 5–30 s apart. They are precipitated by awakening, drowsiness, handling and feeding. The electrophysiological correlate is an electrodecrement, consisting of generalized attenuation of the EEG amplitude with superimposed low-amplitude fast activity, or a high-amplitude slow-wave burst followed by attenuation.

Severe myoclonic epilepsy of infancy (Dravet syndrome)

The EEG at presentation can be normal or display unilateral or diffuse slowing of the background in post-ictal EEGs (Figures 32.20 and 32.21). Photosensitivity has been noted in some patients at an early onset. Rhythmic centro-parietal theta can be seen. As myoclonus occurs, generalized spike/polyspike discharges are seen in association with focal discharges. Atypical absences are accompanied by irregular slow-spike-and-wave discharges.

Malignant migrating partial seizures of infancy

At onset, the background is usually slowed. A fluctuating asymmetry develops with multifocal spikes. The sleep architecture is poorly defined. During seizures, EEG abnormalities affect various areas in consecutive seizures. In sequential seizures the area of ictal onset may shift from one region to another and from one hemisphere to another (Figure 32.22).

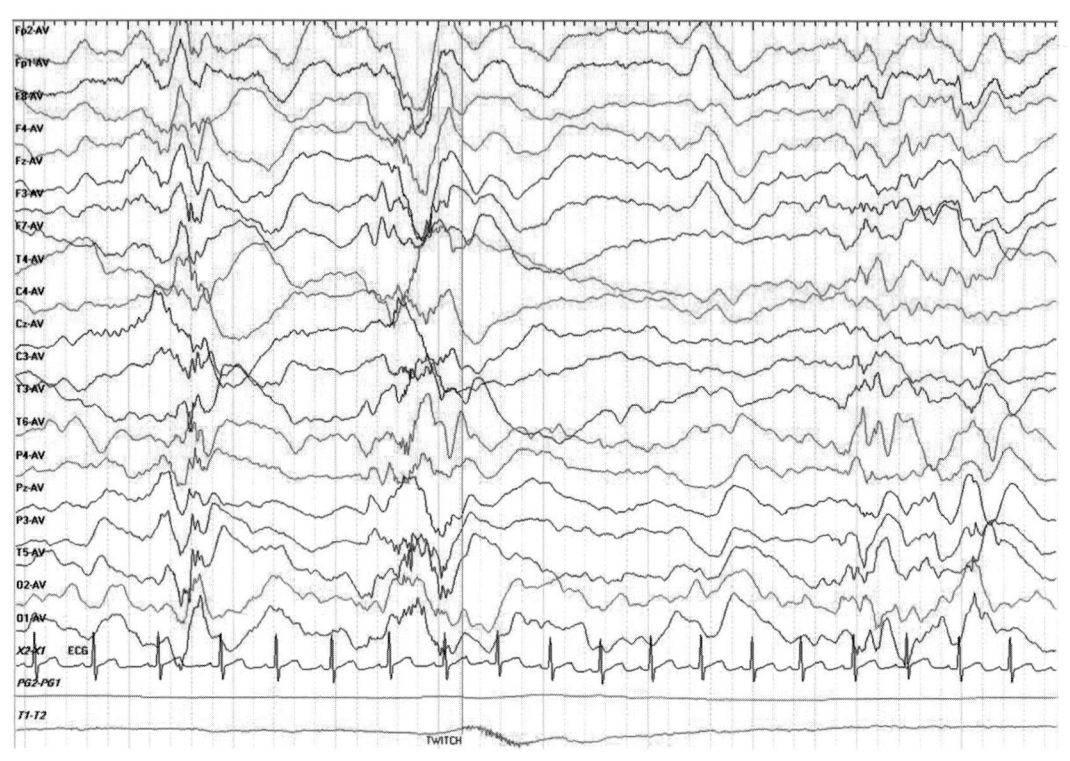

Section 2: Classification and diagnosis of epilepsy

Figure 32.17. EEG and EMG correlate of a spasm.

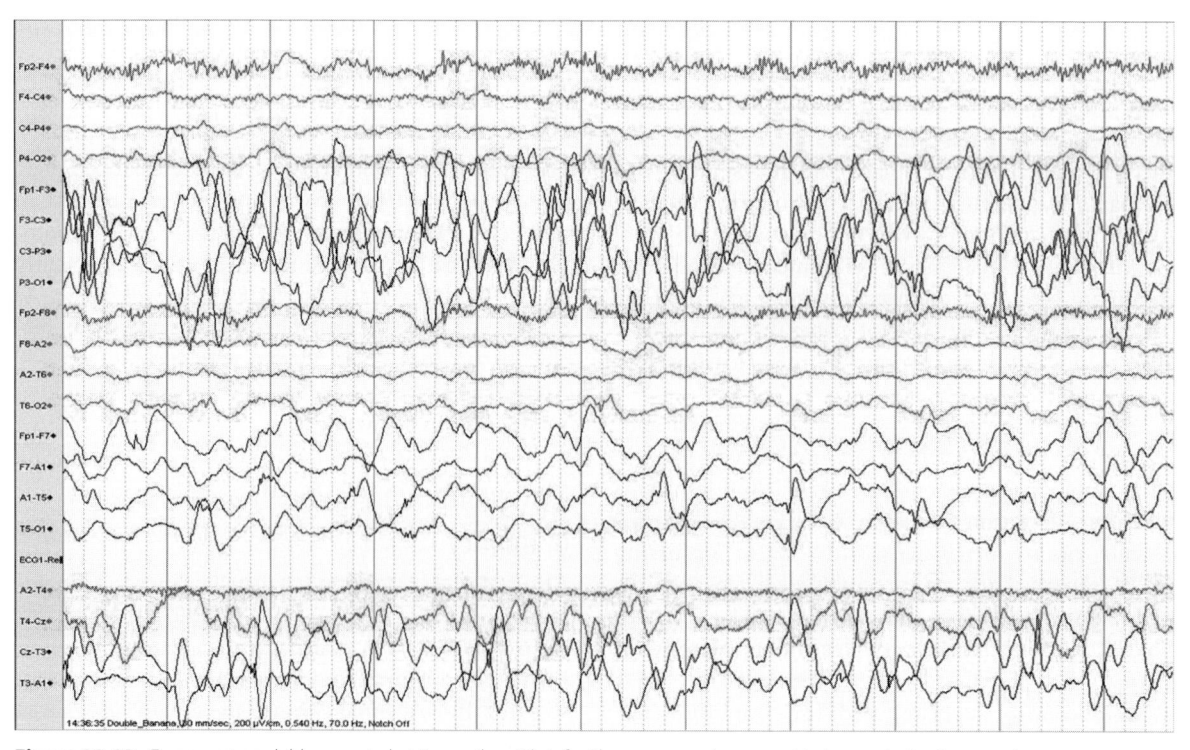

Figure 32.18. Ex-premature child presented at 3 months with infantile spasms and asymmetric hypsarrhythmia secondary to a porencephalic cyst.

Chapter 32: EEG in neonates and children

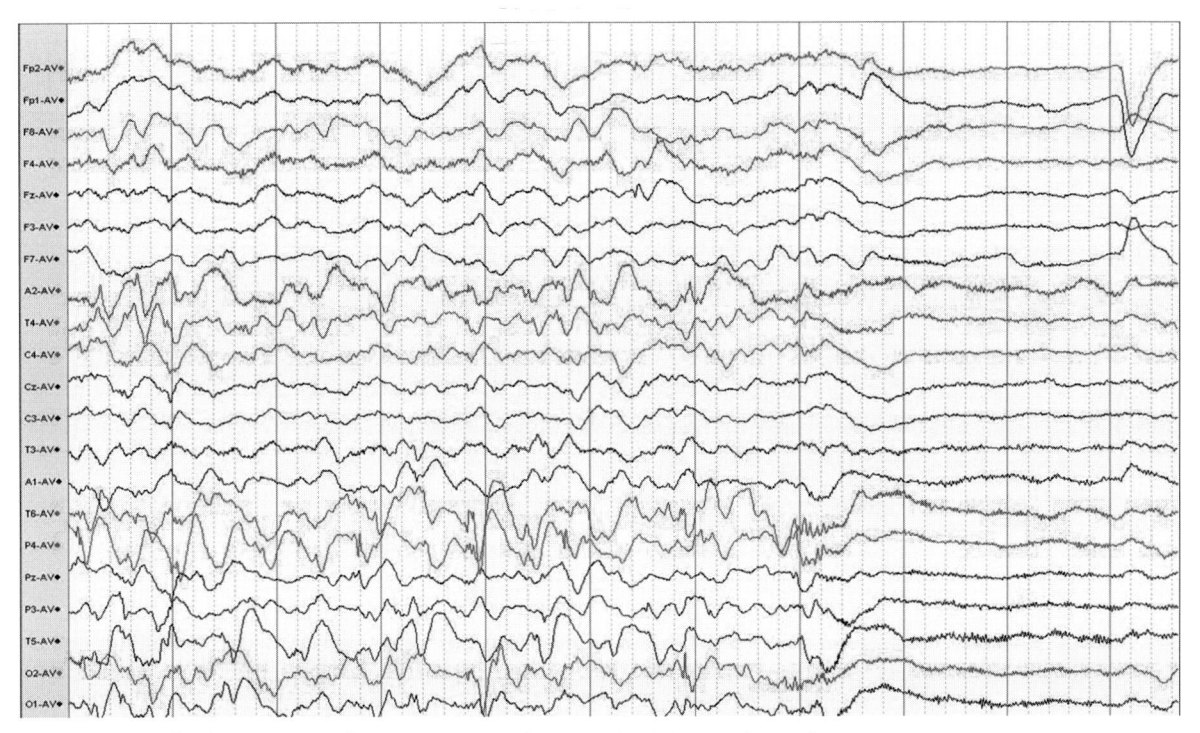

Figure 32.19. Infantile spasms secondary to symptomatic focus over the right posterior quadrant.

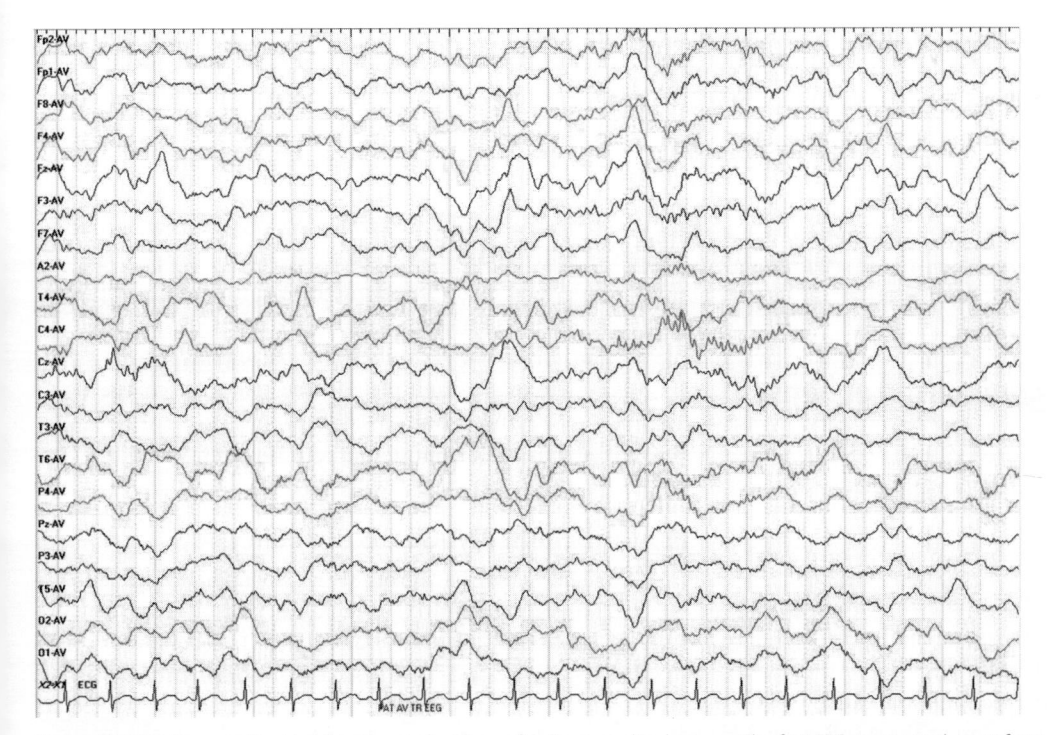

Figure 32.20. Five-month-old child presented with an afebrile generalized seizure. The first EEG was normal, apart from mild right temporal slowing.

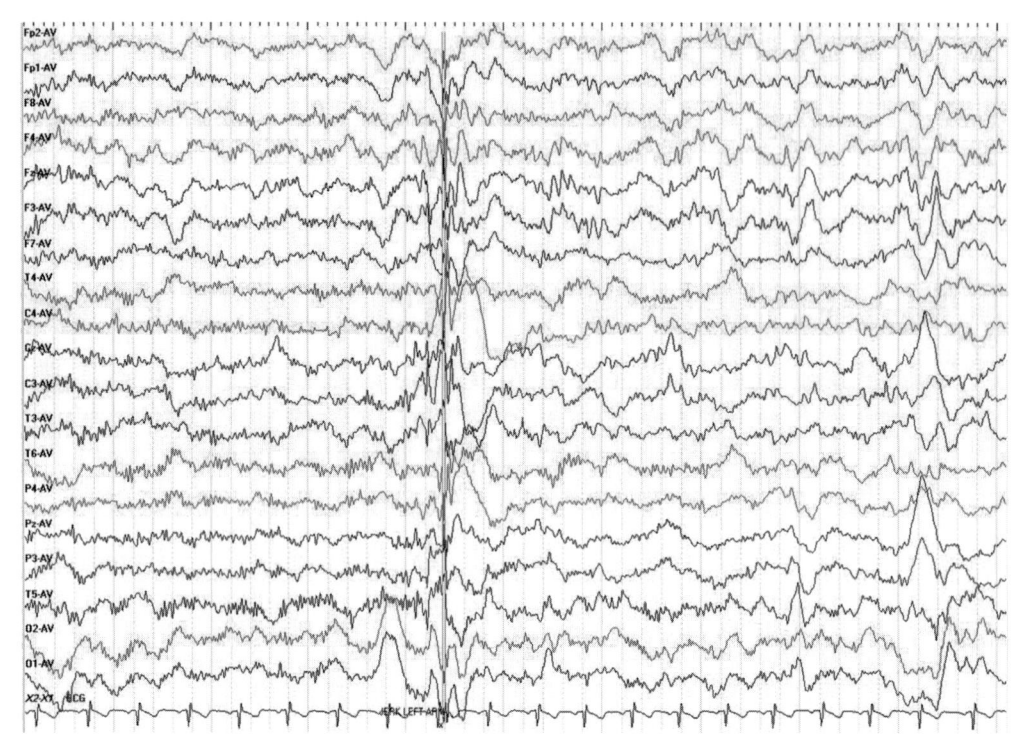

Figure 32.21. Intractable generalized tonic-clonic seizures at 11 months. The patient also developed myoclonus and was positive to SCN1A gene mutation. Third EEG showing generalized spike-and-wave discharges accompanying myoclonus.

Lennox-Gastaut syndrome

EEG abnormalities consist of bursts of diffuse slow-spike-wave discharges during wakefulness. There is activation of discharges in sleep with loss of sleep architecture. During sleep, there are characteristic polyspike-and-wave discharges with generalized low-voltage fast rhythms at 10 Hz (Figure 32.23). Epileptic seizures manifest as tonic, atonic seizures and atypical absences (Figure 32.24).

Idiopathic generalized epilepsy syndromes

Childhood absence epilepsy

Inclusion criteria (Panayiotopoulos, 2007):
- age at onset 4–10 years and peak at 5–7;
- normal neurological state and development;
- seizures are frequent and brief (4–20 s, exceptionally longer);
- EEG: generalized high-amplitude spike-wave discharges (maximum three spikes) at 3 Hz with a gradual slowdown (Figure 32.25).

Exclusion criteria
- other than typical absences such as generalized tonic-clonic seizures or myoclonic jerks prior to or during the active stage;
- eyelid myoclonia, peri-oral myoclonia, rhythmic massive limb jerking and single arrhythmic myoclonic jerks of the head/trunk or limbs;
- mild or no impairment of consciousness during the discharges;
- brief 3–4 Hz spike-wave paroxysms shorter than 4 s, multiple > three spikes; discharge fragmentation, fixed lead;
- visual- or photic-induced seizures.

Benign myoclonus of infancy

The EEG background is normal. Interictal discharges are rare. Myoclonic jerks if recorded are associated with a burst of fast generalized spike/polyspike-and-wave discharges with a frequency higher than 3 Hz lasting for 1–3 s (Figure 32.26). Myoclonus is enhanced during drowsiness and reduced in slow-wave sleep.

Chapter 32: EEG in neonates and children

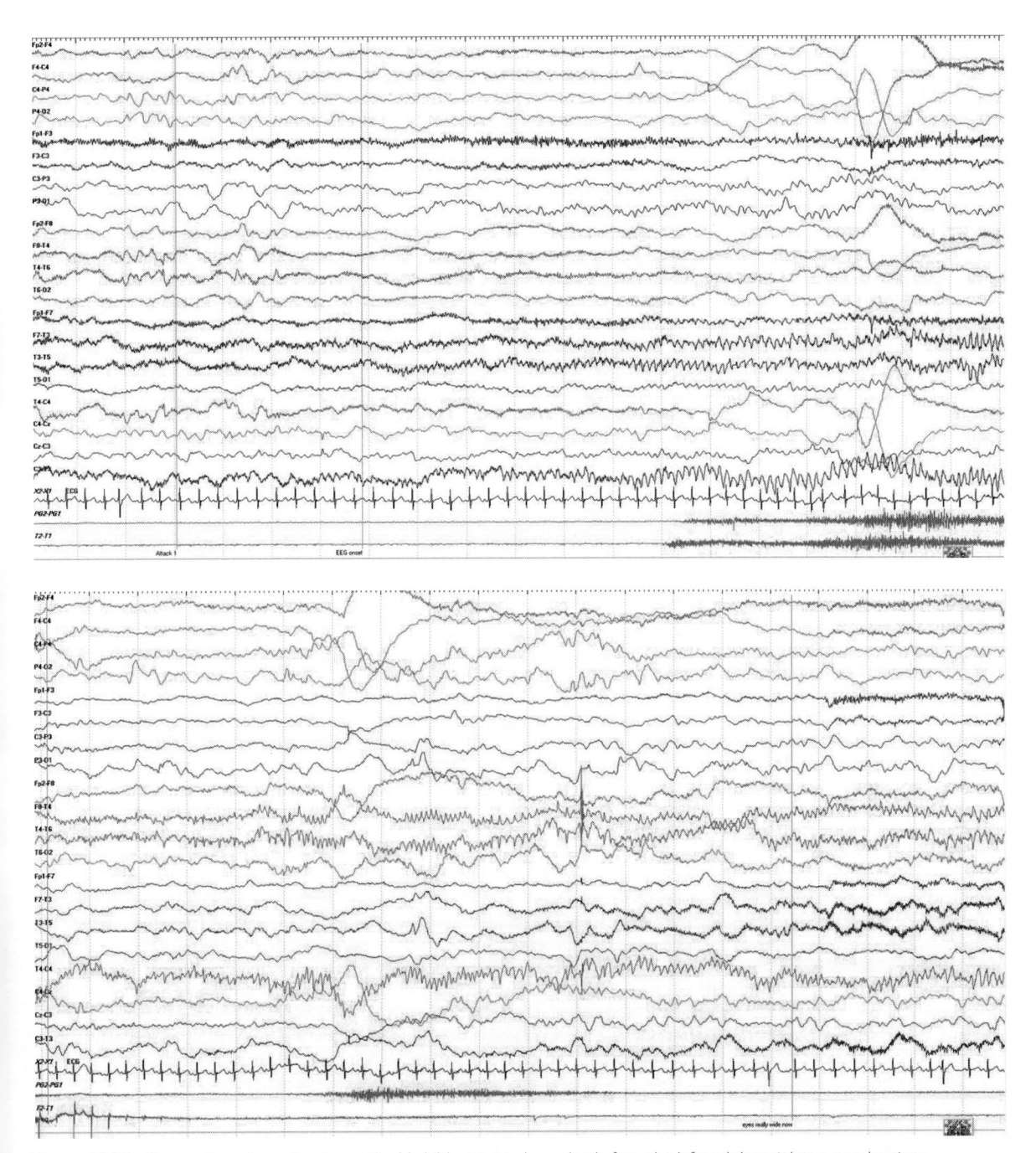

Figure 32.22. Consecutive seizures in a 3-month-old child arising independently from the left and then right temporal regions.

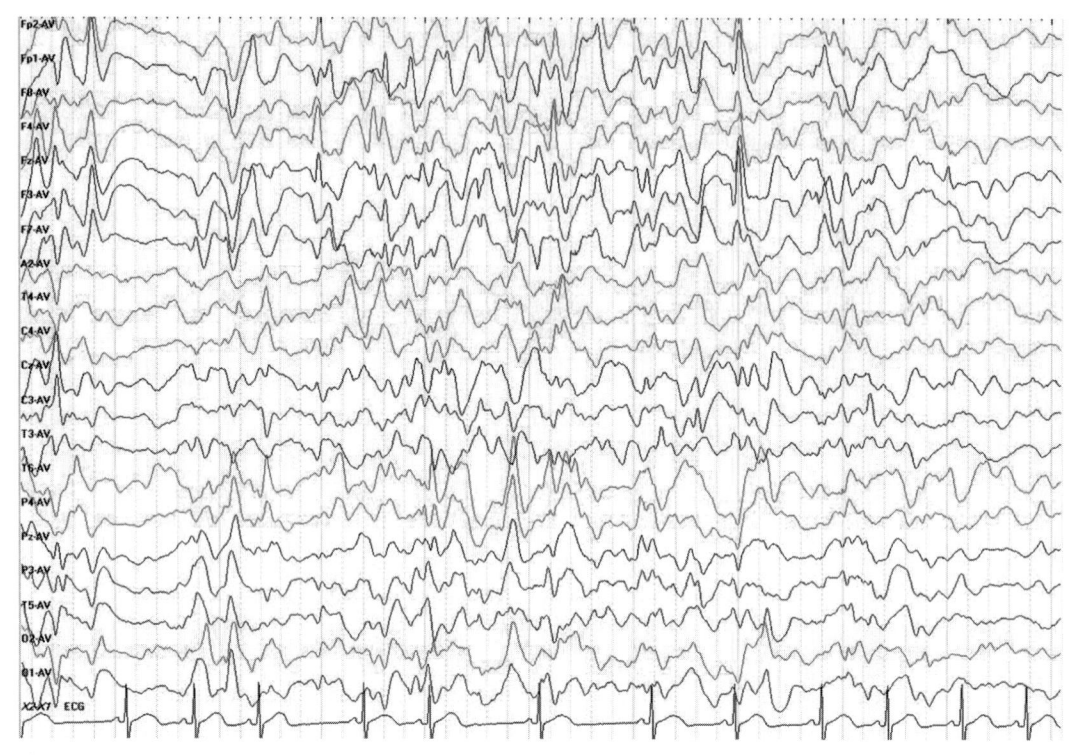

Section 2: Classification and diagnosis of epilepsy

Figure 32.23. Characteristic background abnormality with slow-spike-wave discharges.

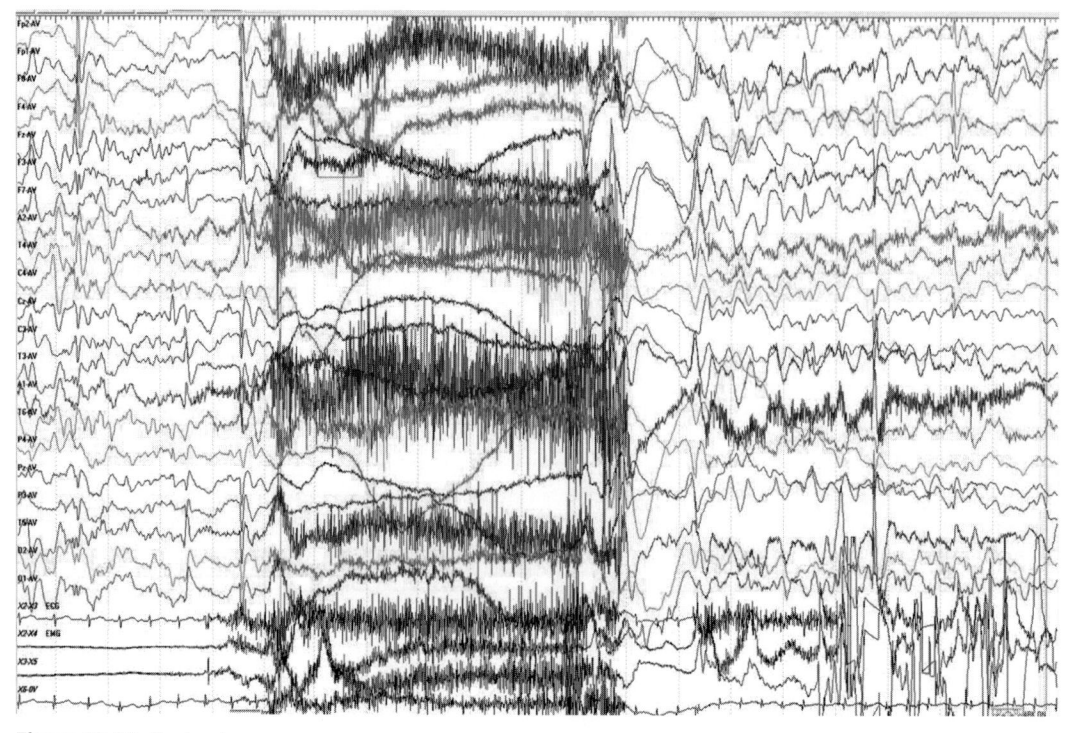

Figure 32.24. Tonic seizure.

Chapter 32: EEG in neonates and children

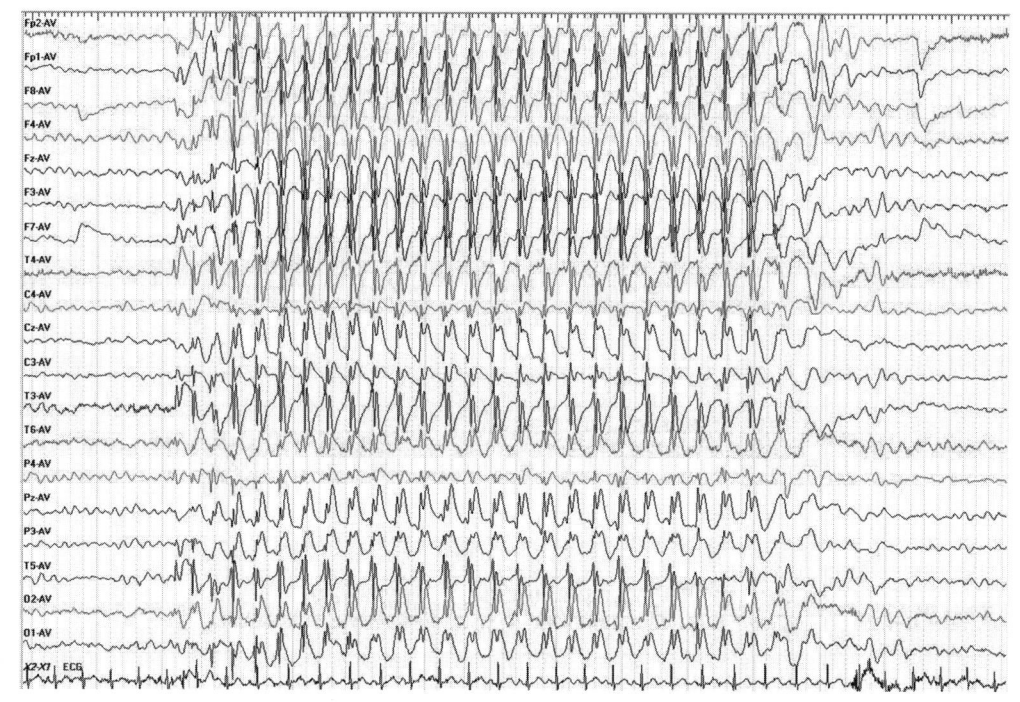

Figure 32.25. Three hertz generalized spike-wave discharges accompanying a clinical absence seizure.

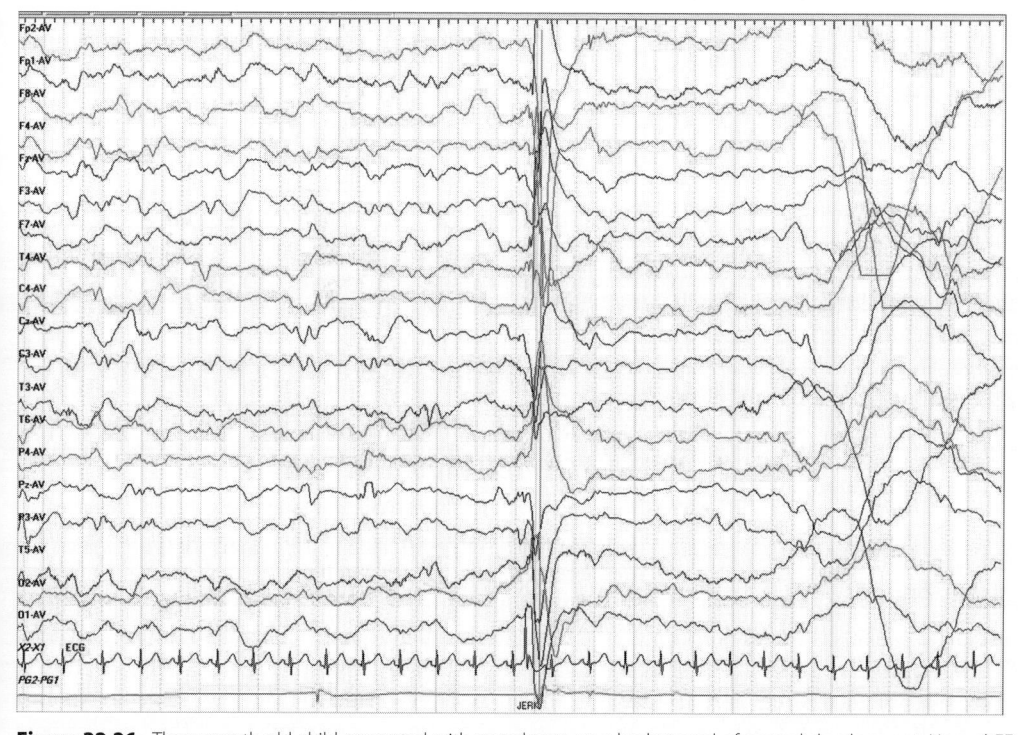

Figure 32.26. Three-month-old child presented with myoclonus on a background of normal development. Normal EEG background with generalized spike-wave discharges accompanying myoclonus.

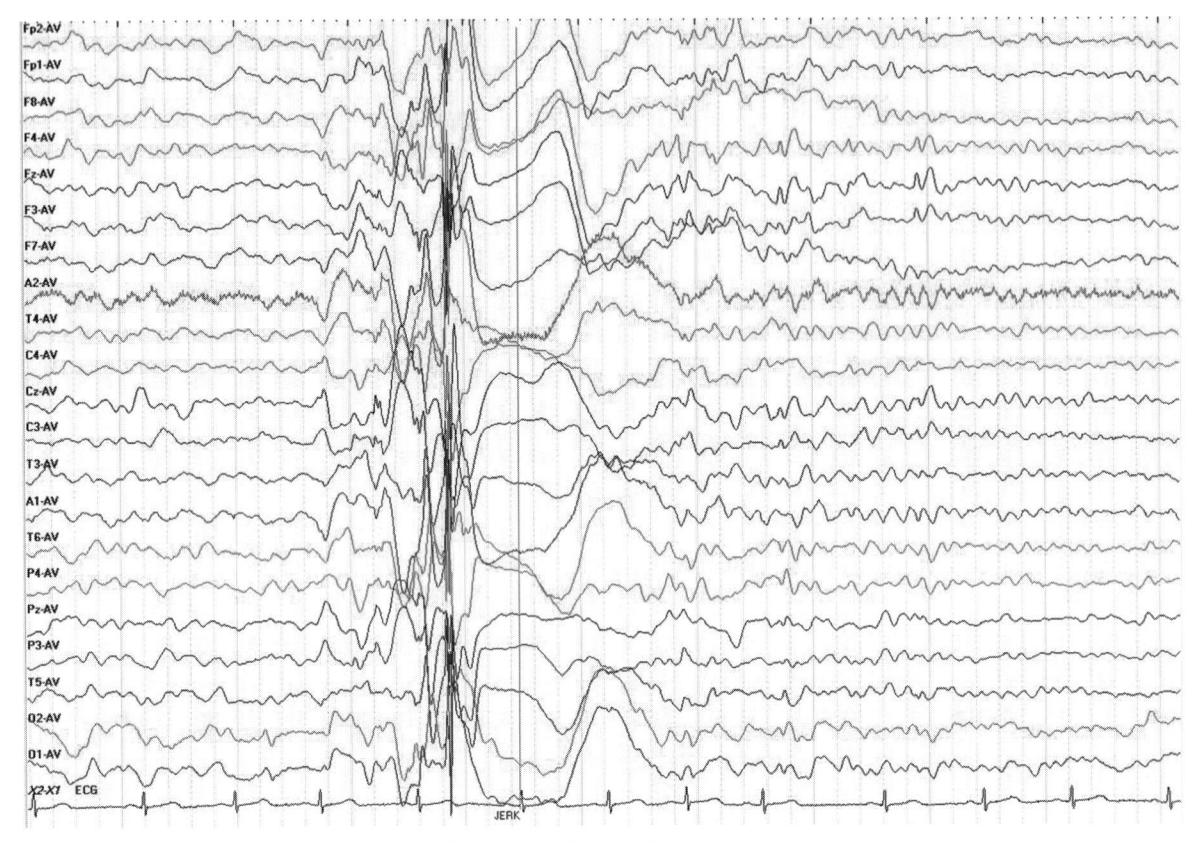

Section 2: Classification and diagnosis of epilepsy

Figure 32.27. Myoclonic jerk followed by atonic drop. Note background theta.

Myoclonic-astatic epilepsy

EEG background may be normal at onset of seizures. A characteristic 4–7 Hz monomorphic diffuse theta is described, with centro-parietal emphasis. Interictal 2–3 Hz bursts of generalized spike/polyspike-and-wave discharges are seen which can be irregular/asymmetric. Activation of spike-and-wave discharges can occur in sleep. Myoclonus can be single or in a series of two to three jerks electrographically accompanied with isolated or bursts of spike-and-wave discharges lasting for up to 6 s. The EMG correlate of the myoclonus is a burst lasting up to 100 ms, followed by a longer silent period 200–500 ms (Figures 32.27 and 32.28).

Juvenile myoclonic epilepsy

The EEG of symptomatic patients is usually abnormal, with bursts of brief 3–6 Hz generalized spike/polyspike-and-wave discharges lasting for 1–4 s. A third of the patients are photosensitive. Focal discharges and abortive generalized discharges are also seen. Myoclonic jerks are bilateral, single or repetitive, arrhythmic, irregular jerks particularly involving the arms, accompanied with a generalized burst of polyspike-and-wave discharge lasting 0.5–2 s (Figures 32.29 and 32.30). Generalized tonic-clonic seizures are seen in 80–90% of patients and less frequent absences are seen in 10–38%.

Idiopathic focal epilepsy syndromes
Benign childhood epilepsy with centrotemporal spikes

There are high-voltage sharp/spike-and-slow wave complexes seen over the centrotemporal/sylvian region. Discharges can be unilateral, bilateral or independently arising from right and left hemisphere. Discharges usually occur in runs or clusters and activate in stages 1–4 of sleep (Figure 32.31). There is a tangential dipole with the negative pole maximum over the centrotemporal region and the positive pole maximum on the frontal region.

Chapter 32: EEG in neonates and children

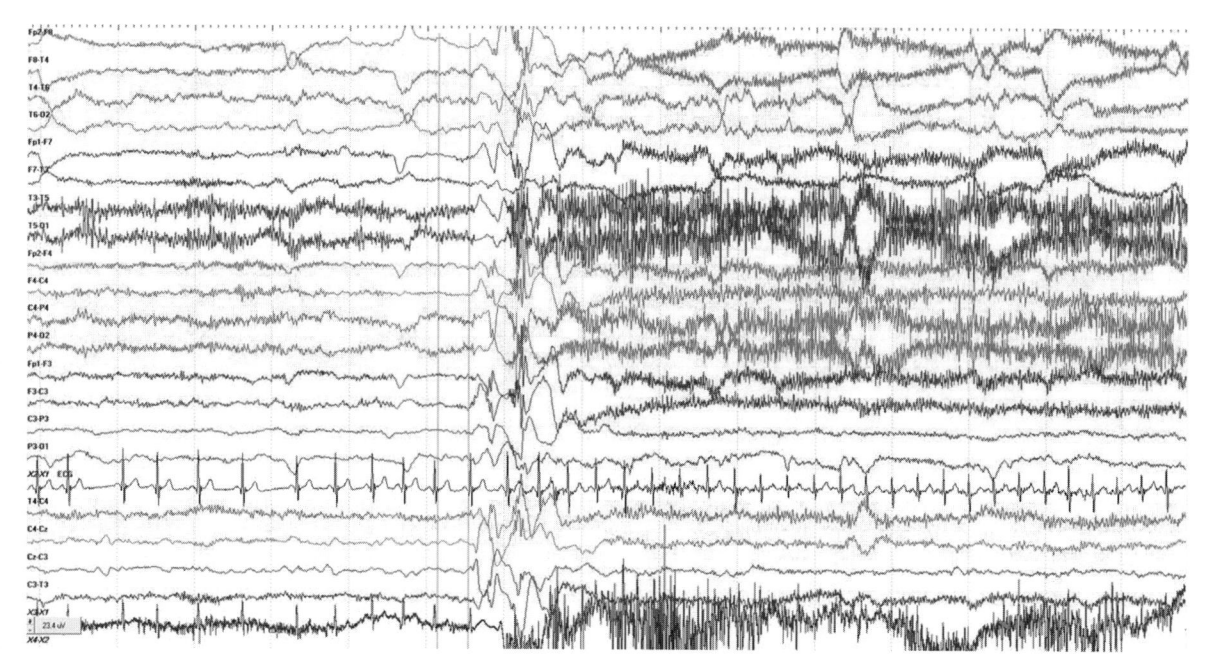

Figure 32.28. Sudden flexion of head and trunk with forward drop. Note silent period in EMG.

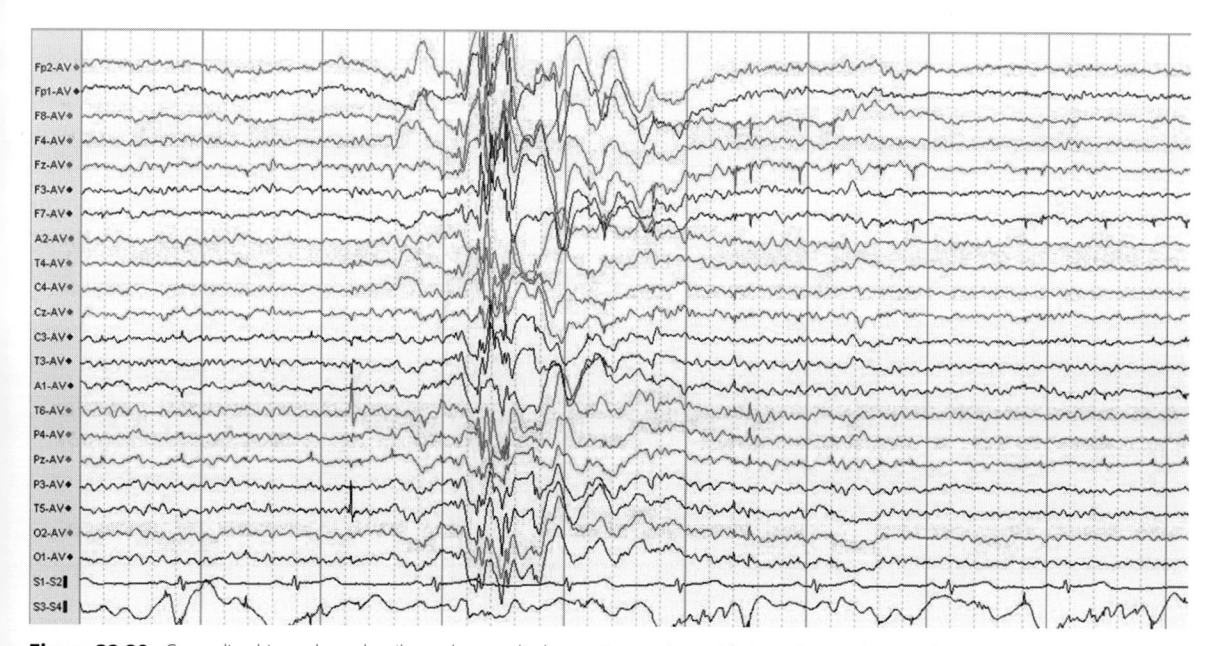

Figure 32.29. Generalized irregular polyspike-and-wave discharges in a patient with juvenile myoclonic epilepsy.

Panayiotopoulos syndrome

An electro-clinical diagnosis as the EEG shows a lot of variability. The background is normal with spikes/spike-and-wave discharges occurring in any location, often changing in foci in follow-up EEGs (Figures 32.32 and 32.33). The characteristic occipital paroxysms are not seen in a third of the patients. Occipital paroxysms show fixation-off sensitivity (activated with elimination of central vision and fixation). Discharges are activated in sleep.

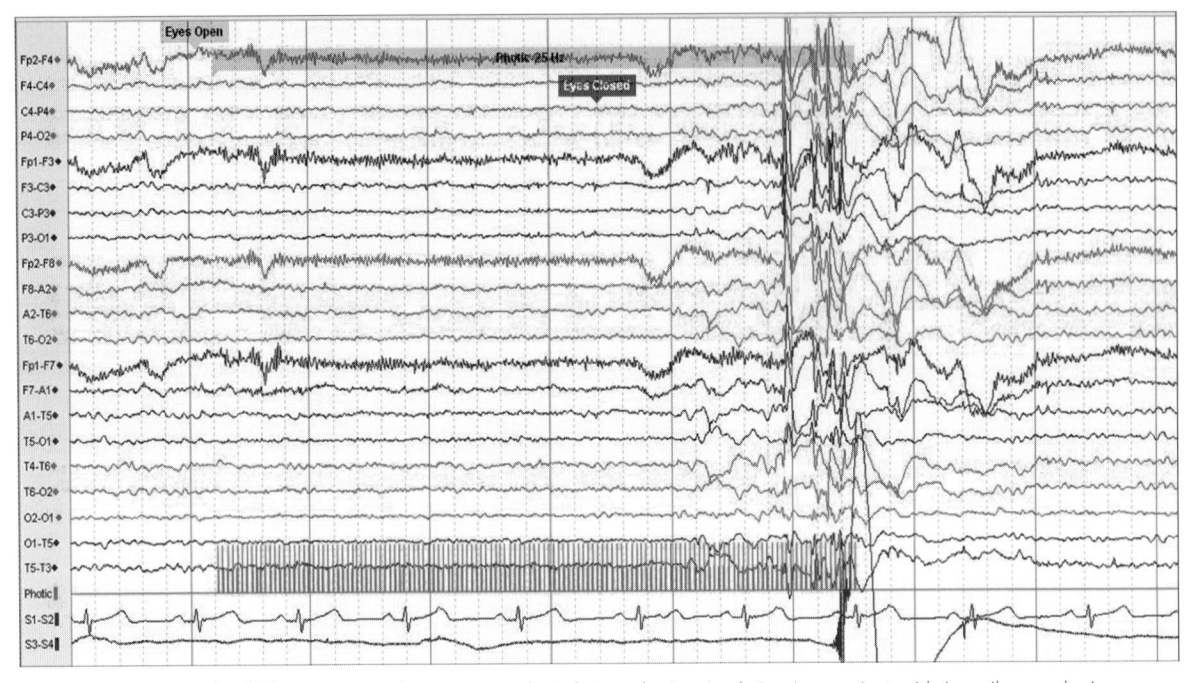

Section 2: Classification and diagnosis of epilepsy

Figure 32.30. Generalized photoparoxysmal response grade 4 during photic stimulation in a patient with juvenile myoclonic epilepsy.

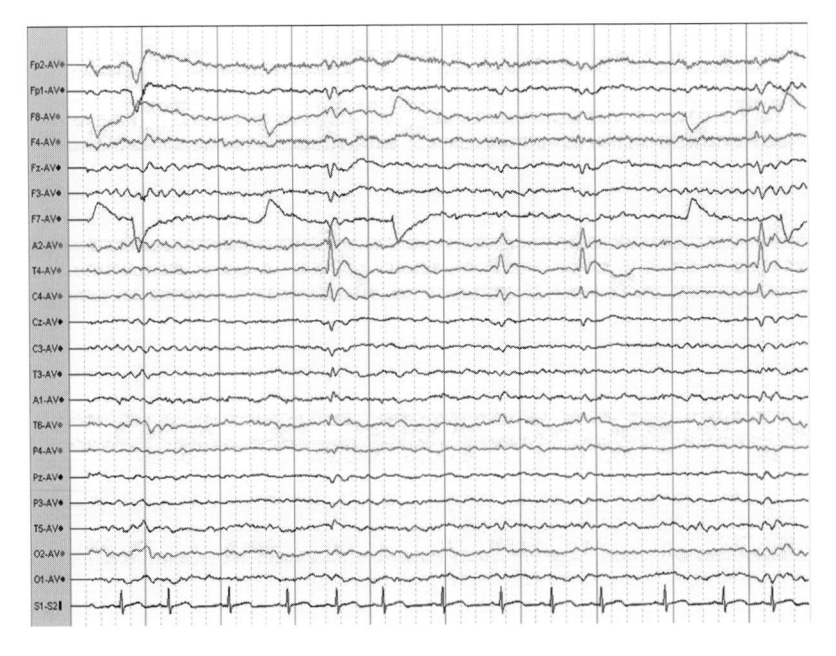

Figure 32.31. Right centro-sylvian spike-and-wave discharges occurring in runs in a patient with benign childhood epilepsy with centrotemporal spikes.

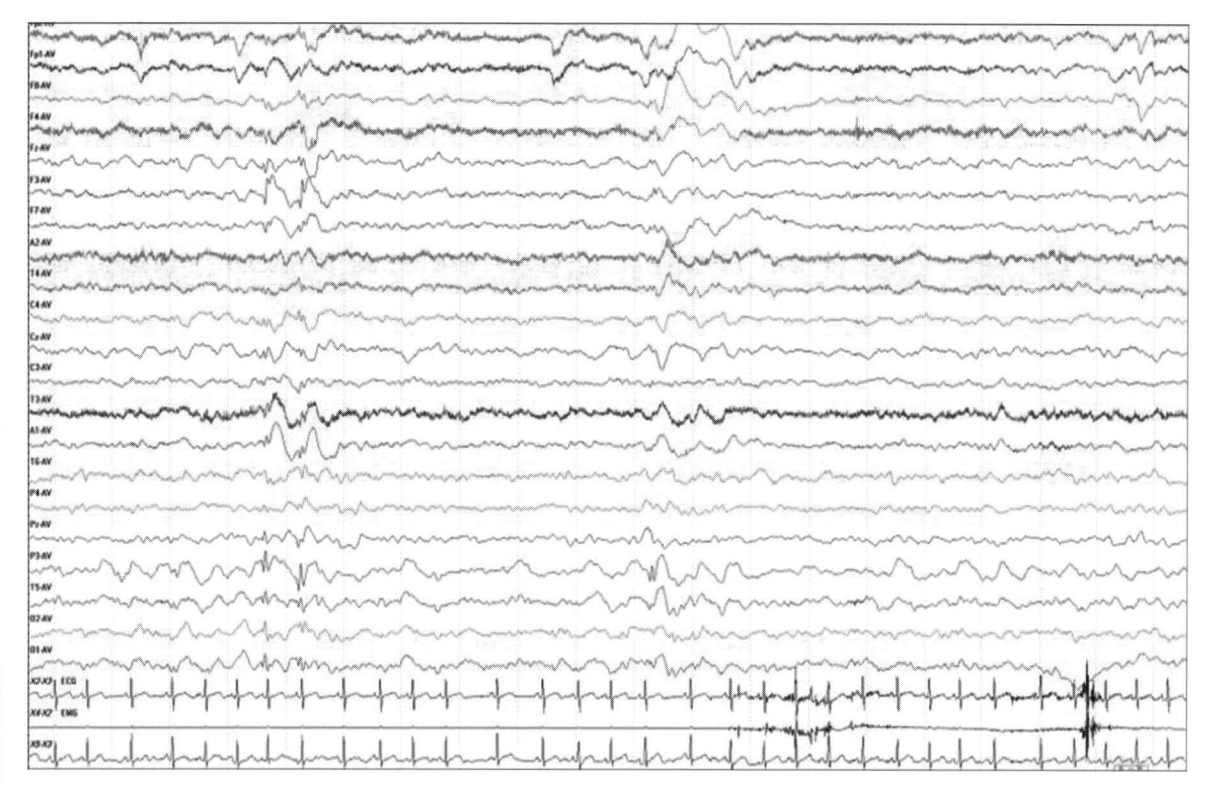

Figure 32.32. A 2.5–year-old girl with a history of two episodes of waking up just after falling asleep, vomiting and eye deviation to one side followed by hemiclonic jerking for 20 minutes. Post-ictal after episode and full recovery after 4–5 hours. The EEG shows left parieto-occipital discharges with anterior spread and activation in sleep.

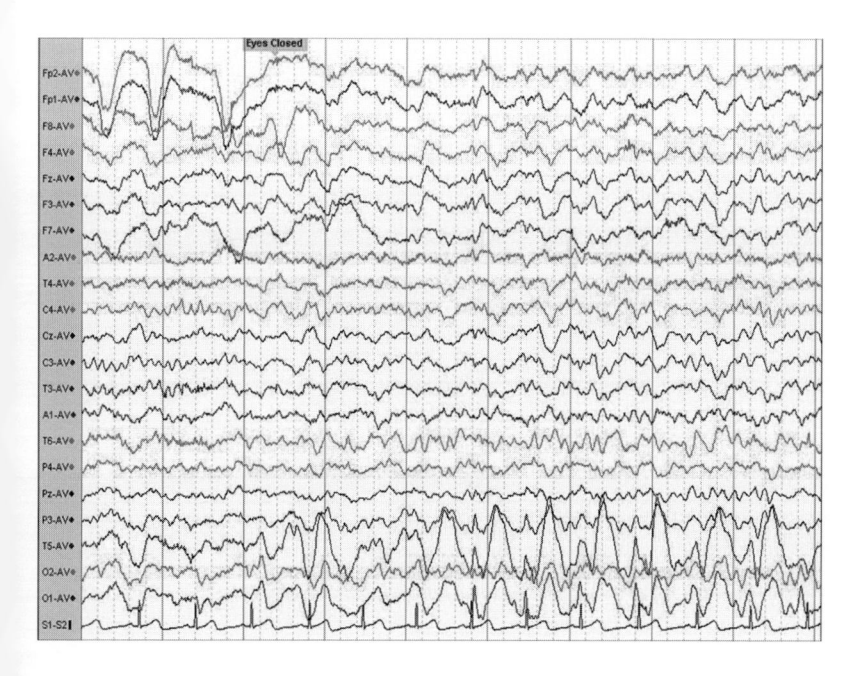

Figure 32.33. Occipital paroxysms.

References

Gibbs FA, Gibbs EL. *Atlas of Electroencephalography. Normal Controls.* Vol 1. Cambridge, MA: Addison-Wesley; 1950.

Jeavons PM, Bower BD. Infantile spasms. In: Vinken PJ, Bruyn GW (eds), *Handbook of Clinical Neurology.* Vol. 15, *The Epilepsies.* pp. 219–34. Amsterdam: North Holland; 1974.

Lamblin MD. EEG in premature and full-term infants: Developmental features and glossary. *Clin Neurophysiol* 1999;**29**:123–224.

Menache CC. Prognostic value of neonatal discontinuous EEG. *Pediatr Neurol*, 2002;**27**:93–101.

Panayiotopoulos C. *A Clinical Guide to Epileptic Syndromes and Their Treatment.* 2nd edn. London: Springer; 2007.

Pressler RM. Early serial EEG in hypoxic ischaemic encephalopathy. *Clin Neurophysiol* 2001;**112**:31–7.

Roger J, Bureau M, Dravet C, *et al. Epileptic Syndromes in Infancy, Childhood and Adolescence.* 3rd edn. London: John Libbey; 2002.

Learning objectives

(1) Understand what constitutes a normal neonatal EEG.
(2) Understand the usefulness of EEG in the diagnosis of
   - neonatal HIE
   - neonatal seizures.
(3) Understand the usefulness of the EEG in the diagnosis of
   - epilepsy syndromes in infancy and early childhood
   - epilepsy syndromes of childhood and adolescence.

Section 2 Classification and diagnosis of epilepsy

Chapter 33
Applications of EEG other than epilepsy

Bidi Evans

Brain disease

The EEG was one of the earliest investigations of the central nervous system and was initially used for many neurological conditions. Most of this early work is now obsolete but there remain some areas, outside epilepsy, where the test is useful and sometimes essential. Some of these conditions resemble epilepsy, or show EEG waveforms resembling those seen in epilepsy, or both. We summarize below the EEG abnormalities seen in conditions other than epilepsy. These conditions are considered in five groups.

Dementia

Dementia is often associated with EEG abnormalities, most commonly a loss of normal background activity and an increase in slower frequencies. This is particularly the case in Alzheimer's disease, where the normal alpha rhythm (8–13 Hz) is replaced with slower activity in the theta and delta range, down to 1 Hz. Vasculo-degenerative dementia also produces EEG slow waves but these are often localized to one or more areas with normal activity between. The EEG in Creutzfeldt–Jakob disease (CJD) is specific and forms an essential part of the investigations for this condition (Figure 33.1). The traces show repetitive high-amplitude biphasic 1/s generalized, long-duration sharp waves. Myoclonus is common in CJD but is not associated with the 1/s sharp waves. A myoclonic jerk may be accompanied by a different generalized epileptiform discharge or may be without any accompanying EEG change. New variant CJD (NVCJD) is clinically similar to CJD but often involves a younger age group. NVCJD is caused by eating meat from cattle infected with bovine spongiform encephalopathy. NVCJD does not show the 1/s sharp waves associated with CJD but the EEG is very abnormal with diffuse slow waves and some ill-defined sharp waves.

In practice one of the most important functions of the EEG in dementia is to distinguish this condition from a psychiatric disorder, where the EEG is essentially normal, although it may be affected by changes due to medication.

Infections of the central nervous system

Encephalitis is associated with marked EEG abnormalities. Acute viral encephalitis shows bursts of high-voltage slow waves mostly between 1–4 Hz and an increase of background slow. The localized necrotizing encephalitis, often associated with the herpes simplex virus, shows a different picture. Very high-voltage slow sharp waves known as periodic lateralized epileptiform discharges (PLEDs) are seen in one frontal or temporal region. This characteristic EEG is diagnostically very useful (Figure 33.2).

One type of encephalitis, sub-acute sclerosing panencephalitis (SSPE), is distinct from all others. This is a dementia of adolescence resulting from persistence of measles virus in the central nervous system. The patient shows repetitive movements, each one associated with an episode of periodic (i.e. regularly repeating) slow waves in the EEG. Later, the background EEG becomes almost flat. This terrible incurable condition had almost disappeared in the UK but will inevitably return with the fall in measles vaccination (Figure 33.3).

Encephalopathy

Encephalopathy can result from any systemic metabolic abnormality such as hypo- or hypernatraemia or uraemia. The EEG shows a generalized increase in slow activity (1–4 Hz) with slowing of the background activity. Uraemia may show epileptiform discharges, occasionally

---

Introduction to Epilepsy ed. Gonzalo Alarcón and Antonio Valentín. Published by Cambridge University Press.
© Cambridge University Press 2012.

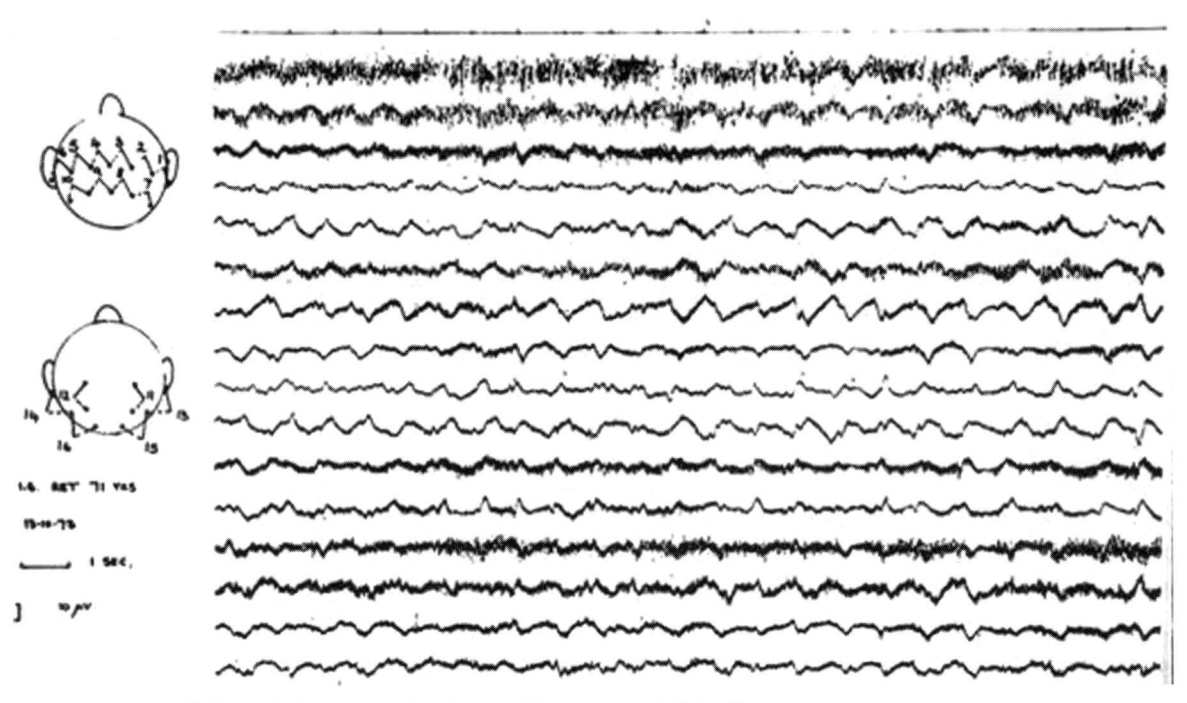

Section 2: Classification and diagnosis of epilepsy

Figure 33.1. Creutzfeldt–Jakob disease. Long-duration slow/sharp waves at 1 Hz in all areas.

resembling absence status. Hepatic encephalopathy has a characteristic EEG in deep coma. The traces resemble those of CJD but the one-per-second slow sharp waves are often triphasic like the letter M or W rather than biphasic as in CJD. Anoxia can produce various abnormalities. Sometimes there is increased slow activity but also epileptiform discharges. Generalized spike-and-slow waves or focal spikes may occur, sometimes on a flat background. Later the traces may become isoelectric (i.e. flat traces, showing no cerebral activity). Toxic poisons such as lead and mercury can produce an encephalopathy. The EEG shows severe generalized nonspecific abnormalities (delta activity at 1–4 Hz and sub-delta activity at less than 1 Hz).

Space-occupying lesions (SOL)

The characteristic EEG of SOL is localized irregular slow activity (delta activity at 1–4 Hz and sub-delta activity at <1 Hz), which is unresponsive and often focal (i.e. arising from a single electrode). The background activity is diminished in the same area. Occasionally an EEG may arouse suspicion in a patient whose illness is not thought to be due to SOL. Some patients with frontal or corpus callosum tumours present as dementia or a psychiatric condition. The EEG findings may lead to further investigation. A cerebral abscess produces very florid localized changes in the EEG whereas the MRI abnormalities may be more diffuse.

Identification of syncope

Syncope can sometimes be difficult to distinguish clinically from epilepsy If an attack occurs during the recording changes in the electrocardiogram are often helpful; there may be slowing of the heart rate or complete asystole. Sometimes heart block can be detected. A prolonged syncopal attack may be accompanied by myoclonic jerks but absence of cerebral discharges and heart rate changes point to the diagnosis. Since syncope may not always be obvious clinically it is important that the EEG is never recorded without a simultaneous electrocardiogram accompanying the trace.

Brainstem death

In the UK, the EEG is not part of the criteria for brainstem death but it may be requested in sensitive

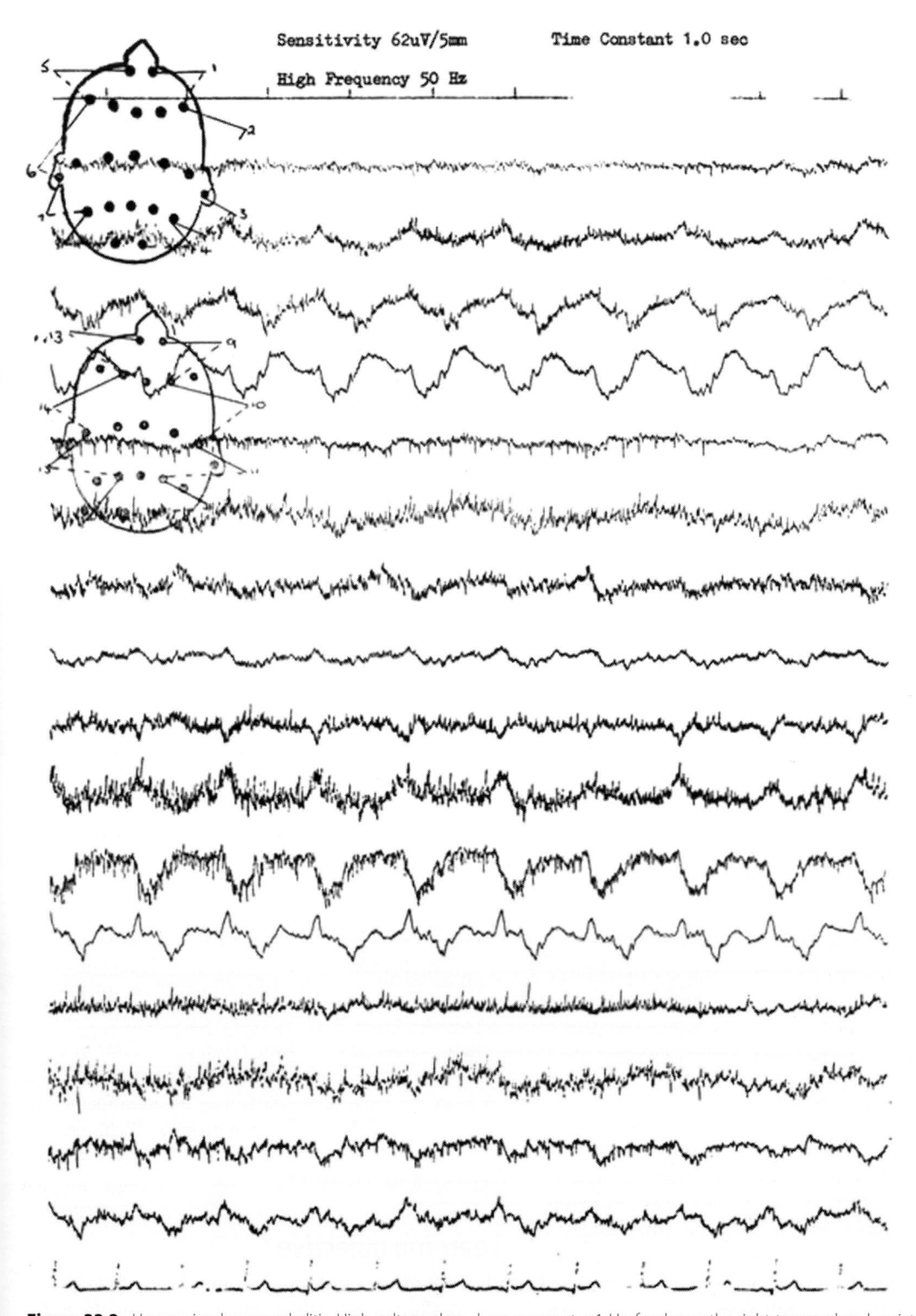

Chapter 33: Applications of EEG other than epilepsy

Figure 33.2. Herpes simplex encephalitis. High-voltage slow sharp waves at <1 Hz, focal over the right temporal and parietal regions.

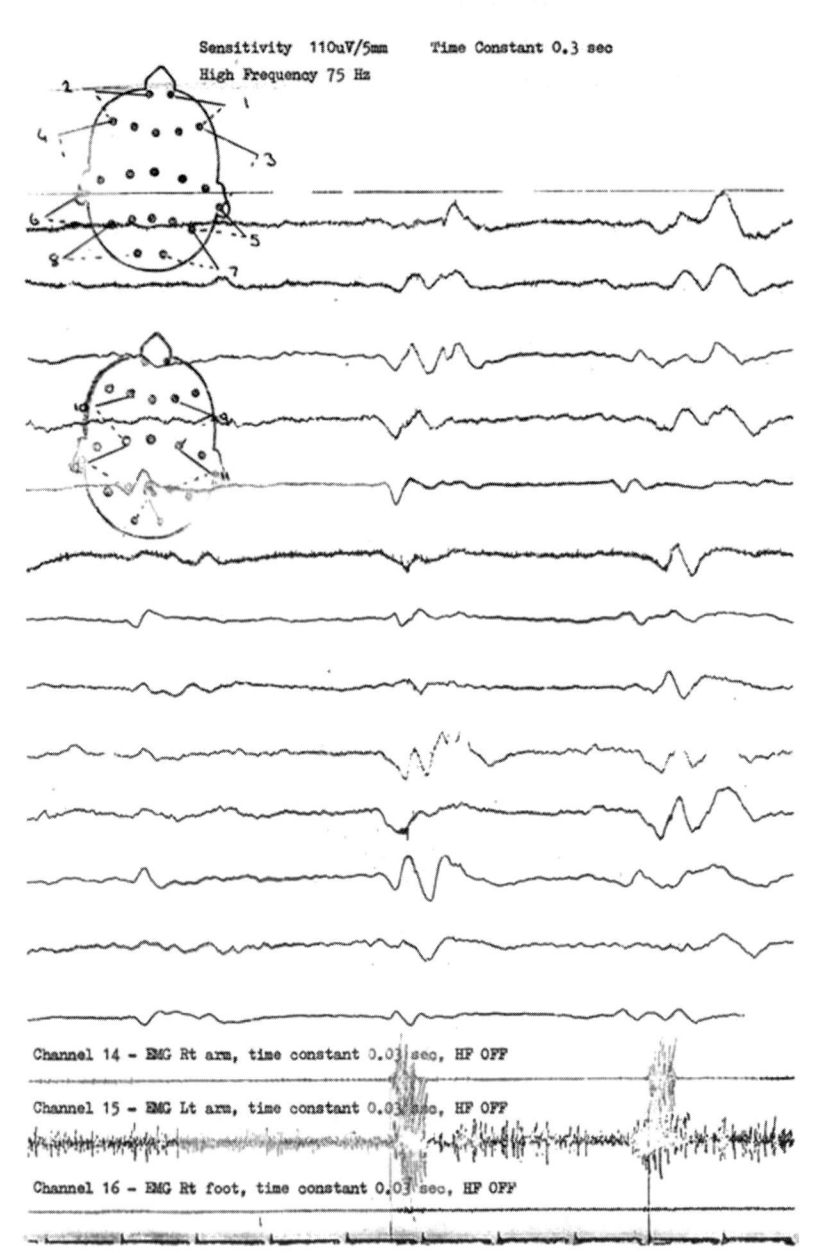

Section 2: Classification and diagnosis of epilepsy

Figure 33.3. Subacute sclerosing panencephalitis (SSPE). High-voltage bursts of slow waves in all areas with almost featureless background. Each burst of slow activity is accompanied by a movement of the right foot (See EMG channel 16).

cases. The purpose of the EEG is to demonstrate an isoelectric (flat) record. This may be very difficult in the milieu of the intensive care unit because of interference. All artefacts should be identified and eliminated if possible but it may be impossible to eliminate all, especially when recording at high gain to detect residual low-voltage activity. Absence of cerebral activity may result from other causes than brain death: sedatives (thiopentone, propofol), a low blood pressure or blood flow or low body temperature may be associated with an isoelectric EEG. Note should be taken of these parameters before recording the EEG.

Learning objective

(1) To understand the significance of the EEG in conditions other than epilepsy and how the EEG can be used to distinguish between epilepsy and other conditions.

Section 2

Classification and diagnosis of epilepsy

Chapter 34

Evoked potentials in epilepsy

Graham E. Holder

Summary

Evoked potentials (EPs) have little role in the direct management of patients with epilepsy. However, as a means of objectively establishing function, and with the ability to demonstrate dysfunction in the absence of symptoms, they do have an important diagnostic role in establishing the nature of the underlying disorder in patients where epilepsy is a symptom of the underlying disease.

Introduction

An evoked potential (EP) is an electrical signal generated in response to an external stimulus. Cortical EP amplitudes are usually much lower than that of background noise (the electroencephalogram, EEG), and signal averaging is usually required to extract the EP from the background EEG. The sensory modalities used are usually visual, auditory or sensory. It is beyond the scope of this chapter to address most aspects of EP recording in detail and the reader is referred to a standard text (e.g. Binnie *et al.*, 2004) for further information. A short discussion follows on the different types of EP, and how they may be used diagnostically in relation to epilepsy.

Basics of visual evoked cortical potentials (VEPs) and electroretinography (ERG)

The recording of the VEP enables assessment both of the primary visual cortex and of the intra-cranial pathways that transfer the information from eye to brain, particularly the optic nerves and the optic chiasm. Scalp electrodes are positioned over the occipital areas, usually O1 and O2, referred to Fz. The patient then views a suitable repetitive stimulus, and computerized signal averaging is used to extract the time-locked VEP from the higher-amplitude spontaneous background activity of the brain in which it is usually concealed. Guidelines for visual system testing have recently been published (Holder *et al.*, 2010).

The form of stimulation most commonly used for diagnostic purposes, because it has a waveform that is very similar in shape, size and timing both within (interocular and interhemispheric) and across a normal population, is pattern reversal, in which the white squares become black, and black squares become white, with no accompanying change in stimulus luminance. The normal pattern-reversal VEP to a checkerboard reversing twice per second (two reversals per second, or 1 Hz) consists of a prominent positive component, P100, at approximately 100 ms preceded and followed by negative components N75 and N135 respectively (Figure 34.1). The patient centrally views the stimulus, which is changing in contrast information but not in overall luminance, and the pattern VEP is therefore dominated by signals relating to the macula, or central retina. Each eye is tested separately. It is therefore possible to compare not only the function of one eye in relation to the other, but also the function of one hemisphere of the brain against the other. It it should be noted that VEP interpretation in interhemispheric comparisons is complex (Holder *et al.*, 2010). Pupillary dilatation is not used.

In addition, the potentials evoked by a diffuse flash stimulus can also be recorded. These, historically, were the first form of VEP to be recorded, but, due to a wide range of shape, size and timing across a normal population, they have limited diagnostic use. They do, however, exhibit very low variability within an individual patient, similar to that of pattern-reversal VEPs, and thus can be used effectively to compare one

---

Introduction to Epilepsy ed. Gonzalo Alarcón and Antonio Valentín. Published by Cambridge University Press.
© Cambridge University Press 2012.

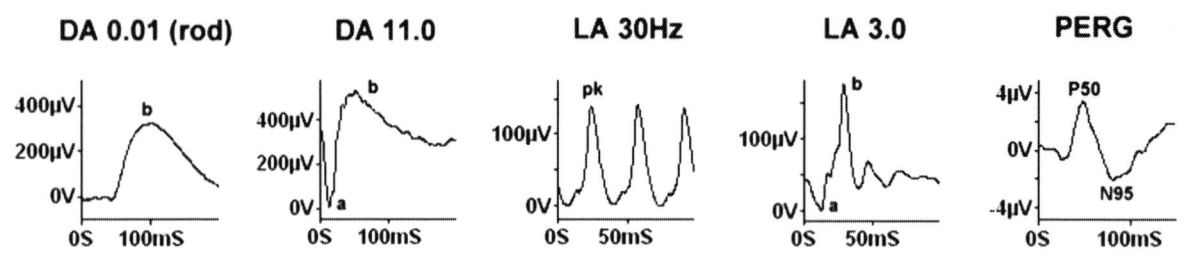

Figure 34.1. A set of ISCEV Standard normal ERGs from an adult subject recorded with gold foil corneal electrodes, Ganzfeld stimulation and a dilated pupil. The numerical values refer to the flash strength in cd·s/m^2. DA, dark adapted; LA, light adapted. PERG, pattern electroretinogram.

eye with the other and one hemisphere of the brain with the other. Because they are generated by a flash of light, the whole of the retina is stimulated, and, consequently, a larger area of the brain is involved.

The (flash) electroretinogram (ERG) is recorded using corneal electrodes and is the mass electrical response of the retina to a luminance stimulus. Changing the adaptive state of the eye and the nature of the stimulus enables the separation of different retinal cell types and layers by utilizing the different functional properties of the retinal rod and cone systems. The stimuli are delivered using a Ganzfeld bowl, an integrating sphere that enables uniform whole field illumination. A Ganzfeld bowl also allows diffuse background illumination for photopic adaptation. Standardization is essential for ERG and the International Society for Clinical Electrophysiology of Vision (ISCEV) defines a standard flash (3.0 cd·s/m^2). A response specific for the rod system is recorded when this flash is attenuated by 2.5 log units, the DA 0.01 response, previously known as the rod, or rod-specific response. This response is generated in the rod ON bipolar cells, and thus acts as a measure of rod system sensitivity. The response to the standard flash under scotopic (fully dark adapted) conditions, with a fully dilated pupil, is the DA 3.0 response, previously known as the Standard or mixed response. It is perhaps this response that many regard as a 'typical' ERG. It consists of two main components, a negative a-wave followed by a larger positive component, the b-wave (see Figure 34.1). There is a contribution from the retinal cone system to this response, but, being recorded under scotopic (dark-adapted) conditions, the rods are highly sensitive and this standard response is dominated by rod-driven activity. In addition, there are perhaps 120 million rod photoreceptors and only 7 million cones. The use of a brighter flash (~11.0 cd·s/m^2; DA 11.0) is 'suggested' in the most recent ISCEV ERG Standard better to view the a-wave, and therefore better to localize dysfunction within the retina. The initial approximately 8 ms of the a-wave arises in relation to hyperpolarization of the (rod) photoreceptors and the slope of the a-wave can be related to the kinetics of phototransduction. The a-wave therefore gives a direct reflection of the metabolic activity taking place in the retinal photoreceptors. In a normal subject, the positive b-wave is larger than the a-wave. The b-wave is generated post-receptorally in the inner nuclear layer of the retina in relation to depolarization of the ON bipolar cells. In general, disease or dysfunction of the photoreceptors or RPE is referred to as outer retinal disease, and disease affecting structures 'downstream' to the photoreceptors as inner retinal disease even though anatomically light passes through the rest of the retina to reach the photoreceptors (anatomically the inner part of the retina).

ERGs that reflect cone system activity are obtained using a rod-saturating photopic background (30 cd/m^2) using superimposed single flash and 30 Hz flicker stimulation (Figure 34.1; LA 3.0, LA 30 Hz). The rod system has low temporal resolution and cannot resolve a fast flickering stimulus, and use of a 30 Hz white flash stimulus, combined with a rod-suppressing background, therefore allows a cone-system specific waveform to be recorded. This response is a more sensitive measure of cone dysfunction than the single-flash cone response, but is generated at an inner retinal level, precluding the distinction between cone photoreceptor and cone inner nuclear layer dysfunction. Rods and short-wavelength cones connect directly to ON bipolar cells; medium and long-wavelength cones additionally connect to OFF bipolar cells. Although there is a demonstrated contribution from hyperpolarizing (OFF) bipolar cells to shaping the photopic a-wave, this component nonetheless has some contribution from cone photoreceptor function, and some localization within the retinal cone system is obtained with the single-flash photopic ERG. The photopic b-wave reflects post-phototransduction activity, and to a short flash stimulus ON and OFF activity within the photopic system is effectively synchronized.

As a mass response of the retina, the macula does not contribute significantly to the (full-field) ERG. Central retinal function can be measured by the pattern ERG (PERG), the response of central retina to a reversing checkerboard similar to that used to evoke the pattern VEP. The PERG is also of great value in the improved interpretation of the pattern VEP by revealing the retinal response to a similar stimulus. It is beyond the scope of this chapter further to address those issues and the reader is referred to a comprehensive review article (Holder, 2001).

The role of VEP and ERG in epilepsy

A small percentage of patients with multiple sclerosis (MS), a central nervous system demyelinating disease, have epilepsy. The incidence of epilepsy is low at 1–8% and it can precede other symptoms. There are problems of co-incidence that preclude accurate assessment of causation. However, when epilepsy does occur in association with MS it may be infrequent and easily controlled; it may rarely, however, be intractable, which can be associated with rapidly increasing disability and has a poor prognosis for survival. Acute symptomatic seizures may occur, usually focally, during acute relapse.

The role of the VEP in the diagnosis of demyelinating disease was defined in seminal series of reports by the Halliday group (Halliday et al., 1972, 1973), and subsequently confirmed in many subsequent publications (reviewed by Holder, 1991). They demonstrated that the pattern VEP was delayed in patients with optic neuritis, the clinical manifestation of optic nerve demyelination; that the delay in optic nerve conduction did not normalize following clinical recovery; and importantly, an observation that fundamentally altered clinical practice at the time, that the pattern VEP could detect sub-clinical optic nerve demyelination in patients with no signs or symptoms of optic nerve disease (e.g. Figure 34.2), and historically occupied an important role in obviating the need for myelography in patients with possible MS presenting with a spinal cord lesion.

Perhaps the main role of the ERG in epilepsy relates to the diagnosis of Batten disease. The neuronal ceroid lipofuscinoses (NCL) are the most common of the neurodegenerative disorders occurring in children and are autosomal recessive in

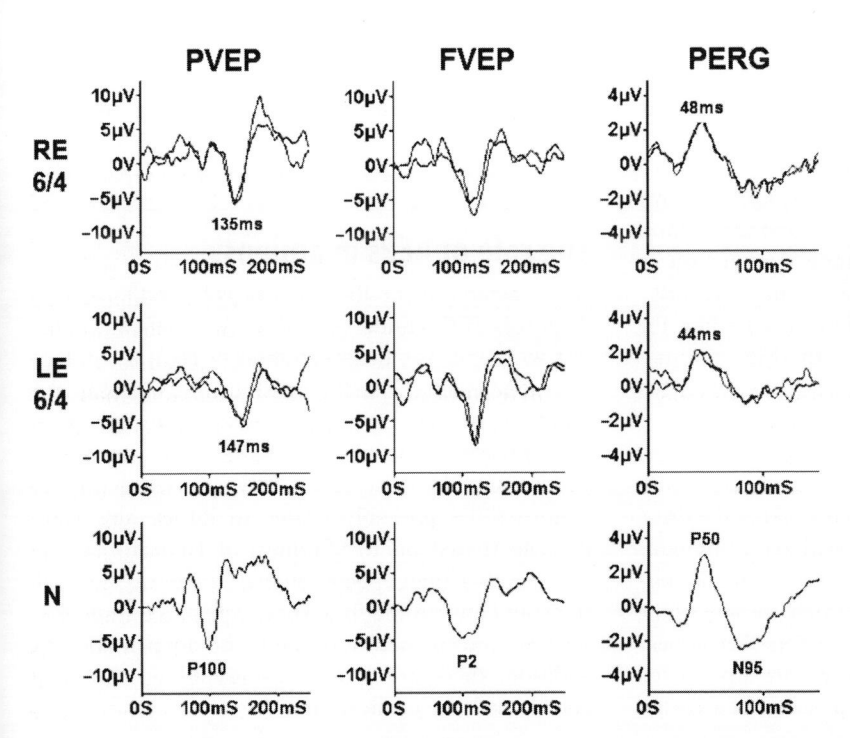

Figure 34.2. VEPs and PERGs from an adult patient with a history of blurred vision in her left eye following a hot bath or exercise, suggestive of Uhthoff phenomenon. There was no relative afferent pupillary defect. The P100 component shows moderate to severe delay in the symptomatic left eye, where reduction in PERG N95 component suggests additional dysfunction at the level of the retinal ganglion cells. There is also moderately severe delay in the asymptomatic right eye, demonstrating the ability of the VEP to detect sub-clinical optic nerve demyelination.

inheritance. Batten in 1903 described two siblings with progressive macular dystrophy and cerebral degeneration and his name has subsequently been associated with the juvenile form of NCL even though the term NCL was not introduced until 1969 by Zemen and Dyken. Clinical features including age of onset and the presence or ultrastructural appearance of this lysosomal storage material that accumulates in these disorders have traditionally classified the NCLs as infantile, late infantile, juvenile and adult. The term Batten disease should refer only to the juvenile-onset form, but this eponym has been applied to all NCLs. The majority of cases of Batten disease are caused by mutations in CLN3, which maps to chromosome 16p21. The primary biochemical defect has not yet been identified, and to date there is no available treatment. Juvenile NCL (jNCL) usually presents with progressive loss of visual acuity between the ages of 4 and 10 years, generally leading to legal blindness within 3 years.

Prompt diagnosis of jNCL is important as it enables families to receive the appropriate counselling and support as early as possible. The diagnosis is based on clinico-pathological findings and can be confirmed by molecular genetic testing. Retinal signs eventually include bull's eye maculopathy, peripheral pigmentary or atrophic changes, disc pallor and attenuation of the retinal arterioles, but at presentation the fundus is often normal or simply shows a bull's eye lesion and thus may be mistaken for an early-onset cone dystrophy. Neurological symptoms including behavioural change, motor disturbance, cognitive impairment and seizures follow the visual symptoms, and the disease characteristically follows an inexorable path to death in the second or third decade. ERGs typically demonstrate a reduction in the b:a ratio under both scotopic (a 'negative ERG' waveform) and photopic conditions, even when the fundus appearance is normal, and the ERG findings usually direct appropriate mutational screening (Weleber et al., 2004; Collins et al., 2006; Figure 34.3).

There is a further role of the ERG in epilepsy. The anti-convulsant drug vigabatrin is associated with visual field loss in 30–40% of patients taking the drug. Although the mechanism of this field loss in humans is far from clearly established, ERGs are often abnormal. Some of the abnormalities, namely the loss of the oscillatory potentials, the small wavelets that appear on the ascending limb of the b-wave, are a predicted consequence of the pharmacological effect of a GABA transaminase inhibitor on the function of the amacrine cells in the retina, some of which are known to be GABA-ergic, and which are involved in the generation of the oscillatory potentials. However, other patients have abnormalities that cannot be so explained, particularly involving the b-wave of the scotopic bright-flash ERG and thus suggesting probable inner retinal dysfunction (Besch et al., 2002; Renner et al., 2006; Audo et al., 2008).

Basics of auditory evoked potentials (AEPs)

Although it is possible to record AEPs that arise in the auditory cortex, from a neurological diagnostic viewpoint it is the brainstem AEP (BAEP) that is the most important. Discussion will be limited to BAEPs. These are recorded as far-field potentials using electrodes situated at each mastoid referred to an electrode at Cz. Click stimuli are used, with a stimulus rate usually between 10 Hz and 20 Hz, and as the BAEP signals are very small, signal averaging is essential, with >1000 stimuli per trial being needed. A series of components (defections) are recorded, with the first five components having a nomenclature of I–V being the most important. The first is mastoid negative, and arises in relation to the volleys generated at the cochlea. Waves II–V are vertex positive. Wave II arises in the proximal portions of the VIIIth cranial nerve prior to entry into the brainstem, wave III arises from the superior olivary complex, wave IV from the lateral lemniscus and wave V from the inferior colliculus. Each ear is stimulated separately.

The role of AEPs in epilepsy

In consideration of the possible role of EPs in the diagnosis of the underlying disorders that can manifest with epilepsy, demonstration of central conduction abnormality with the BAEP can be useful in the diagnosis of MS. In addition, Rodin and colleagues (1982) reported increased I–III and III–V intervals in patients with epilepsy. It was, however, felt that these abnormalities probably related to diffuse structural damage (based on the findings of clinical examination) rather than epilepsy alone. There was no relationship between the frequency, type and duration of seizures and the nature of the BAEP abnormality. In addition, there are possible confounding effects of anti-convulsant medication.

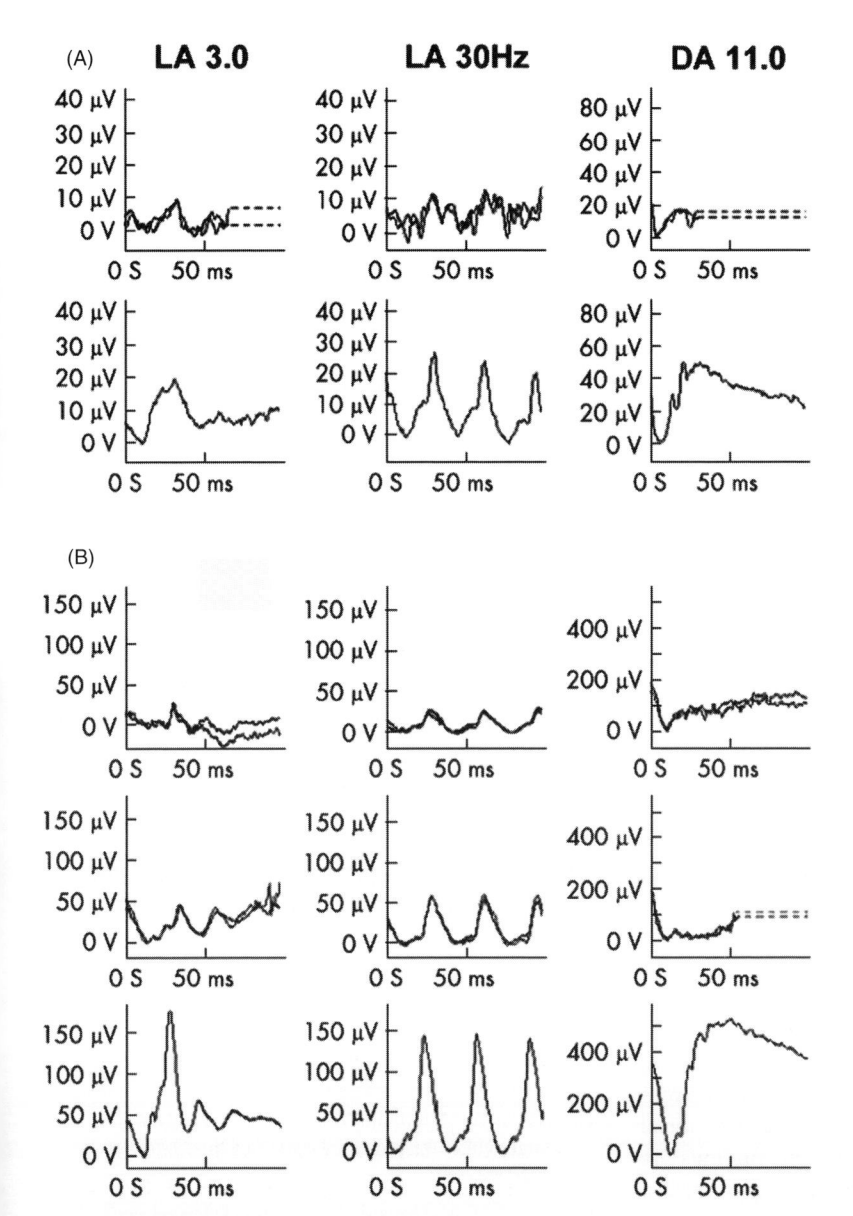

Figure 34.3. (A) ERGs recorded using a surface electrode on the lower eyelid. The upper trace is from a child with Batten disease, the lower trace from a normal child. Note the reduction in the b:a ratio in the photopic single flash ERG; the delayed and reduced 30 Hz flicker ERG; and the profoundly electronegative bright flash dark adapted ERG (maximal). Broken lines have been used to replace blink/eye movement artefact. (B) ERGs recorded using corneal gold foil electrodes. The upper and middle traces are from patients with Batten disease; the lower traces are from a normal subject. The ERG characteristics are similar to those described above with additional amplitude changes in the photopic ERG of the upper patient. Broken lines have been used to replace blink/eye movement artefact. Modified from: Collins et al., 2006.

Basics of sensory evoked potentials (SEPs)

SEPs are usually recorded using upper limb stimulation of the median nerve at the wrist, or with lower limb stimulation of the posterior tibial nerve at the ankle. Scalp electrodes are placed over the sensory areas corresponding to the hand for upper limb stimulation, usually 2 cm posterior and 6 cm lateral to the vertex, but at the vertex for lower limb stimulation. Additional electrodes to record the afferent volleys on upper limb stimulation are positioned at Erb's point and C6/7, but although an electrode at the popliteal fossa can sometimes produce successful recordings, that is less often the case with lower limb than with upper limb stimulation. Stimulation usually takes place at ~3/s with each trial resulting from an average of 300–500 stimulations. A clinical example is shown in Figure 34.4.

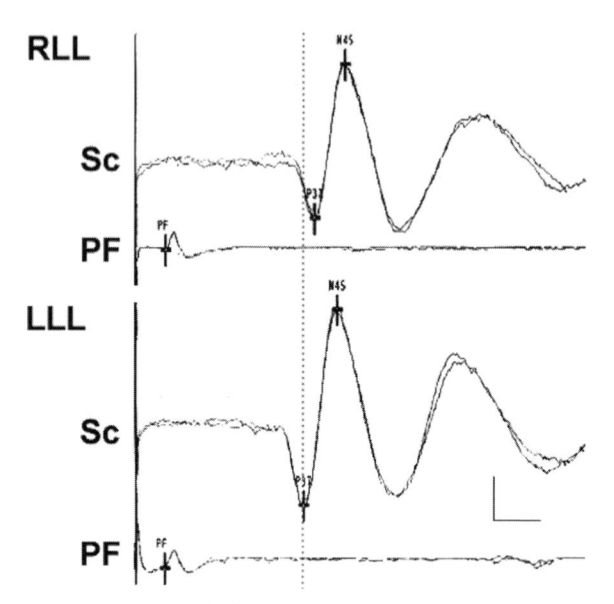

Figure 34.4. Lower limb SEPs in an adult patient with MS. Note the delay in the scalp response to stimulation of the lateral popliteal nerve at the ankle of the right lower limb (RLL). LLL, left lower limb; Sc, scalp; PF, popliteal fossa. Calibration 10 ms, 2 μV for Sc recordings; 10 ms, 5 μV for PF recordings.

The role of SEPs in epilepsy

As with the VEP and the AEP, the SEP has a role in the diagnosis of demyelinating disease. Increased central conduction time can reveal demyelinating lesions of the sensory pathways, even in the absence of symptoms suggesting such involvement. In the upper limb SEPs, the findings are more level-specific, and can localize lesions to the cord or more rostral structures with the Erb's point potential reflecting the afferent volley through the brachial plexus and function distal to the dorsal root ganglion. Lower limb findings are often nonspecific for the level of dysfunction. An example appears in Figure 34.4.

SEPs may also be of some value in patients with myoclonic epilepsy. The presence of 'giant' SEPs was first described by Halliday in 1967. He described supernormal late components, with all earlier components up to N19 being normal. There was some suggestion that this may be related to the severity of the disorder. Later reports (Shibasaki et al., 1978, 1985) also described high-amplitude SEPs in the lipidoses, CJD and post-hypoxic myoclonus, but they were not present in other causes of myoclonus such as midbrain infarction or essential myoclonus.

There is also a possible role for SEPs in the accurate localization of sensory cortex using intraoperative cortical recording (e.g. Wood et al., 1988). Localization of the sensorimotor region by SEP allowed maximal resection of the focus with minimal risk of sensory or motor deficit in patients where frontal or parietal cortex was the primary epileptogenic region in patients with intractable focal epilepsy.

Conclusion

Evoked potential recording contributes little to the management of most patients with epilepsy, but may have an important role in the diagnosis of the underlying disorder when epilepsy is a manifesting symptom.

References

Audo I, Robson AG, Holder GE, Moore AT. The negative ERG: clinical phenotypes and disease mechanisms of inner retinal dysfunction. *Surv Ophthalmol* 2008;**53**:16–40.

Besch D, Kurtenbach A, Apfelstedt-Sylla E, et al. Visual field constriction and electrophysiological changes associated with vigabatrin. *Doc Ophthalmol* 2002;**104**:151–70.

Binnie CD, Cooper R, Mauguiere F, et al (eds). *Clinical Neurophysiology*, vol. 1, pp. 381–401. Revised and enlarged edn. Amsterdam: Elsevier; 2004.

Collins J, Holder GE, Herbert H, Adams GG. Batten disease: features to facilitate early diagnosis. *Br J Ophthalmol* 2006;**90**:1119–24.

Halliday AM. The electrophysiological study of myoclonus in man. *Brain* 1967;**90**:241–84.

Halliday AM, McDonald WI, Mushin J. Delayed visual evoked response in optic neuritis. *Lancet* 1972;**1**:982–5.

Halliday AM, McDonald WI, Mushin J. Visual evoked response in the diagnosis of multiple sclerosis. *Br Med J* 1973;**4**:661–4.

Holder GE. Multiple sclerosis. In Heckenlively JR, Arden GB, eds. *Principles and Practice of Clinical Electrophysiology of Vision*, pp. 797–805. St. Louis: Mosby Year Book; 1991.

Holder GE. The pattern electroretinogram and an integrated approach to visual pathway diagnosis. *Prog Ret Eye Res* 2001;**20**:531–61.

Holder GE, Celesia GG, Miyake Y, Tobimatsu S, Weleber RG. International Federation of Clinical Neurophysiology: recommendations for visual system testing. *Clin Neurophysiol* 2010;**121**:1393–409.

Renner AB, Kellner U, Cropp E, Foerster MH. Dysfunction of transmission in the inner retina: incidence and clinical causes of negative electroretinogram. *Graefes Arch Clin Exp Ophthalmol* 2006;**244**:1467–73.

Rodin E, Chayasirisobhon S, Klutke G. Brainstem auditory evoked potential recording in patients with epilepsy. *Clin Electroencephalogr* 1982;**13**:154–61.

Shibasaki H, Yamashita Y, Kuroiwa Y. Electroencephalographic studies myoclonus. *Brain* 1978;**101**:447–60.

Shibasaki H, Yamashita Y, Neshige R, Tobimatsu S, Fukui R. Pathogenesis of giant somatosensory evoked potentials in progressive myoclonic epilepsy. *Brain* 1985;**108**:225–40.

Weleber RG, Gupta N, Trzupek KM, *et al.* Electroretinographic and clinicopathologic correlations of retina dysfunction in infantile neuronal ceroid lipofuscinosis. *Mol Genet Metab* 2004;**83**:128–37.

Wood CW, Spencer DD, Allison T, *et al.* Localization of human sensorimotor cortex during surgery by cortical surface recording of somatosensory evoked potentials. *J Neurosurg* 1988;**68**:99–111.

Learning objectives

(1) To understand the concept of an evoked potential (EP), including the electroretinogram (ERG).
(2) To receive an overview of how EPs and ERGs are recorded.
(3) To understand the role of EPs in the management of patients with epilepsy.
(4) To understand how EPs help diagnose the underlying disorders that may manifest symptoms of epilepsy.
(5) To recognize some relevant EP and ERG abnormalities.

Section 2 Classification and diagnosis of epilepsy

Chapter 35

Introduction to neuroimaging and relevant anatomical landmarks

Gonzalo Alarcón and Jozef M. Jarosz

Neuroimaging is a rapidly expanding field that progressively allows clinicians and researchers to study structural and functional images of the living brain with increasing precision. A large number of modalities are available, including cross-sectional imaging (computerized tomography or CT, magnetic resonance imaging or MRI), radiographic techniques (angiography, skull X-rays), nuclear medicine (positron emission tomography or PET, single positron emission computed tomography or SPECT) and ultrasound. For each technique, we must know what the images look like, to identify anatomical structures, what the different pathological lesions look like, and their indications and risks.

Each imaging modality has its own peculiarities, pros and cons (see Table 36.1). For instance, bone, calcifications and fresh blood appear bright on CT whereas the ventricles and oedema are seen dark. CT is quick, allows good patient access during the scan and is present in most hospitals. However, CT requires ionizing radiation and achieves only fair tissue contrast.

The most clinically relevant imaging technique at present is structural MRI, which requires no ionizing radiation, achieves much better tissue contrast than CT and is more sensitive to pathology. However, MRI scanning takes longer than CT, is undertaken with poor patient access (difficulties with claustrophobia or patient monitoring), requires a strong magnetic field (contraindicated in patients with pacemakers, aneurysm clips, monitoring leads) and is not available in all hospitals.

Interpreting MRI images can be challenging to the non-expert, in part due to the richness of anatomical detail shown. Figures 35.1 to 35.4 show some of the normal anatomical structures which are often evaluated in patients with epilepsy.

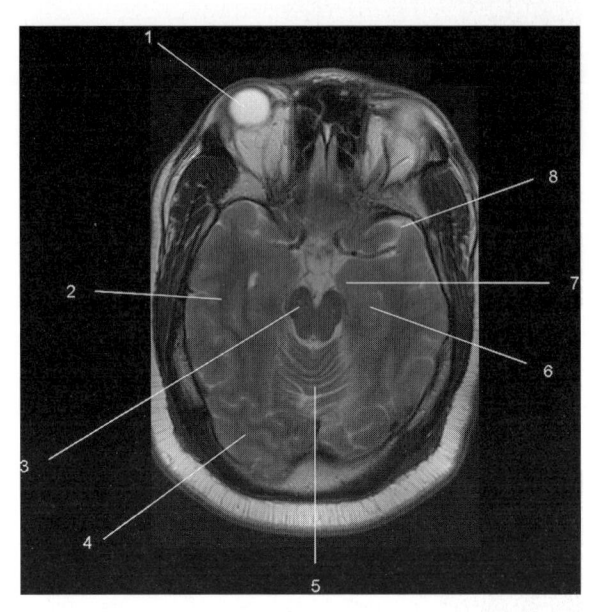

Figure 35.1. Axial T2-weighted image. (1) Right eye; (2) temporal lobe; (3) pons; (4) occipital lobe; (5) cerebellum; (6) hippocampus; (7) uncus; (8) temporal pole.

Learning objectives

(1) To understand the relevance of neuroimaging in epileptology.
(2) To understand the basic differences between the different neuroimaging modalities, in particular between CT and MRI.
(3) To be able to identify basic anatomical structures on sectional brain images.

Introduction to Epilepsy ed. Gonzalo Alarcón and Antonio Valentín. Published by Cambridge University Press.
© Cambridge University Press 2012.

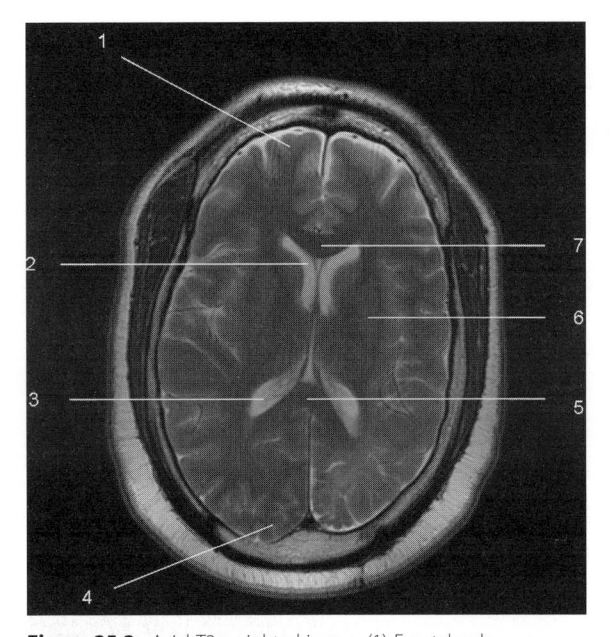

Chapter 35: Introduction to neuroimaging and relevant anatomical landmarks

Figure 35.2. Axial T2-weighted image. (1) Frontal pole; (2) third ventricle; (3) lateral ventricle; (4) occipital pole; (5) corpus callosum (splenium); (6) putamen; (7) corpus callosum (genu).

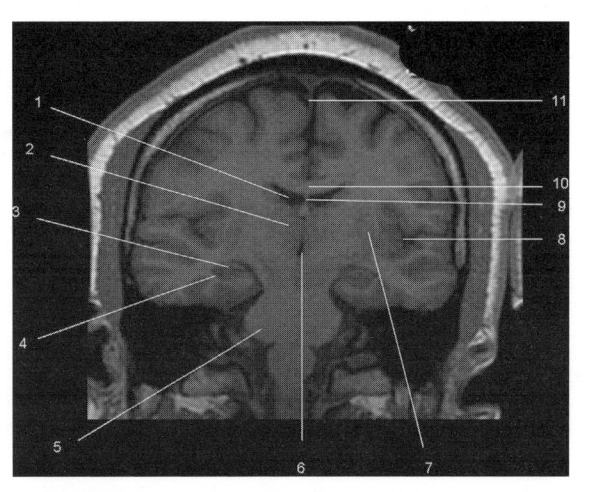

Figure 35.3. Coronal T1-weighted images. (1) Lateral ventricle; (2) thalamus; (3) hippocampus; (4) inferior (temporal) horn of the lateral ventricle; (5) pons; (6) third ventricle; (7) lentiform nucleus (putamen); (8) insula; (9) septum pellucidum; (10) corpus callosum; (11) falx cerebri.

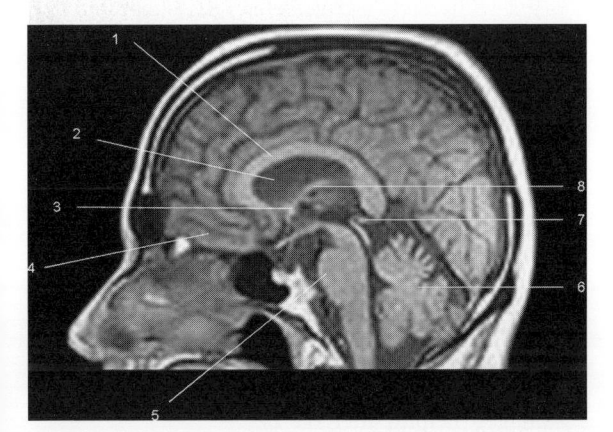

Figure 35.4. Sagittal image near the midline. (1) Corpus callosum; (2) third ventricle; (3) anterior commissure; (4) frontal lobe (orbital cortex); (5) pons; (6) cerebellum; (7) posterior commissure; (8) fornix.

Section 2 Classification and diagnosis of epilepsy

Chapter 36

The role of structural imaging in the assessment of epilepsy

Gonzalo Alarcón, Antonio Valentín, Richard P. Selway and Jozef M. Jarosz

The development of structural brain imaging and, in particular, magnetic resonance imaging (MRI) is probably the single most important recent development in the assessment of patients with symptomatic epilepsy. Structural neuroimaging is expected to be normal in patients with idiopathic epilepsy. Since approximately 30% of patients with epilepsy have idiopathic epilepsy, structural neuroimaging is normal in a significant proportion of patients with epilepsy.

In symptomatic epilepsies, computerized tomography (CT) and MRI are available for structural imaging. Both have specific advantages and disadvantages (Table 36.1), but generally MRI has higher resolution and is considered preferable. In acute neurological insults (head injury, intracranial haemorrhage or encephalitis), CT is acceptable if MRI is not available. Ideally, brain structural MRI should be obtained within 4 weeks in all patients diagnosed with epilepsy except when there is a definite electroclinical diagnosis of idiopathic epilepsy (generalized or focal). MRI is contraindicated if there are intracranial clips or implanted metals because metals can heat up in the brain during MRI acquisition and magnetic metals (basically, those containing iron, such as some steel) can move in the head. Heart pacemaker is also a contraindication for MRI.

CT would be preferable in situations where there are contraindications for MRI. CT may also be preferable in young children not requiring sedation for CT who may need sedation for longer MRI scans.

MRI technology and methodology is still a rapidly evolving field. Interpretation of MRI studies begins with the identification and optimization of the appropriate MRI methods. The typical MRI for epilepsy will be obtained with systems of at least 1.5 tesla (although new systems go up to 3 tesla), and they usually include orthogonal views in two planes as follows:

- coronal T2-weighted images,
- three-dimensional T1-weighted data sets with 1.5 mm or thinner slices, and
- fluid-attenuated inversion-recovery (FLAIR) images (helpful after age 2).

Choice of the appropriate slice orientation is also important. In epilepsy, coronal slices should preferably be perpendicular to the temporal horn and axial slices parallel to the anterior-to-posterior commissural line.

The clinical evaluation of images can be challenging and multidisciplinary involvement is often necessary.

Table 36.1. MRI or CT for epilepsy

MRI	CT
Limited availability	Widely available 24 h/day, 7 days/week
Intimidating environment	Less intimidating
20 min exam time	5 min exam time
No ionizing radiation	Ionizing radiation
Multiplanar	Axial only (except very modern scanners)
Excellent tissue contrast	Moderate tissue contrast

Introduction to Epilepsy ed. Gonzalo Alarcón and Antonio Valentín. Published by Cambridge University Press.
© Cambridge University Press 2012.

Chapter 36: The role of structural imaging in the assessment of epilepsy

Box 36.1. Useful basic rules in interpreting MRI images

- T1-weighted images resemble the real brain (grey matter shows as darker grey and white matter as lighter grey)
- T2-weighted images resemble the negative of the real brain (grey matter shows as lighter grey and white matter as darker grey)
- FLAIR images 'remove' water density such as the cerebrospinal fluid or cysts
- Water appears dark in T1-weighted images and bright (white) in T2-weighted images
- Oedema and gliosis are both bright on T2-weighted images
- Gliosis appears bright in FLAIR images
- Bone is black on all sequences
- Gadolinium-DPTA contrast appears bright on T1-weighted images and can be used with T1-weighted images to reveal lesions associated with breakdown of the blood–brain barrier

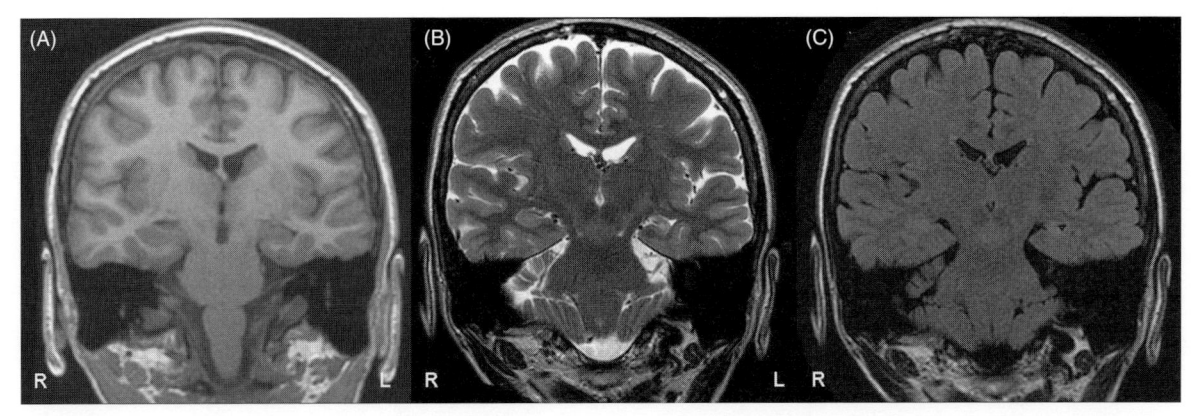

Figure 36.1. Left mesial temporal sclerosis. Note reduction in hippocampal size and destruction of internal hippocampal anatomy in T1-weighted image (A), T2-weighted image (B) and FLAIR image (C).

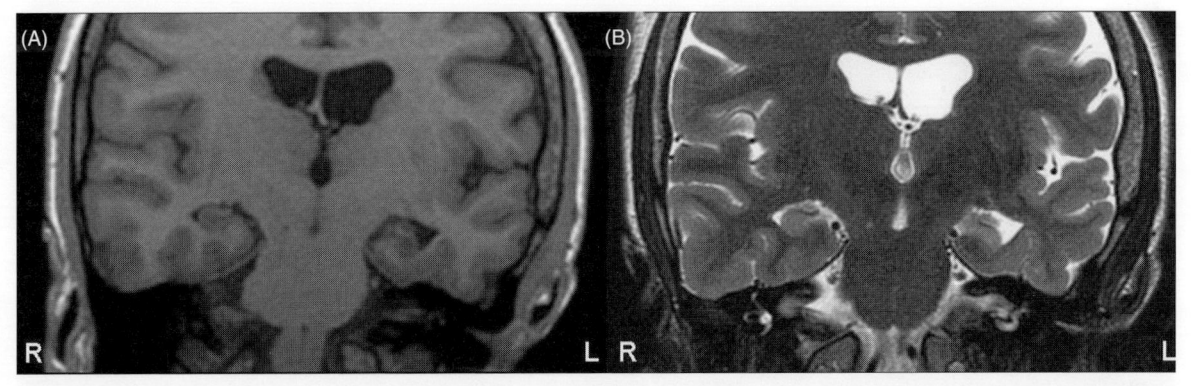

Figure 36.2. Left mesial temporal sclerosis associated with a degree of left temporal atrophy. Note a reduction in the size of the left hippocampus, loss of internal hippocampal structure and increase in size of the temporal horn of the left lateral ventricle.

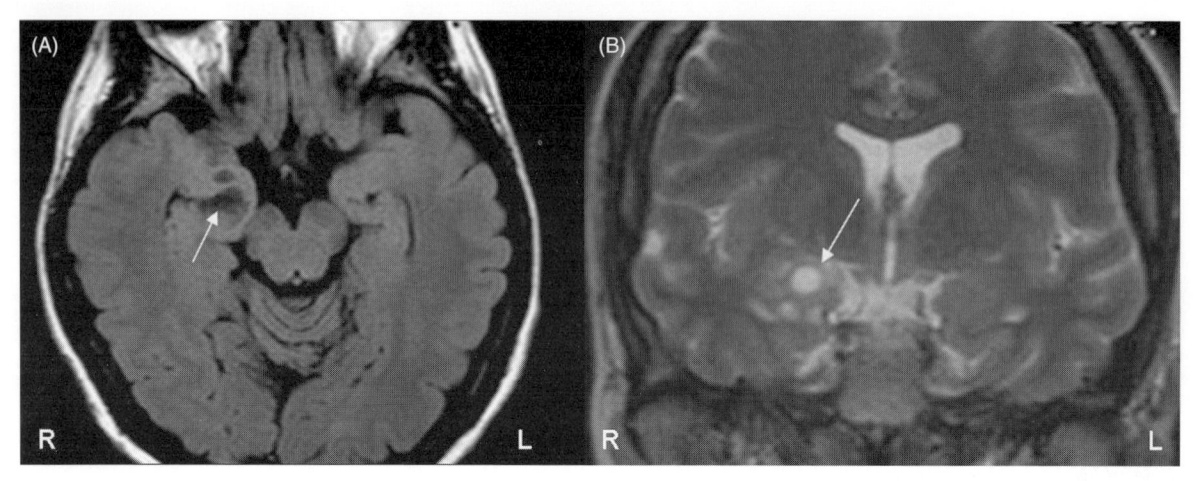

Section 2: Classification and diagnosis of epilepsy

Figure 36.3. Right amygdalar lesion.

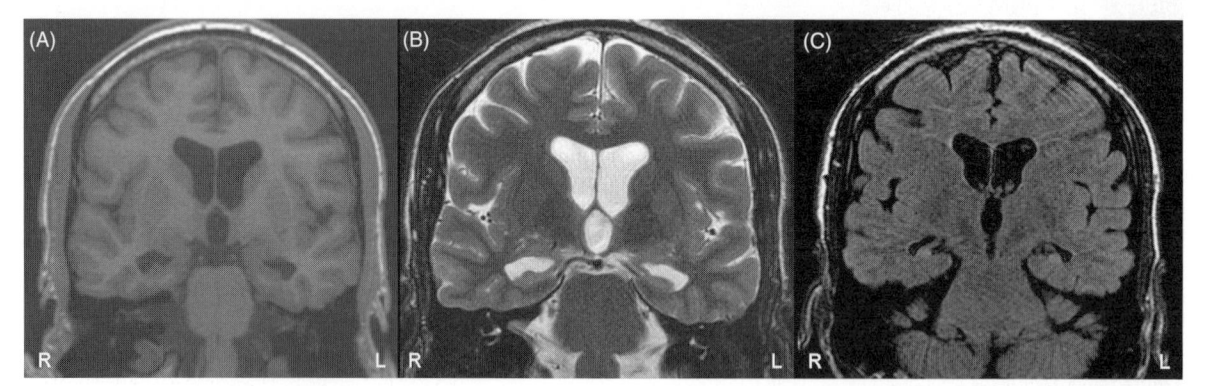

Figure 36.4. Bilateral mesial temporal sclerosis. Note a bilateral marked reduction in hippocampal volume and increase in the size of the temporal horn of the lateral ventricle. On FLAIR there is increased (whiter) hippocampal signal bilaterally, suggesting gliosis (C).

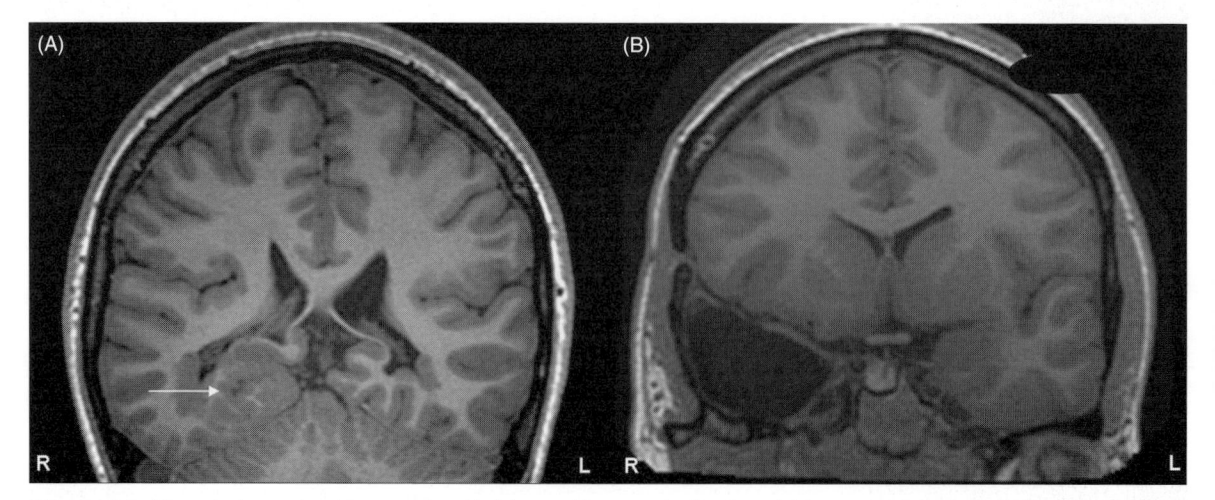

Figure 36.5. Bilateral subependymal heterotopia with right mesial temporal sclerosis and right temporal dysplasia (A). MRI after a right temporal lobectomy (B).

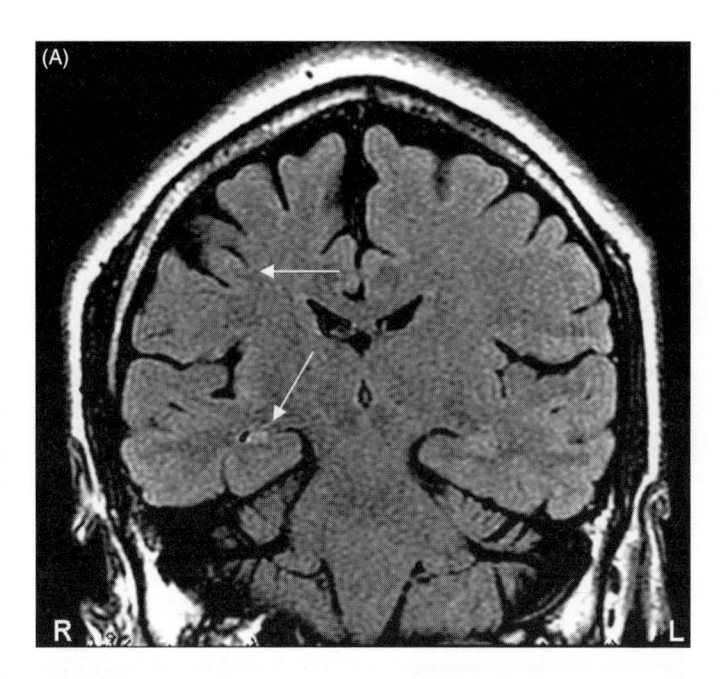

Chapter 36: The role of structural imaging in the assessment of epilepsy

Figure 36.6. Simultaneous presence of two abnormalities on FLAIR image. There is mild focal volume loss of the right parietal lobe, possibly due to encephalomalacia (horizontal arrow), in addition to right mesial temporal sclerosis. Note volume reduction and signal increase in the right hippocampus.

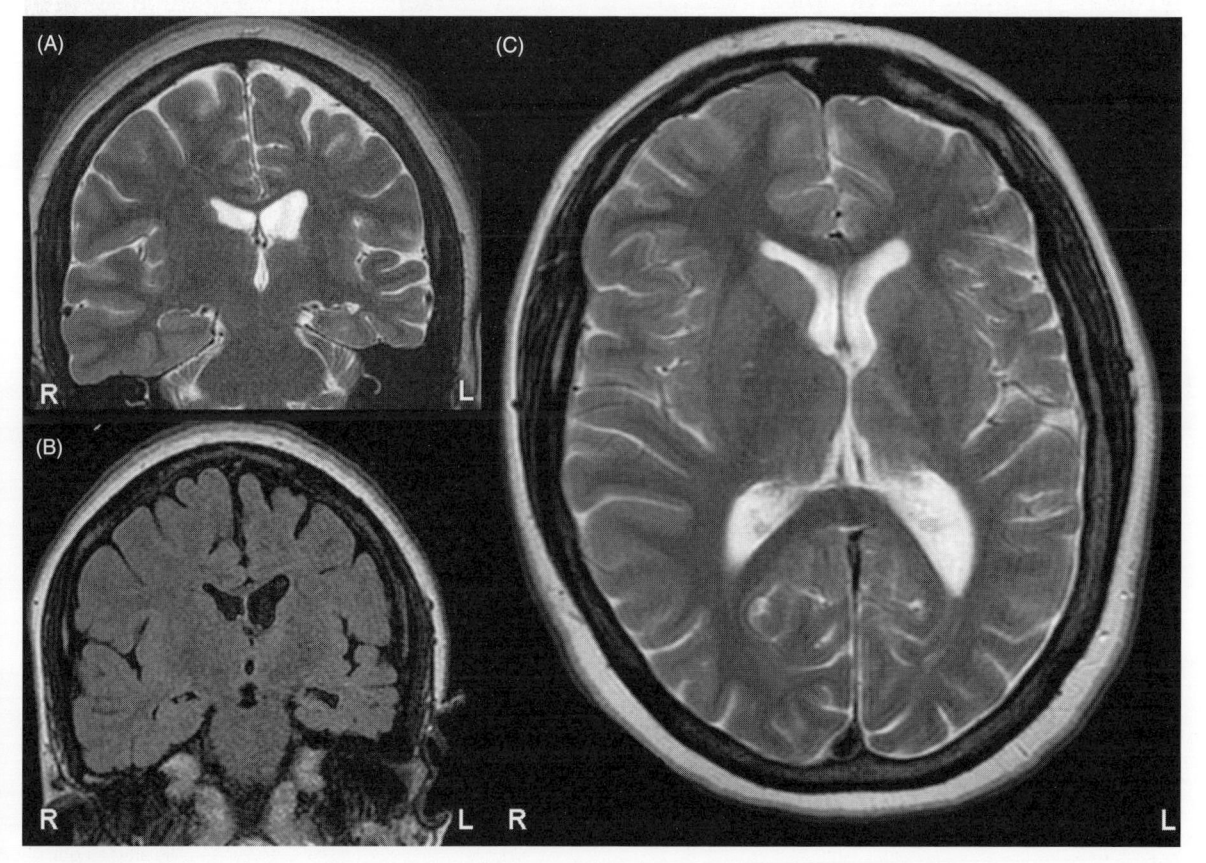

Figure 36.7. Left hemisphere atrophy in a patient with hemiconvulsion, hemiplegia, epilepsy (HHE) syndrome.

229

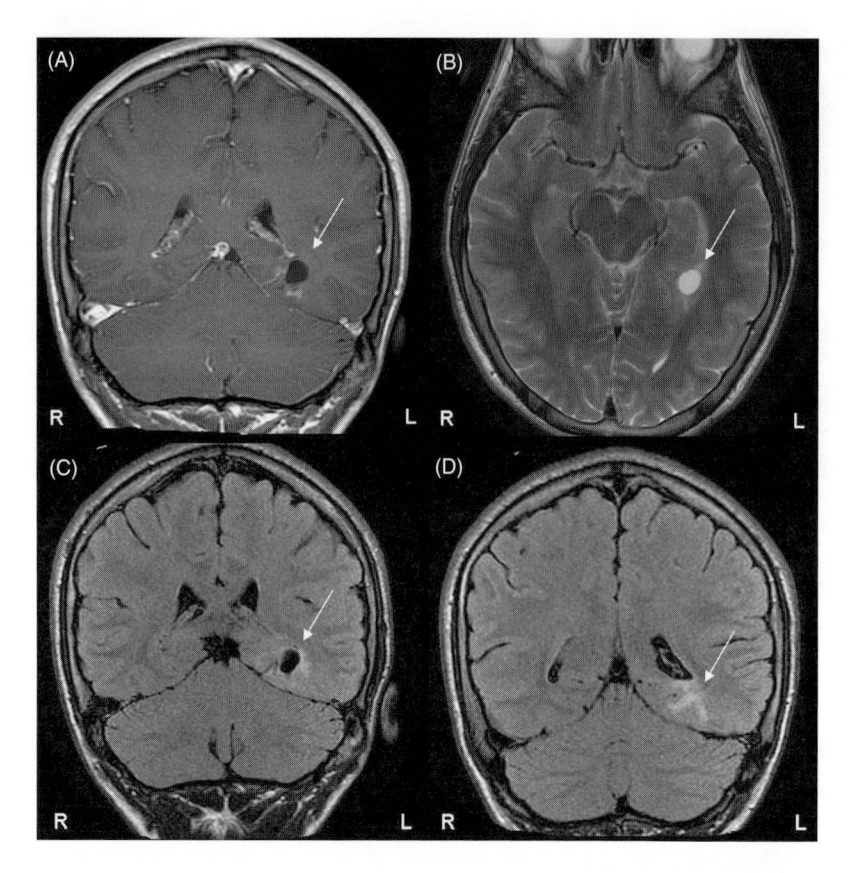

Section 2: Classification and diagnosis of epilepsy

Figure 36.8. Temporal tumour.

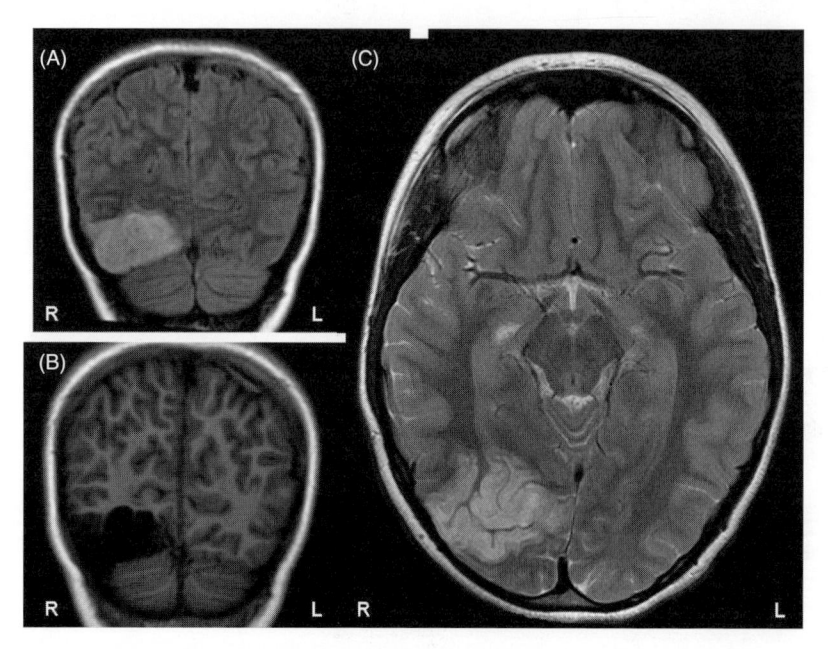

Figure 36.9. Right occipital dysembryoplastic neuroepithelial tumour.

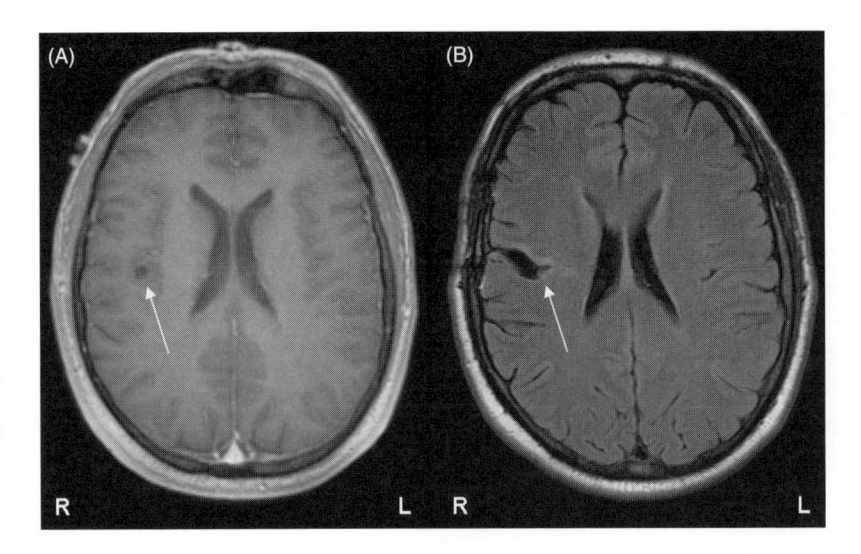

Chapter 36: The role of structural imaging in the assessment of epilepsy

Figure 36.10. Right dysembryoplastic neuroepithelial tumour (A). Patient became seizure-free after lesionectomy (B).

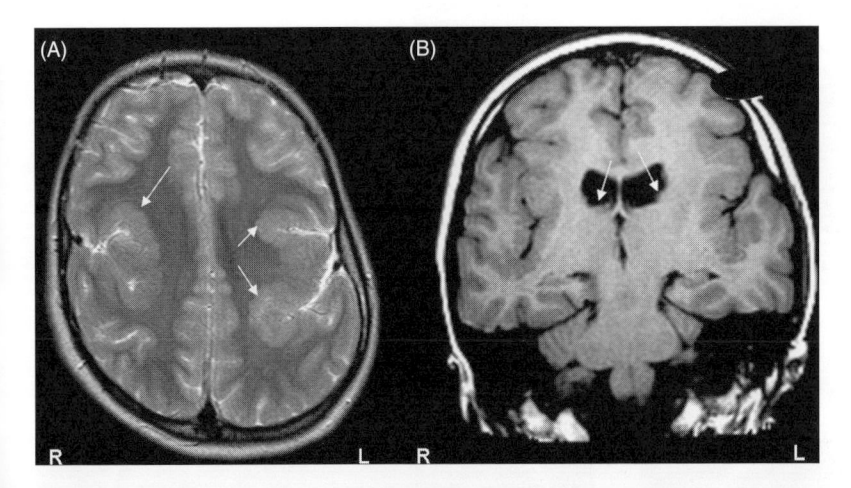

Figure 36.11. Bilateral perisylvian polymicrogiria (arrows in A) and periventricular heterotopia (arrows in B).

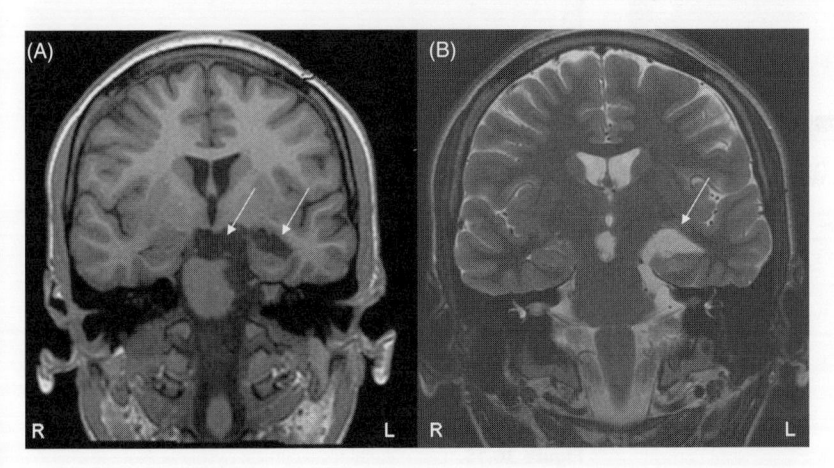

Figure 36.12. Epidermoid affecting medial temporal and brainstem structures.

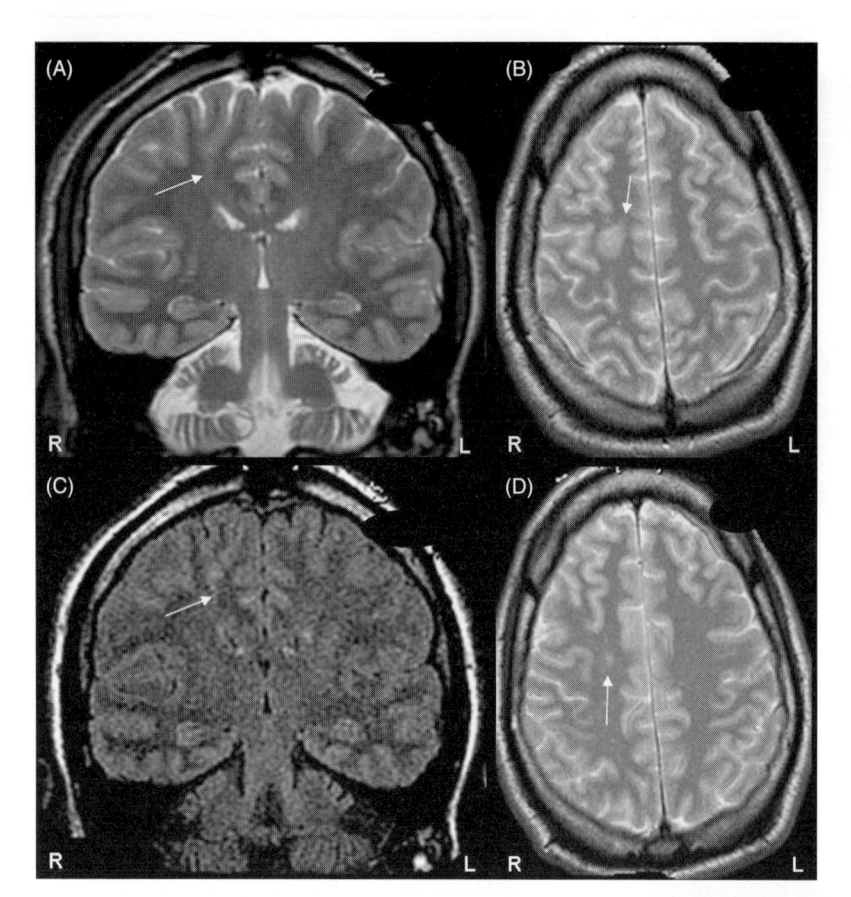

Figure 36.13. Right frontal focal cortical dysplasia. Note subtle tracks of grey matter across white matter (arrows). Note a degree of cerebellar atrophy, possibly due to chronic phenytoin treatment.

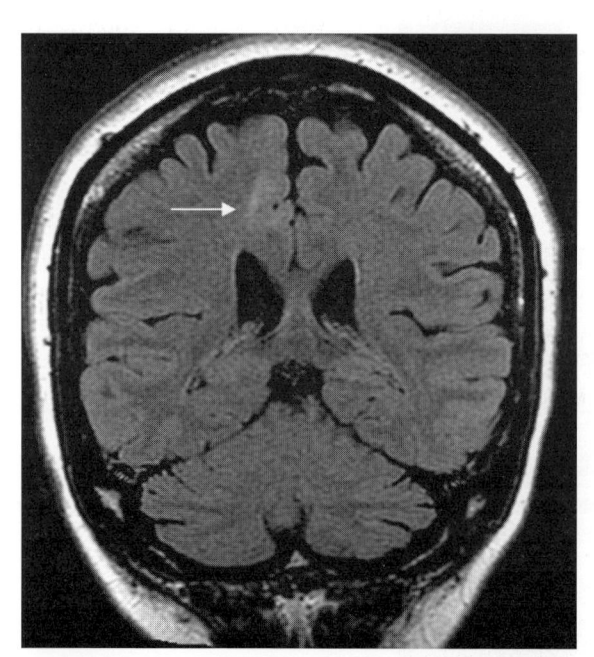

Figure 36.14. Right frontal focal cortical dysplasia. Note cortical thickening and increased signal in the right medial frontal region.

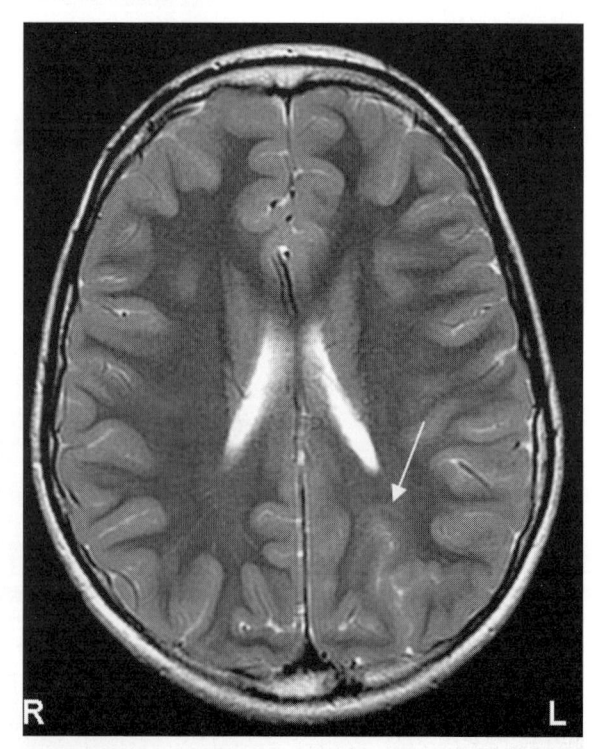

Figure 36.15. Left parietal focal cortical dysplasia. Note thickened gyrus surrounded by linear halo (arrow).

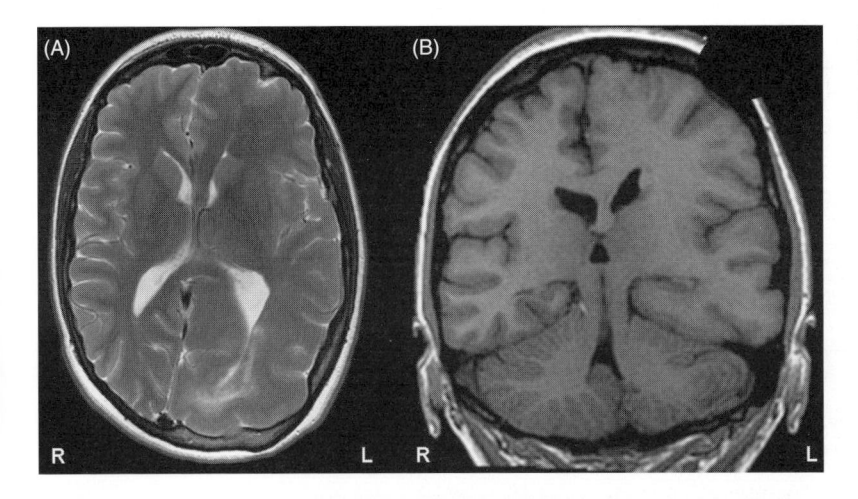

Chapter 36: The role of structural imaging in the assessment of epilepsy

Figure 36.16. Left hemimegalencephaly. Note enlarged left hemisphere with widespread dysplasia, pachygyria and white matter gliosis.

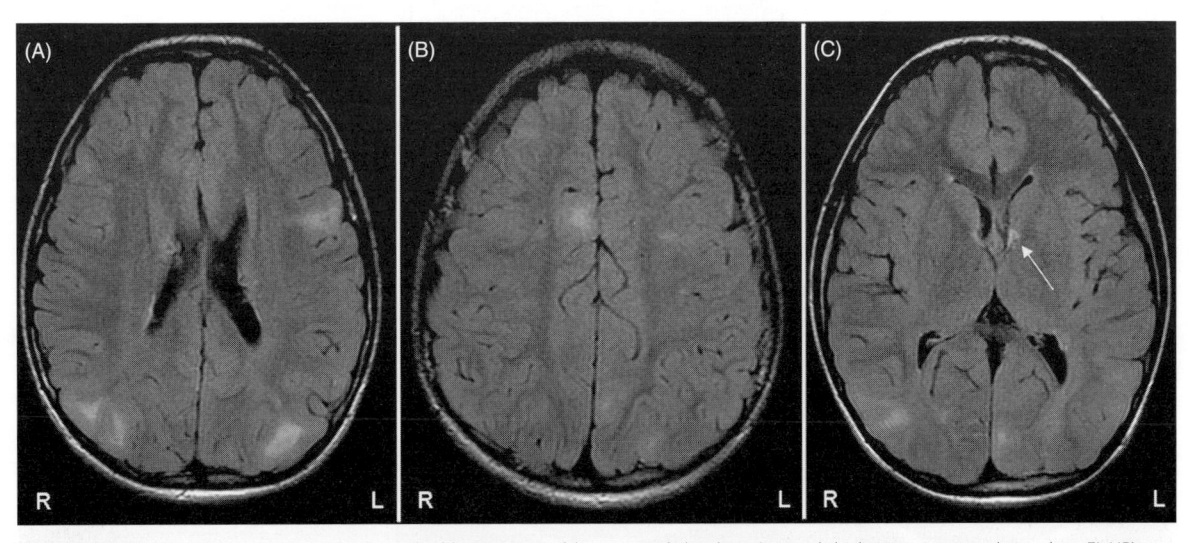

Figure 36.17. Tuberous sclerosis. Multiple cortical lesions resembling cortical dysplasia (cortical thickening, increased signal on FLAIR) and a periventricular tumour (arrow).

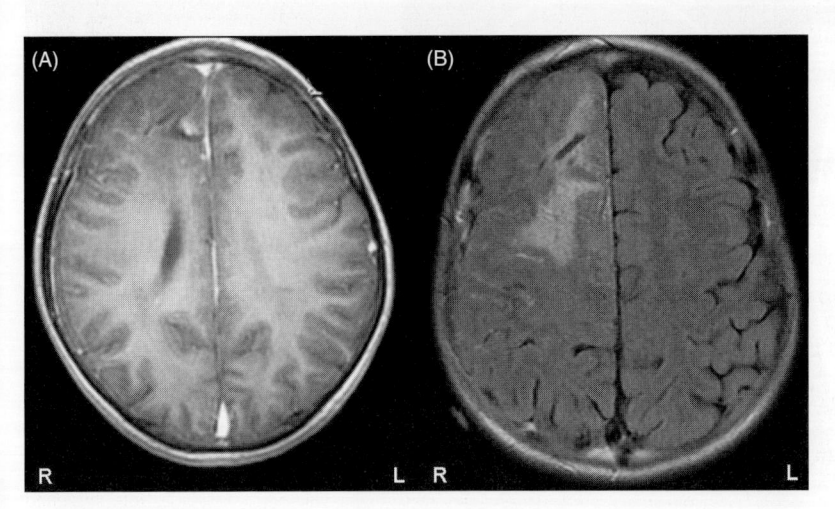

Figure 36.18. Frontal vasculitis.

233

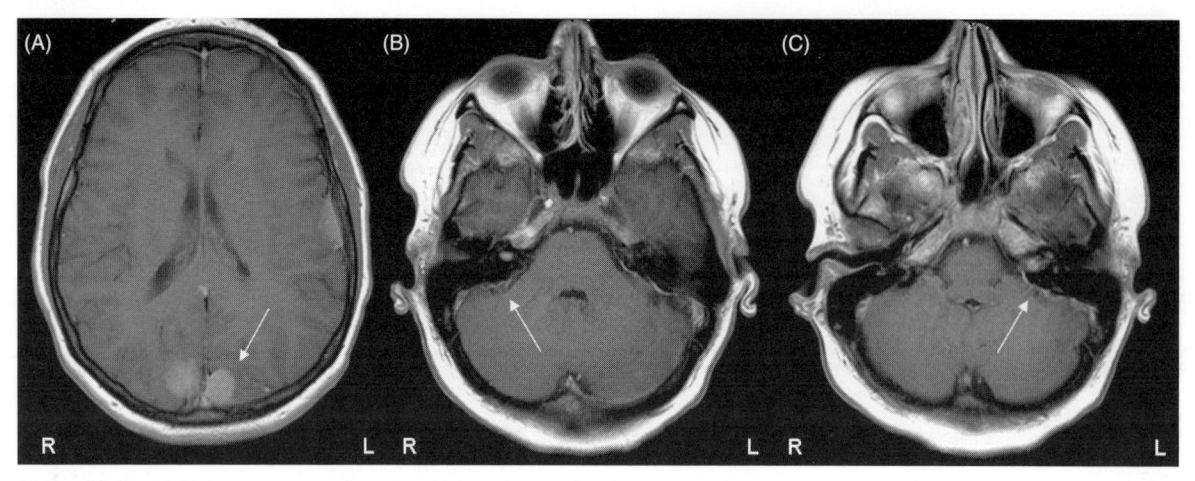

Section 2: Classification and diagnosis of epilepsy

Figure 36.19. Multiple meningiomas (arrow) and bilateral internal auditory meatus lesions in a patient with neurofibromatosis is type II.

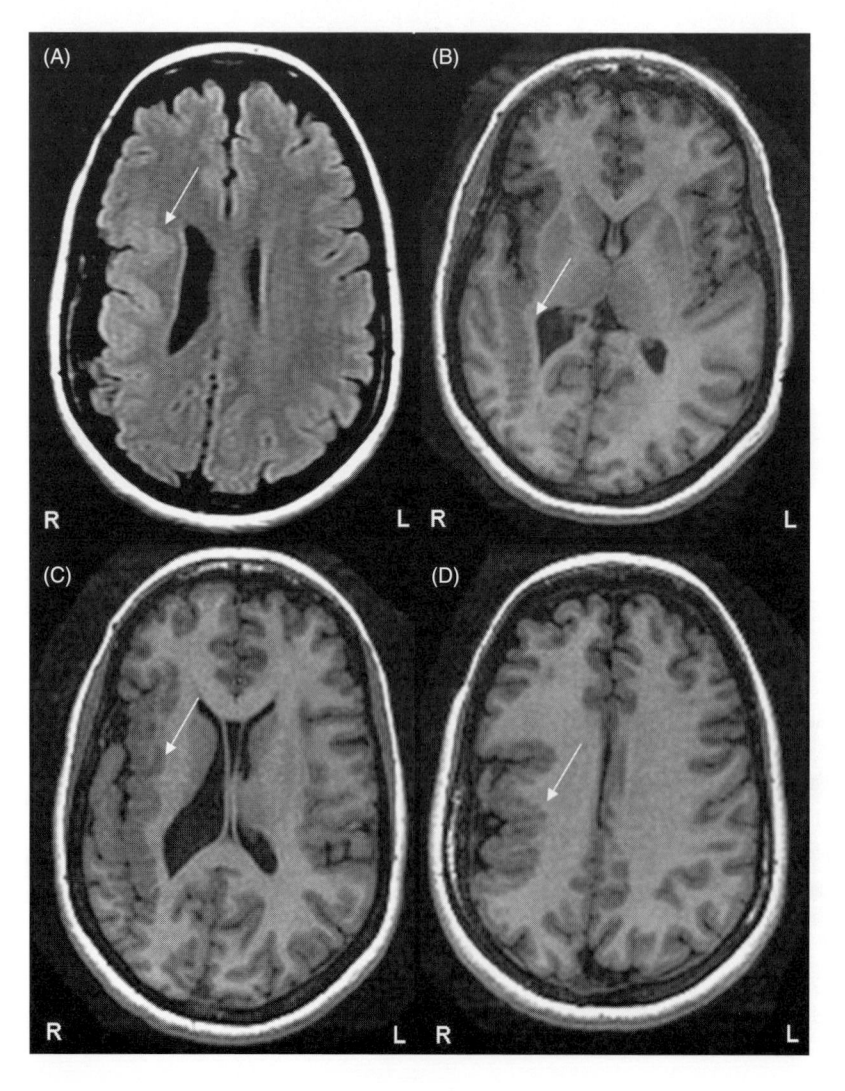

Figure 36.20. Patient with bilateral perisylvian polymicrogyria with extensive polymicrogyria, particularly on the right.

Chapter 36: The role of structural imaging in the assessment of epilepsy

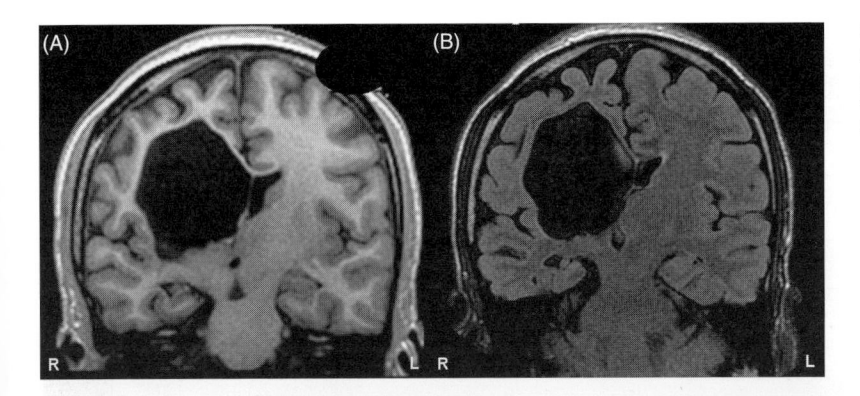

Figure 36.21. Large right hemisphere cyst and right hippocampal sclerosis. The patient had right temporal lobe seizures and became seizure-free following a right temporal lobectomy.

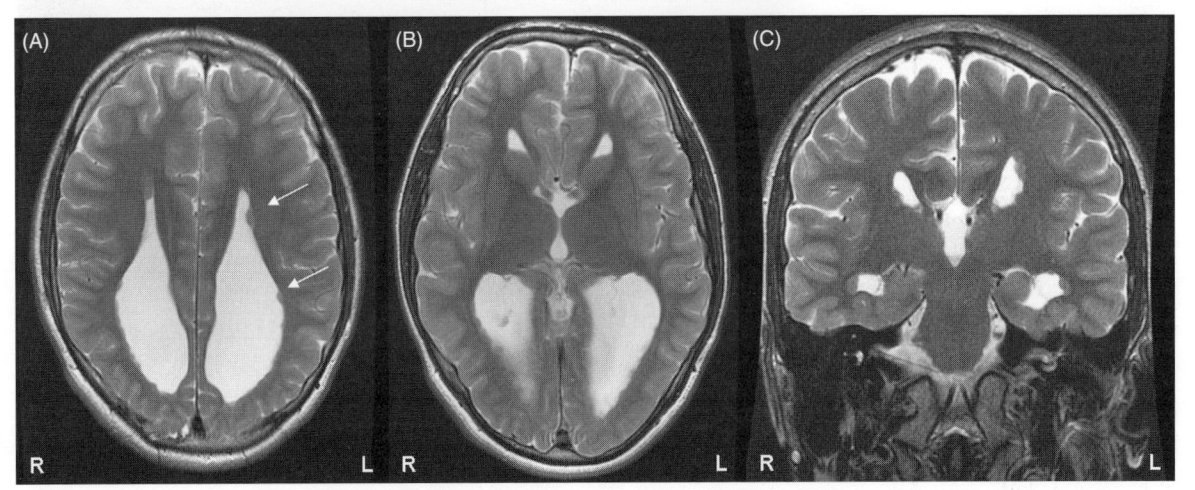

Figure 36.22. Multiple subependymal nodules (arrows) and agenesia of corpus callosum.

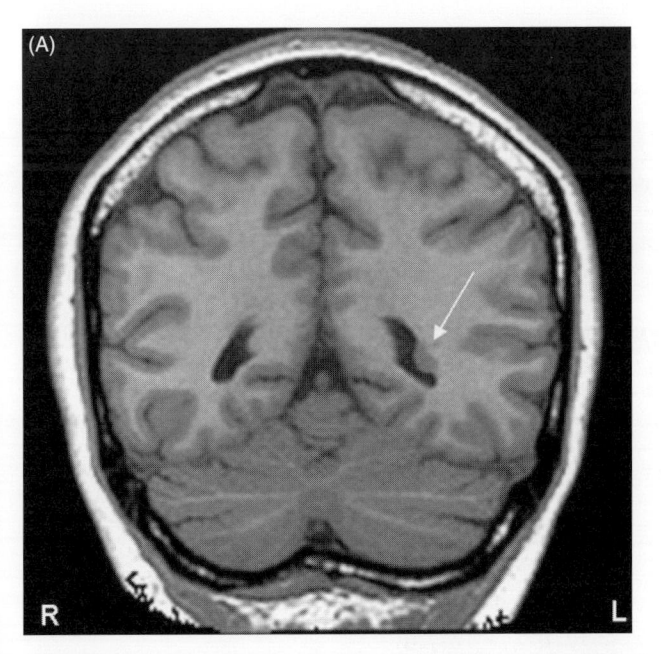

Figure 36.23. Single subependymal nodule in the left lateral ventricle with abnormality in the adjacent white matter.

235

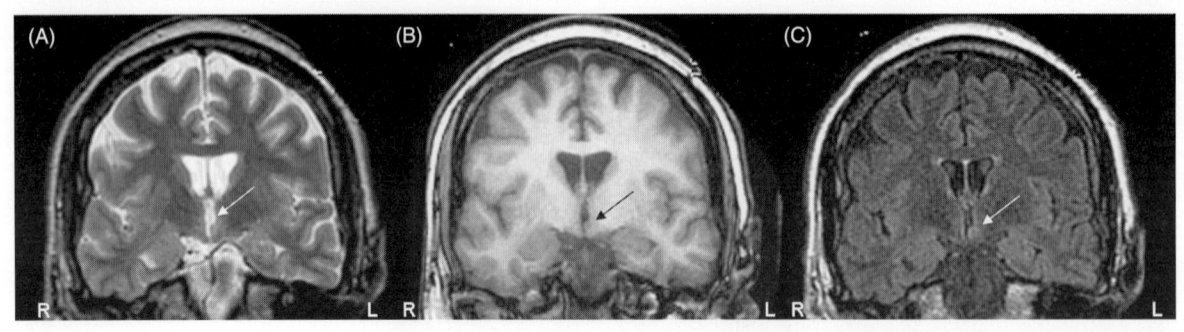

Figure 36.24. Hypothalamic hamartoma (arrow).

Figures 36.1 to 36.24 show examples of structural abnormalities identified on MRI images. Summarized descriptions of changes seen for a variety of pathologies can be seen in the recommended reading below.

Conclusion

MRI is the modality of choice for first-line imaging in epilepsy. Imaging needs to be optimized as there is a wide range of pathology which is often subtle. Hippocampal sclerosis and focal cortical dysplasia are the most common findings in the UK.

Recommended reading

The role of neuroimaging. In Alarcón G, Nashef L, Cross H, Nightingale J, Richardson S, eds. *Epilepsy*, pp. 166–84. *Oxford Specialist Handbooks in Neurology*. Oxford: Oxford University Press; 2009.

Kuzniecky RI, Jackson GD. *Magnetic Resonance in Epilepsy*. 2nd edn. New York: Raven Press; 2005.

Sartor K, Haehnel S, Kress B. *Brain Imaging*, New York: Thieme; 2008.

Learning objectives

(1) To understand the basic indications of CT and MRI.
(2) To know the basic MRI sequences.
(3) To be able to identify clear pathology on MRI images.

Section 2 Classification and diagnosis of epilepsy

Chapter 37

Indications for neuroradiological investigation of epilepsy

Mark P. Richardson

Neuroimaging in epilepsy has a long history, beginning with CT in the 1970s, and advancing rapidly with PET, SPECT and MRI over the next decades. Neuroimaging may be carried out for a number of different reasons: (1) to determine an underlying aetiology especially in newly diagnosed epilepsy, but also in insufficiently investigated chronic epilepsy; (2) to identify factors associated with failure to respond to AEDs, or an unexpected deterioration in seizure control; and (3) as part of detailed evaluation prior to epilepsy surgery.

The ILAE Neuroimaging Commission provided broad guidelines for the neuroimaging investigation of epilepsy in 1997 (ILAE Neuroimaging Commission, 1997). In particular, it was recommended that MRI should be the technique of choice (rather than CT) except in specific emergency situations or if there are contraindications to MRI. It was recommended that neuroimaging should be carried out in all epilepsy patients, except for those with IGE, in the following situations:

- evidence from clinical history or EEG of a focal onset of seizures at any age
- unclassified or apparently generalized seizures beginning in the early years of life or in adulthood
- evidence of a focal fixed deficit on neurological or neuropsychological examination
- difficulty controlling seizures with first-line antiepileptic drugs
- loss of control of seizures with antiepileptic drugs or a change in pattern of seizures, which may imply a progressive underlying lesion.

More recently, the National Institute for Health and Clinical Excellence in the UK published comprehensive guidelines and an evidence review on the management of epilepsy (Stokes *et al.*, 2004). Although a few more years experience with MRI in epilepsy had accumulated, the recommendations were similar. In summary, it was recommended that neuroimaging should be used to identify structural abnormalities that cause certain epilepsies, and that MRI should be the imaging investigation of choice. It was emphasized that MRI is particularly important in those who develop epilepsy before the age of 2 years or in adulthood; in those who have any suggestion of a focal onset on history, examination or EEG (unless there is clear evidence of a benign focal epilepsy syndrome); and if seizures continue in spite of first-line medication. Recognizing that in some instances the underlying diagnosis of recent-onset seizures could be rapidly progressive and potentially life-threatening, it was recommended that individuals requiring MRI should have the test performed soon. These guidelines suggested that neuroimaging need not be routinely requested when a diagnosis of idiopathic generalized epilepsy has been made. The specific role of CT was emphasized: CT should be used to identify underlying gross pathology if MRI is not available or is contraindicated; for children in whom a general anaesthetic or sedation would be required for MRI but not CT; and in an acute situation, CT may be used to determine whether a seizure has been caused by an acute neurological lesion or illness.

New-onset seizures

On first encounter with a person having recent-onset seizures, it may be difficult to be certain whether these are acute symptomatic seizures or the beginning of epilepsy. Furthermore, it is not always possible to assign the patient to a specific epilepsy syndrome immediately. Hence, a pragmatic approach is to arrange neuroimaging for every person with new-onset seizures, unless it is unequivocally clear that the presentation is absolutely typical of benign focal epilepsy or IGE (taking account of all of the syndromic features expected, including age of onset). The imaging modality should be MRI unless there is a specific contraindication. If the contraindication relates to an acute situation, CT should be carried out as urgently as indicated, and MRI should usually be undertaken subsequently once the person is well enough (assuming no other contraindications). Contraindications to MRI will be very familiar to the staff of an MRI unit, and include metallic objects fixed to or within the person, devices, prostheses, body piercings and some cosmetics and tattoos. Many more recent medical devices and prostheses have been carefully designed to be safe in MRI, but this should be specifically confirmed for the device in question, the scanner field strength and the imaging technique to be used.

Pohlmann-Eden and Newton recently reviewed the findings of neuroimaging in new-onset seizures (Pohlmann-Eden and Newton, 2008). The most frequent findings in adults are stroke, brain tumour and neurodegenerative conditions. Hippocampal sclerosis, malformations of cortical development, cavernous angiomas, cortical scars and small benign developmental tumours are less frequent in people with new-onset seizures, but may be seen more frequently in children with new-onset seizures than in adults. Some studies of new-onset seizures find very high rates of structural abnormality on neuroimaging (>50% of people scanned in some studies) whereas other studies find fewer than 10% have abnormalities. This range probably reflects rather different groups in these studies, some being selected from specialist hospital case-series and others from community series. It is notable that studies that have compared MRI with CT have found that even highly sigificant major abnormalities such as malignant brain tumours may be missed with CT but detected with MRI.

Chronic epilepsy

Neuroimaging has a role in the initial diagnostic process for recent-onset seizures, but may often by needed also in chronic epilepsy. Failure to respond to AEDs may indicate an underlying brain abnormality which has not been identified, and which may require treatment on its own merits – for example, a progressive brain tumour, or a focal lesion such as hippocampal sclerosis. Failure to respond to AEDs may also suggest the need to consider epilepsy surgery (evaluation for surgery will always require detailed neuroimaging in a unit experienced in evaluating neuroimaging in epilepsy).

MRI may identify obvious lesions (e.g. hippocampal sclerosis, focal cortical malformations, small tumours such as dysembryoplastic neuroepithelial tumour, cavernous angioma, arteriovenous malformation, malformations of cortical development), but abnormalities can be subtle. In order to detect focal abnormalities, it may be necessary to carry out specific imaging sequences, or to undertake various measurements. The most frequently implemented procedure in this setting is quantitative evaluation of the hippocampus in people suspected to have medial temporal lobe epilepsy. Measurement of T2 relaxation time in the hippocampus, and measurement of hippocampal volume, may allow detection of an abnormality that has escaped visual inspection.

PET and SPECT may be valuable additional investigations in chronic focal epilepsy as part of presurgical evaluation. 18-F fluorodeoxyglucose PET may show regions of reduced glucose uptake in and around the seizure-onset region even in patients whose structural MRI has been entirely normal. Such regions of hypometabolism may then become a target for intracranial EEG evaluation. SPECT can be used to create an image of cerebral blood flow: if the radiotracer is injected during a seizure while the patient is being monitored, an image can be taken after the patient has recovered from the seizure. This ictal SPECT image can be compared with an interictal image taken at a time remote from any seizure to identify brain regions that had an ictal blood flow increase. These regions may also become targets for intracranial EEG evaluation.

Recommended reading

Duncan JS. Imaging and epilepsy. *Brain* 1997; **120**:339–77.

Richardson MP. Epilepsy and surgical mapping. *Br Med Bull* 2003;**65**:179–92.

Richardson MP. Current themes in neuroimaging of epilepsy: brain networks, dynamic phenomena, and clinical relevance. *Clin Neurophysiol* 2010; **121**:1153–75.

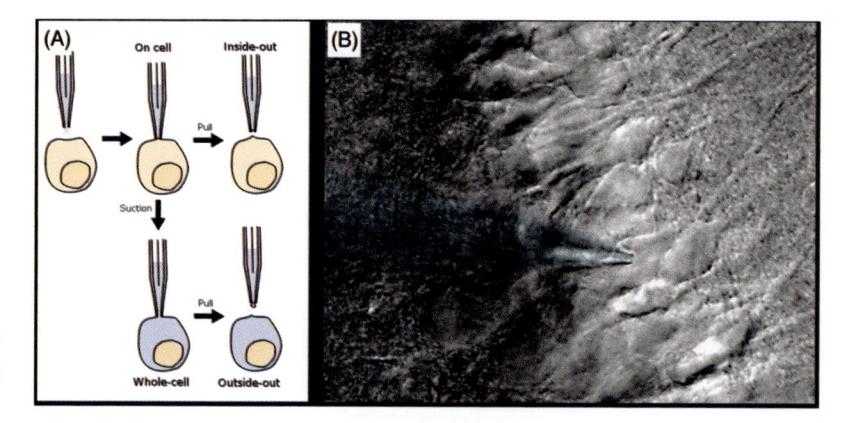

Figure 6.1. (A) Diagram showing different variations of the patch clamp; (B) whole cell recording of a hippocampal neuron. The micropipette in the photograph has been shaded with a blue hue (from Wikipedia).

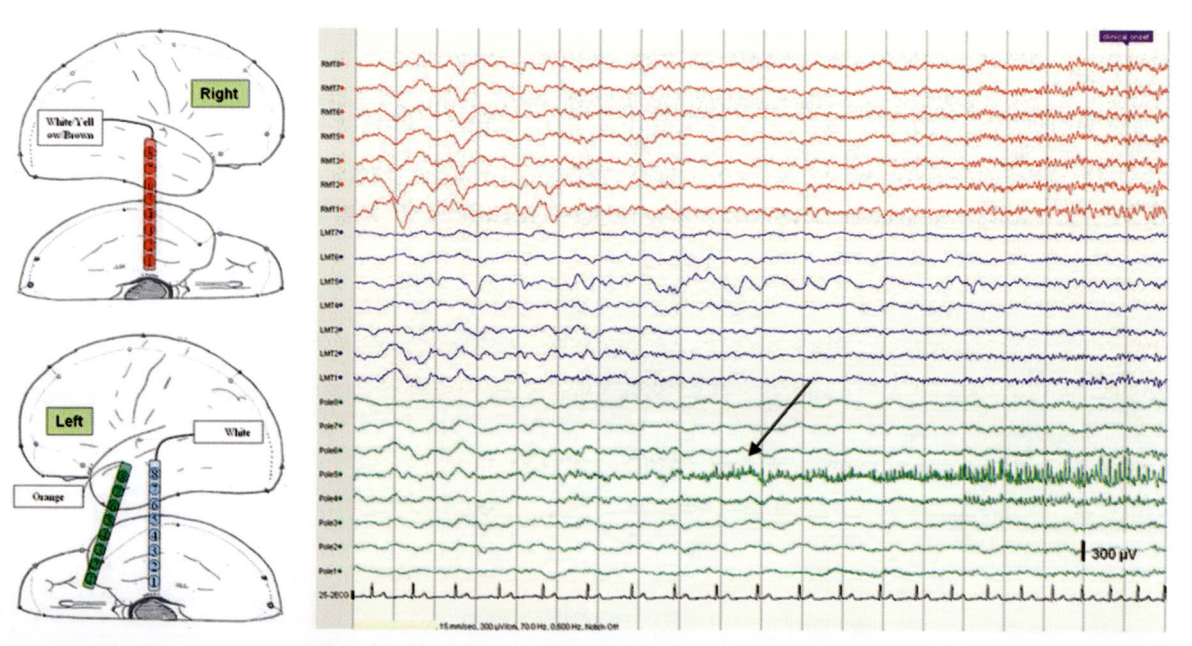

Figure 12.1. Onset of a focal seizure recorded with intracranial subtemporal strips. Note a widespread attenuation of the background activity occurring as rhythmic sharp spike activity occurs at contact 5 of the polar strip.

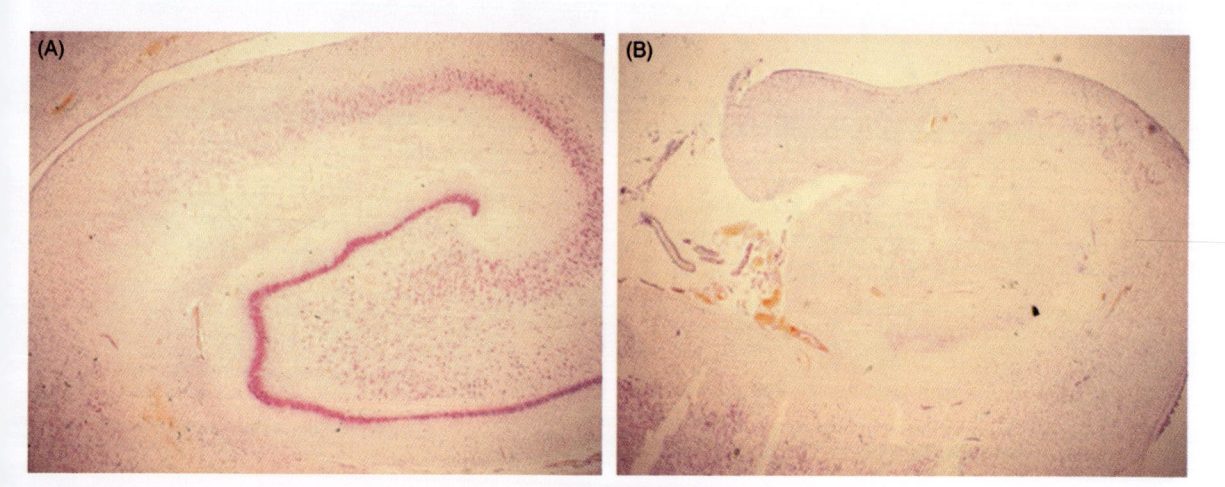

Figure 13.2. Normal hippocampus (A) and severe hippocampal sclerosis (B).

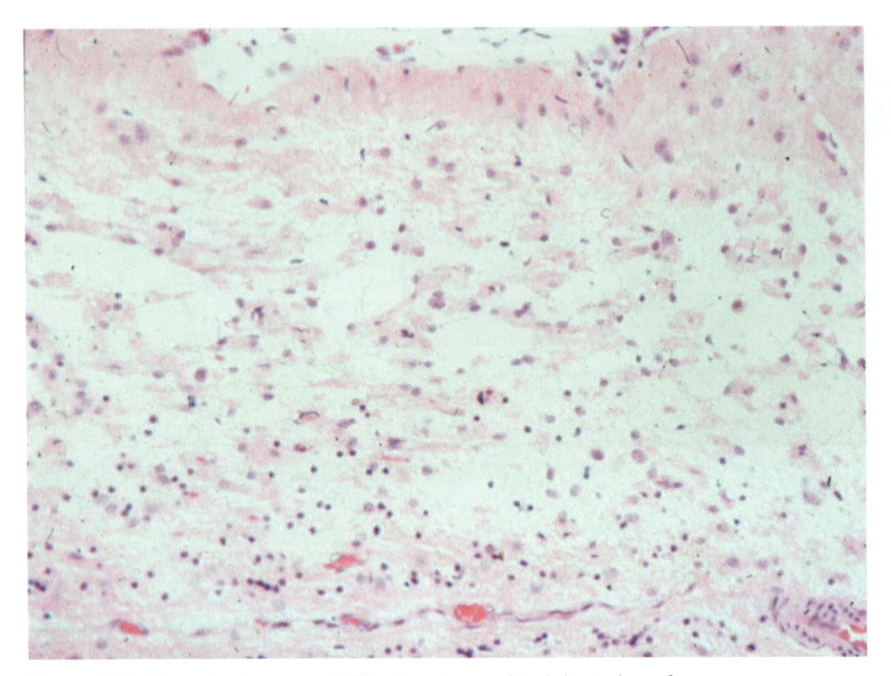

Figure 13.3. Severe laminar necrosis. The tissue is vacuolated due to loss of neurons.

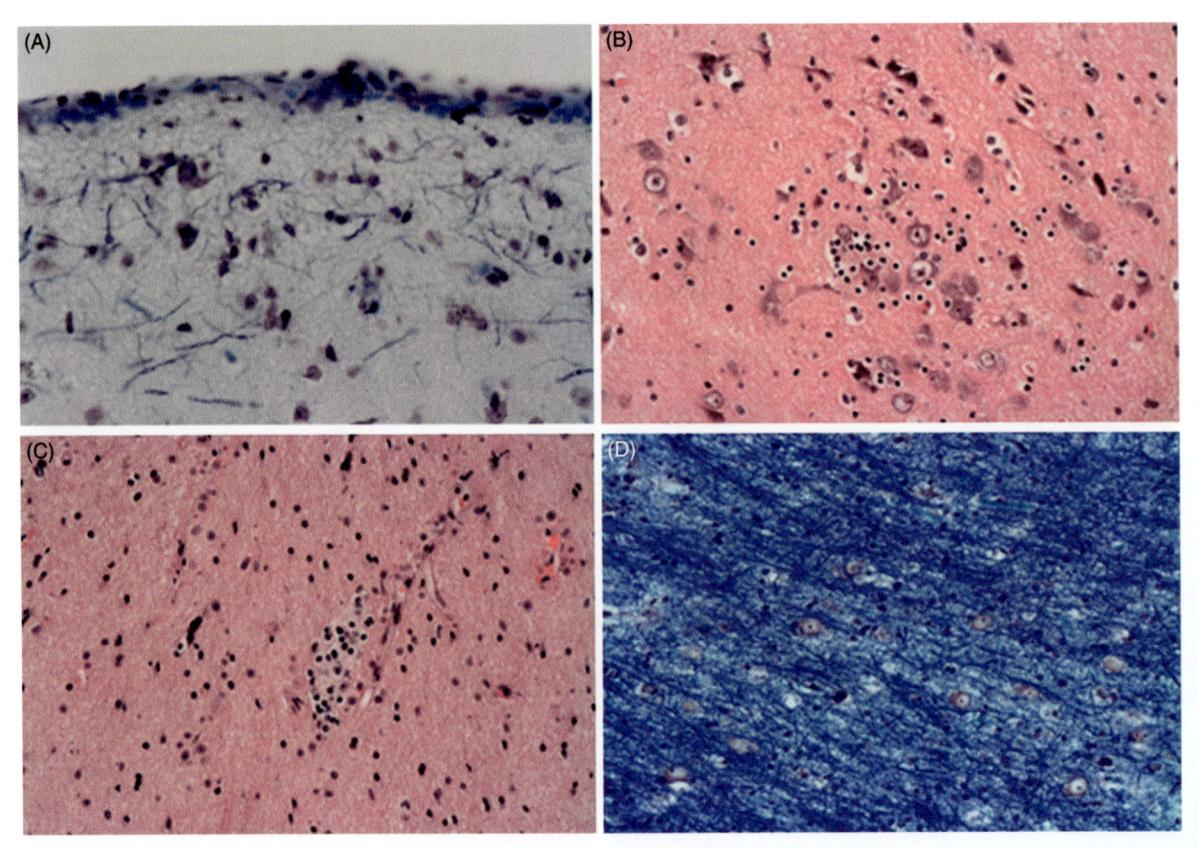

Figure 13.6. MCD. (A) Ectopic neurons and myelinated subpial axons. (B, C) Clusters of immature neurons in the cortex and white matter. (D) Heterotopic neurons in white matter.

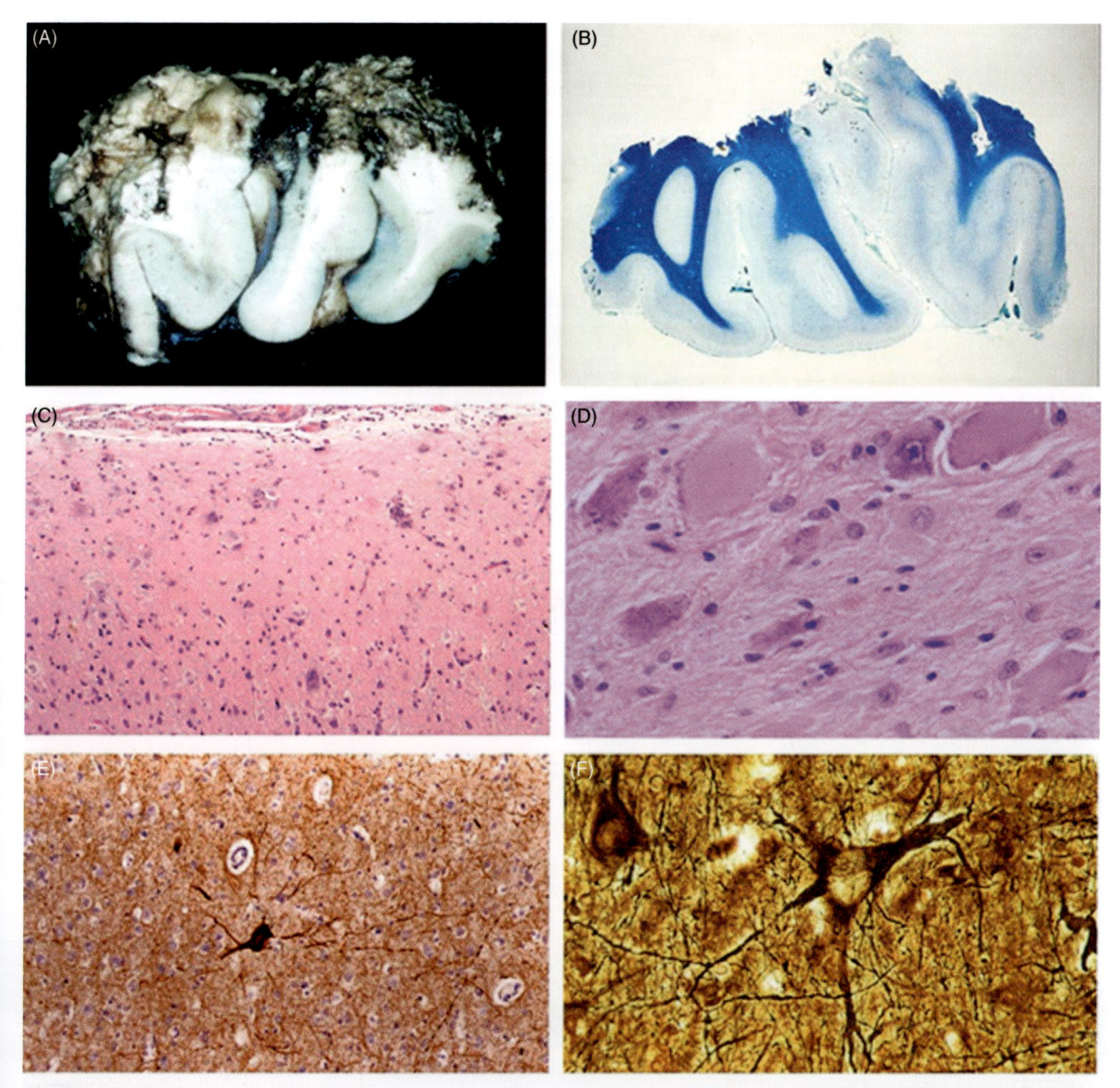

Figure 13.7. FCD type IIB. (A, B) Blurred grey–white matter border in temporal lobectomy specimen (B: LFB/Nissl). (C, D) Abnormal lamination with dysmorphic neurons and balloon cells. Neurofilament (E) and silver stain (F) highlights abnormally oriented neurites in the dysmorphic neurons.

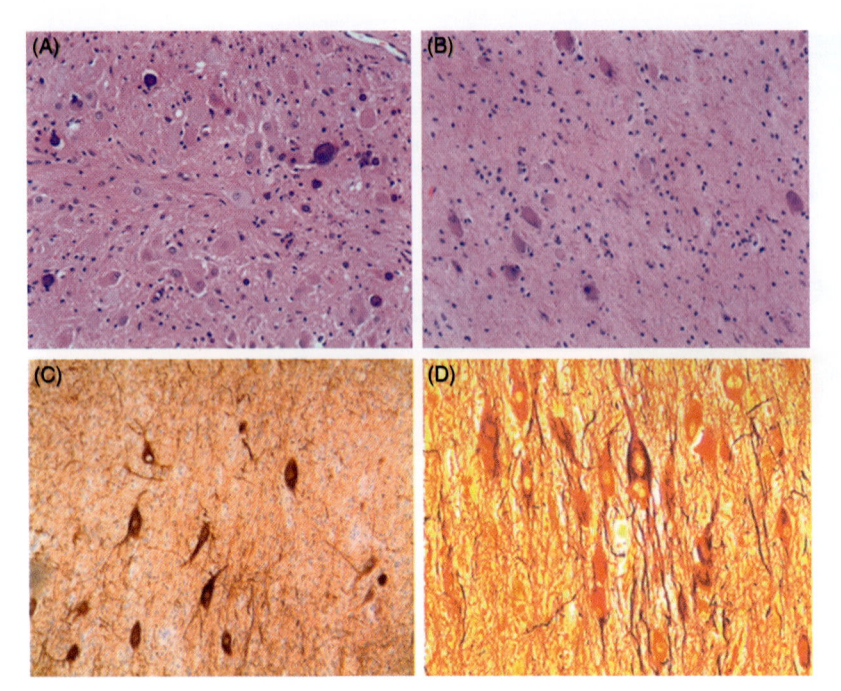

Figure 13.8. Cortical tuber. (A, B) Giant dysmorphic neurons and balloon cells similar to FCD type IIB. Calcification is also noted (A). Neurofilament (C) and silver stain (D) highlights abnormally oriented neurites in the giant neurons.

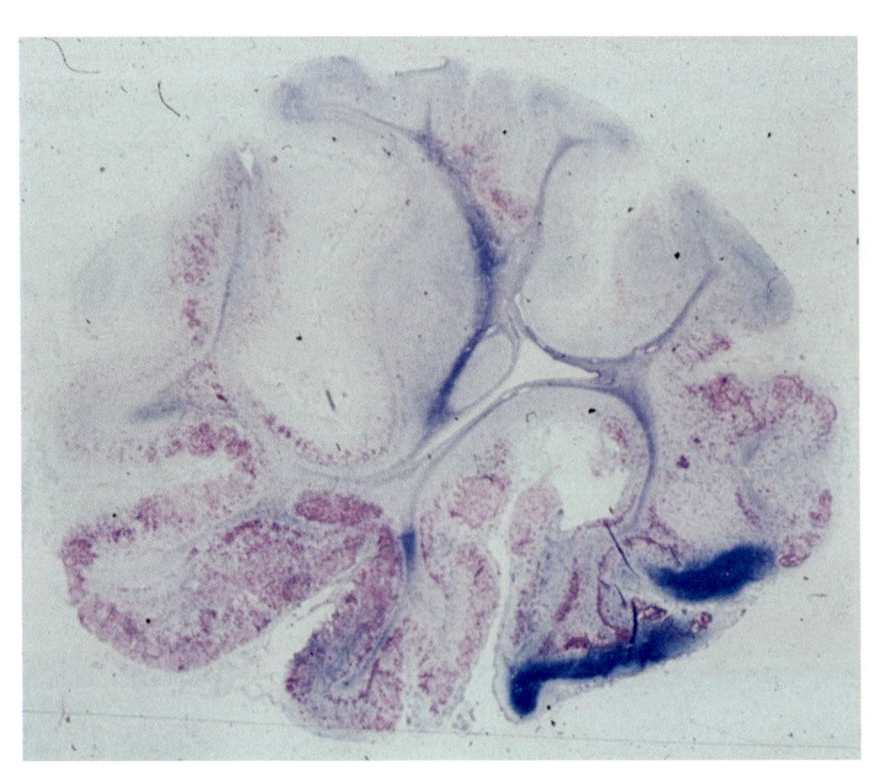

Figure 13.10. Sturge-Weber syndrome. Extensive calcified leptomeningeal deposits.

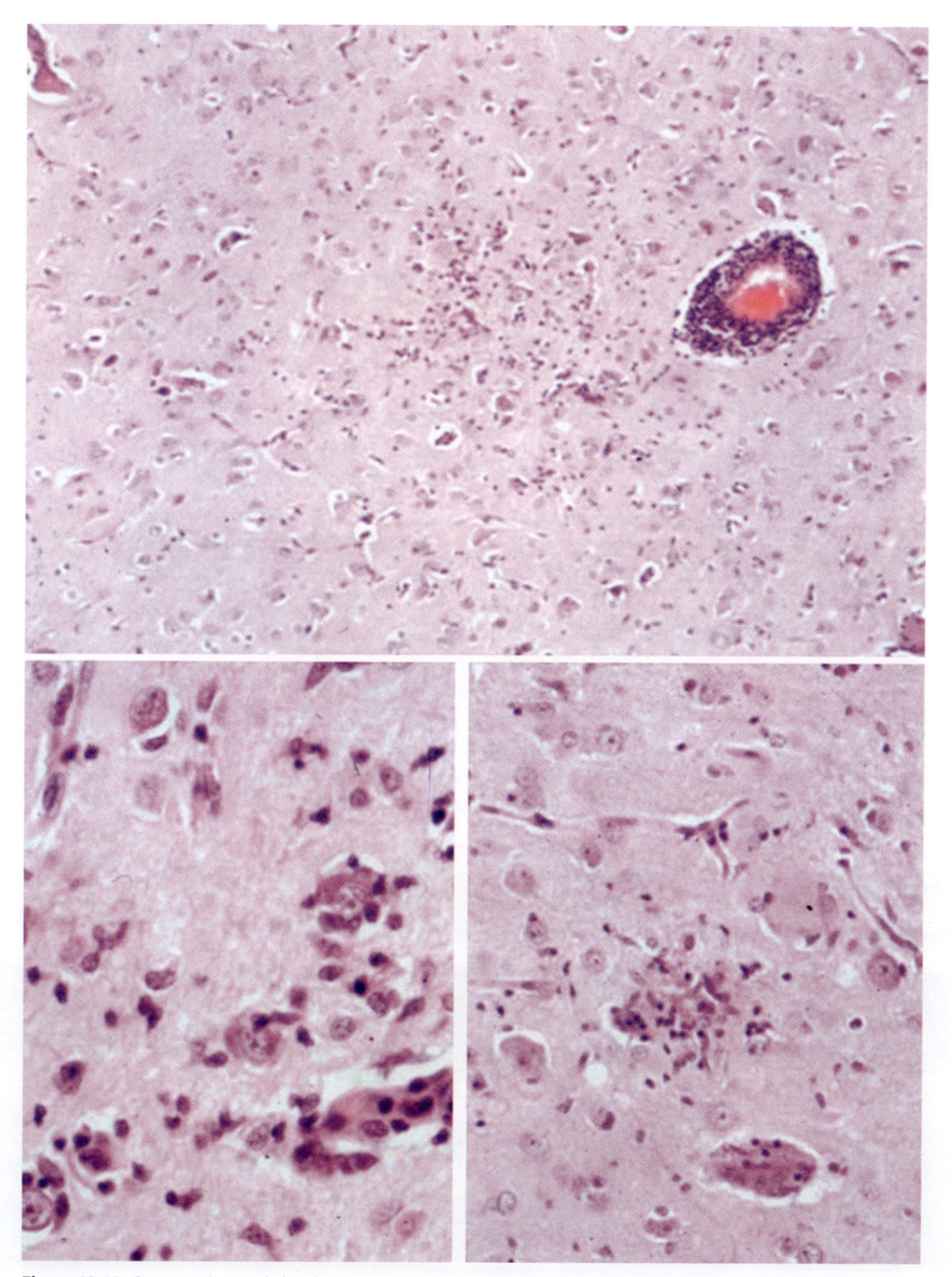

Figure 13.11. Rasmussen's encephalitis showing perivascular lymphocytic inflammation, neuronophagia and microglial nodules.

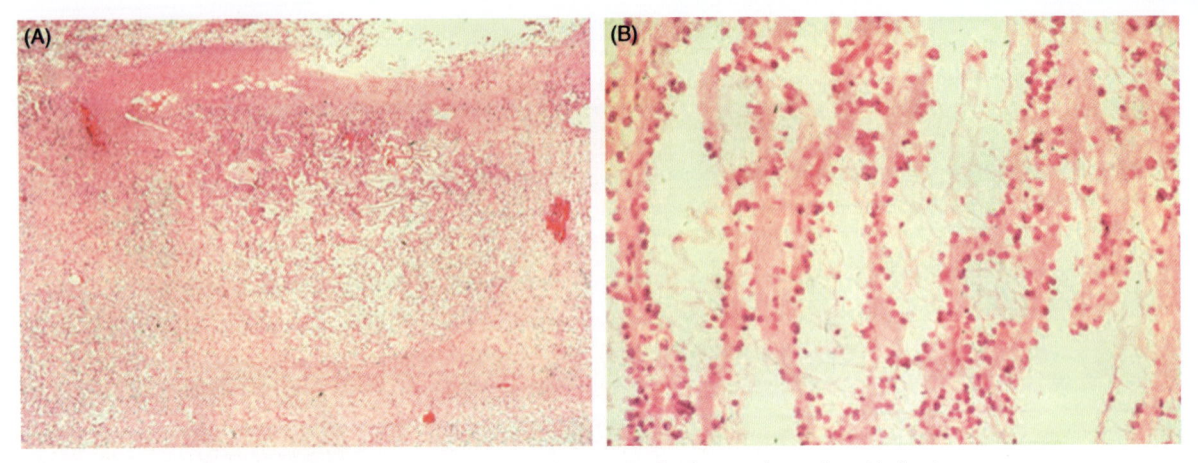

Figure 13.12. DNT. (A) Multinodular intracortical tumour nodules. (B) Specific glio-neural complex with floating neurons.

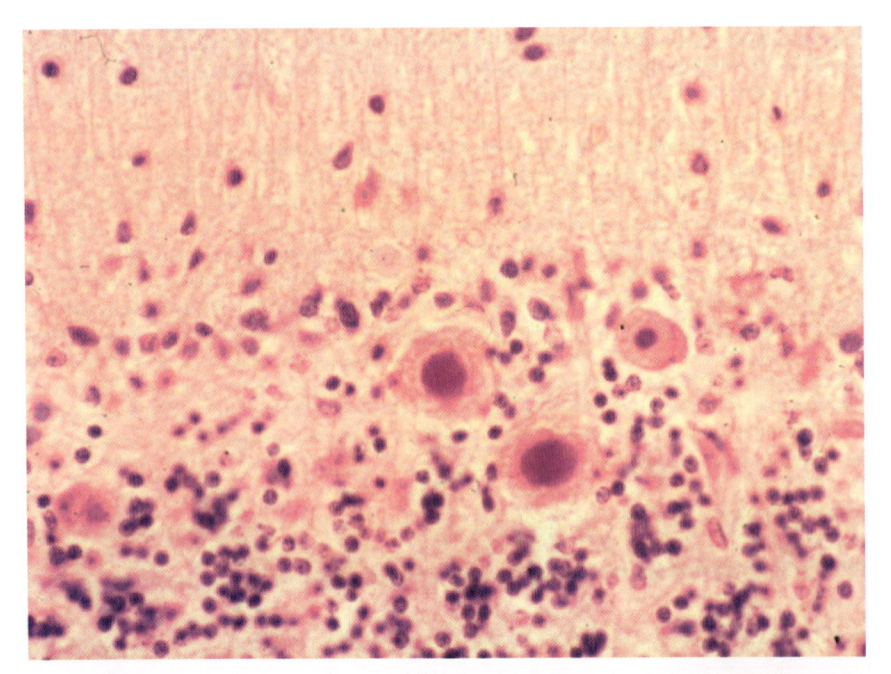

Figure 13.13. Lafora bodies in cerebellum (PAS).

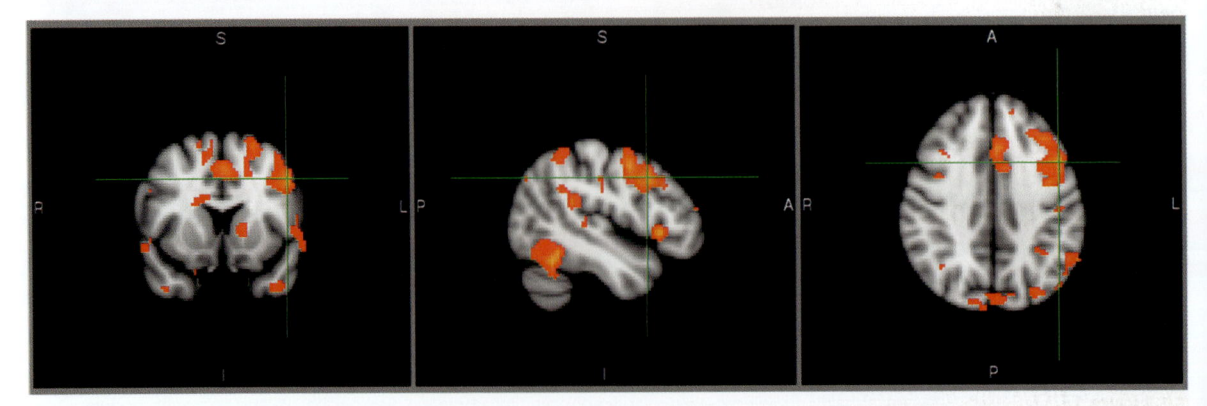

Figure 39.1. A language fMRI study carried out in a patient at King's College Hospital. This patient with frontal lobe epilepsy undertook a 'verbal fluency' task during scanning; this involves silently thinking of as many words as possible beginning with a specified letter. In this case, a normal pattern of left-dominant language activation is seen (red-orange-yellow blobs denote regions significantly active during the task compared with a control condition; brighter yellow indicates stronger activity; R, right; L, left; A, anterior; P, posterior). With thanks to Dr Jonathan O'Muircheartaigh.

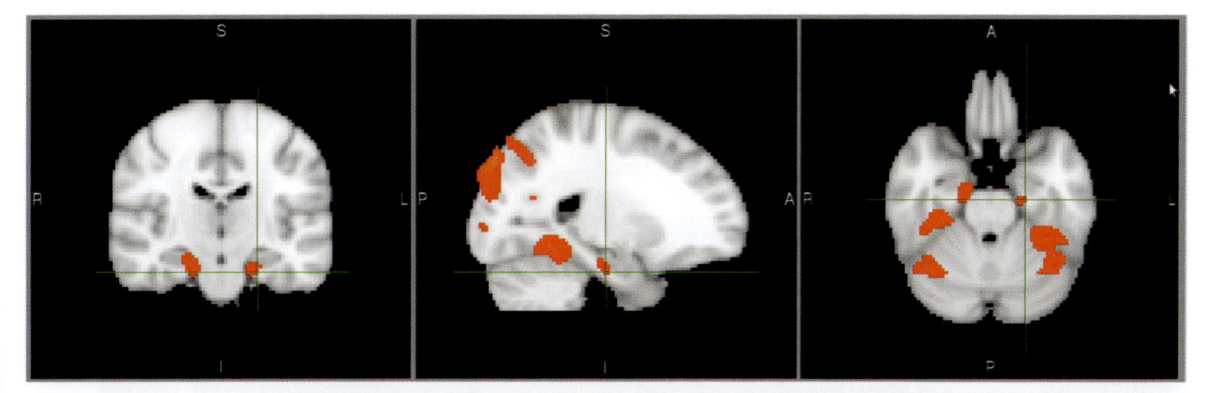

Figure 39.2. A memory fMRI study carried out in a patient at King's College Hospital. This patient with temporal lobe epilepsy undertook a task requiring memorization of a series of pictures. In this case, a bilateral pattern of activity in the mesial temporal lobes was seen, as well as activity more posteriorly in neocortex (red-orange-yellow blobs denote regions significantly active during the task compared with a control condition; brighter yellow indicates stronger activity; R, right; L, left; A, anterior; P, posterior). With thanks to Dr Karren Towgood.

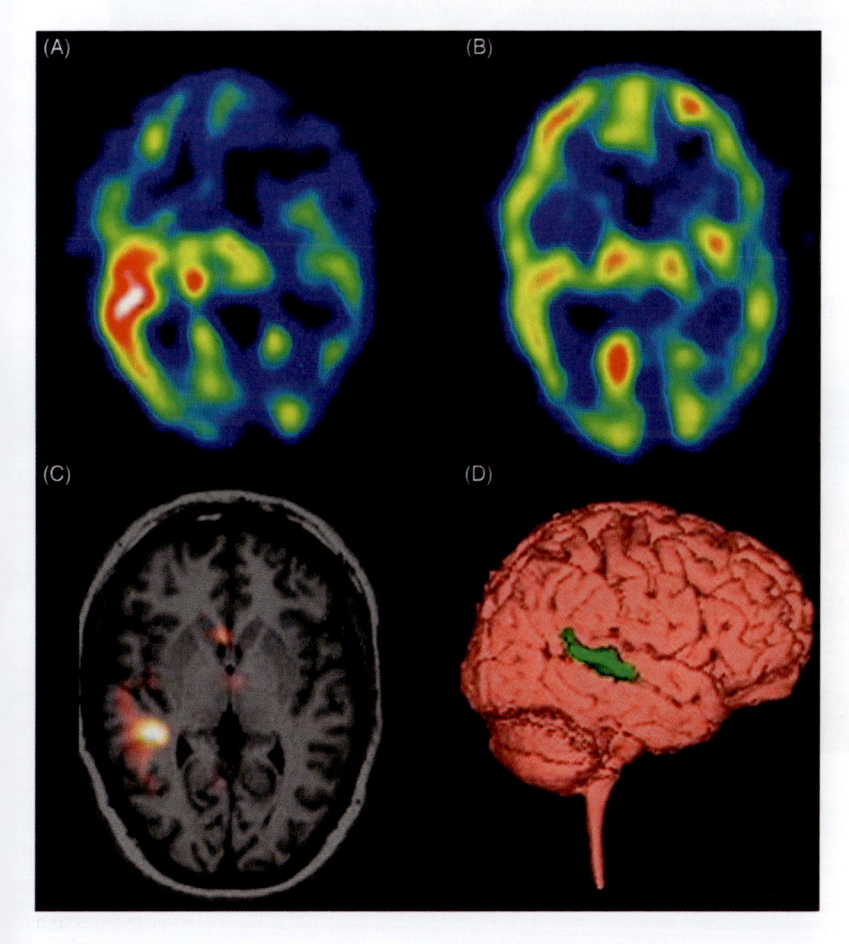

Figure 40.1. Twenty-eight-year-old female patient with refractory complex partial seizures. Semiology included a stereotypic melody followed by altered awareness. MRI was non lesional. Axial ictal SPECT (A) showed a right temporolateral hyperperfusion (red) compared to the interictal SPECT (B). SISCOM in the axial (C) and lateral 3D rendering (D) shows significant (>2 SD) hyperperfusion in the posterior part of the superior temporal gyrus (primary hearing area).

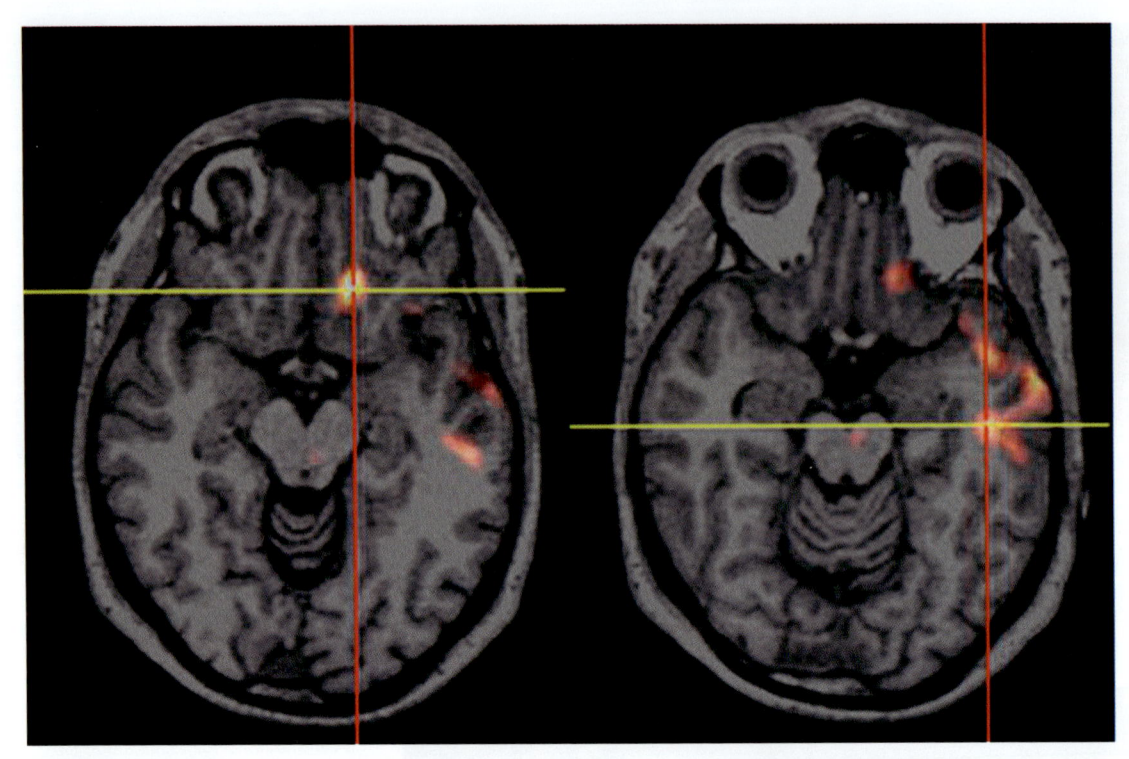

Figure 40.2. Twenty-four-year-old patient with refractory partial epilepsy. Complex partial seizures showed features of temporal lobe and frontal seizures (gestures). MRI was non-lesional and video-EEG monitoring showed left widespread fronto-temporal ictal abnormalities. Ictal SPECT showed left fronto-orbital and left temporal significant hyperperfusion (red/yellow). The patient was implanted with intracranial electrodes covering both areas, which showed seizure onset simultaneously in both areas. In view of these findings, no epilepsy surgical resection was recommended.

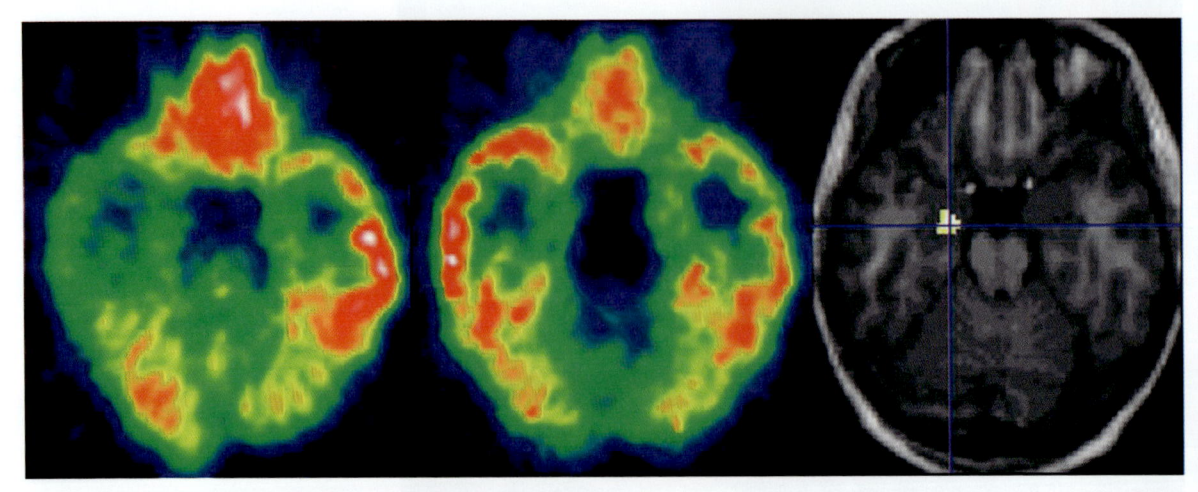

Figure 41.1. Single case comparison in a patient with unilateral hippocampal sclerosis. Comparison FGD-PET (left) reduced in right temporal lobe, flumazenil PET (middle) reductions restricted to mesial temporal structures and statistical comparison of single case FMZ PET versus controls superimposed on T1 volume MRI for illustration purpose.

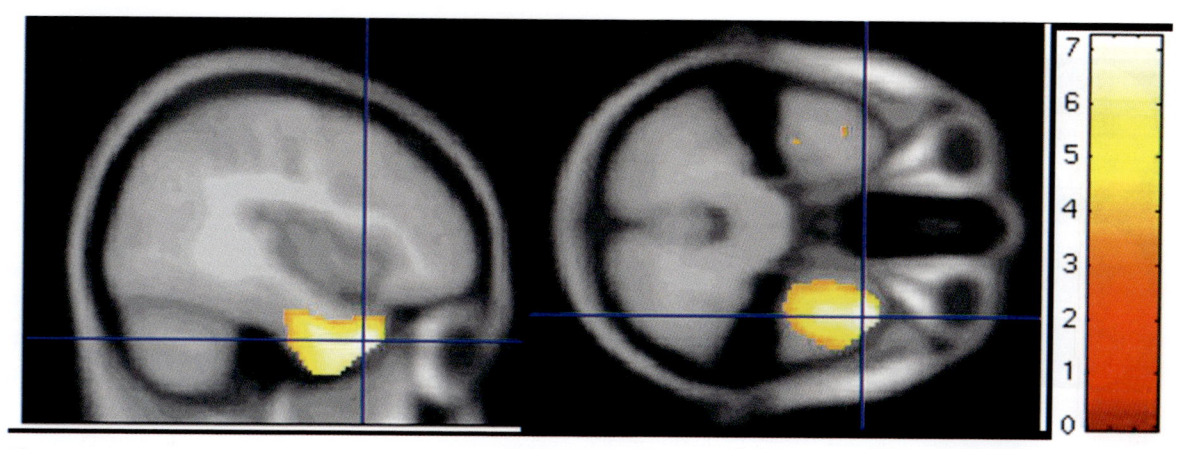

Figure 41.2. SPM comparison of post-ictal versus interictal diprenorphine binding in group of patients with mTLE (Hammers A, Asselin MC, Hinz R, Kitchen I, Brooks DJ, Duncan JS, Koepp MJ. Upregulation of opioid receptor binding following spontaneous epileptic seizures. *Brain* 2007;130(4):1009–16).

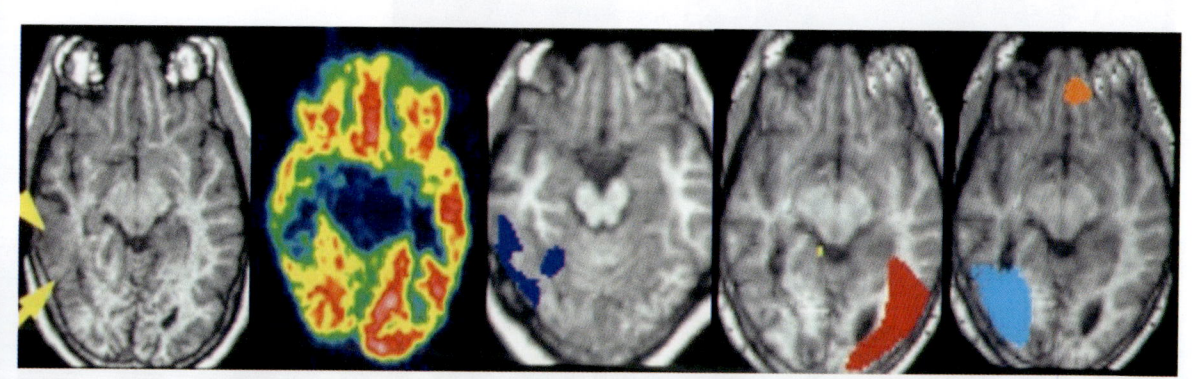

Figure 41.3. From left to right: malformation of cortical development on T1-weighted images (arrows), baseline FMZ PET (2nd panel) showing reduced binding right temporal compared to controls (3rd panel, blue). 4th panel: areas showing significant activation during visual memory task is left, but not right temporo-occipital; 5th panel: area of reduced (light blue) and increased activation (orange) in this patient compared to normal control pattern.

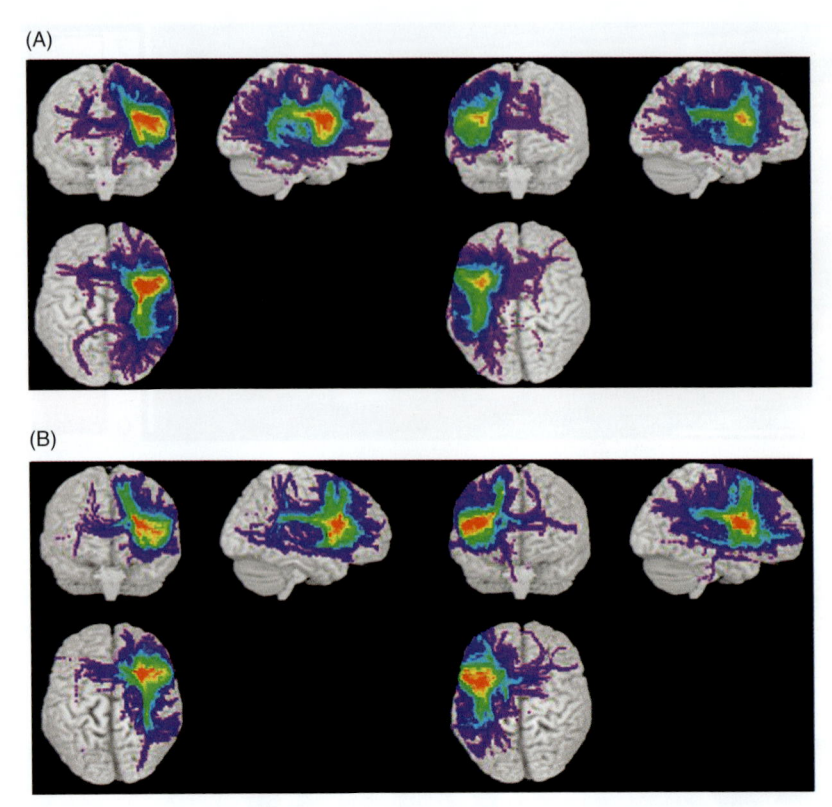

Figure 42.1. (A) Left (left panel) and right (right panel) fasciculus arcuatus in healthy controls. (B) In left TLE, less lateralization of fasciculus arcuatus than healthy controls.

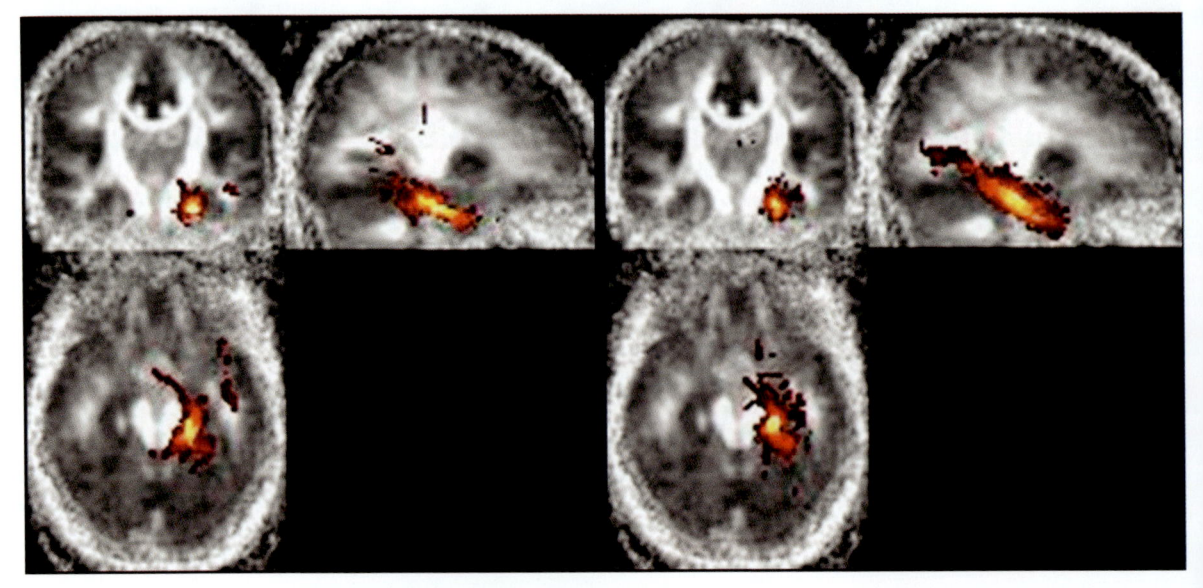

Figure 42.2. Material-specific memory measures correlated with tract volume and FA in right and left TLE.

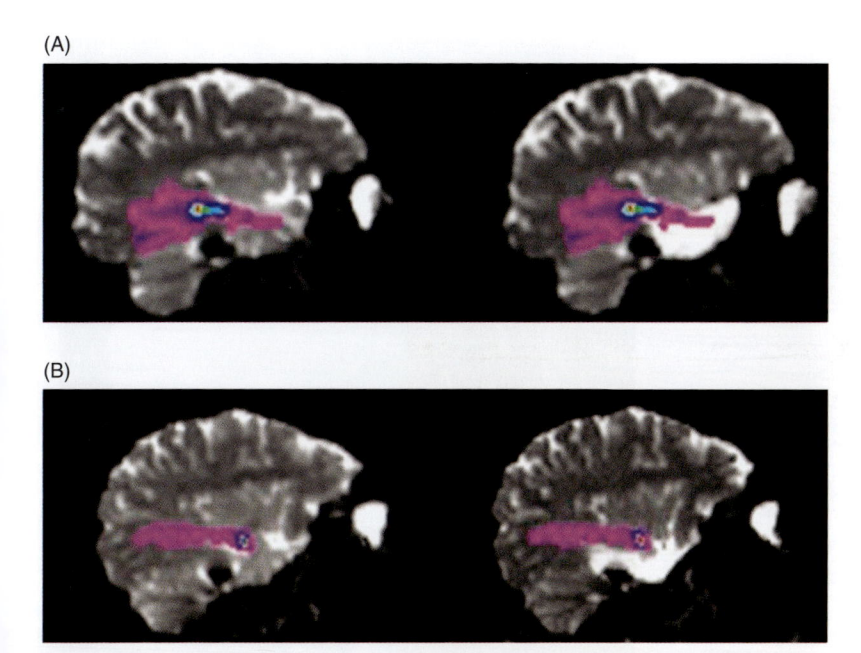

Figure 42.3. (A) Preoperative optic radiation superimposed on preoperative (left panel) and postoperative (right panel) mean high-resolution DTI in a patient with postoperative upper quadrantanopia. (B) Preoperative optic radiation superimposed on preoperative (left panel) and postoperative (right panel) mean high-resolution DTI in a patient without postoperative visual field defects.

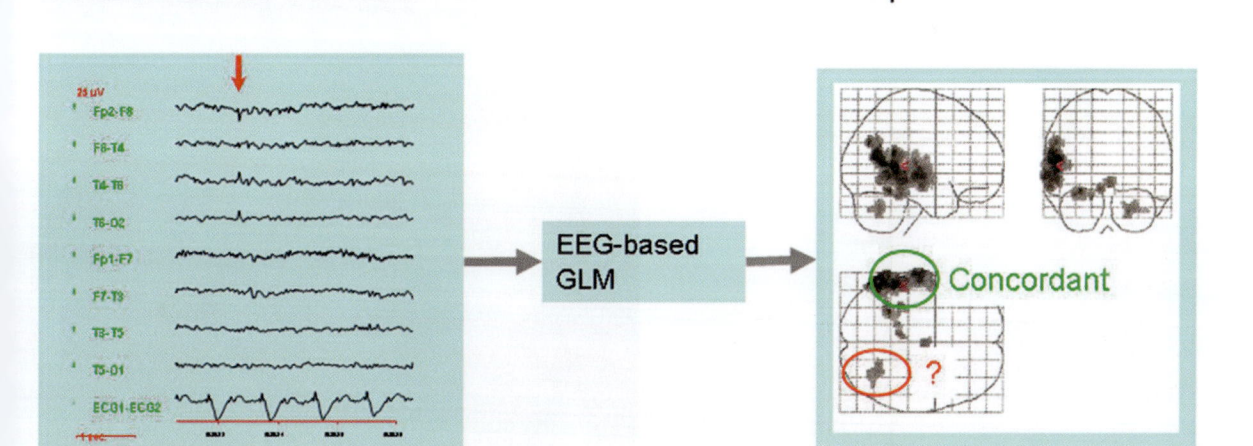

Figure 43.1. Illustration of EEG-correlated fMRI methodology and typical finding in patient with frequent focal spikes. Left: EEG segment recorded during fMRI scanning using special EEG equipment and and processed using dedicated post-processing software. Middle: box representing the conversion of the EEG into a general linear model (GLM) of the fMRI data. Right: resulting BOLD map shows a large cluster in the left temporal region (superimposed on a cartoon brain), concordant with our understanding of the patient's irritative zone, and a contralateral cluster.

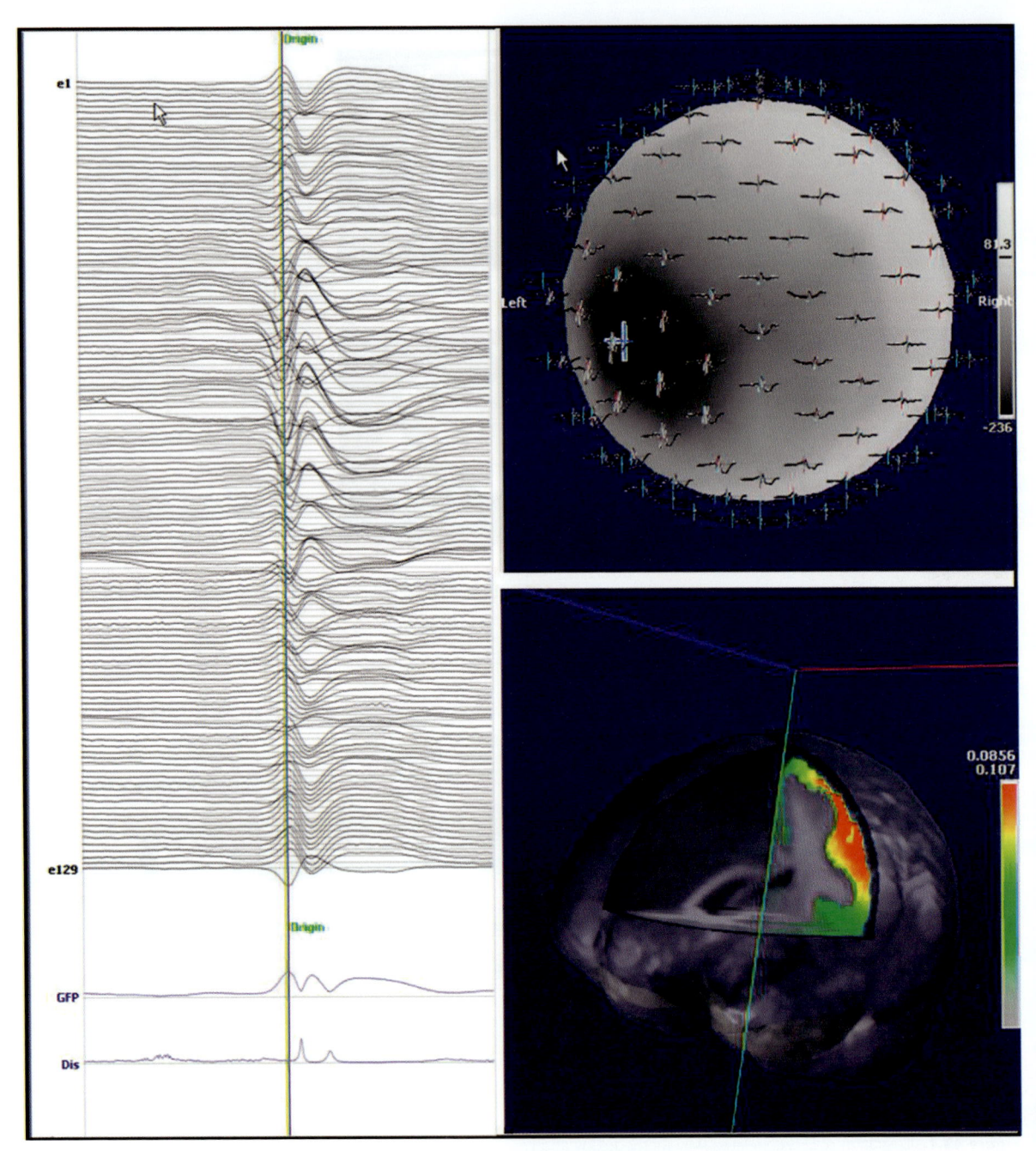

Figure 44.1. Interictal epileptiform transient acquired on a 129-channel EEG system. The averaged waveform (left panel) shows a triphasic sharp wave. The topographic map (top right) shows the field distribution at the first negative peak. The inverse solution at that time-point shows the 3D representation of the active areas within the Montral template MRI, in proximity of the central sulcus.

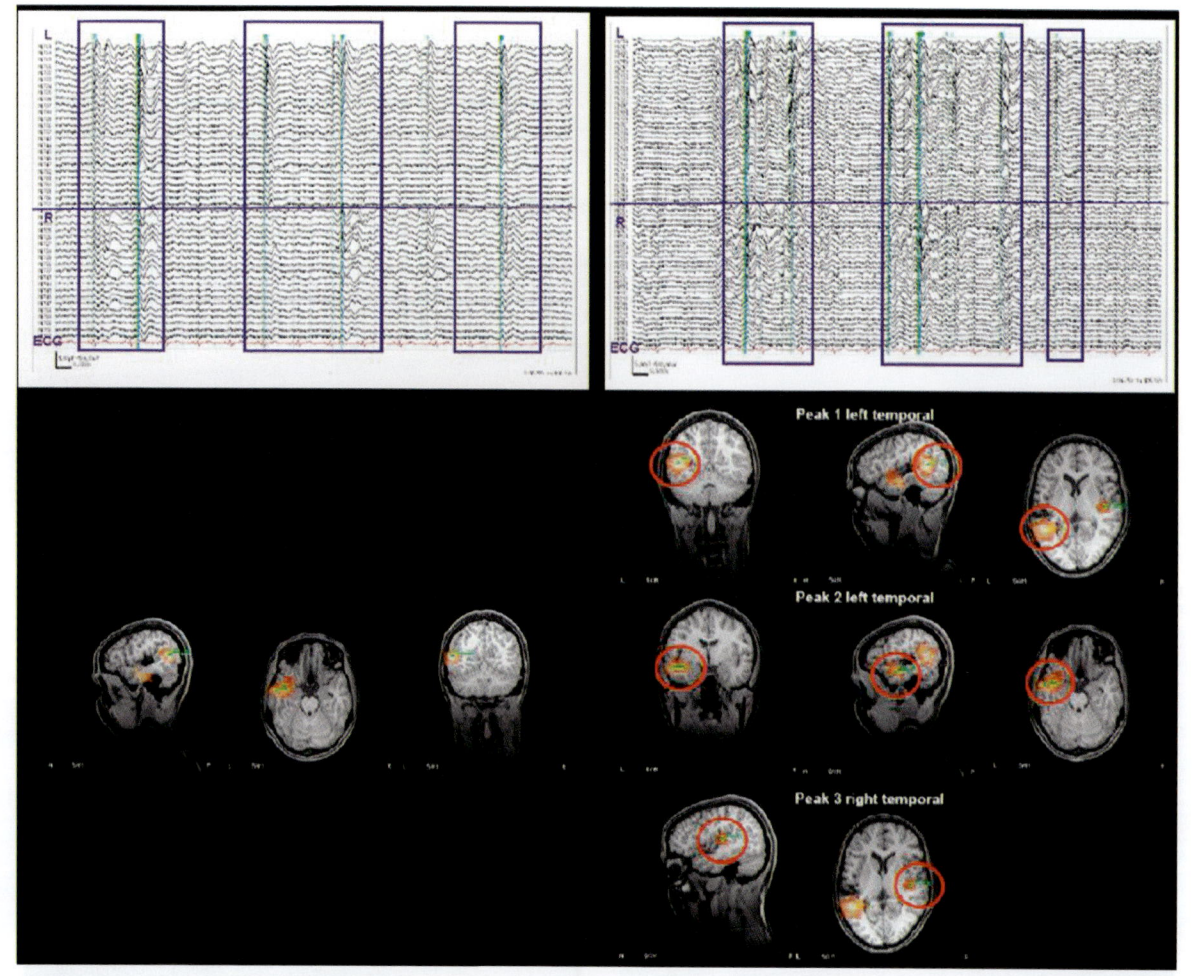

Figure 45.1. MEG recording in a patient with complex partial seizures persisting after surgical removal of a lesion in left temporal lobe. Irritative cortex maps in the neighbouring neocortex of the resected lesion. In colour the activated areas corresponding to the interictal transients which are more consistently unilateral (A) but occasionally show a secondary bilateralization (B).

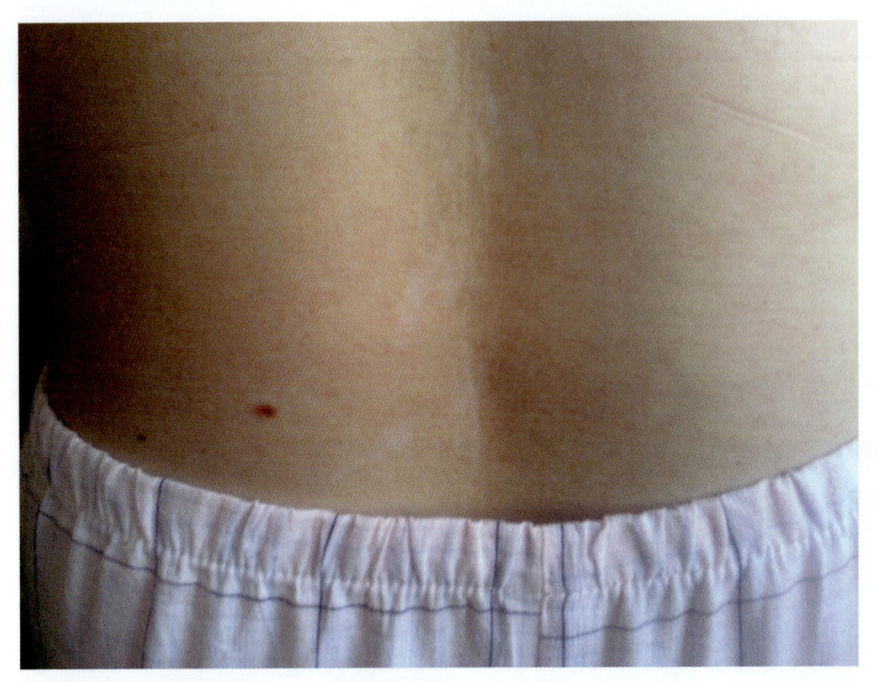

Figure 46.1. Hypomelanosis of Ito. Note hypomelanitic lesions in the lumbar region.

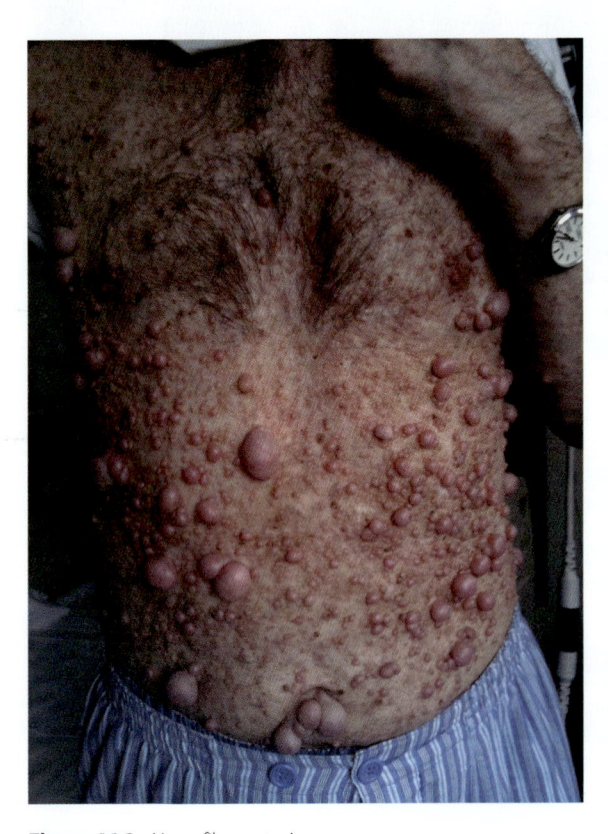

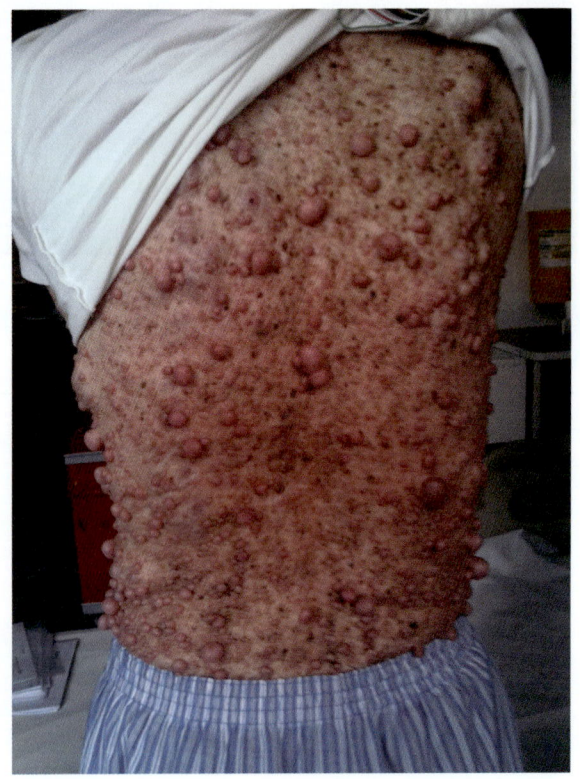

Figure 46.2. Neurofibromatosis.

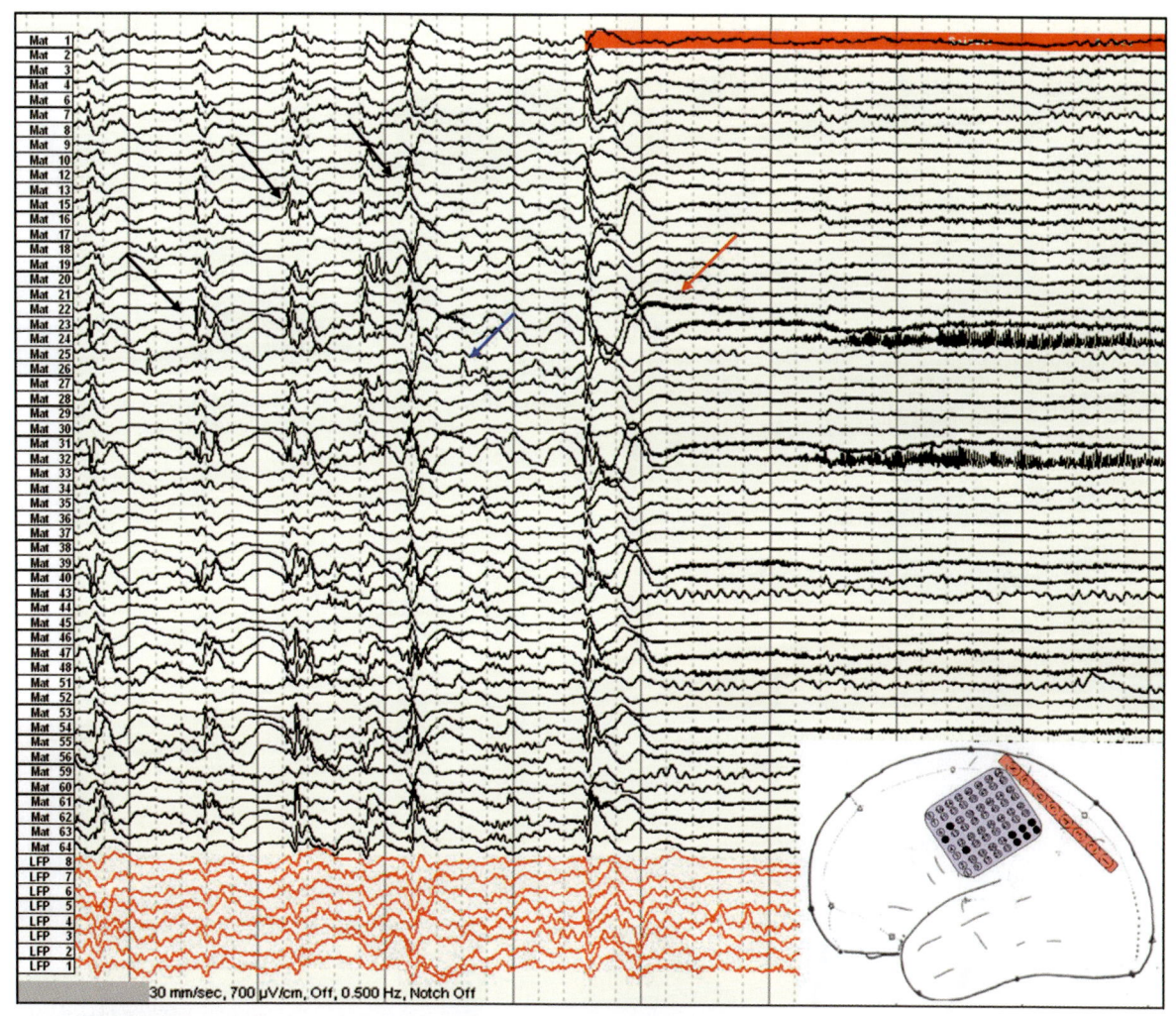

Figure 81.3. Focal seizure onset recorded with a subdural high-density 64-contact mat and an 8-contact subdural strip in a patient with focal cortical dysplasia. Before the seizure, sporadic focal discharges are seen (blue arrow) in addition to nearly continuous more widespread discharges seen at regular intervals (black arrows). During the seizure (top red horizontal bar), there is a diffuse attenuation of the background activity (electrodecremental event) associated with focal fast activity at 71 Hz (red arrow) over the superior two rows of the mat (electrodes 22, 23, 24, 31, 32, 39, 40, 47 and 48 of the mat). Electrode 1 of the mat is the most inferior electrode and electrode 8 is the most anterior.

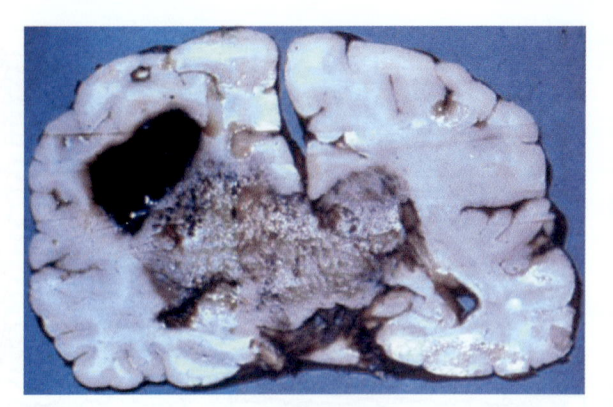

Figure 105.2. Malignant brain tumour (glioblastoma). These lesions cause epilepsy by damaging affected brain structures.

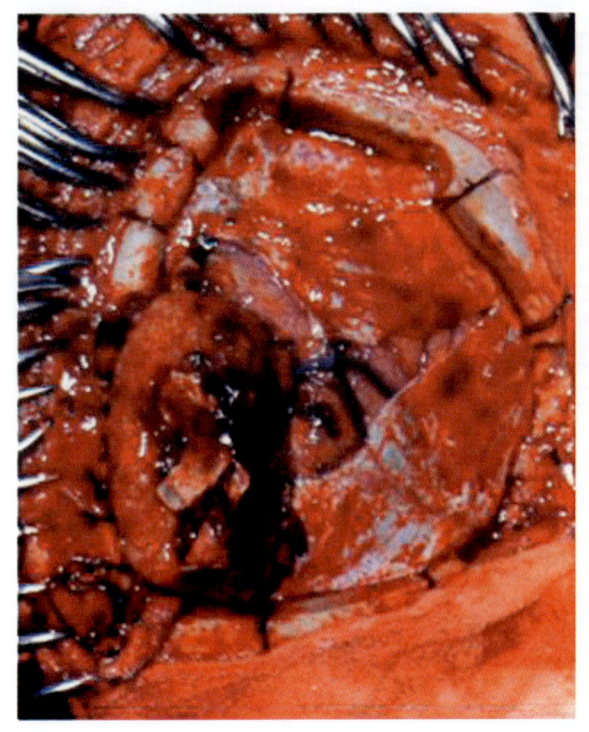

Figure 105.1. Surgical removal of a convexity meningioma. This lesion causes epilepsy by pressure on the underlying cortex.

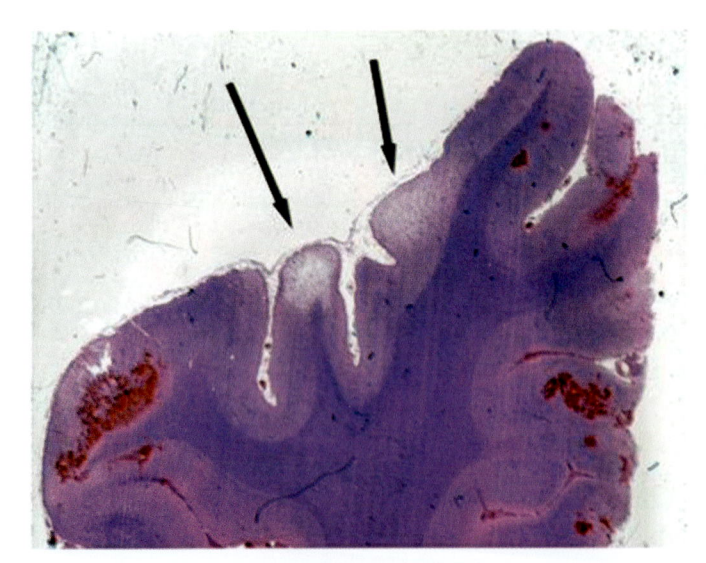

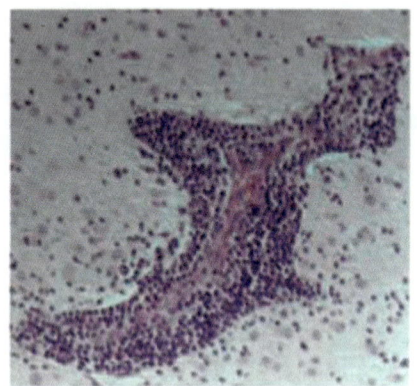

Figure 109.1. Pathological changes in Rasmussen's disease. Left, brain slice showing ischaemic lesions (arrows). Right, photomicrograph showing accumulation of inflammatory cells around a blood vessel.

References

ILAE Neuroimaging Commission. ILAE Neuroimaging Commission recommendations for neuroimaging of patients with epilepsy. *Epilepsia* 1997;**38**(Suppl 10):1–2.

Pohlmann-Eden B, Newton M. First seizure: EEG and neuroimaging following an epileptic seizure. *Epilepsia* 2008;**49**(Suppl 1):19–25.

Stokes T, Shaw EJ, Juarez-Garcia A, Camosso-Stefinovic J, Baker R. *Clinical Guidelines and Evidence Review for the Epilepsies: Diagnosis and Management in Adults and Children in Primary and Secondary Care*. London: Royal College of General Practitioners; 2004.

Learning objectives

(1) To become familiar with guidelines underpinning the use of imaging in epilepsy.
(2) To understand the indications for imaging in new-onset epilepsy.
(3) To understand the indications for imaging in chronic epilepsy.
(4) To become familiar with the indications for different imaging modalities.

Questions

(1) Describe three situations in which neuroimaging is carried out in the evaluation of epilepsy.
(2) In what specific ways do the recommendations of the NICE guidelines (2004) differ from the ILAE guidelines for imaging (1997)?
(3) What are the indications for imaging in new-onset epilepsy?
(4) What are the indications for imaging in chronic epilepsy?
(5) In what situations would CT be used rather than MRI?

Section 2 Classification and diagnosis of epilepsy

Chapter 38

Volumetric MRI and MRI spectroscopy

Andrew Simmons

Magnetic resonance imaging and spectroscopy

Nuclear magnetic resonance (NMR) was first described more than 60 years ago when Bloch and Purcell showed how certain nuclei placed in a magnetic field absorbed energy in the radiofrequency range and re-emitted this energy during their transition back to the relaxed state (Bloch et al., 1946; Purcell et al., 1946). This phenomenon has since revolutionized medical imaging with its application in magnetic resonance imaging (MRI) and magnetic resonance spectroscopy (MRS). MRI produces pictures of 'slices' through the human body with exquisite detail and contrast without the use of radiation, while in vivo MRS provides chemical information from selected areas in a similarly non-invasive way. This chapter describes the principles involved in the two techniques.

Basic principles of nuclear magnetic resonance

Nuclear spin

An atomic nucleus with an odd mass or atomic number exhibits a property termed 'spin'. This spinning positive charge induces a magnetic moment due to the laws of electromagnetism, and can be thought to act like a tiny bar magnet. Hydrogen, ^1H, with its single proton, is the nucleus most commonly used in clinical MRI and MRS.

Hydrogen nuclei in a magnetic field

In the absence of an applied magnetic field a collection of spinning hydrogen nuclei are randomly orientated (Figure 38.1A). When placed in an external magnetic field, however, the magnetic moments of the nuclei are affected by the magnetic field $B0$. Quantum mechanics tells us that a proton can only take up one of two stable states, parallel to the field or antiparallel. These are low and high energy states respectively. A very small excess of nuclei line up parallel to the field to produce a net magnetic moment (Figure 38.1B).

Precession

When placed in a magnetic field the individual hydrogen nuclei do not align perfectly with that field. Instead the influence of B0 produces a 'wobble' in addition to the rotation around their own axis. This is called precession and is similar to the action of a spinning top (Figure 38.1C). The frequency at which the nuclei precess is governed by the Larmor equation, $\omega = \gamma B0$, where ω is the precessional frequency, $B0$ the magnetic field strength and γ is the gyromagnetic ratio, a constant for a given nucleus.

Excitation and resonance

Resonance occurs if a nucleus is exposed to a radiofrequency pulse of energy delivered at its precessional frequency and perpendicular to the main magnetic field by a loop of wire close to the patient. This process is sometimes called excitation because some individual nuclei absorb energy, which causes them to change from the low energy state to the high energy state and thereby reorient the direction of the net magnetization.

Relaxation and detection of the MR signal

The net precessing magnetization induces a voltage in the coil, which is the detected MR signal. The frequency of the signal is the same as the Larmor frequency. When the excitation pulse is switched off the net magnetization realigns with the external magnetic field, and by doing so loses energy. The excited protons return to their equilibrium state by two means. The first is exchange of energy from the nuclei to their surrounding environment

---

Introduction to Epilepsy ed. Gonzalo Alarcón and Antonio Valentín. Published by Cambridge University Press.
© Cambridge University Press 2012.

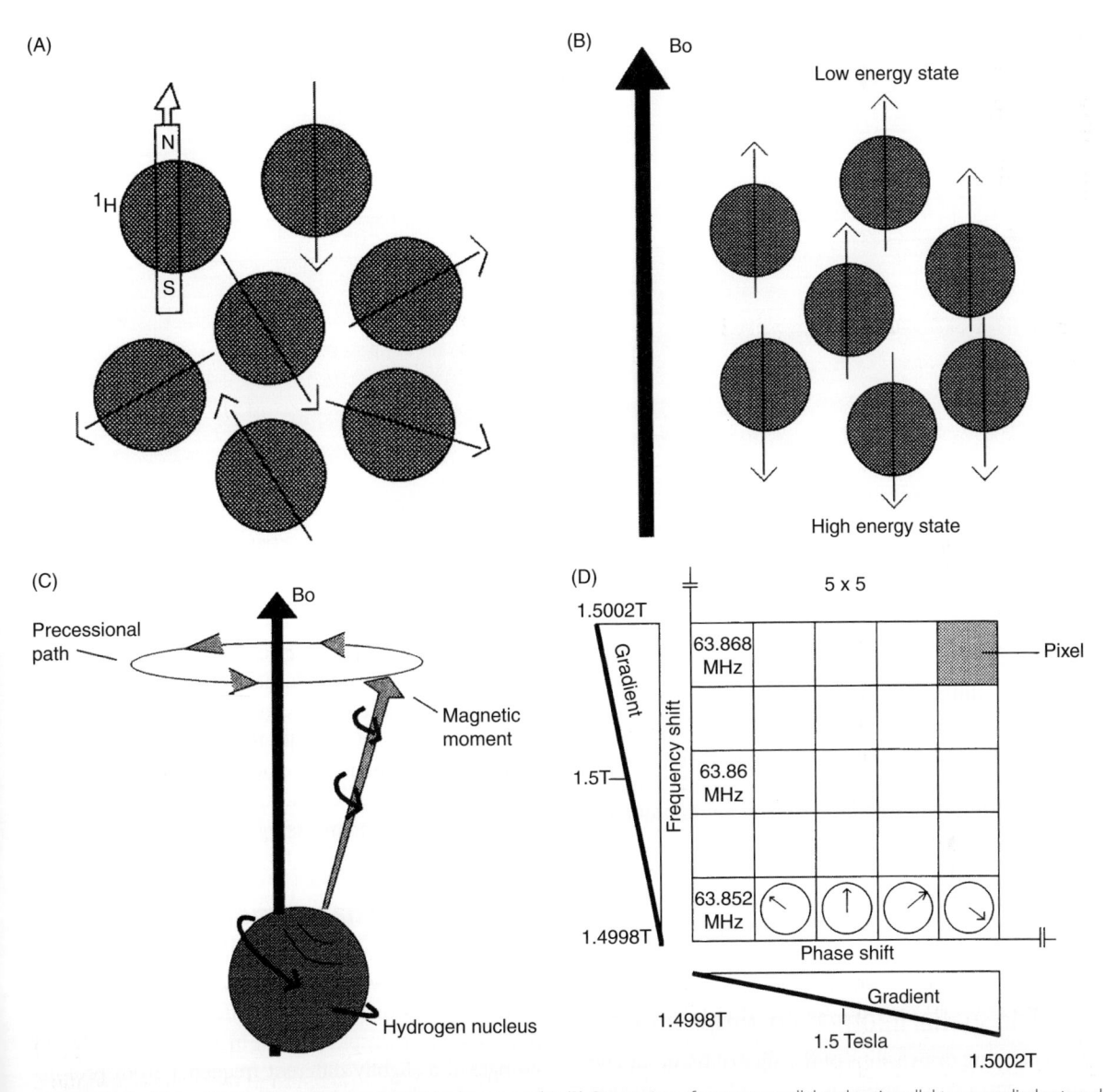

Chapter 38: Volumetric MRI and MRI spectroscopy

Figure 38.1. (A) A collection of randomly oriented hydrogen nuclei. (B) Orientation of protons parallel and antiparallel to an applied external magnetic field with a small excess parallel to the field (the net magnetic moment) (C) Precession of the net magnetic moment which can be considered to be similar to the motion of a spinning top (D) Spatial localization in MRI.

or lattice. This process is called the longitudinal relaxation process or T1 relaxation. At the same time the spins of adjacent nuclei interact and exchange energy with each other. The effect of this interaction is to cause the previously in-phase spins to start to dephase. This dephasing is called the transverse relaxation process or T2 relaxation. By manipulating the timing of the excitation and signal detection the differences in the T1 and T2 times of tissues can be used to produce different image contrast (Figure 38.2A, B).

Magnetic resonance image formation

Magnetic field gradient

In 1973, Lauterbur proposed a way of creating images by combining a strong static magnetic field with a weaker spatially varying field (the gradient field). By applying a varying gradient across a tissue, nuclei will precess at slightly different frequencies dependent on their position due to the different field strengths they encounter.

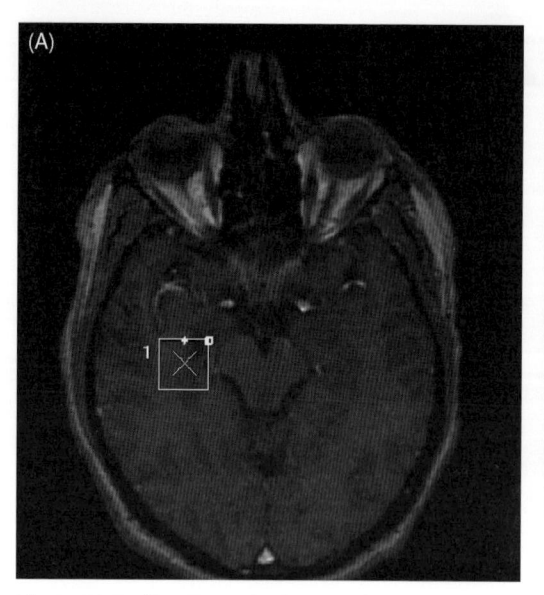

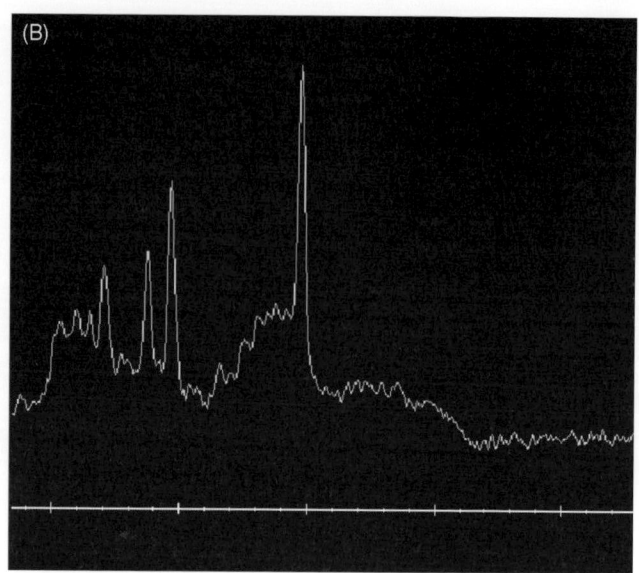

Figure 38.2. (A) A T1-weighted image of the human head. (B) Spectrum from the region of the human brain indicated by the region of interest in (A).

Slice selection

By applying different magnetic field gradients in the x, y and z directions, 3D localization of the MR signal can be obtained. The first gradient switched on is called the slice select gradient. As the gradient is applied nuclei precess at different frequencies. The radiofrequency pulse is then tuned to those precessional frequencies corresponding to the slab of interest, allowing only these nuclei to be flipped into the transverse plane. The resultant signal from this excited slice then needs to be spatially localized in the other two dimensions.

Encoding spatial information within a slice

The remaining dimensions of the slice of tissue can be spatially encoded by applying one gradient to encode the different precessional frequencies of the nuclei and the other to encode the different phase shifts (Figure 38.1D). The resultant digital image is made up of an array of points or pixels assigned different signal intensities relating to the amplitude of signal from each spatial location (Figure 38A).

Volumetric MRI

Volumetric MRI typically provides high-resolution T1-weighted images of the brain with isotropic voxel sizes of approximately 1 mm^3. These images are excellent for visualizing anatomy and are complemented by thicker-slice T2-weighted fast spin echo and/or T2-weighted FLAIR images. The isotropic nature of the T1-weighted volumes allows multi-planar reformatting of the images to best visualize the anatomy in any plane. Clinically these volumetric images are useful for assessing hippocampal sclerosis using a coronal plane oriented along the main axis of the hippocampus or for assessing the structure of subtle cortical malformations or larger abnormalities.

Magnetic resonance spectroscopy

For MRI it is assumed that all hydrogen nuclei resonate at the same precessional frequency. However, different chemical environments subtly affect the precessional frequency. For example, protons in a water molecule will resonate at a slightly different frequency from protons that are part of a fat molecule. This difference in resonant frequencies is termed chemical shift. These frequency differences are expressed in terms of parts per million (ppm) because their differences are relatively small (Hz) in comparison with the total MR frequency (MHz). The chemical shift provides a means of characterizing nuclei based on their chemical environment. Spatial localization for in vivo MRS occurs in a slightly different manner from imaging by exciting three perpendicular slices to produce a single volume of interest where the slices intersect. Figure 38.2B illustrates a spectrum from the left hippocampus. The main peaks are from the biochemicals myoinositol (mI), *N*-acetyl aspartate (NAA), choline (Cho), and creatine/phosphocreatine

(Cr/PCr). The area under the individual peaks reflects the amount of neurochemical present.

NAA is thought to reflect changes in neuronal density or function, and decreased NAA is one of the main findings in both frontal lobe epilepsy and temporal lobe epilepsy, where it can be used to aid lateralization. MRS can also be used to study GABA or lactate.

MRS is used clinically at some hospitals, though its use is not widespread. The clinical focus is normally on NAA for lateralization of temporal lobe epilepsy, where the results are claimed to be as good as other methods for lateralization. This requires good-quality left and right spectra to be routinely acquired, which normally requires a degree of expertise and familiarity with the use of MR spectroscopy.

References

Bloch F, Hanson WW, Packard M. Nuclear induction. *Phys Rev* 1946;**69**:127.

Lauterbur P. Image formation by induced local interaction; examples employing magnetic resonance. *Nature* 1973;**242**:192.

Purcell EM, Torrey HC, Pound RV. Resonance absorption by nuclear magnetic moments in a solid. *Phys Rev* 1946;**69**:37–8.

Learning objective

(1) To understand the basic principles of volumetric MRI and MRI spectroscopy, and their clinical indications and interpretation.

Section 2: Classification and diagnosis of epilepsy

Chapter 39: Functional MRI in epilepsy

Mark P. Richardson

Introduction

Over recent years, functional magnetic resonance imaging (fMRI) is evolving a role in the presurgical evaluation of patients with focal epilepsy. Hitherto, the accepted approach to mapping brain function and dysfunction has usually been confined to the intracarotid amytal ('Wada') procedure (IAP) and electrocortical stimulation mapping (ESM); the latter can be carried out intraoperatively or in the seizure monitoring unit in patients with chronically implanted intracranial electrodes. Both of these procedures are invasive, entail risks to the patient, and IAP can be misleading. Therefore, alternative, preferably non-invasive, tests are needed. In this context, fMRI is emerging as a useful modality of investigation. It has obvious advantages: fMRI uses widely available MRI equipment; it provides information about function of all of the brain, not just the region accessed by ESM; there is no radiation involved; there is extensive experience of fMRI in many basic neuroscience departments which epilepsy units can draw upon (though see below); and fMRI has minimal risks in patients without contraindications.

How does fMRI work? And why is the way it works a problem in patients?

The conventionally established fMRI technique makes use of a physiological phenomenon giving rise to the so-called blood oxygenation-level dependent effect, or BOLD effect. The ability to detect a signal in MRI depends on the magnetization properties of the tissues or structures being imaged. The signal detected from circulating blood alters depending on the ratio of oxyhaemglobin to deoxyhaemoglobin; oxyhaemoglobin gives a stronger signal, therefore tissues with more oxygenated blood appear 'brighter' in fMRI. There is a strong physiological link between neuronal activity and blood flow: as neuronal metabolic activity increases, there is an increase in blood delivery to that region of the brain which outweighs the increased need for oxygen, so that an active brain region will, paradoxically, contain more oxygenated haemoglobin than less active brain tissue. This change in the blood oxygenation level of a brain region as its activity changes is the basis of the ability of fMRI to detect 'active' brain regions. There has been something of a rush to establish fMRI in clinical practice, but there are many problems not yet overcome.

Problem 1: it is not known whether the normal link between neuronal activity and BOLD is the same in pathological brain

Experimental studies in monkeys (Logothetis et al., 2001) have shown that the metabolically demanding processes giving rise to changes in the BOLD signal are probably due to synaptic function rather than due to firing of action potentials; therefore, a change in BOLD signal in a brain region probably reflects alteration in synaptic inputs to neurons in that region, rather than to changes in firing rates alone. It is also well-established that the change in BOLD signal following an instantaneous change in neuronal activity is slow and delayed – although neurons can change their activity levels in milliseconds, blood delivery takes about 10 seconds to change in response, and the change in blood flow is smooth and gradual. Although this physiology of the BOLD effect is established for normal brains, we do not know whether it is the same in pathological brains with epilepsy and treated with AEDs.

Introduction to Epilepsy ed. Gonzalo Alarcón and Antonio Valentín. Published by Cambridge University Press.
© Cambridge University Press 2012.

Problem 2: fMRI images are often subject to distortion, low resolution, signal loss and movement artefact, giving rise to anatomical uncertainties

MRI usually has the advantage of good anatomical resolution. Unfortunately, this does not necessarily apply to fMRI. The images used for fMRI are generally acquired very quickly, in order to track rapid changes in BOLD signal, and these quick acquisitions are of much lower resolution than typical structural MRI. Furthermore, the usual technique used in fMRI (echo-planar imaging) is not good at detecting signal in certain parts of the brain (such as the orbitofrontal cortex and anteromedial temporal lobe). These regions often may also be rather distorted. Hence, unlike structural MRI, fMRI may have uncertainties about exactly where in the brain a signal arises, and indeed whether relevant parts of the brain can be 'seen' at all. A further challenge is that fMRI studies may take several minutes of continuous scanning; most people will move a little during this time, and movements of more than a millimetre or two can give rise to very confusing artefacts.

Problem 3: there is no consensus regarding 'study design' in clinical fMRI

A discussion of study design in fMRI is beyond the scope of this chapter. In brief, fMRI depends on comparing one brain state with another. This is achieved by giving the patient a very carefully designed task to do in the scanner. Usually this will involve watching images on a computer screen projected into the scanner, and making responses using a keypad. Researchers in basic neuroscience have developed extremely sophisticated experiments to identify brain structures involved in complex and subtle psychological or motor tasks. These tasks often produce extremely weak signals, and 'activation' of a part of the brain is often only identifiable by averaging together groups of subjects. Tasks like these are not appropriate for clinical studies – it is essential to use a task which produces brain activation which can be detected in the individual patient. It is equally essential to use a task the patient is capable of following. Although apparently obvious, this requirement is often overlooked: for example, a 'memory' task might be used to study brain activity in patients with memory deficits; however, the memory deficit may make it impossible for the patient to cope with the task. The resulting fMRI images may therefore be uninterpretable – the images will be of the brain regions active when a patient with a memory deficit is struggling to do a memory task he/she cannot do! In summary, a task used for clinical fMRI must be relatively easy, activate brain regions strongly and reliably, and be relevant to the clinical question.

Problem 4: what does brain activity mean? How should statistical thresholds be applied?

fMRI images are usually displayed as bright 'blobs' superimposed on structural MRI images. The bright blobs represent brain regions which changed their activity in a task-dependent way which was unlikely to have been due to chance. A statistical test is used to determine how unlikely it is that the 'activation' was due to chance; often a $P < 0.05$ threshold is used. Experience with fMRI shows that many regions of the brain are activated at this threshold, and relaxing the threshold slightly may reveal much more extensive 'activation'. Basic neuroscience experiments using fMRI go to great lengths to avoid so-called Type I error (in this context, accepting that a brain region was activated when in fact this was a chance effect due to noise or error). The neuroscientist needs to be able to assert that a particular brain region is definitely involved in performing a specific task. Making this assertion will require the neuroscientist to reject brain regions which 'might have been' involved, but at a lower level of certainty. Clinical application of fMRI in epilepsy is usually aiming to determine whether a focal cortical resection would be safe – that is, to work out whether a particular brain function is not in the brain region to be resected. The clinician often needs to be able to assert that a particular brain region is definitely not involved in performing a specific task. Surprisingly, methods to detect lack of activation are very underdeveloped.

fMRI in epilepsy patients

Notwithstanding all these problems, fMRI is rapidly advancing into clinical practice in epilepsy. Personally I believe this rapid advance to be premature, and believe the problems above should be addressed first. In epilepsy clinical practice, in the evaluation of patients with focal epilepsy for possible resection, there are three current scenarios where fMRI may be used.

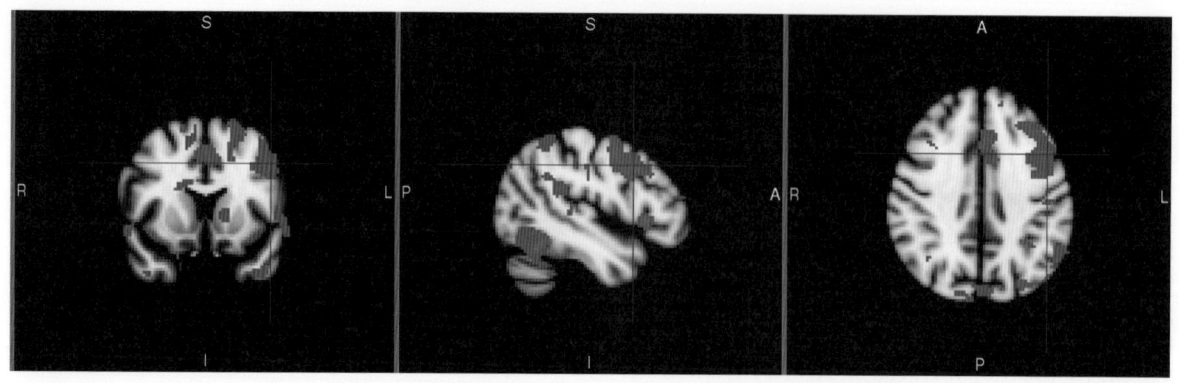

Figure 39.1. A language fMRI study carried out in a patient at King's College Hospital. This patient with frontal lobe epilepsy undertook a 'verbal fluency' task during scanning; this involves silently thinking of as many words as possible beginning with a specified letter. In this case, a normal pattern of left-dominant language activation is seen (red-orange-yellow blobs denote regions significantly active during the task compared with a control condition; brighter yellow indicates stronger activity; R, right; L, left; A, anterior; P, posterior). With thanks to Dr Jonathan O'Muircheartaigh. See colour version in plate section.

Identification of primary sensorimotor cortex

Simple motor or sensory tasks can identify activation in relevant areas of primary sensorimotor cortex with relative ease and these findings are reproducible. Some surgical centres use such information to guide cortical resection and prevent resection of these essential cortical regions.

Lateralization and localization of language

fMRI has been widely applied to studies of language in normal subjects (Figure 39.1). Broad consensus suggests that the normal brain regions involved in language function are widespread, but particularly the left inferior frontal gyrus is activated in many language tasks, e.g. word generation, whereas superior temporal regions predominantly on the left are activated by speech sounds and reading. The left-dominant pattern is typical, but a very small percentage of normal subjects may show a reversed right-dominant pattern. In situations where the IAP is being used to lateralize language function (i.e. to determine which hemisphere is dominant for language), fMRI can provide almost identical information in large case-series (Woermann et al. 2003). However, if the requirement is to precisely localize within a hemisphere exactly which regions of cortex are essential for language function, fMRI is rather less helpful. Compared with ESM, fMRI may identify many brain regions active during language tasks which are not identified by ESM; on the other hand, in one well-designed study (Rutten et al. 2002), there were no brain regions which failed to be activated by fMRI but which were found essential using ESM. In other words, fMRI might be a useful screening test: if there is no fMRI activity in a brain region, then this area may not need to be explored using ESM. In summary, language fMRI in epilepsy patients is feasible, and information from fMRI about language lateralization is robust and reliable; precise localization of language cortex is less certain, however. Studies suggest that language fMRI is improved by repeating several language fMRI studies in each individual rather than relying on one task.

Mesial temporal (memory) function

Promising studies have been published showing that fMRI of memory-related tasks can identify functional activity in mesial temporal lobe regions (Figure 39.2). Undertaken preoperatively in patients who subsequently undergo mesial temporal resections, this activity can predict postoperative memory change. Although these findings are still in need of replication in larger case-series, attempts have been made to optimize memory fMRI for clinical use (Richardson et al. 2006) and it is likely this technique will be further developed for future clinical application.

References

Logothetis NK, Pauls J, Augath M, Trinath T, Oeltermann A. Neurophysiological investigation of the basis of the fMRI signal. *Nature* 2001;**412**(6843):150–7.

Richardson MP, Strange BA, Duncan JS, Dolan RJ. Memory fMRI in left hippocampal sclerosis: optimising

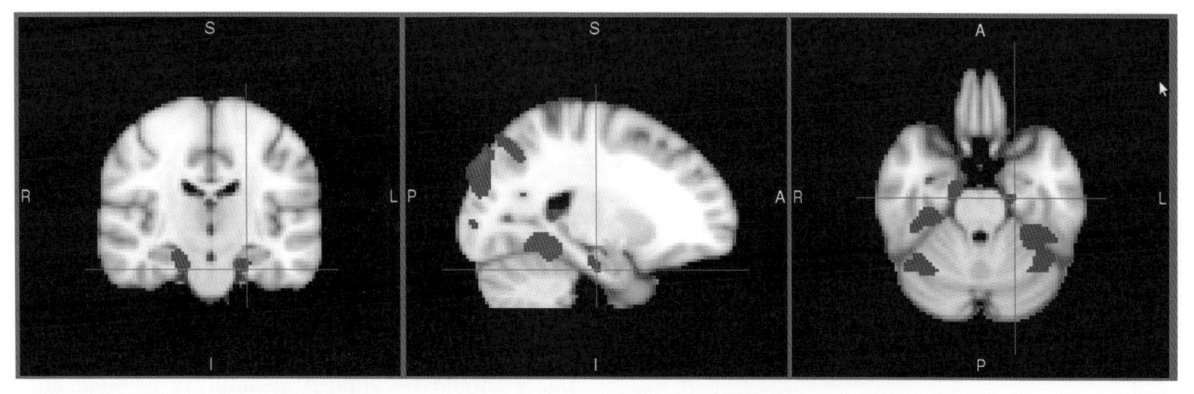

Figure 39.2. A memory fMRI study carried out in a patient at King's College Hospital. This patient with temporal lobe epilepsy undertook a task requiring memorization of a series of pictures. In this case, a bilateral pattern of activity in the mesial temporal lobes was seen, as well as activity more posteriorly in neocortex (red-orange-yellow blobs denote regions significantly active during the task compared with a control condition; brighter yellow indicates stronger activity; R, right; L, left; A, anterior; P, posterior). With thanks to Dr Karren Towgood. See colour version in plate section.

the approach to predicting postsurgical memory. *Neurology* 2006;**66**:699–705.

Rutten GJ, Ramsey NF, van Rijen PC, Noordmans HJ, van Veelen CW. Development of a functional magnetic resonance imaging protocol for intraoperative localization of critical temporoparietal language areas. *Ann Neurol* 2002;**51**(3):350–60.

Woermann FG, Jokeit H, Luerding R, *et al.* Language lateralization by Wada test and fMRI in 100 patients with epilepsy. *Neurology* 2003;**61**(5):699–701.

Learning objectives

(1) To understand the difficulties using fMRI in a patient population.
(2) To become familiar with language fMRI in epilepsy patients.
(3) To become familiar with memory fMRI in epilepsy patients.
(4) To understand the limited but growing role of fMRI in presurgical evaluation.

Questions

(1) What are the problems using fMRI in patients?
(2) What assumptions are made when using fMRI in epilepsy?
(3) Which cognitive functions are typically assessed in epilepsy patients?
(4) Which conventional test or tests could fMRI replace in the future?

Section 2
Classification and diagnosis of epilepsy

Chapter 40
SPECT in epilepsy

T. J. von Oertzen

Background

Single positron emission computed tomography (SPECT) can be used to measure cerebral blood flow (cbf). A radioactively labelled tracer is intravenously injected and in less than 1 minute it binds to the endothelia of the capillaries in the brain, indicating cerebral blood flow. Within 2–6 hours after the injection, the brain can be assessed in the SPECT scanner by reading single positron emissions. The spatial resolution of SPECT is most often around 10–12 mm, at its best 7–8 mm, depending on the camera specifications. SPECT is at most a semi-quantitative method. In contract to PET, absolute quantification is not possible. SPECT is used during presurgical evaluation of patients with refractory epilepsy.

Interictal studies

Interictal SPECT detects local hypoperfusion of the brain, which may represent an area of abnormal brain function and the epileptogenic focus. Despite extensive research conducted in the late 1980s and mid 1990s, the sensitivity and specificity of interictal SPECT remained low. The development of other interictal imaging techniques, particularly MRI and PET, showed much higher sensitivity and specificity. Hence, interictal cbf SPECT has been used progressively less in presurgical evaluation (Duncan, 1997).

Ictal SPECT

Ictal SPECT may detect an area of hyperperfusion, which indicates the seizure-onset zone. The theory is that the hyperexcitability state will require high energy consumption of the cells and subsequently the blood supply will increase in this area. Ictal SPECT was first described in the 1980s (Bonte et al., 1983; Lee et al., 1986). In order to exclusively image the seizure-onset zone and not seizure spread, the tracer should be applied as soon as possible after seizure onset. A second interictal study is used for comparison. The most commonly used tracer, 99Tc HMPAO (hexamethyl-propyleneamine oxime) initially was only available in an unstable preparation. This had to be prepared at seizure onset. Hence, most of the studies from that time showed injection latencies longer than 1 minute after seizure onset. In the mid 1990s a stable HMPAO tracer was developed which allowed shorter injection latencies. Furthermore, 99Tc-ECD (ethyl cysteinate dimer) was developed as an alternative stable tracer (Grünwald et al., 1994). A head-to-head comparison between HMPAO and ECD showed higher brain uptake and lower uptake by the surrounding soft tissue for ECD. Consequently, ECD was regarded as the preferable tracer (O'Brien et al., 1999). However, the study had significant differences in the injection latencies between the groups of stable and unstable tracers used for retrospective comparison.

In the mid 1990s, first attempts were made to use digital subtraction techniques to enhance the sensitivity and specificity of SPECT (Zubal et al., 1995). In the late 1990s a more systematic approach introduced SISCOM (subtracted ictal SPECT co-registered with MRI), which showed superiority for localization over visual inspection (88 vs 42%). The main advantages of this technique are that SPECT images are co-registered in all three dimensions, which allows much better comparison and subtraction of images. Furthermore, fusion onto the MRI allows better anatomical localization (Figure 40.1).

Ictal SPECT, preferably with computational post-processing, has a place in presurgical evaluation of patients with refractory epilepsy. It may be used to

---

Introduction to Epilepsy ed. Gonzalo Alarcón and Antonio Valentín. Published by Cambridge University Press.
© Cambridge University Press 2012.

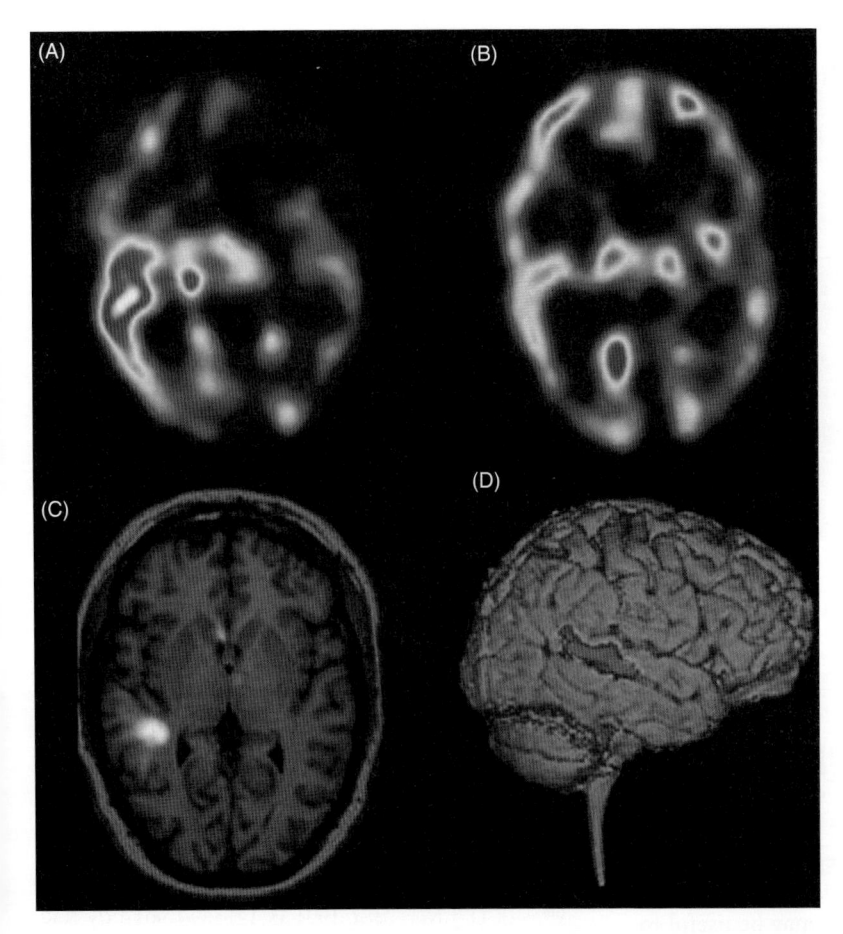

Figure 40.1. Twenty-eight-year-old female patient with refractory complex partial seizures. Semiology included a stereotypic melody followed by altered awareness. MRI was non lesional. Axial ictal SPECT (A) showed a right temporolateral hyperperfusion (red) compared to the interictal SPECT (B). SISCOM in the axial (C) and lateral 3D rendering (D) shows significant (>2 SD) hyperperfusion in the posterior part of the superior temporal gyrus (primary hearing area). See colour version in plate section.

lateralize temporal lobe epilepsy, but, more importantly, it is used in presurgical investigation of extra-temporal epilepsies with discordant results or in epilepsies with non-lesional MRI. Recent studies showed high sensitivity and specificity compared to intracranial ECoG and seizure outcome (Ahnlide et al., 2007; O'Brien et al., 2004; Spanaki et al., 1999; von Oertzen et al., 2006)

Ictal SPECT is extremely time-consuming. The SPECT tracer will be stable for a 6-hour period. The patient has to be closely monitored on video-EEG monitoring to archive short injection latencies and not to confuse ictal and interictal injections (Van Paesschen et al., 2000). Different methods of injecting have been described, including automated injections (Feichtinger et al., 2007; Van Paesschen et al., 2000; von Oertzen et al., 2006). Usually this test will be only be performed during working hours as the SPECT scanner has to be available. It will commonly require several consecutive days of video-EEG monitoring to study a seizure. In our cohort, the mean time to seizure for injection was 2.7 days and 75% of patients were injected, indicating that one quarter did not have a seizure during this period despite drug reduction and subsequent recordings for up to 10 days. Due to these factors, ictal SPECT is most commonly reserved for the most difficult group of presurgical evaluation, i.e. non-lesional and extra-temporal epilepsies (Figure 40.2).

Research

Besides the direct clinical value of localizing the epileptogenic zone, ictal SPECT has been used to study neuronal networks and seizure propagation. In temporal lobe seizures, it showed ipsilateral frontal hypoperfusion (Van Paesschen et al., 2003). Another group showed more widespread changes in hyper- and hypoperfusion depending on injection latency (Blumenfeld et al., 2004). In secondarily generalized seizures, SPECT revealed a network of cortical and subcortical structures. Increased perfusion was shown in subcortical structures

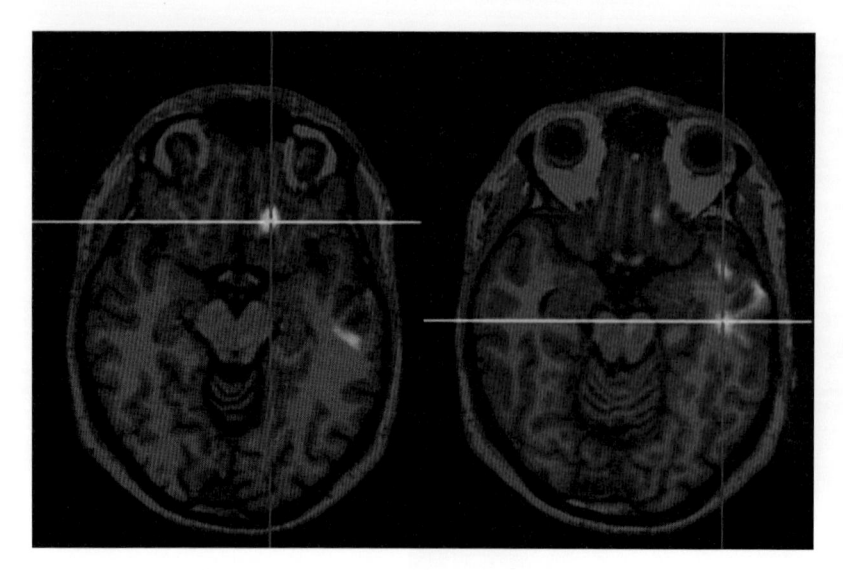

Figure 40.2. Twenty-four-year-old patient with refractory partial epilepsy. Complex partial seizures showed features of temporal lobe and frontal seizures (gestures). MRI was non-lesional and video-EEG monitoring showed left widespread fronto-temporal ictal abnormalities. Ictal SPECT showed left fronto-orbital and left temporal significant hyperperfusion (red/yellow). The patient was implanted with intracranial electrodes covering both areas, which showed seizure onset simultaneously in both areas. In view of these findings, no epilepsy surgical resection was recommended. See colour version in plate section.

(cerebellum, basal ganglia, brainstem and thalamus), along with decreased perfusion in the association cortex (Blumenfeld et al., 2009).

Other applications in epilepsy

In addition to ictal application, SPECT has been used during presurgical evaluation for other purposes. During the Wada test, cbf SPECT represents the brain area perfused if injected together with amobarbital. During intracarotid Wada tests this may be useful to identify bifrontal perfusion and the extent of temporo-mesial perfusion. During selective Wada, this has been proven crucial to identify which brain areas have been perfused (von Oertzen et al., 2000). Furthermore, different tracers such as flumazenil have been used, but quantitative measures with PET have been shown to be superior.

References

Ahnlide JA, Rosen I, Linden-Mickelsson TP, Kallen K. Does SISCOM contribute to favorable seizure outcome after epilepsy surgery? *Epilepsia* 2007;**48**(3):79–588.

Blumenfeld H, McNally KA, Vanderhill SD, et al. Positive and negative network correlations in temporal lobe epilepsy. *Cerebral Cortex* 2004;**14**(8):892–902.

Blumenfeld H, Varghese GI, Purcaro MJ, et al. Cortical and subcortical networks in human secondarily generalized tonic-clonic seizures. *Brain* 2009;**132**(Pt 4):999–1012.

Bonte FJ, Stokely EM, Devous MD Sr, Homan RW. Single-proton tomography study of regional cerebral blood flow in epilepsy. A preliminary report. *Arch Neurol* 1983;**40**(5):267–70.

Duncan JS. Imaging and epilepsy. *Brain* 1997;**120** (Pt 2):339–77.

Feichtinger M, Eder H, Holl A, et al. Automatic and remote controlled ictal SPECT injection for seizure focus localization by use of a commercial contrast agent application pump. *Epilepsia* 2007;**48**(7):1409–13.

Grünwald F, Menzel C, Pavics L, et al. Ictal and interictal brain SPECT imaging in epilepsy using Technetium-99m-ECD. *J Nucl Med*, 1994;**35**(12):1896–901.

Lee BI, Markand ON, Siddiqui AR, et al. Single photon emission computed tomography (SPECT) brain imaging using N,N,N'-trimethyl-N'-(2 hydroxy-3-methyl-5–123I-iodobenzyl)-1,3-propanediamine 2 HCl (HIPDM): intractable complex partial seizures. *Neurology* 1986;**36** (11):1471–7.

O'Brien TJ, Brinkmann BH, Mullan BP, et al. Comparative study of 99mTc-ECD and 99mTc-HMPAO for peri-ictal SPECT: qualitative and quantitative analysis. *J Neurol Neurosurg Psychiatry* 1999;**66**(3):331–9.

O'Brien TJ, So EL, Cascino GD, et al. Subtraction SPECT coregistered to MRI in focal malformations of cortical development: localization of the epileptogenic zone in epilepsy surgery candidates. *Epilepsia* 2004;**45**(4):367–76.

Spanaki MV, Zubal IG, MacMullan J, Spencer SS. Periictal SPECT localization verified by simultaneous intracranial EEG. *Epilepsia* 1999;**40**(3):267–74.

Van Paesschen W, Dupont P, Van Driel G, Van Billoen H, Maes A. SPECT perfusion changes during complex partial seizures in patients with hippocampal sclerosis. *Brain* 2003;**126**(5):1103.

Van Paesschen W, Dupont P, Van Heerden B, *et al.* Self-injection ictal SPECT during partial seizures. *Neurology* 2000;54(10):1994–7.

von Oertzen J, Klemm E, Urbach H, *et al.* SATSCOM – Selective amobarbital test intraarterial SPECT coregistered to MRI: description of a method assessing selective perfusion. *Neuroimage* 2000;12 (6):617–22.

von Oertzen, T. J., Moormann F, Reichmann K, *et al.* Propspective use of SISCOM in presurgical evaluation. *Epilepsia* 2006;47(Suppl 7):343.

Zubal IG, Spencer SS, Imam K, *et al.* Difference images calculated from ictal and interictal technetium-99m-HMPAO SPECT scans of epilepsy. *J Nucl Med* 1995;36 (4):684–9.

Learning objectives
(1) To understand the principle of cbf SPECT.
(2) To understand the use of ictal and interictal SPECT and SISCOM.
(3) To understand the contribution of SISCOM in evaluation for epilepsy surgery.
(4) To be aware of other indications and areas SPECT is used in epilepsy.

Questions
(1) What is cbf SPECT?
(2) What is the advantage of SISCOM compared to EEGfMRI to localize the ictal onset zone?
(3) What is ictal SPECT and SISCOM?
(4) A 34-year-old patient is undergoing evaluation for epilepsy surgery. So far, his MRI was normal, his interictal EEG did not show any epileptiform discharges and ictal EEG in three complex partial seizures did not show seizure onset due to movement artefacts. The seizure video showed a seizure semiology likely to be of frontomesial origin without lateralization. Is a SPECT indicated in this patient? If so, explain why you would consider this and what kind of SPECT you would arrange.

Section 2 Classification and diagnosis of epilepsy

Chapter 41

PET in epilepsy

Mathias Koepp

Introduction

Magnetic resonance imaging (MRI) is generally the imaging method of choice for identifying the structural basis of the epilepsies. MRI has revolutionized the evaluation of patients with epilepsy. Conventional MRI identifies a structural lesion that underlies the etiology of partial seizures in 50–85% of those with medically refractory epilepsy and in 50–70% of newly diagnosed patients, depending on whether the study was hospital- or community-based.

Positron emission tomography (PET) evaluates cerebral glucose metabolism using [^{11}F]fluorodeoxyglucose (FDG), cerebral functions using $H_2^{15}O$ activation studies and receptor systems in the brain. This chapter will show how PET imaging and advanced MRI sequences, in particular tractography, can advance our knowledge about the causes of focal epilepsies.

Methodological considerations

Much progress has been made over the last decade in structural and functional neuroimaging in epilepsy. With increasing resolution of PET cameras and analysis techniques, an underlying structural pathology is readily detectable in more and more patients who are 'MRI-normal'. The location of the epileptogenic zone can be inferred indirectly by defining subtle epileptogenic lesions not visible on MRI, and its relationship with the seizure-onset zone and the region of cortex that generates interictal epileptiform discharges or irritative zone. The epileptogenic lesion does not necessarily completely overlap with the seizure-onset or irritative zone, and may encroach into areas sustaining normal functions or eloquent cortex.

Loss of brain tissue often observed in patients with epilepsy influences the interpretation of 'functional' differences. Only very few studies have employed MRI-based techniques to correct for partial volume effects caused by the limited spatial resolution of PET (Koepp et al., 1998; Hammers et al., 2001a). It is important to know if functional changes are redundant with a simple structural MRI scan or if they yield important additional information.

The 'old' PET tracer: FDG and flumazenil

[^{18}F]FDG PET studies have been less reliable for precise localization of seizure onset than for answering the question of lateralization. The pathophysiology of often widespread interictal hypometabolism in mesial TLE remains incompletely understood. Although reduced glucose metabolism may occur even when quantitative MRI only shows mild hippocampal atrophy, atrophy is a major determinant of cerebral metabolism measured with PET. There have been few studies of newly diagnosed patients; only 20% of children with new-onset epilepsy had focal hypometabolism. A recent [^{18}F]FDG-PET study suggested that interictal hypometabolism reflects the preferential networks involved by ictal discharges and spread pathways. Emotional seizure symptoms correlated with hypometabolism in the anterior part of the ipsilateral insular cortex (Bouilleret et al., 2002) and dystonic posturing was associated with hypometabolism in the contralateral striatum (Dupont et al., 1998).

Comparative PET studies with [^{18}F]FDG and [^{11}C]flumazenil (FMZ), a marker for the functional integrity of the GABAergic inhibitory neurotransmitter system, have shown the area of reduced [^{11}C]FMZ binding to be more restricted than is the area of reduced glucose metabolism in TLE (Henry et al., 1993).

Reduction of [^{11}C]FMZ binding was initially thought to be confined to the sclerotic hippocampus

Introduction to Epilepsy ed. Gonzalo Alarcón and Antonio Valentín. Published by Cambridge University Press.
© Cambridge University Press 2012.

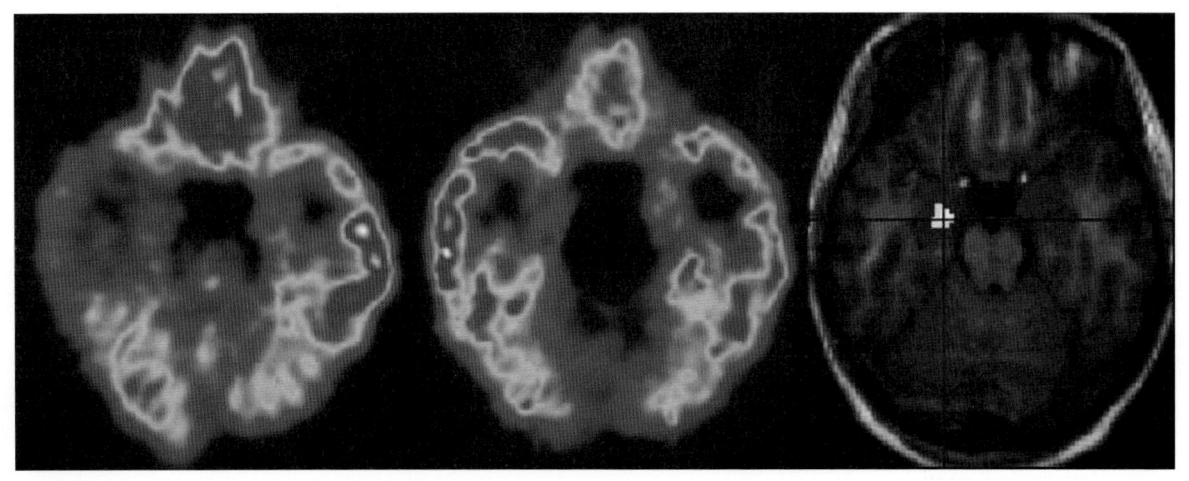

Figure 41.1. Single case comparison in a patient with unilateral hippocampal sclerosis. Comparison FGD-PET (left) reduced in right temporal lobe, flumazenil PET (middle) reductions restricted to mesial temporal structures and statistical comparison of single case FMZ PET versus controls superimposed on T1 volume MRI for illustration purpose. See colour version in plate section.

(Koepp 1996) Correction for partial volume effect increased the sensitivity of [^{11}C]FMZ PET in detection of unilateral hippocampal sclerosis from 65% to 100% with contralateral abnormalities found in a third (Koepp et al., 1997). Loss of GABAA receptor binding was consistently over and above loss of hippocampal volume, indicating that the loss of binding was not simply due to hippocampal atrophy. (Hand 1997; Koepp et al., 1997) In the white matter, [^{11}C] FMZ binding was tightly correlated with the number of heterotopic neurons, determined semiquantitatively ex-vivo in resected specimens (Hammers et al., 2003)

The new PET tracer

New PET ligands for opioid receptors, monoamineoxidase type B activity, serotonergic, cholinergic and glutamatergic neurotransmission have been developed and tested in TLE patients with hippocampal sclerosis providing often redundant information of reduced ligand binding in areas of reduced volume. In general terms, binding increases would be the preferred expression of a disease trait or state, as increases could not be explained by an underlying loss of tissue often observed in epilepsy.

Opiate neurotransmission

Diprenorphine (DPN) is a high-affinity opiate receptor ligand. It has similar in vivo affinities for the three main receptor subtypes: μ, κ and λ. In patients with unilateral temporal lobe epilepsy, there were no significant side-to-side differences in [^{11}C]DPN binding (Mayberg et al., 1991). DPN PET showed a focal increase in opioid receptors in humans in vivo following spontaneous seizures in patients with TLE (Hammers et al., 2007). This latest study provided direct human in vivo evidence for changes in opioid receptor availability over a time course of hours following spontaneous seizures, emphasizing an important role of the opioid system in seizure control.

In an earlier study, higher binding of the μ subtype selective agonist [^{11}C]carfentanyl was seen on the side of the epileptogenic focus in lateral temporal neocortex in the same patients, while binding in the amygdala was decreased. The latter finding might be due to partial volume effects which could be corrected for in contemporary studies. These increases of [^{11}C] carfentanyl binding coincided with areas of hypometabolism seen on [^{18}F]FDG PET. One speculative explanation is that an increase in μ receptors could be in response to endogenous opioids being released post-ictally in an attempt to limit the spread of epileptic activity (Tortella et al., 1985). Temporal neocortical binding increases were also seen using the δ receptor subtype selective antagonist [^{11}C]methylnaltrindole (Madar et al., 1997).

[^{18}F]Cyclofoxy is a specific antagonist at both μ and κ, but not δ receptor subtypes. There was no overall asymmetry in a group of TLE patients, but in some individual patients binding was increased in the ipsilateral temporal lobe (Theodore et al., 1992).

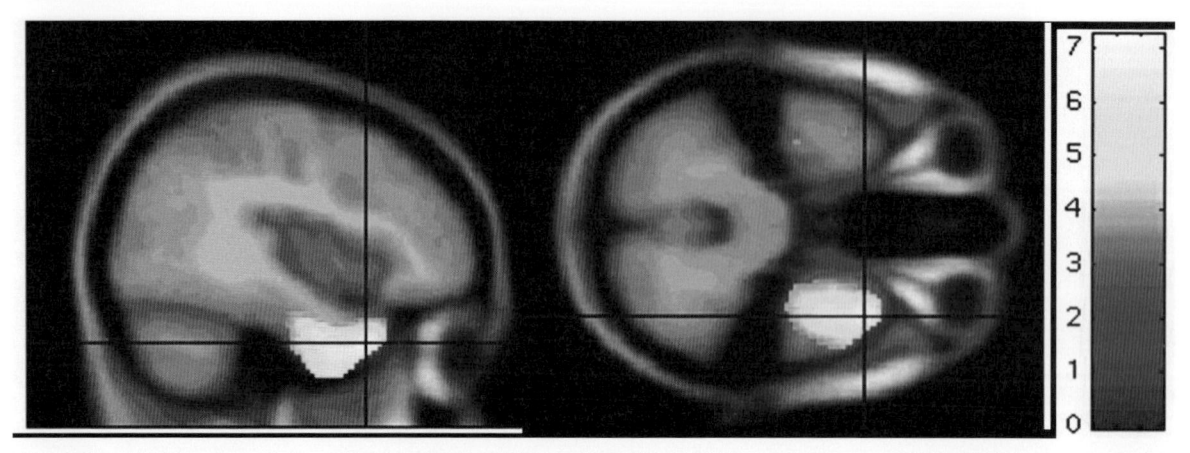

Figure 41.2. SPM comparison of post-ictal versus interictal diprenorphine binding in group of patients with mTLE (Hammers A, Asselin MC, Hinz R, Kitchen I, Brooks DJ, Duncan JS, Koepp MJ. Upregulation of opioid receptor binding following spontaneous epileptic seizures. *Brain* 2007;130(4):1009–16). See colour version in plate section.

Taken together with the temporal neocortical increases of μ receptors described above, this finding would be consistent with a decrease of affinity or number of κ receptors, or with decreased availability of κ receptors through occupation by an endogenous ligand.

Serotonergic neurotransmission

Increased serotonin metabolism has been found in resected specimens from epilepsy patients (Chugani and Chugani, 2000). Tryptophan is the precursor of the neurotransmitter serotonin (5-HT). α-Methyl-L-tryptophan (AMT) is an analogue of tryptophan, and binding levels reflect numbers of serotoninergic neurons. [^{11}C]AMT binding levels reflecting numbers of serotonergic neurons were increased in the ipsilateral hippocampus and positively correlated with the number of interictal epileptiform discharges. Increased binding also occurs when the kynurenine pathway of tryptophan metabolism is pathologically increased. A recent study did not show individual patients' data, but as a group seven unilateral TLE patients with normal hippocampal volumes showed increased [^{11}C]AMT binding in the ipsilateral hippocampus (Natsume *et al.*, 2003). No such group finding was seen in seven unilateral TLE patients with hippocampal sclerosis. The lack of correction for partial volume effects in this study, however, means that hippocampal increases in the sclerotic hippocampus may have been overlooked, and lack of data for individual patients does not allow an estimation of the usefulness of the technique in the presurgical evaluation.

Serotonin (5-HT$_{1A}$) receptors have been investigated in one study with [^{18}F]FCWAY (Toczek *et al.*, 2003). Twelve patients with TLE were correctly lateralized but not localized, including three patients with normal hippocampal volumes. Asymmetry indices for [^{18}F]FCWAY were greater than those for FDG-PET or hippocampal volumes. Another study used the novel 5-HT$_{1A}$ radioligand [^{18}F]MPPF to study nine patients with TLE, compared with 53 controls. Patients had TLE of various aetiologies and all underwent video-EEG evaluation with depth electrodes implanted (Merlet *et al.*, 2004). Binding was reduced in the epileptogenic areas, and the magnitude of decrease was related to both electrophysiological data (greatest in areas of ictal onset and spread) and structural data (greatest in lesions with volume loss, followed by lesions). Binding potential reductions were found in all nine patients; they corresponded to or included the ictal-onset zone in five, propagation areas in two, and were maximal in the onset areas but failed to reach significance in two. In four patients, contralateral abnormalities were seen; in one of these patients who was explored with contralateral depth electrodes, one seizure did start contralaterally. [^{18}F]MPPF PET correctly indicated lateralization in all three patients without lesions on MRI.

Taken together, these studies suggest that 5-HT$_{1A}$ receptor PET could play a role in lateralizing TLE when other imaging modalities are nonconclusive.

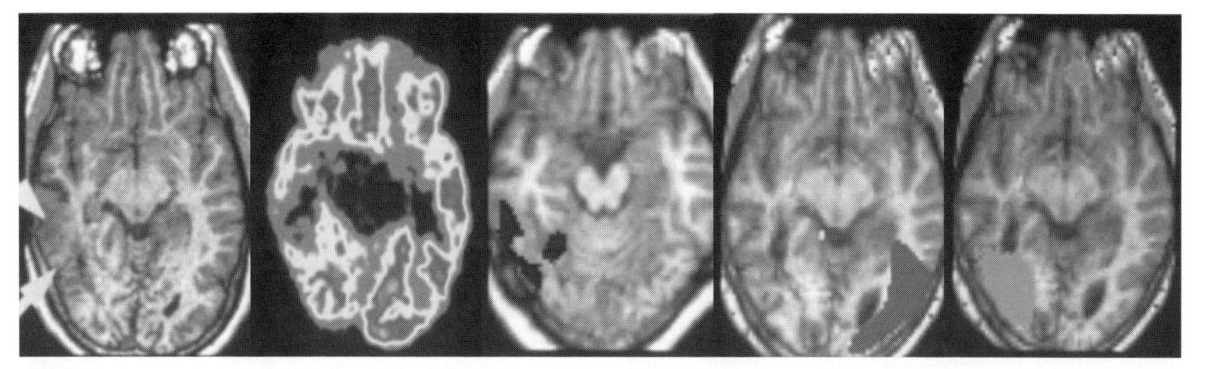

Figure 41.3. From left to right: malformation of cortical development on T1-weighted images (arrows), baseline FMZ PET (2nd panel) showing reduced binding right temporal compared to controls (3rd panel, blue). 4th panel: areas showing significant activation during visual memory task is left, but not right temporo-occipital; 5th panel: area of reduced (light blue) and increased activation (orange) in this patient compared to normal control pattern. See colour version in plate section.

Glutamatergic neurotransmission

[^{11}C]Ketamine, which binds to the open NMDA receptor ion-channel, showed a modest average ipsilateral binding reduction of 14% in mTLE (Kumlien et al., 2001). It is unclear whether the observed modest reduction merely reflects a decrease due to the structural change, or even a true increase per unit of grey matter, which one would have expected in view of the binding site.

In summary, it is unlikely that in mTLE, ligand PET yields information over and above that provided by MRI, but it should be useful in the investigation of patients without MRI signs of hippocampal sclerosis. Imaging of dynamic neurotransmitter changes seems possible, which would reflect synaptic release of endogenous neurotransmitter within epileptogenic networks in response to seizures.

Malformations of cortical development

Malformations of cortical development (MCD) are the second most common cause of refractory epilepsy in adults (Sisodiya, 2004). The imaging diagnosis of MCD requires the use of high-resolution MRI, ideally with multiplanar study. Routine MRI cannot detect or identify all pathologies, or the full anatomical extent may elude routine MRI detection.

Abnormal regions of [^{11}C]FMZ PET binding were frequently more extensive than the abnormality seen with MRI, and were also noted in distant sites which were unremarkable on MRI (Richardson et al., 1996, 1998; Hammers et al., 2001a). Focal increases of [^{11}C]FMZ binding in patients with epilepsy had not been seen in other pathologies. Possible explanations include increased neuronal density, the presence of heterotopic neurons expressing GABA$_A$ receptors, and increased numbers or availability of receptors.

Postoperative seizure freedom is closely related to the complete resection of the whole MCD and identification of widespread or bilateral changes often excludes patients from further presurgical evaluations. Surgery is less successful in these patients than in patients with discrete lesions, most likely because of anatomical and functional abnormalities extending beyond the visible lesions. However, these advanced imaging techniques are very sensitive in detecting subtle lesions without informing about the epileptogenicity of these abnormalities. This is apparent in successful surgery of bilateral MCDs, such as tuberous sclerosis. The detection of more specific neurochemical abnormalities using PET imaging might be helpful in this respect. Elevation of [^{11}C]AMT binding was found in the presumed epileptogenic zone in four of seven adult patients with FCD (Fedi et al., 2001) and, in children with tuberous sclerosis, was only seen in those tubers subsequently shown to be epileptogenic (Fedi et al., 2003).

Some MCDs have intrinsic epileptogenicity and are interconnected with normal brain regions. An important pre-condition for a potential surgical resection of an epileptogenic MCD is that this malformation is not integrated in normal neurological function. Examination of cerebral function using H$_2$^{15}O-PET activation studies provides further evidence for possibly widespread microanatomical disorganization (Richardson et al., 1998).

Tumours

Benign tumours commonly underlie refractory partial seizures. About 20% of adults and children undergoing surgery for chronic epilepsy had a benign tumor, most often localized in the temporal lobe. Dysembryoplastic neuroepithelial tumours (DNTs) are benign developmental tumors causing focal epilepsy with onset before the age of 20, often earlier. Confident differentiation from low-grade astrocytomas and ganglioglioma is not possible by MRI. Even histology may not enable the distinction to be made, especially in small biopsy samples. This is important, as surgery gives effective epilepsy treatment, and adjunctive chemotherapy or radiotherapy is unnecessary. PET typically identified DNTs as single regions of significantly reduced [^{11}C] FMZ binding (Richardson et al., 1998), whereas [^{11}C] methionine uptake was low in DNT's compared to high uptake in gliomas and gangliogliomas (Maehara et al., 2004).

'MRI-negatives'

In about 20% of patients with chronic focal epilepsies high-resolution qualitative and quantitative MRI does not reveal any significant pathology.

[^{11}C]FMZ-PET had a higher yield in detecting abnormalities in binding. Out of 45 published patients with TLE and normal MRI 38 patients (84%) had abnormal [^{11}C]FMZ PET scans, but only in 21 patients (46%) were these abnormalities thought to be surgically useful. In the largest of MRI-negative TLE series, increased [^{11}C]FMZ binding was found in the white matter of 11/18 patients, possibly representing increased density of heterotopic white matter neurons or microdysgenesis (Hammers et al., 2001b). Microdysgenesis is not detectable on MRI, and this new finding may represent the pathophysiological basis of medically refractory TLE cases with normal MRI.

Out of 102 MRI-negative patients with extratemporal seizure origin, 73 patients (71%) showed abnormalities of FMZ binding, but these findings were surgically useful in only 27 patients (26%). In the largest series of MRI-negative patients with seizures of extratemporal origin, abnormal [^{11}C]FMZ binding was found in 33 of 44 patients with significantly increased [^{11}C]FMZ binding in periventricular areas in seven patients (Richardson et al., 1998). The surgical relevance of such findings is still unclear, but they are compatible with an occult migration disorder.

Diagnostic methods with a high sensitivity increase the risk of Type I errors, the positive identification of false abnormalities. Type I errors could cause unnecessary explorations using possibly harmful procedures or even resections. For patients with normal MRI, only postoperative follow-up will provide information about the specificity of the various imaging abnormalities seen. A successful postoperative outcome is less likely in imaging-negative patients. There are only a few studies assessing the significance of contributions from multi-modality imaging in this clinically challenging patient population. These comparisons are usually biased towards the technique the investigators have most experience with. 'Negativity' with a certain imaging tool very much depends on the level of sophistication of its users, and this level varies by technique and research centre.

Recommended reading

Barkovich AJ, Kuzniecky RI. Neuroimaging of focal malformations of cortical development. *J Clin Neurophysiol* 1996;**13**(6):481–94.

Berkovic SF, McIntosh AM, Kalnins RM, et al. Preoperative MRI predicts outcome of temporal lobectomy: an actuarial analysis. *Neurology* 1995;**45**(7):1358–63.

Chassoux F, Semah F, Bouilleret V, et al. Metabolic changes and electro-clinical patterns in mesio-temporal lobe epilepsy: a correlative study. *Brain* 2004;**127**(Pt 1): 164–74.

Daumas-Duport C, Scheithauer BW, Chodkiewicz JP, Laws ER, Jr., Vedrenne C. Dysembryoplastic neuroepithelial tumor: a surgically curable tumor of young patients with intractable partial seizures. Report of thirty-nine cases. *Neurosurgery* 1988;**23**(5):545–56.

Frost JJ, Mayberg HS, Fisher RS, et al. Mu-opiate receptors measured by positron emission tomography are increased in temporal lobe epilepsy. *Ann Neurol* 1988; **23**(3):231–7.

Gaillard WD, Kopylev L, Weinstein S, et al. Low incidence of abnormal (18)FDG-PET in children with new-onset partial epilepsy: a prospective study. *Neurology* 2002; **58**(5):717–22.

Hand KS, Baird VH, Van Paesschen W, et al. Central benzodiazepine receptor autoradiography in hippocampal sclerosis. *Br J Pharmacol* 1997;**122**(2): 358–64.

Koepp MJ, Hammers A, Labbe C, et al. 11C-flumazenil PET in patients with refractory temporal lobe epilepsy and normal MRI. *Neurology* 2000;**54**(2):332–9.

Koepp MJ, Richardson MP, Brooks DJ, Duncan JS. Focal cortical release of endogenous opioids during reading-induced seizures. *Lancet* 1998;352(9132):952–5.

Kumlien E, Hartvig P, Valind S, et al. NMDA-receptor activity visualized with (S)-[N-methyl-11C]ketamine and positron emission tomography in patients with medial temporal lobe epilepsy. *Epilepsia* 1999;40(1):30–7.

Labbe C, Froment JC, Kennedy A, Ashburner J, Cinotti L. Positron emission tomography metabolic data corrected for cortical atrophy using magnetic resonance imaging. *Alzheimer Dis Assoc Disord* 1996;10(3):141–70.

Muzik O, Chugani DC, Chakraborty P, Mangner T, Chugani HT. Analysis of [C-11]alpha-methyl-tryptophan kinetics for the estimation of serotonin synthesis rate in vivo. *J Cereb Blood Flow Metab* 1997;17(6):659–69.

Pennell PB. PET: cholinergic neuroreceptor mapping. *Adv Neurol* 2000;83:157–63.

Ryvlin P, Bouvard S, Le Bars D, et al. Clinical utility of flumazenil-PET versus [18F]fluorodeoxyglucose-PET and MRI in refractory partial epilepsy. A prospective study in 100 patients. *Brain* 1998;121(Pt 11):2067–81.

Savic I, Ingvar M, Stone-Elander S. Comparison of [11C] flumazenil and [18F]FDG as PET markers of epileptic foci. *J Neurol Neurosurg Psychiatry* 1993;56(6):615–21.

Savic I, Thorell JO, Roland P. [11C]flumazenil positron emission tomography visualizes frontal epileptogenic regions. *Epilepsia* 1995;36(12):1225–32.

Sisodiya SM, Free SL, Stevens JM, Fish DR, Shorvon SD. Widespread cerebral structural changes in patients with cortical dysgenesis and epilepsy. *Brain* 1995;118 (Pt 4):1039–50.

Waterhouse RN. Imaging the PCP site of the NMDA ion channel. *Nucl Med Biol* 2003;30(8):869–78.

References

Bouilleret V, Dupont S, Spelle L, et al. Insular cortex involvement in mesiotemporal lobe epilepsy: a positron emission tomography study. *Ann Neurol* 2002;51(2):202–8.

Chugani DC, Chugani HT. PET: mapping of serotonin synthesis. *Adv Neurol* 2000;83:165–71.

Dupont S, Semah F, Baulac M, Samson Y. The underlying pathophysiology of ictal dystonia in temporal lobe epilepsy: an FDG-PET study. *Neurology* 1998;51(5):1289–92.

Fedi M, Reutens D, Okazawa H, et al. Localizing value of alpha-methyl-L-tryptophan PET in intractable epilepsy of neocortical origin. *Neurology* 2001;57(9):1629–36.

Fedi M, Reutens DC, Andermann F, et al. alpha-[11C]-Methyl-L-tryptophan PET identifies the epileptogenic tuber and correlates with interictal spike frequency. *Epilepsy Res.* 2003;52(3):203–13.

Hammers A, Koepp MJ, Richardson MP, et al. Central benzodiazepine receptors in malformations of cortical development: a quantitative study. *Brain* 2001a;124(Pt 8):1555–65.

Hammers A, Koepp MJ, Labbe C, et al. Neocortical abnormalities of [11C]-flumazenil PET in mesial temporal lobe epilepsy. *Neurology* 2001b;56(7):897–906.

Hammers A, Koepp MJ, Richardson MP, et al. Grey and white matter flumazenil binding in neocortical epilepsy with normal MRI. A PET study of 44 patients. *Brain* 2003;126(Pt 6):1300–18.

Hammers A, Asselin MC, Hinz R, et al. Upregulation of opioid receptor binding following spontaneous epileptic seizures. *Brain* 2007;130(4):1009–1016

Henry TR, Frey KA, Sackellares JC, et al. In vivo cerebral metabolism and central benzodiazepine-receptor binding in temporal lobe epilepsy. *Neurology* 1993;43(10):1998–2006.

Koepp MJ, Richardson MP, Brooks DJ, et al. Cerebral benzodiazepine receptors in hippocampal sclerosis. An objective in vivo analysis. *Brain* 1996;119(Pt 5):1677–87.

Koepp MJ, Labbe C, Richardson MP, et al. Regional hippocampal [11C]flumazenil PET in temporal lobe epilepsy with unilateral and bilateral hippocampal sclerosis. *Brain* 1997;120(Pt 10):1865–76.

Koepp MJ, Richardson MP, Labbe C, et al. 11C-flumazenil PET, volumetric MRI, and quantitative pathology in mesial temporal lobe epilepsy. *Neurology* 1997;49(3):764–73.

Koepp MJ, Hand KS, Labbe C, et al. In vivo [11C] flumazenil-PET correlates with ex vivo [3H]flumazenil autoradiography in hippocampal sclerosis. *Ann Neurol* 1998;43(5):618–26.

Kumlien E, Nilsson A, Hagberg G, Langstrom B, Bergstrom M. PET with 11C-deuterium-deprenyl and 18F-FDG in focal epilepsy. *Acta Neurol Scand* 2001;103(6):360–6.

Madar I, Lesser RP, Krauss G, et al. Imaging of delta- and mu-opioid receptors in temporal lobe epilepsy by positron emission tomography. *Ann Neurol* 1997;41(3):358–67.

Maehara T, Nariai T, Arai N, et al. Usefulness of [11C] methionine PET in the diagnosis of dysembryoplastic neuroepithelial tumor with temporal lobe epilepsy. *Epilepsia* 2004;45(1):41–5.

Mayberg HS, Sadzot B, Meltzer CC, et al. Quantification of mu and non-mu opiate receptors in temporal lobe epilepsy using positron emission tomography. *Ann Neurol* 1991;30(1):3–11.

Merlet I, Ryvlin P, Costes N, et al. Statistical parametric mapping of 5-HT(1A) receptor binding in temporal lobe epilepsy with hippocampal ictal onset on intracranial EEG. *Neuroimage* 2004;**22**(2):886–96.

Natsume J, Kumakura Y, Bernasconi N, *et al.* Alpha-[11C]methyl-L-tryptophan and glucose metabolism in patients with temporal lobe epilepsy. *Neurology* 2003;**60**(5):756–61.

Richardson MP, Koepp MJ, Brooks DJ, Fish DR, Duncan JS. Benzodiazepine receptors in focal epilepsy with cortical dysgenesis: an 11C-flumazenil PET study. *Ann Neurol* 1996;**40**(2):188–98.

Richardson MP, Koepp MJ, Brooks DJ, Duncan JS. 11C-flumazenil PET in neocortical epilepsy. *Neurology* 1998;**51**(2):485–92.

Richardson MP, Koepp MJ, Brooks DJ, *et al.* Cerebral activation in malformations of cortical development. *Brain* 1998;**121**(Pt 7):1295–304.

Richardson MP, Hammers A, Brooks DJ, Duncan JS. Benzodiazepine-GABA(A) receptor binding is very low in dysembryoplastic neuroepithelial tumor: a PET study. *Epilepsia* 2001;**42**(10):1327–34.

Shoaf SE, Carson RE, Hommer D, *et al.* The suitability of [11C]-alpha-methyl-L-tryptophan as a tracer for serotonin synthesis: studies with dual administration of [11C] and [14C] labeled tracer. *J Cereb Blood Flow Metab* 2000;**20**(2):244–52.

Sisodiya SM. Malformations of cortical development: burdens and insights from important causes of human epilepsy. *Lancet Neurol* 2004;**3**(1):29–38.

Theodore WH, Carson RE, Andreasen P, *et al.* PET imaging of opiate receptor binding in human epilepsy using [18F]cyclofoxy. *Epilepsy Res* 1992;**13**(2):129–39.

Toczek MT, Carson RE, Lang L, *et al.* PET imaging of 5-HT1A receptor binding in patients with temporal lobe epilepsy. *Neurology* 2003;**60**(5):749–56.

Tortella FC, Long JB, Holaday JW. Endogenous opioid systems: physiological role in the self-limitation of seizures. *Brain Res* 1985;**332**(1):174–8.

Learning objectives

(1) To understand the basic principles of PET.
(2) To know the advantages and disadvantages of the different ligands used.
(3) To know the indications and interpretation of PET in epilepsy.

Section 2**Classification and diagnosis of epilepsy**

Chapter 42: Advanced MRI sequences – diffusion tensor imaging

Mathias Koepp

Introduction

Diffusion-based imaging is an advanced MRI technique which is sensitive to the molecular displacement of water molecules, providing information on the micro-structural arrangement of tissue. Diffusion tensor tractography is an extension of diffusion-based imaging, and can provide additional information about white matter pathways. Despite the need to interpret results carefully, it promises, in combination with other imaging modalities, electrophysiological techniques and clinical data, to increase our understanding of the effects of epilepsy on the structural organization of the brain. Furthermore, this information can also be used to optimize presurgical planning of patients with epilepsy.

The study of the anatomy of white matter pathways is crucial to our understanding of both normal and abnormal brain function. To date, these connections have been studied by way of direct visualization predominantly in animal brain specimens. In view of the intrinsically slow nature of this work, and the difficulties in drawing inferences from animal models, our knowledge of cerebral white matter connections in humans is still very limited. The development of MRI-based tract mapping techniques offers the prospect of non-invasive, in vivo imaging of white matter tracts for the first time. Furthermore, this technique can be employed synergistically with clinical, fMRI, PET and electrophysiological data, in order to obtain insights into both the anatomy and function of these connections. This knowledge has a variety of clinical applications to patients with epilepsy.

The goal of structural MRI in epilepsy patients is to identify those patients suitable for surgery, locate the epileptogenic lesion or zone (by using concurrent clinical, electrophysiological and other imaging data), and resect it, causing minimal damage to eloquent cortex. In patients with cerebral lesions, the localization of cognitive activation may differ from the pattern in normal subjects, and for this reason functional MRI (fMRI) is useful to delineate areas of eloquent cortex such as primary sensorimotor cortex, essential language areas, occipital visual areas and mesial temporal regions crucial for episodic memory. By noting the anatomical relation of these areas to those of planned resection, postoperative complications can be minimized. The use of tractography enables the identification of white matter fibre tracts connecting these eloquent cortical areas to be delineated, so that inadvertent surgical damage can be avoided, thus further reducing postoperative complications. Moreover, this technique also lends itself to an exploration of the reorganization of white matter networks in chronic epilepsy, which may underlie changes in cognitive function.

Background
The biological and physical basis of diffusion-based imaging

In a free medium, the molecular diffusion of water refers to the random translational motion (Brownian motion) of molecules resulting from the thermal energy carried by these molecules. In the brain, diffusion is restricted by intra- and extracellular boundaries, and represents the effects of several variable, independent factors. These include the presence of impermeable or semi-permeable membranes, macromolecules which hinder the diffusion of small molecules, and intra- and extracellular microcirculatory effects. The measurement of water diffusion

---

Introduction to Epilepsy ed. Gonzalo Alarcón and Antonio Valentín. Published by Cambridge University Press.
© Cambridge University Press 2012.

therefore provides a means of probing cellular integrity and pathology.

The principles of diffusion MRI were first developed in vivo in the mid 1980s. In diffusion-weighted imaging (DWI), images are sensitized to the diffusional properties of water by the incorporation of pulsed magnetic field gradients into a standard spin echo sequence. By taking measurements in at least three directions, it is possible to characterize the mean diffusion properties within a voxel in the image by way of a single scalar apparent diffusion coefficient (ADC). Early diffusion studies discovered that ADC measurements depended on a subject's orientation relative to the magnet and gradient coils. White matter tracts parallel to an applied gradient had the greatest ADC whereas those lying oblique or transverse to a gradient had smaller ADC values. This gave rise to the concept of asymmetry of diffusion of molecules in three directions, or 'anisotropy'.

Diffusion tensor imaging (DTI) enables not only the quantification of water molecule diffusion, but also the characterization of the degree and direction of anisotropy. The diffusion tensor is a mathematical construct that can be calculated from a non-diffusion-weighted image plus six or more diffusion-weighted measurements along non-colinear directions. The tensor can be diagonalized to give three eigenvectors, ε_1, ε_2 and ε_3, representing the principal directions of diffusion, and three eigenvalues, λ_1, λ_2 and λ_3, representing the magnitude of diffusion (or the corresponding ADC values) along these directions. The eigenvectors are ordered with decreasing values of their eigenvalues so that ε_1 represents the principal direction of diffusivity, and λ_1 will be the ADC value along ε_1. This corresponds to the maximum diffusion in each voxel regardless of the orientation of the subject's head. Furthermore, a number of diffusion parameters can be derived in each voxel, which are insensitive to subject positioning and fibre tract alignment within the diffusion gradients of the MRI scanner. Mean diffusivity (MD) is a summary measure of the average diffusion properties of a voxel and is equivalent to the estimated ADC over three orthogonal directions. Fractional anisotropy (FA), on the other hand, is an estimate of what proportion of the magnitude of the diffusion tensor is due to anisotropic diffusion. Anisotropy in white matter results from the organization of tissue as bundles of axons and myelin sheaths run in parallel, and the diffusion of water is freer and quicker in the long axis of the fibres than in the perpendicular direction. Malformations or acquired insults cause disruption to the microstructural environment and, more often than not, a subsequent reduction in anisotropy. Such abnormalities may also lead to a reduction in cell density and/or expansion of the extracellular space, resulting in an increase in MD/ADC.

From diffusion tensor imaging to tractography

With conventional MRI, variations in white matter signal are subtle, and white matter tracts cannot be accurately parcellated. In most studies, DTI quantitative measures have been assessed using either region-of-interest or voxel-based analysis. The former has limitations in that it is user-dependent, and has a possibility of error that other fibre tracts, grey matter and CSF or other white matter structures may be included. The latter, though observer-independent, has problems associated with the need for spatial normalization and smoothing due to anatomical variations in ventricular size, gyral patterns, etc. Both methods have limited ability to quantify specific white matter pathways along their entire trajectories. Tractography is an extension of DTI, whereby the directional information obtained in each voxel is used to generate virtual three-dimensional white matter maps. These maps are based on similarities between the diffusion properties of neighbouring voxels in terms of shape (quantitative diffusion anisotropy measures) and orientation (principal eigenvector map). Tractography does not therefore trace fibres in the sense that injected tracers do; rather it demonstrates the path of least resistance to water diffusion.

Methods
Selecting a seed region

In most tractography experiments, start regions are defined using anatomical reference points. As a result, they are susceptible to operator bias, and can introduce a source of variability into tractography results. The combination of fMRI and tractography enables the use of operator-independent placement of seed regions. Furthermore, it offers an opportunity to study the relationship between brain structure and function by providing a selective tracing of white matter pathways within a behaviourally characterized network. In studies of language networks therefore, our group has used verbal fluency, verb generation and reading comprehension paradigms to define functional regions which were then used to generate starting regions for tractography.

Tractography algorithms

A variety of algorithms has been devised to generate white matter maps using the information provided by diffusion imaging. Linear or streamline methods use the orientation of maximum diffusion at each voxel, and are performed by following these orientation estimates to reconstruct pathways that, within a coherent bundle, correspond to the underlying fibre pathway. They therefore define a single route of connection for each start point(s) or region of interest (ROI) from voxel to voxel. These types of streamlined approaches are generally susceptible to errors in the orientation of $\epsilon 1$ due both to noise and to instances where the direction of the underlying tract anatomy is ambiguous or reflects the presence of multiple non-colinear fibre pathways. They assume absolute knowledge in fibre direction at every point with no representation of the uncertainty present in the recovered pathway. An erroneous pathway, due to noise or partial volume effects, is therefore assigned as much significance as 'true' pathways.

For this reason in our laboratory we use a probabilistic tractography approach to exploit the inherent uncertainty in the orientation of ϵ_1 for each voxel to generate maps of connection probability. Orders of uncertainty based upon the anisotropy of the tensor and the relative magnitudes of the eigenvalues are used to generate probability density functions (PDFs) of the result of the diffusion tensor mixture model. These are a means of describing the local uncertainty in fibre orientation. Each PDF is intended to interpret the information from a diffusion imaging acquisition in terms of the likely underlying fibre structure at each point within the brain. The end result is that for every voxel, a distribution of directions rather than a single principal eigenvector is obtained. Any of these points can then be selected as a starting place for running a streamline propagation process. This can be repeated a large number of times (N), and the number of times that any voxel in the brain is encountered over N repetitions provides an index of connectivity for that voxel to the start point, eventually giving a map of probability of connection, or a probabalistic index of connectivity (PICo) to the chosen seed point. The probability of connection in any experiment generally decreases with distance from the start point due to the cumulative effect of the uncertainties in propagation at each step in the streamline process.

The effects of noise on this model are also explicitly simulated and used to analyse the uncertainty associated with the principal diffusion direction of each diffusion tensor. It is observed that this uncertainty, and therefore the distribution of the principal diffusion direction, decreases as the fractional anisotropy increases.

Tract analysis

The tracts generated in individual subjects can be analysed at a qualitative level. Tracts from different individuals can also be combined to generate group maps, which give an indication of how reproducible a given connection is across a population of subjects.

Finally, the white matter tracts can also be used to derive quantitative information, including volume and anisotropy parameters. These can then be compared across groups, or tested for correlations against fMRI or clinical data.

Results

Language – the superior longitudinal fasciculus

Temporal lobe epilepsy (TLE) may be associated with disrupted lateralization of language, and may be further impaired by anterior temporal lobe resections. Indeed selective language deficits have been reported in up to 40% of patients following dominant ATLR. The superior longitudinal fasciculus is known to be a crucial part of the language network, connecting anterior (Broca's) and posterior (Wernicke's) language areas. In a study of 14 patients with unilateral temporal lobe epilepsy and 10 controls, the language paradigms described above were used to generate seed regions for tractography in both Broca's and Wernicke's area. Controls and right TLE patients were found to have a left-lateralized pattern of both language-related activations and associated white matter organization as demonstrated by FA and volume measures. Left TLE patients showed more symmetrical language activations, along with reduced left hemisphere and increased right hemisphere white matter pathways, in comparison with both controls and right TLE patients.

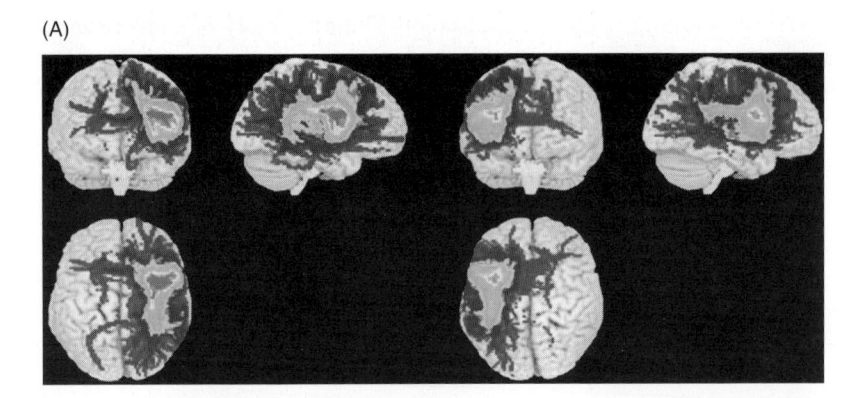

Section 2: Classification and diagnosis of epilepsy

Figure 42.1. (A) Left (left panel) and right (right panel) fasciculus arcuatus in healthy controls. (B) In left TLE, less lateralization of fasciculus arcuatus than healthy controls. See colour version in plate section.

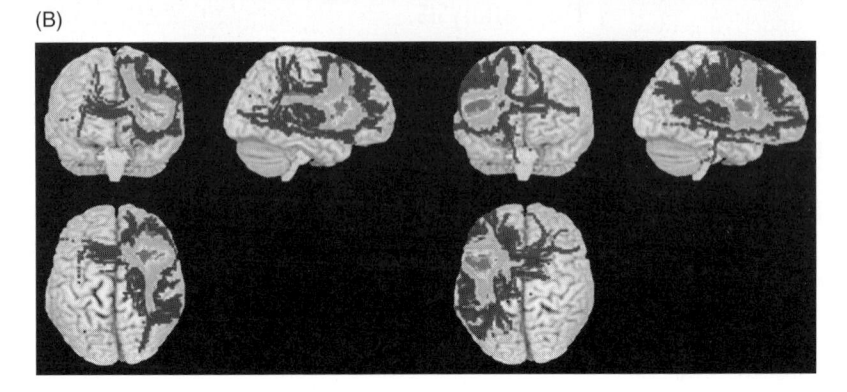

Correlations between measures of structure (FA) and function in both patient groups were found, with subjects with more lateralized functional activation having more lateralized white matter pathways. The findings of this study therefore demonstrate that tractography is able to demonstrate the structural network underpinning the lateralization of language function elucidated by fMRI studies.

Memory – the parahippocampal gyrus

Parahippocampal structures, which are critically implicated in the generation and propagation of seizures in TLE, are also essential for declarative memory. Longitudinal neuropsychological studies have shown that persisting epilepsy is associated with progressive memory impairment. Those who undergo anterior temporal lobe resection (ATLR) are at further risk of memory impairment, the nature of which depends on whether surgery is on the dominant or non-dominant side. Patients typically show a decline in verbal memory following surgery involving the language-dominant hemisphere and deficits in topographical memory following non-dominant temporal lobe resection. Neuropsychological assessment, quantitative MRI and latterly functional MRI (fMRI) indicate the role of the medial temporal lobe structures (MTL) in sustaining material-specific memory functions, and the reorganization of memory that occurs with TLE. These and lesion deficit studies have shown that memory deficit after ATLR is related to the functional integrity of the parahippocampal structures. The strength of connections, or structural connectivity, of the parahippocampal gyrus in TLE has not been evaluated, or related to function.

Our group performed a tractography analysis of diffusion magnetic resonance imaging scans in 18 patients with unilateral TLE undergoing presurgical evaluation, and in 10 healthy controls. An anatomically derived seed region in the anterior parahippocampal gyrus was selected from which to trace the white matter connections of the medial temporal lobe. A correlation analysis was also carried out between volume and mean FA of the connections, and preoperative material-specific memory performance. There was no significant difference between the left- and right-sided connections in controls. In left TLE patients, the connected regions ipsilateral to the epileptogenic region were found to be significantly

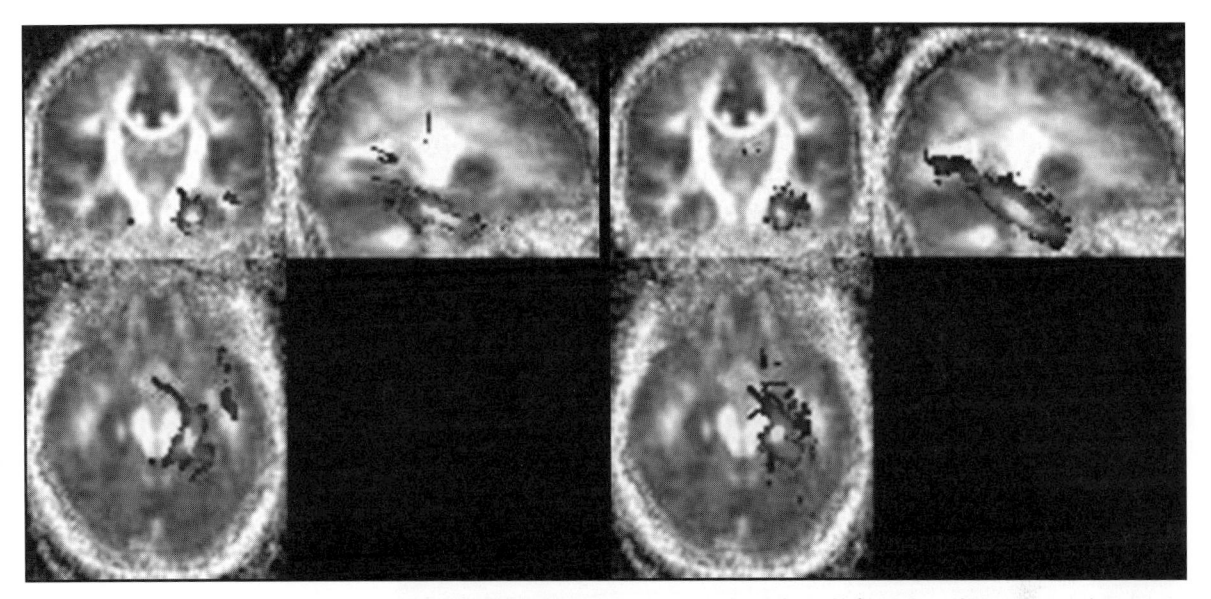

Figure 42.2. Material-specific memory measures correlated with tract volume and FA in right and left TLE. See colour version in plate section.

reduced in volume and mean FA compared with the contralateral region. Significant correlations were found in left TLE patients between left and right FA, and verbal and non-verbal memory respectively. Though there was a trend towards ipsilateral reduction in volume and FA in right TLE patients, this was not significant. Similarly, no correlations between left or right FA and memory measures were found in this group of patients. It is unclear why no differences were seen in right TLE patients. It is possible that the speech-dominant hemisphere has greater and denser connectivity to the rest of the brain, and that it is more sensitive to damage than is the non-speech-dominant hemisphere.

Other groups have assessed other memory structures within the limbic system. Concha *et al.* found that patients with unilateral TLE have bilateral changes in the fornix and cingulum bundle, characterized by impaired tracking of these pathways, and increased mean diffusivity and reduced fractional anisotropy along them. This was thought to be consistent with the degeneration of pathways connecting to the hippocampus. Studies by the same group have assessed the progression of Wallerian degeneration in the limbic structures in patients with refractory epilepsy who have undergone surgical procedures such as corpus callostomy and temporal lobe resections.

Taken together, these results suggest that the use of tractography-derived quantitative measures may have a significant role to play in the longitudinal evaluation of the effects of epilepsy on the brain, and on cognitive functions such as memory and language, particularly when correlated with neuropsychological measures.

Preoperative planning – visual pathways

ATLR can also cause visual field defects (VFDs) in up to 10% of patients. Indeed, in 5% it can be severe enough to render the patient ineligible for a driving licence, despite being seizure-free. Typically, VFDs after ATLR occur in the superior homonymous field contralateral to the resection and are due to disruption of fibres of Meyer's loop. The anterior extent of the Meyer loop is not visualized on conventional imaging and varies from person to person. As a consequence the occurrence and extent of a postoperative VFD cannot be accurately predicted by conventional MRI, or from the extent of resection performed. Tractography has been used to demonstrate the optic radiation in normal subjects, and has been applied to pre- and postoperative surgical patients with arteriovenous malformations and tumours in and around the visual pathways. Kikuta *et al.* carried out pre- and postoperative tractography in 10 such patients, and were able to predict the magnitude of pre- and postoperative visual field loss from the geometrical relationship between the optic radiation and arteriovenous malformation.

A recent study by our group demonstrated its application to temporal lobe surgery for epilepsy. The

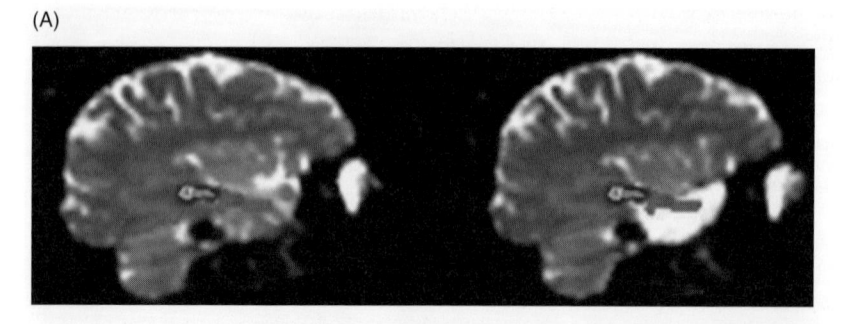

Figure 42.3. (A) Preoperative optic radiation superimposed on preoperative (left panel) and postoperative (right panel) mean high-resolution DTI in a patient with postoperative upper quadrantanopia. (B) Preoperative optic radiation superimposed on preoperative (left panel) and postoperative (right panel) mean high-resolution DTI in a patient without postoperative visual field defects. See colour version in plate section.

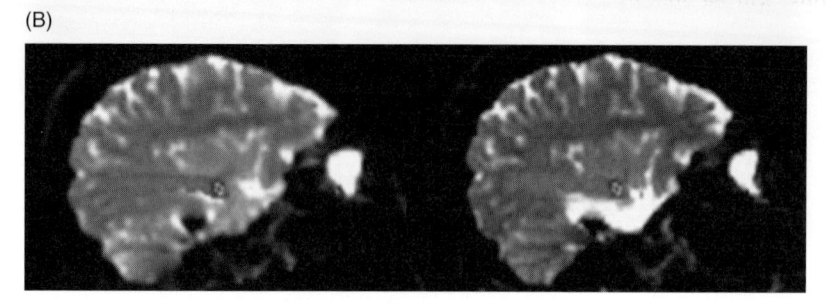

optic radiation was visualized before and after ATLR, and disruption of Meyer's loop was clearly demonstrated in a patient who developed a quadrantanopia.

Future goals

The development of tractography-based techniques is still at a relatively early stage, and several major challenges remain. The most pressing of these is the lack of a single 'gold standard' method of validation. Tractography is essentially a user-defined process, where tracking results may vary according to the algorithm used, size and definition method of a region of interest, FA threshold for termination of tracking, angular threshold, step length and numbers of sampling within a voxel. Despite the concordance of results in areas such as language, and the fact that studies have shown that the technique can reconstruct and be consistent with major fibre tract trajectories, there is a need for robust standardized tests with which to assess the different algorithms and data acquisition techniques. Pre- and postoperative tractography studies in epilepsy surgery may be in a prime position to rectify this problem. The use of tractography together with MEG, fMRI and fMRI-EEG has the potential to provide complementary but equally important information in these patients. Furthermore, concordance of results derived from these techniques in the same patient groups would go some way towards validation of tractography-based techniques.

The other challenges of tractography relate to the quality of data acquisition, and the tracking algorithms. This includes problems such as eddy current distortions, gradient non-linearities, motion artefact, signal loss due to susceptibility variations, and low resolution acquisition. The relatively low signal-to-noise ratio of DTI data introduces errors in the information obtained using it. Signal-to-noise ratio is inversely proportional to spatial resolution, in that increasing spatial resolution (i.e. decreasing voxel size) leads to a reduction in signal-to-noise ratio. Using a higher magnetic field or longer acquisition times can compensate for this loss of signal-to-noise ratio. Even at higher spatial resolutions however, the size of typical imaging voxels is two to three millimetres cubed, so a single voxel could contain thousands of axons. This limited spatial resolution can lead to false positives, and can lead to the false definition of a tract direction in a voxel, especially in the presence of fibres crossing or kissing within individual voxels. In addition, it may also lead to false negatives by ignoring small fibre tracts that may be functionally important.

Despite these limitations tractography is currently the only technique available for tracing white matter pathways in the living brain. Furthermore, as methodological developments occur in orientational and spatial resolution, and in diffusion modelling and tractography algorithms, these limitations should prove less of a problem. By applying tractography both postoperatively and in a longitudinal fashion, it is hoped that tractography-derived data, in synergy with fMRI and neuropsychological data, may provide valuable prognostic information regarding cognitive outcomes in patients with refractory epilepsy. In addition, when the technical challenges of co-registration of preoperative tractography with the T1-weighted MR images are surmounted, preoperative tractography of the optic radiation and other vital white matter connections, will be able to be displayed when planning and undertaking surgical procedures. Further, the advent of perioperative MRI will allow the correction of the movement of tracts caused by craniotomy, and will improve the accuracy of the data, to aid surgical planning and result in a lower risk of postoperative deficits. Ultimately, it is hoped that it may one day be possible to develop potentially novel approaches to functionally disconnect the seizure focus from the surrounding brain.

Conclusion

Neuroimaging has had a dramatic impact in the field of cognitive neuroscience. Knowledge gained or methodological improvements made in the basic application for cognitive neuroscience tends to directly benefit clinical neuroimaging. PET techniques can tell us about how brains of certain epileptic syndromes differ neurochemically from unaffected populations, or they can be used in assessing brain abnormalities in a single patient. These studies highlight the link between abnormal epileptiform activity, network brain activity and cognitive function. In addition to their use for presurgical planning, PET has the potential for contributing to monitoring the course of treatment and prediction of prognosis. For all of these reasons, clinical PET will continue to improve the quality of health care. The strengths and weaknesses of any clinical tool must be fully appreciated by the health-care provider before it can be used routinely and influence the course of treatment.

Recommended reading

Alexander DC. Multiple-fiber reconstruction algorithms for diffusion MRI. *Ann N Y Acad Sci* 2005;**1064**:113–33.

Alexander DC, Barker GJ, Arridge SR. Detection and modeling of non-Gaussian apparent diffusion coefficient profiles in human brain data. *Magn Reson Med* 2002;**48**:331–40.

Catani M. Diffusion tensor magnetic resonance imaging tractography in cognitive disorders. *Curr Opin Neurol* 2006;**19**:599–606.

Concha L, Beaulieu C, Gross DW. Bilateral limbic diffusion abnormalities in unilateral temporal lobe epilepsy. *Ann Neurol* 2005;**57**:188–96.

Concha L, Beaulieu C, Wheatley BM, Gross DW. Bilateral white matter diffusion changes persist after epilepsy surgery. *Epilepsia* 2007;**48**:931–40.

Concha L, Gross DW, Wheatley BM, Beaulieu C. Diffusion tensor imaging of time-dependent axonal and myelin degradation after corpus callosotomy in epilepsy patients. *Neuroimage* 2006;**32**:1090–9.

Guye M, Parker GJ, Symms M, et al. Combined functional MRI and tractography to demonstrate the connectivity of the human primary motor cortex in vivo. *Neuroimage* 2003;**19**:1349–60.

Johansen-Berg H, Behrens TE. Just pretty pictures? What diffusion tractography can add in clinical neuroscience. *Curr Opin Neurol* 2006;**19**:379–85.

Le Bihan D. Looking into the functional architecture of the brain with diffusion MRI. *Nat Neurosci* 2003;**4**:469–80.

Mori S, van Zijl PC. Fiber tracking: principles and strategies – a technical review. *NMR Biomed* 2002;**15**:468–80.

Parker GJ, Alexander DC. Probabilistic anatomical connectivity derived from the microscopic persistent angular structure of cerebral tissue. *Philos Trans R Soc Lond B* 2005;**360**:893–902.

Parker GJ, Haroon HA, Wheeler-Kingshott CA. A framework for a streamline-based probabilistic index of connectivity (PICo) using a structural interpretation of MRI diffusion measurements. *J Magn Reson Imaging* 2003;**18**:242–54.

Powell HW, Guye M, Parker GJ, et al., Noninvasive in vivo demonstration of the connections of the human parahippocampal gyrus. *Neuroimage* 2004;**22**:740–7.

Powell HW, Parker GJ, Alexander DC, et al. MR tractography predicts visual field defects following temporal lobe resection. *Neurology* 2005;**65**:596–9.

Powell HW, Parker GJ, Alexander DC, et al. Abnormalities of language networks in temporal lobe epilepsy. *Neuroimage* 2007;**36**(1):209.

Learning objectives

(1) To understand the basic principles of DTI.
(2) To understand the potential use and the indications of DTI in epilepsy.
(3) To understand the future avenues for DTI development.

Section 2 Classification and diagnosis of epilepsy

Chapter 43

EEG-correlated fMRI in epilepsy

Louis Lemieux

EEG and functional MRI

Electroencephalography (EEG) and functional magnetic resonance imaging (fMRI) are important techniques for the study of the human brain. Features visible on scalp EEG, such as spikes or rhythms, reflect increased synchronization of cortical activity at various spatial scales, ranging from sub-lobar to the entire brain. Crucially, scalp EEG is most sensitive to superficial cortical activity with limited or no sensitivity to events taking place deeper in the brain such as on the medial aspect of the temporal lobe, which are only detectable via propagation to more superficial cortex (Alarcón et al., 1994). EEG can provide specific markers of epilepsy containing localizing information in relation to a brain abnormality responsible for the epilepsy. In patients with drug-resistant epilepsy who may benefit from surgery, EEG recordings are capable of providing very useful information. Although in general spikes may originate from outside the epileptic focus itself, in many cases there is considerable overlap. In theory, spike generator localization can be improved on using computational EEG source reconstruction methods based on assumptions on the form of the EEG generators (Fuchs et al., 2007). Although widely used in research, this type of localization has had limited impact on clinical practice in large part due to uncertainties in the modelling assumptions, and the relatively low yield due to the difficulty in capturing spikes during the 30–60 minute scanning session (similarly to MEG). Therefore, the clinical utility of EEG-based localization remains limited.

Functional MRI, in the form of activation maps derived from series of scans, is a powerful, relatively new tool for visualizing changes linked to epochs of specific brain activity (Goebel, 2007). Two great potential advantages of fMRI over EEG-based localization are its more or less uniform spatial sensitivity and sampling down to a few mm. However, fMRI is limited by other factors such as poor temporal resolution (of the order of seconds) and is subject to numerous artefacts. Perhaps more importantly, fMRI reflects neuronal activity only indirectly, in the form of signals related to the haemodynamic changes that are associated with neuronal activity, namely the blood oxygen-level dependent (BOLD) effect. This phenomenon remains the subject of intense investigation (Shmuel et al., 2006). One of the main features of the BOLD signal is that it involves a period of 15–20 seconds following even the briefest external stimulus. In some circumstances, the BOLD signal decreases following an event. An important aspect of fMRI, quite distinct from most EEG, is its current reliance on correlation with an independent factor, such as external stimulus or task, i.e. precisely timed cues, for acquisition and interpretation. Therefore most fMRI is acquired and analysed in a fashion similar to evoked potential EEG experiments.

Combined EEG and fMRI experiments

It has now been made possible to acquire good-quality EEG and fMRI data simultaneously. Furthermore, work in our group and a few others around the world has shown that paroxysmal activity of the type encountered in patients with epilepsy, such as seizures and focal spikes, could be imaged using fMRI. In view of the way fMRI is usually analysed, based on correlation, this requires data to be collected in at least two experimental states, namely normal background (control state) and paroxysmal ('active' state) in the case of studies in patients with epilepsy, such that each scan in the time series can be labelled as either. Because of

Introduction to Epilepsy ed. Gonzalo Alarcón and Antonio Valentín. Published by Cambridge University Press.
© Cambridge University Press 2012.

Continuous EEG and fMRI:

Spike-related BOLD

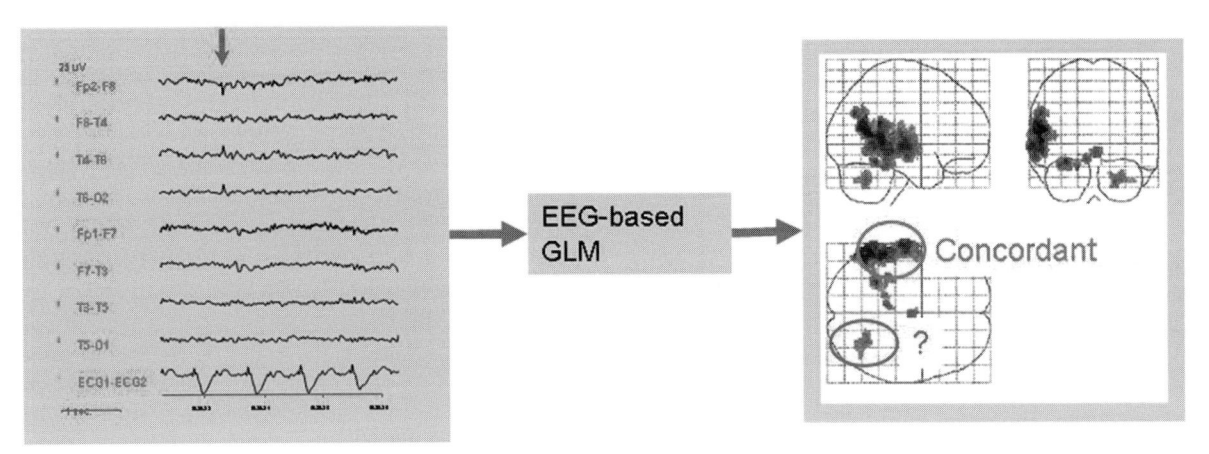

Figure 43.1. Illustration of EEG-correlated fMRI methodology and typical finding in patient with frequent focal spikes. Left: EEG segment recorded during fMRI scanning using special EEG equipment and and processed using dedicated post-processing software. Middle: box representing the conversion of the EEG into a general linear model (GLM) of the fMRI data. Right: resulting BOLD map shows a large cluster in the left temporal region (superimposed on a cartoon brain), concordant with our understanding of the patient's irritative zone, and a contralateral cluster. See colour version in plate section.

the rarity of ictal events and other problems associated with head movement, it is usually neither practical nor safe to aim at imaging seizures in an MR scanner, although there have been a few instances of ictal fMRI in patients with focal epilepsy (Salek-Haddadi et al., 2003). In generalized epilepsy, absence seizures are interesting candidates for imaging. Interictal events, such as focal spikes, occur much more commonly but by definition are devoid of clinical manifestations. Therefore, imaging this type of activity requires the recording of EEG during the fMRI acquisition. This represents a technical challenge because of interactions between the MR scanner and EEG recording equipment, which can result in degradation of image and EEG data quality, and because of patient safety concerns. These have been largely addressed over the last 10 years and have given rise to a specialized type of EEG recording equipment.

In a typical EEG-fMRI experiment, as performed in our centre, an EEG electrode cap is attached to the patient's scalp and to an MR-compatible EEG recording system. One of the main features of this type of system is the lack of ferrous components to avoid mechanical forces turning it into a dangerous projectile and minimizing image quality degradation, and the very high sampling signal rate (and synchronization link to the scanner) necessary to get rid of the artefacts caused in the EEG by the scanning process.

The patient is asked to relax during the 20 to 40 minute scan and no experimental task or stimulus is therefore imposed. Their resulting resting-state fMRI dataset is analysed by categorizing each scan according to the experimental (or brain) state at any given time, which is determined based on the simultaneously recorded EEG and performing a correlation between the fMRI data and the state dependent model. Effectively, scans acquired during or following an EEG event of interest (focal spike, spike-wave complex or run) are compared with those acquired during periods of background activity. Spike-related BOLD maps are obtained following the application of statistical tests to assess the likelihood of chance correlation (Figure 43.1).

The application of EEG-fMRI in epilepsy remains largely exploratory, focusing on investigating the technique's ability to reveal activations in relation to various types of EEG abnormalities and syndromes. The technique has now been applied in more than 300 patients with focal epilepsy in our centre and the main findings can be summarized as follows:

- fMRI of focal spikes provides localizing information (i.e. statistically significant regional BOLD changes) in roughly 60% of cases in which interictal spikes are captured;
- regions of spike-related BOLD increases tend to correspond with the presumed focus;

- regions of spike-related BOLD decreases tend to be remote from the presumed focus;
- BOLD increases in the ipsilateral hippocampus and decreases in the precuneus are commonly observed in relation to temporal spikes;
- the time course of focal spike-related BOLD signal increase is similar to that observed following brief external stimuli or tasks in healthy subjects (Salek-Haddadi et al., 2006).

Although much more work needs to be done to assess the technique's potential clinical value, there are already signs that EEG-fMRI can provide valuable additional information in the presurgical evaluation of patients with drug-resistant epilepsy (Zijlmans et al., 2008; Thornton et al., 2010). In generalized epilepsies, absence seizures and interictal generalized spike-wave discharges have been shown to be characterized by BOLD increases in the thalamus and widespread (though rather variable) cortical decreases (Hamandi et al., 2006). There is increasing interest in the study of seizures using fMRI, with the realization that the main practical concerns (e.g. related to safety, data quality degradation due to motion) can be managed adequately in a significant proportion of patients (Salek-Haddadi et al., 2002; Donaire et al., 2009; Tyvaert et al., 2009; Thornton et al., 2010a) potentially providing important new information about this defining feature of the condition. These unique observations illustrate EEG-fMRI's scientific interest in addition to its potential clinical utility.

References

Alarcón G, Guy CN, Binnie CD, et al. Intracerebral propagation of interictal activity in partial epilepsy: implications for source localisation. *J Neurol Neurosurg Psychiatry* 1994;**57**:435–49.

Donaire A, Bargallo N, Falcon C, et al. Identifying the structures involved in seizure generation using sequential analysis of ictal-fMRI data. *NeuroImage* 2009;**47**:173–83.

Fuchs M, Wagner M, Kastner J. Development of volume conductor and source models to localize epileptic foci. *J Clin Neurophysiol* 2007;**24**(2):101–19.

Goebel R. Localization of brain activity using functional magnetic resonance imaging. In Stippich C, ed. *Clinical Functional MRI*. Berlin: Springer; 2007.

Hamandi K, Salek-Haddadi A, Laufs H, et al. EEG-fMRI of idiopathic and secondarily generalized epilepsies. *Neuroimage* 2006;**31**(4):1700–10.

Niedermeyer E. Epileptic seizure disorders. In Niedermeyer E, Lopes Da Silva F, eds. *Electroencephalography: Basic Principles, Clinical Applications, and Related Fields*. 4th edn. Baltimore: Lippincott Williams and Willkins; 1999.

Salek-Haddadi A, Merschhemke M, Lemieux L, Fish DR. Simultaneous EEG-correlated ictal fMRI. *NeuroImage* 2002;**16**:32–40.

Salek-Haddadi A, Friston KJ, Lemieux L, Fish DR. Studying spontaneous EEG activity with fMRI. *Brain Res Rev* 2003;**43**(1):110–33.

Salek-Haddadi A, Diehl B, Hamandi K, et al. Hemodynamic correlates of epileptiform discharges: an EEG-fMRI study of 63 patients with focal epilepsy. *Brain Res* 2006;**1088**(1):148–66.

Shmuel A, Augath M, Oeltermann A, Logothetis NK. Negative functional MRI response correlates with decreases in neuronal activity in monkey visual area V1. *Nat Neurosci* 2006;**9**(4):569–77.

Thornton R, Laufs H, Rodionov R, et al. EEG correlated functional MRI and postoperative outcome in focal epilepsy. *J Neurol Neurosurg Psychiatry* 2010;**81**(8):922–7.

Thornton R, Rodionov R, Laufs H, et al. Imaging haemodynamic changes related to seizures: Comparison of EEG-based general linear model, independent component analysis of fMRI and intracranial EEG. *Neuroimage* 2010a;**53**:196–205.

Tyvaert L, Levan P, Dubeau F, Gotman J. Noninvasive dynamic imaging of seizures in epileptic patients. *Hum Brain Mapp* 2009;**12**:3993–4011.

Zijlmans M, Huiskamp G, Hersevoort M, et al. EEG-fMRI in the preoperative work-up for epilepsy surgery. *Brain* 2007;**130**(Pt 9):2343–53.

Learning objectives

(1) To understand the concept of fMRI applied to the study of spontaneous epileptic discharges (e.g. spikes) in humans.
(2) To understand the need for and method of EEG recording during fMRI scanning for such studies.
(3) To understand the interest and limitations of this methodology.
(4) To become familiar with the main findings of EEG-fMRI in epilepsy.

Section 2: Classification and diagnosis of epilepsy

Chapter 44: Source localization methods

Stefano Seri and Antonella Cerquiglini

One of the most pressing demands on electrophysiology applied to the diagnosis of epilepsy is the non-invasive localization of the neuronal generators responsible for brain electrical and magnetic fields (the so-called inverse problem). These neuronal generators produce primary currents in the brain, which together with passive currents give rise to the EEG signal. Unfortunately, the signal we measure on the scalp surface doesn't directly indicate the location of the active neuronal assemblies. This is the expression of the ambiguity of the underlying static electromagnetic inverse problem, partly due to the relatively limited number of independent measures available. A given electric potential distribution recorded at the scalp can be explained by the activity of infinite different configurations of intracranial sources. In contrast, the forward problem, which consists of computing the potential field at the scalp from known source locations and strengths with known geometry and conductivity properties of the brain and its layers (CSF/meninges, skin and skull), i.e. the head model, has a unique solution. The head models vary from the computationally simpler spherical models (three or four concentric spheres) to the realistic models based on the segmentation of anatomical images obtained using magnetic resonance imaging (MRI). Realistic models – computationally intensive and difficult to implement – can separate different tissues of the head and account for the convoluted geometry of the brain and the significant inter-individual variability.

In real-life applications, if the assumptions of the statistical, anatomical or functional properties of the signal and the volume in which it is generated are meaningful, a true three-dimensional tomographic representation of sources of brain electrical activity is possible in spite of the 'ill-posed' nature of the inverse problem (Michel et al., 2004). The techniques used to achieve this are now referred to as electrical source imaging (ESI) or magnetic source imaging (MSI). The first issue to influence reconstruction accuracy is spatial sampling, i.e. the number of EEG electrodes. It has been shown that this relationship is not linear, reaching a plateau at about 128 electrodes, provided spatial distribution is uniform. The second factor is related to the different properties of the source localization strategies used with respect to the hypothesized source configuration.

According to these assumptions, source localization methods can be classified as linear or non-linear.

(1) Non-linear (over-determined or dipolar): dipolar models can be efficient reconstruction methods provided the configuration of the electrical potential field can be modelled by a small discrete number of point-like sources. This number (the model order) must be correctly hypothesized a priori by the user (Achim et al., 1991) and has to be less than or equal to the number of electrodes. Methods such as singular value decomposition or principal component analysis can be used to inform this choice. Acceptance of a specific source configuration as a reliable reconstruction is reliant on quantitative measures. One procedure is to iteratively compute possible dipolar source configurations and project these as scalp field potential maps (forward solution). Maps are then compared with the recorded surface potential map to produce a measure of difference between the two (squared error). This process is iterated until a source configuration that minimizes the difference between the computed and original scalp maps is obtained. In this process, the iteration can be trapped in undesirable local minima, resulting in the algorithm accepting a certain location because moving in any direction increases the error of the fit. A further difficulty is that the forward solution requires defining

Introduction to Epilepsy ed. Gonzalo Alarcón and Antonio Valentín. Published by Cambridge University Press.
© Cambridge University Press 2012.

specific features of the compartments (single to multiple concentric sphere vs realistic head models) and conductivity tensor across the compartments (CSF, scalp, skull) for the head model as detailed above. Finally, dipolar estimations are sensitive to the signal-to-noise ratio of the signal, and to low-frequency activity operating more reliably after high-pass filtering and on averaged data.

(2) Linear (under-determined or distributed): unlike dipolar models, linear inverse solutions do not require any a priori assumptions on the number of sources to solve the inverse problem. The entire brain volume is divided into discrete solution points, each one of them characterized by a current density value, and these can be represented overlaid on the patient's MRI (Figure 44.1). This family of methods has seen several computational implementations. The minimum norm solution is the most general formulation. Its main limitation is that it tends to favour superficial sources, with deeper sources incorrectly projected on the surface, ultimately being potentially prone to erroneous interpretations. Researchers have developed a number of algorithms to overcome this problem (FOCUSS, LORETA, sLORETA, LAURA, EPIFOCUS). Clinical validation of these techniques is still limited to small series from few centres, limiting the ability to assess reliably their contribution to the presurgical evaluation. Mesial temporal lobe series have suggested good concordance between intracranial measures and ESI extra-cranial interictal predictions (Lantz et al., 1997). For ictal recordings, separation between origin and propagation is more problematic, even though a 2–3 cm accuracy can be seen as a realistic estimate. Only recently, larger surgical series have been analysed in terms of concordance between the ESI-predicted sources, intra-cranial confirmation and surgical outcome and concordance was found in 93% of the patients. A critical review of the pitfalls and the state of ESI has recently been produced (Plummer et al., 2008).

Other source identification techniques

The application of independent component analysis (ICA; Bell and Sejnowski, 1996) has been used to decompose the EEG into statistically independent sources. The fundamental physiologically plausible assumption of this method is that if different signals belong to different underlying physical processes, they will also be statistically independent. When applied to EEG, this corresponds to hypothesizing that neural ensembles underlying the surface-recorded activity – also called generators or sources – are linearly mixed with background activity and noise in the recorded external signals. While ICA algorithms do not solve the inverse problem, they are able to demix the signal into its underlying components and estimate their amplitude over time. This information can be fed to a further analytical step such as dipolar methods to recover the source position without further a priori assumptions other than the statistical independence of the components, improving the accuracy of the localization. The potential for clinical application of these methods in epilepsy has only recently been explored. One promising application is the identification of sources of ictal EEG activity, although risks of spurious ICA-based localization in the absence of clear focality of seizure onset have been highlighted. In a recent study on patients in phase II presurgical assessment, the method offered promising results in characterizing the seizure onset zone and the propagation pattern of seizures (Patel et al., 2008). Further potential for ICA-based methods is to support the clinical decision of laterality of seizure onset in mesial temporal lobe epilepsy and in supporting localization of interictal epileptiform abnormalities.

An application of radar technology has been proposed to extract spatial filtering on data to discriminate between signals arriving from a location of interest and those originating elsewhere. These methods are known as beamformers (see for review Hillebrand and Barnes, 2005) and try to identify the contribution of a single brain position to the measured field and operate on raw non-averaged EEG/MEG data. Computationally this is achieved by multiplying the measurement matrix (the EEG/MEG time times electrode/sensor data matrix) by a weighting matrix, which passes signals coming from the location of interest, while attenuating signals from elsewhere. Beamformers do not require any a priori specification of the number of active sources and are insensitive to time-correlated sources.

To conclude, the revolution initiated with the development of digital EEG equipment has enabled collaboration between neurophysiologists and scientists from physics and computational backgrounds. This has contributed to the implementation of methods which offer a new window on understanding the origin and time course of brain electrical activity. The methods

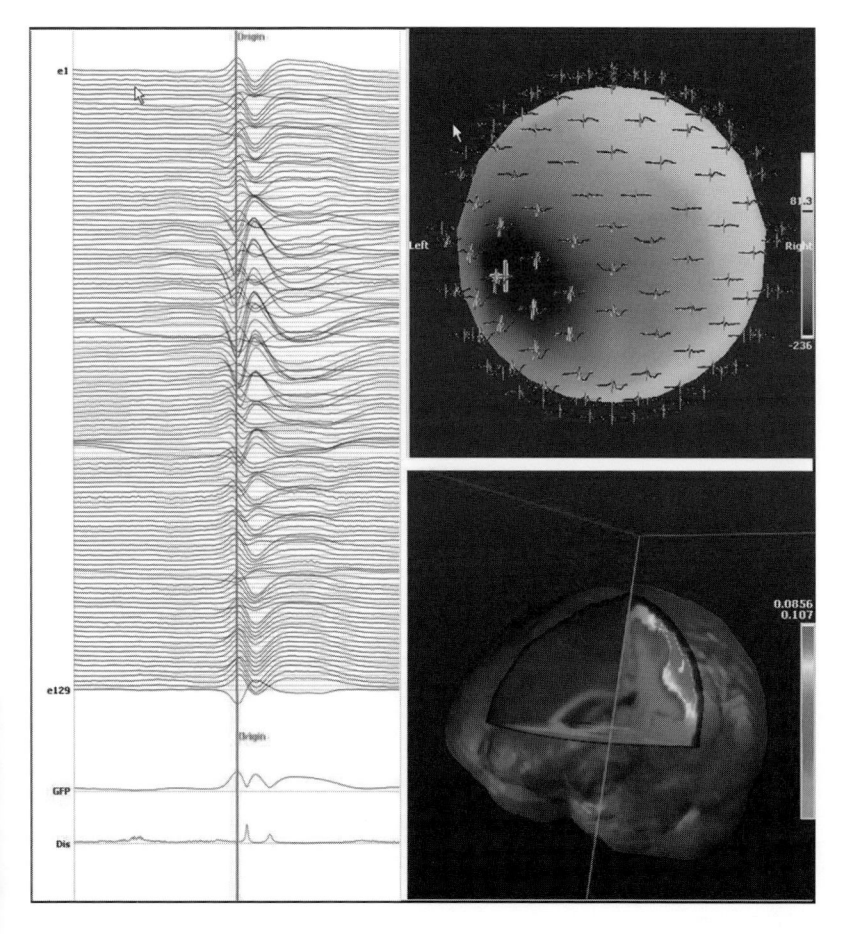

Figure 44.1. Interictal epileptiform transient acquired on a 129-channel EEG system. The averaged waveform (left panel) shows a triphasic sharp wave. The topographic map (top right) shows the field distribution at the first negative peak. The inverse solution at that time-point shows the 3D representation of the active areas within the Montreal template MRI, in proximity of the central sulcus. See colour version in plate section.

presented in this chapter have been mostly applied to 'interictal' EEG and MEG data (the irritative zone). The relationship between this and the epileptogenic zone varies across subjects and needs to be assessed through extensive electro-clinical and imaging evaluation. The clinical application of these techniques is still in its infancy, at least in terms of evaluating the role in pre-surgical assessment of patients with refractory epilepsies, requiring multicentre studies with large numbers of homogeneously acquired and analysed datasets.

References

Achim A, Richer F, Saint-Hilaire JM. Methodological considerations for the evaluation of spatio-temporal source models. *Electroencephalogr Clin Neurophysiol* 1991;**79**(3):227–40.

Bell AJ, Sejnowski TJ. Learning the higher-order structure of a natural sound. *Network* 1996;**7**(2):261–7.

Grave de Peralta Menéndez R, González Andino SL. Some limitations of spatio temporal source models. *Brain Topography* 1995;**7**(3):233–43.

Hillebrand A, Barnes GR. Beamformer analysis of MEG data. *Int RevNeurobiol* (Special volume on Magnetoencephalography) 2005;**68**:149–71.

Lantz G, Michel CM, Pascual-Marqui RD, *et al*. Extracranial localization of intracranial interictal epileptiform activity using LORETA (low resolution electromagnetic tomography). *Electroencephalogr Clin Neurophysiol* 1997;**102**(5):414–22.

Michel CM, Murray M, Lantz G, *et al*. EEG source imaging. *Clin Neurophysiol* 2004;**115**(10):2195–222.

Patel A, Alotaibi F, Blume WT, Mirsattari SM. Independent component analysis of subdurally recorded occipital seizures. *Clin Neurophysiol* 2008;**119**(11):2437–46.

Plummer C, Harvey AS, Cook M. EEG source localization in focal epilepsy: where are we now? *Epilepsia* 2008; **49**(2):201–18.

Learning objectives

(1) To understand the concept of the forward and inverse problems and how they apply to localization of brain electrical activity.
(2) To understand the relationship between scalp recorded activity and the localization of the generators in the brain.
(3) To become familiar with the two main localization strategies (linear and non-linear models).
(4) To understand the limitation of source localization techniques and their potential use in presurgical assessment of refractory epilepsies.

Section 2 Classification and diagnosis of epilepsy

Chapter

45

Magnetoencephalography in epilepsy

Stefano Seri, Jade N. Thai and Paul L. Furlong

Introduction

Magnetoencephalographic (MEG) signals, like electroencephalographic (EEG) measures, are the direct extracranial manifestations of neuronal activation. The two techniques can detect time-varying changes in electromagnetic activity with a sub-millisecond time resolution. Extra-cranial electromagnetic measures are the cornerstone of the non-invasive diagnostic armamentarium in patients with epilepsy. Their extremely high temporal resolution – comparable to intracranial recordings – is the basis for a precise definition of onset and propagation of ictal and interictal abnormalities.

Given the cost of the infrastructure and equipment, MEG has yet to develop into a routinely applicable diagnostic tool in clinical settings. However, in recent years, an increasing number of patients with epilepsy have been investigated – usually in the context of presurgical evaluation of refractory epilepsies – and initial encouraging results have been reported. We will briefly review the principles and the technology behind MEG and its contribution in the diagnostic work-up of patients with epilepsy.

MEG signal

MEG signal measures the net effect of ionic currents flowing in the dendrites of neurons during synaptic transmission. The peak value of each post-synaptic potential is of the order of 10 mV and has a duration of approximately 10 ms. Neurons such as pyramidal cells are aligned with similar orientation in the cortex and therefore their post-synaptic electrical fields sum with increasing area. Typically it is thought to take approximately 50 000 such adjacent neurons, acting in temporal synchrony, to produce a measurable change in the magnetic field outside the head.

EEG signals are produced by 'ohmic' current flow in the head (directly proportional to the potential difference and inversely proportional to the resistance) and therefore sensitive to the conductivity of the brain, skull and extracranial tissue. MEG signal has the advantage of being largely due to neural current generators (apical dendrites) and is relatively insensitive to inhomogeneity of the conductive medium (cerebrospinal fluid, skull, scalp).

According to the 'right-hand grip' rule, a current dipole gives rise to a magnetic field that flows around the axis of its vector component. This relationship is described in http://en.wikipedia.org/wiki/Right_hand_grip_rule. Magnetic fields and electrical potentials are orthogonal to each other.

As a gross generalization, MEG appears to be more sensitive to tangential dipole sources, which lie principally on sulcal walls, and less sensitive to radial sources along gyral surfaces. MEG and EEG are therefore preferentially sensitive to different cortical sources, and arguments on the superiority of one technique over the other are largely undecided (Srinivasan *et al.*, 2006).

The MEG equipment

When compared to the magnetic field of the Earth, MEG signal is extremely weak. This difference has been estimated as a few hundred micro (10^{-3}) tesla for the MEG vs a few hundred femto (10^{-15}) tesla for the Earth's magnetic field. Because of this mismatch, MEG equipment require very expensive shielding of the recording room, using μ-metal (a nickel-iron alloy) in order to screen static and low-frequency magnetic fields. Brain magnetic fields are captured by a large array of sensors (superconductive quantum interference devices or SQUIDs) – of the order of

Introduction to Epilepsy ed. Gonzalo Alarcón and Antonio Valentín. Published by Cambridge University Press.
© Cambridge University Press 2012.

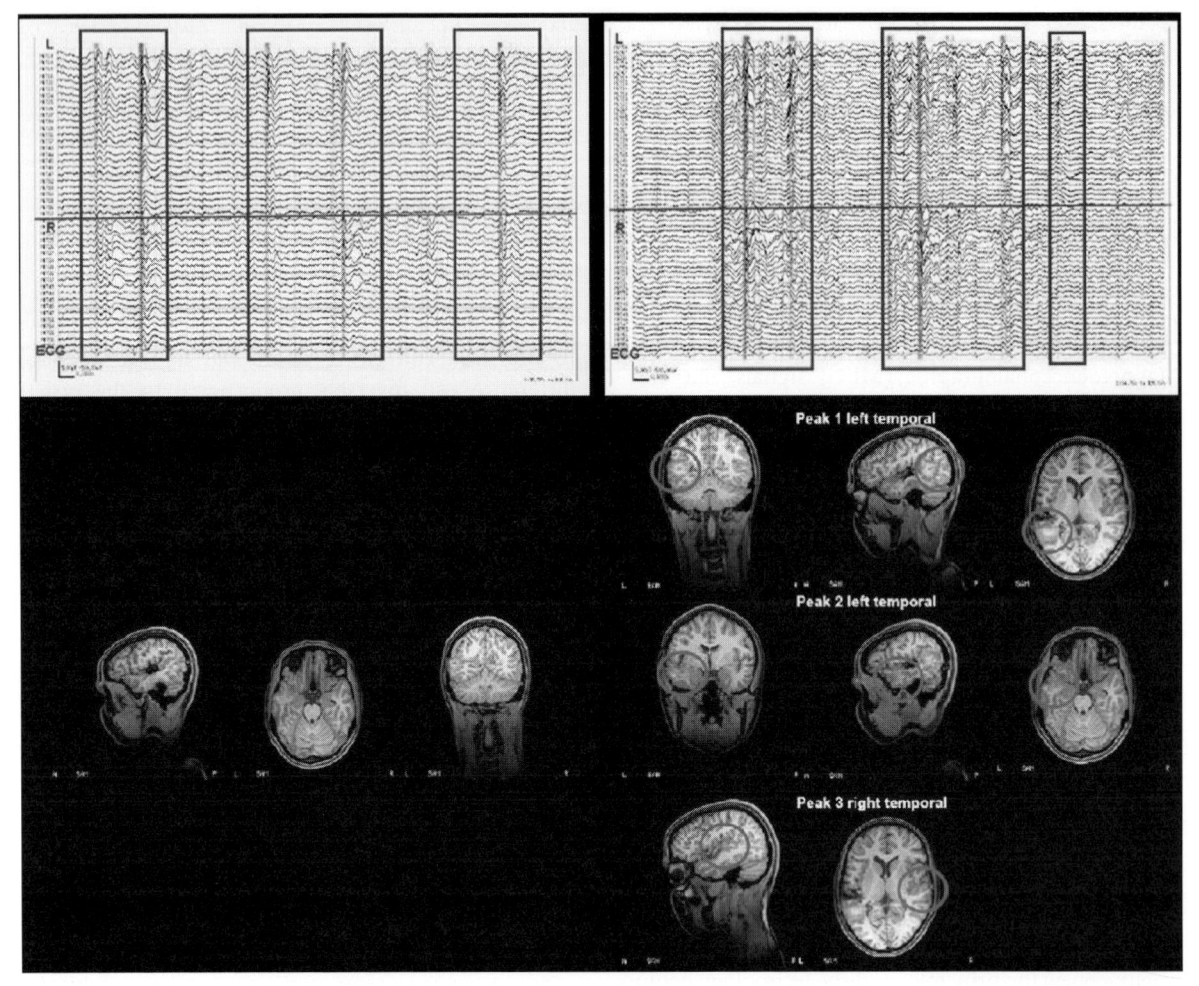

Figure 45.1. MEG recording in a patient with complex partial seizures persisting after surgical removal of a lesion in left temporal lobe. Irritative cortex maps in the neighbouring neocortex of the resected lesion. In colour the activated areas corresponding to the interictal transients which are more consistently unilateral but occasionally show a secondary bilateralization. See colour version in plate section.

200 to 300 – immersed in liquid helium and operating at superconductive temperatures (−270°C) to eliminate impedance. These devices effectively transform changes in current intensity recorded from the scalp surface into voltage changes. Manufacturers have capitalized on relative advantages of two different classes of sensors (magnetometers and planar gradiometers) in the design of their system. The main difference is in the magnitude of the sensitivity decay as a function of distance, which is greater for gradiometers. This results in sources located in the region closest to the sensor giving the largest contribution to the measured field strength.

The voltage at the SQUID level is digitized at a very high sampling rate and presented on a computer screen in a very similar way to modern digital EEG equipment. The very large number of sensors makes it impossible to mentally visualize the field topography, requiring 2D mapping or better source reconstruction techniques. Based on surface magnetic fields, these strategies infer the location and intensity of their intracranial current sources and display them co-registered with the MRI of the individual patient. The most promising family of these algorithms is the so-called beamformer, which estimates the contribution of any given point (commonly called virtual electrode) within the brain to the measured field. Within the beamformers, signal aperture magnetometry (SAM) has been more recently applied in clinical studies. This estimates the time-course of a sufficiently dense structure of virtual electrodes, and allows reconstruction of a reliable picture of the time-varying activation of intra-cranial sources during interictal 'epileptiform' transients in 3D (Figure 45.1).

Relative merits

Magnetoencephalography shares with EEG a high temporal resolution, which makes the two techniques particularly appropriate for use in epilepsy diagnosis. Its millisecond time resolution compares favourably with respect to the hundreds of milliseconds of functional MRI and several minutes of positron emission tomography. Its spatial resolution is obviously much higher than that offered by the commonly used 21-channel EEG and is of the order of 5–10 mm. The accuracy of the source reconstruction is dependent on the spatial sampling and the source configuration. Movement of the patient during the recording is detrimental to the reliability of the source reconstruction strategy to a similar extent as it is for MRI. To minimize this problem, motion correction algorithms have been recently developed. The design and limitation of the equipment (the sensor position is fixed with respect to the head) have limited the possibility of applying MEG activity for long-term recordings and collection of ictal data is limited and by and large anecdotal (Grondin *et al.*, 2006; Paulini *et al.*, 2007).

Most of the available studies have reported encouraging results in the localization of interictal transients in presurgical series. A recent meta-analysis of 192 articles was able to select only 17 in which it was possible to compare presurgical MEG prediction with surgical outcome (Lau *et al.*, 2008). The review highlights the disparity in the spatial sampling, patient age, epilepsy localization, analysis methods and definition of concordance, which makes a definite statement on the usefulness of MEG premature. Our experience on over 100 presurgical patients confirms these findings, with 45% of the patients being very accurately localized and being seizure-free on follow-up with the resected area including the area predicted by MEG, and 35% of the patients showing no interictal transients during the recording session. Further areas of clinical application include identification of eloquent cortex to allow non-invasive language or sensorimotor cortex mapping (Merrifield *et al.*, 2007; Fisher *et al.*, 2008). Prospective, possibly multicentre, studies with stringent and homogeneous diagnostic criteria and a coherent analysis strategy are required before a definite statement on the role of MEG in presurgical assessment can be reliably formulated.

References

Fisher AE, Furlong PL, Seri S, *et al*. Interhemispheric differences of spectral power in expressive language: a MEG study with clinical applications. *Int J Psychophysiol* 2008; **68**(2):111–22.

Grondin R, Chuang S, Otsubo H, *et al*. The role of magnetoencephalography in pediatric epilepsy surgery. *Childs Nerv Syst* 2006;**22**(8):779–85.

Lau M, Yam D, Burneo JG. A systematic review on MEG and its use in the presurgical evaluation of localization-related epilepsy. *Epilepsy Res* 2008;**79**(2–3):97–104.

Merrifield WS, Simos PG, Papanicolaou AC, Philpott LM, Sutherling WW. Hemispheric language dominance in magnetoencephalography: sensitivity, specificity, and data reduction techniques. *Epilepsy Behav* 2007; **10**(1):120–8.

Paulini A, Fischer M, Rampp S, *et al*. Lobar localization information in epilepsy patients: MEG – a useful tool in routine presurgical diagnosis. *Epilepsy Res* 2007; **76**(2–3):124–30.

Srinivasan R, Winter WR, Nunez PL. Source analysis of EEG oscillations using high-resolution EEG and MEG. *Prog Brain Res* 2006;**159**:29–42.

The MEG work at Aston University is supported by the Wellcome Trust, the Dr. Hadwen Trust and the Birmingham Children's Hospital Research Foundation.

Learning objectives

(1) To understand the basic principles of magnetoencephalography.
(2) To understand the potential use and the indications of magnetoencephalography in epilepsy.
(3) To understand the future avenues for magnetoencephalography development.

Section 2　Classification and diagnosis of epilepsy

Chapter 46

History-taking and physical examination in epilepsy

Gonzalo Alarcón

Introduction

Symptoms and signs of epilepsy may be difficult to observe as they can be intermittent and brief. A detailed description of the seizure characteristics from the patient and relatives is necessary, as the initial diagnosis of epilepsy will arise on the basis of a careful clinical history. An important consideration is that history-taking cannot follow strict rules, and that there could be new opportunities arising from casual comments during conversation. For instance, clumsiness during breakfast may point to juvenile myoclonic epilepsy, or frequent distractions at school may point to absence epilepsy.

Background factors in history-taking

- Avoid distracting factors: noise, music, phone calls, frequent interruptions.
- Listen to clinical history and make the patient feel understood.
- Allow time with the patient, even if it is a relatively simple case: dismantling the history to obtain the relevant information can be time-consuming.
- Ask patients to come with at least one seizure witness: a reliable description of the attacks is fundamental to diagnosis. A witness is usually required because patients are often unconscious during seizures and may be unaware of them, apart from the warning sensations (aura) and the symptoms on recovery.
- Consider possible pitfalls of history from witnesses:
  - Descriptions from witsesess can be over-rehearsed or may conform to pre-conceived ideas.
  - Different witnesses can provide contradictory information. Mistaking 'right' and 'left' is relatively common, as witnesses will usually be describing events observed on their 'mirror image'.
  - Descriptions from health professionals are usually of great value. However, they could be misleading, as they can adjust descriptions of what they think 'should be', instead of what actually happened.
  - First-hand witnesses are more reliable than second-hand witnesses.
- Small children usually find it difficult to explain subjective sensations or feelings: auras of fear or strangeness might manifest as sudden unexpected crying, running scared to his/her parents, or the child withdrawing into a corner.
- How to take the clinical history depends on the subject: some subjects are best being listened to, whereas with others it is better to ask direct questions, avoiding medical terms.
- If it is not possible to complete history-taking, try to reschedule an early appointment with other witnesses.

History of the seizures

- Obtain description of each seizure type.
- Obtain description of specific attacks:
  - first seizures: they may differ from others, as in the case of febrile seizures;
  - last attacks witnessed: usually the best remembered;
  - worst seizures: to estimate the scale of the clinical problem, and the risk to life.

Introduction to Epilepsy ed. Gonzalo Alarcón and Antonio Valentín. Published by Cambridge University Press.
© Cambridge University Press 2012.

- Investigate the settings in which attacks tend to occur: it may help in management (to avoid triggers and precipitating factors) and in the diagnosis of non-epileptic attacks. In particular inquire about:
  - Relation to sleep cycle: if attacks occur during sleep, enquire whether they occur at the onset or middle of sleep, or just before awakening or shortly after. Ask if changes in sleep patterns or abrupt awakenings precipitate attacks.
  - Circadian rhythms: inquire whether attacks occur in the morning, evening or randomly, and what the patient is doing at the time of the attacks (resting, exercising, playing, at school, in the bath, fasting, eating, standing, reclining, reading, concentrating, at a computer, watching television, playing video games, bored, emotionally disturbed or engaged in a pleasant occupation).
  - Situations associated with attacks: crowded places, heat, discos, etc.
- Description of the prodrome indicating a possible forthcoming attack:
  - Behavioural changes (such as clumsiness, irritability, sleepiness) which may precede epileptic seizures or migraine by minutes or hours.
  - Hunger, dizziness, sweating, which can suggest hypoglycaemia.
- Description of immediate stimuli having a short-term association with the attacks, which may have diagnostic value:
  - In syncope, sitmuli tend to be blood-letting, sight of blood, injections, prolonged standing in hot or confined places, standing after prolonged sitting or lying down, breath-holding, pain from minor trauma. In some QT syndromes exercise and auditory stimuli are triggers.
  - In reflex epilepsy, stimuli are flashing lights, striped visual patterns, reading, startle (also for hyperekplexia, which is rare).
- Description of auras if present: visceral, motor, sensory, psycho-sensorial. Proper auras suggest focal seizures and they can have a localizing and lateralizing value. However:
  - auras can be present in migraine and syncope;
  - auras may not be as clear in small children, where auras sometimes manifest as screaming, looking terrified, stopping ongoing activity, running to their mother, looking preoccupied or as if the child was concentrating.
- Reconstruction of ictal signs: this may be difficult as many things occur in a brief period of time.
  - Video monitoring in hospital or at home may be helpful.
  - Ask witnesses to mime the attacks, which can reveal subtle clinical details such as posture asymmetries or distinguish jerks from tremor or shivering. Many witnesses will mimic clonic and myclonic jerks fairly accurately.
  - Incontinence and tongue-biting have traditionally been considered as suggestive of epileptic seizures, but are not necessary nor specific. Lateral tongue-biting is unusual in disorders other than epilepsy (occasionally in syncope).
- Duration of attacks:
  - If possible, obtain objective time-clues, as duration is often exaggerated by patients and/or witnesses.
  - Distinguish between seizure duration and the period of post-ictal confusion, sleepiness or headache.
  - The post-ictal phase can show lateralizing signs (Todd's paralysis, aphasia).
- Frequency/pattern of attacks: if asked for the frequency of attacks, many patients would respond 'it depends' or 'not fixed'. Try to establish:
  - frequency for each seizure type
  - average frequency per week
  - highest frequency per week
  - longest attack-free period
  - if attacks occur in clusters
  - relationship between attacks and sleep cycle
  - relationship to menstrual cycle.

History of the patient

Developmental history
- Peri-natal history: delivery, milestones (age of independent walking, first words, school performance).
- Deterioration or arrest of cognitive or behavioural development.
- Changes in performance or loss of skills.

Section 2: Classification and diagnosis of epilepsy

- Previous diseases: meningitis, encephalitis, febrile seizures (length, lateralization, localized post-ictal deficits).
- But beware! Previous history of epileptic seizures does not imply that the present attacks are epileptic. Investigate changes in seizure frequency and characteristics.

History of the epilepsy: try to establish the following:
- Age at onset of seizures.
- Clinical manifestations of the first seizures.
- Investigate whether there are different types of seizures.
- Changes in seizure frequency.
- Detailed drug history: this is essential, often requiring detailed copies of clinical notes. Compile information about all antiepileptic drugs taken (alone or in combination), preferably in chronological order, with starting doses and rates of escalation, maximum doses, duration of treatment, benefits and side effects, and reason for discontinuing. Document previous drug levels and their correlation with attacks.
- Family history of neurological disease and seizures: this is often difficult, and copies of clinical documents such as clinical notes and previous EEG/MRI reports may prove very helpful.

Knowledge of the psycho-social background
- Assess the disruption of day-to-day life for patients and their family caused by epilepsy.
- Epilepsy may be a more severe handicap for active lifestyles.
- Assess the attitudes and help from family members.
- Epilepsy may have an impact on emotional, professional and social status.
- In children, epilepsy affects the patients and their families, and has an impact on school, and on the parents' expectations for the child. Assess how the patient and the family cope with the disease.
- Clinical and management decisions are often guided by social and family assessments.

The physical examination in epilepsy

Physical examination is often normal in epilepsy; however, it should always be carried out as it can be useful in a number of patients.

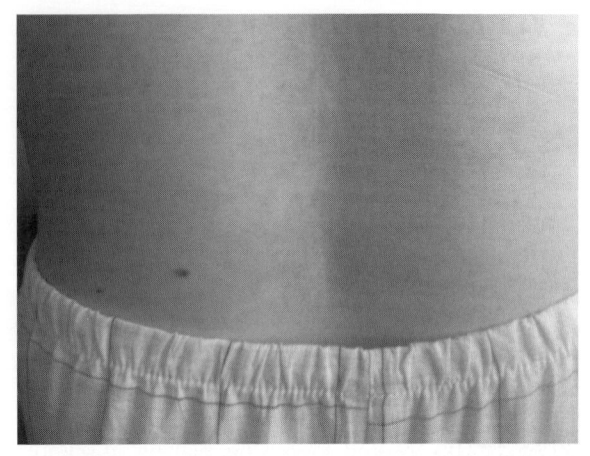

Figure 46.1. Hypomelanosis of Ito. Note hypomelanitic lesions in the lumbar region. See colour version in plate section.

Interictal examination in patients with new seizure presentation

The initial assessment should be based on a general and neurological examination looking for any abnormality suggesting the causes of attacks: abnormal cardiac examination (cardiac syncope), obstructive airway disease (cough syncope), postural hypotension, obtunded patient with focal signs (coning), evidence suggesting hydrocephalus (obstruction of ventricular flow resulting in loss of consciousness), evidence suggesting organ failure associated with metabolic encephalopathy.

Assess abnormalities that may suggest conditions associated with epilepsy. For instance, adenoma sebaceum and retinal tumours in tuberous sclerosis, and short stature or ataxia in mitochondrial disease, linear naevus in the face or abnormal pigmentation in incontinentia pigmenti or Ito's disease (Figure 46.1), café au lait spots in neurofibromatosis (Figure 46.2), facial angioma in Sturge-Weber syndrome, cataracts and fundal cherry spots in the sialidoses, dysmorphic features in Angelman and other paedia-tric syndromes, unusual head shapes in craniosynostosis, hydrocephalus, or meningioma, and features associated with systemic infective, vasculitic or inflammatory diseases such as connective tissue disorders, sarcoidosis or HIV.

Assess neurological or systemic findings indicating early-onset focal encephalic pathology: slight facial asymmetry (unilateral facial weakness is more likely to be observed when people are asked to show their teeth or smile), asymmetry in limb size,

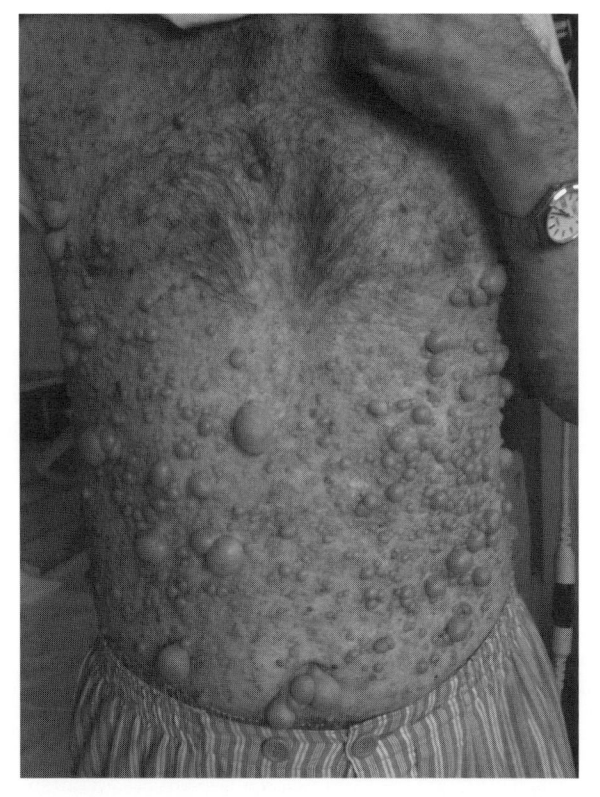

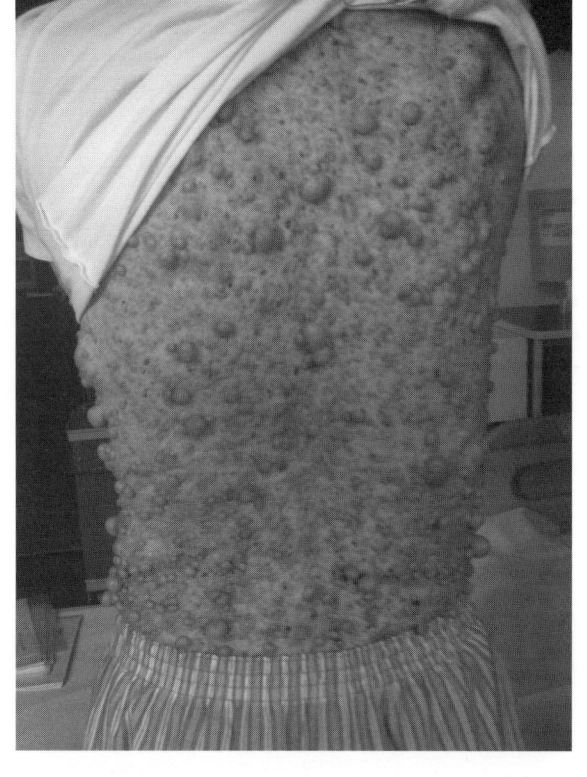

Figure 46.2. Neurofibromatosis. See colour version in plate section.

increased tone or weakness, shift in dominance, unilateral apraxia.

Investigate indications of new focal neurological findings suggesting recent-onset cortical pathology: for instance, a space-occupying lesion may show pyramidal drift or weakness, facial asymmetry, reflex asymmetry, visual field defect or inattention, papilloedema, cortical sensory loss or up-going plantar responses.

Interictal examination in patients with treated epilepsy

In patients with treated epilepsy, clinical examination also assesses:

- Any damage secondary to the epilepsy: evidence of seizure-associated injury and cognitive deficits.
- Side effects of current or previous AED treatment:
  - connective tissue changes such as Dupuytren's contracture, particularly with phenobarbitone
  - reduced verbal fluency and weight loss with topiramate
  - weight gain with gabapentin
- nystagmus, peripheral neuropathy, ataxia, gum disease, hirsutism and coarsening of facial features with phenytoin
- visual field defect with vigabatrin
- weight gain, tremor, hair loss, and motor slowing with high-doses of sodium valproate.

Ictal examination (examination during a seizure)

When assisting a seizure:

- Ensure the person's safety and provide rescue treatment if appropriate (see Chapter 76, 'Epilepsy emergency treatment').
- Examine the patient during the attack for responsiveness and memory.
- Document the attack with special attention to its evolution (see example in Box 46.1). If more than one episode is witnessed, document all in detail. Consider that epileptic attacks are often stereotyped.
- If possible, video the attack as early as possible and continue recording into the post-ictal period.

Video recording allows a careful review and the opportunity to consult other colleagues.

Document your witnessed account of the episode, always describing the following clinical aspects:
- responsiveness/orientation
- abnormal posturing
- speech disturbance
- tonic or clonic convulsions
- loss of tone or fall
- waxing and waning of any convulsive movements
- abnormal movement of eyes, lids, throat (swallowing), mouth (e.g. lip-smacking), limb movement
- plantar responses and pupillary reflexes
- autonomic changes: blood pressure, pulse, colour change, respiration
- how the episode subsides
- presence of confusion, weakness or dysphasia after the event
- evidence of injury, tongue-bite or incontinence.

> **Box 46.1. Example of seizure description**
>
> The patient becomes restless and tells his partner that he is having a seizure. He then becomes vacant and unresponsive. His pulse is regular at around 90 beats per minute. He then says 'Help!' and shows lip-smacking and swallowing movements. His left arm goes stiff for 20 s while he picks at his clothes with the right hand. He then gets up and wanders around the room for 20 s. He gradually comes round and is able to name objects. He recovers fully within 4 min of onset. He confirms that he had his usual warning of a sensation in his stomach followed by a déjà vu feeling shortly before losing awareness.
>
> A clear description such as this suggests a complex partial seizure of right mesial temporal onset in someone who is left dominant for language.

Recommended reading on history-taking

Aicardi J, Taylon DC. History and physical examination. In Engel J Jr, Pedley TA, eds. *Epilepsy: A Comprehensive Textbook*, pp. 805–810. Philadelphia: Lippincott, Raven; 1997.

Alarcón G, Nashef L, Cross H, Nightingale J, Richardson S. *Epilepsy. Oxford Handbook in Neurology*. Oxford: Oxford University Press; 2009.

Recommended reading on physical examination

Smith DF, Appleton RE, MacKenzie JM, Chadwick DW (eds). *An Atlas of Epilepsy*. New York: Parthenon; 1998.

Learning objectives

(1) To understand the relevance of history-taking and physical examination.
(2) To know the different parts of a structured medical history.
(3) To be able to lead history-taking and physical examination for patients with epilepsy.
(4) To be able to evaluate information from history and physical examination.

Section 2 Classification and diagnosis of epilepsy

Chapter 47

The role of video-EEG monitoring in epilepsy

Gonzalo Alarcón

To establish a definite diagnosis of epilepsy, an attack may have to be witnessed with the EEG recorded simultaneously. Due to the intermittent nature of the clinical and electroencephalographic manifestations of epilepsy, this can be difficult unless continuous video-EEG monitoring is used. This is a test of paramount importance in the diagnosis of epilepsy in many situations (see Box 47.1)

> **Box 47.1.** Video-EEG monitoring can be referred to as
> - video monitoring
> - intensive monitoring
> - intensive monitoring in epilepsy
> - epilepsy monitoring
> - video-telemetry
> - telemetry

Video-EEG monitoring consists of continuous recording of the video image of patients simultaneous to their EEG for several hours or days, with the aim of recording the patients' typical seizures. For this test to be successful, seizures have to be sufficiently frequent for a reasonable chance of observing an attack during the necessarily limited period of recording. If the patient has an attack during the recording, the EEG and video image can be played back to allow correlations between clinical and electroencephalographic manifestations. These correlations often allow a definite diagnosis and classification of the epilepsy in patients where other findings such as seizure history and standard EEGs are inconclusive.

The term ambulatory EEG refers to the modality of EEG recording where the patient takes the EEG system with him and can walk freely, carrying out normal everyday activities at home or at work, while the EEG is being continuously recorded, with or without video image.

> **Box 47.2.** Indications for video-EEG monitoring
> - Differential diagnosis: to establish whether the patient's attack is epileptic or non-epileptic (psychogenic seizures, sleep disorders, panic attacks, cardiogenic attacks, faints, movement disorders, etc.)
> - To determine seizure type(s) and classification of epilepsy
> - To estimate seizure frequency
> - To determine precipitants which induce seizures: self-induction, reflex epilepsy, situational factors
> - For presurgical assessment: localization of seizure focus

Diagnosis of epilepsy

A suspicion of epilepsy may arise from events associated with impaired consciousness, temporary mental impairment, dizziness, fear, panic, aggressive outbursts, abnormal movements, behavioural disturbance, fainting or sleep phenomena (somnambulism, apnoea, sudden arousals, night terrors, nightmares, eneuresis, crying and vocalization).

Non-epileptic attacks can be organic or psychogenic. Psychogenic attacks can be panic attacks, abreactive re-enactment of a traumatic event, or conscious or unconscious attempts to simulate epilepsy. In addition, it should be borne in mind that psychological factors can precipitate seizures in patients with epilepsy.

Introduction to Epilepsy ed. Gonzalo Alarcón and Antonio Valentín. Published by CAMBRIDGE UNIVERSITY PRESS.
© CAMBRIDGE UNIVERSITY PRESS 2012.

In the majority of patients, the diagnosis of epilepsy is obtained from an accurate seizure description (often obtained from witnesses) supported by an awake-sleep interictal EEG and imaging. However, in some patients there remains doubt regarding the following:

- whether they suffer from epileptic or non-epileptic attacks;
- the epileptic nature of the attacks is clearly established, but the type of epilepsy and seizures is unclear.

These issues can be established in most patients if attacks are observed during video-EEG monitoring. Since in many cases treatment depends on diagnosis, video-EEG monitoring is sometimes crucial.

In many centres, a main reason for referral for video-EEG monitoring is the differential diagnosis between epileptic and non-epileptic seizures. In interpreting video telemetry it is useful to keep in mind the following:

- in most epileptic seizures, some form of EEG change occurs during the attack;
- exceptions to this rule are some simple partial seizures and some frontal lobe seizures;
- EEG changes during epileptic seizures may not contain epileptiform discharges.

More specific details about EEG changes during epileptic seizures have been described in Chapter 18: 'Clinical use of EEG in epilepsy'.

Diagnosis of psychogenic non-epileptic seizures

Seizures that truly arise out of sleep cannot be psychogenic. In nocturnal non-epileptic seizures, there is usually an interval of some seconds between awakening and seizure onset.

Brief, frequent nocturnal attacks with bizarre frantic movements (automatisms) that may render the EEG unreadable often occur in frontal lobe epilepsy. The strange, violent behaviour of these seizures in the absence of identifiable EEG changes may be misdiagnosed as non-epileptic seizures.

- Prolactin levels: prolactin blood levels can be obtained during or shortly after attacks in order to help establish whether attacks are epileptic or psychogenic. They are not widely used because non-convulsive seizures tend not to elevate prolactin levels, and emotional stress can.

Differential diagnosis of epileptic and non-epileptic seizures is particularly difficult in patients who suffer both. In this scenario, care must be taken not to make assumptions about other attacks from the few seizures recorded during video-monitoring, since observation of a non-epileptic attack does not exclude epilepsy, or vice versa. Careful questioning of patients and relatives should be carried out to disclose the presence of attacks different from those observed and to confirm that the attacks recorded are habitual (see Chapter 56: 'Psychogenic non-epileptic seizures: diagnostic approach').

The clinical manifestations of the attack are often conclusive in establishing whether a seizure is epileptic or not, but may also be misleading. Keep in mind the following:

- Automatisms, swallowing, sialorrhoea, dystonic postures or clonic movements are unlikely to be simulated by patients who have never witnessed true epileptic seizures.
- Clonic convulsions are virtually impossible to replicate in non-epileptic events, as simulated movements tend to have an irregular flapping quality unlike the regular alternating rapid contraction and slower relaxation seen in epileptic clonic movements.
- Epileptic clonus is rather regular with a frequency that often gradually slows down during the course of the seizure.
- Simulated clonus is less regular and does not gradually evolve, but may wax and wane or may stop for a few seconds and then continue, possibly at a different frequency or in different muscle groups ('reprise' phenomenon).
- Cyanosis is rare in non-epileptic seizures but common in tonic-clonic seizures.
- Convulsive movements in non-epileptic attacks might have a non-physiological flavour, such as jerking limited to one arm and the contralateral leg. Movements on either side might occur asynchronously whereas bilateral epileptic clonic convulsions occur simultaneously on both sides. Epileptic clonic movements are brisk, fast, repetitive and regular at about 2–3 Hz, consisting of a fast contraction followed by a more gradual movement in the opposite direction during the

subsequent relaxation. Convulsive movements in non-epileptic attacks are more irregular, less repetitive, with similar speed in both directions, and less brisk, often consisting of trembling, flapping or flailing of limbs.

The inexperienced observer may not appreciate the wide range of ictal manifestations often seen in epileptic seizures. Particularly subject to misinterpretation are the bizarre behaviours often seen in frontal lobe seizures, such as clapping, bicycling movements, playing pat-a-cake, kicking, stamping, running, rocking, pelvic thrusting, swearing.

By contrast, other behaviour is typical of non-epileptic attacks, such as prolonged asynchronous jerking of all limbs in full consciousness, sliding gently off a chair without injury with legs extended, arc de cercle posturing (opisthotonus) or jerking of one arm and contralateral leg (which cannot be explained in terms of ictal physiology). It should be noted that there have been rare reports of reliably documented cases with bilateral tonic-clonic movements or of ictal automatisms without loss of consciousness in epileptic seizures (Alarcón et al., 1998).

Intervention by an observer during a seizure might establish that the event is non-epileptic:

- When a jerking limb is held and its movements restricted by the observer, another limb may begin to shake in non-epileptic attacks.
- A patient staring vacantly may fixate his/her gaze when a mirror is held in front of his/her eyes if the attack is not epileptic.
- Patients in non-epileptic attacks can resist examination, preventing eye-opening or screwing up their eyes if attempts are made by the observer to open them. If their own hand is held above their face and then released, the hand falls deviating to one side, missing the face. Care must be taken to avoid the patient's hand hitting his/her face during this manoeuvre.

No EEG changes should be seen in non-epileptic psychogenic attacks, although sometimes it is difficult to establish the absence of EEG changes due to artefacts. In this case, the presence of alpha activity while the patient is apparently unconscious will establish that the attack is not epileptic.

Attacks of daytime sleep and cataplexy accompanied by the characteristic sleep patterns in the EEG (multiple sleep latency test) allow the diagnosis of narcolepsy (see Chapter 49: 'Sleep disorders simulating epilepsy').

Episodic occurrences of abnormal nocturnal behaviour with normal EEG should raise the question of night terrors, benign myoclonus of drowsiness, sleep apnoea, or restless legs syndrome (see Chapter 49: 'Sleep disorders simulating epilepsy').

Cerebral anoxic episodes can induce EEG changes and, conversely, epileptic seizures can be associated with autonomic changes, including tachycardia, bradycardia and asystole. Thus, the temporal relationship between EEG and ECG changes is crucial in determining the aetiology.

Similarly, EEG changes may occur in hypoglycaemia and hypocalcaemia, and a blood sample may be necessary to establish whether metabolic abnormalities are a possible cause of the attacks.

Video-EEG monitoring with EEG, ECG and sometimes polysomnography can establish the nature of the attacks in around 80% of patients.

Classification of seizures in known epilepsy

The distinction between focal and generalized seizures has implications for medical and surgical treatments. In patients where epilepsy has been confidently diagnosed by history and/or previous interictal EEGs, video monitoring might be necessary to distinguish between absence seizures (spike-and-wave activity) and brief complex partial seizures (focal discharges or diffuse EEG slowing), or between generalized and secondarily generalized tonic-clonic seizures.

Focus localization

Patients suffering from drug-resistant epilepsy may be suitable for surgical resective treatment if a single source is identified as the origin of the seizures. Video monitoring might be necessary to establish whether there is a single focus and where it is (see Chapter 81: 'Preoperative assessment'). Recording of seizures is crucial, but the study of interictal abnormalities might also be helpful. In focal seizures, scalp EEG changes at seizure onset might be lateralized, but more frequently they are bilateral and start after the onset of clinical manifestations (Alarcón et al., 2001). In a relatively small proportion of patients, intracranial electrodes are necessary to identify the focus.

A small proportion of patients assessed for surgery turn out to have non-epileptic attacks, and video-EEG monitoring is essential to categorically confirm the diagnosis of epilepsy in these patients.

Evaluation of clinical syndromes

A number of syndromes can be first identified, or their clinical manifestation fully characterized, after patients have been observed on video-EEG monitoring.

Subtle seizures

Video monitoring can establish the occurrence of seizures not previously recognized or thought to be infrequent, particularly if ictal signs are subtle or consist of normal behaviour (blinking, head movement, smiling, etc.). Subtle events are a particularly frequent problem in neonates and young children who cannot report subjective symptoms, and in older children who are thought to under-perform at school because of suspected frequent absence seizures. Seizures with negative symptoms (aphasia, motor slowing) will not be identified during video telemetry unless the patient is kept active, often by talking to visitors or other patients. The epileptic nature of subtle seizures will only be established by a consistent association with EEG changes.

Estimation of seizure frequency

Estimation of seizure frequency with video-EEG monitoring can be used to adjust medication dosage and the regimen of administration, particularly if seizures are occurring frequently as is in absence epilepsies. In a minority of patients, estimation of seizure frequency may be necessary to establish the efficacy of surgical treatment.

Detection of precipitating factors

Poor response to treatment may be due to external factors precipitating seizures. These can be highly specific, such as in reflex epilepsies (flashing lights, visual patterns, eating, reading, music, calculation), or more general, such as sleep deprivation, alcohol consumption, stress, emotion or menstruation. While some patients have learnt to recognize these factors, in others it might be important to assess such potential precipitating factors. Sometimes ambulatory EEG might be necessary, since the situational factors may be rather specific. For instance, physiological as well as emotional factors can be involved in eating epilepsy, so that the patient may have seizures when eating at home and not at the hospital.

Self-induced seizures in reflex epilepsies might be difficult to recognize in part due to patients' reluctance to discuss their habit. This is particularly common in photosensitive epilepsy, where the proportion of patients who self-induce seizures may be as high as 30%. Manoeuvres used to trigger seizures can be rather subtle, such as slow eye closure with upwards deviation of the eyes, waving the outstretched fingers in front of the eyes while looking at a bright light, or gazing at striped patterns. Where there is doubt as to whether such manoeuvres are the precipitating factor or an ictal phenomenon, the dilemma can be solved by darkening the room, since patients will initially continue to perform the manoeuvre but seizures and EEG discharges no longer occur.

Recommended reading

Binnie CD, Burr W, Stefan H. Epilepsy monitoring. In Binnie C, Cooper R, Mauguière F, *et al.*, eds. *Clinical Neurophysiology* vol. 2, pp. 650–68. Amsterdam: Elsevier; 2003.

References

Alarcón G., Elwes RDC, Polkey CE, Binnie CD. Ictal oro-alimentary automatism's with preserved consciousness: Implications for the pathophysiology of automatism's and relevance to the International Classification of Seizures. *Epilepsia* 1998;**39**:1119–27.

Alarcón G, Kissani N, Dad M, *et al.* Lateralizing and localizing values of ictal onset recorded on the scalp: evidence from simultaneous recordings with intracranial foramen ovale electrodes. *Epilepsia* 2001;**42**:1426–37.

Learning objectives

(1) To understand the technical foundations of video telemetry.
(2) To know the indications of video telemetry in epilepsy.
(3) To be familiar with the interpretation of video-telemetry findings.

Section 2 **Classification and diagnosis of epilepsy**

Chapter 48

Cardiovascular syndromes simulating epilepsy

R. Shane Delamont

Epilepsy syndromes

Epilepsy syndromes depend on which part and how much of the brain are involved in the epileptiform discharges. If one considers cardiovascular syndromes (CVS) mimicking epilepsy, similar arguments apply. Whereas focal areas of cerebral hypoperfusion depend on focal obstruction to cerebral blood flow, the cardiovascular system is involved in the overall supply of blood flow to the cerebral circulation. Consequently, focal events are not seen in association with CVS unless CVS are triggered by seizures.

Cerebral perfusion

The brain has four main arteries: the left and right carotid and vertebral arteries. These arteries are early branches of the aorta or its first major branch, the brachiocephalic artery. The brain itself is very dependent on its blood supply for essential nutrients, particularly glucose and oxygen. In addition, cerebral blood flow is tightly matched to cerebral activity. This is one of the reasons that humans have evolved with such a good blood supply to the brain. Brain activity regulates brain blood supply by a system of autoregulation. Small pial blood vessels are able to constrict and dilate to control cerebral blood flow over a narrow range despite mean arterial blood pressure varying between 50–150 mmHg. This mechanism fails at the extremes and then blood flow is proportional to the mean systemic arterial pressure. At the lower end, circulatory failure is responsible for brain hypoperfusion whilst at the upper end hypertensive encephalopathy develops. This chapter addresses the causes of circulatory failure.

Syncope

Circulatory failure causes the clinical syndrome of syncope (from the Greek for cessation), which is characterized by loss of consciousness and postural tone with collapse and occasionally positive phenomena (jerks, eye rolling, muscle spasms) or incontinence. Incomplete syncope may be associated with weakness, difficulty concentrating, neck pain (classic coat-hanger headache) and described as 'dizziness' or 'light-headedness'. Partial awareness of surroundings will be maintained and prominent visual and auditory symptoms mentioned.

Incidence varies between 3% of men and 3.5% of women. Prevalence increases with age from 0.7% in the fourth decade to 5.6% in those over 75 years of age. Causes vary and are greatly influenced by the general medical state. These factors include the presence of systemic illness, endocrine disease, anaemia, hydration status, timing of last meal and drug use.

Details of the history should include questions about circumstances prior to the attack, about the onset of the attack, the attack (from eye witness), the end of the attack and the background health.

Examination should include looking for orthostatic hypotension, pathological cardiac and vascular murmurs, signs of pulmonary embolus, aortic stenosis, idiopathic hypertrophic cardiomyopathy, myxomas, aortic dissection, autonomic failure, brainstem signs and parkinsonism.

A 12-lead ECG should be performed looking for arrhythmias, acute infarction and cardiac conduction defects. The most important objective is to determine whether syncope is the harbinger of significant underlying disease and the following criteria should be used:

- clear medical reason for admission
- severe injury
- new neurological signs
- a potential cardiac cause:
    - significant past cardiac history

Introduction to Epilepsy ed. Gonzalo Alarcón and Antonio Valentín. Published by Cambridge University Press.
© Cambridge University Press 2012.

- clinical findings suggestive of heart failure, valvular stenosis etc.
- abnormal ECG
- family history of sudden cardiac death
- syncope with palpitations
- syncope during exercise or while lying flat.

Further investigations may be necessary and two commonly used techniques are tilt-table testing to trigger an attack and cardiac loop recording of the ECG (REVEAL®). The former is designed to reproduce an attack alone, whilst the latter is designed to identify cardiac arrhythmias during attacks occurring in the course of normal day-to-day activities.

Neurocardiogenic syncope

This is a triggered reflex designed to re-establish cerebral blood flow. It may have seizure-like features. Triggers include: situations (fear, pain, blood, personal threat, standing, heat, travel, instrumentation), carotid sinus stimulation, micturition, cough, sneeze, defecation, post exercise, swallowing, glossopharangeal neuralgia, wind instrument playing and weightlifting. Consciousness is not abolished as abruptly as with an epileptic seizure. Patients are often able to protect themselves as they slump and can abort attacks short of complete loss of consciousness if they lie down.

The pathophysiology involves a reversal of the normal mechanism for maintaining blood pressure. Normally the baroreceptors in the aorta and carotids control the heart rate and systemic blood pressure through the baroreflex. This causes the heart rate to speed up as blood presure falls and increases sympathetic output to the vascular system, which maintains blood presure. During syncope, at a critical moment as blood pressure falls, the sympathetic output to the vascular system is switched off and there is a large increase in parasympathetic input to the heart, which slows the rate down. In fact, asystole may ensue briefly. During head-up tilts, an attack can be triggered from between 3 to 40 minutes of tilting. Further activation procedures such as the administration of glycerol trinitrate sublingually or lower body suction are sometimes used.

Autonomic failure

In contrast to neurocardiogenic syncope, autonomic failure is associated with chronically impaired sympathetic activity and there can be impaired postural blood pressure response. During head-up tilts there is a gradual decline in blood presure as soon as tilting commences. There may be evidence of other autonomic dysfunction: pupils, loss of heart rate variability, constipation, urinary or sexual dysfunction.

Treatment of syncope

This requires an accurate diagnosis and attention to nonspecific contributors to syncope, avoidance of triggers and advice about first aid measures including lying down, clenching of buttocks and crossing legs when standing and pre-syncope threatens. The evidence for the use of specific pharmacological treatments is lacking. However, a number of agents are used. They include:

- volume expansion with salt loading and fludrocortisone
- the use of β-blockers to reduce cardiac contractility
- midodrine, an α-adrenergic agonist to cause vascular contraction
- serotonin reuptake inhibitors, which modulate the baroreflex if neurocardiogenic syncope is the cause.

Conclusion

Syncope needs to be investigated if recurrent, and an underlying diagnosis reached. Much treatment revolves around education and lifestyle modification but drug modulation is available for recurrent attacks with injury.

Learning objectives

(1) To understand the physiological principles of cerebral perfusion.
(2) To be aware of the cardiovascular syndromes simulating epilepsy.
(3) To understand the criteria used for differential diagnosis between syncope and epilepsy.
(4) To understand the treatment of syncope.

Section 2 Classification and diagnosis of epilepsy

Chapter 49

Sleep disorders simulating epilepsy

Bidi Evans

Introduction

There are two types of sleep, rapid eye movement (REM) sleep and non-REM (NREM) sleep. These arise from quite separate cerebral areas. REM arises in the brainstem from a group of cerebral nuclei, whereas NREM arises from many cerebral areas working in synchrony, including the mid-brain, thalamus, supra-chiasmatic nuclei and cerebral cortex. Sleep onset is through NREM in four stages distinguished by the EEG appearances. Stage 1 shows intermittent alpha (8–13 Hz) and theta (4–7 Hz) activity. Stage 2 is associated with spindles of fast activity (14 Hz) (Figure 15.12) and high-voltage slow components called K-complexes (Figure 15.13). In stage 3 slow activity (delta at 1–4 Hz) increases and, finally, in stage 4 the EEG traces show continuous delta and sub-delta (<1 Hz) activities (Figure 49.1).

Stage 4 sleep continues for about 1 hour before the first period of REM sleep. In REM, the EEG shows low-voltage fast activity, muscle tone is absent and characteristic jerky eye movements are seen. Each REM episode lasts 10–15 min (Figure 49.2).

REM and NREM alternate throughout the night with about four periods of REM, at hourly intervals, the last often on awakening. REM sleep is associated with dreaming.

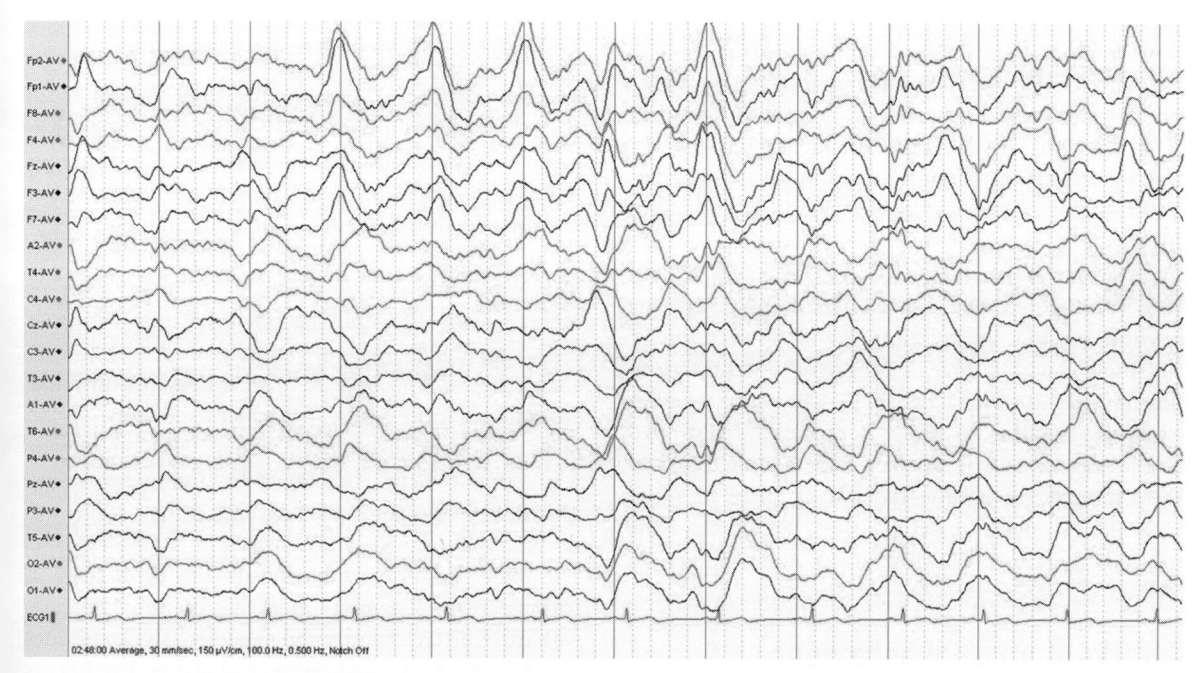

Figure 49.1. Stage 4 sleep of NREM sleep, EEG dominated by delta activity.

Introduction to Epilepsy ed. Gonzalo Alarcón and Antonio Valentín. Published by Cambridge University Press.
© Cambridge University Press 2012.

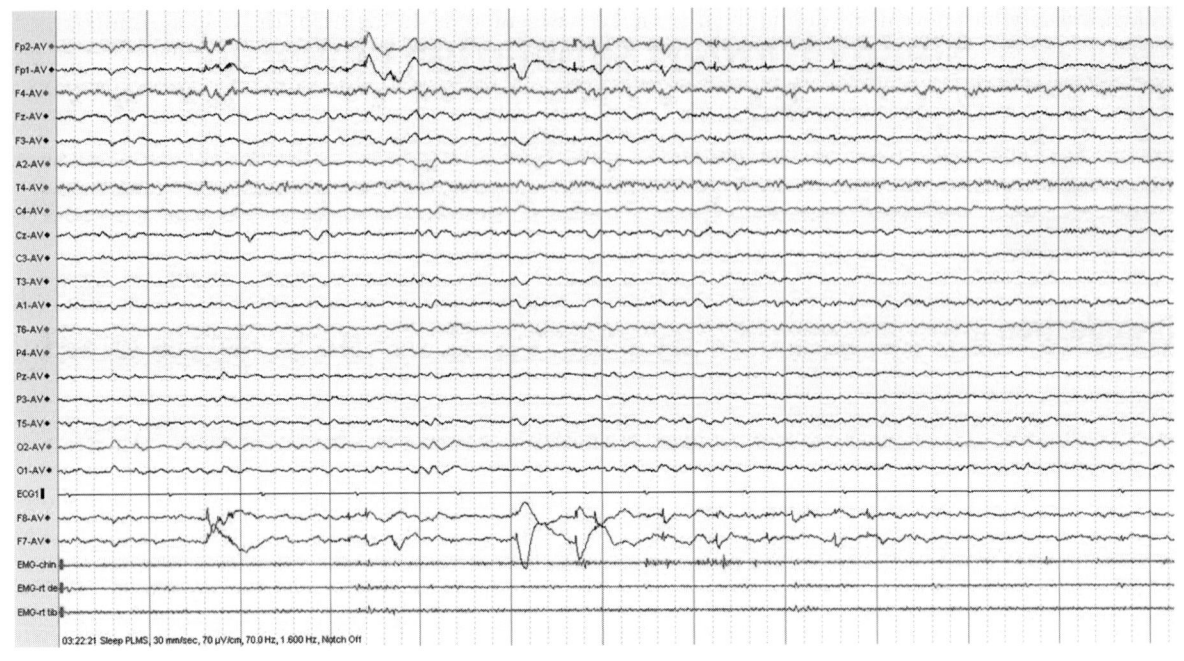

Figure 49.2. REM Sleep. The EEG is dominated by fast activity, and shows rapid eye movements in Fp1, Fp2, F7 and F8. The EMG channels show almost absent muscle tone.

Narcolepsy is a malfunction of REM sleep. It is characterized by excessive daytime drowsiness (EDD), cataplexy (a sudden loss of muscle tone resulting in collapse) and hypnogogic hallucinations (HH), waking dreams. This symptom complex is known as Gelineau's triad. In narcolepsy, the first period of REM is seen within 15 min of sleep onset. The Multiple Sleep Latency Test (MLST; Carskadon et al., 1986) can be used to diagnose narcolepsy in a single daytime session by revealing REM at sleep onset. The method allows three or four naps of natural sleep during waking hours. The EEG will show whether REM occurs within 15 min of sleep onset (determined by the presence of NREM sleep stage 2 in the EEG). If sleep onset REM is observed during three or more naps the diagnosis of narcolepsy is confirmed. The patient may report dreaming during the nap.

Attacks of unusual behaviour

Attacks of unusual behaviour may occur during sleep that can be confused with epilepsy. They may arise in NREM or REM sleep.

Attacks associated with NREM sleep

These episodes are arousal disorders. The level of sleep fluctuates during NREM with occasional awakenings. Sometimes these arousals are incomplete. Arousal disorders are commonest in childhood but may persist into adult life. The commonest is sleepwalking. The patient gets up and wanders round out of contact but rarely dangerous to themselves or others. If the EEG can be obtained it shows stage 2–4 sleep, and the patient can be guided back to bed, where they will go back to NREM sleep. Confusional arousals are more severe; the patient suddenly gets up in a semiconscious state and may fight off anyone who tries to help, sometimes becoming aggressive. The EEG before the attack usually shows stage 1–2 sleep. Night terrors are uncommon and dramatic. The patient arouses suddenly, usually from stage 4, with a scream. There are marked autonomic changes with extreme tachycardia and sweating. These episodes may last some time and cause great alarm. The EEG is difficult to obtain in arousal disorders because the electrodes usually become detached. It is possible to misinterpret an arousal disorder as focal, particularly frontal, epilepsy but movements during them are not stereotyped or dystonic.

Attacks associated with REM sleep

Some individuals are born with a failure to suppress muscle activity during REM. This results in them acting out their dreams. If the dream is a nightmare they can become extremely violent and may attack helpers or try to escape from a window. The condition is called REM sleep disorder (REMSD) and often begins in early life; it may be familial. REMSD can be confused with frontal or temporal epilepsy but movements are never stereotyped or dystonic. A clue to their nature is the timing during the night in relation to REM periods.

Attacks associated with narcolepsy

These may be mistaken for brief generalized seizures. Cataplexy, due to sudden loss of muscle tone, produces a drop attack. Cataplexy commonly occurs in moments of stress or excitement and may be precipitated by a loud noise or laughter. Sleep attacks in narcolepsy may be very sudden, causing the patient to drop unconscious into their food. The long periods of sleep in narcolepsy can be mistaken for post-ictal behaviour. The EEG in narcolepsy is normal but very drowsy, whereas in generalized epilepsy there are often generalized spike-wave discharges in wakefulness but even more so during sleep. The vivid dreams (HH) on awakening in narcolepsy may be confused with a temporal lobe aura.

Other sleep conditions that may be mistaken for epilepsy

Normal sleep events such as hypnic jerks at sleep onset may be mistaken for generalized seizures, especially in infants. The EEG is normal. Movement disorders such as the restless leg syndrome or repetitive movements at night are occasionally confusing but their timing and appearances are typical. Periodic obstructive apnoea is occasionally associated with genuine seizures during the apnoeic phase. These are usually focal in nature and secondary to cerebral anoxia.

Reference

Carskadon MA, Dement WC, Mitler MM, *et al.* Guidelines for the multiple sleep latency test (MSLT): a standard measure of sleepiness. *Sleep* 1986;**9**(4):519–24.

Learning objectives

(1) To be aware of the sleep disorders simulating epilepsy.
(2) To understand the criteria used for differential diagnosis between sleep disorders and epilepsy.

Section 2: Classification and diagnosis of epilepsy

Chapter 50: Psychiatric disorders mistaken for epilepsy

John D. C. Mellers

Introduction

The psychiatric disorder most commonly mistaken for epilepsy is dissociative seizures (psychogenic non-epileptic seizures). Indeed, up to one in five patients referred to specialist clinics with apparently intractable epilepsy will turn out to have this disorder. How to recognize and treat dissociative seizures is accordingly an important subject for all epileptologists and is considered in detail elsewhere in this book (Chapter 56: 'Psychogenic non-epileptic seizures: diagnostic approach'). Less commonly, certain psychiatric disorders with paroxysmal symptoms or behavioural changes may resemble epilepsy and give rise to diagnostic uncertainty. It is this relatively small group of patients that will be considered here.

Why might psychiatric disorders be confused with epilepsy?

What overlap is there between the clinical presentation of epilepsy and psychiatric disorder that might lead to them being mistaken for one another? From a neurological perspective, partial seizures may sometimes present with psychological symptoms that resemble experiences described by psychiatric patients. The so-called 'psychic' aura of partial seizures (ictal fear, altered perception, hallucinations and odd distortions of thinking, seen particularly with temporal and frontal lobe epilepsy) are the most important examples. For the psychiatrist, certain symptoms seen in schizophrenia can ring alarm bells suggesting an epileptic explanation. Olfactory and visual hallucinations are the most common examples, but there are also episodes of 'blankness' or 'confusion' which might simply be related to a person with major psychiatric illness being preoccupied and distracted by their own mental experiences, or alternatively might represent periods of altered consciousness with an epileptic basis. The good news for clinicians is that, despite the scope for confusion between certain psychiatric conditions and epilepsy, in practice the diagnosis is usually very straightforward and is nearly always made on clinical grounds alone. Overall, it is the brief, paroxysmal and highly stereotyped nature of epileptic seizures that help identify them as epileptic. A golden rule in epileptology is that an informant history should always be obtained and this is true even when patients think they are fully conscious throughout their attacks. Often in such cases the eyewitness account will reveal features that make a diagnosis of epilepsy clear.

The psychiatric disorders that most commonly give rise to diagnostic uncertainty are panic disorder, psychosis, attention deficit hyperactivity disorder and depersonalization disorder. Of these, panic disorder is the most common diagnostic problem.

Panic disorder

The cardinal feature of panic disorder is the panic attack. As its name implies, a panic attack is a paroxysmal episode (usually lasting for several minutes) of acute, severe anxiety. It is accompanied by characteristic cognitive symptoms (specific feared consequences such as a fear of suffocation, collapsing or dying), symptoms of physiological arousal (e.g. hyperventilation, tachycardia, perspiration) and usually occurs in specific triggering situations (e.g. crowded or enclosed places). Panic disorder is frequently associated with agoraphobia, an avoidance of these triggering situations, which in its most severe form may lead to the sufferer being housebound. A comparison of panic attacks with partial

---

Introduction to Epilepsy ed. Gonzalo Alarcón and Antonio Valentín. Published by Cambridge University Press.
© Cambridge University Press 2012.

Table 50.1. Comparison of panic attacks and partial seizures with ictal fear

	Panic attacks	Partial seizures with ictal fear
Emotion	'Panic'	Often has unusual, unique quality
Cognitive features	Irrational feared consequences	Rare
Somatic symptoms	Physiological arousal	Physiological arousal also common
Associated features	Agoraphobia common	May have 'seizure phobia'
Situational triggers	Common	Rare
Occurrence in sleep	Rare	Common
Impaired consciousness	No	Common – informant history is critical
Other epileptic features	No	Common – informant history is critical

seizures featuring prominent anxiety (ictal fear) is given in Table 50.1. The cognitive symptoms in panic attacks and their association with specific triggering situations are their most useful hallmarks. Ictal fear occurring as part of a partial seizure usually has a unique quality that is unlike 'normal anxiety': it seems to rise out of the blue for no reason and is usually independent of any environmental triggers. Most importantly, seizures with prominent ictal fear are often complex partial seizures. It is vital therefore that an informant history is obtained, even when the patient believes he/she is fully conscious throughout the episode. Not infrequently the eyewitness will reveal that in fact the patient becomes unresponsive and engages in subtle oroalimentary or gestural automatisms.

Psychosis

Perceptual distortions, illusions, hallucinations and memory flashbacks may occur as ictal phenomena, particularly in temporal and frontal lobe epilepsy. These experiential aura may be highly complex and superficially resemble the sort of hallucinations reported by patients with major psychotic illnesses such as schizophrenia. Certain epileptic aura involving subjective disturbances of thinking may also be reminiscent of psychotic symptoms. 'Forced thinking', for example, in which the patient feels compelled to think about certain restricted topics, and 'evocation of thoughts', in which there is an intrusion of thoughts or stereotyped words or phrases against the subject's will, have some similarity to the passivity phenomena (a sense of being controlled by an external influence) seen with schizophrenia. Speech arrest in epilepsy may resemble schizophrenic thought block. Occasionally, floridly psychotic patients become so preoccupied by their disturbed internal world that they may appear momentarily blank, raising the question of absence or complex partial seizures. While these unusual experiential aura constitute an intriguing neurological model of psychotic symptoms, in clinical practice the distinction between epileptic phenomena and psychosis is almost always straightforward for the reasons already highlighted: experiential ictal symptoms in epilepsy are brief, stereotyped and are usually accompanied by other, more obviously epileptic semiological features. Simple partial status involving experiential aura (aura continua) giving rise to symptoms of more prolonged duration have been reported but these cases are rare and have all had concurrent or previous complex partial seizures, making the diagnosis obvious.

Other psychiatric disorders

In children, absence seizures may be so brief that they are not noticed and the disorder may only come to light when the child is failing at school. As such, the possibility of childhood absence epilepsy must not be forgotten in the evaluation of a child with educational problems. The psychiatric differential in this situation is broad and might include attention deficit hyperactivity disorder, specific learning difficulties, neurodevelopmental disorders and psychosocial difficulties. Careful observation and the EEG will help identify absence epilepsy.

Depersonalization (a sense that the self is changed or unreal) and derealization (a sense of unreality about the external world) are common ictal symptoms and are also seen in a wide range of psychiatric conditions, particularly affective disorders. They are also the core feature of the uncommon depersonalization disorder. In psychiatric conditions, these symptoms are usually of prolonged (sometimes chronic) duration and are associated with other characteristic features of the psychiatric syndrome.

Conclusion

It is obviously important not to miss a diagnosis of epilepsy. But given the far-reaching consequences of this diagnosis (for treatment, employment, driving, lifestyle) it is equally important not to make the diagnosis without firm evidence. Psychiatric conditions may sometimes superficially resemble epilepsy but the correct diagnosis is usually straightforward if the core features of an epileptic seizure are borne in mind. Experiential symptoms in epilepsy are brief, stereotyped and usually accompanied by more obvious epileptic features. An informant history should always be obtained. A 'trial of treatment' with antiepileptic drugs is poor clinical practice and is never a substitute for careful diagnostic work-up.

Recommended reading

Alper K, Devinsky O, Perrine K, Vazquez B, Luciano D. Psychiatric classification of nonconversion nonepileptic seizures. *Arch Neurol* 1995;**52**:199–201.

Mellers JDC. Epilepsy. In David AJ, Fleminger S, Kopelman M, Lovestone S, Mellers JDC, eds. *Lishman's Organic Psychiatry: A Textbook of Neuropsychiatry*. Oxford: Blackwells; 2010.

Seshia SS, McLachlan RS. Aura continua. *Epilepsia* 2005; **46**(3):454–5.

Learning objectives

(1) To be aware of the psychiatric disorders simulating epilepsy.
(2) To understand the criteria used for differential diagnosis between psychiatric disorders and epilepsy.

Section 2 Classification and diagnosis of epilepsy

Chapter 51: Differential diagnosis of epilepsy: migraine and movement disorders

Yvonne Hart

Migraine

As long ago as 1907 Gowers wrote 'Some surprise may be felt that migraine is given a place in the borderland of epilepsy, but the position is justified by many relations, and among them by the fact that the two maladies are sometimes mistaken, and more often their distinction is difficult'.

Similarities include the following:
- both are paroxysmal
- both may involve a spreading aura
- the aura may be followed by a headache
- both may be associated with EEG abnormalities
- there may be other common symptoms, e.g. nausea, dizziness, confusion
- hormonal factors may be triggers for each.

Differences include:
- migraine is not provoked by substances such as bemegride, penicillin and metrazol, which may cause convulsions
- with certain exceptions (such as topiramate and valproate), antiepileptic drugs (AEDs) do not prevent migraine
- most drugs used for migraine treatment do not have an anticonvulsant effect.

The pathophysiological mechanism underlying migraine is thought to be spreading depression of spontaneous EEG activity travelling across the cortical surface at a rate of 2–3 mm/min. This normally reduces susceptibility to seizures, but in animal models in which the brain is pre-treated with acetylcholine or pilocarpine it may instead cause 'spreading convulsion'.

The EEG in migraine may show such changes as posterior slow-wave abnormalities, generalized slow activity, episodic frontotemporal slow activity, and sometimes sharp waves or spike activity.

Clinical differences between migraine and epilepsy

Migraine without aura is characterized by a typically unilateral, pulsating headache, worsened by movement, commonly associated with nausea or vomiting, photophobia and phonophobia. Its differentiation from seizures is usually easy.

Migraine with aura may be more difficult to distinguish from epilepsy, particularly occipital epilepsy. Migraine aura most commonly takes the form of a visual disturbance, though it may take the form of (or progress to) a spreading sensory disturbance, sometimes followed by weakness and dysphasia. The following points may help to distinguish a migraine aura from a focal seizure:

- Migraine auras typically last more than 5 minutes.
- Elementary visual hallucinations may occur in either migraine or epilepsy.
- Black-and-white zigzag linear patterns suggest migraine.
- The location of visual symptoms is often more peripheral in migraine.
- Multicoloured circular patterns suggest an epileptic aura.
- Complex (formed) hallucinations suggest epilepsy.
- Negative symptoms (visual field defect, blindness) are less common in epilepsy whereas positive motor symptoms favour epilepsy.
- Alteration in consciousness is more likely in epilepsy.
- Automatisms favour epilepsy.

Introduction to Epilepsy ed. Gonzalo Alarcón and Antonio Valentín. Published by Cambridge University Press.
© Cambridge University Press 2012.

Is there a link between migraine and epilepsy?

A number of epidemiological surveys have examined the prevalence of migraine in people with epilepsy and vice versa, to see whether there is a link between the two. Such studies have been hampered by the following factors:
- the difficulty and delay in diagnosing either condition (particularly in the case of migraine without aura)
- absence of diagnostic markers
- the high prevalence of both conditions
- the variable age of onset
- interaction of environmental factors
- sex differences in the expression of migraine.

Perhaps as a result, results have varied widely and the situation remains to be resolved. However, Andermann (1987) identified eight situations in which there does appear to be a link between migraine and epilepsy:

(1) Epileptic seizures induced by a classic migraine aura: seizures occurring only immediately after a migraine aura (the so-called 'intercalated seizures').
(2) Epilepsy with seizures no longer triggered by migrainous aura: the occasional development of unprovoked seizures in people with intercalated seizures.
(3) Epilepsy due to gross cerebral lesions caused by migraine: such as seizures due to stroke caused by migraine.
(4) Benign occipital epilepsy of childhood and the spectrum of the occipital epilepsies: Panayiotopoulos syndrome, causing autonomic manifestations such as vomiting, often accompanied by headache and by occipital paroxysms on EEG, and idiopathic childhood occipital epilepsy of Gastaut, with seizures causing visual hallucinations or blindness, sometimes evolving to eye deviation, hemiconvulsion and migrainous headache, may both be misdiagnosed as migraine.
(5) Benign rolandic epilepsy: estimated by some authors to be associated with migraine in 80% of patients, although others have disputed this association.
(6) Malignant migraine, related to mitochondrial encephalomyopathy such as MELAS (mitochondrial encephalomyopathy with lactic acidosis and stroke-like episodes), characterized by the occurrence of migraine, severe epilepsy and progressive neurological deficits.
(7) Migraine attacks following partial complex seizures.
(8) Alternating hemiplegia of childhood: a disorder of children, usually with a family history of migraine, causing paroxysmal hemiplegia, dystonic posturing and headache, sometimes associated with seizures.

Movement disorders

A variety of movement disorders may occasionally be confused with epilepsy, including the following.

Paroxysmal kinesigenic choreoathetosis

Beginning in childhood or adolescence and more common in males, this condition causes brief choreiform or dystonic movements precipitated by sudden voluntary movements or startle. It responds to antiepileptic drugs such as carbamazepine.

Paroxysmal non-kinesigenic choreoathetosis

An autosomal dominant condition with onset usually in infancy. Attacks last 5 minutes to several hours and are precipitated by fatigue, stress, alcohol and caffeine. They do not respond to antiepileptic drugs.

Paroxysmal ataxia and tremor

This may be kinesigenic, usually responding to antiepileptic drugs; non-kinesigenic, often triggered by exercise, fatigue, stress and alcohol, lasting hours, and prevented by acetazolamide; or associated with myokymia and neuromyotonia, when it is usually brief, triggered by exercise, fatigue or stress, and not sensitive to acetazolamide.

Tonic spasms of multiple sclerosis

These are rarely the presenting feature of multiple sclerosis, usually last for seconds to 1 minute, and may respond to low-dose antiepileptic drugs.

Hyperekplexia

A rare, usually familial, condition characterized by hypertonia in infancy and an excessive startle response. This involves forced eye-closure and limb extension followed by stiffness and collapse. The EEG during hyperekplexic episodes is normal. Startle epilepsy is often manifest as asymmetric tonic seizures, although absences, atonic seizures and generalized seizures may sometimes occur.

A number of the paroxysmal disorders described above are now known to be due to mutations in ion channels and related molecules, and it is likely that future genetic advances will clarify the relationship between them. A useful review of current knowledge has been written by Crompton and Berkovic (2009).

References

Andermann F. Migraine and epilepsy: an overview. In Andermann F, Lugaresi E, eds. *Migraine and Epilepsy*, pp. 405–22. Boston: Butterworths; 1987.

Crompton DE, Berkovic SF. The borderland of epilepsy: clinical and molecular features of phenomena that mimic epileptic seizures. *Lancet Neurol* 2009;8:370–81.

Learning objectives

(1) To know the differences and similarities between migraine and epilepsy.
(2) To understand the criteria used for differential diagnosis between migraine and epilepsy.
(3) To be aware of the movement disorders simulating epilepsy.
(4) To understand the criteria used for differential diagnosis between movement disorders and epilepsy.

Section 2 Classification and diagnosis of epilepsy

Chapter 52

Differential diagnosis of epilepsy in children

Elaine Hughes

Differential diagnosis in childhood epilepsy

The starting point for assessment in a child presenting with paroxysmal events is to distinguish epileptic from non-epileptic events. This is not always straightforward. Studies of children referred to tertiary services with a firm diagnosis of epilepsy typically reveal misdiagnosis in 20 – 25%, with implications for medical, educational, emotional and social well-being. In addition to this, even where the epileptic basis of events is not in any doubt, there may be errors in ascertainment of the seizure type or of the epilepsy syndrome which compromise care. The latter problem is not within the scope of this chapter.

At the outset, it is important to try to obtain an eyewitness account of the events, including, where possible, the child's description, alongside medical, developmental and educational history, and general and neurological examination.

Common causes of misdiagnosis include:
- lack of an eyewitness account;
- a past history of febrile convulsions or other seizures leading wrongly to the view that the current events must also have an epileptic basis;
- a positive family history;
- the presence of clonic jerks or incontinence during the event, again leading to the assumption that this inevitably implies an epileptic basis;
- over-interpretation of EEG abnormalities, which is a particular problem in children with pre-existing neurological disorders or developmental delay.

What else could it be?

An awareness of the variety of other conditions that may present as possible epileptic seizures is therefore vital in this situation and it is easiest to consider categories of diagnosis first:

(1) Syncope and related disorders.
(2) Behavioural or psychiatric disorders.
(3) Neurological disorders.
(4) Sleep-related phenomena.
(5) Other, e.g. posturing with gastro-oesophageal reflux (Sandifer syndrome).

Syncope and related disorders

Disorders of orthostatic control include:
- reflex or vasovagal syncope
- drug-induced syncope
- postural orthostatic tachycardia syndrome (POTS)
- multiple system atrophy
- situations where there is autonomic failure.

In infants and children, only the first of these is a common diagnosis, the other conditions being largely confined to adults. Reflex (vasovagal) syncope is common and most readily distinguished by the history of precipitating circumstances; namely, postural, painful or emotional situations. There is the presyncopal phase, which may produce feelings of weakness, accompanied by any or all of the following: pallor, sweating, pupillary dilatation, yawning, hyperventilation, nausea, strange taste, epigastric discomfort or visual distortion. This is followed, if the event progresses, by the syncopal phase, typically with loss of tone, bradycardia and loss of consciousness. More pronounced motor features including eye deviation, clonic jerks or stiffening, which may be asymmetric, and/or urinary incontinence may all cause confusion in diagnosis. Treatment includes discussion of

---

Introduction to Epilepsy ed. Gonzalo Alarcón and Antonio Valentín. Published by Cambridge University Press.
© Cambridge University Press 2012.

precipitants, adequate hydration, treatment of anaemia and improvement in muscle tone, but also reassurance.

Respiratory syncope includes reflex end expiratory apnoeic syncope (previously termed 'blue breath-holding' attacks), the 'fainting lark' or other Valsalva-related syncope, or situations where there is upper airway obstruction.

'Breath-holding' spells occur in 4% of all children aged under 4 years and occasionally older. Approximately 80% of first attacks occur before the age of 18 months and may begin in the newborn period. There is often a family history of similar events in parents in childhood. The cyanotic or blue type – reflex end expiratory apnoea – is the commonest. Episodes are typically provoked by anger or frustration; the child cries, holds their breath in expiration, becomes cyanosed and loses consciousness before recovering spontaneously. Such attacks are terrifying for parents if they are not aware of the benign nature of the episodes in most individuals. The 'pallid' or 'white' breath-holding spells resemble vasovagal episodes, often being provoked by pain, which may be trivial, or by fright or surprise. Loss of consciousness occurs abruptly without the initial phase of distress and is often accompanied by pallor, eye-rolling, extreme stiffening and incontinence.

It is imperative that these benign conditions are distinguished from cardiac syncope where there is an underlying condition that may present with life-threatening events and require urgent intervention. These include syncope secondary to arrhythmias, most often with underlying long QT syndrome, but also with other conditions such as heart block or with anatomical problems such as outflow obstruction or heart muscle disease as in cardiopathy. Although numerically rare in children and adolescents, those with repaired congenital heart disease are at increased risk. Clues to a diagnosis of cardiac syncope include exercise-induced attacks, but emotion, pain or auditory stimuli can also be relevant, so that these conditions are difficult to distinguish on history alone. An ECG with calculation of the corrected QT interval is part of the evaluation in a patient presenting with syncope.

Other rare but important conditions that may mimic epileptic seizures include brainstem syncope in the context of tumour or herniation, which may present as tonic posturing.

Behavioural and psychiatric disorders

These form the second-largest category of mis-diagnosis in most series. It is helpful to separate these into non-epileptic seizures, which have a behavioural basis, and those which are dissociative in nature. The latter have sometimes been termed 'pseudo-seizures', 'psychogenic' seizures or non-epileptic attack disorder (NEAD).

Examples of non-epileptic (behavioural) events include: staring or day-dreaming, isolated clonic jerks, tonic posturing, self-gratification, stereotypies (often seen in children with autism) or episodic rage attacks. Home video recording of events is often the most useful tool to distinguish these events.

Non-epileptic seizures may result from misinterpretation of normal physiological stimuli such as a fluttering sensation in the stomach in the context of anxiety, or from elaboration of a true aura or brief epileptic seizure. Very rarely deliberate simulation of a seizure has been observed but more often the patient is unaware that the events have a psychological basis.

In non-epileptic (dissociative) events, a form of conversion reaction, it has now been appreciated for some time that there is an association in some cases with a background of child sexual abuse. The pattern of attacks may provide a clue to their non-epileptic basis. They are often prolonged, lasting 10 to 15 minutes or more and include non-epileptic movements. The child or adolescent may resist eye-opening and may recall events when they were apparently unconscious and unresponsive to noxious stimuli. Attacks are very rarely associated with injury but may have tongue-biting or incontinence. The frequency is usually unaffected by regular drug treatment but attacks may of course be modified by emergency treatment with benzodiazepines because of their sedative and muscle-relaxant properties. True ictal violence is extremely rare. Assessment may require video-EEG monitoring in order to establish the underlying basis of the attacks with certainty. Alongside this, support from a clinical psychologist with expertise in the management of such disorders may be invaluable.

Neurological disorders

As already highlighted, the diagnosis of paroxysmal events in children with underlying and often complex neurological or developmental disorders can be difficult. In particular dystonic posturing including spasms may occur in children following a hypoxic ischaemic injury and may be difficult to tell clinically from epileptic spasms. Posturing may also be seen in association with underlying gastro-oesophageal reflux (Sandifer syndrome), a common problem in children with neurological disorders, and may improve with management of the reflux. This may also much less commonly be found in neurologically normal children.

Intermittent and recurrent ataxias and other movement disorders such as paroxysmal dyskinesia or choreoathetosis are not usually confused with epileptic seizures. Tics may occasionally be difficult to distinguish initially from myoclonus and hyperekplexia mimics tonic epileptic spasms but both can be separated on electrophysiological terms and appropriate intervention provided.

In otherwise well children the situation is usually easier. Benign paroxysmal vertigo presents in previously well young children with attacks of unsteadiness, pallor, sweating and vomiting. They remain aware throughout and nystagmus may be noticed during attack. Frequency is low at 1–4 per month and the condition is thought to be self-limiting and may be related to paroxysmal torticollis.

Sleep disorders

These are common and may present a diagnostic dilemma.

Primary parasomnias can be divided into those occurring at sleep onset and those on waking, such as rhythmic movements, sleep starts or sleep paralysis. Non-REM sleep disorders comprise the disorders of arousal, namely confusional arousals, sleep terrors and sleep-walking. REM sleep disorders range from the common problem of nightmares to the fortunately rare REM sleep behaviour disorder.

Secondary parasomnias may have a medical basis and include sleep apnoea, asthma and epilepsy where there are nocturnal seizures. Frontal lobe seizures may be difficult to distinguish because the motor manifestations may be unusual. Psychiatric disorders may also present with sleep disturbances but should not usually present diagnostic difficulty.

In all cases it is important to keep an open mind as to the nature of events and to re-visit the diagnosis especially where there is a poor or incomplete response to treatment. The conditions described above include some that are encountered relatively frequently in clinical practice. The list of conditions is not intended to be exhaustive but a starting point for evaluation of children with paroxysmal disorders.

Recommended reading

Fowle A, Binnie C. Uses and abuses of EEG in epilepsy. *Epilepsia* 2000;**41**(Suppl 3):S10–18.

Stephenson JBP. Fits and faints. In *Clinics in Developmental Medicine No. 109*. Oxford: Mackeith Press; 1990.

Thirumalai S, Bassel AK, Toufic F, Gautham S. Video-EEG in the diagnosis of paroxysmal events in children with mental retardation and in children with normal intelligence. *Devel Med Child Neurol* 2001;**43**:731–4.

Learning objectives

(1) To know the paediatric conditions that can resemble epilepsy.
(2) To understand the criteria used for differential diagnosis between such conditions and epilepsy.

Section 2: Classification and diagnosis of epilepsy

Chapter 53: Investigation of newly diagnosed and chronic epilepsy in adults

Robert D. C. Elwes

Seizures can be the symptom of a multitude of disorders. Investigations should be carried out in an orderly manner with a clear view of the management issues that are being addressed, which vary depending on the clinical presentation.

Assessment of acute symptomatic seizures

This usually arises when the patient presents for the first time in the emergency department with a seizure. Alcohol or drug abuse, metabolic disorders or acute neurological disorders such as head injury, brain haemorrhage, meningitis or encephalitis have to be considered. A prodromal illness, a prolonged seizure, focal fitting, failure to recover, post-ictal deficits, papiloedema and neck stiffness may all indicate primary acute neurological disease. Investigations are directed by the clinical findings and include:

- metabolic and drug screens;
- CT scan, which is better than MRI for detecting fractures and bleeding;
- CSF examination if meningitis or encephalitis is suspected.

Cardiology assessment

The commonest differential diagnosis of blackouts is syncope. In adolescents or young adults a diagnosis of vasovagal syncope can be made clinically, is usually benign and further assessment is not needed. In older people, however, syncope carries a significant incidence of morbidity and mortality, and cardiological assessment should be undertaken. A history or clinical signs of cardiac disease and syncope on exercise (long QT syndrome, valvular disease or cardiomyopathy) should also be investigated, usually including cardiology referral. In older people, transient ischaemic attacks may be considered and assessment of the extracranial vessels using carotid ultrasound or angiograph may be needed. The following tests may be needed depending on clinical indication:

- ECG
- 24-hour ECG
- cardiac echo
- tilt test
- carotid ultrasound.

Identification of new/progressive neurological disease

This primarily arises when acute symptomatic seizures have been excluded and the patient is being assessed in the neurology clinic. About 5% of adults with new-onset seizures will have a brain tumour. From an epidemiological perspective, vascular disease in the elderly is the commonest cause of epilepsy. The following tests may be needed depending on clinical indication:

- high-resolution MRI: tumour, vascular disease, arteriovenous malformations, cavernomas, rarer lesional causes such as demyelination, sarcoid, Whipple's disease, lymphoma;
- immunology, see below: small vessel disease/vasculitis;
- chest X-ray: tuberculosis and sarcoidosis;
- X-ray of muscles: neurocystercicosis;
- skull X-ray or CT: brain calcification in coeliac disease, Sturge-Weber syndrome and subepedymal nodules in tuberose sclerosis.

Introduction to Epilepsy ed. Gonzalo Alarcón and Antonio Valentín. Published by Cambridge University Press.
© Cambridge University Press 2012.

Table 53.1. Cumulative utility of clinical assessment, EEG and MRI in 300 cases of new-onset epileptic seizure (adapted from King *et al.* 1998)

Classification	Clinical data only	Clinical and EEG	Clinical and EEG and MRI[a]
Generalized	25 (8%)	69 (23%)	68 (23%)
Partial	116 (39%)	163 (54%)	175 (58%)
Unclassified	159 (53%)	68 (23%)	57 (19%)

[a] Lesional causes identified: tumour, 17; disorders of cortical development, 7; trauma, 6; unilateral hippocampal atrophy, 4; cavernous haemangioma, 2; hydrocephalus and hippocampal atrophy, 2.

Identification of fixed static disease

A detailed evaluation of birth and perinatal history, early developmental milestones and scholastic and employment achievement may give an indication of long-standing brain disorder that has made the person prone to seizures. In the most severe form this may manifest itself by learning difficulties and cerebral palsy. High-resolution MRI is the most important test, which can identify intrauterine or childhood stroke, hypoxic ischaemic injury, malformations of brain development, hydrocephalus or evidence of previous trauma. Areas of atrophy on encephalomalacia may be identified that are of uncertain aetiology but of probable significance.

Routine blood tests

These are performed at the onset of epilepsy as a screen for general health and a baseline for drug treatment. They should be repeated before starting a new drug and at 1–2 year intervals in people on long-term medication. Specific uses include monitoring the following:

- urea: renal failure producing metabolic seizures, effects of renal failure on drug excretion;
- sodium: metabolic cause of seizures/confusion, drug effect of carbamazepine and oxcarbazepine;
- alkaline phosphatase: drug effect with enzyme-inducing AEDs, indicator of liver or bone disease;
- calcium/phosphate: metabolic bone disease from chronic drug toxicity;
- gamma GT, AST, ALT: screen for liver function and general health, especially alcohol abuse; baseline before drug treatment; possible effects of liver disease on drug metabolism;
- vitamin B12 and folate: chronic drug toxicity, especially megaloblastic anaemia with older antiepileptic drugs;
- vitamin D: chronic drug toxicity from drugs producing metabolic bone disease, especially at-risk groups;
- full blood count: drug effects, especially neutropaenia with carbamazepine and low platelets with valproate.

Electroclinical classification of seizures

This is one of the most important functions of the neurologist or epilepsy specialist and is highly dependent on a detailed seizure history and the appropriate use of the EEG. Because of reduced sampling a single EEG in someone with epilepsy will show epileptiform discharges in about 50% of cases. Repeated examinations, especially using sleep activation, increase the yield to about 85%. There remains a small group in whom the EEG is always normal, probably because the focus is restricted in size, medial or inferior.

The utility of EEG and MRI in classifying new-onset epilepsy is well illustrated by a study of new-onset seizures (Table 53.1). From a total of 496 cases with presumed new-onset seizures, 196 were found to have other causes for the attacks, particularly syncope or psychogenic non-epileptic attacks. The utility of clinical assessment, MRI and EEG was assessed in the remaining 300 cases aged over 5 years with unprovoked seizures.

On clinical grounds, 25 were thought to have primary generalized epilepsy due to a history of seizures on awakening, absences or early morning myoclonus. Following a routine EEG, and a sleep recording if the awake EEG was normal, more were found to have generalized spike and wave and the total with generalized epilepsy increased to 69. A large number of the unclassified cases, most of whom had convulsive seizures with no focal features, were found to have an EEG focus and those with partial epilepsy increased from 116 to 163. MRI was important as it revealed a number of lesional causes of significance but the overall effect on classification was rather modest.

Indications for routine and specialist EEG investigations

Most departments will perform a routine EEG as the first investigation and proceed to a sleep recording if this is normal, the classification of the epilepsy remains unclear or a case of chronic epilepsy is being re-evaluated. Advances in technology have made prolonged intensive EEG monitoring much more widely available, which has had a major impact on diagnosis and treatment. Surgical telemetry, with or without intracranial electrodes, remains the most important indication for intensive EEG monitoring. If a diagnosis of non-epileptic seizures is suspected the diagnosis should be confirmed by diagnostic telemetry or outpatient activation clinic.

Structural imaging

MRI and CT remain the mainstay of diagnostic imaging. The latter is of use in acute situations where identification of skull fractures or intracranial bleeding is needed, or to look for cerebral calcification in some cases of chronic epilepsy. Most clinical centres now use a 1.5 tesla MRI with head coils. Even the slightest movement can degrade images, and examination under general anaesthesia may be needed. Higher magnet strengths facilitate specialist techniques such as fMRI but do not greatly increase the yield of diagnostic imaging. Quantification of results such as measuring hippocampal volumes or T2 signal intensity is simple and improves accuracy but is time-consuming and tends to be performed in centres with a research interest in these techniques. In addition to thin T2 coronal and axial slices, the following sequences are particularly helpful in epilepsy:

- FLAIR: helpful in identifying high T2 signal in both grey and white matter, particularly in mesial temporal sclerosis, dysplasia, indolent tumours and encephalomalacia;
- volumetric acquisition: reformatting in multiple planes in diagnostic imaging; base for intraoperative guidance systems; three-dimensional rendering; fusing of images from multiple sources such as functional studies;

Table 53.2. Indications of several EEG technologies

Good indications	Less helpful indications
Routine/sleep standard EEG	
Classification of seizures	Follow-up 'check' EEGs
New-onset epilepsy	Monitoring disease activity
Failure to respond to treatment	Exacerbation of seizures
Drug withdrawal	'Excluding' epilepsy
Ambulatory EEG	
Sleep studies	Non-epileptic attacks
Situational seizures	Presurgical evaluation
Frequency of known event (e.g. absences)	
Telemetry	
Presurgical evaluation	Episodic behaviour disorders
Confirm non-epileptic seizures	Monitoring disease activity
Poor history/documentation of seizures	Inattention or 'absences' in children
Nocturnal episodes/parasomnias	
Document seizure frequency	
Unclassified epilepsy	

- inversion recovery sequences: may help in identifying cavernous haemangiomas.

It is disappointing that many of the sequences such as MR spectroscopy or diffusion-weighted imaging have not become widely accepted clinically useful tools.

Functional imaging

Functional imaging techniques are primarily used in presurgical evaluation and tend to be available in a restricted number of centres with a research interest.

- Functional MRI: lateralizing language function; memory mapping in medial temporal area as an adjuvant or replacement to amytal; motor and language mapping as an adjuvant to invasive assessment.
- Combined fMRI and EEG: under assessment.
- FDG PET: presurgical evaluation, lateralizing TLE or in TLE with normal MRI.

- Ictal SPECT: presurgical evaluation, particularly in extratemporal epilepsy, planning electrode placement, may avoid invasive EEG in some cases.
- MEG: still under assessment. It seems accurate in modelling neocortical foci especially with complex dipoles such as those in Landau Kleffner syndrome and ESES.

Epilepsy with autoimmune disease, progressive deterioration or atypical features

MRI and EEG will identify the aetiology and classify most cases with seizures and epilepsy. The remaining cases who have no past history, normal development and cognition and then epilepsy occurring for no obvious cause may need further investigation. Most do not have a demonstrable structural cause or belong to a recognized childhood epilepsy syndrome. Further evaluation is particularly needed if there is a malignant or progressive course, bouts of status epilepticus, recurrent lesions on imaging, psychosis or neurological or cognitive deterioration. The type of investigation will be dictated by the clinical context or associated features as indicated below. The list emphasizes important causes and does not attempt to include the very large number of other storage disorders, chromosomal or genetic illnesses, degenerative conditions or metabolic disorders where seizures may be a feature.

Epilepsy and autoimmune disease

- Systemic lupus erythromatosis (EEG slowing, psychosis and epilepsy): anti-DNA ABs.
- Antiphospholipid syndrome (stroke, miscarriage, deep venous thrombosis and epilepsy): anti-cardiolipin ABs.
- Limbic encephalitis (confusion, memory loss, frequent seizures, medial temporal MRI lesions, paraneoplastic): anti-voltage-gated potassium channel antibodies.
- Hashimoto's encephalitis (encephalopathy, recurrent status epilepticus, psychosis): anti-thyroid antibodies.
- Anti-NMDA receptor encephalitis (psychosis, seizures, movement disorder, ovarian cancer).
- Anti-GAD antibodies (stiff person syndrome, diabetes, epilepsy)
- Anti-gliadin antibodies (coeliac disease, occipital calcification, possibly mesial temporal sclerosis).

Rarer cases of seizures and epilepsy

- Unverricht-Lundborg disease (stimulus-sensitive myoclonus; photosensitivity, giant evoked potentials): cystatin B (stefin B) (CSTB) gene.
- Mitochondrial cytopathies, MERF (myoclonic epilepsy with ragged red fibres), MELAS (mitochondrial encephalomyopathy, lactic acidosis, and stroke-like episodes, where there is epilepsy and migraine, recurrent MRI lesions, myoclonus, focal motor status, occipital epilepsy): muscle biopsy will show POLG1 mutations.
- Ring chromosome 20 (recurrent nonconvulsive status, subtle nocturnal frontal seizures).
- Sodium channel mutations (early-onset epilepsy, onset after immunization, exacerbations with fever, family history, regression with severe myoclonus in infancy).
- Glucose transporter disorders (early-onset seizures, learning difficulties, movement disorders, worsening with fasting): csf glucose, response to ketogenic diet.
- Porphyria (exacerbations with abdominal pain, psychosis, drug-induced worsening): urinary porphyrin excretion.
- Rett syndrome (girls, learning difficulties, breathing disorders, hand stereotypies, autonomic disorders): MECP2 gene.
- Down syndrome (late-onset myoclonus): trisomy 21.

Epilepsy and progressive cognitive decline

- Lafora body disease (epilepsy and progressive cognitive loss): skin biopsy of sweat glands, polyglucosan: EPM2A gene (the name of this gene stands for epilepsy, progressive myoclonus type 2A, Lafora disease (laforin)).
- Leukodystrophy: very-long-chain fatty acids.
- Storage disorders (white cell enzymes, genetic tests):
  - sialidosis: neuraminidase deficiency
  - Gaucher's: glucocerebrosidasy.
- Neuronal ceroid lipofuscinosis (Kufs): skin/brain biopsy, genetic testing.

- Zellweger syndrome (leukodystrophy, polymicrogyria): PEX gene.
- Action myoclonus–renal failure syndrome (AMRF): SCARB2 gene.
- Other metabolic disorders.

Recommended reading

Duncan JS. Imaging and epilepsy. *Brain* 1997;**120**:339–77.

King MA, Newton MR, Jackson GD, *et al.* Epileptology of the first-seizure presentation: a clinical, electroencephalographic, and magnetic resonance imaging study of 300 consecutive patients. *Lancet.* 1998;**352**(9133):1007–11.

Leen WG, Klepper J, Verbeek MM, *et al.* Glucose transporter-1 deficiency syndrome: the expanding clinical and genetic spectrum of a treatable disorder. *Brain.* 2010;**133**(Pt 3):655–70.

Shahwan A, Farrell M, Delanty N. Progressive myoclonic epilepsies: a review of genetic and therapeutic aspects. *Lancet Neurol* 2005;**4**:239–48.

Vignoli A, Canevini MP, Darra F, *et al.* Ring chromosome 20 syndrome: a link between epilepsy onset and neuropsychological impairment in three children. *Epilepsia* 2009;**50**:2420–7.

Vincent A, Irani SR, Lang B. The growing recognition of immunotherapy-responsive seizure disorders with autoantibodies to specific neuronal proteins. *Curr Opin Neurol* 2010;**23**:144–50.

Learning objective

(1) To know the investigations necessary for the study of epilepsy in adults, their indications and the principles involved in their interpretation.

Section 2 Classification and diagnosis of epilepsy

Chapter 54

The role of investigations in the management of epilepsy in children

J. Helen Cross

There are two main aims to the investigation of epilepsy: firstly to aid in our diagnosis of the epilepsy itself, particularly with regard to the epilepsy syndrome, and secondly to attempt to determine an underlying cause.

The main investigation is of course the electroencephalogram (EEG), but this has to be requested and interpreted appropriately in the context of the clinical history of the individual. Further investigations are directed at determining an underlying cause. Magnetic resonance imaging of the brain has greatly enhanced our understanding of the underlying cause of epilepsy. Many other investigations may be useful, but need to be targeted according to the clinical presentation of the individual.

The role of neurophysiology
The EEG

As indicated above, the EEG is a major contributor to helping in the diagnosis of epilepsy, not necessarily whether an individual has had an epileptic seizure but in trying to diagnose an underlying epilepsy syndrome. The most important part of investigation remains the history, particularly a description from an eyewitness to determine whether events could be epileptic seizures. Thereafter a diagnosis of epilepsy would depend on the recurrent tendency of that individual to have such epileptic seizures. As NICE (2004) has documented, an EEG should be used to support a diagnosis to help determine seizure type and syndrome. It may help to assess the risk of recurrence after a first seizure; however, it cannot be used definitively as such. It is recommended that an EEG should be performed after a second seizure unless evaluated otherwise by a specialist, namely in some circumstances where an individual may warrant an EEG after an initial seizure (e.g. following an initial generalized tonic-clonic seizure in teenage years). EEG should not be used to exclude a diagnosis of epilepsy in cases of probable syncope or in isolation to diagnose epilepsy outside the context of the clinical history.

The EEG may help in several ways to further diagnosis; firstly, if abnormalities are seen consistent with the clinical history. The EEG may be diagnostic if there is documentation of an actual seizure during the procedure. Thereafter we will be looking for patterns on the EEG consistent (spikes, spike-wave activity) with a particular type of epilepsy or syndrome. Changes may also confirm locality in individuals presenting with focal seizures. The EEG may be used in children with an established diagnosis of epilepsy, in particular with relation to frequency of abnormalities that may interfere with cognition, especially during sleep. However, it is imperative that an EEG is viewed and reported by an individual experienced in paediatric EEG in view of developmental changes that take place that may be misinterpreted as abnormal. In general, background frequencies become faster and reach an adult level by the age of 10 years. Furthermore there may be other sharpened or indeed high-altitude slow components that may be a normal variant according to the wake or sleep state of the child and therefore also need to be interpreted in the context of such; in an adult if seen these would be interpreted as abnormal. There are also artefacts that may need to be appropriately recognized. With the use of digital video-EEG in most departments, this helps in diagnosis as the video can be reviewed at a time the EEG has been performed. This is particular relevant in young children where blink and chewing artefacts (sucking artefacts) may mimic discharges. Reported changes should always be interpreted in the context of the clinical presentation.

Introduction to Epilepsy ed. Gonzalo Alarcón and Antonio Valentín. Published by Cambridge University Press.
© Cambridge University Press 2012.

Types of EEG and their use

The most commonly available EEG is of course the routine wake EEG. This is an hour's recording which, in order to be complete, should include provocation techniques, including hyperventilation and photic stimulation. Within the routine EEG, we will be looking for abnormalities supportive of the diagnosis whether this is generalized spike-wave activity, focal epileptiform activity or photic-induced abnormalities. Of course, the situation is eased if we actually document an attack. Further, we would be looking for changes consistent with an epilepsy syndrome diagnosis, for example centrotemporal discharges in a child presenting with nocturnal focal motor seizures (benign epilepsy with centrotemporal spikes). However, as indicated, the routine EEG is not complete without photic stimulation or indeed hyperventilation. Permission is now sought of parents and individuals for these indeed to take place, as in certain sensitive individuals these may lead to provocation of an attack. This has led to some individuals being wary of having such performed, but, as indicated, an EEG cannot be considered as complete without these provocation techniques being undertaken. In children, however, changes seen also need to be interpreted by those experienced in reviewing paediatric EEG. Generalized spike wave induced by hyperventilation must not be confused with the generalized slow activity that is seen in the normal individual. Further, there are grades of photic response and it is only the grade 4 photo (generalized) convulsive response that would be regarded as significant in the context of an individual with epilepsy.

Should an awake EEG be normal and a diagnosis of epilepsy still suspected, then a sleep EEG recording may help. This would again be looking for abnormalities supportive of a diagnosis of epilepsy, perhaps focal abnormalities, increased abnormalities during sleep and therefore also possibly a syndrome diagnosis. A sleep-deprived EEG may enhance abnormalities in the idiopathic generalized epilepsies.

Where there remains diagnostic doubt, it may be that events remain frequent enough (namely several in a 24–48-hour period) that an ambulatory EEG recording may be helpful. This has a more limited electrode placement, but the individual can go home and undertake normal day-to-day activities. These are particularly used to diagnose the nature of events as to whether they are epileptic or not, but has the disadvantage that there is no video to accompany the EEG.

Video-EEG recording, with time-locked video and EEG (video-telemetry), is particularly useful for diagnosing the nature of events and the types of seizures and ultimately is used in presurgical evaluation of individuals to localize seizure onset. It is highly resource-intensive and therefore only available in a limited number of centres.

When requesting an EEG it is absolutely imperative for there to be a question that is being asked, and that it is realistic that this question can be answered. If there is no question that can be answered by performing an EEG then it should not be used. Thereafter interpretation of the results has to be reviewed in the clinical context, to ascertain whether the results support the clinical history and thereafter the specific diagnosis. We have to be very aware of over-interpretation of otherwise normal findings.

Neuroimaging
Structural imaging

Neuroimaging of course remains the standard in the attempt to diagnose an underlying cause of epilepsy. It may in some circumstances contribute to the diagnosis of an underlying syndrome, and also the management of the individual. Magnetic resonance imaging remains the technique of choice, having greatly enhanced our understanding of the structure of the brain, particularly of malformations. There still remains a role for CT scans in certain circumstances. There are other more specialized investigations including functional MRI, SPECT and PET, which have a very specific remit particularly in presurgical evaluation of individuals undergoing consideration for epilepsy surgery.

According to the NICE guidelines (2004) all adults presenting with seizures should have an MRI scan. However, an individual does not routinely require an MRI when a diagnosis of idiopathic generalized epilepsy has been made. It is particularly important for children in those who have developed epilepsy under the age of 2 years, where there is any suggestion of a focal onset to seizures, or in all where seizures continue despite first-line medication.

Magnetic resonance imaging is mainly used for determining structural brain abnormalities. Appropriate protocols should be used to optimize visualization of grey/white matter contrast, and specific structures relevant to epilepsy (e.g. hippocampus). In certain individuals contrast should be given, namely gadolinium, particularly where a cerebrovascular malformation or tumour is suspected. CT scanning may still be useful in circumstances where an urgent scan is required in small children, who may lie still for such a short procedure, but also where lesions involving calcification may be suspected (tuberous sclerosis) or acute bleeding.

The role of functional imaging

There are specialized functional techniques that are used mainly with regard to presurgical evaluation. For example, functional MRI may be used to show functional cortex with regard to language or motor function. Single photon emission computed tomography (SPECT), where a radiolabelled ligand is injected into the bloodstream and preferentially taken up across the blood–brain barrier, showing a cerebral blood flow map, can be useful, but only in a presurgical context. Interictal scans (where the injection is made in between seizures) may be helpful in demonstrating areas that correlate with structural abnormalities. Ictal scans (where the injection is made during the seizure) are more likely to show an area of hyperperfusion, where the seizure arises, especially when compared with an interictal scan. Positron emission computed tomography (PET) scans using labelled fluorodeoxyglucose may show areas of hypometabolism that correlate with areas responsible for seizure onset. This investigation may be useful particularly in young children where lack of myelination through normal development may make it difficult to determine specific lesions on MRI scan. Other ligands may be used but are predominantly used for research purposes again to determine areas possibly responsible for seizure onset.

Other investigations

The degree to which other investigations are performed will be driven by the clinical picture. Decisions about whether such investigations are warranted should be made after discussion with a paediatric neurologist. Genetic evaluation is playing an increasing role in the diagnosis of certain types of epilepsy, particularly in the early-onset epilepsies (Table 54.1). Karyotyping should be considered in all children with early onset of epilepsy and

Table 54.1. When to consider genetic investigation

Girl, early-onset epilepsy, mental retardation	CDKL5, MECP2 PCDH19
Boy, early-onset epilepsy, mental retardation	ARX
Febrile seizures, prolonged, later development of other seizure types, developmental plateau (Dravets, SMEB)	SCN1A
Early-onset epilepsy, developmental delay, dysmorphic, myoclonus	Angelman's
Early onset epilepsy, tonic seizures, possible evolution to infantile sapsms, developmental delay	STXBP1

developmental delay. Certain laboratories will now also perform routine array comparative genomic hybridization (CGH). A request for assessment of mutations in specific genes will currently depend on the clinical presentation, e.g. sodium channel mutations (SCN1A) in children with a phenotype of Dravets syndrome (see Table 54.2).

Whether investigations for neurometabolic or neurodegenerative disorders are performed will also depend on the clinical presentation. Sometimes it can be difficult to determine whether regression or indeed a plateauing of cognitive skills is related to the epilepsy itself or is due to an underlying progressive cause. Clues to this may be in the fluctuating nature and the purely cognitive nature of any fluctuation in such skills, also whether the skills appear to have plateaued rather than truly regressed, all suggesting a relationship to the epilepsy. On examination there may be key features that may help towards deciding whether there is an underlying progressive aetiology, namely:

- whether there is an associated movement disorder;
- whether there has been a change in the developmental age of a child;
- whether there is any evidence of other neurological findings such as an eye-movement disorder or pyramidal signs and the determination whether there has been any evolution to such.

The onset of epilepsy in the first year of life is more highly associated with a progressive or metabolic disorder than later epilepsy onset (see Table 54.2). Therefore, metabolic investigations may be more appropriate if presentation of epilepsy is in the first

Table 54.2. Metabolic and neurodegenerative conditions that may present with epilepsy

Infancy	1–5 years	5–10 years	Adolescence and adulthood
Pyridoxine dependency	Homocysteinuria	SSPE	Progressive myoclonic epilepsy
Non-ketotic hyperglycinaemia	Rett syndrome	HIV	• Lafora body
Biotinidase deficiency	Late infantile NCL	PNDC (Alpers)	• Unverricht-Lundberg
Molybdenum cofactor deficiency	Gaucher's type III	Wilson's	• Sialidoses
Late infantile NCL		Niemann-Pick type C	• PNDC (Alpers)
Menkes syndrome			
Krabbe disease			
Peroxisomal disorders			

year of life rather than in those with a later onset. Thereafter investigations can be targeted according to the clinical presentation. Neurophysiology may also be helpful in that any atypical features of the EEG out of context of any presumed epilepsy syndrome or indeed progressive changes may help target investigations, some of which may be quite invasive.

Recommended reading

The epilepsies: diagnosis and management of the epilepsies in adults and children and young people in primary and secondary care. *National Institute for Health and Clinical Excellence (NICE)* Clinical Guideline **20**, October 2004. http//guidance.nice.org.uk/CG20.

Diagnosis and management of epilepsies in children and young people. *Scottish Intercollegiate Guidelines Network.* www.sign.ac.uk/guidelines/fulltext/81.

Diagnosis and management of epilepsies in adults. *Scottish Intercollegiate Guidelines Network.* www.sign.ac.uk/guidelines/fulltext/70.

Learning objective

(1) To know the investigations necessary for the study of epilepsy in children, their indications and the principles involved in their interpretation.

Section 2: Classification and diagnosis of epilepsy

Chapter 55: Case scenarios in paediatric epilepsy

David McCormick

The aim of this chapter is to outline a number of cases I have personally managed which demonstrate the experience of some children with respect to their seizure conditions. These scenarios underline the importance of appropriate assessment and diagnosis, so that appropriate advice can be given, and effective management implemented.

As outlined elsewhere in this book (Chapter 17), the ILAE classification system is used for classifying seizure disorders, and wherever possible a seizure syndrome diagnosis is also made. However, more recently, the 2001 modification of the ILAE classification system has proposed a multi-axial classification system (www.ilae-epilepsy.org/visitors/centre/ctf/over_frame.html). This enables the inclusion of aetiology and co-morbid conditions, and ensures the inclusion of an accurate description of the seizures and identification of the seizure types (see Table 55.1). This model will therefore be used in the small number of case scenarios which are outlined here. In addition, key lessons or principles from each case are described at the end of each scenario.

Samuel

Samuel was referred at the age of 15 with a recent onset of quite unusual episodes. Approximately five times per day he would have a strange feeling of everything he had read or seen recently becoming very clear to him, everything in his head relating to everything else, or a clear experience that he had seen or heard something before. These sensations were at times associated with nausea, and on one occasion associated with vomiting. When specifically asked, Samuel stated that he could hear other people during the episodes but found it hard to respond to them. Others described him as staring straight ahead,

Table 55.1. Multi-axial classification system

Axis 1	Description of the episodes (e.g. went stiff then had rhythmic jerking of all four limbs)
Axis 2	Naming of seizure types (e.g. generalized tonic-clonic seizures)
Axis 3	Syndrome diagnosis (where possible)
Axis 4	Aetiology (when known)
Axis 5	Co-morbid conditions (e.g. learning difficulty)

looking vacant, and when spoken to saying little other than 'just a minute'.

In the past, Samuel had never been a good school attender, had a tendency towards depression, and had previously been diagnosed with chronic fatigue syndrome. There was no family history of epilepsy but he admitted to quite frequent use of marijuana. His neurological examination was normal. The differential diagnosis was felt to include psychogenic episodes related to anxiety, or drug-induced episodes. Focal-onset seizures of probable temporal lobe origin were also considered in view of the described semiology, and with the relatively short history it was felt that an underlying structural lesion such as a brain tumour needed to be excluded. A standard awake EEG and epilepsy protocol MRI brain scan were therefore requested.

The EEG was found to show sharp waves over the left frontal and mid temporal regions. The MRI brain scan showed an abnormal lesion in the left temporal lobe felt to be consistent with a dysembryoplastic neuro-epithelial tumour (DNET). Adam was commenced on a slow-release form of carbamazepine building to a dose of 400 mg twice daily, at which dose he achieved seizure control unless he was poorly compliant (which he was intermittently). At the time

---

Introduction to Epilepsy ed. Gonzalo Alarcón and Antonio Valentín. Published by Cambridge University Press.
© Cambridge University Press 2012.

of writing, Samuel has not progressed to epilepsy surgery. The multi-axial classification for Samuel is thus as follows:

Axis 1	Unusual sensations involving déjà vu, and connectedness of thoughts whilst appearing vacant to others
Axis 2	Focal-onset seizures of left temporal origin
Axis 3	Symptomatic focal epilepsy
Axis 4	DNET left temporal lobe
Axis 5	Depression and recreational drug use

Key learning points from this case
- Subtle and even poorly described episodes can reflect true seizures as patients may find such sensations very difficult to describe. Pre-existing psychiatric or other chronic health problems should not lead to a less thorough assessment for a possible seizure disorder.
- All patients with probable focal-onset seizure disorders should have appropriate neuroimaging.
- Not all patients with identified structural lesions causing their seizures need to or wish to proceed to an epilepsy surgery programme.

Rubi

Rubi was born at term to a healthy mother and her initial health and development appeared normal. Aged 5 months she had the onset of episodes involving the forward flexion of her head and trunk with her arms held stiff and extended at the elbows. These episodes escalated extremely rapidly to the point where within weeks she was having more than 100 episodes in a day, usually in clusters. Her EEG showed a high-voltage chaotic picture consistent with hypsarrhythmia, but neuroimaging and all metabolic and genetic tests were normal. Rubi was treated with vigabatrin in the first instance, and on failing to respond to this was treated with a course of adrenocorticotrophic hormone injections (ACTH). However, neither agent led to seizure control, and despite subsequently going on to treatment with multiple antiepileptic drugs, implantation of a vagal nerve stimulator, and trial of the ketogenic diet, more than 15 years later Rubi continues to suffer from tonic spasms in clusters. She has developed severe learning difficulties, is wheelchair-bound, is unable to talk and is fed by gastrostomy. The multi-axial classification for Rubi is therefore as follows:

Axis 1	Episodes of forward flexion of head and trunk with stiffening and extension of arms lasting seconds and occurring in clusters
Axis 2	Infantile spasms followed by chronic mature tonic spasms
Axis 3	West's syndrome
Axis 4	No cause identified
Axis 5	Severe developmental delay

Key learning points from this case scenario
- The onset of infantile spasms should be regarded as a medical emergency and appropriate investigation and treatment undertaken straight away. There is some evidence that the early suppression of infantile spasms, when idiopathic, can significantly improve outcome.
- In many patients, the onset of infantile spasms heralds a severe disorder, which will have a major negative impact on the child's subsequent development and quality of life.
- Despite this, use of appropriate medication or non-drug management modalities can improve quality of life in these children.

Sadia

Sadia experienced her first episode aged 3½ when she was sitting on the bed combing her auntie's hair and was felt to be pulling it. On turning around, auntie found her to be staring and unresponsive, Sadia becoming floppy and going blue within 1 minute. She was given mouth-to-mouth resuscitation by her uncle, had recovered by the time she arrived at the accident and emergency department, and was sent home. She had a further such episode the next day when she similarly became blue and lifeless and once again was given mouth-to-mouth resuscitation. On this occasion she took much longer to respond and remained tired and apparently confused for several hours. She was assessed at her local hospital, a seizure considered and an initial EEG found to show runs of epileptiform discharges mainly in the right posterior quadrant. The neurophysiologist reporting the EEG included the comment that the child may be suffering from significant cerebral damage, predominantly occipital. However, Sadia remained well, made normal developmental progress, had a small number of similar episodes, and a subsequent EEG 18 months later showed runs of occipital spikes increasing on eye-closure, suggestive of a benign occipital epilepsy. An MRI brain scan was carried out and found to be normal. Sadia continued to make normal developmental progress and became seizure-free on carbamazepine. A diagnosis of benign childhood epilepsy with occipital paroxysms or Panayiotopoulos syndrome was made. Sadia's multi-axial classification is therefore as follows:

Axis 1	Episodes of floppiness, unresponsiveness, pallor and blueness around the mouth lasting several minutes followed by minutes to hours of drowsiness and confusion
Axis 2	Focal-onset seizure with predominantly autonomic features
Axis 3	Panayiotopoulos syndrome
Axis 4	Idiopathic
Axis 5	Nil

Key learning points from this case scenario

- An adequate knowledge of the wide range of seizure syndromes which can occur in children is necessary if some of the less classic forms of seizure disorder are to be recognized.
- Interpretation of the EEG must always be made in the context of the age of the child and the nature of the events which they have experienced, combined with an adequate knowledge of the literature.
- The identification of a specific syndromic diagnosis can significantly enhance the clinician's ability to give accurate information on treatment and prognosis as well as management of future episodes should they occur.

Teresa

Teresa was born at term to a healthy mother with no immediate concerns after delivery and with age-appropriate early developmental progress. She went on to infants' school and was felt to be an above-average student. By the age of 8 years when she was first seen in the epilepsy clinic there were, however, emerging concerns about her academic progress related to poor concentration and slow processing of information. She appeared to have a normal neurological examination, apart from a slight tendency to hold her right hand fisted and have reduced arm swing on the right. She had been referred for the assessment of possible blank episodes at school, combined with her general fall-off in school performance. An MRI brain scan was carried out and was normal but EEG showed predominantly generalized discharges of 2–3 Hz, enhancing with hyperventilation, and when these discharges were not occurring multifocal spikes were superimposed on the background, maximal in the right temporal region. Treatment was initiated initially in the form of sodium valproate, followed by the introduction of alternative agents, but despite this Teresa had worsening absence seizures, some prolonged, had a further loss of cognitive skills, and fall-off in her spoken communication as well as development of disinhibited behaviour. She began to have absences lasting up to 30 minutes in which she was completely unresponsive, and breakthrough generalized tonic-clonic seizures both by day and by night. The only AED which had a significant impact in terms of seizure control was phenobarbitone but this led to a marked deterioration in cognition. Due to her clinical course, a range of further investigations were carried out which demonstrated no underlying identified neurometabolic condition. Standard karyotype was normal, Fragile X testing was negative, but examination of multiple cells revealed the presence of ring chromosome 20 in a significant proportion. Teresa's multi-axial classification is therefore as follows:

Axis 1	Prolonged episodes of unresponsiveness, some associated with flickering of the eyelids
Axis 2	Atypical absence seizures, focal motor seizures and generalized tonic-clonic seizures
Axis 3	No specific syndromic diagnosis but epileptic encephalopathy identified
Axis 4	Ring chromosome 20
Axis 5	Severe learning difficulties and behavioural disorder

Key learning points from this case scenario

- Any child who has regression in developmental skills or learning should be investigated promptly and rigorously.
- Seizure disorders can present subtly in children on occasions, and subclinical epileptiform discharges can lead to significant deteriorations in cognitive performance.
- An adequate knowledge of potential underlying causes is required if appropriate investigations are to be carried out.
- The identification of a serious underlying disorder such as ring chromosome 20 informs prognosis and expectations regarding the child.
- Patients and their families identified as suffering from serious underlying conditions with an uncertain or potentially negative outcome require significant support and ongoing engagement with clinical services.

Amy

Amy was born to a healthy mother by normal delivery at term and had no perinatal problems or significant illnesses until her presentation. She had made good educational progress until year 6 at school, aged 10, when it was noted that she was having periods of not paying attention well. Subsequently her parents noted her to have some episodes of loss of awareness lasting 10 to 20 seconds, during which her eyes stared straight ahead and her eyelids occasionally flickered. These were seen occasionally in the first instance but over a period of 3 to 4 months increased to 10–20 times per day. On specific questioning, Amy did not remember the episodes but was at times aware that she had missed something, such as part of what her teacher was saying or missing part of a song during choir. Neurological examination was normal. Absence seizures were suspected and an awake EEG was requested. This showed spontaneous bursts of generalized 2.5–3 Hz spike-and-wave discharges, lasting up to 6 seconds without clinical manifestations. On hyperventilation, a persistent run of 2.5 Hz generalized spike-and-wave discharges lasting 20 seconds with clinical absence including cessation of hyperventilation occurred. There was a brief run of generalized spike-and-wave discharges occurring on photic stimulation at 18 Hz, which ceased on cessation of the stimulus. After discussion with Amy and her family, lamotrigine was prescribed and built to the desired dose over a 10-week period. Control of the absences was achieved, and it was then noted that Amy's school performance picked up a little, parents and teachers then coming to recognize that she had been under-performing for at least the last 6 months. The duration of Amy's treatment is yet to be determined. The multi-axial classification for Amy is therefore as follows:

Axis 1	Episodes of staring and being unresponsive, sometimes associated with eyelid flickering lasting up to 20 s
Axis 2	Classic absence seizures
Axis 3	Juvenile absence epilepsy
Axis 4	Idiopathic
Axis 5	Transient fall-off in school performance

Some of the key learning points from this case scenario

- Knowledge of epilepsy syndromes affecting children is vital if appropriate seizure syndrome diagnoses are to be made.
- Syndromic diagnoses can allow accurate prognostic information to be offered and appropriate medication to be prescribed.
- The majority of seizure disorders affecting childhood are well managed, with seizure freedom achieved on a single antiepileptic medication, enabling return to normal quality of life.

In summary

There is an extremely wide range of seizure disorders which can present in childhood, ranging from severe symptomatic seizure disorders reflecting profound underlying pathology to idiopathic seizure disorders in otherwise well children which are relatively easily controlled with medication. Adequate knowledge of this range of seizure disorders is vital if appropriate investigation and management is to be undertaken. The ILAE multi-axial classification allows a framework for the identification and recording of information relevant to the patient. All children presenting with seizures should be treated as individuals, and their management tailored to their individual needs based on underlying conditions, age, family and other social circumstances as well as their point on the education pathway. Long-term management of such children can offer a significant challenge to the clinician but also the potential for significant job satisfaction as the child and their family are supported through the challenges which such seizure disorders bring.

Reference

A proposed diagnostic scheme for people with epileptic seizures and with epilepsy: *report of the ILAE task force on classification and terminology.* www.ilae-epilepsy.org/visitors/centre/ctf/over_frame.html.

Learning objectives

(1) To recognize the importance of the ILAE multi-axial classification system and see its use in real cases of childhood epilepsy.
(2) To 'experience' several presentations and clinical courses of children with seizure disorders representing some of the vast array of these conditions in childhood.
(3) To recognize that adequate assessment and knowledge of epilepsy in childhood is necessary if children with seizure disorders are to be appropriately diagnosed and treated.
(4) To learn from clinical case scenarios regarding the significant impact which seizure disorders can have on the quality of life of children and young people.

Section 2 Classification and diagnosis of epilepsy

Chapter 56

Psychogenic non-epileptic seizures: diagnostic approach

Franz Brunnhuber

Misdiagnosis: facts and consequences

Staring episodes in children: the literature suggests caution in children with staring episodes. In 30% of these children the diagnosis was disproved where there were no initial doubts about the epileptic nature (Uldall *et al.*, 2006).

Costs: the estimated annual medical costs of England and Wales were £29 million, while total costs could reach up to £130 million a year (Juarez-Garcia *et al.*, 2006).

Detainees in police stations frequently claimed to suffer from epilepsy (Beaumont, 2007).

The misdiagnosis rate in epilepsy ranges from 5% by experienced paediatric neurologists to 23% in population-based general practitioners (van Donselaar *et al.*, 2006).

Definition, terminology and classification

'Non-epileptic seizures may be defined as a sudden, usually disruptive, change in a person's behaviour, perception, thinking or feeling that is usually time-limited and resembles, or is mistaken for, epilepsy but does not have the characteristic electrophysiological changes in the brain, detectable by EEG, that accompany a true epileptic seizure' (Betts, 1997). The international classification of diseases (ICD 10) defines dissociation as a partial or complete loss of the normal integration between memories of the past, awareness of identity and immediate sensations and control of body movements. In the following context, non-epileptic seizures are used synonymously with 'psychogenic non-epileptic seizures' or 'dissociative seizures'. They are to be distinguished from factitious disorders, which are characterized by presenting with physical or psychological symptoms or both and the symptoms are produced from a motivation to assume the sick role and differ from malingering in the external gains. Malingering is the conscious and deliberate production, simulation or exaggeration of a symptom for some gain, such as obtaining disability payments. The DSM IV uses the term 'somatization disorder', which originates in the concepts of hysteria: multiple unexplained physical symptoms for which the patient sought treatment or experienced significant social or occupational impairment.

Investigating for psychogenic non-epileptic seizures

What is the rationale for making a diagnosis of non-epileptic seizures? It is commonly accepted that inpatient video-telemetry is the ultimate tool for seizure classification and thus if there is any doubt about the nature of seizures it is widely agreed that the goal standard for making a diagnosis of non-epileptic seizures is the inpatient video-telemetry investigation. This usually requires a hospital admission mostly to a video-telemetry ward. There, a history of the habitual seizures is taken and, when seizures occur, an analysis of the EEG and semiology including an ictal assessment can be provided. A seizure review with the patient and/or the relatives or witness is often necessary. In addition, long-term monitoring allows long-term interictal EEG sampling.

Limitations and pitfalls of video-EEG telemetry

- Simple partial seizures may be EEG-negative (false negative for epilepsy and false positive for NES).

Introduction to Epilepsy ed. Gonzalo Alarcón and Antonio Valentín. Published by Cambridge University Press.
© Cambridge University Press 2012.

Section 2: Classification and diagnosis of epilepsy

Table 56.1. Video-telemetry modalities in the diagnosis of psychogenic non-epileptic seizures

	Inpatient VT	Outpatient VT: day case	Activation clinic
Duration	3–5 days	4–6 h	2 h
Inpatient	+	−	−
Outpatient	−	+	+
Information about VT	+	+	+
Information about activation	−	−	+
History of habitual seizures	+	+	+
Ictal assessment: nurse	+/−	−	+
Ictal assessment: techn.	−	+	+
Ictal assessment and activation: consultant	−	−	+
Analysis of semiology	+	+	+
Analysis of interictal EEG	+++	++	+
Analysis of ictal EEG	+	+	+
Seizure review with relatives	+/−	+/−	+
Main advantage	Gold standard	Outpatient	Outpatient/second chance/opinion
Main disadvantage	Costs/resources/IP	High seizure frequency	Works only in 50%

- Orbitofrontal seizures may be scalp EEG-negative and thus falsely suggest non-epileptic seizures.
- Co-existence of epilepsy: there can be a co-existence of epilepsy and non-epileptic seizures.
- Some patients suffer from rare seizures and an inpatient investigation is not indicated.
- It can be difficult to determine whether an event indeed represents the habitual seizures or is an ad hoc event (false positive).

Video-telemetry modalities in the diagnosis of psychogenic non-epileptic seizures

Table 56.1 summarizes the basic differences, advantages and disadvantages of the various modalities available for video-telemetry (VT). Essentially, during inpatient VT, the patient stays in hospital for 24 hours/day. In patients with several attacks per day, the patient may come to hospital in the morning, have VT for several hours and return home later in the day (outpatient VT). Alternatively, the patient may come to hospital for activation of seizures (activation clinic, see below) which typically only lasts for about 2 hours.

In the context of identifying and classifying non-epileptic seizures, verbal suggestion and/or intravenous saline injections, in an inpatient or outpatient setting, with prolonged video-EEG monitoring is effective in triggering non-epileptic seizures (the so-called 'provocation or activation procedure'). In an outpatient setting, it yields a success rate of 50% of capturing or provoking non-epileptic seizures, and thus ultimately establishing the diagnosis without requiring a hospital admission (Dericioğlu et al., 1999; McGonigal et al., 2004). Intravenous saline injection as a provocation method increases the yield of capturing non-epileptic seizures by 30% in the inpatient setting (Ribaï et al., 1994). To avoid misdiagnosis, careful history-taking and reviewing the 'seizures' in question with the patient and relatives is of utmost importance.

Chapter 56: Psychogenic non-epileptic seizures: diagnostic approach

Protocol for the 'Activation Clinic' at King's College Hospital in London

(1) Patients with assumed non-epileptic seizures are given an outpatient appointment in the 'activation clinic'. They are asked to attend with a relative or friend who has witnessed the seizures in question.

The appointment letter includes information about the purpose of the clinic, which is to identify whether the patient is suffering from non-epileptic seizures, which are usually caused by psychological causes.

Table 56.2. Evidence-based approach to a diagnosis of NES

	Interictal phase	Pre-ictal phase	Ictal phase	Post-ictal phase
State of the patient	Normal and/or psychiatric morbidity (1)	"Wake or sleep" (2)	Responsiveness/ duration (3)	"Wake or sleep" (4)
EEG	Interictal EEG (5)	Wake or sleep (6)	Alpha? Slowing/ artefacts (7)	Alpha, slowing (8)
Semiology/ behaviour	History/questionnaires (9)	Subtle changes (11)	Ictal semiology	Memory/deficit (13)
Heart rate	Baseline (14)	?		Change form baseline (15)
Serum levels	Baseline (16)			Change ? (16)

Table 56.3. Evidence-based approach to the diagnosis of psychogenic non-epileptic seizures (NES) with video-telemetry

Step	Evidence and clinical experience	Reference
1, 9	History and psychiatric co-morbidity: in the interictal state an interview will allow assessment of psychiatric co-morbidity. A detailed seizure description can be obtained from the patient and a witness to ascertain what the habitual seizure type is.	
2	From sleep: less than 1% of NES occur from sleep. In other words if an event occurs from sleep, there is a 99% chance that this is not a NES.	Orbach et al., 2003
3	Responsiveness and duration; it is essential to assess responsiveness during a seizure (unresponsiveness with an alpha rhythm in EEG is diagnostic of non-epileptic). Also NES tend to be longer than epileptic seizures. It would be unusual for an epileptic seizure to last 20 min or longer. See step 6.	
4	Awake or asleep: many patients after epileptic seizures are sleepy and fall asleep. Also patients with NES are found to be 'asleep'. Also see step 6.	
5	Interictal EEG abnormalities: 93% of patients with NES and epilepsy have EEG abnormalities; 54% of patients with NES have EEG abnormalities. Compared to healthy controls patients with NES have 1.8-fold higher rate of EEG abnormalities.	Reuber et al., 2002
6, 7, 8	EEG: awake or asleep: the EEG can unequivocally determine whether the patient is asleep or awake and thus provides a major step in the diagnosis of NES: • NES is suggested if the patient is unresponsive during the event (showing normal wake EEG). • NES is suggested if the patient appears asleep post-ictally while the EEG shows a normal alpha EEG.	Vinton et al., 2004

Table 56.3. (cont.)

Step	Evidence and clinical experience	Reference
	• If the patient hyperventilates during the attack (e.g. in a panic attack) the EEG could show a degree of slowing, particularly over frontal regions, which must not be confused with ictal or post-ictal slowing (see Chapter 18). • Convulsive psychogenic NES show movement artefacts with non-evolving frequency, distinctly different from an ictal EEG pattern.	
11	Subtle behavioural changes: pre-ictally, some subtle changes such as taking off eye-glasses or pushing away the bed or other suble preparatory actions may indicate that the seizure is a NES. This may often be noticeable on careful video review.	
12	Eye-closure occurs: • in 90% of GTCS • in 5% (21/408) of complex partial seizures, eye-closure occurs • in only in 0.5% (2/49) of simple partial seizures. In NES, forceful eye-closure is seen in 41/75 of NES with a clear motor component and in 16/21 of NES with no motor component (unresponsive). Henry-Woodruff sign: deviation of the eyes towards the ground with the patient lying on each side is proposed as a diagnostic sign in psychogenically mediated states resembling coma epilepsy.	DeToledo and Ramsay, 1996 Brunnhuber et al., 2003 Henry and Woodruff, 1978
13	Post-ictal symptoms: Post-ictal headache: 38% of patients with epilepsy and 4% of NES. Post-ictal fatigue: 56% of patients with epilepsy and 13% NES. Post-ictal confusion: No difference between epilepsy and NES.	Ettinger et al., 1999
14	Heart rate: • in 93% of epileptic seizures, heart rate increased at least by 10 bpm • in 49% of seizures, heart rate increase preceded both EEG and clinical onsets • heart rate in staring spells: an increase of 30% compared to the baseline has positive predictive value of 97% to predict epilepsy.	Zijlmans et al., 2002 Opherk and Hirsch, 2002
15, 16	Prolactin: • in NES, prolactin raised in 26% and was raised more than 2-fold (false positive) in all 26% • in epilepsy, prolactin raised in 58% and in 17% raised by 2-fold • we think it is not advisable to use prolactin in differentiating NES from epilepsy.	Shukla et al., 2004

(2) The activation clinic is carried out jointly with a technician. While the physician is taking the history, electrodes are applied and a baseline recording is achieved. During the baseline recording, the patient's carer or witness is asked to wait outside.

(3) Not infrequently, patients have non-epileptic seizures already during the baseline recording when encouraged, and then do not require the activation procedure.

(4) If unsuccessful, a photic stimulation or hyperventilation protocol is applied. The photic stimulation protocol usually involves low-frequency stimulation ranging from 2 to 10 Hz lasting for 4–10 s with closed or open eyes.

(5) If events are recorded, they are then reviewed with the patient's relative. The final diagnosis is not discussed during this appointment but is usually dealt with by the referring consultant.

How to make a diagnosis of non-epileptic seizures

Table 56.2 provides an evidence-based approach to how to reach a diagnosis of non-epileptic seizures using video-EEG telemetry. The rationale is taken from seizure classification in epilepsy. Epileptic seizures are classified according to signs and symptoms in the interictal, pre-ictal, ictal or post-ictal phase. The signs and symptoms in Table 56.2 correlated with the various phases provide an evidence base for a diagnosis of non-epileptic seizures.

References

Beaumont G. Is this epilepsy? *J Forensic Leg Med* 2007;**14**(2):99–102.

Betts T. Psychiatric aspects of nonepileptic seizures. In Engels J, Pedley TA, eds. *Epilepsy: A Comprehensive Textbook*, Ch. 199. Philadelphia: Lippincott Williams & Wilkins; 1997.

Brunnhuber F, Binnie CD, Fowle AJ. Assessment of epilepsy for surgery. In Binnie C, *et al.*, eds. *Clinical Neurophysiology*, vol. **2**, Ch. 6.3, pp. 669–700. Amsterdam: Elsevier; 2003.

Dericioğlu N, Saygi S, Ciğer A. The value of provocation methods in patients suspected of having non-epileptic seizures. *Seizure* 1999;**8**(3):152–6.

DeToledo JC, Ramsay RE. Patterns of involvement of facial muscles during epileptic and nonepileptic events: review of 654 events. *Neurology* 1996;**47**(3):621–5.

Ettinger AB, Weisbrot DM, Nolan E, Devinsky. Postictal symptoms help distinguish patients with epileptic seizures from those with non-epileptic seizures. *Seizure* 1999;**8**(3):149–51.

Henry JA, Woodruff GH. Diagnostic sign in states of apparent unconsciousness. *Lancet* 1978;**2**(8096):920–1.

Juarez-Garcia A, Stokes T, Shaw B, Camosso-Stefinovic J, Baker R. The costs of epilepsy misdiagnosis in England and Wales. *Seizure* 2006;**15**(8):598–605. Epub 2006 Sep 29 Juarez-Garcia A 2006.

McGonigal A, Russell AJC, Mallik AK, Oto M, Duncan R. Use of short term video EEG in the diagnosis of attack disorders. *J Neurol Neurosurg Psychiatry* 2004;**75**:771–2.

Opherk C, Hirsch LJ. Ictal heart rate differentiates epileptic from non-epileptic seizures. *Neurology* 2002;**58**(4):636–8.

Orbach D, Ritaccio A, Devinsky O. Psychogenic, nonepileptic seizures associated with video-EEG-verified sleep. *Epilepsia* 2003;**44**(1):64–8.

Reuber M, Fernandez G, Bauer J, Singh DD, Elger CE. EEG abnormalities in patients with psychogenic nonepileptic. seizures. *Epilepsia* 2002;**43**(9):1013–20.

Ribaï P, Tugendhaft P, Legros B. Usefulness of prolonged video-EEG monitoring and provocative procedure with saline injection for the diagnosis of non epileptic seizures of psychogenic origin. *Epilepsia* 1994;**35**(4):768–70.

Shukla G, Bhatia M, Vivekanandhan S, *et al*. Serum prolactin levels for differentiation of nonepileptic versus true seizures. Limited utility. *Epilepsy Behav* 2004;**5**(4):517–21.

Uldall P, Alving J, Hansen LK, Kibaek M, Buchholt J. The misdiagnosis of epilepsy in children admitted to a tertiary epilepsy centre with paroxysmal events. *Arch Dis Child* 2006;**91**(3):219–21.

van Donselaar CA, Stroink H, Arts WF. How confident are we of the diagnosis of epilepsy? *Epilepsia* 2006;**47**(Suppl 1):9–13.

Vinton A, Carino J, Vogrin S, *et al*. 'Convulsive' nonepileptic seizures have a characteristic pattern of rhythmic artifact distinguishing them from convulsive epileptic seizures. *Epilepsia* 2004;**45**(11):1344–50.

Zijlmans M, Flanagan D, Gotman J. Heart rate changes and ECG abnormalities during epileptic seizures: prevalence and definition of an objective clinical sign. *Epilepsia* 2002;**43**(8):847–54.

Learning objectives

(1) To understand the epidemiology and cost of non-epileptic seizures.
(2) To become familiar with the definitions, terminology and classifications of non-epileptic seizures.
(3) To understand the investigations and diagnostic criteria for non-epileptic seizures and their interpretation in the differential diagnosis of epilepsy.

Section 2 Classification and diagnosis of epilepsy

Chapter 57

Seminar: paediatric EEG reporting session

Ronit Pressler

This is a practical EEG session intending to improve and deepen your understanding of neonatal and paediatric EEG. There are six cases with a brief history – not less or more than what you would usually find on an EEG request form – together with two typical pages of their EEG. You should attempt a brief factual report and a conclusion for each case. The factual describes the EEG including the ongoing activity, normal and abnormal transients, epileptiform activity and possible seizures. In the conclusion, the findings should be put into clinical context including:

(a) summary of findings – normal or abnormal;
(b) ongoing or background activity normal or abnormal for age;
(c) suggestion of diagnosis or differential diagnosis and clinical relevance.

At the end of the chapter you will find a brief solution for each case. It is hoped you will use these cases as a starting point for further reading and discussion.

Case 1

Neonate born at term, cord prolapse, APGAR 1/3/4, cord pH 6.8.

(a) EEG at 24 hours of age, ventilated, sedated, occasional episodes of mouthing, eye blinking and facial twitching.
(b) Same EEG, no clinical correlate.
(c) Same baby, now 9 months of age, episodes of 'startling' and crying, occurring in clusters and without obvious trigger. Neurodevelopment has always been delayed, but more recently there is some regression of motor and social skills.
(d) Same EEG: 'Startle event' (arrow) with sudden extension of arms and flexion of neck (Figure 57.1).

Case 2

Newborn aged 10 days, frequent myoclonic jerks of arms and legs, mainly during sleep.

(a) Wakefulness.
(b) Sleep, arrow marks, symmetrical myoclonic jerk of upper and lower limbs (Figure 57.2).

Case 3

Girl, 3½ years of age. History of three episodes during sleep with crying out, eyes opening and turning, vomiting, then unresponsive for brief time.

(a) EEG during drowsiness.
(b) EEG on passive eye-closure (Figure 57.3).

Case 4

Boy 5 years of age, with history of two nocturnal generalized tonic-clonic seizures and sided Todd's paresis for 24 hours after last seizure.

(a) Wakefulness.
(b) Sleep (Figure 57.4).

Case 5

Boy 10 years of age. Epilepsy with infrequent seizures (simple partial seizures and tonic-clonic seizures) since age 5 years, on sodium valproate. Since onset of epilepsy, considerable behavioural problems and increasing difficulties at school (now statemented).

(a) Wakefulness.
(b) Sleep (Figure 57.5).

Introduction to Epilepsy ed. Gonzalo Alarcón and Antonio Valentín. Published by Cambridge University Press.
© Cambridge University Press 2012.

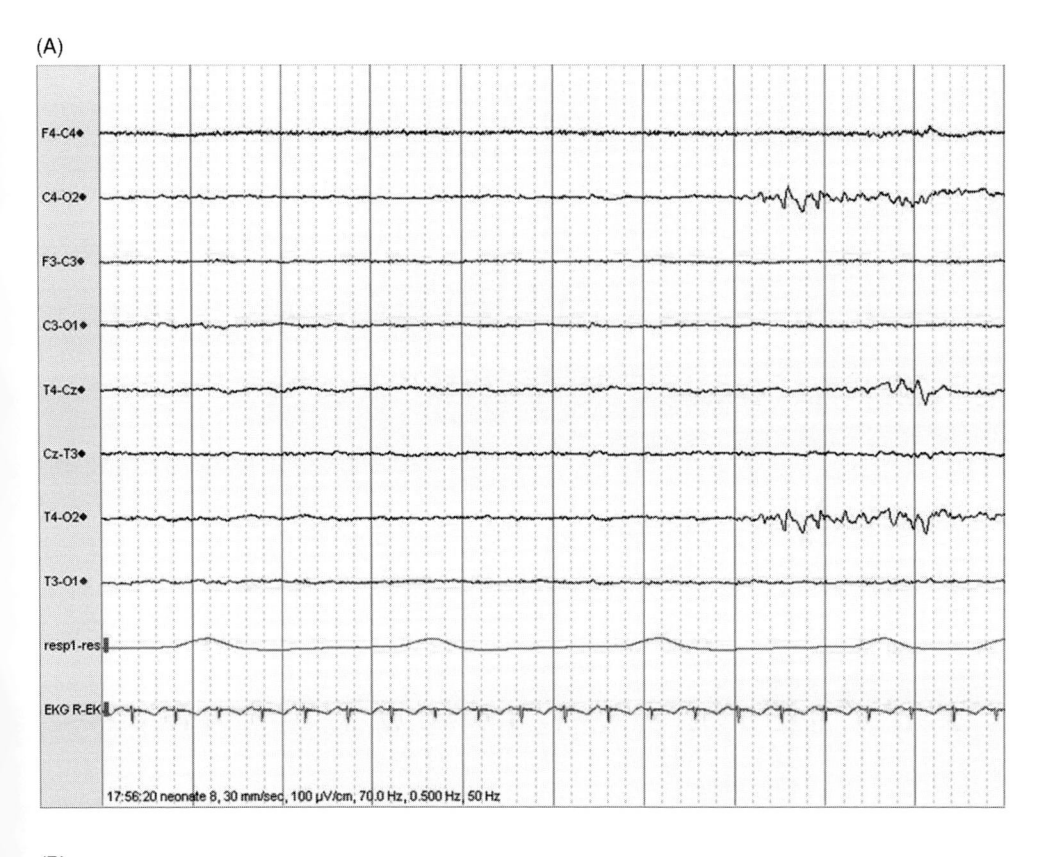

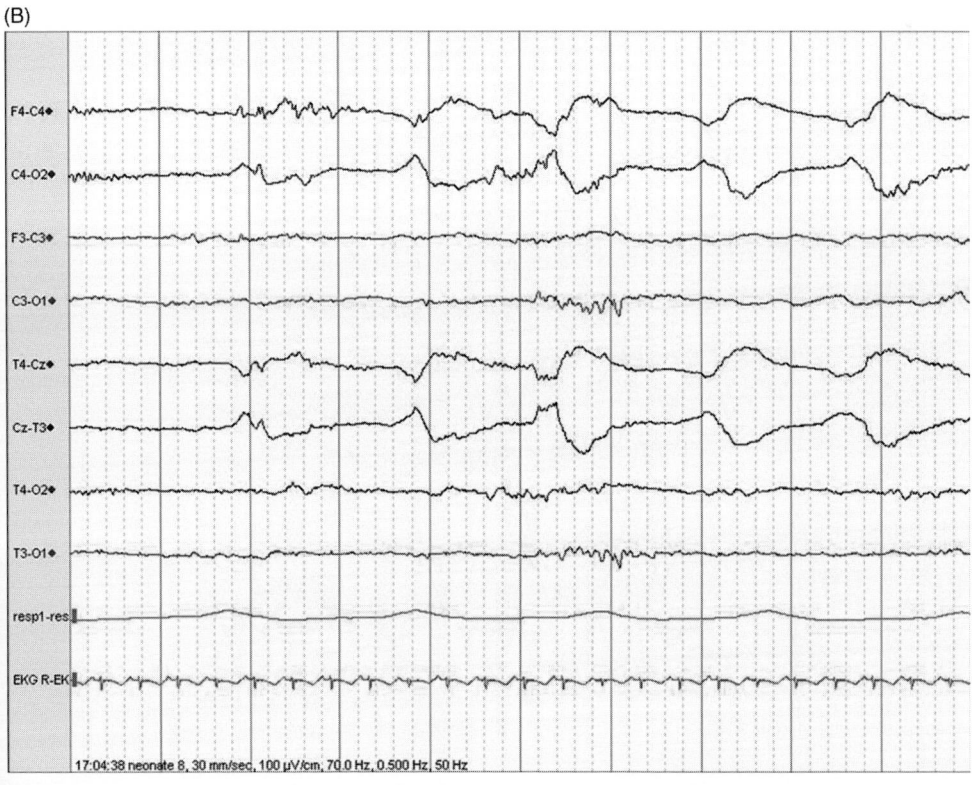

Chapter 57: Seminar: paediatric EEG reporting session

Figure 57.1.

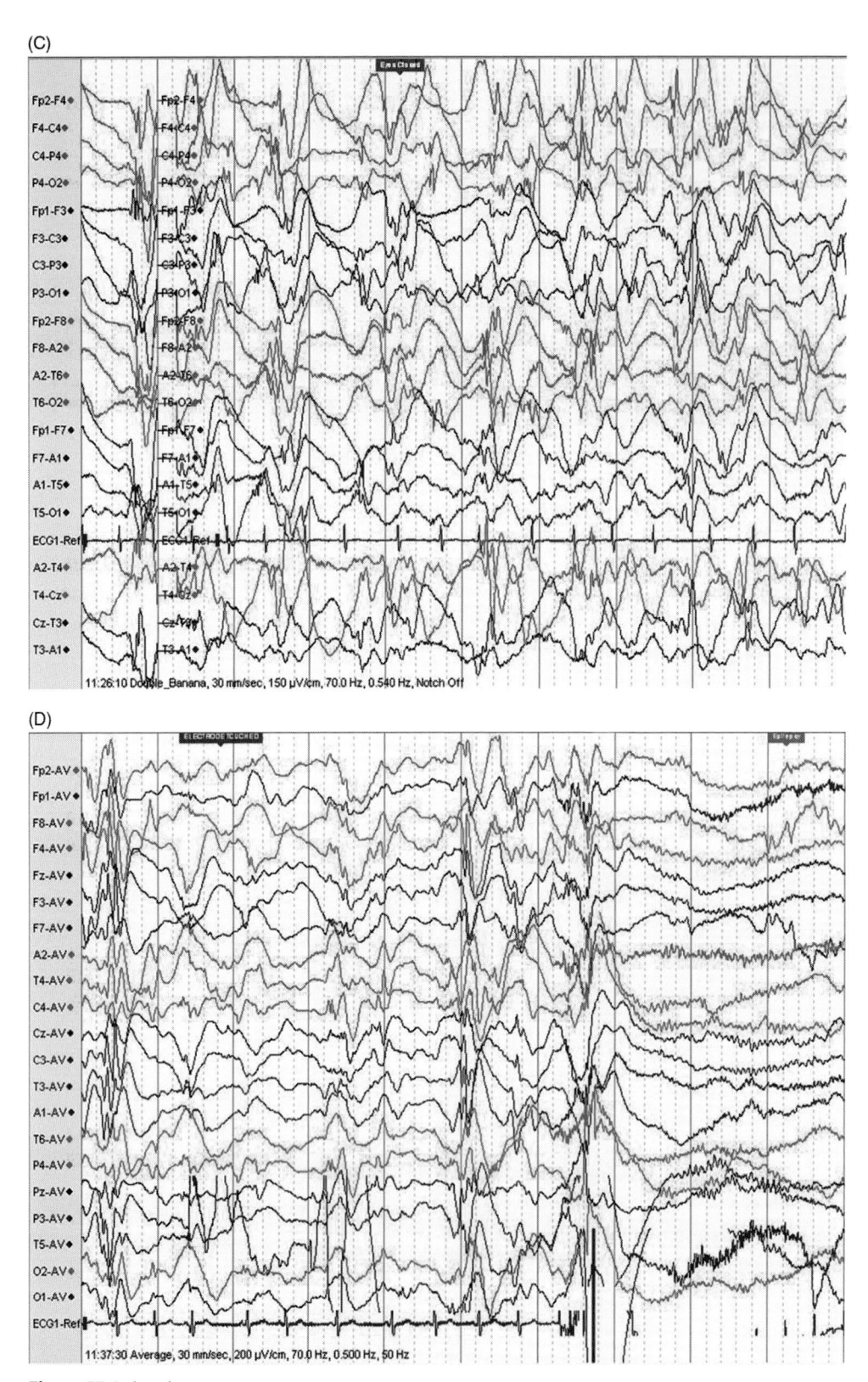

Section 2: Classification and diagnosis of epilepsy

Figure 57.1. (cont.)

Chapter 57: Seminar: paediatric EEG reporting session

(A)

(B)

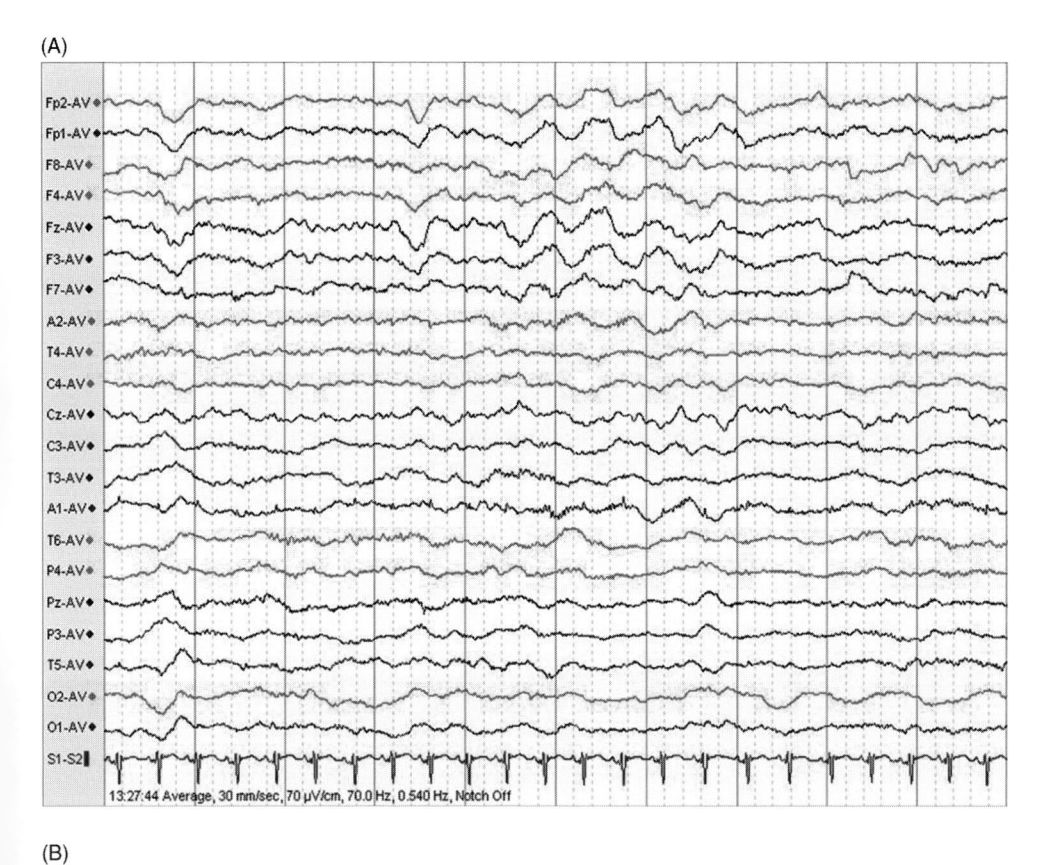

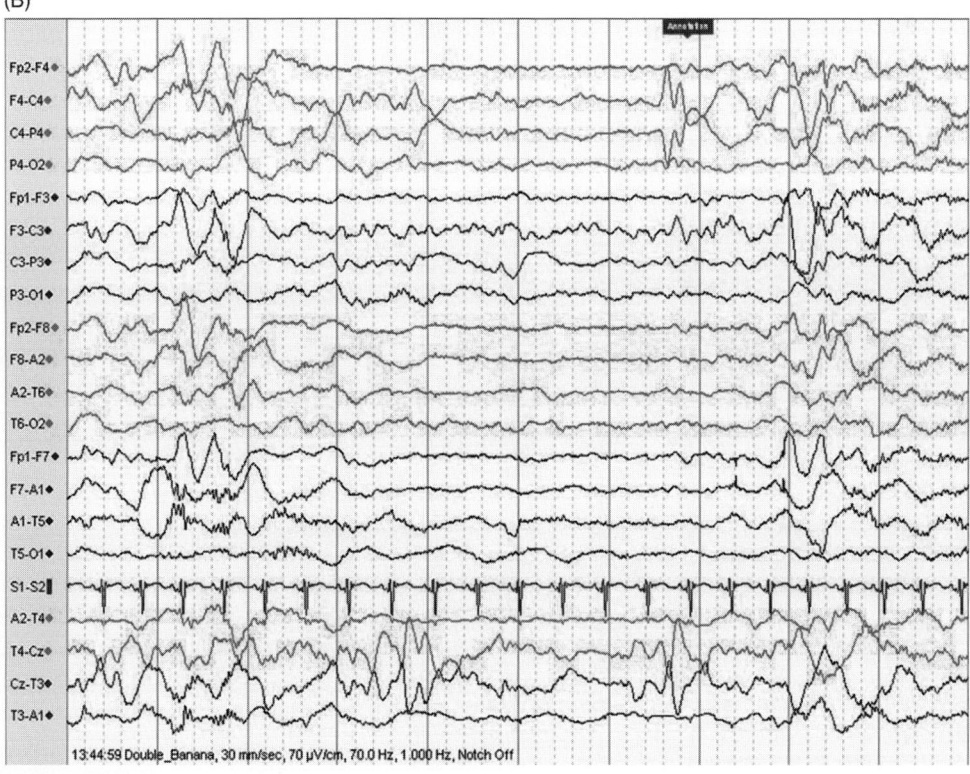

Figure 57.2.

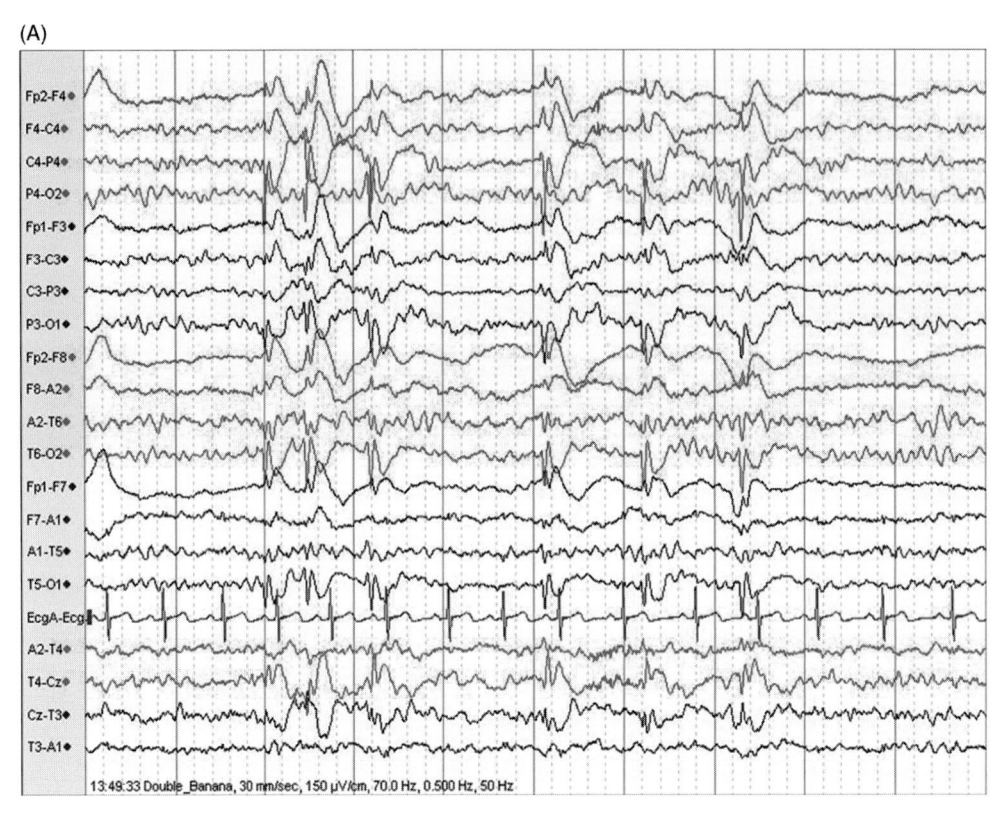

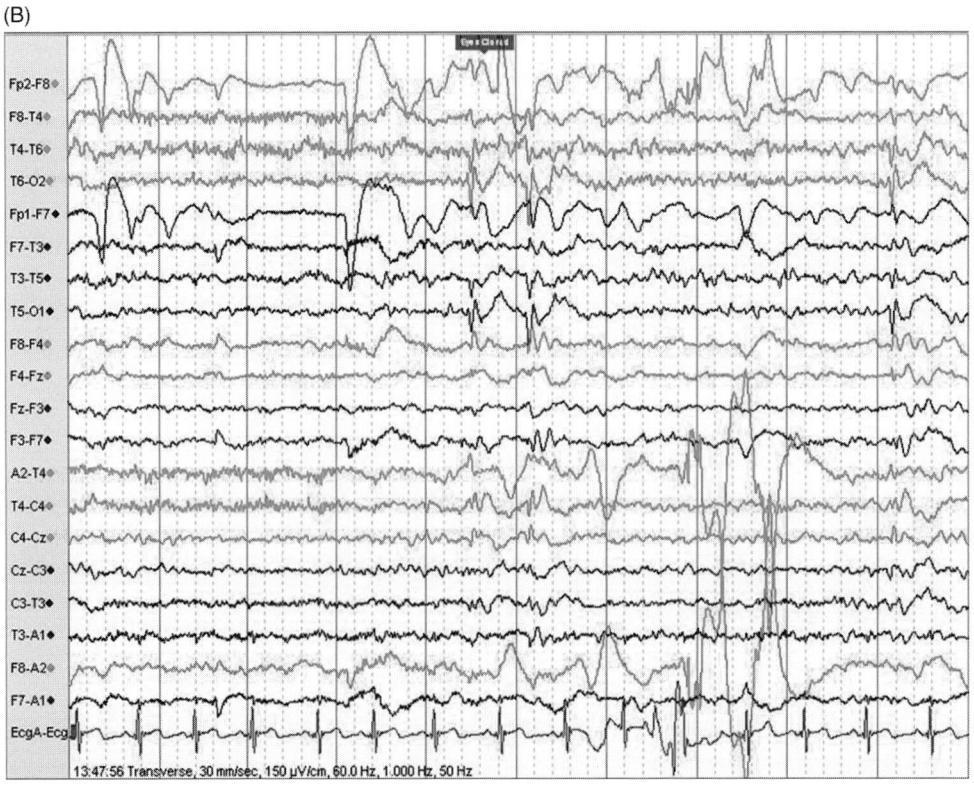

Section 2: Classification and diagnosis of epilepsy

Figure 57.3.

Chapter 57: Seminar: paediatric EEG reporting session

(A)

(B)

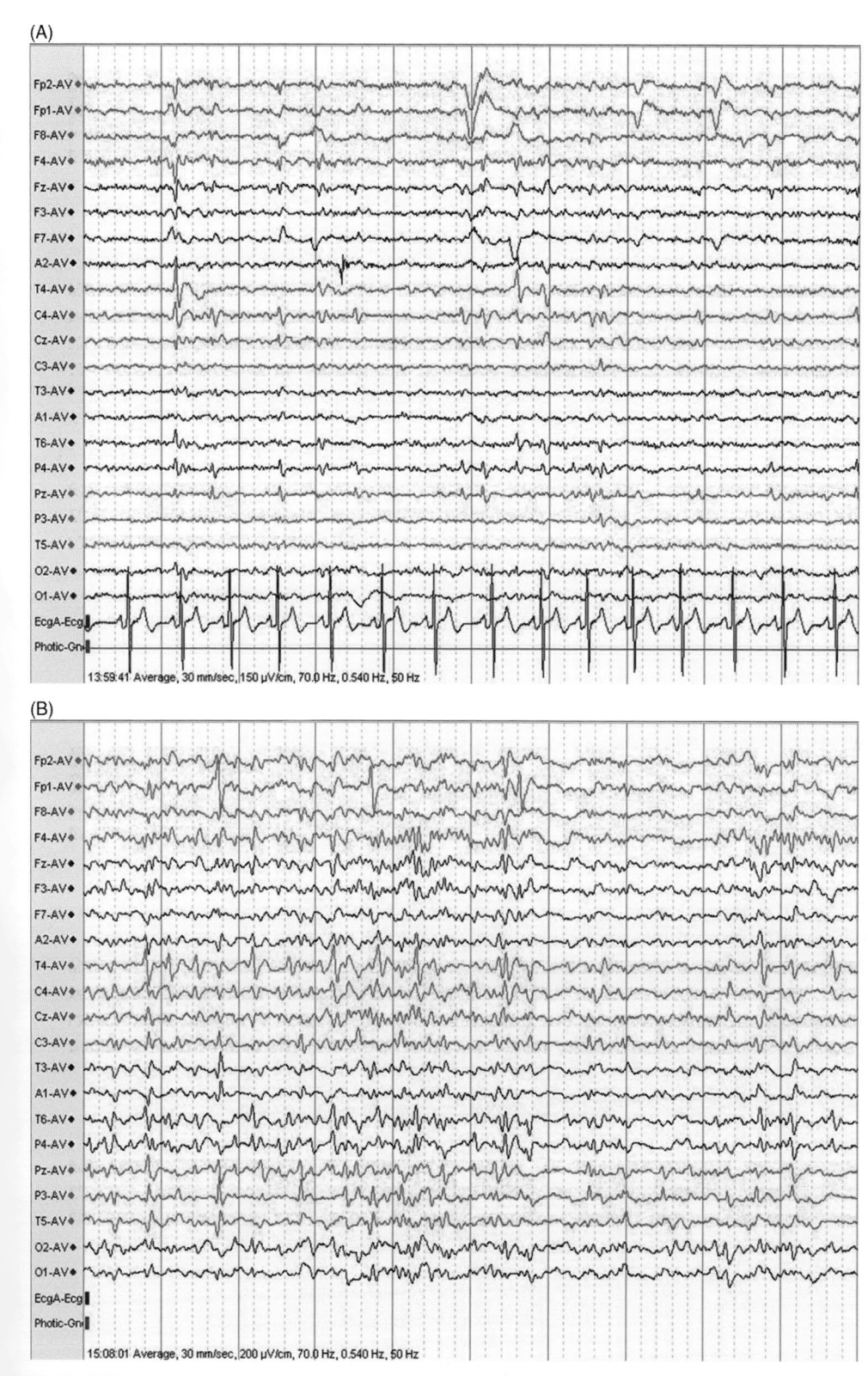

Figure 57.4.

Section 2: Classification and diagnosis of epilepsy

(A)

(B)

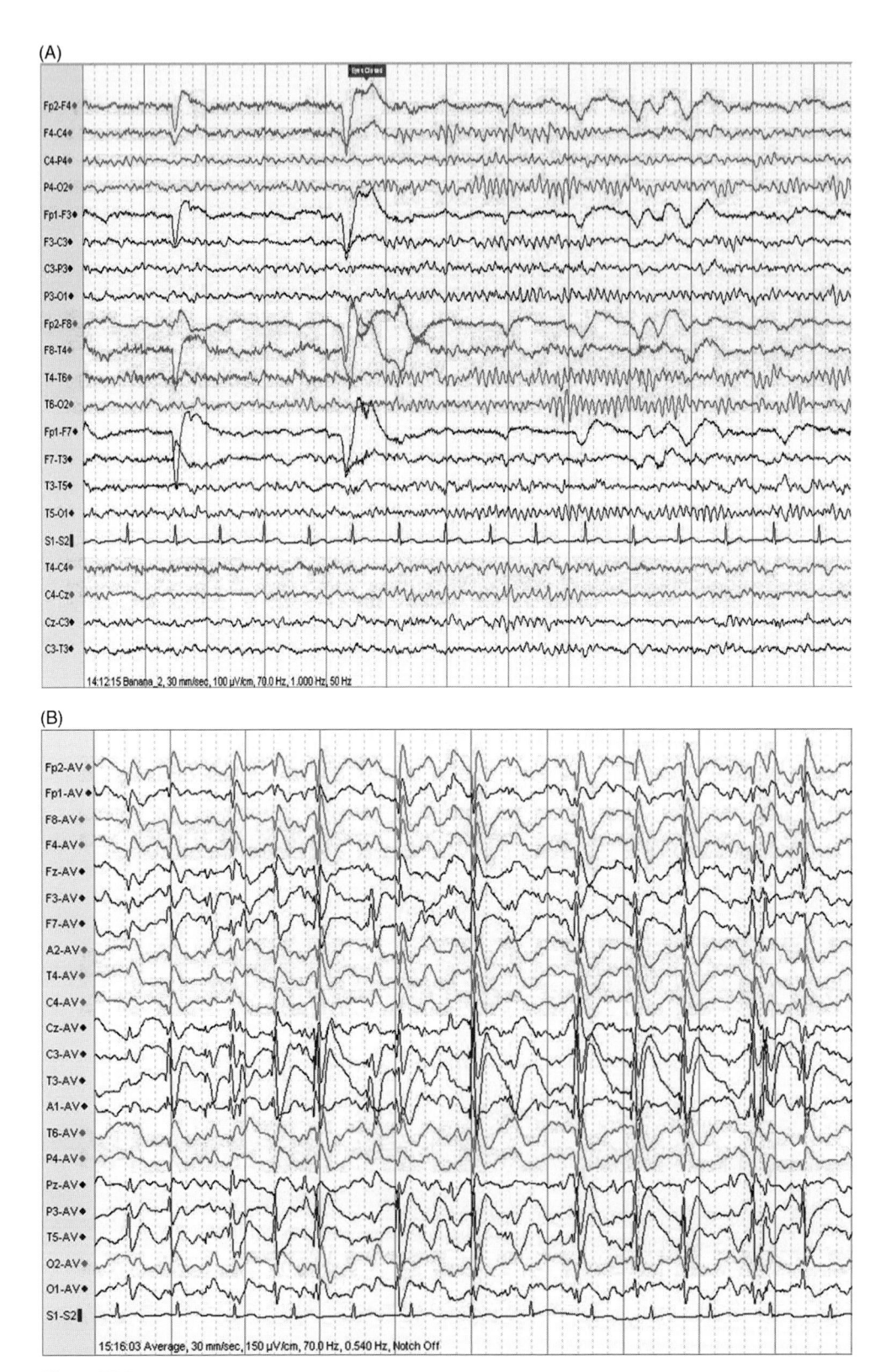

Figure 57.5.

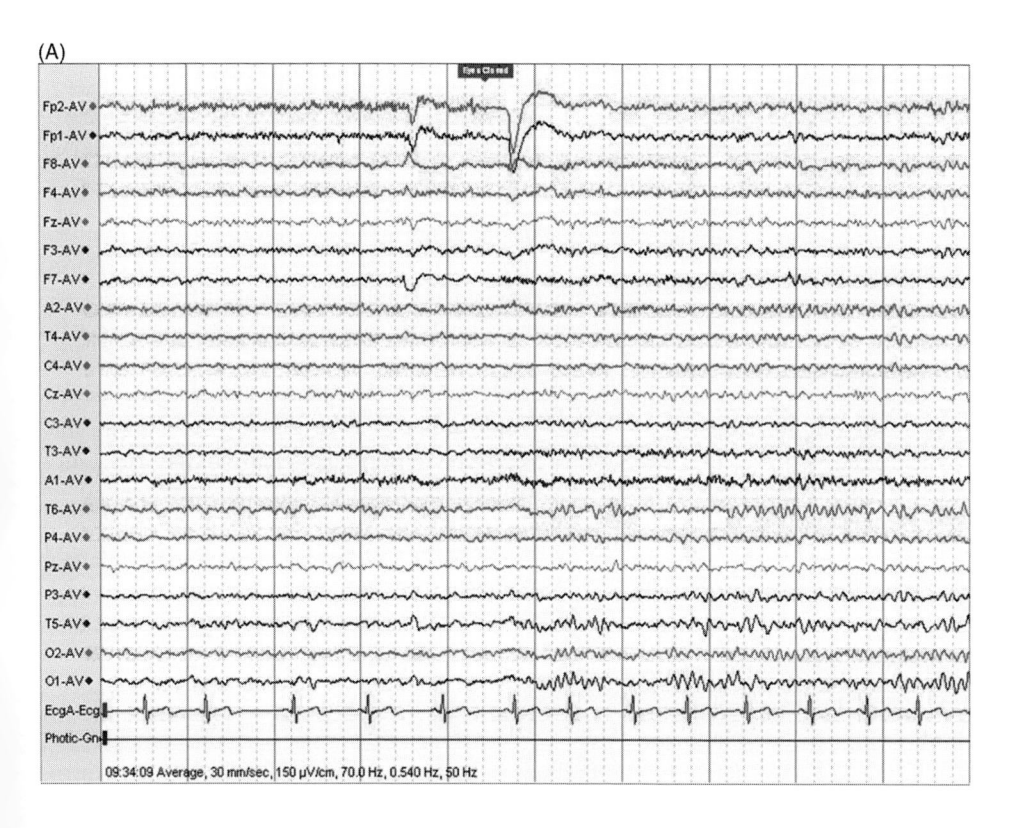

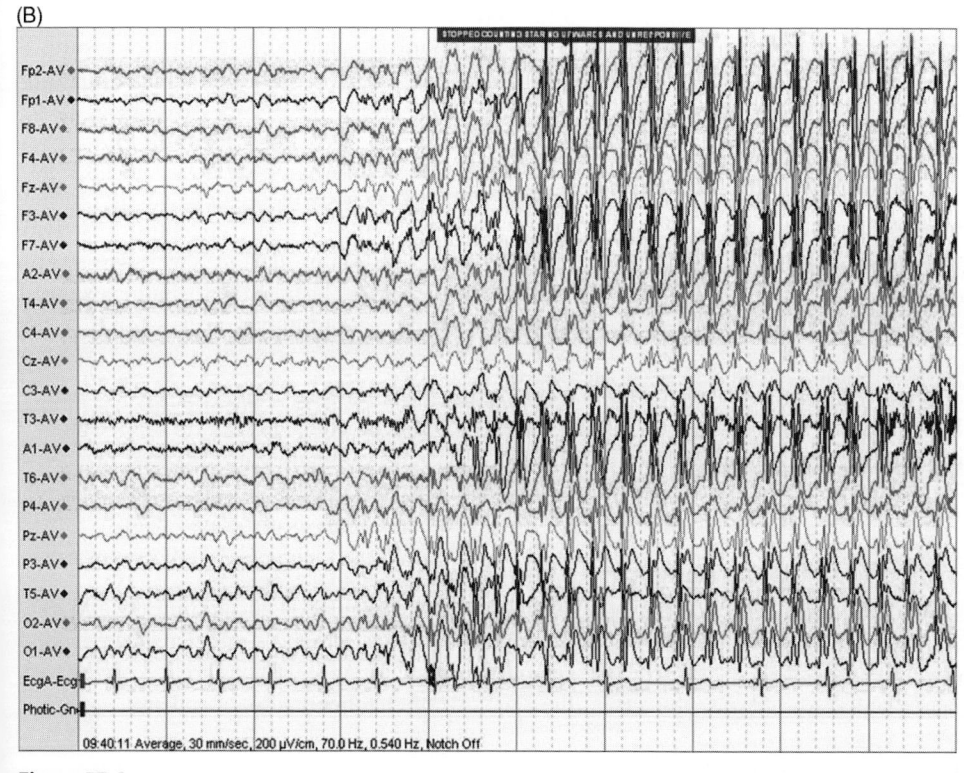

Chapter 57: Seminar: paediatric EEG reporting session

Figure 57.6.

Case 6

Girl aged 6 years, inattentive at school, otherwise normal

(a) Wakefulness, at rest, eye-closure.
(b) Hyperventilation, during which she was asked to count her breaths. She suddenly stops counting, looks upwards and is unresponsive (arrow) (Figure 57.6).

Answers

1 (a) Discontinuous activity with long interburst intervals (>7 s), asynchronous with low-amplitude theta and alpha frequencies over the right, no age-appropriate patterns or transients.

1 (b) Electrographic seizure over mid to right central region.

Conclusion: seizures and very abnormal ongoing activity, in keeping with severe hypoxic ischaemic encephalopathy. Prognosis for neurodevelopment should be guarded.

1 (c) High-amplitude chaotic slow-wave activity with multifocal sharp waves and superimposed low-voltage.

1 (d) During spasm, an electrodecremental event with superimposed fast activity is seen.

Conclusion: grossly abnormal, hypsarrhythmia. Hypsarrhythmia, spasms and regression suggest the diagnosis of West syndrome.

2 (a) Continuous diffuse mixed frequencies (activité moyenne), bifrontal delta activity (anterior slow dysrhythmia).

2 (b) During sleep higher-amplitude delta activity with faster components intermixed, alternating with periods of relative suppression, but >25 µV (tracé alternant). No EEG correlate seen with myoclonic jerk (artefact only).

Conclusion: normal for age. Most likely diagnosis is benign neonatal sleep myoclonus.

3 (a) Frequent high-amplitude spike and slow waves are seen over the occipital regions with a clear right-sided emphasis, with some anterior spread.

3 (b) Passive eye-closure (arrow). On eye closure, posterior alpha rhythm at around 8 Hz is seen, as well as spike and slow waves over occipital regions (left more than right). Note movement artefact (**).

Conclusion: abnormal EEG recording with frequent epileptiform discharges over the occipital regions with right-sided emphasis, provoked by eye-closure. Ongoing activity is normal for age. Together with clinical history these findings are suggestive of early-onset benign childhood epilepsy with occipital paroxysms (Panayiotopoulos syndrome).

4 (a) Sharp waves over right centrotemporal region with bipole (negativity right centrotemporal, positivity mid-frontal).

4 (b) During sleep, discharges become more bilateral and increase in frequency, but not continuous. Normal age-appropriate sleep spindles can be seen (marked with **).

Conclusion: abnormal EEG recording. Ongoing activity is normal for age, normal sleep phenomena. EEG findings indicate benign partial epilepsy with centrotemporal spikes.

5 (a) During wakefulness symmetrical activity, with well-modulated alpha activity on eye-closure.

5 (b) During sleep continuous bilateral high-amplitude sharp slow waves, no normal sleep phenomena.

Conclusion: abnormal EEG recording. During wakefulness normal EEG activity, ongoing activity normal for age. During sleep continuous epileptiform activity (ESES = electrical status during slow-wave sleep). Together with clinical history these findings suggest CSWS syndrome (continuous spikes and waves during slow sleep).

6 (a) During wakefulness symmetrical activity, with well-modulated alpha activity on eye-closure.

6 (b) During hyperventilation abrupt onset of generalized 3 Hz spike-and-slow-wave activity with frontal emphasis associated with behavioural arrest and eye deviation upwards.

Conclusion: hyperventilation elicits clinically and electrographically typical absences. Ongoing background activity is normal for age. Findings are in keeping with the diagnosis of childhood absence epilepsy.

Recommended reading

Drury I. EEG in benign and malignant epileptic syndromes of childhood. *Epilepsia* 2002;**43**(Suppl 3):17–26.

Holmes GL, Moshe SL, Jones HR (eds). *Clinical Neurophysiology of Infancy, Childhood, and Adolescence.* Boston, MA: Butterworth-Heinemann; 2006.

Mizrahi EM. Avoiding the pitfalls of EEG interpretation in childhood epilepsy. *Epilepsia* 1996;**37**(Suppl 1):S41–51.

Pitt M, Pressler R. Neurophysiological testing in the newborn and infant. *Early Hum Dev* 2005;**81**:939–46.

Pressler RM, Binnie CD, Cooper R, Robinson RC (eds). *Neonatal and Paediatric Clincial Neurophysiology.* Amsterdam: Elsevier; 2007.

Tassinari CA, Rubboli G. Cognition and paroxysmal EEG activities: from a single spike to electrical status epilepticus during sleep. *Epilepsia* 2006;**47**(Suppl 2):40–3.

Learning objective

(1) To improve and deepen understanding of neonatal and paediatric EEG interpretation.

Section 3 Epidemiology

Chapter 58: Epidemiology of epilepsy

Gonzalo Alarcón

What is epidemiology?

Epidemiology is broadly defined as the study of factors affecting the health and illness of populations. More specifically, epidemiology studies the definition, causes, risk factors, frequency and natural evolution (natural history) of diseases. In this context, it often provides the foundation for interventions in the interest of public health and preventive medicine.

Objectives of epidemiology with regard to epilepsy

To study the following aspects of epileptology:
- Definition of epilepsy.
- Frequency of epilepsy:
  - Incidence: new cases per year (expensive studies).
  - Prevalence: proportion of cases at a given moment (cheaper studies).
- Causes of epilepsy
- Natural history of epilepsy:
  - Course of epilepsy without treatment.
  - Necessary to establish efficacy of treatments.

Definition of epilepsy

- Propensity to spontaneous epileptic seizures or to epileptic seizures induced by stimuli that do not induce seizures in most people.
- Acute symptomatic seizures should be excluded.

Incidence of epilepsy

Total population studies

- In developed countries:
  - Recurrent unprovoked seizures: 24–53/100 000 persons per year.
  - Single or recurrent unprovoked seizures: 26–70/100 000 persons per year.
- In developing countries:
  - Rural Chile: 114/100 000 persons per year.
  - Tanzania: 77/100 000 persons per year.
  - Ecuador: 190/100 000 persons per year (including acute symptomatic seizures and febrile convulsions).

Age-specific incidence

- In developed countries there are two age peaks:
  - In young age, particularly during the first few months of life. Approximately 50% of cases start in childhood or adolescence.
  - In old age due to stroke.
- In developing countries there is also a peak in young adults.

Gender

No major differences among genders; slightly more frequent in males but not statistically significant.

Seizure types

Partial seizures more frequent in studies in Rochester, Faroe Islands, Chile and Sweden.

Race

- Not much difference in most studies.
- One study showed epilepsy 1.7-times more frequently in black than in white people, which could be explained by lower socioeconomic level (Shamansky and Glaser, 1979)

Introduction to Epilepsy ed. Gonzalo Alarcón and Antonio Valentín. Published by Cambridge University Press.
© Cambridge University Press 2012.

Time trends

In developed countries:
- Overall incidence of epilepsy appears to be decreasing with time, particularly in children.
- Incidence of epilepsy in the elderly is increasing, as populations age and more people survive stroke.

Epilepsy syndromes

- Loiseau *et al.*, *Epilepsia*, 1990, **31**:391–6:
  - Incidence of epilepsy: 24.5/100 000
  - Incidence of idiopathic focal epilepsy: 1.7/100 000 (7%)
  - Incidence of symptomatic focal epilepsy: 13.6/100 000 (56%)
- West syndrome: 2–4/10 000
- Juvenile myoclonic epilepsy: 1–6/100 000 (2.5%)
- Acute symptomatic seizures: 18–40/100 000

Cumulative incidence

Risk of having epilepsy during the mean lifespan of age 80:
- 1.3% in Denmark
- 4% in Rochester

Prevalence of epilepsy

- More studies available than for incidence, as they are easier and cheaper to do.
- Prevalence depends on incidence and chronicity of the condition.
- Difficulty to distinguish mortality from remission.
- Of value in planning health care.
- Prevalence of epilepsy: 2.7–40/1000 people
- Gender: most studies show higher prevalence in males.
- Etiology: the majority of cases (55–89%) have no identified cause.
- Race: in USA more prevalent in black than in white or Hispanic people. Perhaps related to socioeconomic status.

Causes of epilepsy (etiology)

- Clear cause identified in only 30%.
- The most common causes are:
  - in children: associated with neurological deficits from birth and cerebral palsy;
  - in the elderly: cerebrovascular disease;
  - in developed countries: cerebrovascular disease (12% of new cases and 30% of cases with identified cause);
  - in South America: infection of the CNS.
- Other frequent causes: head injury, degenerative brain disease, idiopathic.

Epidemiological study designs to identify risk factors

- Case-control studies: comparison between patients with epilepsy and controls without epilepsy to calculate the 'odds ratio' of developing epilepsy if certain factors are present.
- Retrospective and prospective cohort studies: follow up people with and without a presumably predisposing factor, and study proportions of people who develop epilepsy among those exposed and unexposed to the factor, in order to calculate the 'relative risk' of developing epilepsy in the presence of the specific factor.

Risk factors for epilepsy (Hesdorffer and Verity, 1997)

- Baseline (no risk): 1
- Military head injury: 580
- Civil head injury: severe, 29; moderate, 4; mild, 1.5
- Stroke: 20
- Hypertension: 1.3 (not significant)
- Encephalitis: 13
- Bacterial meningitis: 4
- Alzheimer's disease: 10
- Multiple sclerosis: 4
- Epilepsy in first-degree relative: 3
- Alcohol: 3
- Heroin: 3
- Cannabis: 0.4 (protective)
- Depression: 3.7 (not significant)
- Neuroleptic drugs: 1.3 (not significant)
- Tricyclic antidepressants: 1.5 (not significant)
- Electroconvulsive shock therapy: 1.5 (not significant)

Other risk factors for epilepsy

- No increased risk in head injury with loss of consciousness or amnesia shorter than 30 minutes.

- Family history is an important risk factor.
- Single genes:
  - benign familial neonatal convulsions: dominant linked to chromosomes 20 and/or 8
  - Progressive myoclonic epilepsy: chromosome 21
  - juvenile myoclonic epilepsy: unclear.
- Febrile convulsions (particularly if complex: multiple, focal and > 15 min) are a risk factor for temporal lobe epilepsy (30% of patients with mesial temporal sclerosis have had febrile convulsions) and for epilepsy with febrile seizures plus.
- Brain tumours, particularly in adults.
- Acute symptomatic seizures.

Non-genetic risk factors of childhood epilepsy

- Younger age.
- Febrile seizures, even for idiopathic epilepsy.
- Febrile seizures in the mother.
- Central nervous system infection.
- Learning difficulties.
- Cerebral palsy.
- Pre- and perinatal adverse events are not a risk factor unless associated with learning difficulties or cerebral palsy.
- Postnatal factors: head injury (30%–70% after depressed fractures), no clear risk from vaccination (apart from the risk of fever and associated febrile convulsions).

Recommended reading

Engel J, Pedley TA. *Epilepsy: A Comprehensive Textbook*, pp. 47–86. Philadelphia: Lippincott-Raven; 2007.

References

Hesdorffer DC, Verity CM. Risk factors. In Engel J, Pedley TA, eds. *Epilepsy: A Comprehensive Textbook*, pp. 59–67. Philadelphia: Lippincott-Raven; 1997.

Loiseau J, Loiseau P, Guyot M, *et al.* Survey of seizure disorders in the French southwest. I. Incidence of epileptic syndromes. *Epilepsia* 1990;**31**:391–6.

Shamansky SL, Glaser GH. Socioeconomic characteristics of childhood seizure disorders in the New Haven area: an epidemiologic study. *Epilepsia* 1979; **20**:457–74.

Learning objectives

(1) To understand the concept and objectives of epidemiology.
(2) To know the incidence and prevalence of epilepsy and the factors which determine them.
(3) To understand the differences between case-control studies and cohort studies.
(4) To know the main causes and risk factors for epilepsy.

Section 3 Epidemiology

Chapter 59

Prognosis of newly diagnosed and chronic epilepsy

Gonzalo Alarcón

Prognosis of epilepsy
- Traditionally considered poor.
- In fact, 70–90% become seizure-free with medical treatment.
- Would it have the same prognosis if untreated?
- Prognosis greatly depends on the individual syndromes and causes.

Basic definitions
- Terminal remission: seizure-free period of more than 5 years previous to the most recent follow-up clinic.
- Prognosis: the probability of terminal remission once the diagnosis of epilepsy has been established.

Prognosis after a single seizure
- The risk of recurrent seizures after a single seizure is unclear: 27–81%; hospital-based studies show lower values than community based or studies that include patients after 24 hours of the first seizure, probably because:
- the risk of a second seizure decreases with time after occurrence of a first seizure: importance of including patients in the study immediately after first seizure.

Risk factors for recurrence after a first seizure
- Seizure type: after a partial seizure recurrence is more likely than after a generalized seizure. Nocturnal seizures are also likely to recur.
- Aetiology: recurrence 12 months after first seizure was (Hart *et al. Lancet* 1990;336:1271–4):
  - 100% if congenital neurological deficits
  - 75% after acquired CNS lesions
  - 40% in presence of acute precipitant.
- Head trauma:
  - 2% if mild trauma (amnesia or LOC < 30 min and no cranial fracture)
  - 2–5% if moderate trauma (non-depressed skull fracture, amnesia < 30 min or LOC < 24 h)
  - 12–15% after severe head injury (intracranial bleeding, brain contusions, dural tear, amnesia or LOC > 24 h)
  - 50% after missile or penetrating injury
  - early seizures (within a week) do not presage epilepsy
- Intracranial infection: any infection increases the risk of epilepsy. Postnatal meningitis, brain abscess, and encephalitis increase risk 3-fold.
- Neurological examination: increased risk if abnormal but only in symptomatic epilepsies.
- Family history: debatable, perhaps for idiopathic epilepsies.
- EEG abnormalities: increased risk, particularly for idiopathic epilepsies.
- Early medical treatment: appears to be effective (First Seizure Trial Group, 1993):
  - after 24 months, 26% risk if treated versus 51% if not treated
  - after 12 months, 50% versus 67%
  - after 36 months, 57% versus 78%.
- Sex and duration of first seizure are not associated with particular risks.

Introduction to Epilepsy ed. Gonzalo Alarcón and Antonio Valentín. Published by Cambridge University Press.
© Cambridge University Press 2012.

Natural history of treated epilepsy

- Newly diagnosed epilepsy (two or more unprovoked seizures): medication is usually started.
  - 1 year remission rate: 65–80%.
  - Worse for complex partial than secondarily generalized seizures: remission rate 16–43% versus 48–53%.
  - Worse in the presence of multiple seizure types, neurological deficits, behavioural or psychiatric disturbance.
  - No particular antiepileptic drug is better in the overall population, but individuals or specific syndromes may respond better to some.
- Newly diagnosed epilepsy: remission rates increase with time (Annegers et al., Epilepsy 1979;20:729–37):
  - 42% after 1 year
  - 65% after 10 years
  - 76% after 15 years.
- Chronic epilepsy:
  - 20–30% of patients do not enter remission (confirmed by hospital-based and community studies)
  - only 20% of patients have seizure-free periods
  - only a few become seizure free on antiepileptic drugs.
- Drug withdrawal and seizure relapse: the majority of patients on antiepileptic drugs eventually become seizure-free and drug withdrawal is contemplated. The risk of seizure relapse after drug withdrawal should be evaluated.
  - Risk of relapse: 11–41%.
  - Lower risk in children than in adults.
  - Higher risk of relapse if: long history of seizures, more than one seizure type, structural brain lesion, neurological signs, learning difficulties, history of remissions and relapses, juvenile myoclonic epilepsy, remote symptomatic seizures, EEG abnormalities.

Natural history of untreated epilepsy

Most of what we know on the natural history of epilepsy is from treated patients. The following two burning questions remain unanswered:

- Is there remission without treatment?
- What is the effect of early treatment on prognosis?

Spontaneous remission without treatment

- Similar prevalence of epilepsy in developed (largely treated) and developing (largely untreated) countries, suggesting that remission rates are similar (Osuntokun et al., 1987; Placencia et al., 1992).
- Measured remission rates in developing and developed world are also similar: 40–50%.
- Since epilepsy in the developed world is usually treated and in the developing world is largely untreated, these findings raise the question of whether medical treatment affects prognosis.

Effects of early treatment on prognosis

Initial studies have shown that early treatment of epilepsy may not improve remission rates. Studies in Kenya, Ecuador and Malawi (Sander and Sillanpää, 1997) suggest that around 50% of treated patients remit in the second 6 months after a previous untreated 6-month period. This percentage is similar to the improvement reported in early treated epilepsy. However, this does not exclude an effect on prognosis in specific syndromes.

Prognosis of specific syndromes

Epilepsy prognosis largely depends on the epilepsy syndrome. The prognoses of a few syndromes are summarized below:

- Benign familial (idiopathic) neonatal convulsions ('5th day fits'): only 10% do not show complete remission and continue with epilepsy later in life.
- Neonatal convulsions (occurring within the first 4 weeks of life): these affect 0.5% of infants. Among patients with this syndrome, 30% die within the year; 25% suffer seizures into adulthood or have learning difficulties or spasticity, and only 40% show a full remission. Some poor prognostic factors are: prematurity, early-onset seizures (first 2 days), focal brain lesions, brain malformations, intracranial bleeding, inborn errors of metabolism, and abnormal EEG. Prognosis is usually better in cases where no aetiology is found.
- Idiopathic generalized epilepsies: these are around 33% of all epilepsies under 20, generally with a good prognosis:
  - childhood absence epilepsy (CAE): 80% become seizure-free; poorer prognosis if tonic-clonic convulsions or other seizure types occur;

- juvenile absence epilepsy: slightly worse prognosis than in CAE;
- juvenile myoclonic epilepsy: good response to treatment, but seizures usually recur if treatment stops. It often requires lifetime treatment.
- Epilepsy with generalized tonic-clonic seizures on awakening: seizures remit in most without mental deterioration.
- Idiopathic focal epilepsies: generally good prognosis with complete seizure remission, but it depends on the syndrome. For example, in benign childhood epilepsy with centrotemporal spikes (rolandic epilepsy), only 2% have lifelong seizures. However, in other idiopathic focal epilepsies, up to 10% of patients can have lifelong seizures.
- Symptomatic generalized epilepsies: neurological and/or cognitive impairment is present in 90% of patients. Prognosis depends on the underlying syndrome but can be considered as generally poor:
  - infantile spasms (West syndrome): one in five die, and among survivors, 90% suffer learning difficulties and chronic epilepsy;
  - Lennox-Gastaut syndrome: around 60% of patients suffer status epilepticus (convulsive or non-convulsive); seizure remission occurs in 10%;
  - severe myoclonic epilepsy in infancy: onset in first year of life, showing frequent generalized tonic-clonic and myoclonic seizures. Around 16% of patients die within 10 years of onset, all survivors have uncontrolled seizures, and 90% show severe learning difficulties.
- Symptomatic focal (partial) epilepsies: prognosis depends on the underlying lesion. Poorer seizure prognosis is seen in congenital lesions (malformations, tuberous sclerosis, Sturge-Weber syndrome). Epilepsy surgery can be a treatment option, with excellent response in mesial temporal sclerosis.
- Epilepsia partialis continua (Kojewnikow's syndrome):
  - Rasmussen's encephalitis: progressive, neurological deficits and mental impairment; antiepileptic drugs are generally not effective, and surgical treatment should be considered;
  - dysplastic lesions, tumours, vascular malformations: outcome depending on cause.
- Epilepsy with continuous spike and wave during slow-wave sleep: usually this is a type of symptomatic generalized epilepsy. There is an identifiable cause in 20–30% of cases (meningitis, birth injury, cytomegalovirus infection). It is usually associated with developmental arrest and behavioural difficulties. The EEG abnormality is age-dependent, and seizures remit in a large percentage of patients, although learning and behavioural difficulties tend to persist.
- Landau-Kleffner syndrome (acquired epileptic aphasia): 80% of patients enjoy seizure remission, and 60% have persistent learning (particularly language) difficulties.

References

Annegers JF, Hauser WA, Elveback LR. Remission of seizures and relapse in patients with epilepsy. *Epilepsia* 1979;**20**:729–37.

First Seizure Trial Group. Randomized clinical trial on the efficacy of antiepileptic drugs in reducing the risk of relapse after a first unprovoked tonic-clonic seizure. First Seizure Trial Group (FIR.S.T. Group). *Neurology* 1993;**43**:478–83.

Hart YM, Sander JW, Johnson AL, *et al*. National General Practice Study of Epilepsy: recurrence after a first seizure. *Lancet* 1990;**336**:1271–4.

Osuntokun BO, Adeuja AO, Nottidge VA, *et al*. Prevalence of the epilepsies in Nigerian Africans: a community-based study. *Epilepsia* 1987;**28**:272–9.

Placencia M, Shorvon SD, Paredes V, *et al*. Epileptic seizures in an Andean region of Ecuador. Incidence and prevalence and regional variation. *Brain* 1992;**115**:771–82;

Sander JWAS, Sillanpää M. *Natural History of Epilepsy*. In Engel J, Pedley TA, eds. *Epilepsy: A Comprehensive Textbook*, pp. 69–86. Philadelphia: Lippincott-Raven; 1997.

Learning objectives

(1) To be able to estimate and discuss the overall prognosis of epilepsy.
(2) To be able to estimate and discuss the natural history of treated and untreated epilepsy.
(3) To be able to estimate and discuss the prognosis after a single seizure.
(4) To be able to estimate and discuss the risk factors for recurrence after a first seizure.
(5) To know the prognosis of common specific syndromes.

Section 3 Epidemiology

Chapter 60: Single seizures

Robert D. C. Elwes

Five per cent of the population will have at least one afebrile seizure at some time in their life. In adults presenting to a neurological clinic with a single unprovoked convulsion, the recurrence rate is of the order of 50%. In primary care or in the community recurrence may be higher. Epidemiological surveys in the general population suggest that seizures are recurrent in about 80% of cases. The second seizure follows the first quite rapidly, within a month in one-third and within a year in a further third, and many will have their second seizure before being seen in hospital. The factors predicting a poorer prognosis are broadly the same as those predicting response to treatment and seizure recurrence following drug withdrawal.

Good prognosis

- Acute precipitating event such as psychotropic medication
- One or more months with no recurrence
- Antiepileptic treatment

Poorer prognosis

- Remote symptomatic aetiology
- Structural brain disease
- Neurological deficit
- Focal onset to seizure
- Generalized spike and wave on EEG

Investigations and management

Patients with a single seizure should be assessed in a similar manner to those with new-onset epilepsy. They should be seen in an appropriate hospital department within 1–2 weeks by a physician with neurological training or specialist experience in the assessment of epilepsy. Routine bloods are done to check general health. An MRI should be performed and approximately 5% of cases will be found to have a tumour. If seen acutely and there is a suggestion of head injury or intracranial bleed, CT is helpful. An EEG is obtained to help classify the type of epilepsy. If normal and a clear clinical diagnosis of seizures has been made a sleep recording is indicated. Most patients with absences and those with simple or complex partial seizures will have had multiple attacks when first seen. The great majority of those presenting with a single seizure will have had a tonic-clonic seizure. If the convulsion occurred first thing in the morning, there is a history of early morning myoclonus or absences, then a clinical diagnosis of primary generalized seizure can be made. Many do not give this history and generalized spike and wave on the EEG confirms the diagnosis. Alternatively the EEG may show a clear focal abnormality suggesting that the seizure was in fact secondarily generalized. The EEG is crucial in classifying convulsive seizures and both conclusions may be of help in guiding future drug treatment.

Advice concerning lifestyle issues is important, and similar to that given to those with established epilepsy. In the UK the patient should not drive until seizure-free for a year, regardless of treatment. There may be implications for work and the usual issues concerning safety should be discussed. It is not the practice of neurologists in the United Kingdom to recommend treatment following a first seizure. There is a 50% chance of no further problems and starting treatment may (incorrectly) imply a diagnosis of epilepsy. The person will be exposed to the side effects of medication and stopping the drug in the future may cause a withdrawal seizure, generating problems especially for driving. Randomized studies, however, have shown that treatment reduces the recurrence rate by some 50% and some people may wish to make a different informed

---

Introduction to Epilepsy ed. Gonzalo Alarcón and Antonio Valentín. Published by Cambridge University Press.
© Cambridge University Press 2012.

choice, if for example a further seizure might have serious employment implications or there are adverse prognostic factors. Establishing a first-seizure clinic with an epilepsy nurse specialist to provide information and advice and access to same-day investigations after the clinic appointment can enhance quality of care.

Recommended reading

Elwes RD, Chesterman P, Reynolds EH. Prognosis after a first untreated tonic-clonic seizure. *Lancet* 1985; **2**(8458):752–3

Hauser WA, Kurland LT. The epidemiology of epilepsy in Rochester, Minnesota, 1935 through 1967. *Epilepsia* 1975;**16**(1):1–66.

Kim LG, Johnson TL, Marson AG, Chadwick DW; MRC MESS Study Group. Prediction of risk of seizure recurrence after a single seizure and early epilepsy: further results from the MESS trial. *Lancet Neurol* 2006;5(4):317–22.

Leone MA, Solari A, Beghi E; FIRST Group. Treatment of the first tonic-clonic seizure does not affect long-term remission of epilepsy. *Neurology* 2006; **67**:2227–9.

Marson A, Jacoby A, Johnson A, Kim L, Gamble C, Chadwick D; Medical Research Council MESS Study Group. Immediate versus deferred antiepileptic drug treatment for early epilepsy and single seizures: a randomised controlled trial. *Lancet* 2005;**365** (9476):2007–13.

Learning objectives

(1) To know the risk factors of developing epilepsy after having a single seizure.
(2) To know and be able to discuss the investigations recommended and the management of subjects who have had a single seizure.

Section 3 Epidemiology

Chapter 61: Epidemiology of epilepsy in childhood

Euan M. Ross

Introduction to epilepsy in childhood

Children with epilepsy need high-quality ongoing medical care. The subject keeps advancing but much more is yet to be learnt. Many (perhaps most) parents think that their child is dying when he or she has the first fit. Two points should be kept in mind:

- the causes and types of epilepsy in children differ greatly from those in adults
- the younger the child the greater are these differences.

Epilepsy in infants

Epilepsy occurs most frequently in the first year of life, particularly in the early postnatal weeks. Causes include:

- intracranial infection
- biochemical/metabolic abnormality
- congenital neurological abnormality
- intracranial bleeding.

Young infants are uniquely susceptible to antenatal and birth hazards. The physical nature of the infant brain makes it susceptible to epilepsy, being soft, poorly supported, with fragile blood vessels and poor clotting ability in the premature baby. Infants lack acquired immunological protection and show particular susceptibility to Gram-negative infection.

Particular sensitivity to biochemical imbalances: in particular to changes in calcium and phosphorus ratio, hypomagnesaemia and low blood glucose, especially in the child who grew poorly in utero and those born to mothers with diabetes mellitus. Rarer problems include biotin deficiency, lack of/or insensitivity to vitamin B6, galactosaemia and other metabolic disorders.

In young infants clinical features of the epilepsy seizure may not be as diagnostic as in older children and adults (see Chapter 20: 'Neonatal seizures'). Some forms of epilepsy are not seen in babies (e.g. absence seizures).

Management starts with close observation and recording. Sometimes clinical signs of seizure activity are difficult to detect and may be misinterpreted. The seizures may not be pronounced and may take the form of abnormal eye movements, irritability or very low-grade limb twitching. The following will be necessary:

- accurate, informed observation of the seizures;
- urgent hospital admission to a unit that can perform necessary investigations.

Febrile convulsions

From age 5–6 months to about age 6 years, febrile convulsions affect about 3% of children. These usually are brief generalized seizures, mainly occurring in previously healthy children, though virus infection can often be detected. The fits tend to occur as temperature rises and they rarely last for more than 10 minutes (if longer, seizures may indicate a more serious condition, possibly leading to epilepsy). Full clinical examination is needed. One pressing question – does the child have early signs of meningitis? In practice, meningitis rarely presents with seizures: look for a full fontanelle and keep a careful watch for signs of meningococcal rash, persisting fever and signs of systemic ill health. Emergency lumbar puncture is currently undertaken much less frequently on infants where purely febrile convulsions are diagnosed than in the past.

In two-thirds of affected children, febrile seizures occur once only. There are often difficulties in deciding whether the index fit is truly a febrile fit or the first fit in a child already destined to have an

---

Introduction to Epilepsy ed. Gonzalo Alarcón and Antonio Valentín. Published by Cambridge University Press.
© Cambridge University Press 2012.

ongoing form of epilepsy. The latter is more likely if seizures are multiple, focal or longer than 10 minutes. Fitting in a fully dressed child in itself can raise the temperature.

Infantile spasms

In the age span 6 to 24 months, infantile spasms present in 1 in 3000 to 10 000 children. About half prove to have tuberose sclerosis. The spasm includes characteristic slow but sudden upward jerks of the limbs in an irritable child. Urgent EEG with a characteristic EEG pattern (hypsarrhythmia; Figure 21.1) is needed to help document and diagnose the condition. The condition is readily missed in the early stage. Prognosis is variable and can be followed by brain dysfunction. Older children may develop a broadly similar condition with an even poorer prognosis (Lennox-Gastaut syndrome). After the first 6 months seizures tend to become easier to characterize. The clinician has a duty to classify the epilepsy type according to the current international classification (see Chapter 17).

Epilepsy in children

Non-febrile epilepsy affects about four per thousand children of school age. Of these about:

- One-third can be regarded as having 'active epilepsy', having had a seizure in the past 24 months.
- Two-thirds have been seizure-free in the previous 24 months.
- A fifth can be expected to have multiple disabilities and require special education. For the majority the outcome can be much more promising, with many becoming seizure-free. Problems can include psychological overlay, over-fussing the child, unnecessarily low expectations and over-medication.
- There can be difficulty in knowing when a child should be regarded as having 'grown out' of epilepsy. This decision will become much easier if the cause of the epilepsy is known. Despite newer methods of neurological diagnosis, the proportion of children where the cause of the epilepsy can be determined remains stubbornly around the 50% mark. Hopefully, emerging understanding of genetics will lead to fewer children being labelled as having 'idiopathic epilepsy'.

Commoner causes of non-febrile epilepsy in children

- Congenital abnormality of the brain, often part of a syndrome.
- Post meningitis or encephalitis.
- Bleeding into the brain associated with injury (accidental or non-accidental).
- Epilepsy of a genetic (congenital) type.

History-taking

Often parents and the clinician have not seen the presenting seizure, which may have happened in nursery or been witnessed by a child carer. Try to contact the witness and get as precise a description as possible. Memories soon fade. Where repeated fits occur, a family-made videotape can be a great help in diagnosis. Some clinics lend cameras out to the ever-decreasing proportion of parents who do not have a camera or equipped mobile phone that can record short videos.

Clinical observation

This demands a full (eventually undressed) physical examination so that the skin can be examined in detail. Many children with epilepsy have multiple complex neurological problems. Subtle skin signs can be diagnostic in the index child and sometimes other family members. It is necessary to review the head and body growth chart and school reports as well as observing the child at play, watching specially for abnormal walking and hand use. Fundoscopy is a key to recognizing raised intracranial pressure.

Main types of seizures in childhood

- Generalized motor seizures account for about 50% of cases.
- True absence attacks are much rarer, affecting perhaps 2 or 3%. The EEG helps to determine the type of epilepsy.
- Focal seizures emanating from a limited area of affected brain on the opposite side from the symptoms
- Sleep-associated seizures, such as in benign rolandic epilepsy, in perhaps 15% of epilepsy in teenagers.

There are many other potential differential diagnoses including:

- Temporal lobe epilepsy.
- Seizures induced by flashing lights (photosensitivity): the most common reflex epilepsy.
- Seizures associated with loss of speech in toddlers: Wooster-Drought or Landau-Kleffner syndrome.
- Seizures associated with deteriorating performance include brain tumours and rare degenerative brain disorders.
- Severe myoclonic epilepsy in infancy – otherwise known as Dravet syndrome, which explains some of the previously unexplained serious seizure disorders which present with prolonged seizures in febrile children during their first year. Further details including genetic factors (mutation of sodium channel SCNIA gene) (Chapter 9E, pp. 157–160 in Wallace SJ, Farrell K, 2004).
- Hypoglycaemia (which can be due to alcohol ingestion).

The type of epilepsy

There are many types and subtypes of epilepsy. New variations keep being described. It is most important that the epilepsy be correctly described because effective management and prognostic advice depends on the epilepsy syndrome. If there is any doubt, the child and family must be seen by a paediatrician with specialized skills in epilepsy. Help from a clinical geneticist may also be needed. The extent of investigation required demands a complex mix of skills and experience. Questions must include: Does the child need brain imaging? If so, to what level? The type of equipment used and the skill of those interpreting scans and EEG vary enormously. It is not enough to say 'MRI negative' and feel that the job is done. Normal MRI findings may be different from those found in older children or adults, where the brain is more fully myelinized. This matter is discussed in detail by King and Stephenson (2009).

An EEG when awake may be very different from one done on a sleeping child in terms of findings and interpretation. An electroencephalographer with paediatric experience is required.

Epilepsy emergencies

Status epilepticus: constant seizure state with or without return to consciousness that lasts 30 minutes or more. This condition may be fatal and demands intensive drug treatment in a hospital.

Non-epilepsy seizures

Difficult diagnostic problems can occur in the frequent circumstances when seizures are not seen by the clinician and reliance has to be placed on caretakers. Not by any means are all shaking episodes described by carers actually seizures. At the milder end of the spectrum 'breath-holding attacks' seen in young children may result in seizure-like activity and cause much anxiety which needs to be 'defused'. Rarely, children may be described as having florid seizures, yet investigations including EEG reveal nothing: in such instances, the described seizures tend not to resemble 'true' epilepsy.

Recommended reading

King MD, Stephenson JBP. *A Handbook of Neurological Investigations in Children*. Oxford: MacKeith Press; 2009.

O'Donohoe NV. *Epilepsies of Childhood*. 3rd edn. London: Butterworth Heinemann; 1994.

Panayiotopoulos CP. *Epileptic Syndromes and their Treatment*. 2nd edn. Berlin: Springer; 2007.

Wallace SJ, Farrell K. *Epilepsy in Children*. 2nd edn. London: Arnold; 2004.

Learning objectives

(1) To know the causes of epilepsy in children and infants, and how they differ from those in adults.
(2) To learn the relationship between febrile convulsions and later epilepsy.
(3) To have an overview of the investigations necessary to diagnose epilepsy and find its cause in children and infants.

Section 3 Epidemiology

Chapter 62: Mortality in epilepsy

Lina Nashef

Summary

An excess mortality is observed in cohorts of patients with epilepsy. Most of the early mortality, in the first years after diagnosis, is related to underlying disease causing the epilepsy or associated with it. In addition, there is also a small excess mortality related to the epilepsy itself. This varies depending on the cohort under study.

Background

The study of mortality in epilepsy is not straightforward and there are methodological difficulties, examples of which are listed below:

- While they can provide some information, it is not possible to base studies on death certificates alone as these may not be accurate. In addition, over time, differences in death certification practice occur. For example, before the entity of sudden death in epilepsy was widely recognized, status epilepticus was often assumed and recorded as the cause of death, without sufficient evidence. Furthermore, the diagnosis of epilepsy is not always stated on death certificates.
- Data regarding epilepsy diagnosis or cause of death are often incomplete, particularly in large population-based studies, which are the most representative.
- Definitions in relation to the diagnosis and classification of epilepsy and cause of death vary between studies.
- Many different cohorts have been studied. Results from selected cohorts, where more detailed information about diagnosis and cause of death may be available, are often not applicable to the population.
- Autopsy rates, causes of death and death certification vary between countries.

Standardized mortality ratio (SMR) and proportional mortality

Standardized mortality ratio (SMR): SMR refers to the death rate observed in a given cohort compared to that expected in the general population, standardized for age and sex.

SMR in epilepsy is 2–3-times that in the general population. However, it is much higher in selected cohorts, particularly if the epilepsy is severe and intractable, especially if it is associated with other handicap or disease.

Proportional mortality: the term refers to the proportion of deaths within a give cohort due to a specific cause. In epilepsy, these include:

(a) causes of death which would have been observed anyway in the general population;
(b) additional deaths due to the underlying or associated disease;
(c) deaths due to complications of epilepsy or its treatment.

> **Box 62.1.** How to calculate SMR in a given cohort over a designated period
> - Identify cohort
> - Identify date of entry
> - Identify date of exit (this being date of death, or date person last known to be alive)
> - Calculate person years of follow-up in 5 year age groups for males and females
> - Use death rates from published national statistics over the same time period to calculate expected deaths in each age group
> - Summate for total expected deaths in whole cohort
> - SMR = observed deaths/ expected deaths
> - Define confidence intervals

Introduction to Epilepsy ed. Gonzalo Alarcón and Antonio Valentín. Published by Cambridge University Press.
© Cambridge University Press 2012.

Causes of death in epilepsy

Proportions differ depending on the cohort. Causes of death include, amongst others, cerebrovascular and cardiac diseases, pulmonary diseases (including bronchopneumonia), neoplasms including brain tumours, pneumonia, suicide, traumatic accidents, drowning, status epilepticus, SUDEP (see below) and other seizure-related deaths. Some of these are addressed below.

Suicides

Background suicide rates vary between countries. An excess in suicides in cohorts with epilepsy is reported by some but not all studies. If present, this is likely to be low in population-based studies, with the excess mostly observed in selected cohorts. Those with partial epilepsy, in particular temporal lobe, have a higher associated risk. This suggests that the pathological substrate is a main predisposing factor. Post-temporal lobectomy patients are also at potential risk. Physicians looking after patients with epilepsy need to identify depression and refer/manage those at potential risk. They also need to be aware of the potential of antiepileptic drugs to cause depression and modify drug regimes if an adverse effect on mood is observed.

Treatment of epilepsy

Deaths due to treatment of epilepsy are rare. Examples include severe hypersensitivity reactions, liver or bone marrow failure, and complications of procedures as part of epilepsy surgery.

Seizure-related deaths

These are discussed below and include accidental deaths, status epilepticus, the majority of SUDEP cases and deaths provoked by habitual seizures due to identified co-existing cardiorespiratory disease.

Accidental deaths

These include aspiration, drowning and accidents (trauma or burns). While it is common for mild aspiration to occur, severe aspiration causing death is rare, as is airway obstruction with food bolus.

Drowning is increased in cohorts with epilepsy and, being exposure-dependent, is largely preventable. Patients with epilepsy are advised to avoid waterfronts and ensure appropriate supervision and, where appropriate, use flotation devices during water sports.

Box 62.2. To minimize accidental death in epilepsy, it is advisable to

- Avoid potentially dangerous situations in the event of a seizure, including unprotected heights, waterfronts, unsupervised baths, proximity to fires/heat and dangerous machinery
- Follow driving regulations
- Take care as a pedestrian/cyclist, avoiding traffic
- Consider helmet or wheelchair use in severe epilepsy, particularly where sudden drop attacks occur
- Consider supervision

They are also advised not to have unsupervised baths. A sit-down shower with thermostat water-temperature control is considered safer in epilepsy than baths.

The risk of injury relates to exposure as well as seizure frequency and seizure type, particularly in relation to seizures associated with abrupt falls. Mild injury is common, severe injury much less so and fatalities rare. Epileptic seizures can also cause vehicle driver collapse. Studies vary as to whether epilepsy is associated with an increase risk of serious accidents over the general population. One possible explanation for these variable results is that while risks from seizure-related injury are undoubtedly present, risks from other accidents may be reduced in some group because of caution, life-style restriction or supervision.

Status epilepticus

Status epilepticus is more common in children but mortality is higher in adults. Overall mortality is about 20% and is largely influenced by the cause of the status. Status epilepticus, particularly if convulsive, is a life-threatening medical emergency requiring prompt treatment along pre-defined protocols in high dependency or intensive care units. The following is advised:

- prevention of status whenever possible;
- early prompt treatment of pre-status with individualized guidelines in the community for those known to be risk;
- prompt treatment of established status.

SUDEP – sudden unexpected ('unexplained') death in epilepsy

- Profile: patients with epilepsy sometimes die unexpectedly in benign circumstances without a cause of death found at post-mortem examination. Pulmonary, and sometimes other organ, congestion is often observed. The majority of deaths are unwitnessed: most often the person is found dead in bed. Often, but not invariably, there is evidence suggestive of an epileptic seizure.

- Definitions: a few investigators exclude death in a documented seizure, but most include this within the category of SUDEP. A workable definition is: sudden, unexpected, witnessed or unwitnessed, non-traumatic and non-drowning death in epilepsy, with or without evidence for a seizure and excluding documented status epilepticus, where post-mortem examination does not reveal a cause for death. Where information is incomplete the following useful categories have been proposed: definite SUDEP (sudden death in benign circumstances with no other known cause and autopsy performed), probable (as before but without autopsy), possible, and not SUDEP
- Incidence: rates vary depending on the cohort studied and range from 1:100 person years of follow-up in highly selected intractable surgical cohorts, 1:200–300 in tertiary centres, 1:1000 in unselected cohorts, 0.35/1000 in one population-based study and 1:2,500 in a cohort in remission and < 1:5 000 in an incidence epilepsy cohort.
- Mechanisms: the most likely cause is cardiorespiratory compromise during or shortly after an epileptic seizure. A number of risk factors have been identified in case control studies. The most important is a history of generalized tonic-clonic seizures and uncontrolled epilepsy. Individual susceptibility is not fully explained and risk prediction is difficult.
- Potential for prevention: in addition to prevention of seizures, particularly generalized tonic-clonic seizures, with optimum treatment and by avoiding non-adherence to treatment and seizure triggers, there is some evidence to suggest that supervision gives some protection. There is also evidence of an association with frequent medication changes and polytherapy. While this may be a surrogate for epilepsy severity, on current albeit limited evidence, it is best to avoid (a) very frequent and abrupt medication changes and (b) medication combinations that adversely affect seizure severity or the severity of the post-ictal phase.

Excess mortality in epilepsy: practical implications

Excess mortality in epilepsy has practical implications for clinical management in relation to information provision, treatment decisions and service delivery. It also has medico-legal implications. Guidelines generally advocate more information provision to patients regarding risks associated with epilepsy, including SUDEP, than is commonly practised. This has been subject to debate. The individual with epilepsy is frequently faced with treatment or social choices. An awareness of the risks associated with epilepsy is a prerequisite for informed choice.

Some epilepsy-related deaths, including SUDEP, are potentially preventable. Whenever possible, the physician and patient/carers should work towards:

(a) prevention of injury and drowning;
(b) prevention of seizures and reduction in seizure severity, with optimal and regular treatment;
(c) detection and treatment of psychiatric co-morbidity,
(d) ensuring adequate immediate response to convulsive seizures to minimize cardio-respiratory compromise and risk of injury;
(e) early treatment of status epilepticus and pre-status;
(f) minimizing risk associated with treatment.

Recommended reading

Cockerell OC, Johnson AL, Sander JW, *et al.* Mortality from epilepsy: results from a prospective population-based study. *Lancet* 1994;**344**(8927):918–21.

Hitiris N, Mohanraj R, Norrie J, Brodie MJ. Mortality in epilepsy. *Epilepsy Behav* 2007;**10**(3):363–76.

Lhatoo SD, Sander JW. Cause-specific mortality in epilepsy. *Epilepsia* 2005;**46**(Suppl 11):36–9.

Nashef, Sander JWAS, Shorvon SD. Mortality in epilepsy. In Pedley TA, Meldrum BS, eds. *Recent Advances in Epilepsy 6*. Philadelphia: Churchill Livingstone; 1995.

Nei M, Bagla R. Seizure-related injury and death. *Curr Neurol Neurosci Rep* 2007;7(4):335–41.

Tomson T, Nashef L, Ryvlin P. Sudden unexpected death in epilepsy: Current knowledge and future directions. *Lancet Neurol* 2008;7(11):1021–31.

Learning objectives

(1) To be aware of the methodological difficulties in studying mortality in epilepsy.
(2) To understand the concept and the use of standardized mortality ratio (SMR) and proportional mortality.
(3) To know the causes of death in epilepsy and be able to discuss them.
(4) To understand the concept of excess mortality in epilepsy and its practical implications.

Section 4 **Genetics of epilepsy**

Chapter 63

Introduction to modern molecular genetics: a genetics timeline

Robert Robinson

In order to appreciate recent advances in the genetics of human epilepsy, some understanding of the basic concepts of clinical and molecular genetics is required. These concepts will be illustrated by a review of the scientific advances which have led to our current understanding of the human genome.

In 1859, Charles Darwin published *On the Origin of Species*. Darwin provided evidence for the evolution of species by natural selection, describing how valuable traits become more common in a population. A mechanism for the process of natural selection was described by the Augustinian monk Gregor Mendel, whose work with peas showed that heredity is transmitted in discrete units. These units (subsequently identified as genes) remain discrete entities, even though parental characteristics appear to blend in their offspring. Mendel's laws of heredity introduce the following important concepts:

- Alternative 'alleles' account for variations in inherited characters.
- For each character, an organism inherits two 'alleles', one from each parent.
- If two alleles differ (a heterozygote), then one, the 'dominant allele', is expressed in the organism, whilst the other, the 'recessive allele', has no noticeable effect.
- The two genes for each character segregate during gamete production (meiosis).
- The emergence of one trait will not affect the emergence of another.
- This results in the observed 3:1 ratio between dominant and recessive phenotypes for a single (Mendelian) trait.

DNA was isolated in 1869. In 1879 chromosomes (packages of DNA comprising multiple genes) were observed during cell division, and in 1902 it was observed that the segregation of chromosomes during meiosis matched the segregation patterns of Mendel's genes. Thomas Hunt Morgan's work on fruit flies in 1911 showed that genes are linked together in chromosomes, genes become shuffled (recombine) during meiosis, and distant genes on a chromosome recombine more frequently than nearby genes.

In the 1940's it was shown that DNA is the genetic molecule, and DNA's double helix structure was described by Crick and Watson in 1953. DNA comprises a chain of nucleotides, each of which contains one of four nitrogenous bases (A, C, G, T). In the double helix, A is always paired with T, and G paired with C, so that only half the DNA ladder is a template for copying the whole. DNA polymerase, the enzyme required for DNA replication, was isolated from *Escherichia coli* in 1955.

Sickle cell anaemia was the first disease to be attributed to an alteration in a protein molecule, haemoglobin, in 1956. The first chromosomal abnormality, trisomy 21, was shown to be the cause of Down syndrome in 1959.

In 1961, messenger RNA (mRNA) was shown to be the molecule that takes information from DNA in the nucleus to the protein-making machinery in the cytoplasm. The central dogma of molecular biology, as enunciated by Frances Crick, describes the flow of genetic information from DNA to messenger RNA (transcription) and then to protein (translation). This information is in the form of the genetic code, cracked in 1966 by Nirenberg, Khorana and Ochoa. The four letter alphabet of the nucleic acids in DNA is interpreted three letters at a time. Each set of three letters (a codon) encodes one of the 20 amino acids that form proteins.

Recombinant DNA technology, which involves the joining of DNA from different species and inserting

Introduction to Epilepsy ed. Gonzalo Alarcón and Antonio Valentín. Published by CAMBRIDGE UNIVERSITY PRESS.
© Cambridge University Press 2012.

the hybrid DNA into a host cell, requires the ability to cut DNA at specific short sequences. Restriction enzymes, which recognize sequences known as restriction fragment length polymorphisms (RFLPs), were isolated in 1968, and the first recombinant DNA was produced in 1972.

In 1975, Sanger developed the first methods for rapid sequencing of DNA. The Sanger method is still commonly employed today.

The Huntington disease gene was the first to be mapped to a chromosomal location in 1983. In the same year, the polymerase chain reaction was developed, which allows a specific segment of DNA to be copied billions of times.

The first human genetic map, based on 400 RFLPs, appeared in 1987. Over subsequent years, far more detailed genetics maps have been developed, based first on microsatellites (stretches of DNA with repeated sequences of 2–4 nucleotides) and then on single nucleotide polymorphisms (SNPs), which are variations occurring at a single nucleotide.

The Human Genome Project was launched in 1990, with the aim of sequencing the entire human genome (an estimated 3 billion bases), as well as identifying every gene and characterizing sequence variations. This was a huge and controversial undertaking at the time.

The combination of public and privately funded projects resulted in a working draft of the human genome earlier than predicted in 2000, with a completed human sequence (99%) in 2003. Several model organism genomes were also sequenced, including yeast, *Escherichia coli*, *Mycobacterium tuberculosis*, mouse and rat. The total number of human genes was less than predicted at around 25 000, with alternative splicing resulting in around 100 000 proteins.

Initiatives to establish the genetic and environmental causes of common diseases were launched in 2006. The first high-resolution map of human structural variation in eight human genomes was published in 2008.

The ethical, legal and social implications of the Human Genome Project are complex and continue to be widely debated. Issues such as confidentiality of genetic information, the psychological impact of genetic testing, stigmatization and commercialization of genetic knowledge are important considerations when making use of genome-based knowledge in clinical care.

Learning objective

(1) To understand the basic principles and advances of modern molecular genetics.

Section 4   Genetics of epilepsy

Chapter 64

Methods of molecular genetics

Robert Robinson

Strategies for identification of epilepsy genes

Progress in the identification of epilepsy genes has been largely dependent on the underlying genetic mechanisms involved and the mode of inheritance. The greatest success has been in the mendelian epilepsies, where mutations in a single gene account for segregation of the disease trait. The mendelian epilepsies are most commonly 'symptomatic', with seizures being just one element of a complex neurological phenotype.

The common familial idiopathic epilepsies rarely show a mendelian pattern of inheritance. The mode of inheritance of the idiopathic epilepsies is usually complex, involving multiple gene interactions, age-dependent penetrance and possible environmental modifiers. Gene identification in the idiopathic epilepsies has largely been limited to the rare mendelian idiopathic epilepsies, including benign familial neonatal seizures (BFNS), benign familial neonatal infantile seizures (BFNIS), autosomal dominant nocturnal frontal lobe epilepsy (ADNFLE), generalized epilepsy with febrile seizures plus (GEFS+), autosomal dominant partial epilepsy with auditory features (ADPEAF) and some rare mendelian forms of childhood absence epilepsy and juvenile myoclonic epilepsy.

The strategy applied to the investigation of epilepsy genes clearly depends on knowledge about the underlying genetic architecture. Segregation analysis and family studies of a particular epilepsy syndrome can provide evidence for a genetic basis and the likely mode of inheritance. This will influence the patient resource available for study and the approach to analysis which can be employed. Strategies for the mendelian and non-mendelian 'complex' epilepsies will be considered separately.

Mendelian epilepsies

The technique of positional cloning, which has been successful in the identification of several mendelian epilepsy genes, first requires ascertainment of a single large pedigree or multiple small pedigrees. It is essential that an accurate determination is made of the specific epilepsy phenotype for all affected individuals. DNA must be obtained from both affected and unaffected individuals. The use of cheek swabs or saliva rather than blood for DNA extraction may be more acceptable for small children.

Polymorphic genetic markers distributed across the genome are then 'typed' in all individuals. These markers are selected from one of the human genetic maps discussed in the previous chapter, and may be microsatellites or single nucleotide polymorphisms. Microsatellite marker typing involves amplification of specific sequences in each DNA sample by the polymerase chain reaction, then allele sizing of the PCR products by polyacrylamide gel electrophoresis.

Co-segregation of each polymorphic marker with the disease phenotype is tested by linkage analysis, which provides a map of the strength of genetic linkage across the genome (a genome-wide scan). A single large pedigree or several small pedigrees are required. A 'linked' marker, identified by a high linkage (LOD or logarithm of odds) score, has undergone few recombinations with the causative gene during meiosis and therefore lies on the same chromosomal segment (Figure 64.1). A region of significant linkage on the genetic map is then used

---

Introduction to Epilepsy ed. Gonzalo Alarcón and Antonio Valentín. Published by Cambridge University Press.
© Cambridge University Press 2012.

Section 4: Genetics of epilepsy

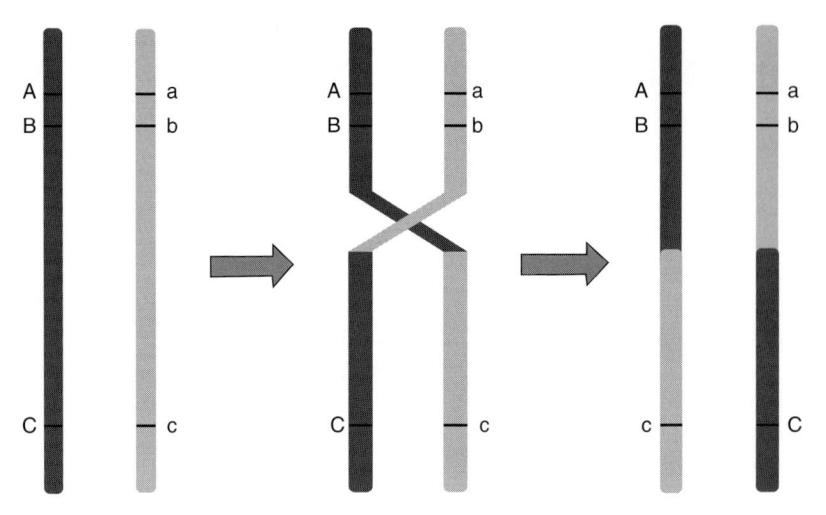

Figure 64.1. Linkage analysis. During prophase of meiosis 1, pairs of homologous chromosomes synapse and exchange segments. Alleles at three loci are shown: A, B, C on the light grey (paternal) chromosome and a, b, c on the white bordered (maternal) chromosome. Recombination between closely spaced loci (A and B) is likely to occur much less frequently than between well-separated loci (A and C). If A is the disease gene and B and C are polymorphic genetic markers, linkage analysis allows the disease gene to be mapped relative to the markers B and C.

to construct a physical map so that coding DNA sequences can be identified and screened for mutations.

An alternative to performing a genome-wide scan is the identification of candidate genes initially, and then testing of each gene for a causative role in the disease by linkage analysis or mutation screening. Candidate genes can be identified in several ways:

- studies on neuronal physiology and mechanisms of seizure generation providing evidence of genes playing a key role;
- genes identified in animal models of human epilepsies;
- genes identified by linkage and association studies in human epilepsies.

Candidates in the symptomatic mendelian epilepsies are usually genes involved in brain development, neuronal survival or energy metabolism. In the idiopathic epilepsies, however, there is strong evidence for the role of ion channels and related proteins in seizure generation. Ion channel defects have now been identified in both human and animal epilepsies.

Once potential causative genes have been identified by either a genome-wide scan or a candidate gene approach, these genes must be analysed for disease-causing mutations. Direct sequencing is just one of several methods available, and those regions of the gene known to be of functional importance are targeted. Sequence variations identified must be carefully evaluated, as many may have no functional significance. Pathogenic mutations usually occur in coding sequences or regulatory sequences, and alter a highly conserved amino acid, splice site or stop codon. Studies of gene expression and protein function are ultimately required to assess the functional significance of a gene mutation.

Non-mendelian epilepsies

Linkage analysis and positional cloning are much less powerful when applied to the epilepsies displaying non-mendelian inheritance. These disorders may result from a number of susceptibility loci, each of relatively small effect, and occurring at relatively high frequency, but the exact value of theses parameters is unknown. Linkage analysis will fail to detect loci exerting a small effect on the disease phenotype, particularly when there is locus heterogeneity (several alternative alleles each with a pathogenic effect). Extended pedigrees do not occur in non-mendelian disorders, and ascertainment of sufficient small pedigrees to provide adequate power to detect linkage is extremely difficult, even with large multinational collaborations.

Association analysis is an alternative strategy often applied to complex diseases, with variable success (Figure 64.2). Association analysis detects non-random associations between a trait and a marker allele (or a cluster of alleles in linkage disequilibrium known as a haplotype). It does not require pedigrees, as control samples can be unrelated individuals from a population, or heterozygous parents of affected individuals (intra-familial association). However the success of association analysis depends on the presence of unique susceptibility alleles (allelic homogeneity) occurring at a relatively high frequency. Extremely large patient cohorts are

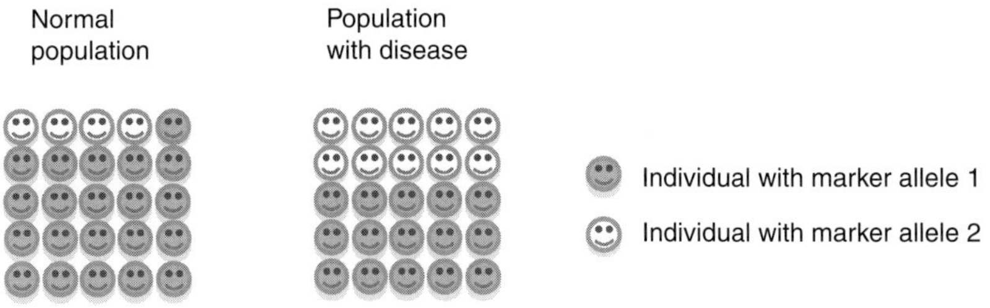

Figure 64.2. Association analysis. A higher than expected incidence of a marker allele (typically a SNP or SNP haplotype) in a disease population suggests that the allele is associated with the disease, and that the marker lies in proximity to a causative gene.

required, and weak associations generated from studies with cohorts of insufficient power are frequently reported but then fail to be replicated.

Learning objective

(1) To understand the present strategies for identification of epilepsy genes.

Section 4 Genetics of epilepsy

Chapter 65

Progress in the genetics of the epilepsies

Robert Robinson

Mendelian epilepsies

As discussed in the previous chapter, the mendelian epilepsies are largely 'symptomatic'. Over 200 mendelian diseases include epilepsy as part of the phenotype. The genetic mutations in these disorders may cause abnormal brain development, progressive neurodegeneration or disturbed energy metabolism, so the mechanism of seizure generation is often indirect.

Abnormalities of brain development are exemplified by the neuronal migration disorders, including lissencephaly (literally 'smooth brain'). The genes identified in the neuronal migration disorders, which include *LIS1*, *DCX*, *FLN1*, *RLN*, *ARX* as well as several genes responsible for the congenital muscular dystrophies, have all been shown to play an important role in the regulation of cortical migration during brain development. Mutations in these genes can interfere with all stages of neuronal migration, causing defects of initiation, ongoing migration, cortical lamination and stop signalling. This results in disruption of cortical organization and neuronal circuitry, often resulting in seizure generation.

Disorders of neuronal survival include the progressive myoclonic epilepsies. These include the neuronal ceroid lipofuscinoses (NCLs), the commonest neurodegenerative disorders of childhood. NCLs are characterized by the accumulation of autofluorescent lipofuscin-like material in the lysosomes of neurons and other cells, and at least seven human genes are known to be responsible.

Epilepsy associated with disturbance of energy metabolism is best represented by the mitochondrial disorders. Characteristic features include ataxia, myopathy, deafness, dementia, multisystem involvement and seizures. Mitochondrial disorders are caused by mutations in both mitochondrial DNA (comprising 37 maternally inherited genes) and nuclear DNA.

Although rare, the idiopathic mendelian epilepsies have provided the major recent advances in the molecular basis of the epilepsies (Table 65.1). The genes identified to date have highlighted several important features of epilepsy genetics:

- Other than *LGI1*, *MASS1* and *ISSX*, all mutations occur in genes encoding ion channels. These genes include both voltage-gated and ligand-gated ion channels.
- The idiopathic mendelian epilepsies demonstrate both locus heterogeneity (mutations in more than one gene causing the same clinical phenotype) and phenotypic heterogeneity (mutations in the same gene causing different clinical phenotypes). For example, GEFS+ can be caused by mutations in either sodium channel or $GABA_A$ receptor genes, whilst mutations in *SCN1A* can result in both GEFS+ and SMEI phenotypes.
- No gene identified in a mendelian epilepsy has been shown to act as a major locus in any non-mendelian epilepsy.

Non-mendelian epilepsies

Success in determining the molecular genetic basis of the common familial epilepsies has been relatively slow. Possible susceptibility genes have been associated with the idiopathic generalized epilepsies, including childhood absence epilepsy and juvenile myoclonic epilepsy, as well as photosensitivity on EEG. These include both ion channel (*CACNA1H*, *GABRD*, *GABRB3*, *CACNG3*) and non-ion channel genes (*BRD2*, *EFHIC*, *NEDD4–2*). Idiopathic partial epilepsies such as benign childhood epilepsy with centrotemporal spikes (BCECTS) and benign childhood occipital epilepsy (BCOE) have also shown

---

Introduction to Epilepsy ed. Gonzalo Alarcón and Antonio Valentín. Published by Cambridge University Press.
© Cambridge University Press 2012.

Table 65.1. Genes identified in mendelian epilepsies

Gene class	Gene	Gene location	Epilepsy syndrome	Inheritance
Voltage-dependent ion channels:				
Sodium channels	SCN1A	2q24	GEFS+/SMEI	
	SCN2A	2q23-q24	GEFS+/BFNIS	AD
	SCN1B	19q13	GEFS+	
Potassium channels	KCNQ2	20q	BFNS	AD
	KCNQ3	8q24		
	KCNA1	12p13	EA1 with partial epilepsy	AD
Calcium channels	CACNA1A	19p13	Generalized epilepsy with ataxia	Sporadic
Chloride channels	CLCN2	3q26	CAE/JAE/JME/EGMA	AD
Ligand-gated ion channels:				
Nicotinic acetylcholine receptors	CHRNA4	20q13.2	ADNFLE	AD
	CHRNB2	1p21		
GABA$_A$ receptor	GABRG2	5q34	GEFS+/SMEI	AD
	GABRA1	5q34	FS with CAE	AD
			JME	AD
Non-ion channel genes:				
Leucine-rich, glioma inactivated protein	LGI1	10q24	ADPEAF	AD
G-protein-coupled receptor	MASS1	5q14	Febrile and afebrile seizures	AD
Aristaless-related homeodomain transcription factor	ARX	Xp22.13	ISSX	X-linked
Serine-threonine protein kinase	CDKL5	Xp22		

GEFS+, generalized epilepsy with febrile seizures plus; SMEI, severe myoclonic epilepsy of infancy; BFNIS, benign familial neonatal infantile seizures; BFNS, benign familial neonatal seizures; EA1, episodic ataxia type 1; CAE, childhood absence epilepsy; JAE, juvenile absence epilepsy; JME, juvenile myoclonic epilepsy; EGMA, epilepsy with grand mal on awakening; ADNFLE, autosomal dominant nocturnal frontal lobe epilepsy; FS, febrile seizures; ADPEAF, autosomal dominant partial epilepsy with auditory features; ISSX, X-linked infantile spasms.

positive associations with genes such as *EFHIC*, *KCND2* and *CACNA1A*. However, genetic association studies have proved difficult to replicate, are usually of insufficient power, and variants rarely show a clear co-segregation with the epilepsy. The extent of heterogeneity in the complex epilepsies is likely to be far greater than the mendelian epilepsies. The exact role of any of these genes in the common familial epilepsies is yet to be determined.

Chromosomal epilepsies

Epilepsy occurs with increased frequency in several chromosomal disorders, where the phenotype results from a gross cytogenetic abnormality. Examples include chromosomal deletions (Wolf-Hirschorn syndrome, 4p deletion), duplications (inverted duplication 15), ring chromosomes (ring chromosome 20) and trisomies (trisomy 21).

The future

The key challenge remains the identification of susceptibility genes for the common familial epilepsies. Technological advances, such as microarray techniques, providing high-throughput sample analysis, will allow more powerful genome-wide linkage and association studies using large numbers of single nucleotide polymorphisms (SNPs) and SNP haplotypes generated by international efforts such as the SNP consortium and the international HapMap project. However the ascertainment of large, well-characterized patient cohorts is essential, and requires multicentre collaborations and partnerships between clinicians and scientist. The benefits will be a greater understanding of the physiological defects in epilepsy, improved diagnosis and new targets for antiepileptic drugs.

Recommended reading

National Human Genome Research Institute, National Institute of Health. http://www.genome.gov/.

Online mendelian medicine in man (OMIM). http://www.ncbi.nlm.nih.gov/sites/entrez.

Robinson R, Gardiner RM Genetics. In Wallace S, Farrell K, eds. *Epilepsy in Children*, p. 29. London: Arnold; 2004.

Learning objective

(1) To know the genes and chromosomes involved in the generation of different epilepsy syndromes.

Section 5 Management of epilepsy

Chapter 66

Neurochemistry of antiepileptic drug action

Brian Meldrum

Introduction

Most current antiepileptic drugs are thought to act either by modifying the function of voltage-gated (VG) ion channels in nerve cell membranes or by altering excitatory or inhibitory synaptic function. GABA-ergic or glutamatergic function can be most readily modified by direct action on the ligand-gated ion channels, but various indirect targets involved in the metabolism or disposition of the neurotransmitter are available.

The pharmacological properties of VG and ligand-gated ion channels are commonly altered in animals or patients with epilepsy. It may therefore be more appropriate to screen potential antiepilepsy drugs (AEDs) in animals with epilepsy (rather than in normal animals with seizures induced chemically or electrically). Similarly it may be more appropriate to analyse the molecular mechanisms of action of AEDs using the abnormal ion channels found in chronic epilepsy.

AED action via voltage-gated ion channels

The excitability of neuronal membranes is dependent primarily on VG ion channels. The largest group of these form a super-family whose members are cation-selective and comprise:

- the voltage-gated Na^+ channels;
- the voltage-gated Ca^{2+} channels (traditionally classified as L-type, P/Q- N- and R- type and T-type);
- the voltage-gated K^+ channels (with more than 70 subtypes).

There are also some channels with less cation selectivity, such as the hyper-polarization-activated cyclic nucleotide-gated cation channels (HCN channels that are Na^+ and K^+ permeable). The VG ion channels are created by alpha subunits with some degree of homology between the different types of VG channels.

Many of the older AEDs and several of the newer ones have potent actions on VG ion channels that are thought to provide a significant part of their AED action.

Voltage-gated sodium channels

There are nine iso-forms of the voltage-gated Na^+ channels. Three of these are prominently expressed in the mature mammalian brain (referred to as Nav1.1, Nav 1.2 and Nav 1.6). They generate both a transient Na^+ current (that underlies the action potential) and a persistent Na^+ current (that contributes to some burst discharges).

Mutations in the alpha or beta subunits of the VG Na^+ channel are associated with various forms of idiopathic generalized epilepsy, including epilepsy with febrile seizures plus.

Actions of AEDs on VG sodium channels

Many AEDs bind to a site on the alpha subunit of voltage-gated Na+ channels (Figure 66.1). Their main effect is to prolong the inactivation phase that follows an action potential. This prolongs the refractory period and slows the maximal firing rate, thereby diminishing high-frequency burst firing. This phenomenon has been most intensely studied for phenytoin and lamotrigine, particularly by studying effects on channels with single site mutations.

Voltage-gated calcium channels

Voltage-gated calcium channels are found in all excitable membranes. They are classified on the basis of their biophysical properties as L, N, T, P/Q and R type channels. T-channels have a low-voltage threshold and play

Introduction to Epilepsy ed. Gonzalo Alarcón and Antonio Valentín. Published by Cambridge University Press.
© Cambridge University Press 2012.

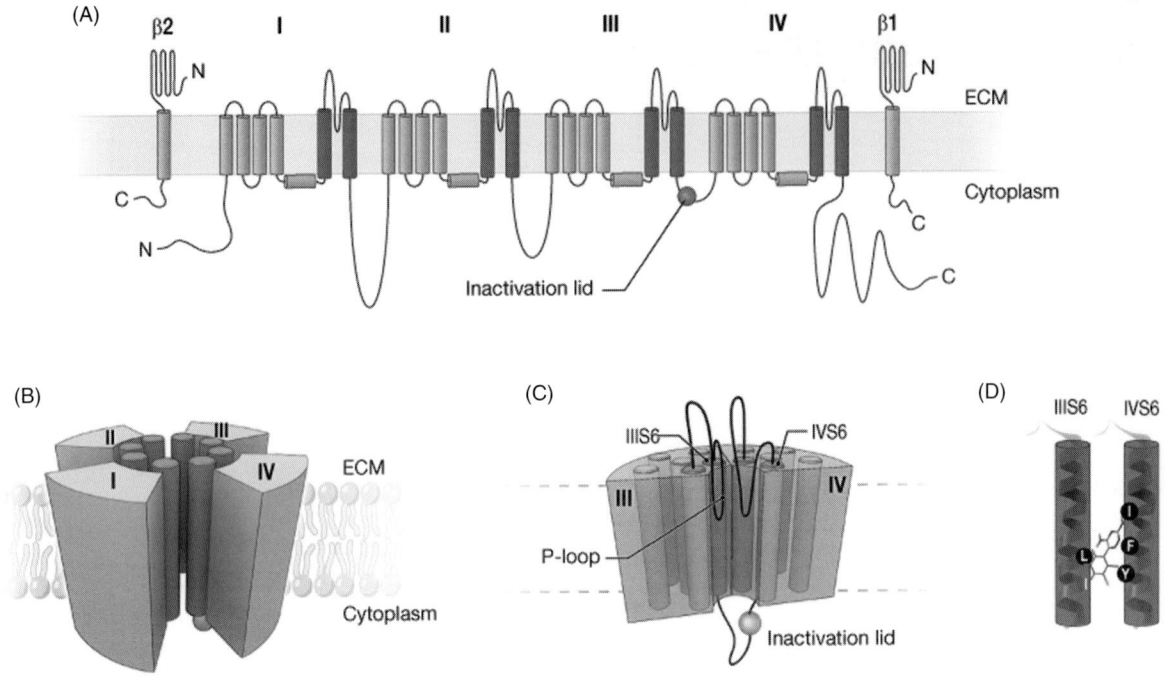

Figure 66.1. The morphology of voltage-gated Na$^+$ channels and the site of AED action. (A) Showing the four domains of the alpha subunit, each with six transmembrane elements, and the beta 1 and beta 2 subunits, each with one transmembrane element. (B) Showing how the S5 and S6 transmembrane elements of domains I–IV form the ion-selective channel. (C) Showing how the p loops between S5 and S6 provide the ion-selective element of the channel. (D) Showing how lamotrigine binds to amino acid residues in III6 and IV6.

a particular role in oscillatory potentials, including those in thalamic and cortical neurons that contribute to the spike-and-wave discharges of absence-type seizures. N, P/Q and R channels occur in pre-synaptic terminals and link the action potential to vesicular neurotransmitter release. The pore-forming alpha-1 subunits of the VG Ca^{2+} channels are homologous with the alpha subunits of the VG Na$^+$ channels.

Mutations in various VG Ca^{2+} channels in mice are associated with absence-like seizure syndromes.

Actions of AEDS on VG Ca^{2+} channels

Ethosuximide and also zonisamide modestly decrease the T-type current in thalamic neurons. This effect is probably sufficient to decrease the oscillatory potentials that contribute to thalamo-cortical spike-and-wave discharges in absence epilepsy.

Gabapentin and pregabalin bind highly specifically to a particular auxiliary subunit of the VG Ca^{2+} channels (the α2-δ-1 and the α2-δ2 subunits). This appears to decrease the currents in N- and P/Q-type channels, diminishing Ca^{2+} entry pre-synaptically and decreasing synaptic release of glutamate.

Lamotrigine is also thought possibly to act via P/Q- and N-type Ca^{2+} channels to decrease synaptic glutamate release.

Voltage-gated potassium channels

Opening K$^+$ channels tends to enhance the resting negative potential and decrease epileptic discharges. Several existing AEDs have been claimed to interact with potassium channels but the significance of any of these effects for AED action has not been established.

A potential AED, retigabine, has broad-spectrum activity in animal models of epilepsy and has been in phase I and II clinical trials. Retigabine has been shown to potentiate a particular K channel (the KCNQ or Kv7 channel). Mutations in subunits of this channel are associated with benign familial neonatal convulsions.

AED action via GABA-mediated inhibitory transmission

GABA is the principal inhibitory transmitter in the brain. It acts on two types of receptor in neuronal membranes, known as GABA$_A$ and GABA$_B$ receptors

Table 66.1. AEDs and their mechanisms of action

AED	Ion channel Na⁺	Ion channel Ca²⁺	GABA GABA_A	GABA Other	Glutamate AMPA/KA	Glutamate NMDA
Phenobarbitone			D,A		++	
Phenytoin	I					
Ethosuximide		T				
Carbamazepine	I					
Valproate	(I)	(T)		?		
Diazepam	(I)		A			
Felbamate	I		A			++
Gabapentin (pregabalin)						
Lamotrigine	I					
Tiagabine				G		
Topiramate			A		++	
Vigabatrin				Tr		
Zonisamide						
Levetiracetam						

A, acting at an allosteric site to potentiate the effect of GABA on chloride conductance; D, acting directly to open Cl⁻ channels in the GABA_A receptor; G, inhibiting the GABA transporter (GAT-1); I, prolonging inactivation of the transient Na⁺ current; PQ, binding to the $\alpha 2\delta$ subunit of VS-Ca²⁺ channels, and decreasing Ca²⁺ entry via P/Q type channels; Sv, acting on a synaptic vesicular protein to modify inhibitory and excitatory transmission; T, decreasing the T-type Ca²⁺ current; Tr, irreversible inhibition of the enzyme GABA-transaminase; (), not proven.

(see Chapter 7). GABA_A receptors enhance Cl⁻ and HCO₃⁻ conductance. This increases the negative membrane potential when the external [Cl⁻] is higher than the internal [Cl⁻]. GABA_A receptors are responsible for fast phasic inhibition post-synaptically and for tonic inhibition extra-synaptically. Differing subunit composition correlates with these differing functions.

GABA_B receptors are metabotropic and can modify K⁺ and Ca²⁺ conductances. They produce slow post-synaptic inhibitory potentials and alter the synaptic release of GABA.

GABA_A receptors and AEDs

Very many AEDs potentiate GABA-mediated inhibition. The commonest mechanism for this is through an action on the GABA_A receptor, either directly causing Cl⁻ channel opening (as with phenobarbitone and chlormethiazole) or potentiating the Cl⁻ channel opening effect of endogenously released GABA. There appear to be many sites on the GABA_A receptor at which such effects can be produced (Figure 66.2). The phenomenon most extensively studied is the action of compounds such as diazepam and clobazam on an allosteric site, often referred to as the benzodiazepine-binding site.

Allosteric modulation via the benzodiazepine site: benzodiazepines and some other anxiolytic compounds bind to an allosteric site on the GABA_A receptor, which involves the alpha and gamma subunits, and potentiates the inhibitory action of GABA. The effect is to increase the number of openings of the Cl⁻ channel produced by a given concentration of GABA. Topiramate and felbamate have also been shown to potentiate the inhibitory effect of GABA in in vitro preparations. These effects differ from those of benzodiazepines, in terms of site and mechanism.

Action of AEDs on GABA re-uptake and further metabolism

GABA is removed from the synaptic cleft by specific transporters in the membranes of astrocytes

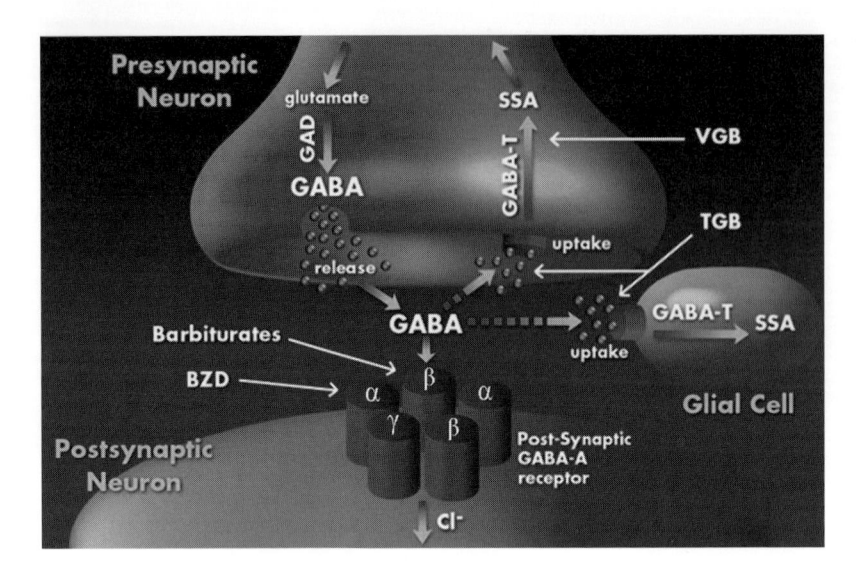

Figure 66.2. Sites at which AEDs potentiate inhibition at the GABA-ergic synapse. Diagram shows a presynaptic terminal and a post-synaptic neuron with a GABA$_A$ receptor molecule.

and presynaptic terminals. There are four such proteins (GAT-1, GAT-2, GAT-3 and BGT-1), each with different regional distribution and with different pharmacology. Tiagabine selectively blocks GAT-1, which is predominantly expressed in the forebrain (cortex and hippocampus). This has the physiological effect of prolonging the inhibitory action of GABA in the synaptic cleft and the pharmacological effect of suppressing cortical and limbic seizures.

The further metabolism of GABA in astrocytes and neurons is initiated by GABA-transaminase, which converts it to succinic semialdehyde (see Chapter 7). Vigabatrin is an irreversible (catalytic) inhibitor of GABA-transaminase that is effective in complex partial seizures and sometimes in Lennox-Gastaut syndrome but can exacerbate absence seizures. It increases the brain content and the extracellular concentration of GABA and increases tonic Cl$^-$ conductance.

GABA$_B$ receptors and epilepsy

Activation of GABA$_B$ receptors by GABA or by an agonist such as baclofen facilitates the occurrence of thalamo-cortical spike-and-wave discharges of the kind seen in absence epilepsy. Antagonists at this site suppress such discharges in animal models of absence epilepsy. This probably explains why some AEDs enhancing the extracellular concentration of GABA (such as tiagabine and vigabatrin) can exacerbate discharges in absence epilepsy.

AED action via glutamatergic excitatory transmission

Glutamate is the principal excitatory neurotransmitter in the brain. It acts via three types of ionotropic receptor known as AMPA, kainate and NMDA receptors and three subtypes of metabotropic receptors (Groups I, II and III).

AMPA and kainate receptors

Agonists at AMPA and kainate receptors cause focal seizures if applied locally to cortical structures and some of them induce limbic seizures if given systemically (kainic acid and domoic acid). Selective antagonists of AMPA receptors are potent anticonvulsants in many animal models of epilepsy, including kindled seizures in rats.

AEDs acting on AMPA and kainate receptors: some barbiturates decrease excitation at AMPA receptors. This may contribute to their AED or anaesthetic action. Topiramate decreases the effect of glutamate on AMPA/kainate receptors, possibly via an action on phosphorylation. One non-competitive AMPA antagonist, talampanel, has undergone successful clinical trials in man.

NMDA receptors

NMDA receptors are involved in post-tetanic potentiation and kindling and are thought to be crucial for learning and epileptogenesis. Compounds that selectively block NMDA receptors are potent anticonvulsants in animal models of epilepsy, especially reflex seizures in rodents and baboons.

AEDs acting on NMDA receptors: felbamate decreases the excitatory effect of glutamate on the NMDA receptor probably through interaction with the glycine site. Some pure NMDA antagonists (such as dizocilpine and CPPene) have been tested in man but have been relatively toxic and ineffective.

Glutamate metabotropic receptors

Agonists at Group I receptors are excitant and some group I antagonists are anticonvulsant. Group II and III receptors are expressed presynaptically and control glutamate release. Some agonists are anticonvulsant. The potential contribution of these phenomena to AED action is not known.

Actions of glutamate antagonists on epileptogenesis

NMDA antagonists if given prior to the kindling stimulus block the kindling process in rodents. This is probably because they greatly decrease the Ca^{2+} entry associated with the after-discharge and this is the important link between the kindling stimulus and the long-term changes responsible for epileptogenesis.

Mechanism of AED action in relation to side effects

There is a clear correlation between the central nervous system side effects of AEDs and their presumed molecular mode of action. Thus AEDs believed to act potently through prolongation of the inactivation phase of the VG Na^+ channel tend to show nystagmus, cerebellar ataxia and dysarthria when given in toxic doses. This would appear to be a result of slowing the maximal firing rate of cerebellar neurons. Drugs potentiating GABA-mediated inhibition tend to induce sedation, muscle relaxation, amnesia and anxiolysis in high dosage. This correlates with the known functions of GABA-ergic pathways. Most drugs acting on VG Na^+ channels can produce a skin rash if treatment is initiated at high dosage, but the mechanism is not understood.

Conclusion

The principal targets of existing AEDs are voltage-gated or ligand-gated ion channels. Among these, the most significant are the voltage-gated Na^+ channels that are the basis of the action potential, and the $GABA_A$ receptors that produce inhibition by opening Cl^- channels. Many AEDs prolong inactivation of the transient Na^+ currents. This effect correlates highly with AED action. Some AEDs also enhance persistent Na^+ currents.

AEDs act on diverse sites on the $GABA_A$ receptor either to directly open Cl^- channels or to potentiate the channel-opening effect of GABA. This action is responsible for much AED action and for some CNS side effects.

A third mechanism of AED action is to decrease excitation either through diminishing the release of glutamate or blocking its post-synaptic effect.

Recommended reading

Meldrum BS, Rogawski MA. Molecular targets for antiepileptic drug development. *Neurotherapeutics* 2007;4:18–61.

National Society for Epilepsy. E-epilepsy. The development of new antiepileptic drugs. http://www.epilepsysociety.org.uk.

Porter RJ, Meldrum BS. Antiseizure drugs. In Katzung BG, ed. *Basic and Clinical Pharmacology*, pp. 379–400. 9th edn. New York: McGraw-Hill; 2004.

Rho JM, Sankar R. The pharmacologic basis of antiepileptic drug action. *Epilepsia* 1999;**40**:1471–83.

Rogawski MA, Löscher W. The neurobiology of antiepileptic drugs. *Nature Rev Neurosci* 2004;5:553–64.

White HS. Comparative anticonvulsant and mechanistic profile of the established and newer antiepileptic drugs. *Epilepsia* 1999;**40**(Suppl 5):S2–10.

Learning objectives

(1) To know the generic and specific mechanisms of action of antiepileptic medication.
(2) To be able to discuss differences and similarities in the mechanisms of action of the different anticonvulsants.
(3) To learn the relevance of the mechanisms of action in the development of new anticonvulsants and in the criteria to combine treatments with approved anticonvulsants.

Section 5 Management of epilepsy

Chapter 67
Antiepileptic drug pharmacokinetics and therapeutic drug monitoring

Philip N. Patsalos

Introduction

The pharmacokinetics of antiepileptic drugs (AEDs) is a crucial consideration when undertaking therapeutic drug monitoring (TDM). Pharmacokinetic considerations include:

(1) Linear pharmacokinetics: most AEDs exhibit linear pharmacokinetics but some show non-linearity, e.g. phenytoin consequent to saturable metabolism and Michaelis-Menten kinetics, gabapentin consequent to dose-dependent bioavailability, carbamazepine consequent to auto-induction and valproic acid consequent to concentration-dependent plasma protein binding;

(2) Inter-individual variability in pharmacokinetics: this is pronounced for clobazam, clonazepam, carbamazepine, felbamate, gabapentin, lamotrigine, phenytoin, tiagabine, topiramate, valproic acid and zonisamide; moderate for ethosuximide, eslicarbazepine acetate, oxcarbazepine, phenobarbital and primidone; slight for lacosamide, levetiracetam, pregabalin and vigabatrin.

(3) Whether active metabolites are produced: occurs with carbamazepine, clobazam, eslicarbazepine acetate, oxcarbazepine and primidone.

Because AEDs are used prophylactically in the management of epilepsy, their efficacy is not readily measured (seizures occur at irregular intervals) and AED-related toxicity is sometimes difficult to detect, TDM has become the surrogate marker of choice in guiding clinical management. This can be attributed to the fact that a serum or plasma concentration (level) measurement reflects patient variability with regard to age, sex, metabolic capacity, co-morbidities and much more. Thus during the past 40 years AED TDM has had a significant impact on the management of patients with epilepsy and this can be attributed in part to our enhanced understanding of AED pharmacokinetics, their relevance to drug therapeutics and the development of robust, reliable and specific analytical methodologies underpinned by appropriate quality assurance schemes. A quality service from an accredited laboratory that provides assay results quickly, preferably within 24 hours of sampling, is important since the most important use of blood concentrations are for dosage adjustments and diagnosing toxicity, when rapid decisions need to be made.

Pharmacokinetics

Pharmacokinetics describes the concentration time-course of a drug and its metabolites (metabolites become particularly important if they are pharmacologically active) in the intact organism and relates to absorption, distribution, metabolism and excretion processes. In contrast pharmacodynamics relates to the efficacy of the drug at its site of action and is directly dependent on the pharmacokinetic characteristics of the drug. Thus knowledge of the pharmacokinetics of a drug can actually change a therapeutic failure into a success.

The time-course of a drug concentration in the circulation will depend on the mode of application. Maximal peak concentrations are achieved after intravenous application and this occurs instantaneously. Plasma concentrations then decline exponentially. After oral ingestion, drug concentrations increase more slowly and attain lower peak concentrations which then decline exponentially. Intermediate time-course patterns are observed after intramuscular and subcutaneous administration. A very important pharmacokinetic parameter is that of the half-life, which

---

Introduction to Epilepsy ed. Gonzalo Alarcón and Antonio Valentín. Published by Cambridge University Press.
© Cambridge University Press 2012.

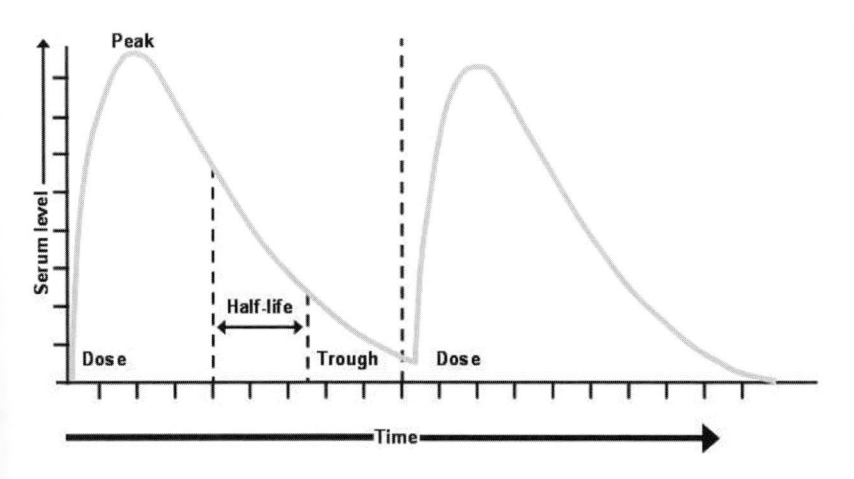

Figure 67.1. Serum concentration versus time curve.

is defined as the time it takes for half the drug concentration to be eliminated from the circulation. Based on the fact that it takes five half-lives for a drug to achieve steady-state plasma concentrations, it is possible to anticipate when the optimum therapeutic response from a particular dose is to occur (Figure 67.1).

During the past 20 years it has become appreciated that there are various pharmacokinetic characteristics that are considered to be ideal for an AED. These include:

- good bioavailability: thus avoiding unnecessarily high doses in order to achieve a desirable therapeutic outcome;
- minimal protein binding: thus avoiding protein binding displacement interactions;
- linear pharmacokinetics: makes dosing and prescribing simpler;
- renal elimination is preferable to hepatic metabolism: this results in less pharmacokinetic variability and also pharmacologically active metabolites are not produced which can complicate therapeutics;
- no drug interactions: consequently one need not consider or worry as to what co-medication the patient is taking today or indeed in the future;
- a half-life (12–24 hours) which allows once or twice a day dosing: patients become non-compliant with more frequent dosing strategies.

Consequently, the emphasis has been to develop new AEDs with better pharmacokinetic characteristics than those AEDs already available and this strategy has been successful in that the top five AEDs (based on 16 pharmacokinetic parameters) are new AEDs (levetiracetam, vigabatrin, gabapentin, pregabalin and topiramate; Table 67.1(1)).

Therapeutic drug monitoring

TDM can be defined as 'the measurement and the clinical use of drug concentrations (levels) in body fluids (usually serum or plasma) to adjust each patient's individual drug dosage and schedule to each patient's individual therapeutic requirement'. In practice it is the patient who is treated and not the concentration, so that the dose of a drug is adjusted, using the drug concentration as a guide, to optimize its efficacy, avoid, minimize or identify toxicity, and detect or confirm poor compliance. It is therefore important to appreciate that TDM begins before a drug concentration is measured and that the measurement itself is only part of the overall process of planning, monitoring, and optimally adjusting the dosage regimen.

The criteria for valid TDM are:

(1) the availability of accurate pharmacokinetic data;
(2) that there is a poor correlation between dose and blood concentrations (i.e. substantial pharmacokinetic variability);
(3) that there is a good correlation between blood concentration and therapeutic effect, toxicity or both, at least within individuals;
(4) a narrow therapeutic index (i.e. the therapeutic dose is close to the dose associated with toxicity); and
(5) the availability of simple, accurate, reproducible and inexpensive analytical assays.

Section 5: Management of epilepsy

Table 67.1. (1) Pharmacokinetic ranking for AEDs

AED	% of perfect score
LEV	96
VGB	96
GBP	89
PGB	89
TPM	79
ETS	77
OXC	77
LTG	73
TGB	67
ZNS	67
PB	58
VPA	52
CBZ	50
PHT	50

Adapted from: Patsalos (2004).

Table 67.1. (2) Some general indications for therapeutic drug monitoring

1. After initiation of treatment (to provide a baseline steady-state concentration).
2. After change in drug dosage, in particular when non-linear kinetics apply (to confirm new drug concentration).
3. At therapeutic failure (to confirm or exclude a pharmacokinetic explanation for uncontrolled seizures or adverse effects).
4. To establish an individual therapeutic concentration range (when a person has attained the desired clinical outcome), which can be used subsequently to assess potential causes of change in response (e.g. a decrease in seizure control or an increase in adverse effects).
5. To identify or control for drug–drug interactions.
6. After a change in drug formulation (including generic substitution).
7. To guide dosage adjustment in patients where potentially important pharmacokinetic changes are anticipated consequent to physiological or pathological changes (e.g. pregnancy, hepatic disease, renal disease and gastrointestinal conditions potentially affecting drug absorption).
8. When poor compliance is suspected.
9. Suspected toxicity.
10. To guide dose adjustment for AEDs with dose-dependent pharmacokinetics (e.g. phenytoin, carbamazepine, valproic acid and gabapentin).
11. The emergency situation (suspected overdose, status epilepticus).

Although none of the AEDs fulfil all these criteria, there are clinical settings where all AEDs can be justifiably monitored. Overall, phenytoin best fulfils these criteria, because its saturable pharmacokinetics makes it very difficult to prescribe the optimum dose without measuring blood concentrations. However, although all AEDs are monitored, some AEDs are more suitable candidates for monitoring than others.

The goal of AED treatment is seizure freedom without side effects. However, even with the introduction of 12 new AEDs since 1989, a significant number of people with epilepsy are still not achieving this goal. TDM can help to improve seizure control in numerous ways and the indications for undertaking TDM are highlighted in Table 67.1(2).

Sampling time

For TDM to be used to maximum utility, it is imperative to have a meticulous dosage history and sampling time. Sampling should be done at steady-state, which occurs at five half-lives after starting treatment or a dose change. For most AEDs, particularly those with short or relatively short half-lives (e.g. carbamazepine, valproic acid, gabapentin, lacosamide, levetiracetam, pregabalin, tiagabine, vigabatrin, lamotrigine and topiramate), it is important to standardize sampling time in relation to dose. For phenobarbital, zonisamide and ethosuximide, the fluctuation in plasma drug concentration during a dosing interval is negligible, because of their long half-lives, and samples can be collected at any time. Sampling before steady-state is achieved will result in an underestimated concentration for that particular dose. Consequently, if a further dose increase is undertaken, this may eventually result in toxicity for the patient. The ideal blood sampling time for all AEDs is immediately before the next oral dose (trough), but if this is not possible, particularly when attending an out-patient clinic, it is desirable to note the sampling time and the time medication was last ingested. In some cases, two blood samples, for example one taken at the time of trough and a second taken at the expected time of peak (or in conjunction with the appearance of symptoms suggestive of transient concentration-related toxicity), could be valuable to optimize the dosing schedule. During overdose, sampling should be undertaken as soon as the patient presents at casualty but repeated sampling might be necessary, depending on the timing of the overdose.

Biological matrixes

Plasma or serum is the matrix of choice for TDM. Although these can be used interchangeably, it is preferable to use one or the other. Other matrixes that have been used include saliva, hair, tears and sweat. Of these saliva is increasingly being used and the reason for this is:

(1) collection of saliva is simple and non-invasive;
(2) it does not require expertise of drawing blood and therefore sampling can be undertaken by patients themselves or by a carer;
(3) it can be especially useful in patients with disabilities and is preferred by children and their parents;
(4) measured concentrations reflect the unbound (pharmacologically relevant) concentration in blood (e.g. carbamazepine, ethosuximide, gabapentin, lacosamide, lamotrigine, levetiracetam, oxcarbazepine, phenytoin, primidone, topiramate and vigabatrin).

Detecting AED non-compliance is important and whilst plasma measurements provide an index of compliance on the preceding 1–3 days, long-term or variable non-compliance is not detectable. However, analysis of AEDs in scalp hair can provide such information because content has been shown to reflect the mean blood concentration profile over a prolonged period prior to sampling, and in addition hair sampling is non-invasive (assuming hair is not at a premium!). Because hair acts as a 'tape recorder', drug concentration in different hair segments may reflect a history of drug ingestion over a period of months or years, depending on the length of hair.

Altered drug binding to plasma proteins

Routine methods for measuring AEDs in plasma do not discriminate between that component that is bound to plasma proteins and that that is in the free (unbound) form. However, only the free drug is biologically active, as it is the only fraction available to move across the endothelium and to equilibrate with the concentration in the interstitial space in the brain. In most situations, the inter-patient variability in the unbound fraction is relatively small, and measurement of total concentrations is more than adequate for clinical purposes. However, if a major change in unbound fraction is expected (or suspected), measuring unbound drug concentrations may be justified. Thus in circumstances in which the free fraction increases, the total drug concentration in plasma will underestimate the amount of free, pharmacologically active drug, and therefore therapeutic and toxic effects will be observed at total drug concentrations which are lower than usual. This is particularly important for AEDs that are extensively bound (>90%) to plasma proteins (e.g. phenytoin and valproic acid) and impairment in the protein binding of these drugs may be caused by hypoalbuminaemia (as observed during pregnancy, old age, liver disease and many other pathological conditions), accumulation of endogenous displacing agents (most notably, in patients with renal insufficiency) and administration of other medications which compete for plasma protein binding sites. In these conditions, interpretation of plasma drug concentration requires special skills.

'Therapeutic ranges' vs 'reference ranges' vs 'individualized therapeutic concentrations'

There is significant confusion regarding the terminology and the concept of the 'reference range' as opposed to the 'therapeutic range'. The 'reference range' is a range of concentrations for a particular drug that is quoted by a laboratory and can be defined as a range of drug concentration providing a lower limit below which a therapeutic response is relatively unlikely to occur, and an upper limit above which toxicity is relatively likely to occur. One needs to be aware that, because of individual variations, some patients might achieve therapeutic benefit below the lower limit of the reference range, might show signs of toxicity below the upper limit of the reference range or, indeed, might have therapeutic benefit without toxic effects above the upper limit of the range. The 'reference range' is not a 'therapeutic range'. The latter can only be determined for the individual patient.

Given the considerable inter-patient variability in the concentration of an AED that produces optimal seizure control, the argument can be made that ultimately AED therapy can be best guided by identification of the 'individualized therapeutic concentration'. The latter is defined as the concentration that has been measured in an individual patient after that patient had been stabilized on a dosage that produced the best response. In a patient who had infrequent seizures before starting treatment, this can only be done after a long period of observation, in order to confirm that remission has been really achieved. Even when an optimal dosage has been established empirically, knowledge of the plasma concentration at which the individual patient has shown a good response provides a useful reference in making management decisions should a modification in clinical status occur over time. An advantage of the 'individualized therapeutic concentration' approach is that it does not rely on fixed 'reference ranges', and can be applied to any AED, including second-generation AEDs, for some of which 'reference ranges' have not yet been clearly defined.

Carbamazepine

Carbamazepine is extensively and variably metabolized, resulting in a poor correlation between dose and plasma concentration. The half-life during long-term treatment is considerably shorter than following a single dose because of auto-induction. The primary metabolite of carbamazepine, carbamazepine-10,11-epoxide, is pharmacologically active and its measurement may be useful in settings where the metabolite is suspected of contributing to carbamazepine-related toxicity.

The unpredictable relationship between dose and carbamazepine concentration, its narrow therapeutic index and the presence of numerous clinically significant drug interactions support the need to individualize and maintain therapy using TDM. Because carbamazepine is associated with significant diurnal oscillation in plasma concentrations, sampling time in relation to dose ingestion is important for the interpretation of the drug concentration. Ideally samples for carbamazepine measurements should be drawn before the morning dose. The reference range for carbamazepine is 17–51 μmol/L (4–12 mg/L; Table 67.2). The upper boundary of the reference range of carbamazepine-10,11-epoxide is 34 μmol/L (8 mg/L).

Eslicarbazepine acetate

Eslicarbazepine acetate is a pro-drug which is rapidly metabolized to eslicarbazepine (also known as S-licarbazepine) and also to two minor metabolites, R-licarbazepine and oxcarbazepine. The role of TDM for eslicarbazepine has not yet been established and a reference range for the drug has yet to be identified. TDM is used to ascertain compliance and also in managing patients that may be overdosed.

Ethosuximide

The elimination of ethosuximide is slow, and its plasma concentration is relatively stable even if the drug is given once a day. The half-life in children is, however, considerably shorter than that in adults. TDM can be useful for individualizing therapy with ethosuximide, although in most cases therapy can be optimized simply on the basis of clinical response and EEG checks. The reference range for ethosuximide is 283–708 μmol/L (40–100 mg/L).

Felbamate

Currently, the use of felbamate is highly restricted due to the risk of aplastic anaemia and hepatotoxicity. Felbamate undergoes metabolism with approximately 50% of an administered dose metabolized to various inactive metabolites, although the atropaldehyde metabolite may be responsible for the development of serious organ toxicity. Protein binding is approximately 25%. The half-life in adults is shortened by enzyme-inducing AEDs. The reference range for felbamate is 126–252 μmol/L (30–60 mg/L).

Gabapentin

The pharmacokinetics of gabapentin can be very variable, which can be attributed to the saturable absorption mechanism from the gut. Gabapentin does not undergo metabolism and is eliminated in the unchanged form via the kidneys. It is not associated with any major pharmacokinetic interactions. Monitoring of gabapentin concentrations may be useful in selected cases. However, because gabapentin has a relatively short half-life, sampling time in relation to dose ingestion is important for the interpretation of the drug concentration. Ideally, samples for gabapentin measurements should be drawn before the morning dose. The reference range for gabapentin is 12–116 μmol/L (2–20 mg/L).

Table 67.2. Characteristics of AEDs

AED	Oral bioavailability (%)	Serum protein binding (%)	Time to peak concentration (h)	Time to steady-state (days)	Half-life (monotherapy) (h)	Half-life (+ enzyme inducers) (h)	Main route of elimination	Pharmacokinetic rating (% of a perfect score)	Reference range[h] (µmol/L)
Carbamazepine	~85	75	4–8[a]	4–7	8–20	5–12	Oxidation	50	17–51
Ethosuximide	100	0	3–7	5–10	40–60	20–30	Oxidation	77	283–708
Felbamate	>90	25	2–6	3–4	16–22	10–18	Oxidation	73	126–252
Gabapentin[g]	<60	0	2–3	2	5–7 15–30	5–7 8–20	Renal excretion	89	12–116
Lamotrigine	100	55	1–3	3–15	(30–90 +VPA)	(15–30 +VPA)	Glucuronide conjugation	73	10–58
Levetiracetam	100	0	1	2	6–8	5–8	Renal excretion and hydrolysis	96	70–270
Oxcarbazepine[e]	100	40	4–6	2–3	8–15	7–12	Keto-reduction, then glucuronide conjugation of MHD	77	12–139
Phenobarbital	100	50	2–8	10–35	50–160	50–160	Oxidation, N-glucoside conjugation, and renal excretion	58	43–172
Phenytoin	100	90	2–8	4–8	7–60[c]	7–60[c]	Oxidation	50	40–79
Pregabalin	100	0	1	2	6–7	5–7	Renal excretion	89	NE
Primidone	100	0	2–5	1–3	4–12	4–12	Cleavage of the pyrimidine ring, oxidation to phenobarbital, and renal excretion	52	23–46
Tiagabine	100	96	0.5–2	2	7–9	2–3	Oxidation	67	53–532[b]
Topiramate	100	15	1–4	4–6	20–30	10–15	Renal excretion, oxidation	79	15–59
Valproic acid	100	78–94[c]	3–6[d]	2–4	11–20	6–12	Oxidation and glucuronide conjugation	52	346–693
Vigabatrin	~60–70	0	1–2	1–2	5–8	5–8	Renal excretion	96	6–279
Zonisamide	>65	60	4–7	5–12	50–70	25–35	Glucuronide conjugation, acetylation, oxidation, and renal excretion	67	47–188

[a] Conventional tablets; [b] nmol/L; [c] concentration dependent; [d] enteric-coated tablets; [e] monohydroxy derivative; [g] decreases with increasing dose; [h] molar digits have not been rounded up or down to ensure precise mathematical correspondence to the mg/L digits. However, laboratories quoting preferentially molar units may decide to round them up or down. NE = not established; VPA = valproic acid.

Lacosamide

Lacosamide is metabolized in the liver to as yet unknown metabolites (60%) and elimination is primarily by renal excretion. Inter-patient variability in pharmacokinetics is considerd to be low. The role of TDM for lacosamide has not yet been established. Nevertheless a reference range for the drug has been identified and it is 40–80 µmol/L (10–20 mg/L).

Lamotrigine

Because of its pharmacokinetic characteristics, TDM is particularly helpful in optimizing lamotrigine therapy. The half-life of lamotrigine is shortened by enzyme-inducing AEDs, is considerably prolonged by valproic acid, and is intermediate in patients treated with both enzyme-inducing AEDs and valproic acid. Lamotrigine clearance is higher in children and somewhat reduced in elderly patients. Furthermore, there are large inter-individual variations in plasma concentrations in patients on monotherapy and its pharmacokinetics are also influenced by pregnancy and oral contraceptives. The reference range for lamotrigine is 10–58 µmol/L (2.5–15 mg/L).

Levetiracetam

Levetiracetam is minimally metabolized, primarily by hydrolysis (non-CYP450 dependent) in whole blood, and is eliminated in the unchanged form via the kidneys. It is not associated with any major pharmacokinetic interactions. Its half-life is shorter in children and somewhat prolonged in elderly patients. Children seem to need higher doses of levetiracetam in mg/kg body weight than adults to achieve a given drug concentration. Although the role of TDM for levetiracetam has not yet been established, it may be useful in ascertaining compliance and managing patients who are overdosed. Because levetiracetam has a relatively short half-life, sampling time in relation to dose ingestion is important for the interpretation of the drug concentration. Ideally samples for levetiracetam measurements should be drawn before the morning dose. The reference range for levetiracetam is 70–270 µmol/L (12 – 46 mg/L).

Oxcarbazepine

Oxcarbazepine, a pre-drug, is rapidly and extensively metabolized to the pharmacologically active monohydroxy metabolite (MHD; 10-hydroxy-carbazepine). Elimination is faster in children (2–6 years) compared with older children and adults and is reduced in the elderly. The metabolism of MHD is enhanced by enzyme-inducing AEDs. The reference range for MHD is 12–139 µmol/L (3–35 mg/L).

Phenobarbital

Phenobarbital is extensively metabolized and its elimination is particularly slow although its half-life is shorter in children than in adults. Some drugs, particularly valproic acid, may increase the plasma concentration of phenobarbital. The relationship between the plasma concentration of phenobarbital and central nervous system adverse effects varies with the development of tolerance. The reference range for phenobarbital is 43–172 µmol/L (10–40 mg/L).

Phenytoin

Whilst all other AEDs are metabolized according to first-order kinetics, phenytoin metabolism follows Michaelis-Menten kinetics, so that even a slight increase in dose (or inhibition of metabolism) may lead to a considerable increase in its plasma concentration and pharmacological effect. This is because the hepatic enzymes responsible for phenytoin metabolism become saturated within the clinically occurring plasma concentration range. Phenytoin is substantially protein-bound and variability in the fraction of unbound drug can have a significant impact on its pharmacological effect. Phenytoin is by far the most interacting of all AEDs and many interactions have been reported, particularly those that lead to an inhibition of phenytoin metabolism. Due to the special pharmacokinetic features of phenytoin, use of this drug is difficult without TDM. The reference range for phenytoin is 40–79 µmol/L (10–20 mg/L).

Pregabalin

Pregabalin does not undergo metabolism and is eliminated in the unchanged form via the kidneys. It is not associated with any major pharmacokinetic interactions. Dose adjustment may be necessary in patients with renal insufficiency. The role of TDM for pregabalin has not yet been established and a reference range for the drug has yet to be identified. TDM is used to ascertain compliance and also in managing patients that may be overdosed.

Primidone

Primidone is rapidly metabolized to phenobarbital and phenylethylmalonamide, which are pharmacologically active and also accumulate during long-term treatment. Primidone also has an anticonvulsant effect. There is significant individual variability in the relationship between primidone dose and the concentration of the drug and its metabolites. Since primidone is metabolized to phenobarbital, most often the phenobarbital concentration is used as a guide to therapy. The reference range for primidone is 23–46 µmol/L (5–10 mg/L).

Rufinamide

Rufinamide is extensively metabolized (98%) by non-CYP dependent hydrolysis to a non-pharmacologically active metabolite (CCP 47292) which is excreted in urine. The role of TDM for rufinamide has not yet been established and a reference range for the drug has yet to be identified. TDM is used to ascertain compliance and also in managing patients who may be overdosed.

Stiripentol

Stiripentol exhibits non-linear (Michaelis-Menton) pharmacokinetics so that its clearance decreases with increasing dose. Because it is is extensively metabolized by CYPs its metabolism is inducible. Furthermore it is a potent inhibitor of isoenzymes and is substantially bound to plasma proteins (99%). These features would suggest that TDM should play a significant role in optimizing stiripentol therapy. However, the role of TDM for stiripentol has not yet been established and a reference range for the drug has yet to be identified. TDM is used to ascertain compliance and also in managing patients who may be overdosed.

Tiagabine

Tiagabine is extensively metabolized and has a short half-life. Clearance is higher in children than in adults, and its metabolism is inducible. There are large intra-individual and inter-individual variations in plasma concentration. It is highly protein-bound and any variability in the fraction of unbound, pharmacologically active drug may be of importance. Information on the usefulness of tiagabine TDM is not available. Nevertheless, its use in ascertaining compliance and managing patients who are overdosed would be helpful, provided that utmost care is placed in ensuring the reliability of the analytical assay. If monitoring were to be undertaken, sampling time in relation to dose is critical because large inter-dose fluctuations in concentrations occur consequent to the short half-life of the drug. Ideally, samples for tiagabine measurements should be drawn before the morning dose. The reference range for tiagabine is 53–532 nmol/L (20–200 ng/mL).

Topiramate

Topiramate is minimally metabolized when administered as monotherapy. However, when prescribed with enzyme-inducing AEDs metabolism becomes a significant feature in its elimination. Importantly it is associated with a wide scatter of plasma concentrations among patients taking the same dose, and wide variation in the relationship between its concentration and therapeutic or toxic effects. Children require a higher dosage in mg/kg body weight than adults to obtain similar plasma concentrations. The reference range for topiramate is 15–59 µmol/L (5–20 mg/L).

Valproic acid

Valproic acid undergoes extensive metabolism by a variety of pathways, including conjugation, β-oxidation and CYP450, and consequently its metabolism is complex, resulting in more than 20 metabolites of which three or four are pharmacologically active. Therefore, inter-individual differences in metabolism are substantial and this results in a poor correlation between the dose and the plasma concentration. Furthermore, enzyme-inducing AEDs lower plasma valproic acid concentrations. Children need higher doses in mg/kg body weight than adults. Valproic acid is highly protein-bound, and the binding is concentration-dependent and saturable. Because valproic acid has a relatively short half-life, sampling time in relation to dose ingestion is important for interpretation of the drug concentration. Ideally, samples for valproic acid measurements should be drawn before the morning dose. The reference range for valproic acid is 346–693 µmol/L (50–100 mg/L).

Vigabatrin

Vigabatrin is not metabolized and is primarily excreted unchanged in urine. A dose reduction is required in patients with impaired renal function. The half-life of vigabatrin is very short and it is not associated with any significant pharmacokinetic interactions. Vigabatrin TDM is not of great value as a guide to therapy due to its irreversible mechanism of action with the long-lasting inhibition of γ-aminobutyric acid (GABA) transaminase, the enzyme responsible for the metabolism of GABA. Consequently the antiepileptic effect of vigabatrin long outlasts its presence in plasma. However, plasma vigabatrin concentrations as a check on recent compliance or for ascertaining toxicity may be useful and the reference range is 6–279 μmol/L (0.8–36 mg/L).

Zonisamide

Zonisamide is extensively metabolized and its metabolism is enhanced by enzyme-inducing AEDs. Compared with adults, children require higher mg/kg doses to attain comparable plasma concentrations. Zonisamide is 50% bound to plasma proteins but shows high-affinity, low-capacity binding to erythrocytes, which can be attributed to high-affinity binding to carbonic anhydrase and other red cell protein components. Consequently haemolysed blood samples can result in spuriously high zonisamide plasma concentrations. The reference range for zonisamide is 47–188 μmol/L (10–40 mg/L).

Conclusions

Whilst the new AEDs do not have ideal pharmacokinetic characteristics, their characteristics are more desirable than those associated with the older AEDs. AED TDM can provide important information in making therapeutic decisions. The reference range should not be considered as a concentration interval appropriate for all patients, but as an expression of the probability of beneficial effects with an acceptable risk of toxicity in a population. Indeed, since the optimal concentration varies between patients, the concept of an individual therapeutic range is advocated. Furthermore, it is increasingly being recognized that the lower limit of the therapeutic range is of little value, because many patients do well with lower plasma concentrations.

Recommended reading

Patsalos PN, Berry DJ, Bourgeois BFD, *et al*. Antiepileptic drugs – best practice guidelines for therapeutic drug monitoring: A position paper by the Subcommission on Therapeutic Drug Monitoring, ILAE Commission on Therapeutic Strategies. *Epilepsia* 2008;**49**:1239–76.

Patsalos PN. Clinical pharmacokinetics of levetiracetam. *Clin Pharmacokinet* 2004;**43**:707–24.

Williams J, Bialer M, Johannessen SI, *et al*. Interlaboratory variability in the quantification of new generation antiepileptic drugs based upon external quality assessment data. *Epilepsia* 2003;**44**:40–5.

Johannessen SI, Bettino D, Berry DJ, *et al*. Therapeutic drug monitoring of the newer antiepileptic drugs. *Ther Drug Monit* 2003;**25**:347–63.

Patsalos PN, Ghattaura S, Ratnaraj N, Sander JW. In situ metabolism of levetiracetam in blood of patients with epilepsy. *Epilepsia* 2006;**47**:1818–21.

Learning objectives

(1) To understand the basic principles of pharmacokinetics.
(2) To understand how absorbtion, protein binding, half-life and elimination affect the action and interaction of the various antiepileptic drugs.
(3) To know the specific pharmacokinetic properties of the different antiepileptic drugs.

Section 5 Management of epilepsy

Chapter 68: Antiepileptic drug trials and their methodology

Graeme J. Sills

Preclinical trials

Introduction

Despite the licensing of more than ten new antiepileptic drugs (AEDs) in the UK since 1989, around 30% of people with epilepsy continue to suffer seizures despite otherwise optimal treatment and still more patients experience side effects from their medication, which impacts on their quality of life. New AEDs are required to meet this therapeutic short-fall.

Drug discovery

Current approaches to drug development in epilepsy include target-orientated design, structural modification and random-screening (Löscher and Schmidt, 1994). Amongst modern AEDs, vigabatrin and tiagabine are the sole products of target-oriented design, exerting their effects on the γ-aminobutyric acid (GABA) neurotransmitter system. Other new drugs are the products of structural modification strategies based on chemical adaptation of neuroactive compounds: gabapentin and pregabalin are analogues of GABA, whereas oxcarbazepine is a carbamazepine derivative. Finally, there are several new AEDs (including lamotrigine, topiramate, levetiracetam and zonisamide) that have arisen from candidate and random screening of libraries of molecules.

Models and methods

The efficacy and neurotoxicity of new AEDs are initially established in a series of experimental models, including the maximal electroshock (MES), subcutaneous pentylenetetrazol (PTZ), and rotarod tests (White et al., 2002; White, 2003). The MES test involves exposing experimental animals to a short electrical stimulus via either corneal or auricular electrodes, and evaluating the ability of a test compound to prevent tonic extension of the hindlimbs. The PTZ test involves the subcutaneous administration of a supramaximal dose of the chemical convulsant PTZ to experimental animals and comparing latency to onset of generalized clonic seizures between control and drug-treated animals. The rotarod test involves placing animals on a 2.5 cm diameter rod rotating continuously at 6 rpm, with neurological impairment identified by the inability of animals to maintain their equilibrium.

Candidate antiepileptic compounds are typically administered orally or intraperitoneally in a volume adjusted according to body weight and species. Data are expressed in a series of values such as median effective dose (ED_{50}), median toxic dose (TD_{50}), time to peak effect (TPE) and protective index (PI), allowing comparison with other AEDs. PIs give a relative measure of the separation between effective doses and those which precipitate side effects. A PI of 1.0 or less is often indicative of little or no efficacy at tolerable doses (White et al., 2002; White, 2003).

The ADD program

The Antiepileptic Drug Development (ADD) program was instituted by the National Institutes of Health (USA) in 1974 and has since screened more than 30 000 compounds submitted by chemists from across the globe. The ADD program comprises four steps: identification, quantification, differentiation and further studies (Krall et al., 1978). Initial identification of efficacy involves MES and PTZ tests in mice and rats. Activity in one or both of these models leads to subsequent quantification of efficacy and neurotoxicity. TPE is established and employed in determinations of both ED_{50} (in MES and PTZ) and TD_{50}

Introduction to Epilepsy ed. Gonzalo Alarcón and Antonio Valentín. Published by Cambridge University Press.
© Cambridge University Press 2012.

(in rotarod) using two species (mice, rats) and two administration routes (oral, intraperitoneal). Differentiation studies involve investigation of efficacy in a host of experimental models, such as the kindled rat, bicuculline and picrotoxin tests, and audiogenic-seizure-sensitive mouse. Compounds may then undergo further studies of their proconvulsant potential, mechanisms of action and potential for tolerance. This characterization provides information about the extent and range of efficacy and neurotoxicity, an indication of PI and preliminary evidence regarding pharmacology, pharmacokinetics, and doses for use in human studies (White et al., 2002; White, 2003).

Predicting clinical activity

The profile of older AEDs suggests that experimental models can forecast clinical activity (White et al., 2002; White, 2003). The MES test identifies efficacy against generalized tonic-clonic seizures, the PTZ model is sensitive to drugs with efficacy against generalized absence seizures, and the kindled rat predicts efficacy in partial seizures. This association does not hold for modern AEDs, several of which possess broad-spectrum clinical activity but are inactive in the PTZ test, while others are effective against PTZ but make clinical absence seizures worse. Current screening procedures may be inadequate: levetiracetam was originally discarded by the ADD program due to lack of efficacy in MES and PTZ models (White, 2003).

Additional investigations

In addition to assessment of efficacy and neurotoxicity, all new drugs are required to undergo detailed toxicological investigation (White et al., 2002). This involves daily oral administration of three different drug doses to two different species (rats, dogs) for a minimum period of 14 days (short-term toxicology) or between 6 and 24 months (long-term toxicology). Toxicology investigations focus on behavioural, haematological and neurological effects, and potential for carcinogenicity. Mutagenic potential is evaluated using the Ames test, and teratogenicity evaluated by examination of the offspring of drug-exposed females.

Future studies

Continued use of old models, such as MES and PTZ, may bias drug discovery towards compounds with mechanisms of action which are identical to those of current AEDs, with little potential benefit for patients with refractory epilepsy. Future screening protocols must be sufficiently sensitive to identify compounds with novel mechanisms and sufficiently flexible to accommodate new models of refractory epilepsy and epileptogenesis in order that novel drug development for epilepsy is targeted at areas of greatest clinical need (White, 2003).

Summary

All new antiepileptic agents undergo rigorous examination in a series of experimental models prior to first human use. Preclinical studies are designed to identify anticonvulsant activity and to quantify efficacy and neurotoxicity. Additional investigations update pharmacology, pharmacokinetics and potential clinical activity. Preclinical toxicology provides essential information about long-term safety. The drug development process in epilepsy must constantly evolve to ensure that future generations of AEDs are superior to current compounds and to prioritize those patients with refractory epilepsy.

Clinical trials

Introduction

After identification of appropriate formulations and reliable manufacturing processes, a fledgling AED is ready for clinical testing. Further development is dictated by regulatory authorities, including the Food & Drug Administration (USA) and European Medicines Agency. Clinical trials are performed out of necessity and are predominantly focused on obtaining approval for marketing. They are performed in series from Phase I to Phase III. A minimum number of trials are required for approval but additional studies may be necessary to clarify unexpected results. This adds to the cost of development, currently around $800 million for each new AED (French, 2006).

Basic principles

Sample size

It is unethical to conduct a trial with insufficient patients to demonstrate a statistically significant effect. In power calculations, investigators select the primary outcome measure and estimate the size of the treatment effect. A power of 90% is employed in regulatory studies, with significance set at $P < 0.01$. Where sample size is unrealistic, it may be necessary to engage more investigators or reduce the number of comparisons.

Inclusion/exclusion criteria

Strict inclusion/exclusion criteria minimizes variability and reduces the likelihood of adverse events being unfairly ascribed to treatment. Patients aged 16 to 65 years experiencing at least four partial seizures per month are typically included in regulatory trials. Children, the elderly, females of childbearing age and individuals with infrequent seizures are routinely excluded. These criteria create an artificial environment in which efficacy is assessed in patients who do not represent the population as a whole (French, 2006).

Randomization

Random allocation of participants minimizes bias and increases the probability that differences can be ascribed to treatment. In its simplest form, effective randomization can be achieved by coin-tossing or rolling a dice. Automated telephone randomization, employing a system of random permuted blocks, is common in regulatory studies.

Blinding

Blinding of trial participants and/or investigators reduces bias. Most regulatory trials are double-blind: neither participant nor investigator knows what treatment has been assigned. Double-blind studies allow objective assessment of response but are problematic when serious side effects occur. On rare occasions, the blind may be broken to determine whether a life-threatening adverse event is treatment-related (French, 2006).

Control

Choice of control can influence outcome of trials. Historical control compares active treatment with a baseline pre-treatment period. Placebo control is preferred for regulatory trials in epilepsy: patients are randomized to treatment with either study drug or an inert tablet (placebo). Dose control compares a full dose of the study drug with a low dose of the study drug or of an alternative AED. Active control is used in monotherapy trials where new drugs are compared head-to-head with established agents (French, 2006; Mohanraj and Brodie, 2003; Schmidt, 2007).

Dose selection

Selecting appropriate doses and titration rates in clinical trials is fundamental to success. Dose selection is continually refined throughout development, from preclinical studies to Phase III trials. Many modern AEDs are used clinically at lower doses and slower titration rates than employed in pivotal trials, because high doses achieved via fast titration are more efficient in providing persuasive short-term efficacy data (Mohanraj and Brodie, 2003).

Analysis

There are two principal approaches to analysis of trial data: intention-to-treat (ITT) and per-protocol (PP). ITT analysis is conservative and expresses efficacy as a percentage of patients taking at least one dose of medication. PP analysis includes only those patients who reach a recognized end point. ITT is preferred by regulators but PP provides more favourable data and is arguably more clinically relevant (French, 2006; Schmidt, 2007).

Section 5: Management of epilepsy

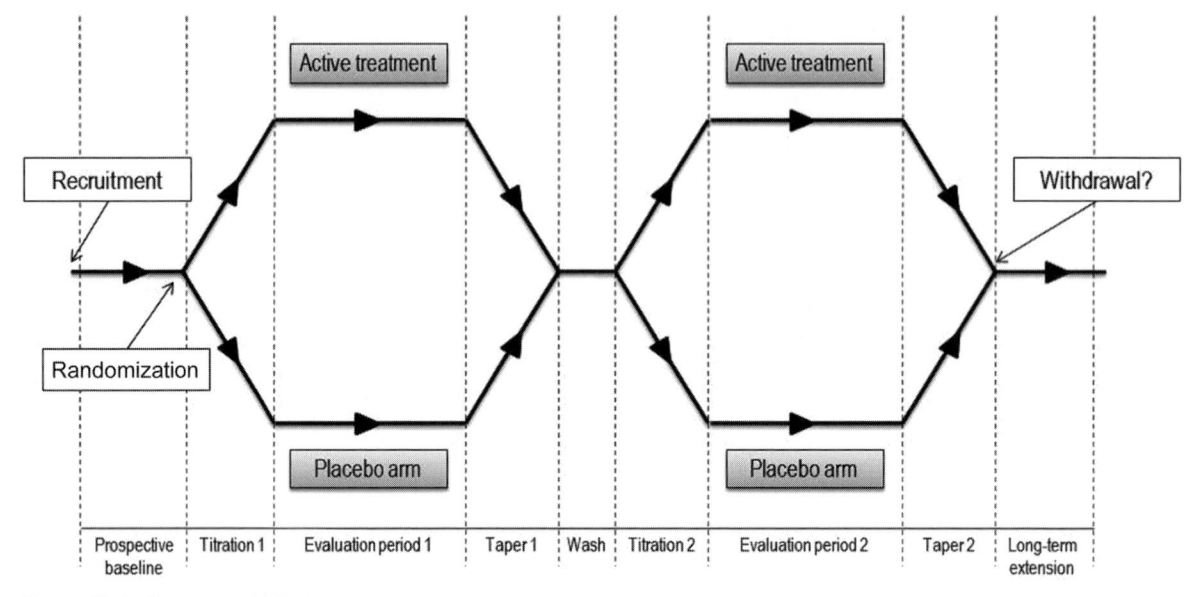

Figure 68.1. Cross-over trial design.

Trial designs

Cross-over studies (Figure 68.1)

Patients are randomized to active drug or placebo, titrated to target dose, and evaluated over a short period (8 to 12 weeks). They are then tapered off initial treatment and titrated to the alternate. Following a second evaluation period, participants are withdrawn or entered into long-term extension. Each subject acts as their own control. Fewer patients are required than in parallel-group trials. However, cross-over studies have a longer duration and do not easily accommodate multiple active drug arms. Drop-outs contribute little to analysis and unblinding is possible when the active drug is more obviously effective than placebo (French, 2006; Mohanraj and Brodie, 2003; Schmidt, 2007).

Parallel-group studies (Figure 68.2)

Patients are randomized to two or more treatment arms, titrated to target dose, and evaluated over a short period (8 to 16 weeks). Thereafter, participants are tapered off their allotted medication and withdrawn or entered into long-term extension. Parallel-group studies can include multiple active drug arms, allowing comparison of multiple doses with a single placebo group. They are relatively short in duration and easily blinded but require large numbers of participants and depend on equitable randomization (French, 2006; Mohanraj and Brodie, 2003; Schmidt, 2007).

Long-term extension studies

Long-term extension studies follow Phase II and Phase III trials. Participants are tapered to a predetermined dose of the active drug, which is subsequently administered on an open-label basis. Those experiencing efficacy in the double-blind phase benefit from continued treatment and those who may have received placebo have an opportunity for active drug exposure. These studies provide the regulators with long-term safety and efficacy data, often in several hundred patients with multiple years of treatment.

Phase I trials

Phase I trials represent first human exposure. They recruit small groups of healthy volunteers and are performed in dedicated trial units. Phase I trials are usually randomized, single- or double-blind, and placebo-controlled. They employ single and multiple dosing schedules and are designed to establish dose range, maximum tolerated dose and pharmacokinetic profile. Simultaneous exposure of multiple volunteers to the highest doses is avoided. Phase I data influence design of subsequent trials, particularly dose selection

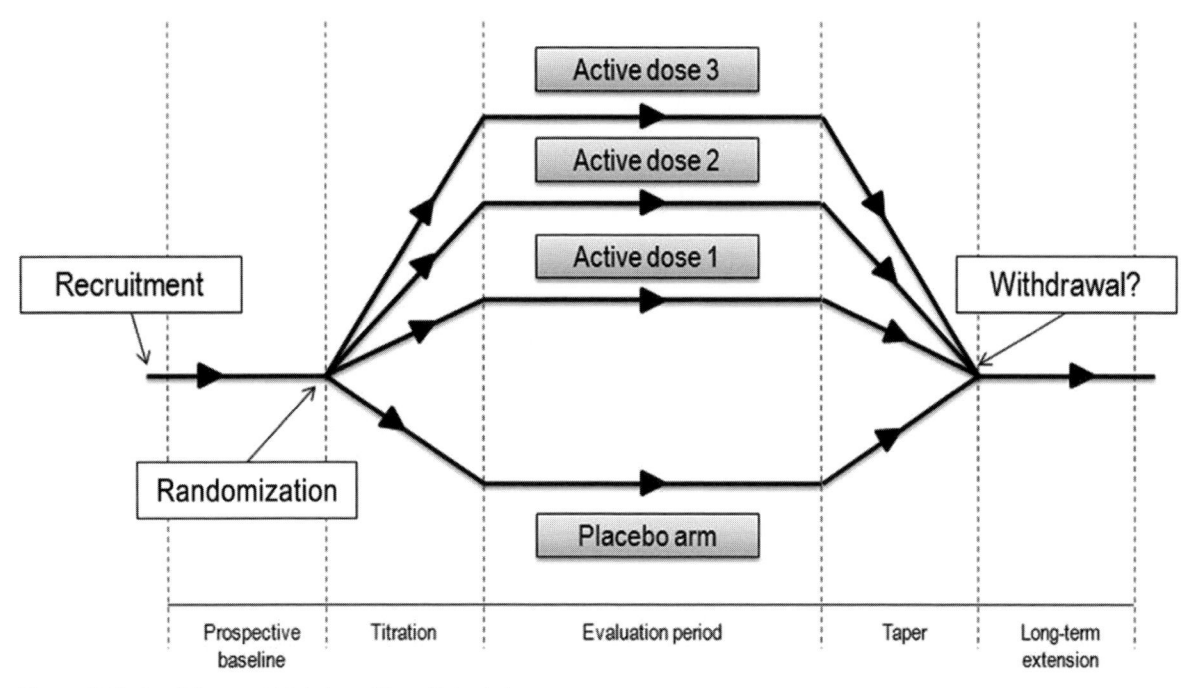

Figure 68.2. Parallel-group trial design with multiple dosing arms.

and dosing interval. If results deviate from expectation, there may be a requirement to reconsider the doses, re-formulate the drug, or abandon development altogether (French, 2006; Mohanraj and Brodie, 2003; Schmidt, 2007).

Phase II trials

Phase II trials represent first use in epilepsy patients. They are randomized, double-blind, placebo-controlled, add-on studies, usually employing a parallel-group design with long-term extension, and recruit several hundred adults with refractory partial epilepsies experiencing at least four seizures per month and taking one to three other AEDs. The objectives are to establish tolerability and safety, explore the pharmacokinetic profile and identify drug interactions. Phase II studies employ fixed doses and fast titration rates, with no inter-individual flexibility, resulting in high incidence of withdrawal due to adverse effects. The short evaluation does not provide any meaningful information on efficacy and safety (French, 2006; Schmidt, 2007).

Phase III trials

At least two Phase III trials (pivotal studies) are required for approval. They each recruit around 1000 patients and are performed as randomized, double-blind, placebo-controlled, add-on studies in adults with refractory partial seizures. The primary objective is to demonstrate superior efficacy of study medication over placebo but they also provide further information on tolerability, pharmacokinetics and drug interactions. Phase III studies generally have a multiple-dosing, parallel-group design, with a single placebo arm, two or three active treatment arms, and long-term extension. They recruit patients with refractory epilepsy, employ fixed doses and fast titration, and provide evidence of efficacy in partial seizures alone (French, 2006; Schmidt, 2007).

Submission and approval

After completion of successful Phase III trials, sponsors prepare a detailed new drug application for submission to regulatory authorities. They are obliged to include data (positive and negative) obtained at all stages of the drug development programme (preclinical and clinical) and to make results of laboratory studies and records of individual clinical trial patients available for scrutiny, if requested. Regulatory review can take upwards of 12 months.

Phase IV studies

Phase IV studies are performed after the new drug is initially licensed as add-on therapy. They focus on issues not addressed in the development programme, such as efficacy for specific syndromes and special populations. Design is variable as studies are not constrained by regulatory requirements. There is little use of blinding or placebo-control because efficacy is already established. Phase IV studies are typically pragmatic and of more clinical relevance than regulatory trials. Investigation of efficacy in other indications (i.e. neuropathic pain, migraine, bipolar disorder) is often undertaken at this stage (French, 2006; Mohanraj and Brodie, 2003; Schmidt, 2007).

Monotherapy trials

New AEDs are initially licensed for adjunctive use only. Manufacturers may seek regulatory approval as monotherapy to increase market-share and encourage first-line use of their compound. The requirements for a monotherapy licence differ between Europe and the USA. With the use of placebo unethical in monotherapy trials, the new drug must show equivalence to an established AED in an active control study (Europe) or demonstrate superiority over an established AED in a low-dose control study (US) (French, 2006; Mohanraj and Brodie, 2003; Schmidt, 2007).

Active control

Active control monotherapy studies compare the efficacy and tolerability of a new AED with an equivalent dose of an established agent in a randomized, double-blind manner. Data are analysed on the basis of 6 and 12 month seizure-free rates and the aim is to show non-inferiority. Carbamazepine is the most common comparator, and studies recruit patients with newly diagnosed partial and/or generalized tonic-clonic seizures (French, 2006; Mohanraj and Brodie, 2003; Schmidt, 2007).

Low-dose control

Low-dose control monotherapy studies compare a therapeutic dose of study drug with a minimally effective dose of an established AED (often 15 mg/kg sodium valproate) in a randomized, double-blind design. Trials recruit patients with refractory partial epilepsy, whose existing medication is tapered-off with the aim of establishing them on the new monotherapy alone. Data are typically analysed by comparing time to nth seizure. Use of low-dose control circumvents the placebo issue, affords some protection against catastrophic seizures and permits demonstration of superiority (French, 2006; Mohanraj and Brodie, 2003; Schmidt, 2007).

Monotherapy studies designed to satisfy the demands of regulatory authorities employ fixed doses and fast titration and do not necessarily allow the demonstration of efficacy in both an ethical and statistically sound manner. Active control studies are unlikely to demonstrate superiority at equivalent doses, whereas low-dose control trials are ethically questionable and recruit a different patient population (refractory epilepsy) from that for which the new drug will be licensed (newly diagnosed epilepsy).

Novel designs

New monotherapy designs can avoid the ethically questionable use of low-dose control, allow demonstration of superiority in practical numbers of patients, and simultaneously satisfy the demands of European and US regulators. A sequential analysis design has recently been used to demonstrate the superior efficacy of carbamazepine over remacemide hydrochloride in a randomized, double-blind trial in newly diagnosed epilepsy (Brodie et al., 2002). This study lasted just 18 months and included efficacy data on 449 patients. Using an active control design would have required more than 1000 patients investigated over a number of years to demonstrate the same effect.

Summary

Clinical development of new AEDs as adjunctive therapy follows a clearly defined path, through a series of trials shaped by the demands of regulatory authorities and desire of sponsors to obtain marketing approval quickly and with minimal expense. Phase I studies demonstrate tolerability and determine dose range, Phase II studies advance knowledge of tolerability and pharmacokinetics, Phase III studies enable demonstration of efficacy, and Phase IV studies provide information about the use of new AEDs in the real world. Monotherapy trials have different challenges, not least of which is the inappropriateness of placebo. Clinical development of novel AEDs is a lengthy and expensive process with no guarantee of success: there is little to suggest that it will become easier in time.

References

Brodie MJ, Wroe SJ, Dean ADP, *et al.* Efficacy and safety of remacemide versus carbamazepine in newly diagnosed epilepsy: comparison by sequential analysis. *Epilepsy Behav* 2002;**3**:140–6.

French JA. Antiepileptic drug development and experimental models. In Wyllie E, Gupta A, Lachhwani DK, eds. *The Treatment of Epilepsy: Principles and Practice*, pp. 645–53. 4th edn. New York: Lippincott, Williams & Wilkins; 2006.

Krall RL, Penry JK, White BG, Kupferberg HJ, Swinyard EA. Antiepileptic drug development: II. Anticonvulsant drug screening. *Epilepsia* 1978;**19**:409–28.

Löscher W, Schmidt D. Strategies in antiepileptic drug development: is rational drug design superior to random screening and structural variation? *Epilepsy Res* 1994;**17**:95–134.

Mohanraj R, Brodie MJ. Measuring the efficacy of antiepileptic drugs. *Seizure* 2003;**12**:413–43.

Schmidt B. Clinical development of antiepileptic drugs in adults. *Neurotherapeutics* 2007;**4**:2–9.

White HS. Preclinical development of antiepileptic drugs: past, present, and future directions. *Epilepsia* 2003; **44**(Suppl 7):2–8.

White HS, Woodhead JH, Wilcox KS, *et al.* Discovery and preclinical development of antiepileptic drugs. In Levy RH, Mattson RH, Meldrum BS, Perucca E, eds. *Antiepileptic Drugs*, pp. 36–48. 5th edn. Philadelphia: Lippincott, Williams & Wilkins; 2002.

Learning objectives

(1) To know the objectives and underlying philosophy of modern drug trial design.
(2) To be aware of the ethical issues underlying modern drug trials.
(3) To know the different stages in drug testing and drug trials involved in the development of new drugs.
(4) To know the different clinical trial designs, their advantages and disadvantages.

Section 5 **Management of epilepsy**

Chapter 69

Treatment with traditional antiepileptic drugs

Robert D. C. Elwes

Effective treatment for epilepsy has been available since the introduction of bromides in the middle of the nineteenth century. This medication was a major therapeutic advance and remained the mainstay until barbiturates were used around the time of the First World War. Ironically they were first introduced because of their known sedative effects but were found to be overall much less toxic than bromides. There are surprisingly good trials in the historical literature suggesting they were of equal efficacy. Phenytoin was introduced around the time of the Second World War and was an important advance. The drug was tested systematically in animal models and was shown to be of equal efficacy to phenobarbitone but less sedative, showing for the first time that these two therapeutic effects could be clearly separated. Valproic acid is an organic solvent and therapeutic effects were discovered by chance. Carbamazepine is related to tricyclic antidepressants and was predicted to have antiepileptic effects from its chemical structure. It quickly became apparent that valproate was highly effective for treating idiopathic generalized epilepsy and clinical trials showed that it was not as good for partial epilepsy. Both of these drugs superseded phenobarbitone and phenytoin as they have fewer long-term chronic toxic effects and appear less sedative. Randomized monotherapy trials in the 1980s, developed by Reynolds, showed, however, that there appeared to be little difference in efficacy for the common seizure types between the standard antiepileptic drugs. Comparative studies with the newer drugs have shown surprisingly similar results. The history of antiepileptic development teaches us that drugs have become less toxic and easier to use but probably not much more effective.

Principles of drug treatment

- Carbamazepine and lamotrigine remain the drugs of first choice for focal epilepsy; contrary to trials evidence, the former may be more effective in partial epilepsy.
- Valproate is the most effective drug for controlling seizures in idiopathic generalized epilepsy.
- For all drugs use a cautious initial dosing (see Table 69.1) to reduce allergic reactions and toxicity.
- About a third of people with new-onset epilepsy have their seizures fully controlled with the starting dose, for example carbamazepine 200 mg bd or phenytoin 100 mg bd. Do not escalate to an arbitrary 'therapeutic' dose; it varies for each person.
- Although once-daily doses can be given for phenytoin, phenobarbitone and valproate, most drugs should be given twice a day.
- Careful increments using the doses in Table 69.1 should be made only in response to further seizures, usually at rates no more quickly than every 1 to 2 months.
- Avoid sudden changes or abandoning a drug too early. A temporary worsening of seizures may be due to not taking tablets or intercurrent illness. Find what is best for each individual, discuss and negotiate and give the drug a proper therapeutic trial.
- Aim for a moderate to high dose if seizures continue; monitoring levels is mandatory for phenytoin and is a useful guide for the other drugs, especially if there is a worry that they are taken irregularly or not at all.
- If there are idiosyncratic intolerable side effects even at low doses switch to another first-line drug given as monotherapy.

Introduction to Epilepsy ed. Gonzalo Alarcón and Antonio Valentín. Published by Cambridge University Press.
© Cambridge University Press 2012.

Chapter 69: Treatment with traditional antiepileptic drugs

Table 69.1. Indications and doses of the standard antiepileptic drugs for the common seizure types and syndromes

Syndrome or seizure type	Drug	Doses in milligrams			
		Initiation dosing	Starting dose	Increments	Moderate to high dose
Partial/secondarily generalized	Carbamazepine	100/100 2 weeks	200/200	200	800–1600
	Lamotrigine	25, 1 week[a] 25/25 25/50 50/50	100/100	50	300–600
	(Phenytoin)	–	100/100	50[b]	300–600
	(Phenobarbitone)	–	30/30	30	120–180
Idiopathic generalized	Valproate	–	400/400	400	1600–2000

[a] Half this dose rate if on valproate; [b] 25 mg increments if phenytoin level is near or in optimum range. Drugs in parentheses are second-line.

- The aim of drug treatment in new-onset epilepsy is complete control of seizures. Do not accept 'occasional' seizures as the therapeutic goal. Using the above regimes with the first-line older antiepileptic drugs, this can be achieved in about 60–70% of cases.
- Once complete control has been obtained full remission off drugs becomes a possibility.

Toxicity

All of the drugs are to some extent sedative and the older drugs, phenobarbitone and phenytoin, are undoubtedly worse than carbamazepine, valproate or lamotrigine. The older drugs are also more prone to produce chronic toxicity (see Table 69.2). Toxic effects are often additive and, unless there has been a clear synergistic effect, drugs should wherever possible be used as monotherapy. Alertness may affect cognition but otherwise the drugs do not seem to produce major changes in memory or intellectual function that can be easily measured. At higher doses a number of nonspecific neurological symptoms such as dizziness, unsteadiness or difficulty with vision appear. Weight gain is particularly associated with valproate but can also occur with the other drugs.

Table 69.2. Chronic toxicity of standard antiepiletic drugs

Toxic effect	Drug	Monitoring
Gum hypertrophy	Phenytoin	–
Hirsuitism, facial coarsening	Phenytoin, phenobarbitone	–
Metabolic bone disease	All enzyme inducers	Calcium, vitamin D, bone scan
Megaloblastic anaemia	Phenytoin, phenobarbitone	Vitamin B12 folate
Peripheral neuropathy	Phenytoin, phenobarbitone	–
Neutropaenia	Carbamazepine	Full blood count

- Lack of major neuropsychiatric side effects (cf. levetiracetam and topiramate)
- Clinical trials suggest broadly equal efficacy to newer drugs
- Much cheaper and usage familiar to most physicians

Advantages of traditional antiepileptic drugs

- Generally well tolerated
- Long-term side effects known (cf. vigabatrin and visual failure)

Disadvantages of traditional antiepileptic drugs

- Major allergic reaction including serum sickness and organ failure can occur (phenobarbitone, phenytoin, carbamazepine and lamotrigine)

- Long-term chronic toxicity, especially phenobarbitone and phenytoin (see below)
- Phenobarbitone and phenytoin more sedative
- Rare severe idiosyncratic reactions (carbamazepine and bone marrow suppression, valproate and liver failure)
- Non-linear kinetics of phenytoin
- Active and toxic metabolites with carbamazepine
- Increased teratogenicity and possible adverse effects on fetal brain development with valproate
- Metabolized by liver microenzyme (phenobarbitone, phenytoin, carbamazepine, lamotrigine)
- Numerous and often unpredictable drug interactions
- Reduces efficacy of contraceptive pill
- Inhibition of metabolism by other drugs producing toxicity
- Interactions between antiepileptic drugs
- Interactions make use of whole groups of other drugs difficult, e.g. anti-retrovirals, immune suppression, cancer chemotherapy
- Affects vitamin B12, folate and vitamin D metabolism
- Affects endogenous and exogenous hormones, e.g. testosterone and thyroxine
- Can precipitate neuropsychiatric porphyrias

Chronic toxicity of barbiturates and hydantoins

- Low vitamin B12 and folate, rarely megaloblastic anaemia
- Metabolic bone disease and altered vitamin D metabolism
- Connective tissue changes, coarsening of face
- Peripheral neuropathy
- Movement disorders

Clinical use of phenobarbitone

The barbiturates are the most sedative of the antiepileptic drugs and will cause behaviour disorders in about 50% of children given the medication. Most adults, however, tolerate barbiturates very well. They act via the chloride ionophore, producing cell hyperpolarization and are broad-spectrum drugs, effective in partial and idiopathic generalized epilepsies. They are cheap and are still one of the most widely used antiepileptic drugs, particularly in developing countries. They are also very effective given as an intravenous bolus for the second-line treatment of status after lorazepam or phenytoin plus diazepam. Along with benzodiazepines they seem to be a medication particularly prone to producing withdrawal seizures as the dose is reduced. There is a long half-life and monitoring antiepileptic drug levels is helpful in both optimizing efficacy and avoiding toxicity. The barbiturates are potent inducers of mixed-function oxidases within the liver and have been widely associated with the various forms of chronic antiepileptic drug toxicity described above. People with bad epilepsy who have failed on some of the newer second-line antiepileptic drugs can on occasion be successfully treated with phenobarbitone.

Clinical use of phenytoin

This drug is particularly effective in symptomatic partial epilepsies. As with carbamazepine and lamotrigine the main mode of action is on the fast sodium channel and in this regard the drugs are related to local anaesthetics. Its principal problem is that liver metabolism saturates, producing non-linear kinetics. Drug levels may suddenly increase with a small dose change, even when the level is in the therapeutic range. This can produce a particularly unpleasant form of toxicity with an acute cerebellar syndrome causing ataxia, nystagmus, dysarthria and disequilibrium. This can undoubtedly on rare occasions be irreversible. Because the drug is also broken down in the liver, interactions precipitating toxicity are possible. The ability to obtain seizure control is very closely related to drug levels and careful adjustment with small doses such as 25 mg to get the level into the top half of the therapeutic range can be of benefit. It has been widely used as an intravenous drug in acute neurological disorders, especially neurosurgery. It is perhaps not the best medication in this regard, as slow intravenous injection is needed with cardiac monitoring, and extravasations during venous injection can cause unpleasant phlebitis. It is widely used in status epilepticus although again similar considerations apply. The drug produces gum hypertrophy and connective tissue changes with coarsening of the facial features, which is particularly unpleasant in young people who take the drug for many years. Its propensity to induce liver enzymes, and therefore markedly reduce the efficacy of other drugs such as steroids, is also a drawback in the treatment of acute disorders.

Clinical use of carbamazepine

This drug is related to the antidepressants in structure, and seems to be very well tolerated by the majority of people with chronic epilepsy. It is probably the most effective drug for focal seizures and most people with chronic epilepsy remain on it as their first-line medication. It is, however, rapidly absorbed, even with the slow-release preparations, which can cause side effects, particularly in the elderly. At higher doses, difficulty with vision causing oscillopsia and unsteadiness is particularly prone to occur intermittently, often 2–3 hours after the first morning dose. This is the commonest sign of impending toxicity. The rash and allergy can be quite severe and for this reason, in addition, careful initial dosing should be used. Severe haematological reactions were reported when the drug first came into use but these now seem less common. A dose-dependent neutropenia, however, is frequently seen. It is often not severe and can be managed expectantly if serial full blood counts show that the change is stable. Hyponatraemia is another common dose-related side effect but again, if mild, asymptomatic and non-progressive, can be safely observed. The drug produces both toxic and active metabolites and therefore serum level monitoring is of much less help than with phenytoin. In the face of continuing seizures, the dose can be gradually increased up to the moderate or high doses indicated in Table 69.1, without the risk of severe or sudden toxicity. It is a strong inducer of liver enzymes but seems to have far fewer of the chronic side effects that are seen with phenytoin or phenobarbitone and is in general very well tolerated. Some have claimed it may have positive psychotropic effects.

Clinical use of sodium valproate

Valproate is an organic solvent and its antiepileptic properties were discovered by chance. It has a completely different simple chemical structure when compared to the other first-line drugs. It still remains the most effective treatment for idiopathic generalized epilepsy. It is not as good as carbamazepine for focal seizures but can, in some people, be an effective second-line treatment for this disorder. The main problem has been an increase in congenital malformations, from about 0.5% in the general population up to 2–4%, compared to a rate of about 1–2% for the other major antiepileptic drugs. Lamotrigine is an alternative for absences and tonic-clonic seizures, but can make myoclonus worse at higher doses. Other effective alternative drugs in idiopathic generalized epilepsy include topiramate, levetiracetam and zonisamide, but the teratogenicity of these has yet to be determined. When it was first introduced, there were a number of reports of liver failure which nearly led to the medication being withdrawn. It became apparent, however, that this was usually in children, often with inborn errors of metabolism and who were taking other antiepileptic drugs in addition that induced liver enzymes. This probably produced a toxic metabolite which was the cause of the liver failure and this complication is now only very rarely seen. Some people with mitochondrial cytopathies are also prone to liver failure with this drug. The drug can also cause pancreatitis. Weight gain is an important side effect and appears to be particularly common in young women. Longer-term use can be associated with polycystic ovaries and infertility. The increased weight is also associated with a higher incidence of hypertension and an anti-insulin effect. Low platelets, hair loss, tremor and bradykinesia are other important dose-related side effects. The drug has a very short half-life, making serum level monitoring of limited use. The drug does, however, have a prolonged pharmacodynamic action and can in fact be given as a single daily dose. Despite all these problems it remains an important drug for the treatment of idiopathic generalized epilepsy and many derive enormous benefit from it. It is also used in symptomatic generalized epilepsies with tonic seizures, atypical absences and drop attacks.

Clinical use of lamotrigine

This was initially developed as an anti-folate medication and found to be effective in epilepsy by screening in animal models. It has a broad spectrum of efficacy, being useful in focal epilepsies and also idiopathic and symptomatic generalized epilepsy. It is, however, not as effective as valproate in idiopathic generalized epilepsy and at higher doses can make myoclonus worse. Whilst clinical trials suggest it is of equal efficacy to carbamazepine in focal epilepsy, patients who fail on lamotrigine and respond to carbamazepine do occur whilst the reverse seems less common. It is, however, very well tolerated and seems to have a particularly low incidence of sedative side effects. It is also well tolerated by people with learning difficulties. Its principal problem relates to a number of metabolic interactions. A very severe rash and allergy, sometimes with serum sickness and organ failure, can occur. This is now rarer with very careful initial dosing at the onset. The breakdown of the drug is inhibited by valproate, which effectively doubles the level of lamotrigine for a given dose. Even more careful initial dosing of lamotrigine is therefore needed in people taking valproate and, similarly, switching these two drugs over has to be done with care. Although widely marketed as a particularly good treatment for women of childbearing age, the contraceptive pill can markedly reduce the level of lamotrigine. It appears to be equally teratogenic to carbamazepine and valproate at moderate doses, and there can be a very marked fall in drug levels in the third trimester. It is perhaps the one drug where prophylactic increase in total dose in the third trimester should be considered, particularly in people with brittle or severe epilepsy. It is also quite markedly concentrated in breast milk. Dose-related toxicity is fairly mild but insomnia can be a problem. It appears to be safe for chronic long-term usage.

Clincial use of ethosuximide

Ethosuximide is highly effective in the treatment of childhood absence seizures. Recent evidence suggest that it is equally as efficacious as valproate and may be better tolerated. Both drugs may be more efficacious than lamotrigine. If the onset of the absence seizures is late, then the risks of convulsive seizures increase and valproate may be a better choice.

Clinical use of benzodiazepines

Benzodiazepines are the most effective drugs for stopping seizures acutely and their principal use is intravenously in status epilepticus. They can, however, be used in chronic epilepsy as an 'escape' medication, given intermittently to treat clusters of seizures or bad seizures occurring in the community. As with status, the indications and usage of individual drugs is dictated by mode of administration and kinetics.

Oral clobazam: this can be given 10 mg once or twice a day for about 3 or 4 days. This is helpful if there is a bad seizure cluster as in catamenial seizures or serial fits with a risk of status. The difficulty with this approach is that on careful review of patient diaries predicting a cluster is often quite difficult. As the drug is stopped, the cluster may be merely postponed.

Rectal diazepam: 10 mg given by this method acts almost as quickly as the intravenous route. It is therefore a very useful emergency treatment for a prolonged seizure if there is no venous access. As with intravenous diazepam the effect does wear off rather quickly.

Buccal midazolam: the same considerations as rectal diazepam apply but this route of administration is more socially acceptable and is now widely replacing rectal diazepam.

Benzodiazepines are not used as a first-line oral drug in epilepsy. They should not, however, be forgotten as a useful adjuvant in chronic epilepsy. A small proportion of people get a dramatic response that is sustained. If nothing has happens at 2 or 3 months or if tolerance occurs, which unfortunately is common, then the drug should be withdrawn. Long-term usage without clear benefit is to be avoided due to tolerance, increasing difficulty of stopping the drug due to withdrawal seizures and possibly reduced efficacy of parenteral benzodiazepines if these are needed in an emergency.

Conclusions

Despite a plethora of new drugs, carbamazepine and lamotrigine remain the drugs of first choice for focal epilepsy. Sodium valproate is also the most efficacious medication in idiopathic generalized epilepsy although care must be exercised in women of childbearing age. All three are relatively non-toxic and careful dose adjustment can be done on clinical grounds. All of the drugs except valproate can cause a rash and sometimes other very severe immune-related idiosyncratic reactions can occur. The older drugs such as phenytoin and phenobarbitone are more sedative and have a problem with long-term chronic toxicity, particularly affecting connective tissues. Phenytoin has nonlinear kinetics and serum level monitoring is mandatory. The induction of liver mixed-function oxidases and the large number of sometimes unpredictable drug interactions are an important drawback of the standard antiepileptic drugs. In the longer term the principal force driving new drug development has been reducing toxicity and greater ease of use, with less evidence of improving efficacy.

Recommended reading

Shorvon SD, Chadwick D, Galbraith AW, Reynolds EH. One drug for epilepsy. *Br Med J* 1978;**1**(6111):474–6.

Elwes RD, Johnson AL, Shorvon SD, Reynolds EH. The prognosis for seizure control in newly diagnosed epilepsy. *N Engl J Med* 1984;**311**:944–7.

Mattson RH, Cramer JA, Collins JF. A comparison of valproate with carbamazepine for the treatment of complex partial seizures and secondarily generalized tonic-clonic seizures in adults. The Department of Veterans Affairs Epilepsy Cooperative Study No. 264 Group. *N Engl J Med* 1992;**327**:765–71.

Heller AJ, Chesterman P, Elwes RD, *et al.* Phenobarbitone, phenytoin, carbamazepine, or sodium valproate for newly diagnosed adult epilepsy: a randomised comparative monotherapy trial. *J Neurol Neurosurg Psychiatry* 1995;**58**:44–50.

Brodie MJ, Dichter MA. Antiepileptic drugs. *N Engl J Med* 1996;**334**:168–75.

Glauser T, Ben-Menachem E, Bourgeois B, *et al.* ILAE treatment guidelines:evidence-based analysis of antiepileptic drug efficacy and effectiveness as initial monotherapy for epileptic seizures and syndromes. *Epilepsia* 2006;**47**:1094–120.

Luciano AL, Shorvon SD. Results of treatment changes in patients with apparently drug-resistant chronic epilepsy. *Ann Neurol* 2007;**62**:375–81.

Marson AG, Al-Kharusi AM, Alwaidh M, *et al.*; SANAD Study group. The SANAD study of effectiveness of valproate, lamotrigine, or topiramate for generalised and unclassifiable epilepsy: an unblinded randomised controlled trial. *Lancet* 2007;**369**(9566):1016–26.

Marson AG, Al-Kharusi AM, Alwaidh M, *et al.*; SANAD Study group. The SANAD study of effectiveness of carbamazepine, gabapentin, lamotrigine, oxcarbazepine, or topiramate for treatment of partial epilepsy: an unblinded randomised controlled trial. *Lancet* 2007;**369**(9566):1000–15.

Learning objectives

(1) To know the principles of drug treatment with traditional anticonvulsants.
(2) To be aware of the indications, toxicity, advantages and disadvantages of traditional anticonvulsants.
(3) To be aware of the principles and practicalities of the clinical use of phenobarbitone, phenytoin, carbamazepine, sodium valproate, lamotrigine, ethosuximide and benzodiazepines.

Section 5: Management of epilepsy

Chapter 70

Treatment with 'new' antiepileptic drugs

Lina Nashef

There are now many licensed antiepileptic drugs (AEDs). The older drugs include phenobarbitone, primidone, phenytoin, carbamazepine, valproate, ethosuximide and benzodiazepines, with the main first-line drugs being valproate and carbamazepine (see previous chapter). The new ones, listed alphabetically, include felbamate, gabapentin, lacosamide, lamotrigine, levetiracetam, oxcarbazepine, pregabalin, rufinamide, tiagabine, topiramate, vigabatrin and zonisamide. Others are about to be licensed (see Chapter 73). How can we make sense of all these drugs? How do we choose one medication over another? What are the characteristics of the ideal antiepileptic drug? How do we view the new AEDs in practice? How do they compare with the older drugs? What of the future?

Background

Ideally, an AED should:

- be effective against a broad range of seizure types and epilepsy syndromes
- be well tolerated in both the short and long term
- have low potential for exacerbating seizures
- have few drug interactions
- have no life-threatening or irreversible side effects and low teratogenic potential
- have a reasonably long half-life.

It should also be affordable. Once beyond its patent, however, generic substitutes usually ensure availability of a cheaper product.

For practical reasons, drug trials before licensing usually first test the efficacy and tolerability of a new AED compared to placebo as add-on treatment in adults with partial epilepsy, usually with pre-set escalation regimes. Thus, for a new AED, an add-on licence in partial seizures only should not be taken to mean lack of efficacy in monotherapy, children or in generalized epilepsy. Information regarding efficacy in other settings may not yet be available. Other trials are sometimes carried out post-marketing which allow extension of the licence, but sometimes, and where appropriate, use in clinical practice extends to other indications before this takes place. A relatively limited number of trials involve 'head-to-head' comparisons between AEDs. These are often underpowered and designed to demonstrate non-inferiority across a predefined clinical difference in response. Their utility in guiding choice is therefore limited. Additionally, pre-licensing studies allow for a drug to be licensed, but do not sufficiently inform clinical use, which evolves post-marketing. Yet, dose regimens used in such studies are often included, as recommended dosing schedules, in the data sheet and drug formularies. Most often, and with experience, new AEDs are in practice introduced more slowly than recommended in these schedules, sometimes with different dose ranges than originally quoted. Long-term efficacy is often unknown, although, in recent years, this has been partly redressed by studies reporting retention figures over the first few years of use. Finally, a word of caution! We cannot assume that a newly licensed drug is safe. First, person numbers and duration of use included in pre-licensing drug trials are too small to exclude major life-threatening side effects, which, although rare, may still be of clinically relevant frequency. Second, trial duration is usually insufficient to identify long-term side effects. With regard to the former, a recently licensed AED should not be offered in preference to an old one unless sufficient person-years of experience have accumulated. In those unresponsive to established AEDs, it may be offered before sufficient experience has accumulated only if the risk of the epilepsy is felt to outweigh the, as yet,

---

Introduction to Epilepsy ed. Gonzalo Alarcón and Antonio Valentín. Published by Cambridge University Press.
© Cambridge University Press 2012.

> **Box 70.1.** 2004 NICE guidelines (www.nice.org.uk/CG020NICEguideline)
>
> Newer AEDs are recommended:
> - For adults who have not benefited from treatment with the older AEDs (e.g. carbamazepine or sodium valproate)
> - When the older AEDs are unsuitable because:
>   - of contraindications
>   - of potential interactions with other drugs (notably oral contraceptives)
>   - they have been poorly tolerated by the person with epilepsy
>   - the person is a woman of childbearing potential

poorly defined risk of the new drug. Vigilance regarding short- and long-term side effects is required.

NICE and AEDs

Many of the available studies were reviewed by NICE in 2004. On the basis of this, NICE concluded that, in general, there were no clear advantages of the new drugs over the old, but allowed for their use in certain circumstances, with a form of words which can be interpreted as somewhat non-restrictive (see Box 70.1). Currently clinicians, at least in the UK, may use a new or old AED as first-line treatment.

Meta-analyses and Cochrane reviews

Meta-analyses and Cochrane reviews of the results of drug trials comparing new AEDs have been carried out and reported on by Chadwick, Marson and colleagues. In a review, and because of overlapping confidence intervals, 'no conclusive evidence of a difference in efficacy or tolerability between these AEDs was derived, even though the apparently most effective agent (topiramate) may be twice as effective as the apparently least effective agent (lamotrigine). Comparative randomized studies are needed to further evaluate these drugs'(Chadwick *et al.*, 1996). Whereas the observation above is that such differences have not been proven conclusively, this and similar statements have unfortunately been sometimes misrepresented as indicating that there are no significant differences between the AEDs looked at in terms of efficacy and tolerability. Such a conclusion does not concur with clinical experience, nor with the findings of the SANAD (Marson *et al.*, 2007a, 2007b) study, comparing new and old AEDs in new-onset epilepsy.

New-onset epilepsy

In new-onset epilepsy, which is reportedly generally easy to control in some two-thirds of cases, most AEDs, if appropriate to the epilepsy syndrome, have a reasonable likelihood of being effective. If the syndrome is not well-characterized, and especially if the patient is young, a broad-spectrum AED is preferred. In the patient group of new-onset epilepsy, the choice of medication, appropriate to the syndrome, will depend more on short- and long-term safety and tolerability, ease of use, low interactions, the profile of the drug, the profile of the patient and affordability. The results of the SANAD study, an open pragmatic randomized multi-centre study, favoured valproate in generalized epilepsy (Marson *et al.*, 2007a) and lamotrigine in partial epilepsy (Marson *et al.*, 2007b) amongst the drugs studied. There are a number of limitations to this study, an inevitable one of which is that it did not include all new AEDs. In any case, choice of AEDs should be individualized. For example, there are concerns about valproate in pregnancy, and suitable alternatives need to be considered first in women of childbearing age.

Intractable epilepsy

In those with intractable epilepsy, with limited response to previous AEDs, efficacy becomes paramount although the other factors still need to be taken into account. In such cases the prognosis for seizure freedom with each new AED tried is small, although significant improvement can be observed. The somewhat dire pessimism of one earlier study in terms of medication changes in those who have not responded to the first few AEDs or combinations offered was not supported by a more recent study, which clearly reported better results, albeit modest. Nevertheless, it is important that patients' and clinicians' expectations in this situation are realistic (Mohanraj and Brodie, 2006; Luciano and Shorvon, 2007).

Where are we now?

Individual 'new' AEDs are listed below with some main features, advantages and disadvantages, described including how narrow- or broad-spectrum a medication is, a key consideration in selecting an AED. Where in the pecking order a particular AED lies evolves with time and experience and depends not only on its profile, but also on how it compares with other available AEDs. Of the new AEDs, lamotrigine and levetiracetam are widely used. Both have had very successful advertising campaigns. An advantage of lamotrigine is good tolerability, particularly in terms of its cognitive and cosmetic profile, resulting in it being used early, often as first line. Advantages of levetiracetam are its lack of interactions, its efficacy against myoclonic jerks and that it has proved effective in a proportion of previously intractable patients as add-on therapy. As with all other AEDs, both have limitations (see below). Oxcarbazepine is similar to carbamazepine with better tolerance when first introduced and with no autoinduction. Topiramate is effective and broad spectrum, but is less well tolerated than some other AEDs. It is often not selected early, although its tolerability in monotherapy is better than in polytherapy. Zonisamide shares some similarities with topiramate, but seems better tolerated in moderate doses. It is also broad-spectrum despite having a licence only for focal seizures. It can be effective in IGE including intractable absences, for example, a group that can be difficult to treat. Gabapentin and pregabalin share similarities, with pregabalin the more potent. Both have a licence in pain and pregabalin is also licensed for anxiety. Both, however, can be associated with weight gain. Tiagabine has been used less than some of the other AEDs, in part because of other considerations at the time it was licensed. Although it can be associated with non-convulsive status, it can be effective in focal seizures. Lacosamide has a licence for partial epilepsy as an adjunctive treatment and appears reasonably well tolerated without significant interactions. The niche-licence of rufinamide in Lennox-Gastaut may be extended to partial seizures. Vigabatrin and felbamate have major side effects and use is very restricted. Information about teratogenicity remains limited in new AEDs apart from lamotrigine, which has a low malformation rate, comparable to carbamazepine, and is safer in pregnancy, in terms of teratogenicity, than valproate. Information about levetiracetam teratogenicity is still limited but an initial report seems promising, although this still needs to be confirmed with larger patient numbers. Safety cannot be assumed for the others at the present. All pregnant women on AEDs should be appropriately counselled prior to conception and, in the event of pregnancy, encouraged to contact one of the pregnancy registers (in the UK: www.epilepsyandpregnancy.co.uk). See also Chapter 97: 'Management of epilepsy in women'.

The greater choice of available AEDs in general, whether new or old, is an advantage. However, we cannot predict an individual patient's response to an AED with any certainty. The process of finding the most suitable AED, or AED combination, for an individual from the many options available can be lengthy and demanding of the patient and of resources. It is also often not rigorously addressed or documented, nor indeed completed. It is hoped that developments in the future, whether in relation to pharmacogenomics or surrogate markers of efficacy, can simplify this process. For the present, a well-characterized epilepsy syndrome, good knowledge of the patient and his or her priorities, and a good knowledge and experience of the use of all available AEDs, new or old, with careful review/documentation of previous AED use and outcome, as well as reasons for clinical decisions, are all needed to navigate this process. Support for the patient while medication is introduced is also needed.

Selected features of some of the new AEDs, listed alphabetically

See more details in Summaries of Product Characteristics on www.medicines.org.uk.

Felbamate. Site of action: NMDA receptors, sodium channels. Effective; broad spectrum; significant drug interactions; in view of risk of aplastic anaemia and liver failure, has restricted licence in some countries only.

Gabapentin. Site of action: possibly calcium channels. Narrow spectrum for focal epilepsy syndromes; can exacerbate generalized syndromes including myoclonus; low interaction profile: reasonably well tolerated; weight gain; more use in pain; competes with amino acids for transport mechanism with decreased bioavailability with higher doses.

Lacosamide. Site of action: sodium channels; also binds collapsin response mediator protein-2 (CRMP-2). Licence for focal epilepsy syndromes; low interaction profile: reasonably well tolerated; contraindicated with peanut allergy. Can prolong PR interval. Intravenous preparation available.

Lamotrigine. Site of action: sodium channels. Reasonably broad spectrum with efficacy against focal and generalized seizures, but not as broad spectrum as valproate; can exacerbate generalized syndromes, particulary myoclonic; some support for use as first-line monotherapy in focal or generalized epilepsy; wide dose range and half-life between individuals; half-life prolonged by valproate and reduced by enzyme-inducing AEDs; clinically significant reduction in levels by contraceptive pill and in pregnancy; reasonably well tolerated with generally good cognitive profile; slow introduction essential to minimize allergies and hypersensitivity reactions, so unsuitable if quick effect required; insomnia; low teratogenicity.

Levetiracetam. Site of action: synaptic vesicle 2A. Effective; reasonably broad spectrum with efficacy against focal and generalized seizures but perhaps not as broad spectrum as valproate in idiopathic generalized syndromes; particularly effective in myoclonus; covers many seizure types; low interaction profile; also available intravenously; side effects include headache, low mood, irritability and depression, both on introduction and with chronic treatment. Intravenous preparation available.

Oxcarbazepine. Site of action: mainly sodium channels. Effective; narrow spectrum for focal epilepsy; similar to carbamazepine and possibly equally effective; a good choice in those whose epilepsy responds to carbamazepine and who are intolerant of it; possibly greater occurrence of hyponatraemia; drug interactions present; not really new as licensed many years ago in some countries, but pregnancy data nevertheless limited.

Pregabalin. Site of action: calcium channels. Narrow spectrum for focal epilepsy syndromes; can exacerbate generalized syndromes including myoclonus; more potent than predecessor gabapentin; also has licence for generalized anxiety disorder and pain (so, like gabapentin, quickly achieved large number of person-years of exposure); dose-related weight gain; dizziness.

Rufinamide. Site of action: sodium channels. Niche-licence in Lennox-Gastaut syndrome with studies showing significant reduction in drop attacks; data also support efficacy in focal epilepsy as add-on treatment.

Tiagabine. Site of action: inhibits GABA re-uptake. Narrow spectrum for focal epilepsy syndromes. Can precipitate nonconvulsive/absence status.

Topiramate. Sites of action: sodium and calcium channels, GABA, AMPA. Effective; broad spectrum with efficacy against focal and generalized seizures including myoclonus; better tolerated in monotherapy than polytherapy but side effects not infrequent; associated with weight loss, risk of kidney stones, rarely acute glaucoma, neuropsychiatric side effects, cognitive side effects including reduction in verbal fluency; pregnancy data still limited; thus, though effective, not first line.

Vigabatrin. Site of action: inhibition of GABA transaminase. Effective; narrow spectrum, effective in focal epilepsy syndromes, although tolerance may develop. However, because of visual field defects, new use is restricted to West syndrome by specialists. For those already on it, who are aware of the risks, and nevertheless wish to stay on it, regular monitoring of visual fields is mandatory.

Zonisamide. Mechanism of action: uncertain; possibly sodium and calcium channels/GABA/glutaminergic inhibition. Effective; broad spectrum with efficacy against focal and generalized seizures, including absences; very long half-life; sulphonamide derivative, so risk of hypersensitivity/rashes; other side effects include weight loss, risk of kidney stones, effect on blood count and cognitive; pregnancy data lacking despite licence in Japan some 20 years ago.

References

Chadwick DW, Marson T, Kadir Z. Clinical administration of new antiepileptic drugs: an overview of safety and efficacy. *Epilepsia* 1996;**37**(Suppl 6):S17–22.

Luciano AL, Shorvon SD. Results of treatment changes in patients with apparently drug-resistant chronic epilepsy. *Ann Neurol* 2007;**62**(4):375–81.

Marson AG, Al-Kharusi AM, Alwaidh M, et al.; SANAD Study group. The SANAD study of effectiveness of valproate, lamotrigine, or topiramate for generalised and unclassifiable epilepsy: an unblinded randomised controlled trial. *Lancet* 2007a;**369**(9566):1016–26.

Marson AG, Al-Kharusi AM, Alwaidh M, et al.; SANAD Study group. The SANAD study of effectiveness of carbamazepine, gabapentin, lamotrigine, oxcarbazepine, or topiramate for treatment of partial epilepsy: an unblinded randomised controlled trial. *Lancet* 2007b;**369**(9566):1000–15.

Mohanraj R, Brodie MJ. Diagnosing refractory epilepsy: response to sequential treatment schedules. *Eur J Neurol* 2006;**13**(3):277–82.

National Institute for Health and Clinical Excellence. *Newer Drugs for Epilepsy in Adults*. NICE Technology Appraisal Guidance no. 76. London:

Section 5: Management of epilepsy

National Institute for Health and Clinical Excellence; 2004. Available from: http://www.nice.org.uk/TA076.

Learning objectives

(1) To know the principles of drug treatment with new anticonvulsants.

(2) To be aware of the indications, toxicity, advantages and disadvantages of new anticonvulsants.

(3) To be aware of the principles and practicalities of the clinical use of newly approved antiepileptic drugs.

Section 5 Management of epilepsy

Chapter 71: Pharmacological interactions

Philip N. Patsalos

Introduction

Antiepileptic drugs (AEDs) administered as monotherapy regimens can make approximately 70% of newly diagnosed patients with epilepsy seizure-free. For the remainder, a combination of two or more AEDs may be required to optimize seizure control and consequently the potential for drug interactions is considerable, and such interactions may have a profound impact on the well-being of patients.

Mechanisms of drug interactions

Interactions can be divided into two types, pharmacokinetic and pharmacodynamic. Pharmacokinetic interactions, which represent the largest category of AED interactions, are associated with a change in plasma drug concentration, are readily identifiable and are the consequence of a change in the absorption, distribution, metabolism or excretion of the affected drug. Pharmacodynamic interactions take place directly at the site of action and result in a modification of the pharmacological effect without any change in drug concentrations. The effects of the interacting drugs can be additive (when they equal the sum of the effects of the individual drugs), synergistic (when the combined effects are greater than expected from the sum of individual effects) or antagonistic (when the combined effects are less than additive). Pharmacodynamic interactions can be adverse (when the increase in toxicity is greater than any gain in anticonvulsant activity) or beneficial (when therapeutic effects are additive or synergistic, and toxic effects are less than additive). Pharmacodynamic interactions are less well-recognized and are usually concluded by default when a change in the clinical status of a patient consequent to a drug interaction cannot be ascribed to a pharmacokinetic mechanism.

Pharmacokinetic interactions

Interactions affecting drug absorption

Interactions at the absorption level are uncommon in AED therapy. One example is the impaired phenytoin absorption which is seen when the drug is given together with certain nasogastric feeds.

Displacement from plasma protein binding

Interactions between two drugs for binding sites on plasma proteins are common but in quantitative terms these are only important for drugs which are more than 90% bound to plasma proteins (e.g. phenytoin, valproic acid).

The displacement of protein-bound phenytoin by valproic acid typically results in a fall in total phenytoin concentration while the concentration of free, pharmacologically active, phenytoin is unaltered because the liver metabolizes any transient increase in free concentration that occurs. In some patients, a modest rise in free phenytoin concentration may actually be seen, due to a concomitant inhibition of phenytoin metabolism by valproic acid or, possibly, a transient displacement of phenytoin from tissue binding sites, which may be associated occasionally with signs of phenytoin toxicity. The most important implication of this interaction, however, is that the 'therapeutic' range of total plasma phenytoin concentrations is shifted towards lower values.

Metabolic drug interactions

Induction and inhibition of drug metabolism represent by far the most important mechanisms of pharmacokinetic interactions with AEDs. Enzyme induction, primarily by carbamazepine, phenytoin, phenobarbital and primidone, is the consequence of an increase in

---

Introduction to Epilepsy ed. Gonzalo Alarcón and Antonio Valentín. Published by Cambridge University Press.
© Cambridge University Press 2012.

the synthesis of certain drug-metabolizing isoenzymes in the liver resulting in an increase in enzyme activity and an increase in the rate of metabolism of drugs which are substrates of those enzymes, leading to a decrease in plasma concentration of the affected drug. If the affected drug has an active metabolite, this complicates the interaction because induction can result in increased metabolite concentration and possibly an increase in drug toxicity. Because enzyme induction requires synthesis of new enzymes, the time course of induction (and its reversal upon removal of the inducer) is gradual and dose-dependent and relates to the rate of enzyme synthesis and degradation and the time to reach steady-state concentrations of the inducing drug.

Enzyme inhibition is the process by which a drug or its metabolite(s) blocks the activity of one or more drug-metabolizing enzymes, resulting in a decrease in the rate of metabolism of the affected drug and an increase in plasma concentrations of the affected drug and, possibly, clinical toxicity. Inhibition is usually competitive in nature and dose-dependent, and tends to begin as soon as sufficient concentrations of the inhibitor are achieved, with significant inhibition being often observed within 24 hours after addition of the inhibitor.

In recent years, the prediction of metabolic interactions has become more feasible because the isoenzymes responsible for the metabolism of individual drugs have been characterized. The primary enzyme system responsible for the metabolism of AEDs is the cytochrome P450 (CYP) in the liver. Three isoenzymes (CYP2C9, CYP2C19 and CYP3A4) are of particular importance in relation to AED interactions. Databases listing substrates, inhibitors and inducers of different CYP isoenzymes provide an invaluable resource in helping the physician to predict and to avoid potential interactions. For example, knowledge that carbamazepine is an inducer of CYP3A4 allows one to predict that it will reduce the plasma concentration of CYP3A4 substrates such as ethosuximide and tiagabine.

Another enzyme system that is important with regard to AEDs is that of the uridine glucuronyl transferases (UGTs) that catalyse the process of glucuronidation. UGT1A4 isoenzyme plays an important role in the glucuronidation of lamotrigine, whereas UGT1A3 and UGT2B7 catalyse the glucuronide conjugation of valproic acid. These glucuronidation processes are susceptible to inhibition and induction.

Interactions affecting renal excretion

Agents which cause alkalinization of urine enhance the elimination of phenobarbital by reducing the reabsorption of this acidic drug from the renal tubuli. There are no other examples of major AED interactions involving renal excretion processes.

Pharmacodynamic interactions

Clinical evidence does indicate that some AED combinations are more beneficial than others. For example, valproic acid and ethosuximide in combination can lead to control of absence seizures in patients refractory to either drug given alone. Lamotrigine and valproic acid in combination show remarkable effectiveness against refractory complex partial seizures and absence seizures. Patients receiving this combination, however, may also experience increased toxicity, particularly hand tremor, that requires adjustment in the dosage of both drugs. Other AED combinations for which favourable pharmacodynamic interactions have been claimed include carbamazepine with valproic acid, valproic acid with clonazepam, carbamazepine with vigabatrin, lamotrigine with vigabatrin, lamotrigine with topiramate, lamotrigine with gabapentin and vigabatrin with tiagabine.

Interactions between different AEDs

The propensity for AEDs to interact pharmacokinetically with other AEDs is substantial, and by far the most interacting AEDs are phenytoin, carbamazepine, valproic acid and phenobarbital. Gabapentin, levetiracetam, pregabalin and vigabatrin are the only AEDs that are not associated with such clinically significant interactions. The probability of a drug interaction occurring and the associated clinical consequences are dependent on a number of factors (Box 71.1). A comprehensive summary of pharmacokinetic interactions between AEDs is given in Table 71.1. Those that are most relevant clinically are discussed briefly below.

Carbamazepine

Carbamazepine, phenytoin, phenobarbital and primidone are potent inducers of various CYP isoenzymes and they also induce UGT and epoxide hydrolases. As a result, these compounds stimulate the metabolism of other concurrently administered AEDs, most notably valproic acid, tiagabine, ethosuximide, lamotrigine,

Chapter 71: Pharmacological interactions

Box 71.1. Factors that affect the clinical significance of a metabolic interaction
- The nature of the interaction – is the drug a substrate, an inhibitor or an inducer of the isoenzyme?
- The spectrum of isoenzymes that are induced or inhibited by the interacting AED.
- The potency of the inhibition/induction – a potent effect will result in a more substantial interaction affecting most patients.
- The extent of metabolism of the substrate through the particular isoenzyme – if the affected enzyme is only responsible for a small fraction of the drug's clearance, its inhibition is not going to result in a substantial interaction. Conversely, enzyme induction may increase the activity of the affected enzyme several-fold, and therefore it may increase substantially the total clearance of the drug.
- The saturability of the isoenzyme – isoenzymes that are saturable at drug concentrations encountered clinically are more susceptible to significant inhibitory interactions.
- The presence of pharmacologically active metabolites – such metabolites complicate the outcome of a potential interaction, and may themselves act as enzyme inducers or inhibitors.
- The therapeutic window of the AED – interactions affecting AEDs with a narrow therapeutic window are more likely to be of clinical significance.
- The concentration of the affected AED at baseline – any change in plasma AED concentration will have deleterious consequences if the baseline concentration is near the threshold of toxicity. In contrast if the baseline concentration is very low, an increase in efficacy may occur and a favourable therapeutic outcome may result.
- The genetic predisposition of the individual patient – subjects who show deficiency of a genetically polymorphic isoenzyme (e.g. CYP2C19) will not exhibit interactions mediated by induction or inhibition of that isoenzyme.
- The susceptibility and the sensitivity of the individual in relation to adverse effects – as a patient group the elderly are more susceptible to interactions because they are more likely to receive multiple medications. Also, the elderly are more sensitive to the adverse effects of drugs.

topiramate, zonisamide, oxcarbazepine and its active monohydroxy-metabolite, felbamate and many benzodiazepine drugs. The metabolism of carbamazepine itself can be markedly stimulated by co-administration of phenytoin or barbiturates.

In patients taking carbamazepine, administration of valproic acid may lead to an increase in the concentration of the active metabolite carbamazepine-10,11-epoxide through inhibition of the enzyme epoxide hydrolase, without any marked changes in the concentration of the parent drug. Valpromide, an amide derivative of valproic acid that is considered to be a valproic acid pro-drug, also inhibits epoxide hydrolase but the effect is much more pronounced than that seen with valproic acid. Thus, addition of valpromide to the therapeutic regimen of a patient stabilized on carbamazepine results in up to 8-fold increases in carbamazepine-10,11-epoxide concentrations and, frequently, signs of toxicity. For patients treated with carbamazepine, valpromide and valproic acid should not be used interchangeably.

Eslicarbazepine acetate

Phenytoin can increase the clearance of eslicarbazepine and decrease eslicarbazepine serum levels by 31–33%. A similar effect can occur with carbamazepine and indeed may occur with phenobarbital and primidone.

Ethosuximide

Carbamazepine, phenytoin, phenobarbital and primidone enhance the metabolism of ethosuximide, resulting in lower plasma concentrations.

Gabapentin

Gabapentin does not undergo metabolism but is instead excreted in urine in the unchanged form. Also, it is not bound to plasma albumin. Consequently, gabapentin is not expected to be associated with any significant pharmacokinetic interactions and indeed to date none have been described.

Lacosamide

Lacosamide undergoes moderate (60%) hepatic metabolism by non-CYP-dependent enzymes. Consequently, lacosamide is not expected to be associated with any significant pharmacokinetic interactions and indeed to date none have been described.

Table 71.1. Expected changes in plasma concentrations when an antiepileptic drug (AED) is added to a pre-existing AED regimen

	Pre-existing AED														
	PB	PHT	PRM	ETS	CBZ	VPA	OXC	LTG	GBP	TPM	TGB	LEV	ZNS	VGB	STP	RFN
PB	—	PHT↑↓	NCCP	ETS↓	CBZ↓	VPA↓	H-OXC↓	LTG↓	↔	TPM↓	TGB↓	↔	ZNS↓	↔	STP↓	RFN↓
PHT	PB↑	—	PRM↓ PB↑	ETS↓	CBZ↓	VPA↓	H-OXC↓	LTG↓	↔	TPM↓	TGB↓	↔	ZNS↓	↔	STP↓	RFN↓
PRM	NCCP	PHT↑↓	—	ETS↓	CBZ↓	VPA↓	?	LTG↓	↔	TPM↓	TGB↓	↔	ZNS↓	↔	STP↓	RFN↓
ETS	↔	↔	NA	—	↔	VPA↓	NA	NA	NA	NA	NA	NA	NA	NA	?	?
CBZ	↔	PHT↑↓	PRM↓	ETS↓	—	VPA↓	H-OXC↓	LTG↓	↔	TPM↓	TGB↓	↔	ZNS↓	NA	STP↓	RFN↓
VPA	PB↑↑	PHT↑↓*	PB↑↑	ETS↑↓	CBZ-E↑	—	H-OXC↓	LTG↑	↔	TPM↓	↔	↔	↔	NA	?	RFN↑↑
OXC	PB↑	PHT↑	?	?	CBZ↓	↔	—	LTG↓	NA	?	?	NA	NA	NA	?	?
LTG	↔	↔	NA	NA	↔	↔	NA	—	NA	NA	NA	↔	ZNS	NA	?	?
GBP	↔	↔	NA	NA	↔	↔	NA	NA	—	NA	NA	↔	NA	NA	?	?
TPM	↔	PHT↑	↔	NA	↔	VPA↓	?	?	NA	—	?	NA	NA	NA	?	?
TGB	↔	↔	↔	NA	↔	↔	NA	NA	NA	NA	—	NA	NA	NA	?	?
LEV	↔	↔	↔	NA	↔	↔	NA	↔	NA	NA	NA	—	NA	NA	?	?
ZNS	↔	↔	NA	NA	CBZ↑↓	?	?	↔	NA	NA	NA	NA	—	NA	?	?
VGB	PB↓	PHT↓	PRM↓ PB↓	NA	CBZ↓	↔	NA	NA	NA	NA	NA	NA	NA	—	?	RFN↓
STP	PB↑	PHT↑	PRM↑ PB↑	?	CBZ↑↑	VPA↑	?	?	?	?	?	?	?	?	—	?
RFN	?	?	?	?	?	?	?	?	?	?	?	?	?	?	—	—

CBZ, carbamazepine; CBZ-E, carbamazepine-10,11-epoxide; ETS, ethosuximide; GBP, gabapentin; H-OXC, 10-hydroxy-oxcarbazepine (active metabolite of OXC); LTG, lamotrigine; OXC, oxcarbazepine; PB, phenobarbital; PHT, phenytoin; PRM, primidone; RFN, rufinamide; STP, stiripentol; TGB, tiagabine; TPM, topiramate; VPA, valproic acid; VGB, vigabatrin; ZNS, zonisamide. NA, none anticipated; * free (pharmacologically active) concentration may increase; NCCP, not commonly co-prescribed; ↔, no change; ↓, a usually minor (or inconsistent) decrease in plasma concentration; ↓↓, a usually clinically significant decrease in plasma concentration; ↑, a usually minor (or inconsistent) increase in plasma concentration; ↑↑, a usually clinically significant increase in plasma concentration.

Lamotrigine

Enzyme-inducing AEDs (carbamazepine, phenytoin, phenobarbital and primidone) enhance the metabolism of lamotrigine so that its dosage requirement is significantly increased.

Valproic acid, in contrast, inhibits the metabolism of lamotrigine, resulting in significant increase in plasma lamotrigine concentrations. When valproic acid is co-ingested with an enzyme-inducing AED, enzyme induction and enzyme inhibition tend to cancel each other out, and the rate of lamotrigine metabolism will approach that seen in patients on lamotrigine monotherapy.

The introduction of lamotrigine in a patient already taking valproic acid should be undertaken with caution, using a low starting dose (in adults, 25 mg on alternate days) and a slow dose escalation rate to avoid problems related to a fast increment in plasma lamotrigine concentration, particularly skin rashes. However, there is no risk of rash if valproic acid is introduced in a patient already stabilized on lamotrigine, although in such a patient a reduction in the dosage of lamotrigine (as a rule of thumb, by about 50%) is advisable as soon as the dosage of valproate reaches, in an adult, about 250–500 mg/day.

Levetiracetam

Levetiracetam is minimally metabolized by hydrolysis in blood, which is not CYP-dependent. Also, it is not bound to plasma albumin. Consequently, levetiracetam is not expected to be associated with any significant pharmacokinetic interactions and indeed to date none have been described.

Oxcarbazepine

Oxcarbazepine is a pro-drug and is rapidly metabolized to a 10-hydroxy metabolite which is responsible for the pharmacological action of oxcarbazepine. The metabolism of the 10-OH metabolite is enhanced by the enzyme-inducing AEDs, resulting in lower plasma concentrations and typically requiring higher doses of oxcarbazepine to be prescribed.

Phenobarbital

By far the most important interaction affecting phenobarbital is that of inhibition of its metabolism by valproic acid. On average, the increase in plasma phenobarbital concentration after addition of valproic acid is of the order of 30–50%, but inter-individual variability is considerable and a reduction in phenobarbital (or primidone) dosage by up to 80% may be required to avoid side effects, particularly sedation and cognitive impairment.

Phenytoin

Phenytoin has some rather unusual and unique pharmacokinetic characteristics that make it particularly susceptible to interactions. These include saturable metabolism and the fact that it is only weakly bound to CYP isoenzymes (CYP2C9 and CYP2C19 responsible for ~80% and ~20% of metabolism respectively). Consequently it is the most interacting AED that is available in clinical practice. Oxcarbazepine is a weak inhibitor of the CYP2C19 isoenzyme and as a result oxcarbazepine, particularly when used at high dosages (> 1800 mg/day), may increase plasma phenytoin concentrations by up to 40%. Carbamazepine may also cause a modest increase in plasma phenytoin concentration, but this interaction is inconsistent. Topiramate is also a weak inhibitor of CYP2C19, which might explain its ability to increase plasma phenytoin concentrations in a small subset of patients.

Pregabalin

Pregabalin does not undergo metabolism but is instead excreted in urine in the unchanged form. Also, it is not bound to plasma albumin. Consequently, pregabalin is not expected to be associated with any significant pharmacokinetic interactions and indeed to date none have been described.

Primidone

Because primidone is primarily metabolized to two pharmacologically active metabolites, phenobarbital and phenylethylmalonic acid, with the former being the principal metabolite, the interactions that can be expected with primidone are those observed with phenobarbital.

Rufinamide

Rufinamide is extensively metabolized by non-CYP-dependent hydrolysis and is minimally bound to plasma albumin (~34%). Consequently, rufinamide is not expected to be associated with any significant pharmacokinetic interactions. Nevertheless, valproic acid increases (~42%) whilst phenytoin, primidone, phenobarbital, carbamazepine and vigabatrin decease (25–46%) rufinamide plasma concentrations. In addition, plasma phenytoin concentrations are increased (~21%) when co-ingested with rufinamide.

Stiripentol

Stiripentol undergoes metabolism which is saturable and also it is substantially bound to albumin (99%). In addition it is a potent inhibitor of CYP isoenzymes. These features would suggest that stiripentol is highly interacting and indeed that is the case. The enzyme-inducing AEDs enhance the metabolism of stiripentol whilst stiripentol inhibits the metabolism of numerous AEDs (carbamazepine, phenytoin, phenobarbital, primidone, clobazam), resulting in elevated plasma concentrations.

Tiagabine

Tiagabine is extensively metabolized and is substantially bound to plasma albumin (96%). When co-prescribed with enzyme-inducing AEDs, tiagabine plasma concentrations are significantly reduced, necessitating higher tiagabine doses so as to maintain seizure control. Plasma protein binding displacement interactions with valproic acid and salicylic acid have been described but their clinical significance has yet to be ascertained.

Topiramate

Topiramate is minimally metabolized in the liver (~40%) and its protein binding is 10%. However, when co-prescribed with enzyme-inducing AEDs, topiramate metabolism becomes an important feature in its elimination and typically topiramate plasma concentrations decline by 50%, requiring higher doses of topiramate.

Valproic acid

Among commonly used AEDs, valproic acid stands out by far for its ability to act as an inhibitor of drug metabolism and increasing plasma concentration (e.g. phenobarbital, lamotrigine). In contrast, plasma concentration of valproic acid can be reduced on average by 76%, 49% and 66% in patients co-medicated with phenobarbital, phenytoin and carbamazepine respectively.

Vigabatrin

Vigabatrin does not undergo metabolism but is instead excreted in urine in the unchanged form. Also, it is not bound to plasma albumin. Consequently, vigabatrin is not expected to be associated with any significant pharmacokinetic interactions. However, vigabatrin can decrease the plasma concentration of phenytoin through an unidentified mechanism.

Zonisamide

Zonisamide is metabolized in the liver by CYP-dependent isoenzymes and consequently the enzyme-inducing AEDs will enhance its metabolism, resulting in lower plasma zonisamide concentrations.

Conclusions

Interactions between AEDs are numerous and multiple drug therapy should only be considered when it is clearly indicated. Most patients with epilepsy can be best managed with a carefully individualized dosage of a single AED. Whilst it is impractical to memorize all known interactions it is important to be aware of the most important interactions and to understand their underlying mechanisms so as to be able to anticipate the consequence of the interaction and to plan any corrective action (e.g. altered dosing requirements). Most interactions are metabolically based and can be predicted from knowledge of the isoenzymes responsible for the metabolism of the most commonly used drugs and the effects of these drugs on the same isoenzymes.

If a pharmacokinetic interaction is anticipated, monitor, if appropriate, the plasma concentration of the affected drug. Be aware that under certain circumstances (e.g. in the presence of drug displacement from plasma proteins) routine total drug concentration measurements may be misleading and patient management may benefit from monitoring of free drug concentrations. In some cases, dosage adjustments may have to be implemented at the time the interacting drug is added or removed.

Recommended reading

Johannessen Landmark C, Patsalos PN. Drug interactions involving the new second- and third-generation antiepileptic drugs. *Expert Rev Neurotherapeut* 2010;**10**:119–40.

Patsalos PN. *Anti-epileptic Drug Interactions. A Clinical Guide.* Guildford: Clarius Press; 2005.

Patsalos PN, Froscher W, Pisani, F, van Rijn CM. The importance of drug interactions in epilepsy therapy. *Epilepsia* 2002;**43**:365–85.

Patsalos PN, Perucca E. Clinically important interactions in epilepsy: general features and interactions between antiepileptic drugs. *Lancet Neurol* 2003; **6**:347–56.

Learning objectives

(1) To know the distinction between pharmacodynamic and pharmacokinetic interactions.
(2) To be aware of the mechanisms responsible for drug interactions.
(3) To know the most common clinically significant interactions between antiepileptic drugs.

Section 5 **Management of epilepsy**

Chapter 72: Monotherapy or polytherapy?

Edward H. Reynolds

Introduction

Polytherapy has characterized the treatment of epilepsy throughout the ages, the more so as prior to the introduction of bromides in 1856 the many medications utilized were of doubtful antiepileptic efficacy. Paradoxically in the twentieth century, with the availability of drugs of proven efficacy, the phenomenon of polytherapy has flourished, especially in Western countries. In a study of 15 centres in four European countries, including the UK, the mean number of drugs per patient was 3.2, of which 84% were antiepileptic (see Reynolds and Shorvon, 1981).

Reasons for polytherapy (Box 72.1)

Epilepsy is predominantly a disorder of early life, commencing before the age of 20 in approximately three-quarters. Although some syndromes, especially in childhood, have a good prognosis, many others, especially those with partial seizures with or without secondary generalization, brain pathology, learning and/or psychosocial disabilities and a long history of seizures, often have a poor prognosis, needing long-term or even lifelong treatment. Even patients who experience complete remission of seizures for up to 5 years on treatment have a relatively high relapse rate of 20–40% on withdrawing medication, especially in the presence of the above adverse prognostic factors. Furthermore some of the relapses are due to withdrawal seizures, because of insufficient caution in reducing medication, thus perpetuating treatment, very often with polytherapy.

Other very important contributions to polytherapy are the increasing numbers of new antiepileptic drugs (AEDs), especially in the late twentieth century (see Table 72.1), inadequate information about the comparative efficacy of individual drugs or drug combinations, and therefore the choice of drugs, and finally a serious lack of guidelines on the limits of antiepileptic drug therapy. Prior to the 1970s there had hardly ever been a controlled trial of an antiepileptic drug and none in newly diagnosed epileptic patients. New drugs were always evaluated by adding them to chronic patients on one or more other drugs, and the only restraint on polytherapy was the occurrence of acute symptoms of toxicity, which were more likely on polytherapy (Reynolds, 1975).

Problems associated with polytherapy (Box 72.2)

From the 1960s onwards there was increasing awareness that long-term AED therapy was commonly associated with previously unsuspected chronic toxicity, sometimes subtle cognitive and behavioural effects or subtle metabolic effects (e.g. liver enzyme induction, folic acid or vitamin D deficiency). Much of this chronic toxicity was related to polytherapy and could be reduced or avoided with monotherapy (Reynolds, 1975). At the same time, the introduction of techniques for blood level monitoring of the

> **Box 72.1.** Reasons for polytherapy (Reynolds and Shorvon, 1981)
> - Early age of onset of seizures
> - Poor long-term prognosis in many patients
> - Prolonged medication
> - Recurrence on drug withdrawal
> - Many available drugs (including combined formulations)
> - Poor drug evaluation (trials in chronic patients)
> - No guidelines to limits of therapy (other than toxicity)

Introduction to Epilepsy ed. Gonzalo Alarcón and Antonio Valentín. Published by Cambridge University Press.
© Cambridge University Press 2012.

Chapter 72: Monotherapy or polytherapy?

Table 72.1. Standard and new antiepileptic drugs

Drug	Date of introduction	Optimum blood level range (μg/ml)
• Phenobarbitone	1912	20–40
• Phenytoin	1938	10–20
• Carbamazepine	1965	5–10
• Valproate	1967	50–100
• Clobazam	1975	–
New drugs		
• Lamotrigine	1990	5–15
• Oxcarbazepine	1990	As for carbamazepine
• Gabapentin	1994	–
• Topiramate	1995	–
• Tiagabine	1996	–
• Levetiracetam	1999	–
• Zonisamide	2000	–
• Pregabalin	2004	–

Vigabatrin (1989) and felbamate (1993) have been withdrawn due to unacceptable side effects.

Box 72.2. Problems associated with polytherapy (Reynolds and Shorvon, 1981)
- Chronic toxicity
- Drug interactions
- Failure to evaluate individual AEDs
- Exacerbation of seizures

standard drugs phenobarbitone, phenytoin, carbamazepine and valproate stimulated an enormous literature on drug interactions between AEDs and between AEDs and non-AEDs, some of which could lead to loss of seizure control, some to increased toxicity and some of little consequence. The widespread practice of polytherapy also undermined the possibility of evaluating the comparative efficacy and toxicity of individual drugs, especially as monotherapy. Finally there was growing evidence that unrestrained polytherapy could actually exacerbate epilepsy in some patients.

Unnecessary polytherapy

A common cause of polytherapy in the past was the utilization of combined capsules or tablets of two or more drugs, e.g. phenobarbitone and phenytoin, even at the start of antiepileptic therapy. This was usually in the unsubstantiated belief either that combinations of two (or more) drugs had a synergistic antiepileptic effect or that the summation of modest doses of two drugs would enhance efficacy, while limiting toxicity with either drug, concepts that are still misguidingly promoted today, especially by the pharmaceutical industry, under the umbrella of 'rational polytherapy'.

In retrospective and prospective studies of chronic adult epileptic patients on two drugs, it was noted that the addition of the second drug resulted in at least 50% improvement in seizure control in only approximately one-third. In the majority, seizure control was unchanged and in about 10–20% it was worse. At the same time in the 1970s and 1980s several studies of cautious reduction of polytherapy to optimum monotherapy, guided by AED monitoring, greatly improved cognitive and social function, especially alertness, concentration and mood, in most chronic patients, while actually improving seizure control in about one-third. In most patients, seizure control was unchanged and in only one-quarter were seizures worse, necessitating continuation of polytherapy (Reynolds and Shorvon, 1981).

Monotherapy in newly diagnosed patients

As the evidence grew that much polytherapy in chronic patients was unnecessary, unhelpful and quite often harmful, the availability of blood level monitoring of standard first-line AEDs greatly facilitated the evaluation of optimum monotherapy, especially in newly diagnosed adults and children.

The first studies were undertaken at King's in the mid-1970s and were rapidly replicated in the UK and other countries. It was soon apparent that in previously untreated patients with at least two or more generalized seizures or partial seizures with or without secondary generalization, 70–80% entered 1 or 2 year remission on carefully monitored optimum monotherapy with phenobarbitone, phenytoin, carbamazepine or valproate. The great majority of these patients went on to longer-term remission. Late relapses were rare. The policy was to begin with small doses of the initial drug and only to increase the dose gradually, if necessary into the optimum blood level range, if seizures recurred despite good compliance. Poor compliance is a major issue in the development and perpetuation of polytherapy. Failure of optimum monotherapy in 20–30% usually occurred within the first 2 years of therapy and was very often followed by chronic epilepsy. The main causes of failure of monotherapy were poor compliance and the presence of brain pathology. Thus partial seizures are usually slightly more difficult to control than generalized seizures, as is also apparent in chronic patients. These observations were also gradually replicated in children with similar types of epilepsy (Reynolds and Shorvon, 1981; Perucca, 1997).

The success of monotherapy with several drugs in most newly diagnosed patients posed the difficult question: which is the drug of first choice for such patients? In the 1980s and 1990s several large prospective randomized pragmatic long-term studies failed to show any significant differences in efficacy between the standard drugs, phenobarbitone, phenytoin, carbamazepine and valproate, in adults or children presenting with untreated generalized or partial seizures, excluding myoclonus or other childhood syndromes, e.g. absence seizures. Of the four drugs phenobarbitone, including primidone, was less well tolerated than the other three. Overall, however, nine out of ten patients tolerated the first drug administered (Mattson et al., 1992; Heller et al., 1995; de Silva et al., 1996).

Should the 20–30% of newly diagnosed patients who fail to respond to optimum monotherapy be treated with alternative monotherapy or, as in the past, by the addition of a second drug? There has been no definitive study of this question. Open practical experience suggests that relatively small numbers of patients subsequently become seizure-free by adding a second (or third) drug or by switching to alternative monotherapy (Kwan and Brodie, 2000). In the only controlled trial, the probability of remaining seizure-free over the next year was 16% for patients given a second drug and 14% for those switched to alternative monotherapy (Beghi et al., 2003).

Over a 15-year period prior to 2004, ten new AEDs became available in the UK, mainly as adjunctive therapy in adults with chronic epilepsy resistant to monotherapy with one of the standard drugs (Table 72.1). These drugs have rarely been compared with one another and no important differences have been found. Clobazam, however, initially has a more dramatic effect in chronic epilepsy, which unfortunately is subsequently reduced in some by tolerance to the drug.

More recently attempts have been made to compare some of these new drugs with the older standard drugs as initial monotherapy in newly diagnosed patients. In a large multicentre prospective randomized pragmatic controlled trial of newly diagnosed patients with partial seizures with or without secondary generalization, the standard drug, carbamazepine, was compared with the new drugs gabapentin, lamotrigine, oxcarbazepine and topiramate. No clinically important differences between the drugs were found but lamotrigine was viewed as the most suitable alternative to carbamazepine in such patients (Marson et al., 2007). In a similar trial in newly diagnosed patients with generalized seizures, valproate was utilized as the standard drug for comparison with lamotrigine and topiramate, as all three are thought to possess 'broad-spectrum' activity. Valproate was slightly more efficacious than lamotrigine and better tolerated than topiramate, and was therefore viewed as still the drug of first choice, except in women of childbearing age, where the potential for teratogenicity may lead to consideration of one of the alternatives (Marson et al., 2007). It is worth noting that blood level monitoring of the newer drugs is hardly ever studied or utilized and therefore comparative studies of new against standard drugs have not employed such monitoring, unlike the comparative studies of standard drugs as monotherapy, described earlier.

Conclusions

Monotherapy with one of the standard drugs is recommended in newly diagnosed patients: i.e. carbamazepine, valproate, phenobarbitone or phenytoin for partial seizures with or without secondary generalization; or valproate, phenobarbitone or phenytoin in idiopathic generalized epilepsy. The choice will be influenced by considerations of toxicity and costs, as well as efficacy, and will vary in different countries depending especially on availability and costs. Of the newer drugs, lamotrigine is a suitable alternative in both groups.

In patients who fail to respond to the optimum use of the first drug, an alternative or additional drug can be considered, but the choice of drug combinations is bewildering (Reynolds, 2006). An alternative is simpler and associated with less toxicity. In those minority of patients in whom seizure control improves with an additional drug it is usually unclear whether improvement is due to the combination or to the second drug.

In chronic patients, every effort should be made to avoid or reduce unnecessary, harmful or irrational polytherapy and to be aware of the limits of modern AED therapy. The availability of blood level monitoring of drugs greatly assists this process, especially in identifying poor compliance, a major issue contributing to polytherapy.

References

Beghi E, *et al.* on behalf of BASE study group. Adjunctive therapy versus alternative monotherapy in patients with partial epilepsy failing on a single drug; a multicentre, randomised, pragmatic controlled trial. *Epilepsy Res* 2003;**57**:1–13.

de Silva M, *et al.* Randomised comparative monotherapy trial of phenobarbitone, phenytoin, carbamazepine, or sodium valproate for newly diagnosed childhood epilepsy. *Lancet* 1996;**347**:709–13.

Heller AJ, *et al.* Phenobarbitone, phenytoin, carbamazepine, or sodium valproate for newly diagnosed adult epilepsy: a randomised comparative monotherapy trial. *J Neurol Neurosurg Psychiat* 1995;**58**: 4–50.

Kwan P, Brodie MJ. Early identification of refractory epilepsy. *N Eng J Med* 2000;**342**:314–19.

Marson AG, *et al.* on behalf of the SANAD study group. The SANAD study of effectiveness of carbamazepine, gabapentin, lamotrigine, oxcarbazepine or topiramate for treatment of partial epilepsy; and of valproate, lamotrigine or topiramate for generalised and unclassifiable epilepsy: an unblinded randomised controlled trial. *Lancet* 2007;**369**:1000–15 and 1016–26.

Mattson RH, *et al.* Comparison of carbamazepine, phenobarbital, phenytoin and primidone in partial and secondarily generalised tonic-clonic seizures. *N.Eng. J.Med.* 1985;**313**:145–51.

Perucca E. Anti-epileptic drug monotherapy versus polytherapy: the ongoing controversy. *Epilepsia* 1997; **38**(Suppl 5).

Reynolds EH. Chronic antiepileptic toxicity; a review. *Epilepsia* 1975;**16**:319–52.

Reynolds EH. Treating refractory epilepsy in adults. *BMJ* 2006;**332**:562.

Reynolds EH, Shorvon SD. Monotherapy or polytherapy for epilepsy? *Epilepsia* 1981;**22**:1–10.

Learning objective

(1) To know the indications, advantages and disadvantages of monotherapy or polytherapy in the treatement of epilepsy.

Section 5

Management of epilepsy

Chapter 73

Antiepileptic drugs currently under development

Philip N. Patsalos

Introduction

Epilepsy, the propensity to have seizures, is the most prevalent neurological condition, with a prevalence of 600 000 persons in the UK (50 million worldwide) and an incidence of 30 000 per year (80 per day). It affects 1 in 200 adults and 1 in 100 children and has a mortality of 1000 persons per year. Despite the introduction into clinical practice of 12 new antiepileptic drugs (AEDs) during the past 15 years, these drugs, whilst making some patients seizure-free, have had no significant impact on the prognosis of intractable epilepsy. Thus, the treatment of patients with intractable epilepsy still relies on the development of new AEDs and the need for new AEDs is substantial. The need is for new drugs with novel therapeutic targets that are more efficacious, that have improved side-effect profiles and better pharmacokinetic characteristics. AEDs that improve the prognosis of epilepsy, that prevent epileptogenesis and the secondary cerebral damage which occurs in epilepsy, and that prevent mortality in those patients at increased risk of premature death, particularly sudden unexplained death, are particularly needed. Drugs that prevent the development of epilepsy following head injury, neurosurgery and in particular stroke are also very much needed.

There are currently numerous molecules that are in development as potential novel AEDs and these are summarized in terms of their mechanism of action, pharmacokinetic and interaction profiles.

Brivaracetam
Mechanism of action

Brivaracetam is an analogue of levetiracetam and its mechanism of action is similar in that it acts via a synaptic vesicle protein 2A (SV2A) which is thought to assist with the coordination of synaptic vesicle exocytosis and neurotransmitter release. However, brivaracetam is more potent than levetiracetam.

Pharmacokinetics

After oral ingestion, brivaracetam is rapidly and almost completely absorbed. It exhibits linear pharmacokinetics with a volume of distribution (Vd) of 0.6 L/kg and is minimally bound to plasma proteins (<20%). Brivaracetam is eliminated primarily by metabolism, by hydrolysis and cytochrome P4502C-mediated hydroxylation (CYP2C), to various inactive metabolites. Whilst brivaracetam renal clearance is low, that of the metabolites is high. The terminal half-life ($t_{1/2}$) of brivaracetam is ~8 hours.

Drug interactions

Brivaracetam interacts with carbamazepine in that AUC (area under the concentration versus time curve) values are reduced by ~13% and carbamazepine epoxide (the pharmacologically active metabolite of carbamazepine) concentrations are increased 2.5-fold. Interactions with other AEDs have yet to be investigated.

2-Deoxy-D-glucose
Mechanism of action

2-Deoxy-D-glucose is taken up into cells by normal glucose transport mechanisms, but unlike glucose cannot undergo metabolism and thereby acts as an inhibitor of glycolysis, which results in an anticonvulsant action and it is through this mechanism that 2-deoxy-D-glucose is considered to act.

Introduction to Epilepsy ed. Gonzalo Alarcón and Antonio Valentín. Published by Cambridge University Press.
© Cambridge University Press 2012.

Pharmacokinetics

2-Deoxy-D-glucose is rapidly absorbed and distributed after oral administration, with peak plasma concentrations occurring at 0.5–1 h, and a half-life of 5–10 h. As an analogue of glucose, 2-deoxy-D-glucose freely passes the blood–brain barrier and is delivered preferentially to brain regions in response to energy demand, specifically regions with circuitries generating seizures.

Drug interactions

The drug interaction profile of 2-Deoxy-D-glucose is at present unknown.

Fluorofelbamate
Mechanism of action

Fluorofelbamate is an analogue of felbamate which has been designed to have the clinical efficacy of felbamate but without its adverse effects (aplastic anaemia and liver toxicity). Preliminary data suggest that fluorofelbamate acts, at least in part, by decreasing responses to γ-aminobutyric acid (GABA,) kainite and N-methyl-D-aspartate (NMDA), and by reducing voltage-dependent sodium currents.

Pharmacokinetics

Data are very limited. Fluorofelbamate is rapidly absorbed (T_{max} 1.1 h) and undergoes metabolism by pathways that are different to that of felbamate. An elimination $t_{1/2}$ of ~16.7 h has been reported.

Drug interactions

The drug interaction profile of fluorofelbamate is at present unknown.

Ganaxolone
Mechanism of action

Ganaxolone is chemically related to progesterone but seems to be devoid of any hormonal activity. It is a member of a novel class of neuroactive steroids, called epalons, which allosterically modulate the $GABA_A$ receptor complex via a unique recognition site.

Pharmacokinetics

Ganaxolone is rapidly absorbed (T_{max} – 1–3 h), after oral ingestion with a high-fat meal. Plasma concentrations increased essentially dose-dependently and subsequently declined bi-exponentially with a terminal $t_{1/2}$ of 37–70 h. Plasma concentration versus time profiles after multiple doses of ganaxolone did not suggest any significant accumulation. There is no gender difference with respect to its pharmacokinetic characteristics. However, fasting significantly reduces the absorption of ganaxolone. It is highly bound (> 99%) to plasma proteins. Ganaxolone is metabolized to yet unknown metabolites which are eliminated from plasma at a rate 3–6-times the terminal $t_{1/2}$ of ganaxolone.

Drug interactions

Preliminary trials have not identified any potential significant drug interactions with concomitant AEDs.

JZP-4
Mechanism of action

JZP-4 (3-(2,3,5-trichlorophenyl)pyrazine-2,6-diamine) is a structural analogue of lamotrigine and is a potent sodium (Nav1.2A and Nav1.3) and high-voltage activated calcium (types N, L and P/Q) channel blocker.

Pharmacokinetics

In healthy volunteers, orally administered JZP-4 was rapidly absorbed and eliminated primarily by metabolism. Excretion of JZP-4 in urine is low, with less than 0.1% of the administered dose recovered in urine as unchanged JZP-4.

Drug interactions

In vitro studies show that JZP-4 has no inhibitory effect on CYP 2E1 and a weak inhibitory effect on CYP1A2, CYP2A6, CYP2B6, CYP2C8, CYP2C9, CYP2C19, CYP2D6 and CYP3A4. Additionally, JZP-4 had no significant inhibitory effect on UDP-glucuronosyltransferase (UGT) enzymes UGT1A1, UGT1A4 or UGT1A9 and minimal effects on UGT1A6, UGT2B7 and UGT2B15. JZP-4 did not induce CYP1A2 or CYP3A in isolated human hepatocytes.

Retigabine (D-23129)
Mechanism of action

The action of retigabine is via multiple mechanisms, the primary mechanism being an activation of KCNQ2 and KCNQ2/3 neuronal potassium channels. Secondary mechanisms include: potentiation of GABA-evoked currents via an action on $GABA_A$ receptors containing β2 or β3 subunits; blocks the 4-aminopyridine-induced synthesis of neuroactive amino acids; and stimulates de novo synthesis of GABA.

Pharmacokinetics

Retigabine is rapidly absorbed ($T_{max} < 1.6$ h) after oral ingestion and its pharmacokinetics are linear after both single and repeat administration. Food co-ingestion does not affect the absorption of retigabine. Its binding to plasma proteins is <80%. Retigabine is primarily metabolized by N-glucuronidation and acetylation to two inactive N-glucuronide metabolites and an N-acetyl metabolite that demonstrates minimal pharmacological activity. The $t_{1/2}$ of retigabine is ~8 h.

Drug interactions

Retigabine does not affect the pharmacokinetics of valproic acid, topiramate, phenytoin, phenobarbital or carbamazepine. However, retigabine increases lamotrigine clearance by 20%. The pharmacokinetics of retigabine are unaffected by valproate or topiramate but retigabine clearance is increased (30%) by phenytoin and carbamazepine. Also, retigabine AUC values are increased by 10% after single-dose administration of phenobarbital.

Safinamide (FCE 26743; PNU-151774E; NW-1015)

Mechanism of action

Safinamide, (S)-(+)-2-(4-(3-fluorobenzyloxy)benzylamino)propanamide methansulfonate, acts via an action on site 2 of the sodium channel. It is also considered to modulate calcium currents and to inhibit MAO-B activity.

Pharmacokinetics

In healthy volunteers, safinamide is rapidly absorbed, with peak concentrations occurring within 2 h of oral ingestion. A high-fat meal delays absorption without affecting the extent of absorption. Safinamide is 92% bound to plasma proteins. Plasma safinamide concentrations increase linearly with dose and the elimination half-life is 21–23 h.

Drug interactions

In vitro studies suggest that safinamide has no inducing or inhibiting activity on the different CYP isoenzymes that are known to be involved in the metabolism of other AEDs. Nevertheless, plasma safinamide concentrations have been reported to be decreased in patients co-prescribed enzyme-inducing AEDs such as carbamazepine and phenobarbital.

Seletracetam (ucb 44212)

Mechanism of action

Seletracetam is an analogue of levetiracetam that binds with higher affinity than levetiracetam to the SV2A binding site.

Pharmacokinetics

Seletracetam is rapidly absorbed ($T_{max} < 1$ h) and is associated with linear pharmacokinetics. Its Vd is 0.6 L/kg and it is minimally bound (<10%) to plasma proteins. Seletracetam is eliminated by metabolism (hydrolysis) and excretion in urine, primarily as unchanged drug (30%) and an acidic metabolite (ucb-101596–1; 60%) which is not pharmacologically active. The $t_{1/2}$ of seletracetam is ~8 h.

Drug interactions

The drug interaction profile of seletracetam is at present unknown.

T2000

Mechanism of action

T2000 (1,3-dimetoxymethyl-5,5-diphenylbarbituric acid) is a pro-drug rapidly metabolized to monomethoxy-methyl-5,5-diphenylbarbituric acid (MMMDPB) and 5,5-diphenylbarbituric acid. The mechanisms of action of 5,5-diphenylbarbituric acid, the metabolite best-characterized pharmacologically, resemble those of both phenytoin and barbiturates.

Pharmacokinetics

In healthy subjects, the pharmacokinetics of T2000 and its primary metabolites 5,5-diphenylbarbituric acid and MMMDPB show near linearity up to 1200 mg/day dosing, with steady-state concentrations achieved within 2 weeks. Because food enhances the absorption of T2000, the compound is usually ingested with food. Plasma protein binding values for T2000, 5,5-diphenylbarbituric acid and MMMDPB are 67%, 35% and 51%, respectively and mean terminal half-lives are in the range 9–29 h, 27–65 h and 8–27 h, respectively. CYP2C19 and CYP2C9 are involved in the metabolic processes.

Drug interactions

In vitro studies using human liver microsomes indicate that MMMDPB is a competitive inhibitor of CYP2C19 and CYP2C9 and that 5,5-diphenylbarbituric acid is a competitive inhibitor of CYP2C9 and CYP3A4. Additionally, 5,5-diphenylbarbituric acid and MMMDPB are potent inducers of CYP3A4.

Talampanel (LY300164; GIKY 53773)
Mechanism of action

Talampanel is a selective non-competitive antagonist at the AMPA (a receptor subtype of glutamate) receptor site with very weak affinity for benzodiazepine receptors.

Pharmacokinetics

Talampanel is rapidly absorbed (T_{max} < 2.5 h). Binding to plasma proteins is ~75%. Although its metabolic pathways have not been completely characterized in man, acetylation appears to be an important route. Thus, acetylation status is likely to impact on the metabolism of talampanel and potentially a 2-fold difference in talampanel concentrations can be expected. The elimination of talampanel is probably via a combination of first-order and capacity-limited processes. The $t_{1/2}$ of talampanel is 6–8 h.

Drug interactions

Talampanel has been shown in an in vitro setting to be an irreversible inhibitor of CYPA3 and consequently it would be anticipated that talampanel may inhibit the metabolism of CYP3A substrates such as carbamazepine. Indeed carbamazepine plasma concentrations are elevated during carbamazepine and talampanel co-administration. In patients with epilepsy the clearance of talampanel is enhanced by hepatic enzyme-inducing AEDs (carbamazepine and phenytoin) whilst it is decreased by valproic acid.

Tonabersat (SB-220453)
Mechanism of action

Tonabersat ((3S-cis)-N-(6-Acetyl-3,4-dihydro-3-hydroxy-2,2-dimethyl-2H-1-benzopyran-4-yl)-3-chloro-4-fluorobenzamide) represents a 'first-in-class' neurotherapeutic agent that does not act via any established anticonvulsant mechanism. Instead, tonabersat selectively and specifically binds to a unique stereoselective site in the CNS, thought to be at the neuronal gap junction.

Pharmacokinetics

After oral ingestion of a single dose (2–80 mg), tonabersat is rapidly absorbed with a median T_{max} of 0.5–3 h. Absorption is delayed by a high-fat meal (T_{max} is extended by approximately 3 h) but food has no effect on the extent of absorption. Peak plasma concentrations were generally dose-proportional between 2 mg and 40 mg. Tonabersat is highly bound to plasma proteins (98%) and undergoes metabolism by cytosolic carbonyl reductase enzymes to a reduced ketone, with negligible amounts excreted in urine unchanged. Tonabersat plasma concentrations decline in a bi-exponential manner with mean terminal half-life values of 24–40 h.

Drug interactions

The drug interaction profile of tonabersat is at present unknown.

Valrocemide (N-valproyl-glycinamide; TV 1901)
Mechanism of action

The mechanism of action of valrocemide is unknown; an effect on GABA or glutamate-sensitive ion channels has been ruled out.

Pharmacokinetics

Valrocemide is rapidly absorbed and its plasma protein binding is <25%. The $t_{1/2}$ is 6.4–9.4 h after single dose administration and 7.2–8.5 h after multiple dose administration. Approximately 20% of administered dose is excreted unchanged, 40% is in the form of valproyl glycine and 4–6% is valproic acid.

Drug interactions

In vitro studies using CYP isoenzymes suggest that significant drug interactions with other AEDs should not be anticipated. Nevertheless, higher valrocemide clearance and shorter valrocemide $t_{1/2}$ values were observed in those patients on enzyme-inducing AEDs (phenytoin and carbamazepine).

YKP3089

YKP3089 is a novel compound with broad-spectrum anticonvulsant activity.

Mechanism of action

The mechanism of action of YKP3089 is at present unknown.

Pharmacokinetics

In healthy volunteers, YKP3089 shows linear pharmacokinetics over a large dose range (5–750 mg), with a median T_{max} of 1.5–3.5 h. Co-ingestion with a high-fat meal had no significant effect on the pharmacokinetics of YKP3089. Its elimination half-life is 30–75 h.

Drug interactions

The interaction profile of YKP3089 is at present unknown.

Conclusions

Seizure freedom with no side effects for all patients is the treatment aim in epilepsy. However, despite the euphoria, the new AEDs have not met expectations and more new AEDs are required. Drug development is now increasingly targeted at differing pathophysiological and chemical mechanisms and some of the AEDs in development act via novel targets and unique mechanisms. Additionally many of these drugs have more desirable pharmacokinetic characteristics and have a lower propensity to interact with concomitant medications.

Recommended reading

Bialer M, Johannessen SI, Kupferberg HJ, *et al*. Progress report on new antiepileptic drugs: a summary of the Eighth Eilat Conference (EILAT VIII). *Epilepsy Res* 2007;**73**:1–52.

Bialer M, Johannessen SI, Levy R, *et al*. Progress report on new antiepileptic drugs: a summary of the ninth Eilat Conference (EILAT IX). *Epilepsy Res* 2009;**83**:1–43.

Kwan P, Brodie MJ. Emerging drugs for epilepsy. *Expert Opin Emerging Drugs* 2007;**12**:407–22.

Learning objective

(1) To know the mechanisms of action, pharmacokinetics and main interactions of antiepileptic drugs currently under development.

Section 5 Management of epilepsy

Chapter 74 Antiepileptic drug withdrawal

R. Shane Delamont

Background

Antiepileptic drug (AED) withdrawal arises commonly in clinical practice. It is necessary to distinguish between complete withdrawal and partial withdrawal. The evidence base for deciding the benefits and risks for complete withdrawal is not strong and rests on several studies from the eighth and early ninth decade of the twentieth century. The evidence for partial withdrawal is even less complete and merges with management of risks and benefits of partial treatment and side effects.

The relapse rate of seizures after stopping AEDs varies in studies from 20 to 41% of patients followed up over a 2-year period. The rate of relapse is lower in children (20%) than adults (41%). It should be noted that the relapse rate in adults on continued treatment over a 2-year period is 22%, though the severity of the seizures was not described.

Clinical markers for increased risk of seizures in adults include a diagnosis of juvenile myoclonic epilepsy and the presence of a structural lesion, often seen on imaging. In children, the additional presence of persisting generalized epileptiform discharges on EEG despite treatment also predicts a reduced chance of successful AED withdrawal.

Most relapses (75%) occur within a 6-month period after withdrawal of AEDs.

Clinical practice

Whether AEDs are withdrawn depends on an assessment of the risk/benefit ratios between continued AED treatment and non-drug treatment. This assessment is carried out by the patient, carers and treating doctor and may take a number of years.

There needs to be an understanding of the risks of recurrent seizures for health, injuries, deaths including SUDEP, social structures, restricted educational and work choices and driving regulations. This needs to be balanced with the risks of ongoing AED intake. Some of these risks are known but there are undoubtedly some that are not. The history of AED treatment shows us that some side effects may take many years to be recognized in clinical practice, an example being osteoporosis associated with enzyme-inducing AED not being recognized for 50 years after the initial licensing of phenytoin in 1937.

AEDs have many side effects that patients find hard to tolerate. They include difficulty in concentrating, headache, neurocognitive slowing, drowsiness, behavioural changes, mood disturbance, weight changes and skin and hair alterations.

AEDs also have long-term side effects which patients may not be fully aware of but which do need to be taken into account. These include alterations in hepatic enzyme function with consequences for bone, endocrine and drug metabolism, fertility for both men and women, renal function and renal calculi and cosmetic and neurological side effects.

AEDs, when taken during pregnancy and while breast-feeding, carry risks to the developing fetus and child, and minimizing these risks is a frequent reason for drug withdrawal or minimization.

The social implications of AED withdrawal need to be explored before making a decision. Education, driving, work and leisure are the four major factors to be considered and their importance changes as the age of the patient increases. Education, preparing a career and not driving are the major factors in children. For young adults, establishing a career and family, driving and leisure are considered more important. The long-term consequences of taking these drugs is more likely to be a factor for considering withdrawal, while in the older population this is less of an issue.

Introduction to Epilepsy ed. Gonzalo Alarcón and Antonio Valentín. Published by Cambridge University Press.
© Cambridge University Press 2012.

Finally, the importance of tailoring the decision to the patient and arriving at a joint decision is emphasized.

Recommended reading

Sirven J, Sperling MR, Wingerchuk DM. Early versus late anti-epileptic drug withdrawal for epilepsy in remission. *Cochrane Database Syst Rev* 2001;3:CD001902. DOI: 10.1002/14651858.CD001902,

Britton JW. Antiepileptic drug withdrawal: literature review. *Mayo Clin Proc* 2002;7:1378–88.

Learning objective

(1) To know the objectives, indications, protocols and risks of antiepileptic drug withdrawal.

Section 5 Management of epilepsy

Chapter 75: Behavioural effects of antiepileptic drugs

Frank M. C. Besag

Introduction

Cognitive and behavioural effects of antiepileptic drugs are of major concern. It is surprising that the quality of the literature in this field is generally poor.

Confounding factors affecting behaviour

Antiepileptic medication is only one of many causes of behavioural disturbance in people with epilepsy. Both individual drug adverse effects and drug interactions can cause behavioural change. Particular attention has been drawn to the much-debated concept of alternative or reciprocal psychosis: the psychosis is worse when the seizure control is better and vice versa. The EEG equivalent is forced normalization: the EEG is more normal during periods of psychosis and less normal when the patient is not psychotic. If an alternative psychosis occurs after the prescription of an antiepileptic drug, the psychosis might be ascribed to that particular drug when it would have occurred with any antiepileptic drug that controlled the seizures. Abrupt seizure control might increase the risk.

Post-ictal psychosis can occur in some people after a seizure or cluster of seizures. Seizures could worsen as a delayed effect of withdrawal of a previous antiepileptic drug or because the introduced drug actually exacerbated seizures. The psychosis might be attributed to the drug when it has nothing to do with the drug itself: it is a result of the increased seizures.

Subtle seizure activity can affect behaviour in a number of ways, as described elsewhere by the current author (Besag, 2002). An increase in epileptiform discharges can cause transitory cognitive impairment, which can be frustrating and lead to the behavioural disturbance. Some drugs precipitate nonconvulsive status epilepticus, which can present with gross behavioural change.

In people with learning disability, adverse effects such as diplopia and dizziness may present as 'behavioural disturbance' if the individual is unable to express himself or herself verbally. The 'behavioural disturbance' is an attempt to communicate the distress caused by the adverse effect and is not a direct behavioural effect of the drug. An important confounding factor in people with learning disability and severe epilepsy is the 'release phenomenon': if there is a sudden improvement in the seizure control, the person may become more able without knowing how to use their new-found ability well. The correct management is not to stop the drug but to provide the necessary social-skills training to enable the individual to use their 'released' abilities to good advantage and in a socially acceptable way.

Antiepileptic drugs can have very different behavioural effects in children from those in adults but very few well-performed studies have been carried out in children.

Older drugs

Phenytoin, phenobarbitone, primidone and ethosuximide have been associated with behavioural problems. Phenobarbitone has been associated with gross behavioural disturbance in children. There have been reports of psychosis with ethosuximide but this is probably an uncommon adverse effect. Primidone has also been associated with behavioural disturbance: 'mysoline madness'. It has been suggested that phenytoin might be associated with cognitive problems and it might, consequently, be expected to be

Introduction to Epilepsy ed. Gonzalo Alarcón and Antonio Valentín. Published by Cambridge University Press.
© Cambridge University Press 2012.

associated with behavioural problems. Evidence for these effects in the older drugs is very limited.

Well-established drugs

Sodium valproate and carbamazepine are used therapeutically in psychiatric practice as mood-levelling drugs. They are not generally implicated in causing deterioration in behaviour. Valproate is said sometimes to be associated with irritability in children. It rarely causes severe sedation but this seems to be an idiosyncratic effect; it is not generally considered to be a sedative drug.

Newer drugs

Vigabatrin, lamotrigine, gabapentin, topiramate, tiagabine, oxcarbazepine, levetiracetam, zonisamide, pregabalin, rufinamide, lacosamide, stiripentol and eslicarbazepine are currently licensed in the UK/Europe. Felbamate is licensed in the USA but not in the UK/Europe. The behavioural effects of most of the newer antiepileptic drugs have been extensively reviewed by the current author elsewhere (Besag, 2001).

Vigabatrin

Psychosis occurs at a rate of 2–4%, much higher than the placebo rate. The psychosis may be an 'alternative psychosis' – see earlier. Depression also occurs more frequently than with placebo. A rate of around 12% has been reported. There have been anecdotal reports of gross behavioural disturbance in children treated with vigabatrin. The high prevalence of visual field constriction with vigabatrin has overtaken concerns about other adverse effects; use of this drug has fallen sharply.

Lamotrigine

There are no convincing reports of behavioural disturbance apart from in adults with pre-existing learning disability, possibly reflecting the 'release phenomenon' described earlier.

Gabapentin

There are some reports of behavioural disturbance in children.

Topiramate

Reported rates of psychosis are 3.7–12%. One study reported a 10.7% rate of affective disorder in patients treated with topiramate (Mula *et al.*, 2003). There have also been reports of aggressive behaviour, irritability, agitation, anger, hostility and anxiety. The author's own group confirmed that topiramate was associated with behavioural disturbance in children with learning disability, in contrast to gabapentin and lamotrigine, for which no similar effect was shown. High starting dose and rapid titration are associated with the higher rates of psychiatric disorder. Cognitive adverse effects, particularly related to expressive speech, can occur. Difficulties with expressive speech could precipitate behavioural problems, especially in people with learning disability who already have limited cognitive resources.

Tiagabine

There are no convincing reports of psychosis or affective disorder. There have been several reports of nonconvulsive status epilepticus. There have also been some reports of small numbers of subjects with aggression and irritability.

Oxcarbazepine

This does not seem to be associated with psychosis, depression or mania. Hyponatraemia is more common than with carbamazepine. This might lead to lethargy and consequent behavioural disturbance.

Levetiracetam

Rates of psychosis and affective disorder are similar to those for placebo. There are some reports of emotional lability, hostility and nervousness, and of behavioural disturbance in children but the quality of the data is questionable.

Zonisamide

There have been several reports of psychosis, depression and mania. Agitation, irritability and nervousness have also been reported in small numbers. The evidence is generally of very limited quality. There has been a suggestion from at least one report that patients with psychiatric disorders might improve, particularly those with bipolar affective disorder.

Pregabalin, rufinamide, lacosamide, stiripentol and eslicarbazepine

There are insufficient data to allow authoritative comment to be made at this stage.

Felbamate

There have been a few isolated reports of psychosis in the literature. Behavioural disturbance has been listed as a relatively common reason for withdrawal. This drug has been associated with anxiety, anorexia and insomnia. There have also been suggestions that there might be significant improvement in social and cognitive function but these improvements might have been related to seizure control. The potentially fatal adverse effects of aplastic anaemia and hepatotoxicity have overshadowed concern about psychiatric and other adverse effects.

Conclusions

Phenobarbitone and the benzodiazepines can have a disinhibiting effect in children. Vigabatrin and topiramate are associated with psychosis and affective disorder but low starting doses and slow escalation can reduce the psychiatric adverse effects, certainly for topiramate. There are many reports of behavioural adverse effects with other antiepileptic drugs but the validity of these reports is questionable, in view of the large number of potentially confounding factors. In general, starting at a low dose and escalating slowly can avoid many of the adverse effects.

References

Besag FMC. Behavioural effects of the new anticonvulsants. *Drug Safety* 2001;**24**(7):513–36.

Besag FMC. Subtle cognitive and behavioural effects of epilepsy. In Trimble M, Schmitz B, eds. *The Neuropsychiatry of Epilepsy*, pp. 70–80. Cambridge: Cambridge University Press; 2002.

Mula M, Trimble MR, Lhatoo SD, Sander JW. Topiramate and psychiatric adverse events in patients with epilepsy. *Epilepsia* 2003;**44**(5):659–63.

Learning objectives

(1) To be aware of the confounding factors affecting the study of the behavioural effects of antiepileptic drugs.
(2) To know the behavioural effects of antiepileptic drugs associated with treatment or withdrawal of the different antiepileptic drugs.

Section 5 Management of epilepsy

Chapter 76: Epilepsy emergency treatment

Frank M. C. Besag and Gonzalo Alarcón

Non-medical management of seizures, by Gonzalo Alarcón

What to do during a convulsive seizure (patient unresponsive, stiff or jerking)

During the seizure, the main aim is to prevent danger and injury:

(1) Make sure that the patient does not hit furniture, walls or other objects while jerking.
(2) Remove patient from the road, from the edge of cliffs or from platforms.
(3) Do not try to move them unless in danger.
(4) Prevent aspiration of secretions: during convulsive seizures the reflex involved in swallowing is abolished, and mouth secretions can be aspirated (risk of pneumonia).
   (a) Put the patient in the recovery position
   (b) If a mechanical aspirator is available, aspirate secretions from the mouth
   (c) If the seizure occurs in hospital, depending on patient's colour and duration of attack, it may be appropriate to give oxygen
(5) Do not restrict movement in convulsive seizures: it can induce joint dislocations and bone fractures.
(6) Make sure airway is clear: uncovering face, removing objects from mouth (even dentures if possible).
(7) Do not introduce objects inside the patient's mouth to prevent tongue-biting:
   (a) Patient's teeth can be broken.
   (b) Your own fingers can be bitten.
   (c) Most likely, patients will bite their tongue or cheek anyway.
(8) Do not automatically call an ambulance straight away in patients with known epilepsy as most seizures stop spontaneously in 2–3 minutes.
(9) An ambulance should be called if:
   (a) A convulsive seizure occurs for the first time (patients need to be assessed for possible underlying neurological or other causes).
   (b) The seizure does not stop spontaneously within 5 minutes.

What to do during a complex partial seizure or prolonged epileptic absence (patient vacant or confused, unresponsive or partially responsive, and may have automatisms)

Again, the main aim is to prevent danger and injury by:

- Preventing patients from getting into dangerous situations such as walking onto the road, falling off platforms in train or underground stations, grabbing knives or other dangerous tools, pouring boiling water onto themselves or others, getting burned with hot irons, etc.
- Gently directing them to safety, as some patients may show resistive aggression if forcibly restricted in the ictal and post-ictal phase.
- Recording the precise behaviour during the seizure and its evolution as it may later aid classification of seizure type and assess the patient's cognitive state:
  - Ask patients where they live, where they are.
  - Ask them to name an object shown to them (watch, tie, coin, key, etc.).
  - Ask them to remember a number.
  - Carry on with the assessment even if the patient is unresponsive.

Introduction to Epilepsy ed. Gonzalo Alarcón and Antonio Valentín. Published by Cambridge University Press.
© Cambridge University Press 2012.

- Carry out this assessment periodically in order to evaluate the evolution of the seizure and whether the patient is recovering.
- Record evidence of word-finding difficulty as the patient recovers as this may suggest dominant hemisphere lateralization of the seizure.

What to do during very brief seizures (absence seizures, myoclonic jerks, atonic and some tonic seizures)

- Myoclonic jerks, atonic and tonic seizures are momentary or last for a few seconds, whereas absence seizures can last up to 30 seconds or longer.
- No specific treatment is required by the observer, except in patients who suffer drop attacks (tonic or atonic seizures) resulting in injuries, which may require specific treatment (stop nose bleeding, suture cuts, etc.).

What to do during a simple partial seizure (patient fully conscious)

- Just wait! Simple partial seizures are not life-threatening and many remit spontaneously. Prolonged simple partial seizures may require treatment depending on the individual case.
- Reassure patient and keep patient under close observation in case the seizure evolves into more severe seizure types (complex partial or convulsive seizures).

Once the seizure has stopped

- Simple partial seizures, absence seizures, myoclonic jerks, atonic and brief tonic seizures are usually followed by quick recovery and do not usually require specific action.
- Complex partial and convulsive seizures usually last for 2–3 minutes and are followed by a period of gradual recovery. The patient may be still unconscious immediately after a convulsive seizure and is vulnerable during this period. Seizures are often followed by a relatively long period of confusion (post-ictal confusion), which can last from a few minutes to several hours. During this period patients gradually recover their cognitive skills.
- It is important to make sure that breathing pattern and colour recover and patients should be monitored until they become fully alert.
- Analgesia may be required as they may complain of headache.
- During post-ictal confusion, patients must be under close observation, as they might wander about aimlessly, sometimes getting themselves into dangerous situations. If disturbed, they might push you away or become mildly aggressive, so leave them alone if they are safe, but keep an eye on them.
- If patients are sleepy or tired, find a place for them to rest.
- Do not give the person anything to eat or drink until fully recovered.
- Do not attempt to bring them around.
- Keep the person under observation until fully recovered.

If the seizure is not stopping

- If the seizure is prolonged, or the patient suffers a cluster of seizures without regaining consciousness in the period between seizures, patients should be taken to hospital. This situation, status epilepticus, is a medical emergency.

Emergency treatment of prolonged seizures, by Frank Besag

There are two situations that are likely to require urgent medical attention possibly in hospital: significant injury in a seizure or a prolonged seizure. Prolonged seizures can result in permanent brain damage. What type of seizure can result in damage? What is meant by prolonged in this context? What treatment needs to be given and how promptly does it need to be given? Status epilepticus may be defined as ongoing seizure activity lasting 20 minutes or more. In theory there are as many types of status epilepticus as there are types of seizures but the type of status epilepticus that causes particular concern, in terms of the possibility of brain damage, is the type that involves ongoing unconsciousness. This important subgroup is often termed 'convulsive status epilepticus', although it is possible to have a partial clonic seizure with retention of consciousness. The convention in the remainder of this chapter will be to use the term 'status epilepticus' (without any preceding adjective such as nonconvulsive or partial) to imply the condition in which unconsciousness continues.

There is good experimental evidence to suggest that toxic chemicals are produced after about 20 minutes of status epilepticus and that these could, at least in theory, cause brain damage. Because of this, many clinicians would recommend that the condition should be terminated before it has reached 20 minutes duration. This implies emergency intervention well under 20 minutes. The usual convention is to treat if the seizure-state with unconsciousness has continued for 5 minutes and does not appear to be resolving. Status epilepticus, as just defined, covers at least two situations. The first is an obvious ongoing seizure, usually a tonic-clonic seizure, although, as already stated, rarely a tonic seizure. The other situation is repeated seizures without recovery of consciousness. Failure to recover consciousness between the seizures probably implies ongoing epileptiform activity. What is meant by 'unconsciousness' in this situation? The important factor is for the carer to use common sense but a reasonable guide to level of consciousness is that if the patient does not make at least a semi-purposeful response to a painful stimulus then they are probably unconscious. The painful stimulus usually employed is either pinching the earlobe or rubbing knuckles firmly on the sternum. A purposeful response to this painful stimulus would be if the patient pushed the examiner's hand away. A semi-purposeful response is if the patient's hand clearly moves in the direction of the painful stimulus in a consistent way, although not quite managing to push the hand away. A generalized extensor response is not a semi-purposeful response, as such a response is possible in an unconscious patient.

To ensure that treatment is given in time to terminate the condition well under 20 minutes, out-of-hospital treatment is often required. Rectal diazepam is the established treatment. This is typically given in a dose of up to 0.5 mg/kg in a child. In an adult, the usual convention is to give 10 mg and, if the seizure does not stop after about 5 minutes, to repeat with a further 10 mg dose. If the seizure has not terminated within a further 5 minutes then a third dose may be given, provided the adult weighs at least 60 kg. It is strongly recommended that an ambulance be summoned urgently after the first dose, in most cases.

The exception might be if the patient is known to be liable to status epilepticus and has always responded promptly to the emergency treatment in the past. Each patient should have a clear treatment plan that is reviewed if circumstances change.

What can go wrong? In young, otherwise well patients, rectal diazepam is unlikely to cause serious adverse effects. However, individual exceptions may occur. The most likely adverse events are respiratory depression and cardiovascular collapse. How should these conditions be managed? In either case, urgent medical attention should be summoned. If the patient is out of hospital, this implies calling an ambulance.

If the patient has stopped breathing or if respiration is inadequate, mouth-to-mouth ventilation should be given. This is a simple and effective procedure. Everyone who is trained in giving rectal diazepam (or one of the other similar options – see later) should be trained in mouth-to-mouth ventilation.

If cardiovascular collapse occurs, the patient should be placed head down with the lower limbs elevated while urgent assistance is awaited. It is unlikely that full-scale cardiopulmonary resuscitation will be required, although in exceptional cases it might.

It should be emphasized that the foregoing comments on dosage and adverse effects of rectal diazepam apply to young, otherwise healthy patients. The elderly may be much more susceptible to the adverse effects of benzodiazepines, and much smaller doses with much closer monitoring may be required.

What other out-of-hospital treatments are available? Some patients, especially children with a history of failing to respond to benzodiazepines or having adverse effects to them, may be prescribed rectal paraldehyde. This can be given by trained carers but special precautions apply. In particular, the paraldehyde should not be administered if it is discoloured because this implies that it may have degraded into toxic products. In the past, it was recommended that the paraldehyde be administered using a glass syringe because it could dissolve plastic syringes. Modern standard syringes can be used but it would be advisable to administer the paraldehyde promptly after having drawn it into the syringe. Paraldehyde is often mixed with oil for administration because of concerns about rectal ulceration, although the current authors have never adopted this procedure. There are theoretical considerations that suggest that absorption might be slower. The paraldehyde can be administered through a short rubber tube which can be flushed with tap water after the administration.

More recently, buccal midazolam has been used to treat status epilepticus (Scott *et al.*, 1999; McIntyre *et al.*, 2005). This is much more convenient than rectal diazepam and appears to be at least as effective. The usual dose is up to 0.3 mg/kg. A commercial product intended for buccal administration ('Epistatus') is now available. Although this is a highly convenient and apparently effective treatment, it should be noted that midazolam is not licensed for the treatment of status epilepticus in the UK and that the buccal route for midazolam is also not licensed.

Nasal midazolam has also been advocated as an emergency treatment for status epilepticus. There are theoretical reasons suggesting that absorption via the nasal route might be more rapid than via the buccal route. However, there are practical considerations that make the buccal route more convenient: the mouth is a larger orifice, making administration easier, and nasal breathing may discharge some of the administered midazolam if it is given into the nose.

Conclusions

Emergency out-of-hospital treatment is relatively easy and can be highly effective in preventing permanent brain damage in the small group of patients who are susceptible to prolonged status epilepticus. However, it is strongly recommended that the treatment only be given by properly trained carers who are both confident and competent.

Recommended reading and references

Shorvon S. *Status Epilepticus: Its Clinical Features and Treatment in Children and Adults*. Cambridge: Cambridge University Press; 1994.

Scott RC, Besag FMC, Neville BGR. Buccal midazolam and rectal diazepam for treatment of prolonged seizures in childhood and adolescence: a randomised trial. *Lancet* 1999;**353**:623–6.

McIntyre J, Robertson S, Norris E, *et al.* Safety and efficacy of buccal midazolam versus rectal diazepam for emergency treatment of seizures in children: a randomised controlled trial. *Lancet* 2005;**366**(9481): 205–10.

Learning objectives

(1) To know what to do if a person has an epileptic seizure.
(2) To know when a seizure is considered too long.
(3) To know what to do if a seizure becomes too long.
- When and how to dispense diazepam, rectal paraldehyde or buccal midazolam.
- When to call an ambulance and to send patient to hospital.

Section 5 Management of epilepsy

Chapter 77

Clinical neuropsychological evaluation

Robin G. Morris

The main tools of clinical neuropsychology evaluation are standardized assessment procedures that have been developed specifically to produce reliable estimates of mental abilities. The procedures are developed to measure particular functions (for example, memory or language ability). They are then used to test the function of sets of normal individuals in order to provide a statistical basis for calibrating the procedures as a measure of level of ability and provide a rigorous approach for determining neuropsychological impairment.

Neuropsychological assessment of people with epilepsy tends to take place in four main contexts:

(1) To aid with presurgical evaluation of people, a neuropsychological assessment is used to supplement investigations concerned with determining side and site of the epileptic focus (Jones-Gotesman et al., 2000). Here the neuropsychological profile of the person may provide some information concerning localized functional disturbance, including lateralization (i.e. determining which side of the brain is dysfunctional and hence may have the epileptic focus). In addition to this, the neuropsychological assessment may be used in part to provide some prediction about the likely functional outcome of surgery and the particular profile associated with either seizure or neuropsychological outcome.

(2) In the same context, it is used to monitor the outcome of neurosurgery, by combining the presurgical assessment with a follow-up postsurgical evaluation. Here the assessment can help determine whether perceived changes in function are corroborated by objective neuropsychological assessment results. They also provide a way of monitoring surgical procedures and provide a broader perspective on their efficacy in addition to seizure outcome. The success of surgical outcome is measured not just in terms of seizure control, but also whether there has been relative preservation of function, including mental ability.

(3) The neuropsychological assessment can be used to determine the specific side effects of antiepileptic drugs and also monitor improvements or deterioration in neuropsychological function following changes in drug treatment.

(4) Within a rehabilitation setting, neuropsychological assessments can help provide information concerning the strengths and weaknesses of a person's abilities that can be used to help with developing strategies to promote everyday function.

The first three uses are mainly carried out in specialist clinical neurosciences centres with access to clinical neuropsychologist epilepsy experts. For neurorehabilitation, in the UK this may be done either in community-based neurorehabilitation teams, if there is significant brain abnormality or damage, or in specialist rehabilitation settings for people with epilepsy.

An assessment may be tailored to the person with epilepsy, following up particular aspects of functioning, often based on what is known already about brain abnormality. This tends to follow what is known about the brain basis for mental function, with particular areas of investigation explored relating to brain regions. For example, in temporal lobe epilepsy, language and memory may be assessed more comprehensively. In cases of patients with frontal lobe epilepsy, there is an emphasis on tests relating to this brain area, including what are termed executive functions, the control mechanisms that coordinate and sequence mental operations. The main areas of

Introduction to Epilepsy ed. Gonzalo Alarcón and Antonio Valentín. Published by Cambridge University Press.
© Cambridge University Press 2012.

Table 77.1. Brain areas that might be implicated in different types of neuropsychological functions

Function	Brain regions
Memory	Mesiotemporal, retrosplenial, thalamic and mammillary bodies • Verbal memory associated with language dominant hemisphere • Visuospatial memory associated with non-dominant hemisphere
Attention	Generalized, anterior cingulated
Executive	Prefrontal cortex
Visuospatial	Left and right parietal regions
Language	Dominant hemisphere posterior frontal, superior temporal, inferior parietal
Motor	Motor cortical, supplementary or premotor areas

neuropsychological function that are covered are intelligence, memory, executive functioning, attention, visuospatial abilities, language and motor skills (Table 77.1).

In addition, there are global attributes concerning neuropsychological function and these include intelligence, an aggregate of all mental abilities, and processing speed, the speed at which mental operations can be performed.

A neuropsychological assessment usually includes some baseline assessment of intelligence. The most widely used procedure is the Wechsler Adult Intelligence Scale (WAIS), with the most recently available version the WAIS-IV. This is a comprehensive set of tests encompassing major components of intelligence and has been shortened into abbreviated versions, including the commonly used Wechsler Abbreviated Scale for Intelligence (WASI). A major distinction in intelligence is between verbal and performance intelligence. The former is mainly to do with verbal knowledge and verbal reasoning or the ability to hold in mind verbal information whilst processing it, whilst the latter combines non-verbal problem-solving with measurement of the speed at which information may be processed. A comparison between verbal and performance intelligence can provide an indication as to whether there are more subtle signs of dominant hemisphere dysfunction affecting language, in which case verbal intelligence may be lower than performance intelligence.

The intellectual assessment may provide a comparison against which to judge specific impairment in a range of functions, as listed in Table 77.1, each of which has specific tests to measure them.

A frequently impaired function in epilepsy is memory, particularly in relation to temporal lobe epilepsy. Here tests are used which distinguish between verbal and non-verbal memory function and within this specific types of memory are measured. For example, it has been found that lists of word pairs (verbal paired associate learning) or learning lists of words as procedures are more sensitive specifically to left hippocampal lesions than attempting to remember short stories (story recall) (Loring *et al.*, 2008). In contrast, non-verbal memory procedures have been developed to determine the ability to draw from memory simple or more complex line drawings. Specialized tests are used to measure attentional, executive, visuospatial, language and motor functioning.

Important considerations are made in conducting a clinical neuropsychological assessment and some of these are summarized by Baker and Goldstein (2004). For example, if the goal of the assessment is to help lateralize neuropsychological impairment, it is important to use a range of tasks rather than relying on a single measure, which may be unreliable. In addition, it is important to take into account a number of factors that might affect neuropsychological performance. These include the age of onset of the epilepsy, duration of the epilepsy and whether the person has had recent clinical seizure activity, and their current medication. Additionally, a person's mood state may affect neuropsychological function, particularly when a person has clinical levels of depression or anxiety. In the context of rehabilitation, the assessment has to be integrated with a range of person factors that might determine final outcome and may include epilepsy and non-epilepsy variables. For example, assessment could include changes in seizure activity or medication, which can influence a person's social function and how this interacts with their social environment. It should be borne in mind that neuropsychological performance in a clinical environment may not be consistent with the difficulties faced by a person, because of the number of intervening or mediating variables that affect everyday performance. A general principle is that people with epilepsy who have neuropsychological deficits can be greatly helped by time spent to explore and help explain their nature by a skilled clinical neuropsychologist with expertise in this area.

References

Baker GA, Goldstein LH. The dos and don'ts of neuropsychological assessment of epilepsy. *Epilepsy Behav* 2004;5:S77–80.

Jones-Gotesman MJ, Harnadek CS, Kubu CS. Neuropsychological assessment for temporal lobe epilepsy. *Can J Neurol Sci* 2000:27(1):S39–43.

Loring DW, Strauss E, Hermann BP, *et al*. Differential neuropsychological test sensitivity to left temporal lobe epilepsy. *J Int Neuropsychol Soc* 2008:14:394–400.

Learning objectives

(1) To know the principles and objectives of neuropsychological evaluation.
(2) To know the indications, methods and assessment of neuropsychological evaluation in epilepsy.

Section 5 Management of epilepsy

Chapter 78

Neuropsychological effects of antiepileptic drugs

Laura H. Goldstein

Introduction

Neuropsychological impairments in people with epilepsy may be associated with a number of factors including the location and aetiology of the underlying epileptogenic lesion, the age at onset, type and frequency of seizures, and the presence/absence of interictal epileptiform activity. Additionally, antiepileptic drugs (AEDs) may also affect cognitive functioning since AEDs may affect normal neuronal function and lead to psychomotor slowing, attentional impairments and memory dysfunction (Motamedi and Meador, 2004). AEDs have differing modes of action and the cognitive profile associated with specific AEDs has been investigated to differing degrees and with varying rigour. Further difficulties in evaluating cognitive effects of AEDs arise from the extent to which they reduce seizure occurrence and how well this is controlled for experimentally.

Evaluating the evidence

Studies of the neurocognitive effects of AEDs have been undertaken in patients and healthy controls. It has been suggested that studies likely to give the most valid and reliable data are those conducted on patients that (Vermeulen and Aldenkamp, 1995):

(1) examine only the effects of monotherapy
(2) include only seizure-free patients
(3) employ a repeated-measures design (so that individuals act as their own controls) in a parallel groups or cross-over design
(4) use fully random treatment allocation to groups when comparing the effects of different AEDs
(5) employ a no-treatment control group to assess practice effects on cognitive scores

(6) are statistically sound
(7) are not overinclusive in terms of outcome measures to prevent Type 1 errors.

Therefore, the results of less well-designed studies should be interpreted with caution. Unfortunately, many studies do not meet the gold standard of a double-blind randomized cross-over study where patients are randomly assigned to treatment or placebo conditions with a wash-out period between the two drugs (Vermeulen and Aldenkamp, 1995).

Neuropsychological effects of AEDs

Kwan and Brodie (2001) highlight the importance of considering whether increased cognitive impairment in the case of polytherapy, as opposed to monotherapy, is purely additive or due to pharmokinetic interactions. They also indicate that consideration should be paid to whether blood serum drug concentrations are within standard limits, since high drug concentrations may be associated with impaired cognitive functioning. In addition, titration rates for drugs, e.g. for topiramate, may be important in minimizing adverse cognitive effects (Aldenkamp *et al.*, 2003).

Older AEDs

While most of the older and well-established AEDs have been associated with adverse cognitive or behavioural effects, phenobarbital is thought to have the most negative profile in terms of cognitive and behavioural change (Kwan and Brodie, 2001; Motamedi and Meador, 2004). Benzodiazepines (especially clonazepam) are also associated with more marked cognitive dysfunction (Kwan and Brodie, 2001; Motamedi and Meador, 2004). Despite early views that carbamazepine might have very few negative

Introduction to Epilepsy ed. Gonzalo Alarcón and Antonio Valentín. Published by Cambridge University Press.
© Cambridge University Press 2012.

consequences, comparisons between several older AEDs suggest broadly comparable neuropsychological effects (Kwan and Brodie, 2001).

Newer AEDs

Of the newer AEDs, lamotrigine has been shown to have a positive cognitive profile but insufficient definitive data are considered to be available about the cognitive sequelae of gabapentin and tiagapine (Aldenkamp et al., 2003). Oxcarbazepine is felt to have a good neuropsychological profile in adults (Aldenkamp et al., 2003). Topiramate, however, has been shown to have a range of adverse effects, including reductions in verbal IQ, verbal learning and verbal fluency (Thompson et al., 2000), and more generally impairing executive function and working memory tests (Kockelmann et al., 2004). Topiramate has been associated with greater executive dysfunction than tiagabine (Fritz et al., 2005) or lamotrigine (Blum et al., 2006). Additionally, patients taking a combination of topiramate and sodium valproate had a more impaired cognitive profile than those taking topiramate with lamotrigine (Kockelmann et al., 2004). Recently, zonisamide monotherapy has been associated with impaired verbal recall, divided attention and verbal fluency in a dose-related manner, with impairments persisting after a year (Park et al., 2008).

Further considerations

Motamedi and Meador (2004) highlight the heightened susceptibility of older adults to possible adverse neuropsychological effects of AEDs. They suggest that, in the face of normal age-related memory changes, further impact on memory by AEDs may influence older adults' ability to tolerate a drug. They also highlight the potential susceptibility of children to the neuropsychological consequences of AEDs due to their ongoing neurodevelopment, although they conclude that long-term effects of AEDs on cognition in children are not well understood.

In addition, to adverse neuropsychological effects of AEDs, increasing interest is being paid to the psychotropic effects of AEDs, e.g. Ettinger (2006); mood may affect subjective impressions of cognitive functioning and AED-altered mood may conceivably influence cognitive test performance (Motamedi and Meador, 2004). The psychotropic effects of AEDs may influence patients' tolerance of them. Thus, the choice of AED needs to include a consideration of its potential effects on both mood and behaviour (Ettinger, 2006).

Conclusion

Since many factors may influence cognitive function in people with epilepsy, neuropsychological effects are only one of the many sets of variables that may influence AED choice (Park et al., 2008). Much may also depend on the person's everyday life demands, the importance of adequate seizure control and the psychotropic effect of the drug.

References

Aldenkamp AP, De KM, Reijs R. Newer antiepileptic drugs and cognitive issues. *Epilepsia* 2003;**44**:21–9.

Blum D, Meador K, Biton V, et al. Cognitive effects of lamotrigine compared with topiramate in patients with epilepsy. *Neurology* 2006;**67**:400–6.

Ettinger AB. Psychotropic effects of antiepileptic drugs. *Neurology* 2006;**67**:1916–25.

Fritz N, Glogau S, Hoffmann J, et al. Efficacy and cognitive side effects of tiagabine and topiramate in patients with epilepsy. *Epilepsy Behav* 2005;**6**:373–81.

Kockelmann E, Elger CE, Helmstaedter C. Cognitive profile of topiramate as compared with lamotrigine in epilepsy patients on antiepileptic drug polytherapy: Relationships to blood serum levels and comedication. *Epilepsy Behav* 2004;**5**:716–21.

Kwan P, Brodie MJ. Neuropsychological effects of epilepsy and antiepileptic drugs. *Lancet* 2001; **357**:216–22.

Motamedi GK, Meador KJ. Antiepileptic drugs and memory. *Epilepsy Behav* 2004;**5**:435–9.

Park S-P, Hwang Y-H, Lee H-W, et al. Long-term cognitive and mood effects of zonisamide monotherapy in epilepsy patients. *Epilepsy Behav* 2008;**12**:102–8.

Thompson PJ, Baxendale SA, Duncan JS, et al. Effects of topiramate on cognitive function. *J Neurol Neurosurg Psychiatry* 2000;**69**:636–41.

Vermeulen J, Aldenkamp AP. Cognitive side-effects of chronic antiepileptic drug treatment: a review of 25 years of research. *Epilepsy Res* 1995;**22**:65–95.

Learning objectives

(1) To be aware of the methods available for evaluating the evidence on the neuropsychological effects of antiepileptic drugs.
(2) To know the most common neuropsychological effects of the different antiepileptic drugs.

Section 5 Management of epilepsy

Chapter 79

The Wada test (intra-arterial amobarbital procedure)

Robin G. Morris

Introduction

The Wada test was developed as a procedure to aid in presurgical planning mainly for people undergoing neurosurgical treatment for temporal lobe epilepsy. It was originally devised by Jules Wada and developed at the Montreal Neurological Institute. It became adopted widely in centres specializing in epilepsy neurosurgery and in recent years there has been debate about in what circumstances it should be used (see for example Baxendale et al., 2008; Paolicchi, 2008).

The procedure

The most widely used procedure involves inserting a cannula or catheter into the internal carotid artery via initially the femoral artery. Angiography is then used to visualize the blood vessels supplied by the internal carotid artery, checking for correct placement and also to screen for arteriovenous abnormality. A barbiturate, usually sodium amytal, is then injected to shut down brain function in the majority of one brain hemisphere. At this point, neuropsychological procedures are used to test language, memory and motor functioning pertaining to the contralateral (non-injected) hemisphere. By repeating the procedure it is possible to compare functioning for each brain hemisphere.

Interpretation

In relation to temporal lobe epilepsy there are several types of information that can be gained by using the Wada procedure:

Lateralizing language function

Language is mainly dominant (localized) in the left hemisphere in a high proportion of right-handed people (about 97%), with the remainder showing mixed dominance or mainly right dominance (3%). For people who are left-handed language dominance is less predictable, with about 70% showing left dominance and 30% with mixed or right dominance. The Wada test provides the gold standard technique for determining language dominance. To test language dominance, aphasiology tests of naming, comprehension, repetition and reading may be used for each independent brain side. For unilateral dominance, impairment in language functioning (dysphasia) is seen only with the ipsilateral injection, whilst for mixed dominance it is seen in a milder form for both injections.

Determining language lateralization can serve two main purposes in relation to neurosurgical pre-evaluation in temporal lobe epilepsy. First, it can help predict the risk of post-surgical dysphasia if the operation is in the same hemisphere as language representation, in particular where the surgical procedure may impinge on posterior lateral regions of the temporal lobe which are involved in language comprehension. This purpose has reduced in importance somewhat as alternatives to the large en bloc resection for temporal lobe epilepsy have been developed. A more specialized use is where surgery is planned for epileptic foci in potential language zones, in which the Wada test forms a useful adjunct to intra- or extra-operative electrical stimulation. A second use is in interpreting the neurological significance of preoperative neuropsychological tests (see Chapter 77). The latter, for example, may produce neuropsychological profiles that suggest weaknesses in verbal functioning. Combining this information with knowledge about language dominance can provide some information concerning lateralized brain dysfunction.

Left and right brain support for memory

The temporal lobe contains key structures that support memory function, including the hippocampus

---

Introduction to Epilepsy ed. Gonzalo Alarcón and Antonio Valentín. Published by Cambridge University Press.
© Cambridge University Press 2012.

and surrounding perirhinal, entorhinal and parahippocampal cortices. Whilst there is some left specialization for verbal memory and right for visual or spatial memory, the brain can be seen as having the memory system duplicated, with one system on each side. Because of this feature, it is possible to severely damage the functioning of memory on one side of the brain without producing profound amnesia (Lacruz *et al.*, 2004). Neurosurgical procedures that remove hippocampal and associated cortical tissues on one side rely on the fact that the other side will continue to be able to support memory function. In conditions such as temporal lobe epilepsy, the latter is not necessarily the case, for example, where there is bilateral pathology affecting both hippocampi. The Wada test was developed further to test memory function on the side contralateral to neurosurgery. The main method is to inject the side ipsilateral to the proposed side for neurosurgery, and then present material, later on seeing whether it can be remembered. If the ability to remember falls below a certain threshold the test is seen as suggesting contralateral damage affecting memory, with the patient at risk for significant postoperative memory difficulties. A subsidiary use is to help determine the side of seizure focus. Here the notion is that if one particular side has the focus, this side should also provide worse support for memory. Injection of the contralateral side, hence forcing the person to rely on this side for memory, should produce worse memory performance than injecting the ipsilateral side. By extrapolating backwards from Wada results it is possible to make some prediction about side of seizure onset. This technique has been found to produce seizure focus lateralization predictions better than, for example, structural magnetic resonance imaging (Akanuma *et al.*, 2003). A recommended main use is for the clinician to take notice if the lateralization indication is at odds with other findings (for example EEG), perhaps suggesting that for a particular patient, additional methods should be used to investigate the side of seizure focus.

Controversies about use and alternatives

The Wada test has a small but significant risk of complication, with an estimated 1% risk of a neurological sequelae. Alternatives such as functional magnetic resonance imaging (fMRI) to determine language lateralization have been proposed and some have questioned the necessity to use the procedure to guard against the possibility of postoperative amnesia with the development of modern neuroimaging and EEG techniques that can more accurately ascertain lateralized pathology. Nevertheless, it is still widely used. fMRI has been found not to be completely accurate in determining language lateralization and shows relatively poor accuracy for individual patients in terms of determining unilateral integrity of memory structures. Whilst more research into fMRI techniques is clearly warranted and may lead to significant improvements, it has not replaced the Wada test. The clinical question has now become what type of patients warrant the Wada test, with a tendency to use it with more complicated cases, for example, where the baseline risk of post-surgical memory impairment is increased due to possible bilateral pathology.

Recommended reading

Akanuma N, Alarcón G, Lum F, *et al*. Lateralising value of neuropsychological protocols for presurgical assessment of temporal lobe epilepsy. *Epilepsia* 2003;**44**:408–18.

Meador KJ, Loring DW. The Wada test for language and memory lateralisation. *Neurology* 2005;**65**:659.

Lacruz ME, Alarcón G, Akanuma N, *et al*. Neuropsychological effects associated with temporal lobectomy and amygdalo-hippocampectomy depending on Wada test failure. *J Neurol Neurosurg Psychiatry* 2004;**75**:600–7.

Baxendale S, Thompson PJ, Duncan JS. The role of the Wada test in the surgical treatment of temporal lobe epilepsy: an international survey. *Epilepsia* 2008; **49**(4):715–20.

Paolicchi JM. Is the Wada test still relevant? Yes. *Arch Neurol* 2008;**65**(6):838–40.

Learning objectives

(1) To know the objectives of the Wada test.
(2) To become familiar with how a Wada test is performed.
(3) To know the indications of the Wada test.
(4) To know how to evaluate results from the Wada test.
(5) To be aware of the current international discussions on the utility of the Wada test.

Section 5 Management of epilepsy

Chapter 80

General principles of surgical treatment

Richard P. Selway

Most conventional epilepsy surgery is classified as resective: i.e. the epileptic focus in the brain is identified by detailed preoperative tests, and then that portion of the brain is removed ('resected'). There are other surgical techniques in which the general function of the brain is changed in an attempt to improve the epilepsy; this is known as functional surgery. These include multiple subpial transection, corpus callosotomy and various forms of electrical stimulation.

Resective surgery

This forms the main component of epilepsy surgery.

Who is a potential surgical candidate?

Candidates for surgery will have stereotyped partial seizures. This implies the likelihood of a single localized focus within the brain. Patients with idiopathic generalized epilepsies or multifocal epilepsies are not suitable for resective surgery.

The seizures should have proved to be medically intractable. How this is defined is slightly open to debate but epilepsy for 2 years which has continued despite trying at least two appropriate antiepileptic drugs (AEDs) in appropriate doses is unlikely to achieve full control with further drug manipulation, and could be considered for surgical investigation. In practice most patients have tried many AEDs and suffered epilepsy for decades before surgery is considered.

A low IQ has previously been regarded as implying a widespread brain problem, rather than a single limited focus, and therefore dissuading one from pursuing surgery. However, it is clear that severe epilepsy itself in early life can affect the IQ even if caused by very focal lesions and such patients may benefit greatly from surgery.

Patients with psychosis are generally not regarded as surgical candidates although some will suffer psychiatric disturbance only in the context of seizures (e.g. post-ictal psychosis). In such cases surgery may still be considered.

Defining the focus

Having selected a patient with intractable partial seizures, it is necessary to define the region of seizure onset. In the vast majority of patients successfully treated, a structural lesion is found and it is this that produces the epilepsy. The central tenet of resective surgery is that complete removal of the responsible lesion is the most likely way of achieving seizure freedom.

Investigations therefore include:

- detailed structural imaging of the brain: best carried out by magnetic resonance imaging (MRI).
- Electroencephalography (EEG), which may detect focal disturbances in background rhythm if there is an extensive abnormality of the underlying brain, or epileptogenic discharges. Such interictal abnormalities may help to suggest that a known structural abnormality is the source of the epilepsy but they are rarely sufficient on their own to confirm the region of seizure onset.
- video-telemetry, in which a patient is continually monitored by EEG and video-camera over several days in hospital, which allows spontaneous seizures to be recorded and studied. This provides much more robust evidence of the region of seizure onset.

In many cases these tests, together with a detailed history from the patient and relatives, are sufficient

---

Introduction to Epilepsy ed. Gonzalo Alarcón and Antonio Valentín. Published by Cambridge University Press.
© Cambridge University Press 2012.

to confirm that a lesion visible on an MRI is the probable source of the seizures. If findings are not conclusive, there are a number of supplementary tests which can help, such as:

- Psychometric tests: tests of memory and cognitive function can define specific functions which are under-performing relative to the rest. This can suggest specific regions of the brain as sites of pathology, and therefore possible regions of seizure onset.
- Positron emission tomography (PET) scanning: a radio-isotope test showing functional activity of the brain. Sites of pathology tend to show reduced cerebral metabolism.
- Ictal SPECT (single proton emission computed tomography): a radio-isotope is injected at the very start of a spontaneous seizure and tends to concentrate in the region of seizure onset. A subsequent scan can demonstrate this.

Defining the risks of surgery

Having identified a likely focus for the seizures, it is necessary to make an assessment of the risks of removing that region. All neurosurgery carries risks from the anaesthetic, postoperative bleeding or infection. However, when a piece of cerebral cortex is removed this may be a region which also serves important functions, even if it also produces the epilepsy. Frequently, a knowledge of anatomy allows one accurately to predict that a lesion can be resected without significant loss of function. If the region of seizure onset is close to 'eloquent' cortex, i.e. the primary motor, sensory or speech areas, then more accurate definition may be required. This can be achieved through placement of intracranial electrodes. These can record the region of seizure onset much more precisely than scalp electrodes but also can be used to map the regions of cortical function. This is done in an awake patient on the telemetry unit. Brief electrical stimulation is applied to adjacent pairs of electrodes on the cortical surface and clinical responses are observed. This can allow very accurate definition of regions subserving motor, sensory or speech relative to the region of seizure onset. If such eloquent areas are remote from the region of seizure onset then resection can safely be carried out. If the regions coincide, then resection will produce a deficit. Sometimes a limited deficit is an acceptable price to pay for epilepsy control but such decisions need to be carefully discussed with the patient.

Functional surgery

If a patient suffers severe epilepsy but is not suitable for resective surgery, it may be appropriate to consider functional procedures.

Multiple subpial transactions (MST)

If a focus can accurately be defined, but resection is not indicated because it is situated in an eloquent area, such as a primary speech or motor region, then MST may be used. This is based on the fact that functional units in the cortex are arranged in columns perpendicular to the brain surface. Epilepsy tends to spread across the cortex, using fibres parallel to the surface, which seem to be much less important to essential functions. MST consists of multiple transverse cuts across the surface of the brain in the epileptic focus, dividing these intracortical fibres through which the epilepsy spreads. This seems to improve epilepsy control without major disruption of function. It is less effective than resection of the brain, however.

Corpus callosotomy

This is an operation dividing the main white matter pathway joining the two hemispheres of the brain. It is used in cases where a single focus cannot be identified and where frequent partial seizures rapidly spread bilaterally, causing the patient to fall. Such 'drop attacks' can result in frequent injury. The callosotomy prevents the rapid spread of the seizure, hopefully preventing the fall. Total callosotomy is associated with a 'disconnection syndrome' in which functions in the two hemispheres have difficulty in integrating properly. Usually an anterior 2/3 callosotomy is performed to reduce this effect. Callosotomy may actually increase partial seizures but often improves drops and quality of life substantially.

Learning objectives

(1) To know the patient selection criteria for epilepsy surgery.
(2) To be aware of the general principles of presurgical assessment.
(3) To be aware of the risks of surgery.
(4) To know the possible surgical strategies.

Section 5 **Management of epilepsy**

Chapter 81

Preoperative assessment

Gonzalo Alarcón

Who can be operated on and when to suggest surgery

Before surgery can be performed for the treatment of epilepsy, detailed preoperative assessment has to be carried out in order to confirm the nature of the attacks, and to establish whether there is a single source for the patient's seizures and where it is.

The general admission criteria for patients to enter a programme for preoperative assessment of epilepsy are the following:

- Reliable diagnosis of intractable epilepsy: there should be no doubt that attacks are epileptic, the possibility of attacks being non-epileptic seizures should be ruled out, the patient must have been on appropriate medication at the correct doses for at least 2 years without adequate seizure control, and the patient must have been compliant with medication.
- Seizures should be disabling: seizures should pose an obstacle to the patient's lifestyle, capabilities and aspirations, because of the nature, timing and/ or frequency of seizures.
- The patient has resources to cope with assessment: patients should be able to tolerate the procedures, have realistic expectations about the results, and be able to accept failure of surgery.
- Absence of general contraindications to neurosurgery.

For specific admission criteria, see Box 81.1.

Surgical strategies

The overview of surgical strategies is detailed in Chapters 80 ('General principles of surgical treatment') and 82 ('Surgical techniques').

Purpose of presurgical assessment

The main reasons for the presurgical assessment are:

- to confirm that the patient suffers from epileptic seizures;
- to identify the brain source for the patient's typical seizures;
- to decide whether the severity of epilepsy warrants surgery;
- to assess the risks of surgery: particularly identifying the functionality of the area which is planned to be resected;
- to identify whether there are contraindications for surgery;
- to decide the type of surgical procedure: resection of a lesion (lesionectomy), wider resection (such as temporal lobectomy), multiple subpial transection of the affected region (if the area is functionally active), callosotomy, hemispherectomy, hemispherotomy;
- to identify the risks of surgery: particularly the function of the area which the surgeon plans to resect.

Clinical contraindications to surgery for epilepsy

- Severe depression: some surgical procedures (temporal lobectomy, particularly on the right) have been associated with depression.
- Chronic psychosis: although post-ictal or ictal psychosis is not a contraindication.
- General contraindications for neurosurgery.

Introduction to Epilepsy ed. Gonzalo Alarcón and Antonio Valentín. Published by Cambridge University Press.
© Cambridge University Press 2012.

Box 81.1. Specific admission criteria for surgical assessment programme

General criteria for admission:
- Reliable diagnosis of intractable epilepsy:
  - Attacks are epileptic, no pseudoseizures (or pseudoseizures distinguishable from epileptic seizures and the latter being the major cause of morbidity – the conditions frequently co-exist).
  - Failure of appropriate medication
  - Patient is compliant.
- Seizures of such a frequency and nature that they are disabling, having regard to the patient's lifestyle.
- No other contraindication of surgery, for example a coagulation defect.

Criteria for investigation for resective surgery:
- Partial (focal) seizures, whether or not secondarily generalized.
- Does not fulfil criteria for hemispherectomy and hemispherotomy as detailed in the next section.
- Full scale IQ generally not <70: a low IQ used to be regarded as a contraindication as it suggested a widespread brain dysfunction. This criterion is less rigidly applied nowadays, as it is recognized that focal lesions may cause severe epilepsy and affect IQ.
- Age generally not >55: again this is less frequently applied nowadays as outcome seems only slightly less favourable in the over 55s.
- Patient has emotional resources to cope with the procedures and possible inoperability.

Note:
- A single interictal EEG focus is not a requirement.
- Psychiatric or behavioural disorder is not an automatic exclusion criterion.
- If patient does not satisfy the criteria for resective surgery, apply selection criteria for hemispherectomy or callosotomy as detailed next.

Criteria for hemispherectomy and hemispherotomy:
- Long-standing unilateral hemispheric damage evidenced by hemiplegia, and brain imaging.
- Partial seizures, whether or not secondarily generalized, arising from the diseased hemisphere.

Criteria for callosotomy:
- Generalized seizures, particularly atonic or tonic seizures, causing injury, in the context of partial or symptomatic generalized epilepsy.
- This may be a preferred solution in patients with unilateral hemisphere disease, not severe enough for hemispherectomy.
- Associated partial seizures, if any, are not amenable to resective surgery.

Criteria for VNS:
- Ineligibility for all the above, or a <50% probability even of palliation.
- Arguably, all possible callosotomy candidates.

Reprinted from Binnie CD and Polkey CE (1992). Surgery for epilepsy. *Recent Advances in Clinical Neurology*, 7, 55–93, with permission from Elsevier.

Presurgical assessment

The principal methods that can be used during the surgical assessment are:
- Proper and complete medical history, including review of old notes.
- Seizure description, including witnesses' reports.
- Neuropsychiatric and neuropsychological assessment.
- Neuroimaging: mainly structural MRI, but may include CT, PET and SPECT.
- Interictal scalp EEG: awake and sleep.
- Ictal scalp EEG: video telemetry.
- Magnetoencephalography.
- Amytal test.
- Video-EEG telemetry with intracranial electrodes: ictal and interictal.
- Electrical stimulation of the brain to assess cortical excitability (SPES)
- Functional mapping:
  - non-invasive, e.g. fMRI
  - invasive: during video-EEG telemetry with intracranial electrodes
  - during surgery under local anaesthetic.
- Intraoperative electrocorticography (ECoG)

The underlying philosophy of surgical assessment for resective surgery is based on the following aspects.

- Resective surgery in epilepsy is unlikely to have a good outcome unless resected tissue is both functionally and structurally abnormal.
- Evidence from all presurgical procedures should converge onto a single brain region.
- If evidence is not convergent, an explanatory hypothesis must be proposed and tested, or resective surgery abandoned.

Medical history

Apart from the general issues regarding history-taking in epilepsy (see Chapter 46: History-taking and physical examination in epilepsy'), special emphasis should be placed on the description, frequency and severity of each seizure type, with the purpose of identifying both the source of the patient's seizures and the impact of seizures in the patient's life. In addition, the patient's educational and working history should be carefully documented to estimate the handicap associated with epilepsy, which could in part be reversed by surgery.

Seizure semiology

- The area responsible for seizures can be lateralized to a hemisphere by studying the clinical features of seizures alone in around 78% of patients.
- Although history-taking is a cornerstone in epileptology, seizure semiology is most accurately studied by observing videos of seizures.
- Often video recording from each seizure must be seen several times before a complete description can be made.
- The main lateralizing and localizing signs are:
  - dystonic posturing, suggesting contralateral onset
  - unilateral automatisms, suggesting ipsilateral onset
  - ictal speech, suggesting onset in the non-dominant hemisphere
  - forced head version (slow, gradual, sustained and extreme rotation of the head), suggesting onset contralateral to the side towards which the head rotates (patient looks away for focus)
  - unilateral clonic movements, suggesting contralateral onset
  - preserved consciousness with automatisms (very rare), suggesting right hemisphere onset
  - blinking, suggesting occipital seizures
  - unilateral blinking, suggesting ipsilateral onset
  - vomiting, suggesting right temporal seizures
  - retching, suggesting an insular onset
  - post-ictal dysphasia, suggesting onset in the dominant hemisphere
  - Todd's paralysis (post-ictal unilateral paralysis or weakness), suggesting contralateral onset
  - post-ictal nose wiping, suggesting ipsilateral temporal onset
  - rhythmic ictal nonclonic hand (RINCH) automatisms, which consist of finger rolling movements, suggesting contralateral temporal onset.
- Auras (simple partial seizures) have the following value:
  - déjà vu (feeling that what is happening has already happened) suggests medial temporal onset
  - epigastric rising sensation suggests medial temporal onset
  - hearing sounds or melodies suggests lateral temporal onset
  - unilateral tingling suggests contralateral onset close to somatosensory area
  - elementary visual symptoms (flashing lights, circles, colours) suggest occipital onset
  - unilateral elementary visual symptoms suggest contralateral occipital onset
  - complex visual hallucinations suggest occipital, parieto-occipital or frontal onset
  - thought disorder (e.g. thought implanted in someone's head) suggests frontal onset.

Neuropsychiatric assessment

- Neuropsychiatric assessment is essential before surgery because there is high psychiatric co-morbidity in patients with epilepsy. Treatable conditions should be identified and treated before surgery.
- Psychiatric morbidity is not per se a contraindication for surgery, particularly if symptoms are related to seizures (peri-ictal), which may be relieved by surgery.

Neuroimaging

- Neuroimaging has become paramount in the surgical assessment of patients with epilepsy.
- MRI is the main imaging modality.

- MRI should include coronal (perpendicular to the long axis of the temporal horn/hippocampus) and T1- and T2-weighted images (preferably with a volumetric T1W acquisition with partitions of 1 mm or less). FLAIR images are also helpful, particularly to look for subtle grey matter and subcortical white matter high signal associated with focal cortical dysplasia and the high signal seen in hippocampal sclerosis.
- CT is occasionally useful as an adjunct to MR to show calcified lesions (tumours such as oligodendrogliomas, phakomatoses such as tuberous sclerosis) and in an emergency. CT is also useful after surgery (to show surgical complications or electrode positions).
- Eighty-five per cent of patients with intractabale epilepsy show a structural abnormality on neuroimaging. However, the absence of a structural abnormality on neuroimaging does not rule out surgery, as the source of seizures may be identified with intracranial electrodes (Alarcón et al., 2006).

Quantification of MR images (hippocampal volume, hippocampal T2 measurements)

This may be helpful but is time-consuming to perform in every patient. For more details, see Chapter 38 ('Volumetric MRI and MRI spectroscopy').

Positron emission tomography (PET)

Fluoro-deoxyglucose (FDG) is the most commonly used PET tracer. The vast majority of PET studies are interictal, since it is unlikely that patients have seizures during the period of PET acquisition. Between 60 and 90% of patients with temporal lobe epilepsy show unilateral temporal hypometabolism on the side of seizure onset (Figure 41.1). Hypometabolism tends to be more widespread than the structural lesion, often involving most of the affected temporal lobe. In frontal lobe epilepsy, hypometabolism is reported to be lower, in the region of 60% or less of patients. For more details, see Chapter 41 ('PET in epilepsy').

Single proton emission tomography (SPECT)

The most commonly used tracer is 99mTc-HMPAO (99mTc-hexamethylpropylamine oxime). SPECT studies can be interictal, ictal or post-ictal. Since the tracer fixes in the brain shortly after intravenous injection, the technique has relatively high temporal resolution and can image seizures if injected shortly after seizure onset. This can be achieved in combination with video telemetry. Ictal SPECT shows appropriately lateralized hypermetabolism in 97% of temporal lobe seizures and in 92% of extratemporal seizures, the interpretation being dependent on timing of injection in relation to seizure onset. For more details, see Chapter 40 ('SPECT in epilepsy').

Neuropsychology

- Neuropsychological assessment may demonstrate a lateralized functional deficit associated with epileptogenesis (Akanuma et al., 2003).
- A discrepancy of more than 15 points between the verbal and performance (non-verbal) IQ suggests a lateralized dysfunction and hence unilateral pathology. A depressed verbal IQ suggests pathology in the dominant hemisphere for language (usually the left). A depressed non-verbal IQ would suggest pathology in the non-dominant hemisphere (usually the right).
- Differences between verbal and non-verbal memory scores have similar implications.
- The lateralizing value of verbal and non-verbal IQ differences is particularly high in right-handed patients because approximately 96% of right-handed patients have language on the left hemisphere. The lateralizing value of IQ difference is much lower in left- or mixed-handed patients, because only 70% have language on the left hemisphere. These figures apply to patients with late brain damage; for those with early damage, the figures fall to approximately 80% and 30% respectively.
- Preoperative IQ and memory have prognostic value: the patients with higher IQs tend to show higher postoperative deficits – possibly because they had more to lose.

Interictal scalp EEG

The principles of EEG interpretation are described in Chapters 14 ('Introduction to the electroencephalogram(EEG)') and 18 ('Clinical use of EEG in epilepsy'). With regard to presurgical assessment it is helpful to keep in mind that:

- patients assessed for surgery are only very rarely photosensitive;

- sleep is useful because it can enhance epileptiform discharges or demonstrate new foci;
- the incidence of bilateral independent epileptiform discharges in temporal lobe epilepsy is around 40% and their presence should not preclude surgery. Discharges are usually more prominent in the epileptogenic side, particularly during sleep.

Magnetoencephalography

This technique is gaining acceptance and is discussed in Chapter 45 ('Magnetoencephalography in epilepsy').

Ictal scalp EEG

Analysis of the EEG during a seizure (ictal EEG) may be of value in determining the side and site (i.e. laterality and localization) of the seizure focus.

- Since seizures are not usually seen during standard EEG recordings, video telemetry is often necessary to obtain recordings during seizures.
- EEG changes associated with seizures can be ictal or post-ictal. Ictal changes can consist of flattening of the EEG (electrodecremental event), low-amplitude fast activity (10–20 Hz), rhythmic sharp waves or spikes, or slowing in the delta or theta ranges (Alarcón *et al.*, 1995).
- EEG changes can be absent during simple partial seizures, and less commonly during frontal seizures.
- The initial ictal changes can be unilateral or bilateral. If unilateral and focal, they have localizing and lateralizing value (Figures 18.13 and 18.14). If the first scalp EEG changes are bilateral, they should not preclude surgery (Alarcón *et al.*, 2001). This is because seizures may still have a focal origin, although EEG changes may be seen on the scalp only after bilateral propagation has occurred. Intracranial recordings may be necessary to show a focal onset.

As it is important to establish whether there is a single site of onset, several seizures should be recorded during video telemetry (preferably five or more). In order to increase the chance of recording several seizures, activation procedures such as one-night sleep deprivation can be carried out, or AED medication may have to be reduced or withdrawn. Reductions in AED medication should be carried out slowly (over 2–3 days or longer) to reduce the risk of triggering status epilepticus or withdrawal seizures, which may show an anomalous onset or rapid generalization, making it difficult to localize seizure onset.

The amytal test (carotid amobarbital test, Wada test)

The interpretation and discussion of the Wada test for resective surgery are discussed in Chapter 79.

In patients with generalized epileptiform discharges with suspected secondary bilateral synchrony (discharges arising from one hemisphere and rapidly generalizing), the amytal test can be used to establish which is the hemisphere that drives the discharges. When the driving hemisphere is anaesthetized, discharges disappear bilaterally. On the other hand, when the driven hemisphere is anaesthetized, discharges disappear only on the injected side. Since secondary bilateral synchrony is generally studied in children with behavioural problems who have generalized spikes mainly during sleep, the amytal test to study this phenomenon is best performed under general anaesthesia. Extensive adjustments of the levels of anaesthesia might be necessary to induce a regular rate of generalized discharges. If generalized discharges still fail to occur, methohexital (a rapid-acting barbiturate) can be administered intravenously at progressively higher doses (up to 70–75 mg) until electrocerebral silence is observed on the EEG. Under such conditions, 'primary epileptogenic foci' show more resistance to synaptic blockade. The hemisphere showing epileptiform activity that disappeared latest and/or reappeared earliest after injection is considered as the driving hemisphere. These pharmacological tests are sometimes carried out as part of presurgical assessment in patients with Landau-Kleffner syndrome where multiple subpial transection of the perisylvian cortex is contemplated to treat acquired aphasia. Discharge latency analysis has been recently used to confirm findings from the amytal test (Martín Miguel *et al.*, 2011).

Intracranial EEG recordings

In patients where seizure semiology, neuroimaging findings, neuropsychological testing, scalp interictal and ictal EEG abnormalities converge to suggest a single region as the source of seizures, surgery can be undertaken. If evidence is not convergent, an explanatory hypothesis must be proposed and tested,

Section 5: Management of epilepsy

or resective surgery abandoned. Often, such an explanatory hypothesis can be tested by implanting electrodes close to the candidate site(s) for seizure onset. Compared to scalp electrodes, intracranial electrodes allow recording of much larger EEG signals from a much smaller region of brain with fewer muscle artefacts.

Once the patient recovers from electrode implantation, standard video telemetry is carried out with the intracranial electrodes to record the EEG until sufficient numbers of seizures are recorded. This is often referred to as chronic or subacute intracranial recordings (as opposed to the acute recordings obtained during intraoperative ECoG; see Chapter 88).

It has been claimed that recent advances in MRI technology will eventually abolish the need for chronic intracranial recordings. While improved imaging, particularly MRI, has undoubtedly been a major advance in epilepsy surgery, our experience in recent years is that intracranial recordings continue to be indicated in a proportion of patients. As with any diagnostic test, improvements in MRI sensitivity will necessarily be associated with increments in the number of true and false positive detections. In some patients multiple lesions are detected, raising the question of whether there is a single focal seizure onset and, if so, which lesion generates seizures. In other patients, mild non-specific unclear abnormalities can be seen, raising doubt as to whether they are indeed epileptogenic.

Several types of intracranial electrodes are available:

Foramen ovale electrodes

These are multicontact electrode bundles that can be inserted through the foramen ovale under fluoroscopic control and under general anaesthesia. The deepest contacts lie close to medial temporal structures. Removal does not require general anaesthesia. Because no craniotomy or burr holes are required for their implantation, they are often considered less invasive than subdural and depth electrodes. However, the use of these electrodes has declined as they are rather disagreeable, often irritating the trigeminal nerve while implanted. See Figure 81.1.

Subdural electrodes

These come as groups of electrodes arranged in either mats (grids) or strips (Figure 81.2). For simplicity, each electrode within a mat or strip is called a contact. Mats are arrays of contacts. Strips are single rows of contacts. Contacts are embedded in Silastic® or

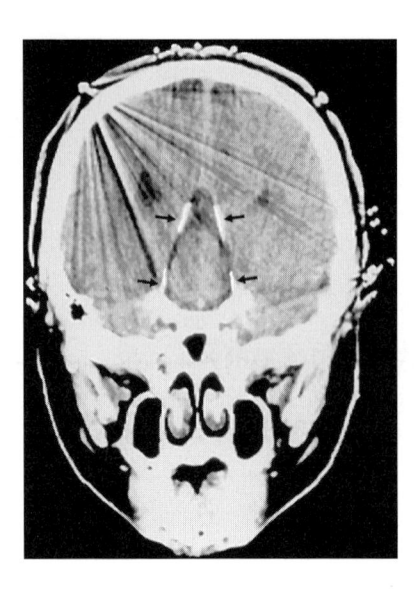

Figure 81.1. CT showing implanted foramen ovale recordings and typical inteictal recordings.

Teflon® sheets. Each contact typically has 5 mm diameter and contact centres are located 1 cm apart. Mats need to be introduced through a craniotomy, and can be placed under the dura over the cerebral convexity, or carefully inserted between brain and dura (at some risk of venous bleeding). Mats are suitable for functional mapping with electrical stimulation or with evoked responses to sensory stimulation. Strips come in single rows, typically of four or eight contacts, and several can be inserted through a burr hole. If inserted through a burr hole anterior to the ear, an eight-contact strip can be slipped under the temporal lobe and provide excellent recording from the parahippocampal gyrus. Used in this way, they serve a similar purpose to foramen ovale electrodes. General anaesthesia is required for insertion and removal. Strips can be combined with mats to cover the cerebral convexity and, if inserted parasagittally, the medial aspect of the cerebral hemispheres.

Depth (intracerebral) electrodes

These are multicontact electrode bundles that can be inserted stereotactically through the brain under neuroimaging control. They provide excellent recordings from deep brain regions (hippocampus, amygdala, cingulum) with some simultaneous EEG sampling from more superficial regions. See Figure 81.2.

Epidural peg electrodes

These consist of a stainless-steel disc mounted in a mushroom-shaped Silastic® support.

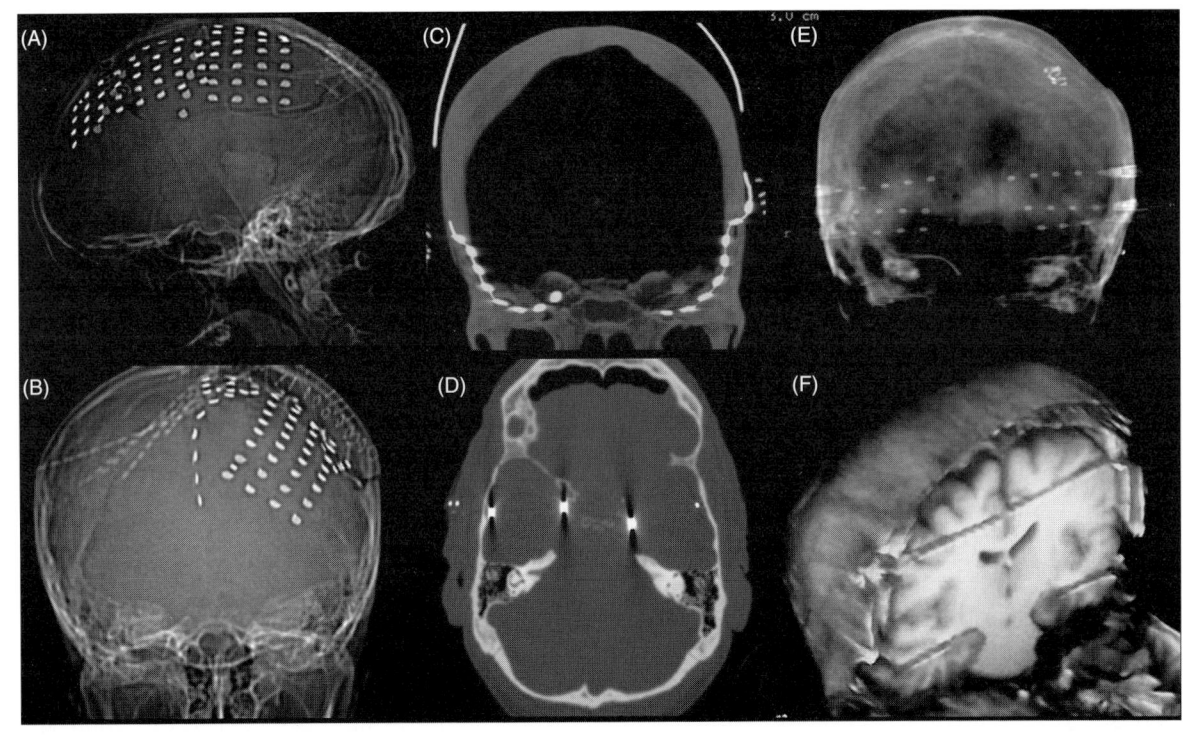

Figure 81.2. Implanted subdural mats over frontocentral regions (A, B), subtemporal strips (C, D) and intracerebral depth electrodes over temporal (E) and frontal and temporal regions (F).

They can be fixed on a burr hole with the top of the mushroom outside the skull. They are useful in addition to other intracranial electrodes when it is found during recording that an additional area needs exploring.

Indications for implantation of intracranial electrodes

The following three resective procedures can be performed without the need to employ intracranial electrodes:

- Lesionectomy: patients with a discrete, cerebral, non-atrophic lesion demonstrated by neuroimaging at a non-functionally eloquent site, with location concordant with seizure semiology, topography of interictal discharges, topography of ictal onset on scalp EEG, distribution of background abnormalities in the interictal EEG, and neuropsychological findings.
- Temporal lobectomy: patients with a consistent, single, temporal site of seizure onset on scalp EEG telemetry, concordant with seizure semiology, distribution of background abnormalities in the interictal scalp EEG, neuroimaging, and neuropsychological findings.
- Hemispherectomy: see Chapter 82 ('Surgical techniques').

Patients not fulfilling these criteria can have studies with intracranial electrodes.

These are patients where a hypothesis is available to explain findings to date, particularly any non-convergence of evidence from different tests, and this hypothesis is testable with intracranial electrode implantation.

The choice and placement of intracranial electrodes depend on the working hypothesis with regard to the site of seizure onset. As intracerebral (depth) electrodes are perceived to be more invasive than subdural recordings, the latter are generally preferred if possible. When temporal lobe seizures are suspected, but laterality is uncertain, recordings with bilateral eight-contact subtemporal strips inserted through fronto-temporal burr holes can be carried out. If this procedure yields inconclusive results, a second intracranial recording can be performed with bilateral temporal intracerebral electrodes. When seizures are thought to arise from the frontal lobes, but laterality is uncertain, bilateral intracerebral electrodes can be used. When the seizures are thought to arise from the cerebral convexity, from peri-central regions or from the supplementary motor area, mats or strips can be used, usually implanted unilaterally. Resective surgery can be excluded if:

- the EEG shows predominantly generalized interictal EEG discharges in the absence of a discrete lesion on neuroimaging;
- independent sites of electrographic seizure onset are demonstrated in more than one lobe;
- generalized discharges are seen at or immediately preceding clinical seizure onset;
- a site of seizure onset is identified which could not be resected without unacceptable complications, and is unsuitable for multiple subpial transaction;
- bilateral or multilobar seizure onset is seen with intracranial recordings and no clear alternative hypothesis exists for further studies with intracranial recordings.

Complications of intracranial electrodes

The main complications are infection and cerebral haemorrhage. The likelihood of complications from intracranial recordings is roughly proportional to the number of electrodes implanted. We have found <2% risk of permanent neurological deficits. Transitory deficits and complications are more common (almost 5%). Transmission of Creutzfeldt–Jakob disease has been reported but can be avoided by disposing of used electrodes.

Chronic implantation of mats can be associated with leakage of cerebrospinal fluid that can be managed by keeping the head high and changing the head bandage regularly. Mat recordings appear to have a 0.85% risk of infection, which can be reduced with prophylactic antibiotics, minimizing duration of implantation and passing the cables through the scalp at a point far from the craniotomy. Frank meningitis or encephalitis is rare.

Depth electrodes have a very low risk of infection, a 1.9% risk of haemorrhage with transitory deficits and a 0.8% risk of haemorrhage with permanent deficits.

Interpretation of intracranial recordings

Epileptiform discharges recorded interictally with intracranial electrodes are larger, sharper and occur more frequently than those seen on the scalp. Each patient usually exhibits several patterns of epileptiform discharges occurring independently at different sites, often including the hemisphere opposite to seizure onset (Figure 81.3). For this reason, interictal activity recorded with intracranial electrodes should be interpreted cautiously. Ictal changes consist of flattening of the ongoing EEG (electrodecremental event), low-amplitude fast activity (10–60 Hz), rhythmic sharp waves or spikes, or slowing in the delta or theta ranges. Fast activity appears to be the pattern with the highest localizing value (Figure 81.1). Generalized electrodecremental events (diffuse flattening of the EEG) are common at seizure onset but should not discourage surgery, since they do not seem to be associated with worse outcome if there are other focal features (Figure 81.3). Any other form of changes occurring diffusely at seizure onset would suggest that the seizure is generalized or, more commonly, electrodes are not placed at the site of seizure origin.

Functional mapping

If the proposed resection is close to an area relevant for vital functions (motor, sensory or speech areas), the risk of major postoperative functional deficits can be reduced by accurate identification of such functional areas with the purpose of avoiding their resection. The role of functional MRI for this purpose is still undetermined. At present, functional mapping can be reliably obtained in patients with intracranial electrodes. Sensory areas can be plotted from sensory evoked potentials recorded with mat electrodes. Alternatively, functional regions can be identified by electrical stimulation in the conscious patient. Mapping can be obtained intraoperatively or during chronic recordings in telemetry. Constant current electrical stimulation of progressively increased intensity and duration is used (up to 6-s trains of electrical pulses, up to 10 mA, 1 ms bipolar pulses at 50 Hz). Pairs of adjacent electrodes are used to deliver current. Stimulation of the somatosensory area induces tingling, numbness or other paraesthesiae in the corresponding cutaneous region. Stimulation of the motor strip is associated with focal twitches or sustained contraction of the corresponding muscle group(s). Stimulation of the speech area induces speech arrest.

Electrical stimulation that induces the patient's habitual auras or seizures can be used to aid in the identification of areas responsible for spontaneous seizures.

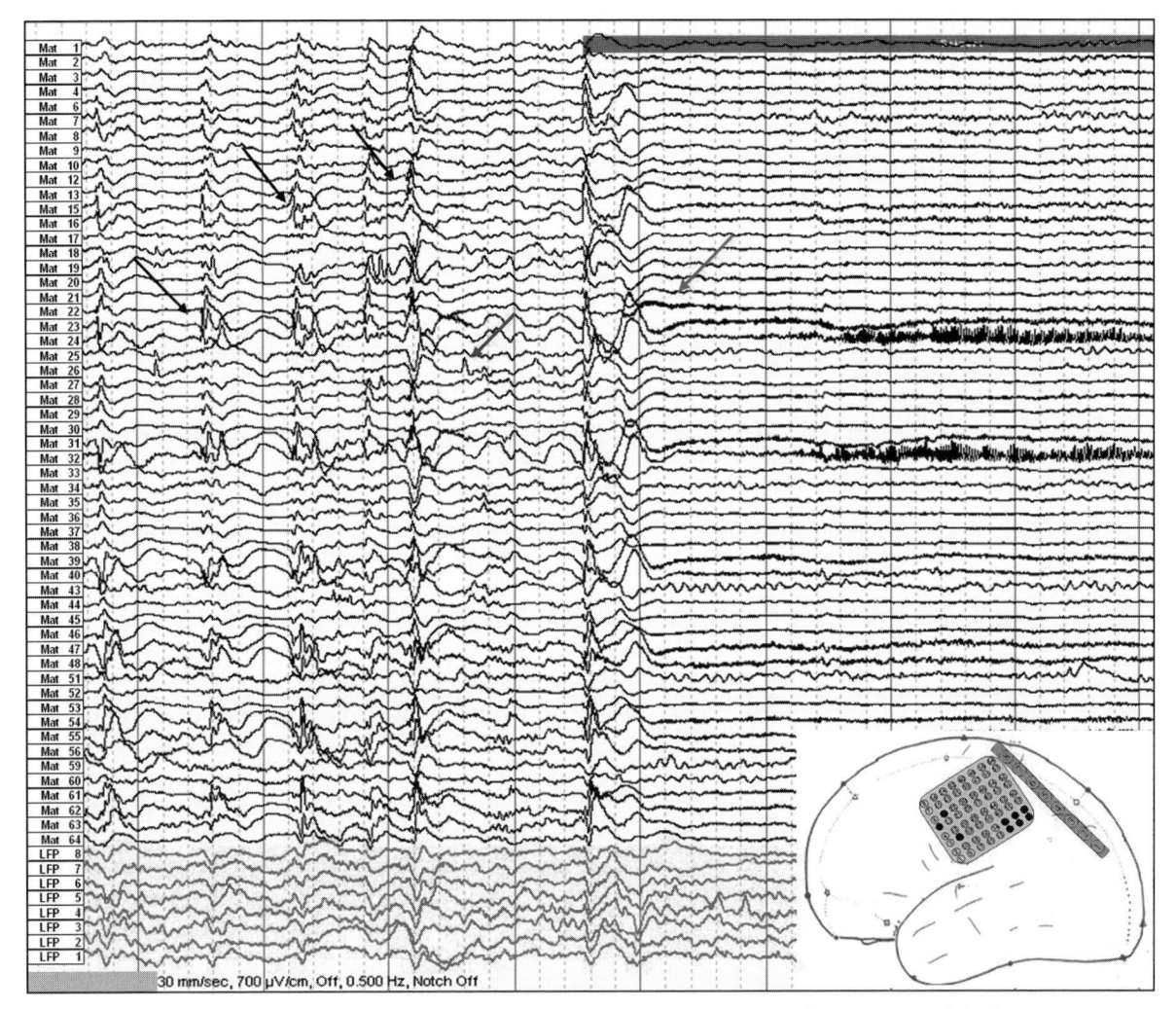

Figure 81.3. Focal seizure onset recorded with a subdural high-density 64-contact mat and an 8-contact subdural strip in a patient with focal cortical dysplasia. Before the seizure, sporadic focal discharges are seen (blue arrow) in addition to nearly continuous more widespread discharges seen at regular intervals (black arrows). During the seizure (top red horizontal bar), there is a diffuse attenuation of the background activity (electrodecremental event) associated with focal fast activity at 71 Hz (red arrow) over the superior two rows of the mat (electrodes 22, 23, 24, 31, 32, 39, 40, 47 and 48 of the mat). Electrode 1 of the mat is the most inferior electrode and electrode 8 is the most anterior. See colour version in plate section.

Phased evaluation

Surgical assessment requires a multidisciplinary team and the interpretation of multiple tests of increasing complexity and invasiveness. See Box 81.2 and Figure 81.3.

Misconceptions about presurgical assessment in epilepsy surgery

The following misconceptions are commonly held and are not necessarily true:

'Neuropsychology is unnecessary': this is simply not true! Neuropsychology is a functional diagnostic method of clear value:

- VIP-PIQ asymmetries >15 suggest lateralized dysfunction.
- Memory asymmetries have similar implication.
- Amytal test + VIP has a lateralizing value of 80% (Akanuma et al., 2003).

'A normal MRI makes the patient inoperable': this is not always true, other tests can accurately localize! In

> **Box 81.2. Phases of investigation for possible surgical treatment***
>
> **Phase Ia:** baseline outpatient investigations routinely performed on referral
> - Clinical assessment
> - High-resolution MRI with FLAIR
> - Routine and sleep EEG
>
> **Phase Ib:** further non-invasive investigations
> - Scalp telemetry
> - Neuropsychology
> - Volumetric MRI
> - FDG-PET
> - Flumazenil PET
> - Ictal SPECT
>
> **Phase IIa:** minor invasive procedures
> - Telemetry with subdural strips
> - Telemetry with foramen ovale electrodes
> - Carotid amylobarbital test (Wada test)
>
> **Phase IIb:** major invasive procedures
> - Telemetry with subdural or depth (intracerebral) electrodes
>
> *Reprinted with permission from Binnie C, Cooper R, Mauguière F, et al. (eds.) (2003). *Clinical Neurophysiology*, vol 2. Elsevier Science B.V., Amsterdam © 2003, with permission from Elsevier.

our centre, 85% of patients with intractable epilepsy show a structural abnormality on neuroimaging. However, the absence of a structural abnormality on neuroimaging should not discourage surgery, as often the source of seizures can be identified with intracranial electrodes (Alarcón et al., 2006).

'Multiple lesions makes the patient inoperable': often only one lesion is epileptogenic! This question more commonly arises with the modern improvements in MRI sensitivity, which has increased the number of true and false positives.

'Bilateral independent temporal interictal discharges mean bilateral independent seizures and precludes surgery': bilateral independent discharges are commonly seen during presurgical assessment, particularly with intracranial electrodes. The incidence of bilateral independent scalp epileptiform discharges in temporal lobe epilepsy is around 40%. However, most patients with bilateral independent interictal temporal discharges have unilateral seizures! Bilateral independent discharges have the following implications:

- Discharges are usually more prominent in the epileptogenic side, particularly during sleep.
- Seizure onset is more likely to occur on the side where spikes are most frequent (Blume et al., 2001).
- Seizure control is better the greater the degree of lateralization of bilateral independent discharges (Chung et al., 1991).

'All epileptic seizures show EEG abnormalities on the scalp': many simple partial seizures (particularly those with phychic, nonspecific or cognitive features) and some frontal seizures do not show clear EEG changes on the scalp. In simple partical seizure this is due to selective involvement of localized deep regions, whose EEG signals do not reach the scalp. Some frontal lobe seizures do not show EEG changes due to muscle and movement artefacts.

'A diffuse onset on the scalp EEG means that there is no focal onset and assessment should be abandoned': this is simply not true, because intracranial recordings can show a focal onset! Among presumed temporal lobe seizures, approximatelly 67% show bilateral or diffuse onset on the scalp, whereas on simultaneous foramen ovale recordings, 64% show a clear focal mesial temporal onset (Alarcón et al., 2001).

'Assessment should be abandoned in the presence of non-convergent information among tests': not so, but a feasible explanation must exist or be searched for.

'A diffuse electrodecremental event at seizure onset precludes surgery': not if there are focal features! About one-third of focal seizures show an initial diffuse electrodecremental event, followed by focal fast or rhythmic theta activities (Alarcón et al., 1995).

'Resective surgery is the only worthwhile intervention': there are a number of treatment alternatives to resection which can be effective: vagus nerve stimulation, multiple subpial transections, hemispherotomy, callosotomy and deep brain stimulation. They are discussed in Chapters 82 ('Surgical techniques'), 85 ('Vagus nerve stimulation') and 86 ('Brain stimulation for the treatment of epilepsy').

Chapter 81: Preoperative assessment

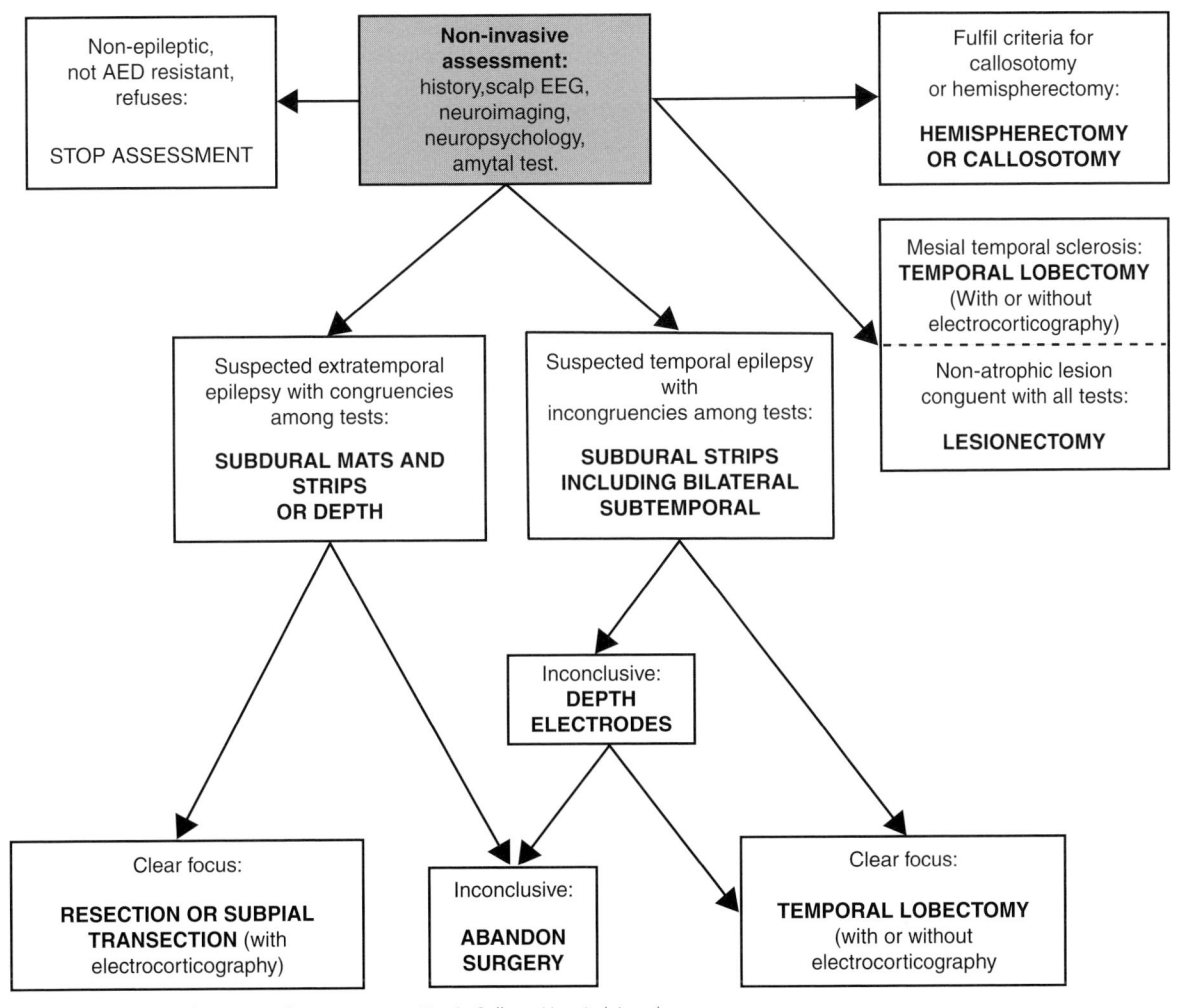

Figure 81.4. Flow of presurgical assessment at King's College Hospital, London.

References

Akanuma N, Alarcón G, Lum F, et al. Lateralising value of neuropsychological protocols for presurgical assessment of temporal lobe epilepsy. *Epilepsia* 2003;**44**:408–18.

Alarcón G, Binnie CD, Elwes RDC, Polkey CE. Power spectrum and intracranial EEG patterns at seizure onset in partial epilepsy. *Electroencephalogr Clin Neurophysiol* 1995;**94**:326–37.

Alarcón G, Kissani N, Dad M, et al. Lateralizing and localizing values of ictal onset recorded on the scalp: evidence from simultaneous recordings with intracranial foramen ovale electrodes. *Epilepsia* 2001;**42**:1426–37.

Alarcón G, Valentín A, Watt C, et al. Is it worth pursuing surgery for epilepsy in patients with normal neuroimaging? *J Neurol Neurosurg Psychiatry* 2006; **77**: 474–80.

Blume WT, Holloway GM, Wiebe S. Temporal epileptogenesis: localizing value of scalp and subdural interictal and ictal EEG data. *Epilepsia* 2001;**42**:508–14.

Chung MY, Walczak TS, Lewis DV, Dawson DV, Radtke R. Temporal lobectomy and independent bitemporal interictal activity: What degree of lateralization is sufficient? *Epilepsia* 1991; **32**:195–201.

Martín Miguel MC, García Seoane JJ, Valentín A, et al. EEG latency analysis for hemispheric lateralisation in Landau-Kleffner syndrome. *Clin Neurophysiol* 2011;**122**:244–52.

Section 5: Management of epilepsy

Learning objectives

(1) To know the criteria for patient selection for epilepsy surgery.
(2) To know the objectives of presurgical assessment.
(3) To know the contraindications for epilepsy surgery.
(4) To be aware of the general strategy for presurgical assessment.
(5) To know the indications, advantages, limitations and evaluation of the different diagnostic methods used in presurgical assessment.
(6) To be aware of common misconceptions about presurgical assessment in epilepsy surgery.

Section 5 Management of epilepsy

Chapter 82

Surgical techniques

Richard P. Selway

Surgery for mesial temporal sclerosis

The commonest resective procedures in epilepsy surgery are temporal lobe resections, where the mesial structures are removed. The main indication is mesial temporal sclerosis (MTS), although frequently this pathology may have been surmised by intracranial electrode recording rather than demonstrated on MRI scan, or some other focal pathology may involve these structures.

Broadly these operations may be divided into en bloc resections and selective amygdalo-hippocampectomy (Figure 82.1). It is clear that the hippocampus and para-hippocampal gyrus should be removed. Most surgeons will include the inferio-lateral portion of the amygdala. The amount of temporal neocortex removed depends on the approach taken.

There is no concensus as to the 'best' surgical approach for MTS and related disorders. This remains a controversial topic. Anterior temporal lobectomy (ATL) involves the removal of the anterior temporal neocortex, providing good access to mesial structures, which are then excised en bloc. Selective amygdalo-hippocampectomy (sAH) involves dividing but preserving cortex overlying medial temporal structures to obtain 'keyhole' access to the mesial structures. Table 82.1 compares the two approaches. Results from large surgical series suggest that the key to good surgical outcome seems to be the degree of resection of the hippocampus and parahippocampal gyrus. Both sAH and ATL seem to produce similar long-term seizure outcome. Moreover, despite over half a century of postoperative neuropsychological assessment, there is no consensus as to which is the best approach.

In temporal lobe surgery where the preoperative target is less precise (e.g. MRI negative with anterior neocortical seizure onset) then intraoperative electrocorticography (ECoG) is helpful in 'tailoring' the extent of neocortical resection (see Chapter 88).

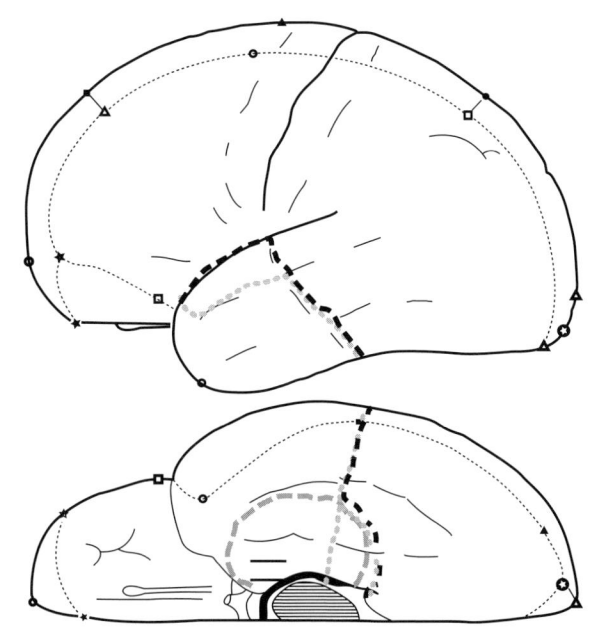

Figure 82.1. Temporal resections. The lines show the limits of resections for selective amygdalo-hippocampectomy (dark grey hatched line), and en bloc temporal lobectomy in the dominant (thick dotted line) and non-dominant (black dashed line) hemispheres.

Lesionectomy

One of the central tenets of epilepsy surgery is that complete resection of the pathological lesion is associated with excellent seizure outcome. For example, there is good evidence that resection of a cortically based cavernous haemangioma (cavernoma) is not

---

Introduction to Epilepsy ed. Gonzalo Alarcón and Antonio Valentín. Published by Cambridge University Press.
© Cambridge University Press 2012.

Table 82.1. Comparison of advantages and disadvantages of anterior temporal lobectomy versus selective amygdalo-hippocampectomy

Anterior temporal lobectomy	Selective amygdalo-hippocampectomy
Technically easier	Surgically more challenging
Less retraction on remaining brain: implying less collateral damage	Less normal tissue removed
En boc pathology specimen	Small fragments for diagnosis
? Benefits for verbal function (no Broca's area frontal retraction)	? Benefits for verbal memory due to less lateral cortex resection

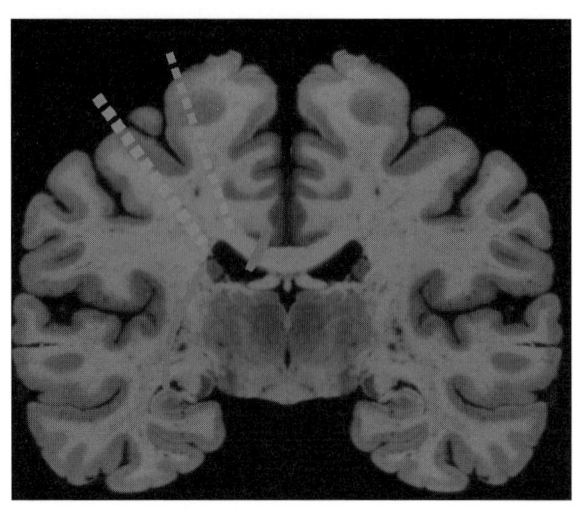

Figure 82.2. Hemispherotomy. Entry into the ventricular system is carried out between the dotted lines. Fibre tracts are then divided along the full lines.

sufficient but that the surrounding blood-stained brain should also be removed to obtain the greatest chance of a seizure-free outcome. In non-eloquent areas of cortex, complete excisions of focal lesions are often feasible. Frequently, however, the extent of the resection is limited by the potential for neurological deficit and the surgical plan may need to be a compromise between the two. Incomplete resections of whichever epileptogenic lesion one is considering are often associated with good or excellent outcome but, particularly in focal cortical dysplasia, there are reports that partial resection can worsen the patient's epilepsy.

In order to optimize the resection size while minimizing the risk of neurological deficit several techniques are available. Preoperatively obtaining as much data as possible about the region of seizure onset and the relative location of functional cortex is crucial. This may require intracranial EEG studies with ictal recordings, and cortical stimulation with mapping as well as structural (MRI) and functional (e.g. ictal SPECT, functional MRI) imaging. With this information, a careful discussion with the patient is required to agree the degree of risk appropriate to the planned surgery: a conservative resection if the risks are high and the epilepsy 'bearable', or an aggressive resection if it is agreed that the neurological deficit is likely to be a price 'worth paying' for the loss of seizures. A good example is that it is frequently agreed that an occipital resection for focal cortical dysplasia has a good chance of achieving excellent seizure results and that the inevitable hemianopia is an acceptable cost. By contrast only the most severe epilepsy would justify resection of primary speech or upper limb motor areas although even this might be appropriate in the catastrophic life-threatening epilepsy syndromes. Intraoperatively, the use of image guidance allows lesions to be resected with considerably more accuracy and confidence. To optimize the resection of the irritative zone (i.e. the areas showing inteirctal discharges), ECoG can guide the initial resection margins, and post-resection recordings can allow small residua to be detected and removed. Finally, if preoperative investigation suggests a lesion closely adjacent to highly eloquent brain, then surgery under local anaesthetic can provide the most accurate distinction. Such awake surgery is taxing for both patient and surgeon, and is much less frequently adopted now that preoperative investigation is so much improved. The most frequent indications are for lesions with vague borders such as dysplastic regions close to the primary motor cortex of the hand or to speech areas.

Hemisphere procedures

In patients with severe epilepsy arising in a previously damaged hemisphere, resection or disconnection of that hemisphere may be an extremely effective therapy. Anatomical hemispherectomy produces a large space inside the skull. This is associated with the risk of haemorrhage into the cavity and long-term repeated minor injury to the remaining brain with the eventual development of superficial cerebral haemosiderosis. This may lead to a gradual dementing process. Various modifications have been developed in which the intracranial space is reduced either by stitching the dura of the resected hemisphere down to the midline (Adams's technique), or by disconnecting regions of the affected hemisphere without removing them (hemispherotomy). In the De la Lande hemispherotomy, for example, the corpus callosum is divided throughout its full length and then the white matter surrounding the thalamus is divided from within the ventricle. This leaves the whole hemisphere in place, retaining its blood supply but preventing it from communicating with the rest of the brain or body. Hemispherotomy procedures have proven to be a considerable advance over the hemispherectomies as they are associated with lower blood loss, quicker recovery and shorter hospital stay. Seizure results seem to be similar whichever procedure is used.

Learning objective

(1) To be familiar with the different surgical techniques used in epilepsy surgery and to be able to discuss their principles, indications, pros and cons.

Section 5 Management of epilepsy

Chapter 83

Outcome of surgery

Charles E. Polkey

It is difficult to obtain Class I evidence for surgical treatments because it is difficult to devise true control groups in trials of surgical operations. Randomly assigning patients to a control group, in whom the surgical operation is delayed for 1 year after the decision has been made that this is appropriate treatment, is an accepted way of overcoming this problem. This was accepted in 2003 by the Quality Standards Subcommittee of the American Academy of Neurology when they agreed on the basis of Class I and Class IV evidence that patients with partial complex seizures should be referred for presurgical evaluation (Engel et al., 2003)

Operations for epilepsy are of two kinds: resective, operations which remove part of the brain responsible for the epilepsy, and functional, operations which attempt to change the way that epilepsy affects the brain. The outcomes from these two procedures are different: resective surgery makes 20–80% of patients seizure-free, depending upon the syndrome and the operative procedure, whereas functional operations render around 2% of patients seizure-free.

Resective surgery

The perfect outcome from resective surgery is complete freedom from seizures, without any additional deficit, neurological, cognitive or psychiatric. This is a counsel of perfection and two schemes of outcome are commonly used. One was proposed by Engel in 1985 (Table 83.1) and the other by the International League Against Epilepsy (ILAE) in 2001 (Table 83.2).

There are minor complications of resective surgery, resolving within 3 months, and major complications persisting beyond 3 months and affecting activities of daily living. A study, between 1990 and 1995, of 449 resective procedures with at least 2 years follow-up revealed minor complications in 8.9% and major complications in 3.1% (Guldvog et al., 1991). Mortality from resective surgery comprises early mortality within 1 month (0–1%) of surgery and late mortality. In our recent series of temporal lobe resections late mortality was 5.6%; 13 deaths were epilepsy-related and six were classified as sudden death in epilepsy (SUDEP).

Engel describes four surgically remediable syndromes, mesial temporal lobe epilepsy (MTLE), lesional partial epilepsies, diffuse hemispheric syndromes and secondarily generalized epilepsies. In the commonest resective procedure, temporal lobe resection, outcome, with regard to seizure control, depends in part on the procedure, but to a greater extent on the pathology, which differs with age. The commonest cause of MTLE is mesial temporal sclerosis, the pathology in 50% of cases in mixed series falling to 30% in children less than 12 years old. In series of temporal lobe resections published during the last two years around 80% of patients are substantially seizure free. A series of 399 patients with MTLE, described in 2006, showed a fall in seizure-free patients from 82% at 6 months after surgery to 72% at 10 years. The principal complications of temporal lobe resection, a homonymous hemianopia or a hemiplegia, depend upon experience and in long-standing centres are less than 1%. The cognitive effects of temporal lobe resection, mainly deterioration in recent memory, are to some extent predictable. Whether a more limited, selected, resection such as selective amygdalo-hippocampectomy can reduce deterioration in verbal memory remains unresolved. A paranoid-type psychosis follows less than 1% of operations, and depression, associated with non-dominant resections, perhaps in as many as 30% of patients. Extensive studies of quality of life after this surgery have shown

---

Introduction to Epilepsy ed. Gonzalo Alarcón and Antonio Valentín. Published by Cambridge University Press.
© Cambridge University Press 2012.

Table 83.1. Engel outcome groups 1993

Outcome		Definition
Group	**Subgroup**	
I Free of disabling seizures[a]	a b c d	Completely seizure free since surgery Non-disabling simple partial seizures only since surgery Some disabling seizures since surgery but free of disabling seizures for two years Generalized convulsion with antiepileptic drug withdrawal only
II Rare disabling seizures	a b c d	Initially free of disabling seizures but rare disabling seizures now Rare disabling seizures since surgery More than rare disabling seizures after surgery but rare disabling seizures for at least two years Nocturnal seizures only
III Worthwhile improvement	a b	Worthwhile seizure reduction Prolonged seizure-free intervals amounting to greater than half the follow-up period but not less than 2 years
IV No worthwhile improvement	a b c	Significant seizure reduction No appreciable change Worse

[a] Excludes early postoperative seizures, i.e. first few weeks.

Table 83.2. ILAE outcome groups 2001 (Weiser et al., 2001)

Outcome class	Definition
1	Completely seizure-free, no auras
2	Only auras, no other seizures
3	One to three seizure days per year ± auras
4	Four seizure days per year to 50% reduction in baseline ± auras
5	More than 50% reduction to 100% increase in baseline ± auras
6	More than 100% increase in baseline ± auras

that only patients who are seizure-free, or virtually so, show any improvement, with a better chance of employment, completing education and forming a stable relationship.

Lesional partial epilepsies are found in all parts of the cerebral cortex. The success of resections depends upon the nature of the lesion and the area in which it is located. If the lesion can be completely removed, seizure-free rates of 45% are obtained for extrafrontal resections and up to 69% for frontal lobe resections. Complications depend upon the location of the lesion: those in functionally eloquent areas pose more risk, which can be minimized by using appropriate preoperative investigations and perhaps local anaesthesia.

Diffuse hemispheric syndromes include several scenarios such as early vascular damage, cortical migration disorder including hemimegalencephaly, Rasmussen's disease and other conditions such as Sturge-Weber syndrome. The technique must allow adequate removal or disconnection. Modern techniques of hemispherotomy minimize blood loss and shorten operating time, making it possible to operate on younger patients (Delalande and Dorfmuller, 2008). Around 75% of patients are seizure-free, except in hemimegalencephaly, where it is around 65%. When seizure control is good there is often an improvement in behaviour and reduction in AED usage. Early and late mortality are low, about 1.5%. Hydrocephalus occurs in 4–19%. Increased neurological deficit is rare but often the addition of a homonymous hemianopia is justified.

The fourth group of patients with secondarily generalized epilepsy have, as it were, occult focal epilepsy and fall into the groups already described. The hypothalamic hamartoma presents with two epilepsy syndromes. One is relatively benign, presenting late with gelastic seizures. The more malevolent form presents in infancy with multiple seizure types, delayed development and a severe behaviour disorder. Open resection using the transcallosal approach has a high success rate. Follow-up from Melbourne and Phoenix indicates 52–54% seizure-free and an over 90% reduction in 24–35% (Rosenfeld and Feiz-Erfan, 2007). Complication rates are very low except for persisting short-term memory problems in 8–14%. A stereo-endoscopic approach from Paris results in 48.5% seizure-free; there were complications in two cases, both involving a pterional approach. The best candidates had type 2 lesions largely confined to the third ventricle. The latest study of gamma knife surgery for these patients suggests that 59.2% had a satisfactory result with regard to seizure control, behaviour and cognitive effects. The results of all kinds of surgery to this lesion are determined by the size and situation of the lesion and more than one approach may be needed.

Stereotactic radiosurgery chiefly using the Leksell Gamma Knife has been used to treat epilepsy. In the latest reports of cases of mesial temporal sclerosis 65% of the patients were seizure-free. During the 2-year interval before seizures are controlled, there may be problems with brain swelling and a significant increase is partial seizures. Complications, apart from visual field defects, are few but the numbers are small. The target and dose have to be precise and treatment will fail if these are inappropriate. The use of gamma knife surgery for hypothalamic hamartoma depends upon the site and size of the hamartoma and is probably best for type 1 or type 2. Callosotomy using a gamma knife has been reported but the series are small and outcome is indifferent and probably inferior to that achieved by conventional techniques.

Reoperation is necessary in around 5% of any surgical series. The literature is diverse in the range of cases covered, the methods of investigation and the outcome. In general reoperation is less successful than the initial operation; the patients should be investigated with the same rigour as new cases and the possibility of seizure freedom is less than in initial operations, in temporal lobe cases for example around 50–60%.

Functional surgery

For functional procedures the standard measure of success is a 50% reduction in the patient's pre-treatment seizure frequency. Discrete lesioning using stereotactic positioning and radiofrequency lesioning has been largely abandoned. Disconnection, if hemispherotomy is excluded, comprises callosotomy and multiple subpial transection. Callosotomy is a well-established procedure applied to a heterogeneous group of patients. Recent publications reflect earlier results with a good relief of drop attacks and generalized seizures. There is a greater than 50% relief in at least 75% with drop attacks and 35–80% for generalized seizures. Complication rates have fallen, with permanent complications reduced to less than 4%. Some believe that a complete callosotomy is more effective in seizure control without introducing additional physical or cognitive defects.

The reported results of MST are variable. A meta-analysis in 2002 of 211 patients suggested that the results for MST alone, and when combined with resection, gave an excellent result in over 70% of patients, with new neurological deficits in about 20% (Spencer et al., 2002). In Landau-Kleffner syndrome it has been shown to be an effective strategy for improving behaviour and expediting speech recovery.

Indirect brain stimulation, using the vagus nerve, was first introduced in 1990 and has been used extensively since. A large number of studies now available indicate that a 50% reduction in seizure frequency occurs in up to 40% of patients with reduction in severity or side effects of seizures in a further 20%. Improvements in QOL and cognition are also described. Side effects are few and mortality from what is essentially a simple surgical procedure is low. Children appear to benefit more than adults and there is some evidence that patients with Lennox-Gastaut syndrome do better than average. At present the results of direct brain stimulation, using both open-loop and closed-loop systems, are experimental.

Conclusions

(1) Resective surgery produces seizure freedom in 20–80% of patients with low mortality and morbidity.
(2) Hemispherotomy is an effective treatment in patients with diffuse hemispheric syndromes.
(3) Functional surgery is less effective but can still give useful seizure control and improved quality of life.
(4) Stimulation techniques are available, VNS is established and direct brain stimulation remains an experimental technique.

References

Delalande O, Dorfmuller G. [Parasagittal vertical hemispherotomy: surgical procedure]. *Neurochirurgie* 2008;**54**(3):353–7.

Engel J Jr, Wiebe S, French J, *et al.* Practice parameter: temporal lobe and localized neocortical resections for epilepsy: Report of the Quality Standards Subcommittee of the American Academy of Neurology, in Association with the American Epilepsy Society and the American Association of Neurological Surgeons. *Neurology* 2003;**60**(4):538–47.

Guldvog B, Loyning Y, Hauglie Hanssen E, Flood S, Bjornaes H. Surgical versus medical treatment for epilepsy. I. Outcome related to survival, seizures, and neurologic deficit. *Epilepsia* 1991;**32**:375–88.

Rosenfeld JV, Feiz-Erfan I. Hypothalamic hamartoma treatment: surgical resection with the transcallosal approach. *Semin Pediatr Neurol* 2007;**14**(2):88–98.

Spencer SS, Schramm J, Wyler A, *et al.* Multiple subpial transection for intractable partial epilepsy: an international meta-analysis. *Epilepsia* 2002; **43**(2):141–5.

Wieser HG, Blume WT, Fish D, *et al.* ILAE Commission Report. Proposal for a new classification of outcome with respect to epileptic seizures following epilepsy surgery. *Epilepsia* 2001;**42**(2):282–6.

Learning objectives

(1) To be aware of the difficulties in studying surgical outcome.
(2) To be familiar with the scales used to quantify surgical outcome.
(3) To be able to estimate the chances of favourable/poor outcome for the different varieties of resective and functional surgery.

Section 5 Management of epilepsy

Chapter 84: Epilepsy surgery in children

Charles E. Polkey

Epilepsy surgery in children, those aged less than 18 years at operation, is based upon a number of considerations other than pharmaco-resistance, as set out in the ILAE Subcommission's report in 2006 (Cross et al., 2006). The presentation of localization-related epilepsy in childhood is more heterogeneous than in adults and the electroclinical syndrome may evolve rapidly. Severe epilepsy in childhood can have significant effects on cognitive function and behaviour. The functional plasticity of the child's brain can facilitate neurological and cognitive recovery after surgery. It has been claimed for many years, perhaps without objective evidence, that early intervention would minimize the social and educational disadvantages of uncontrolled epilepsy. For these reasons, intervention may need to be undertaken earlier than in adults. A clear understanding between the family and the multidisciplinary team is important, as advocated by Taylor et al.(1997).

The data from the ILAE Subcommission's report show that the commonest pathological substrates in children are congenital rather than secondarily acquired lesions and the majority of operations (71%) are resective rather than functional. Cortical neuronal migration disorder is the major pathology in epilepsy surgery in children. This entity is itself very heterogeneous and when bilateral or diffuse may be difficult or impossible to treat surgically. The location of these lesions also varies; although frontal and temporal lobe resections predominate these are less than in adults and offset by hemispherectomy and multilobar resections, which comprise 25.8% of their operations. The use of callosotomy has fallen sharply (3.1%) with the availability of vagus nerve stimulation. This latter procedure should be applied with the same rigorous criteria as other procedures.

Because of the nature of the pathology, the investigation of children in a presurgical assessment programme varies from that in adults. The same ILAE study shows that intracranial electrodes were used by 90% of the centres and were employed in 27% of patients and in 33% of patients who underwent resective surgery. In MRI positive cases, electrodes were used for seizure localization, functional localization and language mapping. There was a clear age difference. Patients who were 4 years old or less at surgery tended to have cortical dysplasia, hemimegalencephaly or tuberose sclerosis as the underlying pathology and underwent large resective operations. Patients aged between 8 and 18 years were more likely to undergo lobar or focal resections and the pathology was tumours, cortical dysplasia or mesial temporal sclerosis. More detailed data are available in the ILAE report (Harvey et al., 2008).

Outcome

Mortality is low but increases in younger patients and with larger resections. Excessive blood loss, leading to hypervolaemia and coagulability problems, fluid balance and temperature control are potential dangers. Hard figures are difficult to find. In small series, mortality is often low or zero but in larger series of hemispherectomy, for example, it may rise to 3–6% (Jonas et al., 2004).

In resective operations, neurological deficit relevant to the locus of the surgery can be expected, and to some extent can be predicted by appropriate preoperative tests such as fMRI or direct or indirect cortical stimulation. Younger patients have more potential for recovery. Cognitive changes vary and to some extent depend upon the underlying

---

Introduction to Epilepsy ed. Gonzalo Alarcón and Antonio Valentín. Published by Cambridge University Press.
© Cambridge University Press 2012.

Table 84.1. Aetiology and operative procedures in 543 children operated in 2004 (ILAE data from 20 programmes; Harvey et al., 2008)

Aetiology	
Cortical dysplasia	42%
Tumour	19%
Stroke and atrophy	10%
Rasmussen's disease	3%
Sturge-Weber syndrome	3%
Vascular lesions	1.5%
Operations	
Lobar and focal resections – frontal and temporal	42%
Hemispherectomy	16%
Multilobar resections	13%
Vagus nerve stimulator	16%

pathology. For example, patients with hemimegalencephaly or extensive cortical dysplasia may fail to show cognitive or behavioural improvement even when there is good seizure control. Outcome, with regard to seizure control, is the same or better than in adults. The complete removal of the epileptogenic area or structural lesion is the key to seizure freedom. Recent series report 82% and 74% of children in Engel I (seizure-free) for temporal lobe resections. The outcome from frontal lobe seizures varies between 25% and 60% dependent upon the pathology, type of resection, etc. A Bonn series of 32 children and adolescents shows 65% seizure-free. Favourable factors were a tailored resection and a structural lesion other than gliosis. All seven patients with low-grade tumours were seizure-free (Kral et al., 2001). Seizure freedom in resections from other extratemporal regions depends upon the nature of the pathology and completeness of resection. Between 60% and 80% of patients are seizure-free after hemispherectomy or allied procedures, depending upon the underlying pathology.

Hypothalamic hamartoma is a rare condition which can present in infancy with a catastrophic illness of multiple seizure types, developmental delay and behavioural problems; as well as later with complex partial seizures against a normal background. The best solution for the first group is transcallosal resection, which has a 53% chance of rendering the patient seizure-free and a further 30% of a 90% reduction, although with a 12% chance of persisting memory problems (Rosenfeld and Feiz-Erfan, 2007).

Other solutions include disconnection, radiosurgery or radiofrequency ablation, which are less effective but less risky.

There are three functional operations which are used. Multiple subpial transection is used in a number of situations, but is most effective in the rare condition of Landau-Kleffner syndrome where, after appropriate presurgical assessment, there is a high chance of reversing the aphasia to an acceptable, but not normal, level (Irwin et al., 2001).

Callosal section has been largely abandoned in favour of vagus nerve stimulation.

Vagus nerve stimulation is applied to a varied paediatric population even when patients have exhausted pharmacological and other surgical possibilities. Recent studies suggest that it is an effective treatment, reducing seizures by 50% in 40–50% of patients, and in many series reduction by 70 – 90% is reported especially after prolonged treatment (Alexopoulos et al., 2006). Analysis of other factors such as structural lesions or epilepsy syndrome has given mixed results. A comparison of vagus nerve stimulation and callosotomy has shown that both are equally effective (You et al., 2008). Complications of vagus nerve stimulation are as expected, with infection, fracture of the stimulating leads, etc. totalling about 10%. Stimulation-related effects are similar to those reported in adults, with hoarseness being the commonest.

Conclusions

(1) There is a wide range of drug-resistant epilepsy syndromes in children which differ significantly from those in adults.
(2) Developmental considerations modify the management of these patients, in some situations making it more urgent.
(3) There is an appropriate range of resective surgery which can be proposed after appropriate and rigorous presurgical assessment.
(4) This surgery produces freedom from seizures in 40–80% of the patients depending upon the pathology and procedure, and with acceptably low mortality and morbidity.
(5) There are functional procedures which are less effective than resective surgery; the most commonly employed is vagus nerve stimulation.

References

Alexopoulos AV, Kotagal P, Loddenkemper T, Hammel J, Bingaman WE. Long-term results with vagus nerve stimulation in children with pharmacoresistant epilepsy. *Seizure* 2006;**15**(7):491–503.

Cross JH, Jayakar P, Nordli D, *et al.* Proposed criteria for referral and evaluation of children for epilepsy surgery: recommendations of the Subcommission for Pediatric Epilepsy Surgery. *Epilepsia* 2006;**47**(6):952–9.

Harvey AS, Cross JH, Shinnar S, Mathern BW. Defining the spectrum of international practice in pediatric epilepsy surgery patients. *Epilepsia* 2008;**49**(1):146–55.

Irwin K, Birch V, Lees J, *et al.* Multiple subpial transection in Landau-Kleffner syndrome. *Dev Med Child Neurol* 2001;**43**(4):248–52.

Jonas R, Nguyen S, Hu B, *et al.* Cerebral hemispherectomy: hospital course, seizure, developmental, language, and motor outcomes. *Neurology* 2004;**62**(10):1712–21.

Kral T, Kuczaty S, Blumcke I, *et al.* Postsurgical outcome of children and adolescents with medically refractory frontal lobe epilepsies. *Childs Nerv Syst* 2001;**17**(10): 595–601.

Rosenfeld JV, Feiz-Erfan I. Hypothalamic hamartoma treatment: surgical resection with the transcallosal approach. *Semin Pediatr Neurol* 2007 Jun;**14**(2):88–98.

Taylor DC, Cross JH, Harkness W, Neville BG. Defining new aims and providing new categories for measuring outcome of epilepsy surgery in children. In Tuxhorn I, Holthausen H, Boenigk H, eds. *Paediatric Epilepsy Syndromes and their Surgical Treatment*, pp. 17–25. London: John Libbey; 1997.

You SJ, Kang HC, Ko TS, *et al.* Comparison of corpus callosotomy and vagus nerve stimulation in children with Lennox-Gastaut syndrome. *Brain Dev* 2008; **30**(3):195–9.

Learning objectives

(1) To be aware and be able to discuss the differences in epilepsy surgery for adults and for children.
(2) To know the indications of epilepsy surgery in children.
(3) To know the surgical techniques most often used in children.
(4) To be aware of the outcome of epilepsy surgery in children.

Section 5 **Management of epilepsy**

Chapter 85

Vagus nerve stimulation

Richard P. Selway

Vagus nerve stimulation (VNS) is a palliative treatment for severe intractable epilepsy when there is inadequate control with drugs and brain surgery is not possible. It requires an implanted pacemaker-like device that supplies electrical stimulation to the vagus nerve in the neck.

It was first noted experimentally in dogs that stimulation of the vagus nerve desynchronizes the EEG. Subsequent work showed both a reduction in epileptiform features on experimental animals' EEG and also a reduction in seizures. The technique was introduced to human epilepsy practice in the mid 1990s.

The mechanism of action is unclear. There is evidence of effects on the main norepinephric and serotoninergic systems of the brain, which seem to be mediated through afferent fibres within the vagus, carrying the impulses to the brainstem. This seems to activate the raphe nuclei, releasing serotonin widely throughout the brain, and the locus coeruleus similarly releasing norepinephrine. These appear to have a nonspecific effect on the cortex, subtly changing the neurochemical environment in a way which may reduce seizures.

Implantation is a minor surgical procedure that can even be done as a day case. A pacemaker box is placed under the skin of the chest wall just below the collar bone, and the wire, again under the skin, is coiled around the vagus nerve on the left side of the neck.

After implantation the device is activated at a low setting and the amplitude is gradually increased over subsequent weeks as an out-patient. Even low levels of stimulation produce some effects on the nerves to the larynx, with a sensation being felt in the throat and a slight hoarseness of voice. This tends to settle quickly but prevents immediate activation of the device at higher settings. Typically stimulation is provided for 30-second periods every 5 minutes. Continuous stimulation appears to damage the nerve so is not used. Over subsequent months the stimulation parameters are adjusted in the light of seizure history to optimize the effect for that individual.

Adverse effects include infection (~1%), which may result in the device needing to be removed, and vagus nerve damage (<1%) leading to hoarse voice, cough and shortness of breath (both dependent on stimulation settings). In patients with swallowing problems this aspect may rarely be exacerbated by VNS.

Once adjustments to the stimulator have been achieved, about 45% of patients will enjoy a halving of their seizures or better while about 70% gain some benefit. Interestingly there seem to be improvements in mood, memory and learning associated with VNS that are independent of the effect on the epilepsy. This means that the treatment is particularly helpful in children and adults with learning disability or in whom depression has been a problem. VNS seems to have a similar degree of benefit irrespective of the seizure type or syndrome. Case selection is based on the fact that epilepsy has proven refractory to a number of appropriate AEDs and direct brain surgery is not feasible. Patients need to be aware that seizure freedom is unlikely with VNS (~2–5%) and that patience is required to optimize the stimulation parameters. The maximum effect may take 1 year to achieve.

Learning objective

(1) To know the indications, the principles of implantation and outcome of vagus nerve stimulation for the treatment of epilepsy.

Introduction to Epilepsy ed. Gonzalo Alarcón and Antonio Valentín. Published by Cambridge University Press.
© Cambridge University Press 2012.

Section 5 Management of epilepsy

Chapter 86
Brain stimulation for the treatment of epilepsy

Richard P. Selway

Epilepsy is a condition mediated through electrical changes in the cerebral cortex, so it is logical to use electrical stimulation in an attempt to treat it. Apart from vagus nerve stimulation, which has an established place in the palliative treatment of refractory epilepsy, no other electrical stimulation technique has yet advanced beyond the experimental phase.

Stimulation may be applied as an open-loop method, in which it is delivered according to predetermined parameters, or closed-loop, in which the device detects changes in the brain activity and applies stimulation dependent on that activity. Most systems that have been used are open-loop. Closed-loop is more complex, requiring both a method of detecting a seizure (or ideally the pre-seizure state) and the ability to deliver a stimulus to abort the event. There are currently few outcome data on closed-loop devices in humans.

Continuous open-loop systems deliver a constant electrical stimulus either at high frequency (typically above 50 Hz), which is thought to deactivate the neurons, or low frequency (usually less than 10 Hz), which may produce a mixture of activation and inhibition.

Stimulation may be applied directly to the cortex, to the cerebellum or to deep brain nuclei, e.g. caudate, thalamus or subthalamic nucleus.

Human studies of brain stimulation for epilepsy have tended to be small-scale and difficult to interpret.

Cortical stimulation: electrodes placed on the epileptic focus, especially in the hippocampus, do seem to have beneficial effects although not as great as the effect of resection. It may prove to have a role in patients whose focus is within eloquent cortex.

Caudate stimulation: low-frequency stimulation has been used in the management of refractory status epilepticus.

Subthalamic nucleus (STN): stimulation at this site has been used for some time in the treatment of Parkinson's disease, so the surgical technique is well established. It seems also to induce some benefits in epilepsy through activation of the nigral contol of epilepsy system, involving the superior colliculus, STN and thalamus, reducing cortical excitability. There are good animal data to support this target.

Thalamic stimulation (Figure 86.1): both the centro-median and anterior nuclei have been used as targets in the treatment of epilepsy. The SANTE (anterior nucleus) study in North America is the only large study of brain stimulation and shows modest benefit (Fisher *et al.*, 2010). Centro-median stimulation may have particular benefits in the generalized epilepsy syndromes.

Cerebellar stimulation: both cerebellar cortex and deep nuclei have been targeted. Many patients have been treated previously but its role is not clear as yet.

Recommended reading
Lüders HO. *Deep Brain Stimulation and Epilepsy*. London: Martin Dunitz; 2004.

Reference
Fisher R, Salanova V, Witt T, *et al.*; SANTE Study Group. Electrical stimulation of the anterior nucleus of thalamus for treatment of refractory epilepsy. *Epilepsia* 2010;**51** (5):899–908. Epub 2010 Mar 17.

Learning objective
(1) To know the indications, the principles of implantation and outcome of deep brain stimulation for the treatment of epilepsy.

Introduction to Epilepsy ed. Gonzalo Alarcón and Antonio Valentín. Published by Cambridge University Press.
© Cambridge University Press 2012.

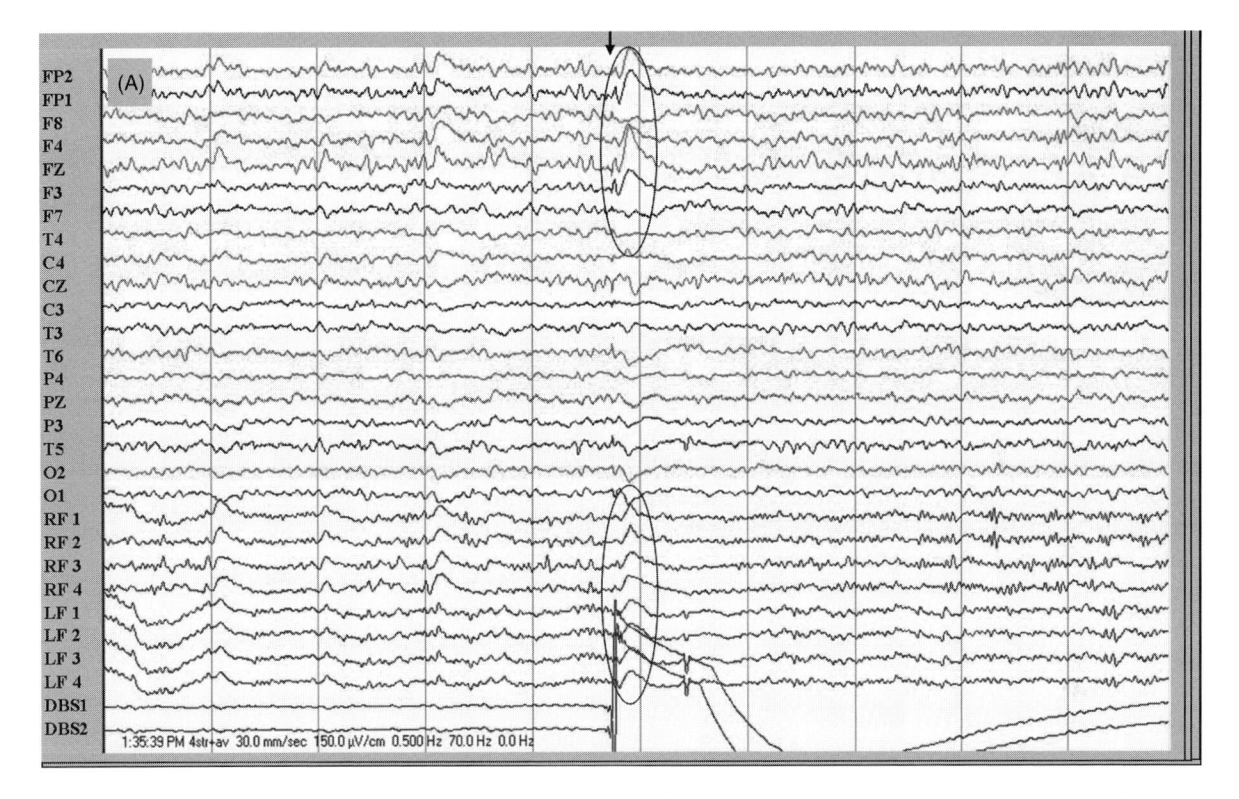

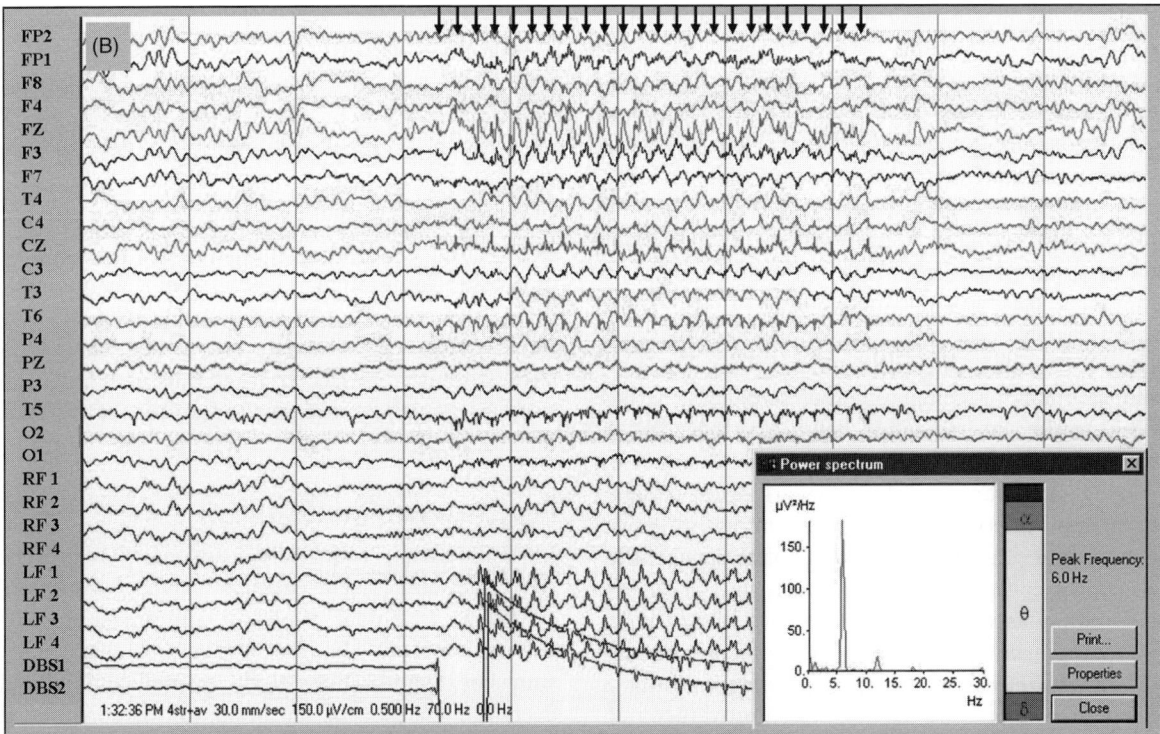

Figure 86.1. Cortical responses to electrical stimulation of the left centromedial nucleus of the thalamus. (A) Frontal responses (circled) to a single 1 ms electrical pulse (arrow). (B) Recruiting responses: repetitive stimulation at 6 Hz (arrows) applied to the centromedial nucleus induces cortical responses with left frontal emphasis. DBS, deep brain stimulation electrodes; RF, right frontal subdural strip; LF, left frontal subdural strip (illustration kindly provided by Drs Valentín and Alarcón).

Section 5 Management of epilepsy

Chapter 87: Diagnosis and treatment of hypothalamic hamartomas

Nandini Mullatti

Hamartomas of the hypothalamus (HH) are rare developmental malformations. The hypothalamus is a small organ, 4 ml in volume, located below the thalamus, on either side of the third ventricle. Despite its small size, the hypothalamus governs all the major 'vegetative' functions of the body, including the sleep–wake cycle, appetite control, body temperature control, sexual drive and development and reproduction, as well as emotions (fear, rage, pleasure, reward). It governs the hormones secreted by the pituitary gland by various hormone-releasing factors. Hamartomas are non-progressive malformations of 'normal neurons' arranged haphazardly, and the presence of these hamartomas in aberrant locations (e.g. hypothalamus) creates a syndrome which is variable but can include precocious (early) puberty, gelastic seizures and a refractory seizure syndrome with multiple seizure types.

The gelastic or laughing seizures are a clinical curiosity often seen in HH. Gelastic seizures can begin very early in life, even in the neonatal period, and are not always recognized as seizures. If precocious puberty intervenes, however, investigation with an MRI scan usually reveals the presence of HH. As the seizure syndrome evolves, gelastic seizures are recognized as 'lacking in mirth', and may develop additional motor or complex partial semiology. It has been proven, by implanting depth electrodes in the HH and by ictal SPECT, that the HH is the source of gelastic and other seizures. Particularly when the epilepsy and precocious puberty begin early, severe behavioural problems are a significant management issue. The epilepsy syndrome evolves into refractory polymorphous epilepsy with multiple seizure types occurring many times per day. With the appearance of this symptomatic generalized epilepsy, about a third of patients also develop learning difficulties.

There is also significant psychiatric co-morbidity. It is the severity of the refractory epilepsy and behavioural problems that often leads to the search for therapeutic surgical options.

Diagnosis

Diagnosis is based on the MRI scan in the context of the typical clinical syndrome. The HH is usually small (0.5–3 cm) usually hypo- or isointense on T1-weighted images and hyperintense on T2-weighted images occurring in the region of the mamillary bodies.

Management

Medical treatment

Precocious puberty, when it occurs in isolation, is safely controlled by long-acting gonadotropin-releasing hormone agonists. In a minority of patients, usually with late onset (i.e. late teens or adult life), the epilepsy may be mild and manageable with antiepileptic drugs alone. In this group of late-onset epilepsy with HH, associated morbidity, for example evolution into symptomatic generalized epilepsy, does not seem to occur, and cognitive abilities are generally preserved. Puberty has already occurred by late teens and thus is no longer an issue. These patients are able to lead productive lives, including having employment and families.

Resective surgical treatment

In the patients with early-onset epilepsy in HH, refractory and severe seizures may require more aggressive treatment aimed at either resection or destruction of the HH. This is inevitably challenging, since the hypothalamus itself is small and located deeply in the base of the brain, and is surrounded

---

Introduction to Epilepsy ed. Gonzalo Alarcón and Antonio Valentín. Published by Cambridge University Press.
© Cambridge University Press 2012.

Chapter 87: Diagnosis and treatment of hypothalamic hamartomas

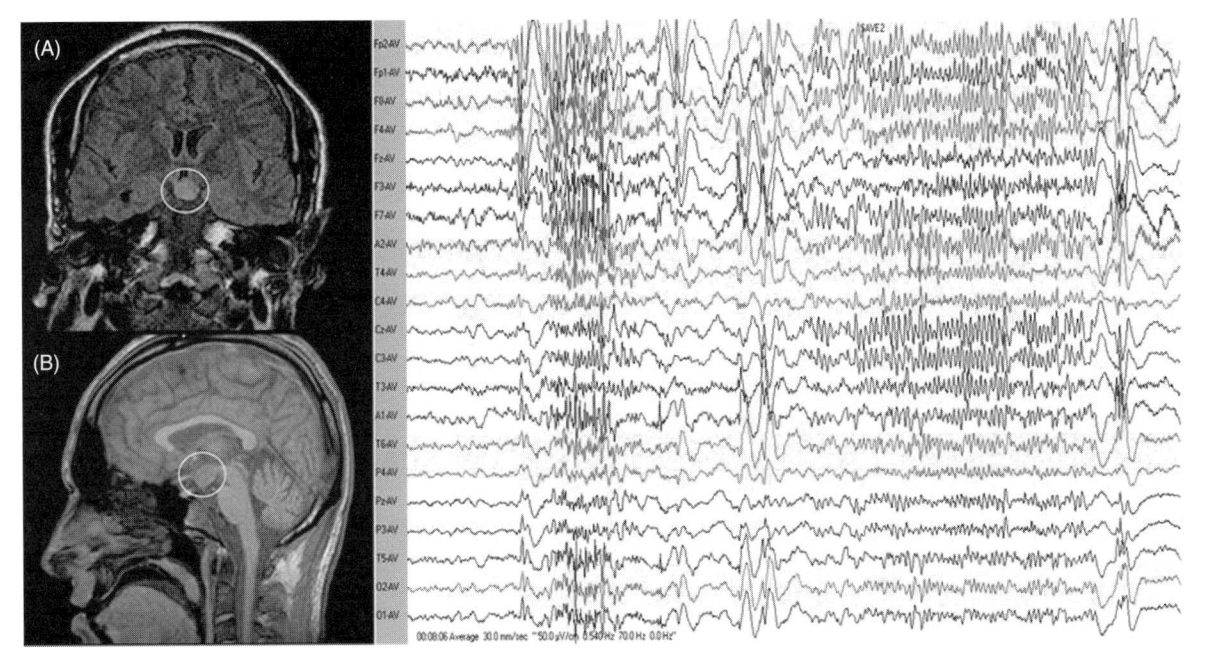

Figure 87.1. Hypothalamic hamartoma (encircled) and seizure.

by important neural and vascular structures. To complicate matters, HH are also usually small, and difficult to delineate intraoperatively (i.e. it is impossible to visually identify at surgery the limits betwen the hamartoma and the normal hypothalamus). Injury to the hypothalamus, resulting in neuroendocrine dysfunction, is a common sequela of open resective surgery. Rosenfeld and Kerrigan, presenting the operative experience using the transcallosal approach, show, respectively, that 52–54% are 100% seizure-free and 24–35% have >90% seizure reduction (Feiz-Erfan et al., 2005). However, there appears to be an 8–14% risk of persisting memory problems. The surgery should ideally be performed in the early years of childhood, before symptomatic generalized epilepsy develops and developmental delay and behaviour problems are established.

Non-resective surgical treatment

The following non-resective surgical techniques should also be considered:

- Gamma knife irradiation: this involves delivering a very high dose but focused irradiation to the HH. Régis et al. reported a prospective trial of sixty patients with HH of whom 59% showed excellent outcome, becaming completely seizure-free (37%) or continuing with only rare non-disabling seizures (22.2%), associated with dramatic behavioural and cognitive improvement (Régis et al., 2006). For reasons that are not completely understood, it can take up to 12–18 months for the destructive effect of radiation to be complete, and during this process the epilepsy might worsen for a period of time.
- Stereotactic thermocoagulation: in this technique, a thermocoagulating electrode is placed stereotactically, under local anaesthesia, following confirmation of seizure onset from the HH using depth EEG electrode recordings. The HH is then coagulated with heat of between 60 and 80°C for about 30 seconds each time. In our experience, this technique is safe and efficacious in reducing seizure burden. The challenge with thermocoagulation is to get the patient seizure-free. This has been achieved by Japanese authors who reported their experience with 25 patients, of whom 19 (76%) became seizure-free (Kameyama et al., 2009).

References

Feiz-Erfan I, Horn EM, Rekate HL, et al. Surgical strategies for approaching hypothalamic hamartomas causing gelastic seizures in the pediatric population:

445

transventricular compared with skull base approaches. *J Neurosurg* 2005;**103**(Suppl 4):325–32.

Kameyama S, Murakami H, Masuda H, Sugiyama I. Minimally invasive magnetic resonance imaging-guided stereotactic radiofrequency thermocoagulation for epileptogenic hypothalamic hamartomas. *Neurosurgery* 2009;**65**(3):438–49; discussion 449.

Mullatti N, Selway R, Nashef L, *et al.* The clinical spectrum of epilepsy in children and adults with hypothalamic hamartoma. *Epilepsia* 2003;**44**(10):1310–19.

Régis J, Scavarda D, Tamura M, *et al.* Epilepsy related to hypothalamic hamartomas: surgical management with special reference to gamma knife surgery. *Childs Nerv Syst* 2006;**22**(8):881–95. Epub 2006 Jun 29.

Learning objective

(1) To know the different types of hypothalamic hamartomas, their clinical manifestations and how to diagnose and treat them.

Section 5 Management of epilepsy

Chapter 88: Intraoperative (acute) electrocorticography (ECoG)

Gonzalo Alarcón

Once a patient has been found suitable for resective surgery or for multiple subpial transection, and the general location of the procedure has been decided, it is possible to further define the surgical procedure at the time of surgery. This can be achieved with intraoperative EEG recordings obtained with electrodes in contact with the cortex in the operating theatre (intraoperative electrocorticography or ECoG; Figures 88.1 and 88.2). ECoG recordings can be obtained under general or under local anaesthesia. The latter allows functional mapping to localize motor, sensory or language areas in the operating theatre.

Electrocorticographic recordings are obtained covering most of the area around the proposed surgical procedure. The following general considerations apply:

- The purpose of ECoG recordings is to intraoperatively guide cortical resections or transections according to interictal abnormalities.
- Practically relying on interictal discharges or focal slowing.
- Slowing is often difficult to assess due to general anaesthesia.
- Ictal findings are unlikely to occur.

Generally, post-resection or post-transection ECoG recordings should be carried out to confirm the abolition of discharges following the procedure. If discharges remain, the procedure should be extended if safely possible. Nevertheless, a number of issues regarding the interpretation of the ECoG are still unsettled:

- Effects of generalized anaesthesia on discharges.
- Is excision of all discharge areas necessary? If not, should resection be guided by the:
  - extent of epileptiform discharges
  - incidence of epileptiform discharges
  - amplitude of epileptiform discharges.
- Which is the utility of activation procedures?
- Is excision of all discharging areas necessary?
- What is the value of residual spikes?
- How to interpret ECoG findings in different lobes.

Effects of general anaesthesia on discharges

Epilepsy surgery can be performed in an awake patient (which allows functional mapping with electrical stimulation) or, more frequently, under general anaesthesia.

During awake craniotomy, patients are usually sedated with propofol during the craniotomy. Thereafter, propofol infusion is discontinued and the patient is allowed to awaken. Propofol is an ideal agent for this purpose because its pharmacokinetic properties permit quick awakening of the patient on the operating table, allowing functional mapping of the cortex with cortical stimulation.

ECoG during general anaesthesia can be challenging, and the most adequate anaesthetic agent has to be chosen between alfentanil, fentanyl, remifentanil, sevoflurane, isoflurane, propofol and methohexitone. Many anaesthetic drugs used in ECoG-guided epilepsy surgery may suppress epileptiform activity, and induce initially diffuse EEG slowing, and then burst-suppression patterns as anaesthesia deepens. For instance, there are reports of propofol suppressing spontaneous epileptiform activity during seizure surgery, while others describe propofol-induced epileptiform activity. Inhalation anaesthetics, such as isoflurane or sevoflurane, have been reported to suppress spike activity in the ECoG, but this effect is

---

Introduction to Epilepsy ed. Gonzalo Alarcón and Antonio Valentín. Published by Cambridge University Press.
© Cambridge University Press 2012.

Section 5: Management of epilepsy

(A)

(B)

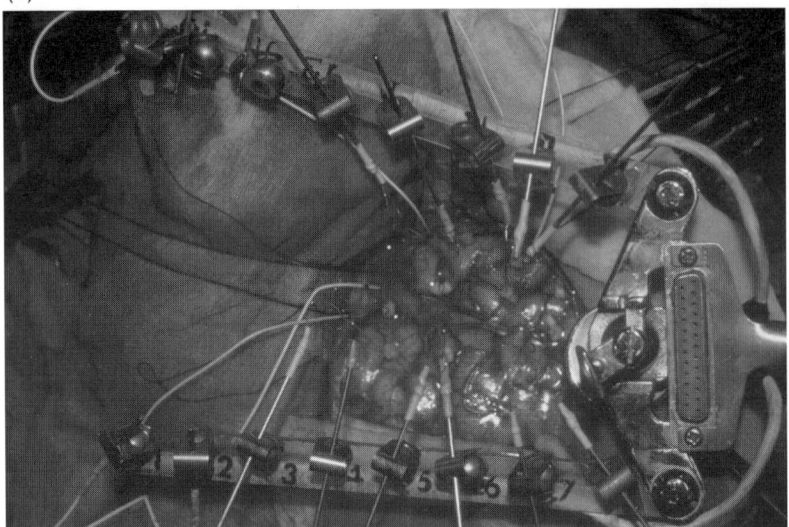

Figure 88.1. Recording electrocorticography in the operating theatre. (A) Electrodes are positioned in direct contact with the cortex.
(B) Surgeon (Professor CE Polkey, left) and neurophysiologist (Professor CD Binnie, right) jointly interpret ECoG recordings on an analog EEG machine to decide the limits of the resection in the late nineties.

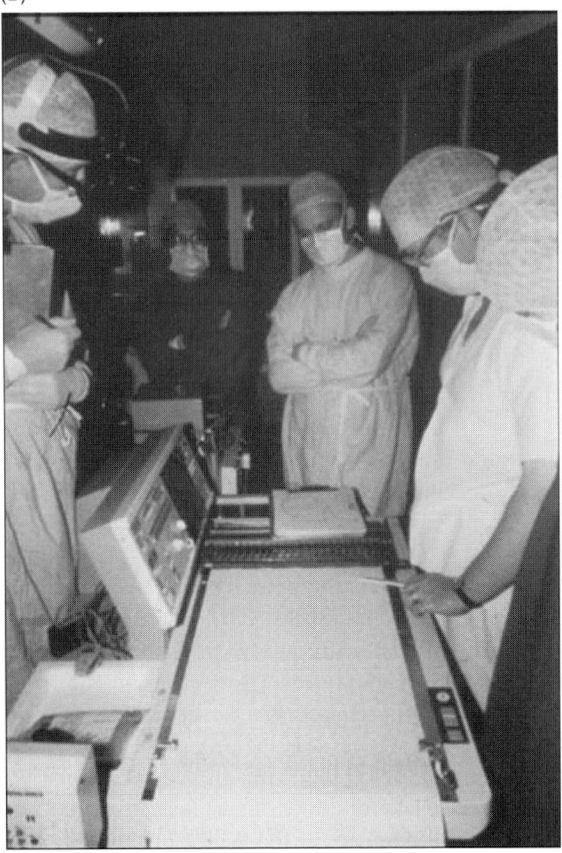

Chapter 88: Intraoperative (acute) electrocorticography (ECoG)

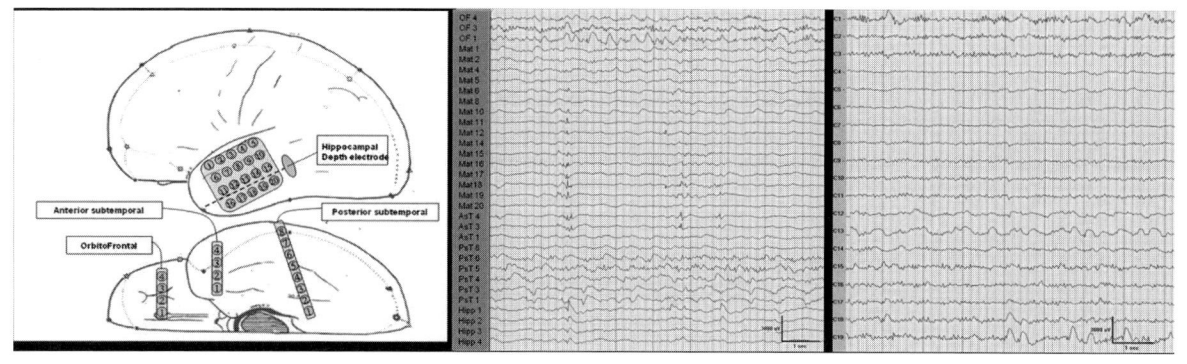

Figure 88.2. Typical ECoG recording in a patient with mesial temporal sclerosis. The electrocorticography was recorded with a lateral temporal mat, orbital and subtemporal subdural strips and a hippocampal electrode introduced in the temporal horn of the lateral ventricle via a lateral temporal incision (left). The pre-resection recording showed frequent anterior subtemporal and inferior lateral temporal epileptiform discharges, occurring independently or in association with positive spikes at the hippocampus (centre). No discharges are seen after resection (right).

dose-dependent. In our experience at King's College Hospital, we have found that both sevoflurane and isoflurane are the most adequate anaesthetic agents during ECoG. If epileptiform discharges are not detected, spike activity can be induced by the administration of thiopentane, methohexital, etomidate or alfentanil.

Value of activation procedures

If epileptiform discharges are not seen, they can be induced by reducing the levels of anaesthesia, or by progressive injection of thiopentone (25 mg every 20 s, up to 250 mg in adults). This is useful, particularly when few discharges are seen on the baseline record. Initially there is activation of one or more interictal foci. Later, burst-suppression patterns are readily seen at higher thiopentone doses. During flattening, the most epileptogenic cortex is thought to be located where discharges disappear last and reappear first.

Is excision of all discharging areas necessary?

- Controversial.
- Supported by Wyllie et al. (1987).
- Unnecessary for Montreal School.
- Discharge rate < 1 per 4 min predicts poor outcome (McBride et al., 1991).
- Discharges confined to resected tissue uncorrelated with outcome (McBride et al., 1991).
- In temporal lobe epilepsy, amygdalo-hippocampectomy is effective even though discharges are recorded outside this region.
- Distinction between primary and propagated spikes (Penfield and Jasper, 1954): the primary discharges that should be resected are those:
  - associated with a structural lesion
  - underlying background abnormality
  - sharpest spikes: sharpness loss with propagation (also suggested by McBride et al., 1991; Alarcón et al., 1994).
- Resection of leading spikes is correlated with good outcome (Alarcón et al., 1997).

Value of residual discharges

- Regarded as unfavorable for Montreal School.
- Significant but weak association with poor outcome.
- Spikes at insula could be ignored (Silfvenius et al., 1964).
- Post-resection discharge rate not significant (McBride et al., 1991).
- Percentage of discharges remaining <50% correlated with good outcome (McBride et al., 1991).

ECoG in temporal lobe surgery

- In mesial temporal sclerosis (MTS), discharges commonly occur independently in the hippocampus and in subtemporal cortex, and less commonly in lateral temporal cortex.
- Positive hippocampal spikes can be recorded introducing an electrode in the temporal horn of the lateral ventricle.

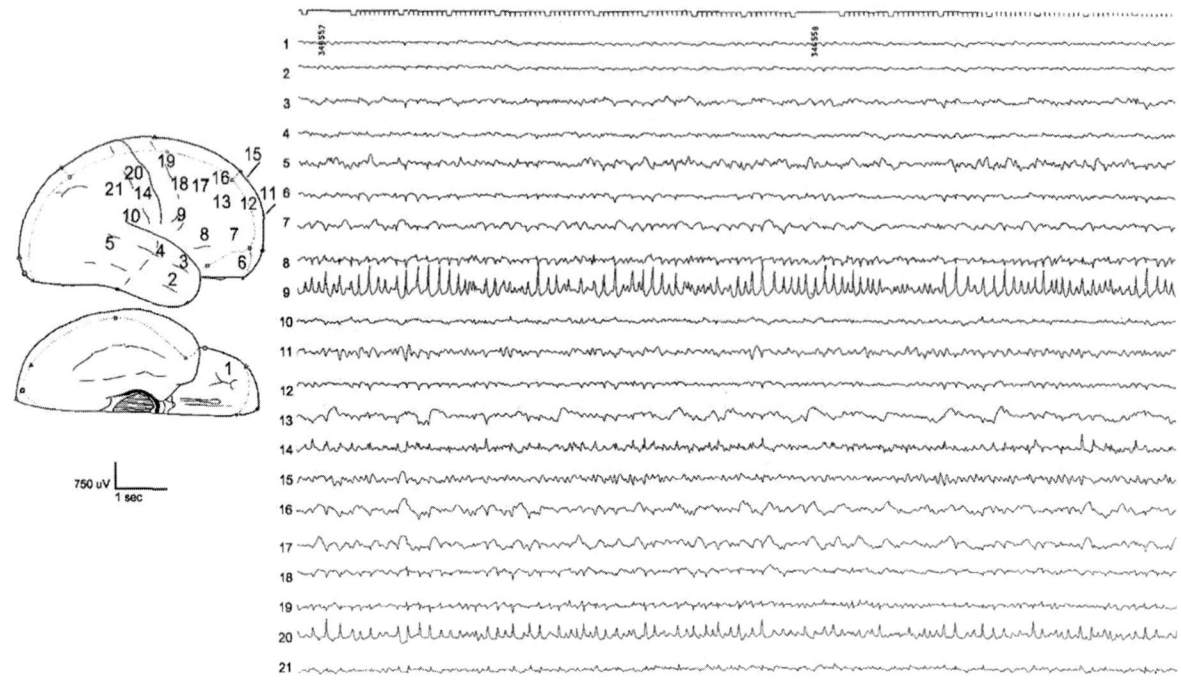

Figure 88.3. Continuous rhythmic sharp discharges in a patient with focal cortical dysplasia (reproduced with permission from Ferrier CH, Alarcón G, Engelsman J, Binnie CD, Koutroumanidis M, Polkey CE, Janota I, Dean A. Relevance of residual histologic and electrocorticographic abnormalities for surgical outcome in frontal lobe epilepsy. *Epilepsia* 2001:42:363–71, Figure 5.2).

- In some centres, ECoG is considered unnecessary in MTS because temporal resections tend to be standardized.
- We find that in a small proportion of patients with MTS, resections should be extended backwards because of posterior leading spikes.

ECoG in frontal lobe surgery

- Frontal lobe epilepsy is often refractory to medical treatment.
- Seizure control after surgery is poorer than for temporal lobe surgery (only around 55% improve compared to around 80% in temporal lobe epilepsy).
- A focal abnormality in neuroimaging and its complete removal are predictive of favourable outcome (Ferrier *et al.*, 1999; Wennberg *et al.*, 1999).
- How can we guide surgery when the lesion cannot be completely excised?:
  - Involvement of eloquent areas
  - Multifocal abnormalities
- Seizure patterns (bursts of fast activity, bursts of rhythmic spikes or continuous rhythmic discharges; Figure 88.3) were associated with cortical dysplasia, which is the underlying pathology in nearly 50% of frontal resections (Ferrier *et al.*, 2001).
- Prognostic factors (Ferrier *et al.*, 2001)
  - Abolition of seizure patterns after resection was associated with favourable outcome.
  - Incomplete removal of the lesion did not preclude favourable outcome.
  - Persistence of sporadic spikes did not associate with poor outcome.
- Conclusion
  - Abolition of seizure patterns should be sought to improve outcome.
  - Abolition of sporadic spikes and complete removal of histological abnormalities appears unnecessary for favourable outcome.

New developments

The development of single-pulse electrical stimulation (SPES) raises the question of whether SPES can be used reliably under general anaesthesia to:

- guide electrode implantation for chronic recordings
- guide resection during electrocorticography.

References

Alarcón G, Guy CN, Binnie CD, *et al.* Intracerebral propagation of interictal activity in partial epilepsy: implications for source localisation. *J Neurol Neurosurg Psychiatry* 1994;**57**:435–49.

Alarcón G, García Seoane JJ, Binnie CD, *et al.* Origin and propagation of discharges in the acute electrocorticogram: implications for physiopathology and surgical treatment of temporal lobe epilepsy. *Brain* 1997;**120**: 2259–82.

Ferrier CH, Alarcón G, Engelsman J, *et al.* Relevance of residual histologic and electrocorticographic abnormalities for surgical outcome in frontal lobe epilepsy. *Epilepsia* 2001;**42**:363–71.

Ferrier CH, Engelsman J, Alarcón G, Binnie CD, Polkey CE. Prognostic factors in presurgical assessment of frontal lobe epilepsy. *J Neurol Neurosurg Psychiatry* 1999;**66**:350–6.

McBride MC, Binnie CD, Janota I, Polkey CE. Predictive value of intraoperative electrocorticograms in resective epilepsy surgery. *Ann Neurol* 1991; **30**:526–32.

Penfield W, Jasper H. *Epilepsy and the Functional Anatomy of the Human Brain.* London: J. & A. Churchill; 1954.

Silfvenius H, Gloor P, Rasmussen T. Evaluation of insular ablation in surgical treatment of temporal lobe epilepsy. *Epilepsia* 1964;**5**:307–20.

Wennberg R, Quesney LF, Lozano A, Olivier A, Rasmussen T. Role of electrocorticography at surgery for lesion-related frontal lobe epilepsy. *Can J Neurol Sci* 1999;**26**:33–9.

Wyllie E, Lüders H, Morris HH 3rd, *et al.* Clinical outcome after complete or partial cortical resection for intractable epilepsy. *Neurology* 1987;**37**:1634–41.

Learning objectives

(1) To understand the general principles and considerations regarding ECoG recordings and their interpretation.
(2) To be aware of the effects of anaesthesia and activation procedures.
(3) To know the predictive ECoG features in temporal and frontal lobe epilepsy.

Section 5: Management of epilepsy

Chapter 89

Single-pulse electrical stimulation

Antonio Valentín

It is widely accepted that a successful outcome of resective epilepsy surgery depends on the localization of nervous tissue that is structurally and functionally abnormal. Recent developments in medical imaging provide a powerful means to localize structural lesions. However, the need for identification of functional abnormalities still requires scalp, and sometimes intracerebral, recordings of seizure onset. The success of surgical procedures depends on the identification of an 'epileptogenic zone' which is defined as that region of tissue the removal (or disconnection) of which is both necessary and sufficient to abolish seizures (Lüders et al., 1992). An important cause of poor outcome is probably failure to identify the epileptogenic zone. No single set of criteria defines this zone since its location is inferred from clinical, imaging and electrophysiological findings. Both ictal and interictal electrographic abnormalities may be found; sometimes these are of localizing value, sometimes not, probably because the characteristic epileptiform activity is rapidly propagated from one region to another (Alarcón et al., 1994).

To address this problem, we have studied cortical excitability using single-pulse electrical stimulation (SPES) at the Department of Clinical Neurophysiology at King's College Hospital. The method measures cortical excitability by recording intracranial EEG responses to single electrical pulses (1 ms, 4–8 mA) directly applied to the cortex via intracranial electrodes implanted during presurgical assessment of patients with epilepsy. We have described two main types of responses to SPES. When normal cortex was stimulated, 'early responses' (ER) were elicited consisting of one sharp and slow transient, usually starting immediately after the stimulus. ER can be used to study brain connectivity (Lacruz et al., 2007). In addition to ER, we have also described abnormal responses to SPES that occur with a delay longer than 100 ms from stimulation, the 'late responses' (LR) which appear to be related to cortical epileptogenesis. LR are of two types: (a) 'delayed responses' (DR), SPES responses resembling spikes, occurring more than 100 ms after the stimulus, usually seen at the areas where seizure onset is recorded; DRs often resemble in morphology and topography the patient's spontaneous interictal discharges; (b) 'repetitive responses' (RR), consisting of a train of repeated early responses, lasting 1 s or longer. We have observed delayed responses in temporal and frontal epilepsies, whereas repetitive responses appear to be restricted to patients with frontal seizures. The onset of spontaneous seizures tends to occur in areas where delayed responses to SPES were recorded and close to areas whose stimulation induced repetitive responses. We have generically called such areas 'abnormal SPES areas' (Valentín et al., 2002, 2005a, 2005b; Flanagan et al., 2009).

A number of important practical implications derive from these results. As delayed and repetitive responses to SPES can predict interictally the topography of seizure onset, they have a potential use in clinical practice. Indeed, in temporal lobe epilepsy, delayed responses were virtually as reliable in the identification of epileptogenic cortex as the study of seizure onset (Valentín et al., 2002, 2005b). In addition, a problem commonly encountered when interpreting intracranial recordings in frontal lobe epilepsy is that seizure onset is sometimes detected by many electrodes simultaneously (regional or diffuse onset). Such a widespread seizure onset may be due to the existence of a large epileptogenic zone or, alternatively, to rapid propagation of ictal activity from a more discrete seizure onset located distant from any recording electrode. Each of these interpretations has

Introduction to Epilepsy ed. Gonzalo Alarcón and Antonio Valentín. Published by Cambridge University Press.
© Cambridge University Press 2012.

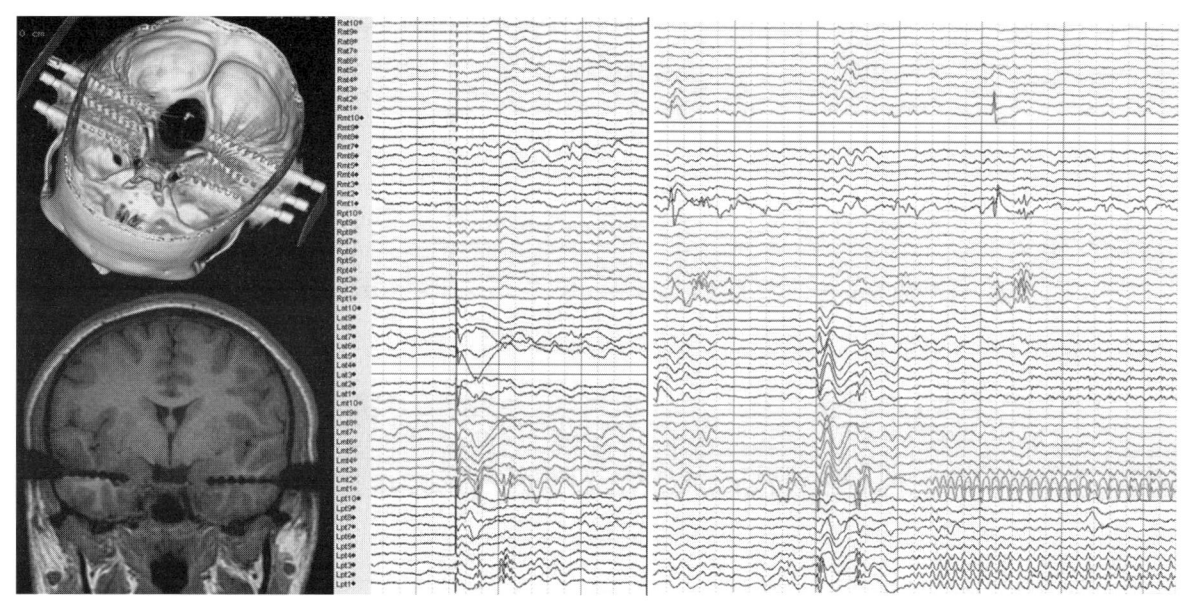

Chapter 89: Single-pulse electrical stimulation

Figure 89.1. Stimulaton of electrodes 3 and 4 (flat lines in the left EEG traces) of the left anterior temporal depth electrode bundle induces delayed responses, which are nearly identical to the onset of spontaneous seizures (right EEG traces) in a patient with intracerebral depth electrodes. For each bundle, electrode 1 is deepest. The vertical line across the left EEG traces is the stimulation artefact.

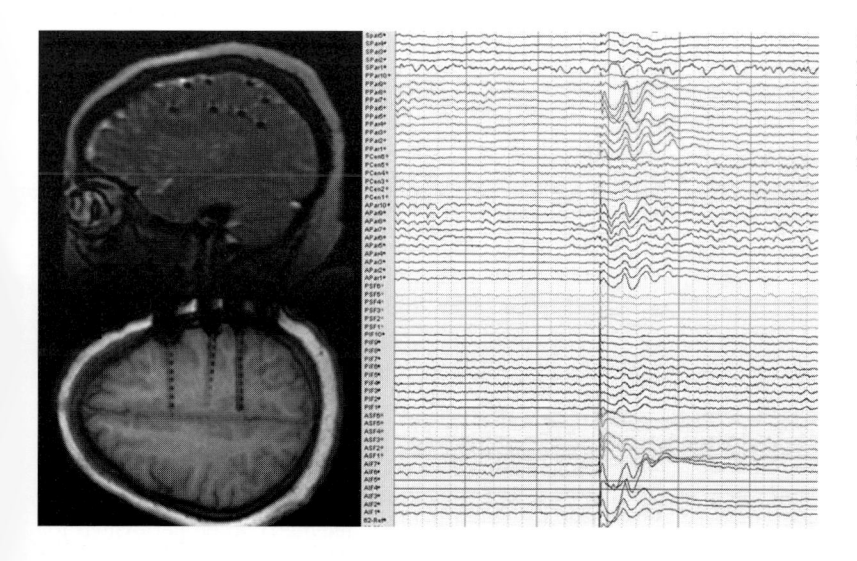

Figure 89.2. Repetitive responses seen when stimulating the anterior inferior frontal bundle (electrodes 4 and 5) in a patient with right frontal and parietal depth electrodes. The vertical line is the stimulation artefact.

distinctly different clinical implications and SPES can help in distinguishing between them. The existence of late responses related to the area of seizure onset would imply that this area is epileptogenic, and that its removal would increase the likelihood of seizure control after surgery (Valentín et al., 2005b). In contrast, the absence of late responses would suggest that seizures arise from remote areas, and the patient may not benefit from surgery of the recording areas.

Two different pathophysiological mechanisms could be the basis of repetitive and delayed responses. Repetitive responses seem to be induced when the epileptogenic area is stimulated, and consist of the repetition of the initial normal early response. Therefore, repetitive responses may arise from the immediate activation of a cortical (or thalamo-cortical) loop at the stimulated cortex, which triggers a re-entry of neuronal activity resulting in repetition of the initial response. The fact that repetitive responses were widespread (sometimes bilateral) but induced by focal stimulation of one frontal lobe might be explained by a cortico-subcortical loop. This is further supported by the finding that subcortical structures appear to have more connections with frontal than temporal cortices (Velasco et al. 2000). We hypothesize that in normal cortex the mechanisms responsible for repetitive responses do not exist or are suppressed by inhibition. Delayed responses are more difficult to explain due to their long and variable delay (100 ms to 1 s). As delayed responses are seen in areas involved at seizure onset and their morphology resembles that of interictal discharges, they could be explained by the presence of a cortical loop in the epileptogenic cortex lasting for some hundreds of milliseconds (Valentín et al., 2002). This loop would be activated by afferents from the stimulated cortex allowing for a build-up of activity or recruitment of neurons until an epileptiform discharge is triggered. The efficacy of such neuronal recruitment would depend on neuronal and/or glial mechanisms that determine excitability of the epileptogenic region. Thus, both delayed and repetitive responses could be due to an abnormal control of cortical activity, probably due to an altered balance between excitation and inhibition. A finding that supports this hypothesis is that responses to SPES resembling repetitive and delayed responses have been seen in animal models with altered balance between excitation and inhibition, such as in in vitro experiments with disinhibited neocortical slices (Chagnac-Amitai and Connors, 1989), in hippocampal slices exposed to Mg^{2+}-free medium (Kohling et al., 2000) and after local injection of tetanus toxin (Jefferys, 1989; Empson et al., 1993).

We have identified three practical limitations to SPES. About 25% of patients experienced brief ipsilateral pain, or facial twitches, clearly related to each pulse when medial temporal structures were stimulated through subtemporal strips. This effect was sometimes disagreeable and the intensity of stimulation had to be reduced, thus decreasing the sensitivity of SPES. The second limitation arises in patients who have nearly continuous epileptiform discharges, such as some patients with focal cortical dysplasia. Since the morphology and topography of DR are often similar to those of spontaneous epileptiform discharges, it can be practically impossible to identify them in the context of continuous spiking. Third, at present SPES can only be carried out in patients assessed with intracranial electrodes, and shares with such recordings their limitations in spatial sampling and applicability. Whether transcranial magnetic stimulation can be applied across the scalp to study cortical excitability in wider patient groups remains to be established. However, an initial study on EEG responses to TMS has shown that this technique can identify epileptogenic cortex and might substantially improve the diagnosis of focal epilepsy, particularly, if combined with standard EEG studies (Valentín et al., 2008).

Conclusion

Single-pulse electrical stimulation is on present evidence a safe and reliable technique for identifying the epileptogenic zone, as evidenced by the close relationship between the topography of abnormal SPES areas and the location of electrographic seizure onset, surgical outcome and pathology. The presence of late responses has been found useful in confirming findings from other diagnostic tests, in disclosing the existence of multiple potentially epileptogenic areas, in establishing whether seizures arise from regions close to the recording electrodes or are propagated from elsewhere, and in identifying epileptogenic cortex in patients who have none or few seizures during telemetry. At the least, by providing additional evidence it may reduce the need to capture seizures, allowing invasive EEG telemetry to be performed for shorter periods. Potentially, SPES might replace ictal recording as a method to localize epileptogenic cortex, as SPES could be used intraoperatively to identify epileptogenic cortex immediately before resective surgery. The technique may also prove of value during electrode implantation to determine whether the sites chosen are likely to lie within the epileptogenic zone.

References

Alarcón G, Guy CN, Binnie CD, *et al*. Intracerebral propagation of interictal activity in partial epilepsy: implications for source localisation. *J Neurol Neurosurg Psychiatry* 1994;**57**:435–49.

Chagnac-Amitai Y, Connors BW. Synchronized excitation and inhibition driven by intrinsically bursting neurons in neocortex. *J Neurophysiol* 1989;**62**:1149–62.

Empson RM, Amitai Y, Jefferys JG, Gutnick MJ. Injection of tetanus toxin into the neocortex elicits persistent epileptiform activity but only transient impairment of GABA release. *Neuroscience* 1993;**57**(2):235–9.

Flanagan D, Valentín A, García Seoane JJ, Alarcón G, Boyd SG. Single-pulse electrical stimulation helps to identify epileptogenic cortex in children. *Epilepsia* 2009;**50**:1793–803.

Jefferys JG. Chronic epileptic foci in vitro in hippocampal slices from rats with the tetanus toxin epileptic syndrome. *J Neurophysiol* 1989;**62**:458–68.

Kohling R, Vreugdenhil M, Bracci E, Jefferys JG. Ictal epileptiform activity is facilitated by hippocampal $GABA_A$ receptor-mediated oscillations. *J Neurosci* 2000;**20**:6820–9.

Lacruz ME, García Seoane JJ, Valentin A, Selway R, Alarcón G. Frontal and temporal functional connections of the living human brain. *Eur J Neurosci* 2007;**26**:1357–70.

Lüders H, Awad I, Burgess R, Wyllie E, Van Ness P. Subdural electrodes in the presurgical evaluation for surgery of epilepsy. *Epilepsy Res* 1992;**5**:147–56.

Valentín A, Anderson M, Alarcón G, *et al*. Responses to single pulse electrical stimulation identify epileptogenesis in the human brain in vivo. *Brain* 2002;**125**:1709–18.

Valentín A, Alarcón G, García-Seoane JJ, *et al*. Single-pulse electrical stimulation identifies epileptogenic frontal cortex in the human brain. *Neurology* 2005a;**65**:426–35.

Valentín A, Alarcón G, Honavar M. Single pulse electrical stimulation for identification of structural abnormalities and prediction of seizure outcome after epilepsy surgery: a prospective study. *Lancet Neurol* 2005b;**4**:718–26.

Valentín A, Arunachalam R, Mesquita-Rodrigues A, *et al*. Late EEG responses triggered by transcranial magnetic stimulation (TMS) in the evaluation of focal epilepsy. *Epilepsia* 2008;**49**:470–80.

Velasco M, Velasco F, Velasco AL, *et al*. Acute and chronic electrical stimulation of the centromedian thalamic nucleus: modulation of reticulo-cortical systems and predictor factors for generalized seizure control. *Arch Med Res* 2000;**31**:304–15.

Learning objectives

(1) To understand the concept of single-pulse electrical stimulation (SPES).
(2) To understand how SPES is performed.
(3) To recognize the waveforms seen in a normal SPES.
(4) To identify the epileptogenic waveforms (late responses) of SPES.
(5) To understand the actual clinical use of SPES.
(6) To understand the possible future clinical uses of SPES and other techniques of brain stimulation.

Chapter 90: Ketogenic diet in the management of childhood epilepsy

J. Helen Cross

The ketogenic diet (KD) is a high-fat diet designed to mimic the metabolic effects of starvation. It is not a new treatment for epilepsy; it has been used for almost 100 years. It was determined at an early stage that starvation may alleviate seizures. The ketogenic diet was born after consideration of how the metabolic effects of starvation could be produced through a diet high in fat. For many years the classic ketogenic diet was used, namely based on the ratio of fat to carbohydrate (including protein (3 or 4:1)) in the diet. However, with the advent of anticonvulsants, the diet gradually went out of favour as it was expected all would respond to medication. It was soon apparent this was not the case but the diet remained in low favour as it was perceived to be unpalatable and high in side effects. In 1971 Huttenlocher reported the use of medium-chain triglyceride, an oil more ketogenic per calorie than standard fat, and its use within a diet permitting the greater bulk of other foods, the medium-chain triglyceride (MCT) diet. Over the years a major deterrent to use of the KD has been the lack of systematic data on efficacy, but this has recently been rectified.

There have been numerous cohort studies over the years that have suggested the diet to be effective. This aside, a systematic review of studies in 2000 revealed only 11 studies, nine of which were from one single institution and all of which were uncontrolled. There have been some large open-label studies reporting consecutive children demonstrating efficacy, with as many as 31% achieving more than 90% seizure reduction of seizures. However, a further systematic review in 2006 again emphasized the lack of randomized controlled data. The first randomized controlled trial was reported in 2008 where children resistant to medication were randomized either to receiving a ketogenic diet or to no change in treatment. This showed from an intention to treat analysis at 3 months 38% to have experienced more than a 50% reduction in seizures, compared to only 6% of controls, reaching significance (Neal et al. 2008). This demonstrated a similar efficacy rate in trials of other newer antiepileptic drugs in drug-resistant epilepsies. Anecdotal reports have shown there may be specific efficacy in certain epilepsy syndromes, namely myoclonic-astatic epilepsy and Dravet syndrome.

The original randomized controlled trial also examined the efficacy of the MCT diet vs the classical diet (based on a ratio of fat to carbohydrate, including protein) and showed no difference in responder rates at 3, 6 or 12 months (Neal et al. 2009). The KD cannot be considered a 'natural diet' as it has side effects like any medication. Most of the side effects demonstrated, however, can be alleviated by manipulation of the diet. Within the randomized controlled trial there were 10 withdrawals by 3 months for a variety of different reasons, including vomiting, diarrhoea, constipation, increased seizures, behaviour through to extreme drowsiness. There were similar numbers of different adverse tolerabilities and indeed withdrawal between the classic and the MCT diet. Other side effects that have been reported have included renal stones. Younger non-ambulant children appear to be more susceptible to this. There is also an increased risk of bruising. This appears to be due to prolonged bleeding times but there is no evidence of vitamin deficiency. Cholesterol rises with either diet. Interestingly the MCT diet does not lead to a rise in triglycerides whereas the classic diet does. There has been further work on growth. A large study showed that with increasing time after starting the diet, growth velocity appears to deviate away from the norm for the age and this is most prominent in the younger children.

Introduction to Epilepsy ed. Gonzalo Alarcón and Antonio Valentín. Published by Cambridge University Press.
© Cambridge University Press 2012.

There is some debate as to how long an individual may stay on the ketogenic diet. Certainly it is thought that after a 2-year period one would attempt to withdraw the diet though anticonvulsants that may not have been effective could have been withdrawn prior to this time. However, each individual child has to be considered in their own right and if the diet still appears to be effective then there is no reason why the diet cannot be continued. The risk/benefit to longer-term use in each child needs to be considered.

The diet is resource–intensive, requiring high dietetic and paediatric neurology input. Further, there are few health economic data on which to base conclusions. Consequently the diet has not been widely available for use. This aside, the diet is palatable. and effective, now widely used around the world, and can be administered within different cultures. There are also suggestions that other more modified versions of the diet such as the modified Atkins or the low glycaemic index (GI) diets could also be as useful, especially in teenagers and even adults. More recently a consensus document was put together to give guidance about implementation, those who could benefit from the diet and appropriate versions of the diet to be used in view of the fact that there are not enough data available to provide evidence-based guidelines (Kossof *et al.* 2008).

Recommended reading

Cross JH, Mclellan A, Neal EG, *et al.* The ketogenic diet in childhood epilepsy – where are we now? *Arch Dis Child* 2010;**95**:550–3.

Keene DL. A systematic review of the use of the ketogenic diet in childhood epilepsy *Pediatr Neurol* 2006;**35**:1–5.

Kossoff EH, Zupec-Kania BA, Amark P, *et al.* Optimal clinical management of children receiving the ketogenic diet: recommendations of the international ketogenic diet study group. *Epilepsia* 2008;**47**:1–14.

Matthewsfriends.org.

Neal EG, Chaffe HM, Schwartz RH, *et al.* The ketogenic diet for the treatment of childhood epilepsy: a randomised controlled trial. *Lancet Neurol* 2008; 7:500–6.

Neal EG, Chaffe HM, Schwartz RH, *et al.* A randomised controlled trial of classical and medium chain triglyceride ketogenic diets in the treatment of childhood epilepsy. *Epilepsia* 2009;**50**:1109–17.

Learning objective

(1) To know the indications, the principles and outcome of the ketogenic diet for the treatment of childhood epilepsy.

Section 6
Epilepsy in specific circumstances

Chapter 91

Reflex epilepsies

Michalis Koutroumanidis

Reflex epileptic seizures are those consistently elicited by a specific stimulus (Beaumanoir *et al.*, 1989; Wieser, 1998; Zifkin, 1998). They are determined by two factors: (a) the stimulus; and (b) the response.

The stimulus

All sensory modalities may act as a stimulus, though in humans visual are by far more common. The stimulus evoking the abnormal response is specific for a given patient and may be simple (e.g. flashes of light, elimination of visual fixation, or tactile stimuli) or complex (coloured pictures, eating). Stimuli may be extrinsic, as in the above examples, proprioceptive (e.g. movements), or involve higher brain function, emotions and cognition (e.g. thinking, music, arithmetic) (Box 91.1). The duration of the stimulus to elicit an abnormal response may be brief or

---

Box 91.1. Stimulus-sensitive epilepsies and the responsible stimuli (Beaumanoir *et al.*, 1989; Zifkin, 1998)

I. Somatosensory stimuli

(1) Exteroceptive somatosensory stimuli
   a. Benign childhood epilepsy with somatosensory evoked spikes
   b. Sensory (tactile) evoked idiopathic myoclonic seizures in infancy
   c. Tapping epilepsy
   d. Tooth-brushing epilepsy
(2) Proprioceptive somatosensory stimuli
   a. Seizures induced by movements
   b. Seizures induced by eye closure and/or eye movements
   c. Paroxysmal kinesiogenic choreoathetosis
(3) Complex proprioceptive stimuli
   a. Eating epilepsy

II. Visual stimuli

(1) Simple visual stimuli
   a. Photosensitive epilepsies
   b. Pattern-sensitive epilepsies
   c. Fixation-off sensitive epilepsies
   d. Scotogenic epilepsy
   e. Self-induced photosensitive epilepsy
   f. Self-induced pattern-sensitive epilepsy
(2) Complex visual stimuli and language processing
   a. Reading epilepsy
   b. Graphogenic epilepsy

III. Auditory, vestibular and olfactory stimuli
   a. Seizures induced by pure sounds or words
   b. Musicogenic epilepsy (and singing epilepsy)
   c. Olfactorhinencephalic epilepsy
   d. Eating epilepsy triggered by tastes
   e. Seizures triggered by vestibular and auditory stimuli

IV. High-level process-induced seizures (cognitive, emotional, decision-making tasks and other complex stimuli)
   a. Thinking (noogenic) epilepsy
   b. Reflex decision-making epilepsy
   c. Epilepsia arithmetica (mathematica)
   d. Emotional epilepsies
   e. Startle epilepsy

Introduction to Epilepsy ed. Gonzalo Alarcón and Antonio Valentín. Published by Cambridge University Press.
© Cambridge University Press 2012.

prolonged. Simple, unstructured sensory stimuli generally provoke fast, within seconds, EEG or clinical response. More complex triggers that involve specific cognitive activities often require many minutes of exposure to activate abnormal responses.

The response

The response may consist of combined clinical and EEG manifestations, EEG only or clinical manifestations without conspicuous electrical changes on the surface EEG. The response may be limited to the stimulus-related brain region or may be much wider or rapidly generalize. Inter-individual responses to the same stimulus vary widely. The induced seizures may be generalized such as typical or atypical absences, myoclonic jerks and generalized tonic/tonic-clonic, or they may be partial such as visual, motor or sensory. Generalized tonic-clonic seizures may be either primarily generalized, or secondarily generalized to a partial, simple or complex seizure, or may follow a cluster of absences or myoclonic jerks. Myoclonic jerks are by far the most common type of stimulus-elicited seizures. They may be manifested in the limbs and trunk or localized in a specific muscle group, such as in the jaw muscles (reading epilepsy) or the eyelids (eyelid myoclonia with absences).

References

Beaumanoir A, Gastaut H, Naquet R. *Reflex Seizures and Reflex Epilepsies*. Geneve: Editions Medecine et Hygiene; 1989.

Wieser HG. Seizure induction in reflex seizures and reflex epilepsy. *Adv Neurol* 1998;75:69–85.

Zifkin BG. *Reflex Epilepsies and Reflex Seizures*. New York: Lippincot-Raven; 1998.

Learning objective

(1) To know the definition and classifications of reflex epilepsies.

Section 6 Epilepsy in specific circumstances

Chapter 92: Photosensitive and language-induced seizures and epilepsies

Simeran Sharma, Mark Stevenson and Michalis Koutroumanidis

Photosensitive epilepsy

Definition

'Photosensitive epilepsy' (PE) is a broad term comprising all forms of epilepsies in which seizures are triggered by visual stimulation and does not correspond to a particular epileptic syndrome. Thus, patients with syndromes of idiopathic generalized epilepsies (IGE) or patients with symptomatic epilepsies such as Lafora's disease may have seizures elicited by photic stimulation. In humans, photosensitivity is generated in the occipital lobes and it is therefore regional (occipital) epilepsy.

Laboratory (EEG) and clinical photosensitivity

Flashing lights (intermittent photic stimulation) are routinely used during EEG recordings to study photosensitivity. Responses to photic stimulation in their mildest form consist of posterior abnormalities (occipital spikes, often time-locked to the flash, or slow waves intermixed with small, larval spikes). They may spread variably forwards, or present as generalized photoparoxysmal responses (GPPR) when they cover the whole of the cerebrum. GPPR are highly (90–95%) associated with clinically evident epileptic disorders (Harding and Jeavons, 1994). Flashing frequencies of 18–20 Hz are generally the most effective to induce GPPRs.

Prevalence

Photosensitive epilepsy affects 1 in 4000 of the population (5% of patients with epileptic seizures), two-thirds are women (video-game-induced seizures occur more often in men) and the onset has a peak age at 12–13 years (Harding and Jeavons, 1994). Amongst patients with GPPR and seizures, 42% have photically induced seizures alone (pure photosensitive epilepsy), 40% have spontaneous and photically induced seizures and the remaining 18% have spontaneous seizures only. The overall annual incidence of cases with a newly presenting seizure and unequivocal photosensitivity in Great Britain was 1.1 per 100 000 (5.7 per 100 000 in the age group from 7 to 19 years). This means that photosensitivity is found in 2% of patients of all ages presenting with seizures and 10% of patients presenting with seizures in the age range 7–19 years (Quirk et al., 1995).

Precipitants

Precipitants include television viewing, video games, visual display units of computers, discotheques and natural flickering lights such as those in between trees or reflecting from water surfaces. Sleep deprivation increases the propensity to photosensitivity.

Pure photosensitive epilepsy

Seizures are always photically induced without spontaneous, unprovoked seizures. Generalized tonic-clonic seizures are reported far more commonly (87%) than absences (6%), partial seizures (2.5%) or myoclonic jerks (1.5%). However, mild myoclonic jerks or absences elicited by lights may escape attention, and are frequently discovered on video-EEG. The resting EEG is usually normal (apart from discharges on eye-closure in about a fifth of these patients), seizures are usually infrequent and prognosis is often excellent. Avoidance of precipitating factors may be the only effective/required treatment.

Introduction to Epilepsy ed. Gonzalo Alarcón and Antonio Valentín. Published by Cambridge University Press.
© Cambridge University Press 2012.

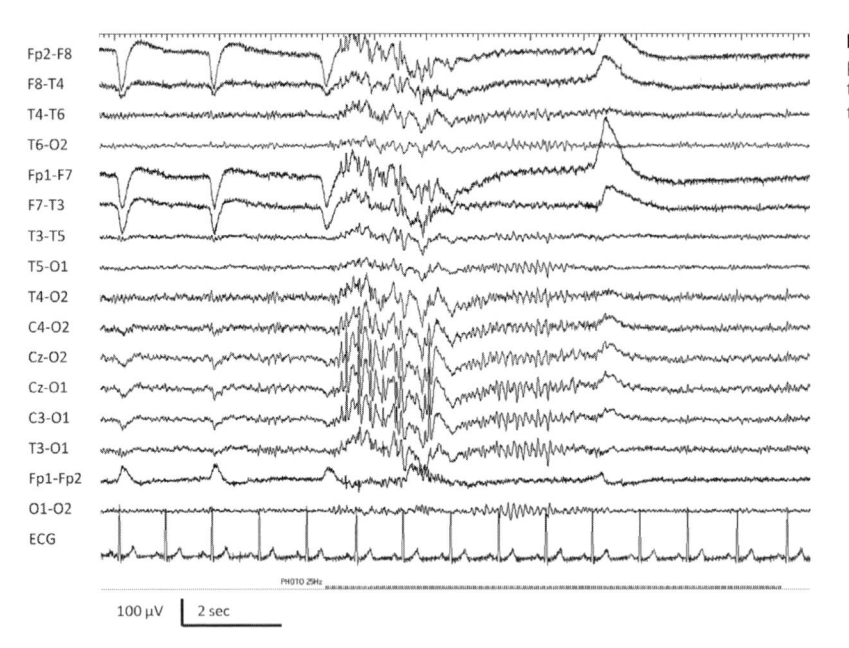

Figure 92.1. Generalized photoparoxysmal response at 25 Hz. It is triggered when eyes are open and seems to stop on eye-closure.

Photosensitivity and epilepsy syndromes

A quarter of patients with spontaneous seizures and EEG photosensitivity suffer from idiopathic generalized epilepsy. The main syndromes associated with photosensitivity are:

- benign myoclonic epilepsy in infancy
- childhood and juvenile absence epilepsies (CAE and JAE)
- juvenile myoclonic epilepsy (JME)
- eyelid myoclonia with absences
- IGE with GTCS only
- epilepsy with myoclonic-astatic seizures
- severe myoclonic epilepsy of infancy (Dravet syndrome, SMEI)
- symptomatic and idiopathic photosensitive occipital lobe epilepsies
- progressive myoclonic epilepsies (PME) including neuronal ceroid lipofuscinoses, Lafora's disease, Unverricht-Lundborg and MERRF syndrome.

Visual stimuli

Seizures may be triggered by visual stimuli other than flashing lights, as described below.

Video game (VG) sensitive seizures

Here, photosensitivity is also a major precipitant, but VG-induced seizures may also occur in non-photosensitive patients with idiopathic generalized epilepsies where sleep deprivation, fatigue, cognitive activities, decision-making and praxis alone or in combination may elicit an epileptic seizure. Provoked seizures can apparently be generalized (absences, jerks and generalized tonic-clonic seizures) or focal (occipital visual with late temporal lobe features due to ictal propagation forwards). Scenes with flashing lights, particularly with bright red colours, appear to be most effective in inducing seizures.

Pattern-sensitive epilepsy

Pattern seizure sensitivity, confirmed with specific EEG testing, is closely related to photosensitivity. Thus, patterns alone appear to be less epileptogenic than photic stimuli. They work most effectively in combination with intermittent light. Nearly all patients with clinical pattern-sensitivity epilepsy show photoparoxysmal discharges on appropriate intermittent photic stimulation testing. Conversely, of clinical photosensitive patients 30% are also sensitive to stationary and 70% to appropriately vibrating patterns of stripes. Pattern sensitivity depends on the spatial frequency, orientation, brightness, contrast and size of the stripes.

Fixation-off sensitive epilepsies

Fixation-off sensitivity (FOS) denotes the form/forms of epilepsy and/or EEG abnormalities that are elicited by elimination of central vision and fixation. Scotosensitive epilepsy implies seizures and EEG abnormalities induced by the complete elimination of retinal light stimulation; most cases described as scotosensitive are probably FOS (Panayiotopoulos, 1998).

Idiopathic photosensitive occipital seizures (IPOS) and epilepsy (IPOE)

The defining symptom is seizures of occipital symptomatology that are elicited by flickering lights, often of television, computer screens or video games. Elementary visual hallucinations predominate either alone or with progression to other manifestations, due to anterior spread and secondarily generalized convulsions (Guerrini *et al.*, 1995). Spontaneous occipital or other types of generalized seizures may co-exist in the less pure forms.

Visually induced occipital seizures are thought to represent a minority of the seizures provoked by photic and other visual stimuli, but prevalence may be higher than currently appreciated: for example, 49 of 88 (56%) children in whom the type of the provoked seizure (by the infamous incident of 'pocket monsters') was known had focal seizures (Takada *et al.*, 1999).

Treatment

In patients with pure photosensitive epilepsy, avoidance and protection from the provocative stimulus may be effective. Patients should maintain the maximum comfortable viewing distance from the TV screen, which is 4–5 times the diagonal measurement of the screen, in a well-lit room with a table lamp close to the screen, use the remote control, and avoid prolonged watching particularly if sleep-deprived and tired. Polaroid sunglasses may protect from flickering sunlight. Monocular occlusion can protect against sudden exposure to flickering lights. Conditioning treatment may be successful.

When drug treatment is deemed necessary, sodium valproate is the first choice, and levetiracetam may also be effective.

References

Guerrini R, Dravet C, Genton P, *et al.* Idiopathic photosensitive occipital lobe epilepsy. *Epilepsia* 1995;**36**:883–91.

Harding GFA, Jeavons PM. *Photosensitive Epilepsy*. London: MacKeith Press; 1994.

Panayiotopoulos CP. Fixation-off, scotosensitive, and other visual-related epilepsies. *Adv Neurol* 1998;**75**:139–57.

Quirk JA, Fish DR, Smith SJ, *et al.* First seizures associated with playing electronic screen games: a community-based study in Great Britain. *Ann Neurol* 1995;**37**:733–7.

Takada H, Aso K, Watanabe K, *et al.* Epileptic seizures induced by animated cartoon, 'Pocket Monster'. *Epilepsia* 1999;**40**:97–1002.

Learning objective

(1) To know the definition, prevalence, precipitants, classification, clinical manifestations, diagnosis and management of reflex epilepsy.

Section 6 Epilepsy in specific circumstances

Chapter 93 Audiogenic epilepsies

Nicholas Moran

Audiogenic epilepsy (AE) is an unusual category of reflex epilepsy. In the reflex epilepsies, seizures are habitually provoked by an external stimulus or, less commonly, an internal mental process. The seizure types in the reflex epilepsies are various and do not differ from spontaneous seizures. For this reason, the reflex epilepsies are classified by the class of triggering stimulus, e.g. photosensitive (see above), somatosensory (e.g. touch), audiogenic (sound), thinking, praxis (certain actions), reading (see above), thinking (e.g. mental arithmetic), eating, hot water. The stimulus may be a simple elementary one (e.g. flashing light or a tone) or complex with a relatively elaborate specific pattern (e.g. a certain tune or a certain type of music). Particularly in the complex reflex epilepsies, there may be a time interval between the stimulus onset and that of the seizure (latency). In addition, in some cases, a seizure may be provoked by anticipation of the stimulus.

Although AE is only infrequently encountered by the clinician, it is of theoretical importance in that there are several robust animal models of AE that provide insight into mechanisms of epilepsy and antiepileptic drugs. However, it should be appreciated that these animal models are independent of the forebrain and no analogous human condition is recognized.

Strictly speaking, reflex epilepsy can only be correctly diagnosed where seizures are exclusively provoked by stimuli. Often, however, an individual may have a mixture of spontaneous and reflex seizures. In this case, reflex epilepsy is not present but reflex seizures are listed as a seizure type.

There are three categories of human AE: startle, musicogenic and psophogenic. In psophogenic (also known as otogenic) epilepsy the stimulus is a simple sound, e.g. police sirens, independent of startle. Psophogenic epilepsy has only very rarely been reported in humans and is not discussed further here. Startle and musicogenic epilepsy are discussed below.

Startle epilepsy

The most frequent trigger is a sudden, unexpected sensory stimulus, most commonly a sound. It is important to note that the immediate seizure trigger is thought to be the set of proprioceptive signals resulting from the startle response, i.e. the stimulus provokes a normal, physiological startle response but the afferent return from this motor response triggers a seizure.

Startle epilepsy/seizures are most commonly symptomatic in association with conditions such as perinatal brain damage, Lennox-Gastaut syndrome, Down syndrome, Sturge-Weber syndrome or Tay-Sachs disease. However, occasionally there is no associated neurological condition.

Usually startle seizures are tonic; less commonly, atonic or complex partial.

Musicogenic epilepsy

This is an example of complex reflex epilepsy. Seizures are triggered by music (usually listening to it but also playing instruments or thinking or dreaming about music). Musicogenic epilepsy/seizures are rare. Around half of individuals with musicogenic seizures also have spontaneous seizures. It is overrepresented in musical individuals. Typically, the seizure type is complex partial with a right or left temporal lobe focus, and the semiology includes prominent autonomic features. Often, there is a delay between the stimulus and seizure onset.

It has not proved possible to identify any elemental feature of music that is responsible for seizure

---

Introduction to Epilepsy ed. Gonzalo Alarcón and Antonio Valentín. Published by Cambridge University Press.
© Cambridge University Press 2012.

provocation, e.g. rhythm or timbre. In some cases, one tune may be exclusively the trigger whereas in others it may be classes of music (particularly affective, e.g. melancholyic pieces). There is some evidence that the most important proving feature may be the affective response to music.

Resective surgery may be successful in selected cases.

Conditions that may be mistaken for audiogenic epilepsy

Cataplexy is a cardinal feature of the disease narcolepsy. In cataplexy there is a loss of muscle tone of varying severity. At its mildest there may be just dropping of the jaw and/or head or there may be total collapse. Such attacks are usually triggered by strong emotion, e.g. exhilaration, amusement, anger, surprise, or exertion.

Tullio's phenomenon: vestibular hypersensitivity to sound causing oscillopsia (visual field appears to oscillate), unsteadiness and vertigo in response to loud external sounds or the subject's own voice. Causes include dehiscence of the roof of the superior semicircular canal, perilymph fistula, Meniere's syndrome, vestibulofibrosis, Lyme disease.

Hyperekplexia is a condition characterized by an excessive startle response. It is usually hereditary. An excessive startle response may also occur in acquired conditions, e.g. stiff person syndrome. In the latter, there may be repetitive jerking resembling convulsions.

Coffin Lowry syndrome: a rare X-linked condition characterized by skeletal abnormalities and learning difficulties. Some patients also display collapses provoked by unexpected stimuli including sound. The nature of these events is uncertain.

Audiogenic epilepsy models in rodents

In contrast to epileptic seizures in humans, seizures in rodents with AE are initiated in the inferior colliculus of the midbrain, a structure subserving auditory processing. Most strains of mice and rats are susceptible to audiogenic seizures (AGS). Resistant strains are rendered prone to AGS by exposure to an acoustic insult in a critical period of postnatal development and are otherwise neurologically intact. In contrast, in genetically prone strains no priming is needed and AGS can occur as early as 3 weeks of age.

Recommended reading

Aguglia U, Tinuper P, Gastaut H. Startle-induced epileptic seizures. *Epilepsia* 1984;**25**:712–20.

Gastaut H, Tassinari CA. Triggering mechanisms in epilepsy. The electroclinical point of view. *Epilepsia* 1966;**7**:85–138.

Manford MR, Fish DR, Shorvon SD. Startle provoked epileptic seizures: features in 19 patients. *J Neurol Neurosurg Psychiatry* 1996;**61**:151–6.

Pittau F, Tinuper P, Bisulli F, *et al.* Videopolygraphic and functional MRI study of musicogenic epilepsy. A case report and literature review. *Epilepsy Behav* 2008;**13**: 685–92.

Ross KC, Coleman JR. Developmental and genetic audiogenic seizure models: behavior and biological substrates. *Neurosci Biobehav Rev* 2000;**24**:639–53.

Zagury S, Maury JA, Jomini-Jalanti RM. Partial sensitive epilepsy triggered by a pure sound. A case report. In Beamanoir A, Gastaut H, Naquet R, eds. *Reflex Seizures and Reflex Epilepsies*, pp. 251–4. Geneva: Editions Medecine et Hygiene; 1989.

Zifkin BG, Zatorre RJ. Musicogenic epilepsy. In Zifkin BG, Andermann F, Beaumanoir A, Rowan AJ, eds. *Reflex Epilepsies and Reflex Seizures: Advances in Neurology*, vol. **75**, pp. 273–81. Philadelphia: Lippincott-Raven; 1998.

Learning objective

(1) To know the definition, prevalence, precipitants, classification, clinical manifestations, diagnosis, differential diagnosis and management of audiogenic epilepsy.

Section 6 Epilepsy in specific circumstances

Chapter 94

Reading epilepsy

Michalis Koutroumanidis

Description

Reading or language-induced epilepsy is a form of complex reflex epilepsy in which all or almost all seizures of the affected patients are precipitated by reading and other linguistic activities. In the vast majority of patients, seizures are myoclonic and affect the jaw, propagating to the upper limbs in some cases, but in few they are strictly focal, manifested with alexia or dyslexia. There is only one case report with reading-induced absences (Koutroumanidis et al., 1998)

Prevalence

Reading or language-induced epilepsy is rare, with fewer than 150 patients reported in the literature. Amongst these, there are only five patients with focal seizures.

Ictal semiology

Reading epilepsy is a distinctive form of idiopathic reflex epilepsy. The clinical manifestations are elicited by silent or aloud reading and consist of brief myoclonic jerks mainly restricted to the masticatory, oral and perioral muscles. They are described as clicking sensations and occur a few minutes to hours after starting reading, particularly aloud. Consciousness is not impaired but if the patient continues reading, jaw jerks become more violent, spread to trunk and limb muscles or generate other seizure manifestations before a generalized tonic-clonic seizure develops. In the focal form, patients present with prolonged alexia with varying degrees of dysphasia.

Treatment

Avoidance of stimuli may be a practical difficulty. However, seizures are usually well controlled with clonazepam or sodium valproate.

Reference

Koutroumanidis M, Koepp MJ, Richardson MP, et al. The variants of reading epilepsy. A clinical and video-EEG study of 17 patients with reading-induced seizures. *Brain* 1998;**121**:1409–27.

Learning objective

(1) To know the definition, prevalence, precipitants, classification, clinical manifestations, diagnosis and management of reading epilepsy.

Introduction to Epilepsy ed. Gonzalo Alarcón and Antonio Valentín. Published by Cambridge University Press.
© Cambridge University Press 2012.

Chapter 94: Reading epilepsy

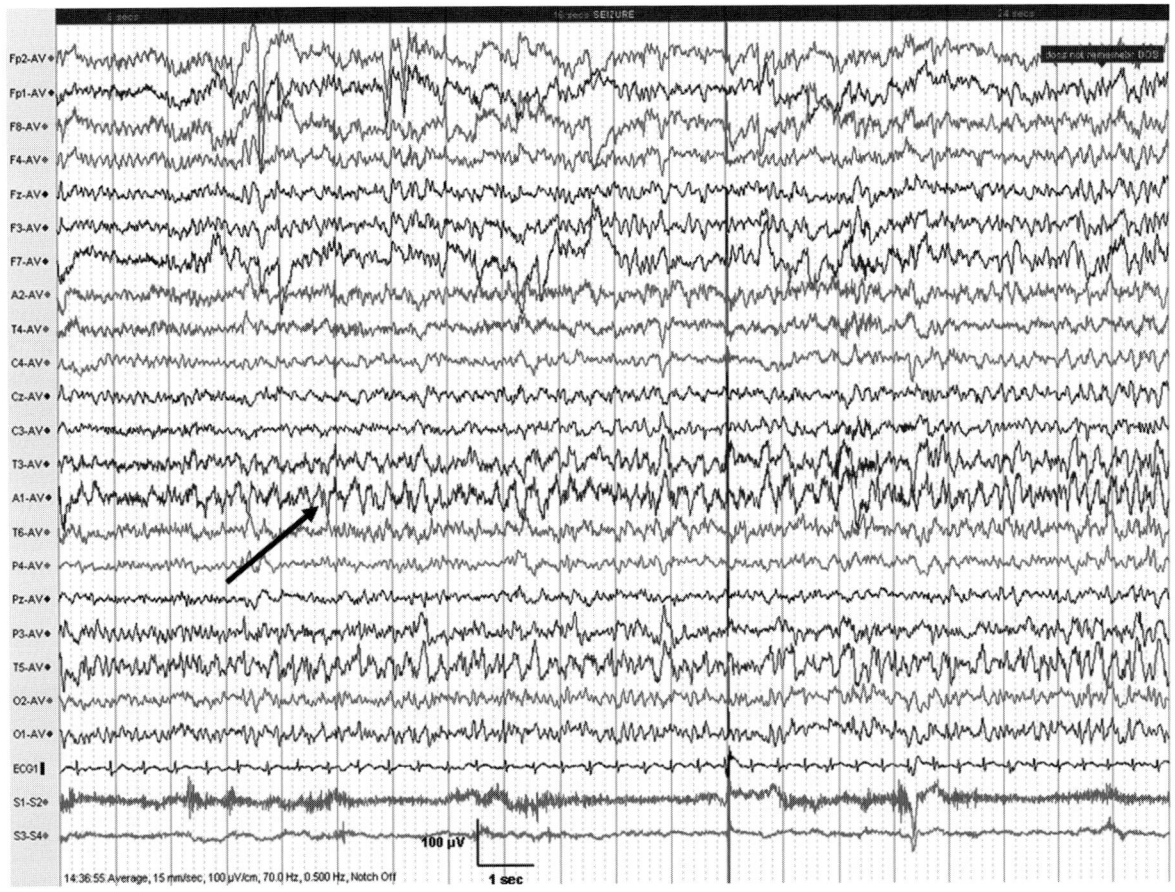

Figure 94.1. Reading induced a focal seizure of left posterior and mid temporal onset (arrow) manifesting with dyslexia (reproduced with permission from Osei-Lah AD, Casadei A, Richardson MP, Alarcón G. Focal reading epilepsy – a rare variant of reading epilepsy. A case report. *Epilepsia* 2010;**51**:2352–5).

Section 6 Epilepsy in specific circumstances

Chapter 95

Status epilepticus: classification and pathophysiology

Matthew Walker

Introduction

Seizures are, for the most part, self-terminating, but on occasions they can persist, leading to status epilepticus. The first definitions of status epilepticus were restricted to tonic-clonic seizures, but at the Marseilles Colloquium in 1962 status epilepticus was redefined so that it depended on the persistence of the seizure rather than its form. The definition was 'a condition characterized by epileptic seizures that are sufficiently prolonged or repeated at sufficiently brief intervals so as to produce an unvarying and enduring epileptic condition'. This definition introduces two aspects that remain contentious, first the duration of a seizure before it becomes 'enduring' and second the concept of status epilepticus as 'unvarying'. Although the length of time that a seizure or series of seizures have to continue before being classified as status epilepticus is to an extent arbitrary, most would accept a limit of 30 minutes. Treatment, however, should begin at an earlier time point to prevent the progression to established status epilepticus (see Chapter 96: 'Status epilepticus: diagnosis and management'). More importantly, as will become apparent, status epilepticus is anything but an 'unvarying' condition, and is perhaps best considered a condition with a number of distinct physiological and pharmacological stages.

Epidemiology

Status epilepticus is a common condition with an incidence of 10 to 60 per 100 000 person-years, depending on the population studied (the higher incidence is in people from poorer socioeconomic background). Over half the cases of status epilepticus occur in people without a prior history of epilepsy and it is critical to identify the underlying cause.

Infections with fever are the most common cause of status epilepticus in children, whilst in adults cerebrovascular accidents, hypoxia, metabolic causes and alcohol are the main acute causes. In people with epilepsy, status epilepticus is commonly precipitated by drug withdrawal, and reintroduction of the withdrawn drug can lead to a rapid resolution of the episode. Status epilepticus is recurrent in over 10% of people, emphasizing the need to have a protocol in place to prevent further episodes of status epilepticus. The prognosis of status epilepticus is related to aetiology; however, the prognosis of certain conditions such as stroke is worse if associated with status epilepticus. The mortality for status epilepticus is 10–20% and is higher in the elderly. If people prove resistant to first-line therapies the mortality increases to approximately 50%. People who survive status epilepticus may be left with permanent neurological and cognitive deficits. Furthermore acute symptomatic status epilepticus results in the development of chronic epilepsy in over 40%.

Classification

The early classifications of status epilepticus classified by seizure type (e.g. simple partial status epilepticus, complex partial status epilepticus etc.), but this failed to include many other forms of status epilepticus such as electrical status epilepticus during slow-wave sleep. More recently a classification based upon age of onset has been proposed (Box 95.1).

Status epilepticus as a staged phenomenon

Status epilepticus can be staged by EEG findings, progressive systemic physiological compromise,

---

Introduction to Epilepsy ed. Gonzalo Alarcón and Antonio Valentín. Published by Cambridge University Press.
© Cambridge University Press 2012.

> **Box 95.1.** Revised classification of status epilepticus
>
> **Status epilepticus confined to early childhood**
> - Neonatal status epilepticus
> - Status epilepticus in specific neonatal epilepsy syndromes
> - Infantile spasms
>
> **Status epilepticus confined to later childhood**
> - Febrile status epilepticus
> - Status in childhood partial epilepsy syndromes
> - Status epilepticus in myoclonic-astatic epilepsy
> - Electrical status epilepticus during slow-wave sleep
> - Landau-Kleffner syndrome
>
> **Status epilepticus occurring in childhood and adult life**
> - Tonic-clonic status epilepticus
> - Absence status epilepticus
> - Epilepsia partialis continua
> - Status epilepticus in coma (subtle generalized tonic-clonic seizure)
> - Specific forms of status epilepticus in mental retardation
> - Syndromes of myoclonic status epilepticus
> - Non-convulsive simple partial status epilepticus
> - Complex partial status epilepticus
> - Status epilepticus confined to adult life
> - De novo absence status of late onset

progressive neuronal damage and progressive drug resistance.

In animal models of status epilepticus, an EEG progression has been noted: first there are discrete seizures, then merging of the discrete seizures, continuous seizure discharge, and lastly periodic epileptiform discharges. These stages may be relevant to human status epilepticus because often there is a premonitory phase (before established status epilepticus) of increasing seizure frequency and the end-stages of status epilepticus are often marked by periodic epileptiform discharges, probably representing neuronal damage.

The systemic effects of convulsive status epilepticus can be divided into early and late stages. The initial consequence of a prolonged convulsion is a massive release of plasma catecholamines, which results in an increase in heart rate, blood pressure and plasma glucose. During this stage the increase in cerebral blood flow more than matches the increased brain metabolism. After 60–90 minutes (earlier in the elderly), the status epilepticus may then enter a second late phase in which there is a fall in blood pressure, and a loss of cerebral autoregulation resulting in the dependence of cerebral blood flow on systemic blood pressure (a combination that can result in cerebral ischaemia). Severe metabolic derangements can also occur, in particular hypoglycaemia, hyponatraemia and acidosis.

Independent of the physiological compromise, status epilepticus can result in neuronal death. This is secondary to the excessive activation of glutamate receptors and the consequent accumulation of calcium within neurons that can lead to mitochondrial failure, free-radical generation and also programmed cell death. This cell death is time-dependent (i.e. the longer status epilepticus continues the more cell death occurs) and occurs even if there are no overt clinical signs of seizure activity (i.e. it can occur with electrical status epilepticus alone). Targeting of the pathways involved can prevent some of this damage.

Lastly there is progressive resistance of status epilepticus to antiepileptic drugs. This is partly due to upregulation of multidrug transporter proteins but predominantly occurs due to internalization of synaptic $GABA_A$ receptors (so profoundly decreasing the response to benzodiazepines).

Conclusion

Status epilepticus can be a devastating condition with a high morbidity and mortality. It is a condition that varies with time, emphasizing the need for rapid treatment. Further status epilepticus is an appreciable brain insult resulting in not only neuronal death, but also channel/receptor changes (both acute and chronic), synaptic reorganization and increased neuronal excitability; all of these may contribute to later consequences such as neurological deficit/cognitive decline and the development of epilepsy.

Recommended reading

Chen JW, Wasterlain CG. Status epilepticus: pathophysiology and management in adults. *Lancet Neurol* 2006;5(3):246–56.

Section 6: Epilepsy in specific circumstances

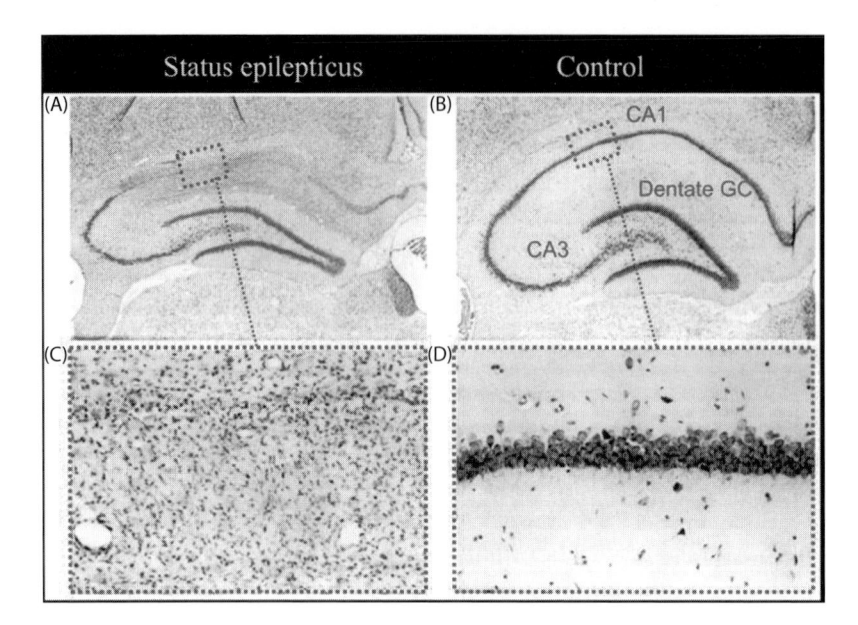

Figure 95.1. Neuronal damage with status epilepticus. Three hours of status epilepticus without systemic compromise results in considerable neuronal damage in the hippocampus (A) and especially CA1 region (C), which shows a microglial reaction. Controls (B, D) are presented for comparison

Meldrum BS. Concept of activity-induced cell death in epilepsy: historical and contemporary perspectives. *Prog Brain Res* 2002;**135**:3–11.

Walker MC, Shorvon SD. Emergency treatment of seizures and status epilepticus. In Shorvon SD, Perucca E, Engel J, eds. *Treatment of Epilepsy*. 3rd edn. Oxford: Wiley-Blackwell; 2009.

Learning objectives

(1) To understand the spectrum and epidemiology of status epilepticus.
(2) To be familiar with the mechanisms and aetiology of status epilepitcus.
(3) To understand that status epilepticus varies over time.

Section 6 Epilepsy in specific circumstances

Chapter 96

Status epilepticus: diagnosis and management

Matthew Walker

Diagnosis

Although the diagnosis of status epilepticus would appear to be straightforward, in an audit of patients transferred in apparently refractory status epilepticus, almost half did not have status epilepticus but rather had pseudostatus epilepticus (psychogenic non-epileptic seizures). Psychogenic attacks (dissociative seizures) can be differentiated by their semiology (such as poorly coordinated thrashing, back arching, eyes held shut and head rolling), by clinical signs (responsive pupils, flexor plantar responses) and, if necessary, by EEG. Serum prolactin plays no role, as it can increase in a variety of circumstances and can normalize during prolonged seizure activity.

Conversely non-convulsive status epilepticus can be difficult to diagnose. As seizures continue, the clinical manifestation can become more subtle, so that, for example, people with absence status epilepticus may complain of 'feeling strange' and complex partial status epilepticus may manifest as a change in personality, varying degrees of confusion or an apparent prolonged (>20 minutes) post-ictal period. Possibly up to 8% of people in coma in an ITU without a prior history of epilepsy or seizures are in non-convulsive status epilepticus. Clues that someone is in nonconvulsive status epilepticus include fluctuations in pupillary size, nystagmus and stereotypical motor manifestations, but an EEG is almost always necessary to confirm or refute the diagnosis. Even with an EEG, the diagnosis may not be straightforward. EEG criteria for a diagnosis of non-convulsive status epilepticus include at least one of the following:

(1) unequivocal electrographic seizure activity;
(2) periodic epileptiform discharges or rhythmic discharge with clinical seizure activity;
(3) rhythmic discharge with either clinical or electrographic response to treatment.

Principles underlying treatment

As was discussed in the previous chapter, status epilepticus is a staged phenomenon and one of the critical aspects of the treatment of status epilepticus is to treat in a staged fashion. Status epilepticus can be divided into a premonitory phase (increasing seizure frequency with less recovery between), established status epilepticus (continuous seizure activity for 30 minutes), late stages (resistance to first-line therapies, continuous seizure activity for more than 1 hour). Another principle that governs treatment is the pharmacokinetics of acutely used antiepileptic drugs. When given acutely, antiepileptic drug concentration-time curves have a rapid redistribution phase (during which the drug distributes from the blood to fat/muscle) and a slower elimination phase. With lipid-soluble drugs, the redistribution phase can predominate and so determine the apparent half-life. However, with repeated boluses, the peripheral compartment becomes saturated, so there is loss of the redistribution phase, resulting in higher peak concentrations and a slower apparent half-life (dependent on the elimination half-life). Diazepam has a redistribution half-life of less than 30 minutes and an elimination half-life of over 30 hours. Therefore, given acutely, diazepam has an apparent half-life of 30 minutes but repeated boluses would lead to higher peak levels and prolongation of the apparent half-life, eventually to 30 hours. Thus repeated boluses lead to progressively greater sedation and more prolonged action, potentially resulting in hypotension and cardiorespiratory arrest. Lastly, EEG is necessary for

---

Introduction to Epilepsy ed. Gonzalo Alarcón and Antonio Valentín. Published by CAMBRIDGE UNIVERSITY PRESS.
© CAMBRIDGE UNIVERSITY PRESS 2012.

Section 6: Epilepsy in specific circumstances

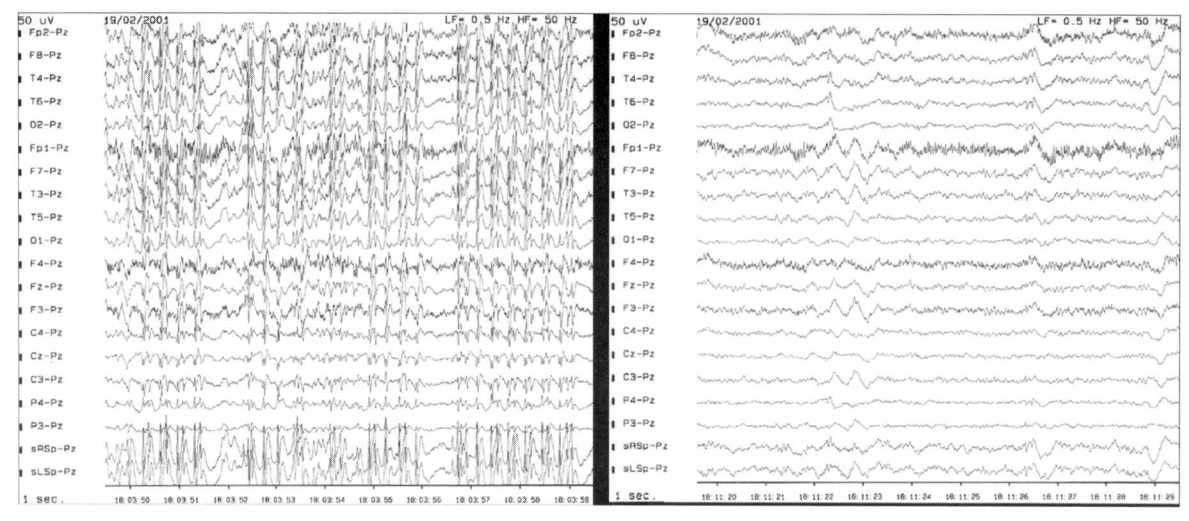

Figure 96.1. Complex partial status epilepticus in a woman with right hippocampal sclerosis: before (left) and then 1 minute after 20 mg intravenous diazepam (right). After the diazepam, the EEG is dominated by post-ictal slow and the woman remains confused.

monitoring all forms of status epilepticus as the natural progression of status epilepticus is to minimal or no clinical manifestations.

Randomized clinical trials in status epilepticus

There have been eight randomized studies of intravenous drug treatment in status epilepticus. These studies have methodological problems, including different definitions of status epilepticus, different doses of drugs and varying outcome measures. These studies have compared lidocaine against placebo, lorazepam against diazepam, phenobarbital against diazepam and phenytoin, intramuscular midazolam against intravenous diazepam, four different intravenous treatment regimens (lorazepam, phenytoin alone, diazepam and phenytoin, and phenobarbital), valproate against phenytoin and valproate against intravenous diazepam in refractory status epilepticus. Very few conclusions can be drawn from these studies: lidocaine is effective in the treatment of status epilepticus; lorazepam and diazepam are equally effective although more patients required additional antiepileptic drugs if given diazepam; lorazepam is more effective than phenytoin alone, and no particular drug or drug combination has significantly more side effects, including respiratory depression. Overall drug choice is perhaps not as important as having a protocol so that adequate doses of antiepileptic drugs are given rapidly.

Drug treatment of convulsive status epilepticus
Premonitory phase

Prior to status epilepticus becoming established (people with repeated seizures or with prolonged seizures), there is a wealth of data indicating that rectal diazepam can prevent the progression to status epilepticus, and can be used safely in the community. More recent evidence in children indicates that buccal midazolam may be a superior alternative.

Established status epilepticus

Once status epilepticus has become established, rapid administration of an intravenous therapy is required. At this stage, intravenous access is necessary, blood should be taken, fluids should be administered and glucose/thiamine may be given if hypoglycaemia is suspected. Oxygen should be administered because of the respiratory depression that occurs in status epilepticus.

At present lorazepam is the drug of choice as it has a long redistribution half-life (3–10 hours) and so is less likely to result in rebound seizures. If the first bolus (usually 4 mg in an adult) fails, then a second bolus can be given followed by a loading dose of phenytoin (20 mg/kg infused at a maximum rate of 50 mg/min).

Refractory status epilepticus

If convulsive status epilepticus has not responded to the first-line treatments above and has continued for 60–90 minutes, then people will be entering a phase of physiological compromise, neuronal damage and increasing drug resistance. At this stage the patient should be transferred to an ITU and given anaesthetic (propofol, thiopentone/pentobarbital or midazolam) to stop seizure activity. Pressor therapy may be necessary at this stage to maintain blood pressure. Phenytoin adminstration should be continued. The patient should be loaded with phenobarbitone. Once all seizure activity has stopped for more than 24 hours and provided there are adequate blood levels of antiepileptic drugs, then the anaesthetic can be slowly withdrawn. Should status epilepticus recur, other drugs can be tried, but at this stage good clinical trials are lacking. Nevertheless, there are anecdotal reports supporting the use of valproate, topiramate, levetiracetam and steroid treatment (especially if an autoimmune disorder is suspected).

Drug treatment of non-convulsive status epilepticus

There is some controversy concerning the degree of neuronal damage that occurs with non-convulsive status epilepticus, and consequently how aggressively it should be treated. There is no evidence of neuronal damage in typical absence status epilepticus, which responds very well to oral or intravenous benzodiazepines. Complex partial status epilepticus (CPSE) is more difficult, and the outcome depends upon circumstance. Patients with epilepsy who have complex partial status epilepticus usually respond well to treatment with an intravenous benzodiazepine and, if they have repeated episodes, then oral clobazam (or oral diazepam) is an alternative in the community. Benzodiazepines can however increase mortality in the critically ill elderly who have CPSE and in this population, an alternative such as intravenous valproate could be considered. In both these instances, there is rarely justification to progress to anaesthesia and ITU. Conversely patient in coma, who have CPSE have a very poor outcome and aggressive treatment in this group is probably justified, although good clinical trials are lacking.

Conclusion

Misdiagnosis of status epilepticus is not uncommon. Status epilepticus is over-diagnosed in convulsive status epilepticus and under-diagnosed in non-convulsive status epilepticus. EEG plays a critical role in diagnosis and monitoring of treatment. Staged protocols should be in place for convulsive status epilepticus and, in view of the high complication rate of refractory status epilepticus, transfer to ITU is necessary. Treatment of non-convulsive status epilepticus remains controversial, but should be governed by underlying cause and the state of the patient.

Learning objectives

(1) To understand that treatment of status epilepticus occurs in a staged fashion.
(2) To realize the complex issues concerning treatment of non-convulsive status epilepticus.

Section 6 Epilepsy in specific circumstances

Chapter 97

Management of epilepsy in women

Gonzalo Alarcón

There are specific problems in the management of women with epilepsy which are related to their role in reproduction, potentially affecting nearly half of patients with epilepsy. Maternal epilepsy is the commonest neurological problem in pregnancy and affects 3–4 per thousand pregnancies. As treatment with antiepileptic drugs is likely to be necessary for long periods, the possibility of pregnancy should be considered in any woman of childbearing age with epilepsy. The following are specific issues which may be relevant to women with epilepsy:

- interaction of hormonal contraceptives with AEDs
- contraceptive methods in women with epilepsy
- teratogenicity induced by antiepileptic drugs
- investigations during pregnancy
- hyperemesis
- the effects of seizures on the fetus
- the effect of pregnancy on seizures
- management of a first fit in pregnancy
- pseudoseizures in pregnancy
- epilepsy during delivery: effects on mother and infant
- the use of vitamin K in the infant
- breastfeeding in women with epilepsy
- post-partum maternal epilepsy
- hereditary risks
- counselling
- catamenial epilepsy
- the menopause and bone density in women with epilepsy.

A detailed discussion on the management of these issues is beyond the scope of this book, as there are excellent reviews in the literature. I would like to suggest the following:

- O'Brien MD, Guillebaud J. Contraception for women taking antiepileptic drugs. *J Fam Plann Reprod Health Care* 2010;**36**(4): 239–42.
- O'Brien MD, Gilmour-White SK. Management of epilepsy in women. *Postgrad Med J* 2005;**81**:278–285.

Learning objectives

(1) To be aware of the contraceptive methods acceptable in women with epilepsy and their interactions with antiepileptic drugs.
(2) To know the risk of teratogenic effects associated with taking antiepileptic drugs during pregnancy.
(3) To be aware of the investigations to be requested during pregnancy.
(4) To know the management of hyperemesis during pregnancy in patients with epilepsy.
(5) To know the effects of maternal fits on the fetus.
(6) To know the effects of pregnancy on seizures.
(7) To know the principles of the management of a first fit in pregnancy.
(8) To know the effects on mother and infant of epilepsy during delivery.
(9) To know the principles and indications of the use of vitamin K after birth in newborns from mothers with epilepsy.
(10) To know the effects on the newborn of breastfeeding when taking antiepileptic drugs.
(11) To be aware of the issues regarding safety for the newborn from a parent with epilepsy.

Introduction to Epilepsy ed. Gonzalo Alarcón and Antonio Valentín. Published by Cambridge University Press.
© Cambridge University Press 2012.

(12) To know and be able to discuss the hereditary risks of epilepsy in offspring of patients with epilepsy.
(13) To be aware of counselling issues to be discussed in women with epilepsy contemplating becoming pregnant.
(14) To be aware of catamenial epilepsy and its management.
(15) To be aware of the effects of the menopause on seizures and of the issues related to treating epilepsy during the menopause and monitoring bone density.

Section 6 Epilepsy in specific circumstances

Chapter 98

Catamenial seizures

Nandini Mullatti

Catamenial epilepsy refers to the exacerbation of epileptic seizures with the hormonal fluctuations of the menstrual cycle. A reasonable working definition would be an increase of 2-fold over baseline frequency of seizures.

The typical menstrual cycle consists of a 28-day cycle. Menstruation commences at the onset of the cycle and this is initiated by the fall in oestrogen and progesterone levels. Levels of oestrogen and progesterone rise again with ovulation, but oestrogen rises more than progesterone, resulting in a raised oestrogen/progesterone ratio. A similar event occurs just before menstruation (Figure 98.1).

It has been shown that the hormone oestrogen is proconvulsant. It inhibits γ-aminobutyric acid (GABA), potentiates glutaminergic transmission and increases neuronal metabolism and discharge rates. Oestrogens promote kindling in experimental as well as clinical seizure occurrence (Herzog et al., 1997). Progesterone, on the other hand, has anticonvulsant properties. Its metabolites have a barbiturate-like action on the GABA-chloride channel. Further, progesterone reduces neuronal metabolism and discharge rates, and suppresses kindling, epileptiform discharges and experimental as well as clinical seizures.

Catamenial exacerbation of seizures occurs in three phases of the menstrual cycle (Figure 98.1):

- The perimenstrual phase (C1) is thought to be due to the reduction of the antiseizure effects of progesterone, and the premenstrual fluid retention causing dilution and drop in AED levels. Additionally, since both AEDs and oestrogen/progesterone are metabolized by the same hepatic microsomal systems, reduction of levels of these hormones may result in more AEDs being metabolized.

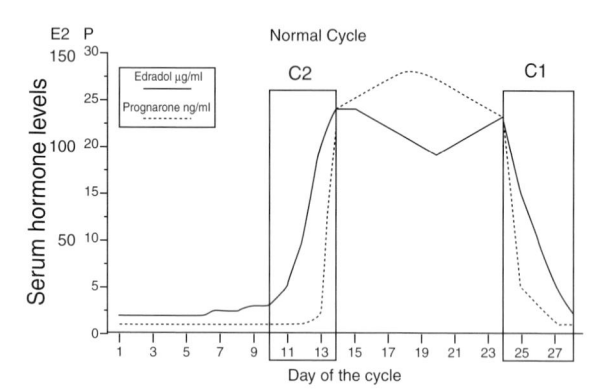

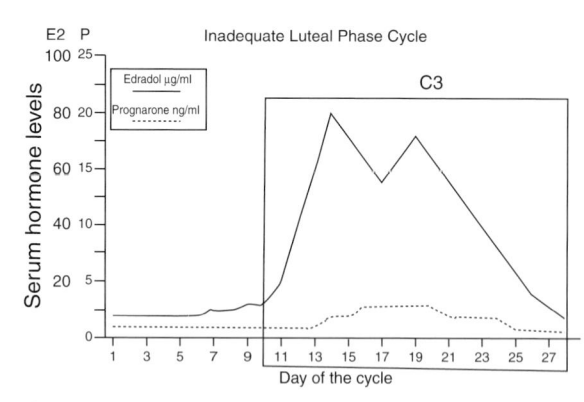

Figure 98.1. Three proposed patterns of catamenial epilepsy: perimenstrual (C1) and periovulatory (C2) exacerbations during normal cycles and entire second half of the cycle (C3) exacerbation during inadequate luteal-phase cycles.

- Mid-cycle exacerbation (C2 pattern) is due to the pre-ovulatory surge of oestrogen, unaccompanied by an increase in progesterone, with a resultant elevation of the oestrogen/progesterone ratio.
- In the C3 phase, oestrogen levels are high but progesterone levels low in the second half of the

Introduction to Epilepsy ed. Gonzalo Alarcón and Antonio Valentín. Published by Cambridge University Press.
© Cambridge University Press 2012.

cycle, and this again facilitates an increase in seizures in the second half of the cycle.

Management

It is important to chart menstruation and seizures on a calendar to establish the pattern of clustering. If a catamenial exacerbation is established, treatment is based on the pattern.

- For perimenstrual exacerbation, therapeutic options include slightly increasing the AED dose perimenstrually or, preferably, adding clobazam 10 mg at night during the perimenstrual period. Acetazolamide 250 mg three times a day is also helpful due to its mild diuretic and anti-seizure effects.
- For periovulatory exacerbation, mid-cycle supplementation of clobazam would be of benefit.
- For the C3 pattern caused by an inadequate luteal phase, an intermittent perimenstrual progesterone supplement is suggested, or a synthetic progestogen during days 10 to 26 of the menstrual cycle. A combined oral contraceptive pill (COCP) may be prescribed.

Reference

Herzog AG, Klein P, Ransil BJ. Three patterns of catamenial epilepsy. *Epilepsia* 1997;**38**(10):1082–8.

Learning objective

(1) To know the definition, epidemiology, pathophysiology and management of catamenial epilepsy.

Section 6 Epilepsy in specific circumstances

Chapter 99 The management of epilepsy in children

David McCormick

Accurate diagnosis is the starting point for effective management of any condition, and it is imperative that, before any course of management for epilepsy is entered into, the diagnosis of a seizure disorder is confirmed. Secondly, as epilepsy is a large group of conditions, rather than just one condition, any management offered must be appropriate to the type of seizure disorder diagnosed. Specificity of diagnosis may range from at its most simple classification only, for example focal onset seizures of left temporal origin, to specific seizure syndrome diagnoses such as benign epilepsy with central temporal spikes (BECTS) or juvenile myoclonic epilepsy (JME).

It is important to recognize that the management of epilepsy in children is far more than simply the prescription of appropriate antiepileptic medication. Not all seizure disorders will warrant antiepileptic medication treatment, for instance where seizures are very infrequent or mild, and/or where they are likely to cease spontaneously, such as in BECTS. It is vital for the management of all seizure disorders in childhood and adolescence, however, that the child and family are appropriately educated. This should include information on the nature of the seizure disorder diagnosed, appropriate safety measures to be put in place, first-aid and emergency seizure management, any lifestyle alterations required, and the impact of the seizure disorder on education. Failure to address these issues may lead to additional stress, which could in itself lead to additional seizures, and could have a significant negative impact on both the safety and quality of life of the patient and their family.

When deciding whether to use antiepileptic medication, several aspects of the child's seizure disorder should be considered:

- How severe are the seizures?
- How frequent are the seizures?
- What is the likely long-term outcome of this seizure disorder?
- Are the seizures likely to have a negative impact on the child's learning and behaviour?
- Could the antiepileptic drugs prescribed have a negative impact on the child's learning and behaviour?
- Do the seizures pose a significant safety risk for the child?
- Is there a significant risk of episodes of status epilepticus?
- Is there a significant risk of sudden unexplained death in epilepsy (SUDEP) if the seizures are not controlled?

The National Institute for Health and Clinical Excellence (NICE) recommends that 'Treatment with antiepileptic drugs (AED) therapy is generally recommended after a second epileptic seizure' (NICE, 2004). This is because some children may present with a single seizure only, and never go on to have another one. As epilepsy can be defined in very short form as 'recurrent seizures', it is only at the point of occurrence of a second or more seizure that the condition can be diagnosed. However, some children will present with a prolonged and severe episode of status epilepticus, or following a single seizure be found to have an identified underlying EEG abnormality or structural change in the brain, and in these children ongoing AED treatment should be considered (NICE, 2004, section 4.8.19).

For those children who have had two or more seizures, the nature of the seizures must be considered. Treatment may not be necessary on severity grounds after two absence seizures or two partial seizures in the context of BECTS, but the situation for two generalized tonic-clonic seizures may be quite different. However, even with two generalized tonic-clonic seizures, if these

---

Introduction to Epilepsy ed. Gonzalo Alarcón and Antonio Valentín. Published by Cambridge University Press.
© Cambridge University Press 2012.

are spaced a significant time apart, for instance more than 1 year, the potential benefit of suppressing seizures through AED usage must be weighed up against potential adverse effects in the context of seizures which appear to be likely to occur very infrequently. The doctor, along with the patient, must ask themselves: 'Is it worth taking this medication every day for the next year when another seizure is unlikely to occur in this time period anyway?' Such considerations must always be weighed against safety, which must be the patient's and the doctor's first priority. In general, it is recommended to consider regular treatment after the first bout of status epilepticus, and to consider regular treatment after a second (afrebile) seizure, unless there is a very long interval between seizures, the epilepsy is likely to have a benign outcome regardless of intervention, or the seizures themselves are not considered to be intrusive enough to justify treatment.

When planning antiepileptic drug treatment for children, the goals of treatment must be clearly identified. The optimal outcome is a seizure-free child with no adverse effects, who is able to reach their optimal potential with regard to their developmental, educational, social, behavioural and emotional well-being. Should this not be possible, the aim should be to lower seizure frequency and/or ensure that seizures are less intrusive, preferably in the absence of adverse effects. If adverse effects cannot be avoided completely, these should be managed so that they are minimized as much as possible and tolerable to the patient. It should go without saying that keeping the patient safe is one of the key goals of treatment.

When introducing an AED, several key principles should be followed. Always begin with a single medication, appropriate to the condition being treated, starting at a low dose and titrating upward slowly. Drugs for children must be prescribed according to the size of the child, usually on a milligram per kilogram basis. In general, the advised rate of increase for medications by the pharmaceutical companies is faster than is appropriate for or tolerated by children. Patients should be given written information on the way the medication will be stepwise increased, and advised to stop increasing the medication once seizure control is achieved. Thus the aim is to titrate the medication up to the lowest dose necessary to control seizures. Should the medication be titrated to maximum tolerated or recommended dose but seizure control not be achieved, the preferable course of action is to withdraw the first medication and substitute another medication. It is vital to avoid, unless absolutely necessary, the use of multiple medications for patients, as this may have a negative impact on patient well-being and as a result quality of life is likely to be higher on monotherapy than on polytherapy. Once seizure control is achieved, it must be recognized that children grow and gain weight with time, and serial adjustments of the dose to keep the milligram per kilogram dose stable may be necessary.

With regard to specific antiepileptic medications, apart from the use of bromide in the mid nineteenth century, the medications used today date back nearly 100 years, to the first use of phenobarbitone in 1912. Phenytoin was introduced in 1938, carbamazepine in 1952 and sodium valproate in 1963. These four older medications still form a major proportion of the antiepileptic drugs prescribed today. However, the last 30 years has seen an explosion in drug development for the treatment of epilepsy, as more and more pharmaceutical companies have entered into the development of medications for the treatment of this chronic condition. This has led to the development and introduction of a significant number of key 'new' medications which have enabled the improvement of seizure control and led to an improvement in quality of life for many children and young people suffering from epilepsy.

When considering which specific medication to choose, consider the following points:

- seizure type and/or syndromic diagnosis;
- other medical conditions and expected side-effect profile;
- potential interactions with other medications the child may be taking;
- the speed at which the medication can be introduced and how urgent it is to achieve seizure control;
- the ability of the child to take the available formulations of the medicine, as well as the impact of dosage interval on the child and family's life;
- the need for drug level monitoring (blood tests can be a very negative experience for children);
- the ability of the family to comply with the proposed course of treatment;
- the evidence for efficacy in this age group and seizure type.

When looking at evidence for efficacy in the treatment of specific seizure types or syndromes in childhood, evidence can be at times sadly lacking. Until recently, pharmaceutical trials often excluded children or excluded children who had significant additional disabilities such as learning difficulty. Only recently has legislation been introduced requiring the trialling of AEDs on children where such a potential market exists. Since July 2008, any company that applies to the European Medicines Agency (EMEA) to market a new drug must include a paediatric investigation plan or obtain a waiver if a drug is not suitable for children (Sinha, 2008). In addition, many trials are aimed at demonstrating the safety and efficacy of an individual medication, and very few compare medications on a 'head to head' basis.

The most common form of trial encountered in the AED literature is the adding on of a new agent to current AEDs for patients with refractory partial seizures. The outcome measure is often the 'responder rate', a measure of the proportion of patients whose seizures are reduced by 50% or more. Whilst such reduction in seizure frequency could have a valuable impact on quality of life, a much higher impact will be achieved by seizure freedom, but relatively few papers focus on this as the key outcome measure. Quite often in paediatric epilepsy management practice, evidence is gained over time from trials of new AEDs in adults, and there is a delay before these medications are trialled in children, usually in relatively low numbers at first. It would be far more preferable for these medications to be appropriately and rigorously trialled in the paediatric age group from the outset.

In treating complex conditions such as epilepsy, it is preferable for doctors to have guidelines outlining standard practice in their region as agreed by their peers and experts in the field. Within my own practice, I refer to the South East Thames Paediatric Epilepsy Interest Group (SETPEG) guidelines (www.setpeg.co.uk), which have been developed over a period of years from available evidence in the literature, NICE guidelines, and shared consultant experience. Based on these guidelines, when considering the treatment of focal onset seizures in childhood, the first-line agent suggested is carbamazepine. Second-line agents recommended for the treatment of such seizures are lamotrigine, sodium valproate, topiramate or levetiracetam. It should be noted that, in one of the few head-to-head trials which examined the use of alternative medications for the management of seizures in children (and in adults), lamotrigine was found to be as effective for focal-onset seizures in childhood as carbamazepine, but had fewer side effects. It may therefore move towards becoming a first-choice medication in the near future (Marson et al., 2007). Third-line agents for partial seizures in children from the SETPEG guidelines include clobazam, gabapentin and phenytoin, with medications such as phenobarbitone and vigabatrin relegated to fourth-line choice because of their potential significant serious adverse effects.

For generalized seizures, it is recommended that sodium valproate is the first-line choice. However, because of the recognized increased risk of teratogenicity in women taking sodium valproate, and the fact that many children may remain on the same medication into their teenage years and even adulthood when suffering from chronic seizure disorders, sodium valproate is usually avoided in girls aged 10 or older. In this age group lamotrigine is the preferred first-line agent. Second-line agents include the use of ethosuximide (for absence seizures) and lamotrigine (where sodium valproate has been tried first). Topiramate, clobazam and clonazepam are listed as third-line agents. Levetiracetam is also recognized as showing some efficacy in generalized seizures in childhood, and is now licensed for adjunctive use for this purpose in the UK from age 4 years. Acetazolamide is a possible fourth-line agent. Carbamazepine is contra indicated in idiopathic generalized epilepsy as there is significant evidence that it can worsen this condition, such as in absence seizures (Parker et al., 1998), or even lead to the occurrence of additional seizure types such as myoclonus. Other considerations when choosing AEDs for generalized seizure disorders include the possibility that myoclonic jerks may be worsened by medication such as gabapentin, vigabatrin and lamotrigine.

In line with these recommendations, the National Institute for Health and Clinical Excellence has recommended that the newer drugs for the management of epilepsy in children (such as lamotrigine, oxcarbazepine, topiramate, etc.) are used for the management of epilepsy in children who have not benefited from treatment with the older antiepileptic drugs such as sodium valproate or carbamazepine, or for whom these older drugs are unsuitable. This is relevant to the cost of management of epilepsy in addition to the evidence base for medication choice. For example, in a report from April 2004 (Perucca, 2004), NICE recommended that whereas the newer drugs accounted to 20% of the total drugs prescribed for adults with epilepsy in 2002, they contributed to 69% of the total cost. The committee considering this matter for the National Institute of Clinical Excellence considered that the evidence from randomized trials comparing newer and older antiepileptic drugs as monotherapy did not suggest differences in their overall effectiveness in seizure control, nor adequate evidence with respect to the incidence of adverse effects to support a conclusion that the newer drugs were generally associated with an improved quality of life. The committee considered, therefore, at that time that it was not possible to conclude that any of the newer antiepileptic drugs were likely to be more cost-effective than the older agents.

The usual practice in the management of childhood epilepsy is to continue medication for at least 2 years after the patient has become seizure-free. Once such seizure freedom has been achieved, it can be difficult to determine whether this is as a result of ongoing efficacy of the AED, or whether the child has outgrown the seizure disorder. In general, other than in some specific idiopathic generalized epilepsies, repeating the EEG is not informative in making this decision. It is appropriate at this time to consider a trial of withdrawal of medication. When withdrawing antiepileptic drug medication in childhood, one should seek to do so when the child is in optimum health, as minimally stressed as possible, and at a time when this is not going to interfere significantly with key moments in education such as examinations. Whilst there is no significant evidence that gradual withdrawal leads to less likelihood of seizure recurrence than more rapid withdrawal, antiepileptic drug medications can have a range of effects on the patient, and rapid withdrawal should be avoided where possible. It is standard practice for medications other than phenobarbitone and benzodiazepines to withdraw the medication over a period of 6–12 weeks in gradual decrements. If seizures recur, the patient should be advised to go back on to the dose which they were taking immediately before seizure recurrence occurred. They may, therefore, remain on medication for a further period, but at a lower dose than previously. If a patient is on multiple antiepileptic drugs and has been seizure-free for 2 years or more, only one medication should be withdrawn at a time, and a reasonable interval left between withdrawal of one drug before considering withdrawal of the next in order to ensure that the patient remains seizure-free on the decreased medication regime. Phenobarbitone and benzodiazepines (such as clobazam and clonazepam) require weaning over a longer period because of possible withdrawal reactions and seizures.

With regard to antiepileptic drug level monitoring, NICE guidelines advise that regular blood test monitoring is not recommended as routine practice for children (NICE, 2004, section 4.8.26C). This should only be done if clinically indicated and recommended by the specialist managing the child. In practice, it is usually only necessary to monitor the levels of three antiepileptic drugs, namely phenytoin, phenobarbitone and carbamazepine. A clear correlation is established between AED level and efficacy for these agents, and in addition there is clear evidence demonstrating that high levels correlate with adverse effects. Phenytoin has saturable pharmacokinetics, variable bioavailability across a range of formulations, and absorption affected by a range of factors such as enteral feeds. As such, levels within the bloodstream can be unstable and unpredictable, and as high levels can lead to increased seizures or chronic adverse effects, levels must be monitored regularly. Phenobarbitone has more predictable pharmacokinetics, but doses required may vary between individuals, and if seizure control has not been achieved then the level should be checked to determine whether it is within the therapeutic range. High doses/levels can also cause significant sedation or negative impact on mood and behaviour and this should be looked for. Carbamazepine has predictable, first-order pharmacokinetics. If the patient is seizure-free and adverse-effect-free, then there is no need to check the level. Levels should be checked if maximum calculated doses have been prescribed but seizure control has not been achieved, if compliance is being questioned, or if significant adverse effects are being experienced. With the exception of phenobarbitone and phenytoin, however, if the patient is well and seizure-free, there is no need to measure the AED level.

In summary, the management of epilepsy in children involves a great deal more than simply the prescription of antiepileptic drugs. It should include appropriate education and advice for the child and family, appropriate modifications of lifestyle as well as appropriate safety measures, advice on the emergency management of seizures, and consideration of the impact of the epilepsy on all aspects of the child's life, including their education and social and emotional well-being. An accurate diagnosis of epilepsy and the type of epilepsy or seizure syndrome is necessary if medication is to be chosen correctly. The decision to treat or not to treat seizures must take into account a number of factors including seizure frequency and severity, and the possibility of any significant adverse effects from the medication. The choice of which AED to use must be based on evidence for efficacy in this seizure type and age group, and is best directed by appropriate guidelines constructed from the available evidence, national recommendations and the experience of expert peers. Medications should be started singly, increased slowly, and remain at the minimal dose required to achieve seizure control. Should the first agent not prove effective, this should be withdrawn and an alternative agent introduced, polytherapy only entered into when necessary. When seizure control of 2 years or more has been achieved, drug withdrawal should be considered, and this carried out in a stepwise fashion at an optimal time. Regular monitoring of the patient is important within the child epilepsy clinic, but in general (with a small number of exceptions) antiepileptic drug level monitoring is not necessary. The aim of the management of childhood epilepsy is to achieve seizure control with minimal adverse effects, thus enabling the child to achieve the best possible quality of life in the context of their seizure disorder.

References

Marson AG, Al-Khanasi AM, *et al*. The SANAD trial of effectiveness of carbamazepine, gabapentin, lamotrigine, oxcarbazepine or topiramate for treatment of partial epilepsy: an unblended randomised controlled trial. *Lancet* 2007;**369**(9566):1000–15.

NICE Guidance. The epilepsies: the diagnosis and management of the epilepsies in adults and children in primary and secondary care. October 2004. www.guidance.nice.org.uk/CG20, section 4.8.18.

Parker AP, Agathonikou A, Robinson RO, Panayiotopoulos CP. Inappropriate use of carbamazepine and vigabatrin in typical absence seizures. *Dev Med Child Neurol* 1998;**40**(8):517–19.

Perucca E. NICE guidance on newer drugs for epilepsy in adults. *BMJ* 2004;**328**(7451):1273–4.

Sinha G. Drugs for kids: EU law mandates drug testing in children. *J Natl Cancer Inst* 2008;**100**(2):84–5.

www.setpeg.co.uk.

Learning objectives

(1) To recognize that the management of seizure disorders in children covers many areas and does not relate solely to the prescription of medication.
(2) To understand the key factors informing the decision whether or not to start antiepileptic medication for children.
(3) To understand the key principles guiding prescription of antiepileptic medication in children, including choice of medication, regime, duration of treatment and medication withdrawal.
(4) To understand current advice with respect to antiepileptic medication blood level monitoring.
(5) To recognize the need for established guidelines with respect to antiepileptic medication management.

Section 6 Epilepsy in specific circumstances

Chapter 100: Learning and educational issues in epilepsy

Corina O'Neill

While many patients with epilepsy have an excellent outcome, for some people it is a chronic condition that can impact on all aspects of their lives, including their learning and behaviour. It is important to consider the complex relationship between epilepsy and 'learning' and how this may impact on quality of life and social outcomes for people with epilepsy. Social outcomes for patients with epilepsy compare unfavourably relative to controls (Binnie et al., 2007). Undoubtedly educational and learning issues are crucial factors contributing to these outcomes (Camfield et al., 1993). Quality-of-life studies indicate the contribution of associated learning and behaviour difficulties to lower quality-of-life scores in patients with epilepsy.

Epidemiology

Approximately 30% of children with epilepsy have learning disability, i.e. IQ lower than 70. Studies have shown, however, that up to 60% of children experience some difficulties with learning, which indicates significant underachievement even for those with 'normal IQ' (Rutter et al., 1970; Binnie et al., 2007).

Learning disability

Epilepsy has a higher prevalence among those with underlying learning disability and neurological conditions. Many in this group will have symptomatic epilepsy with underlying brain damage from various causes such as hypoxic ischaemic injury, disordered brain development or metabolic or genetic conditions. Associated conditions in this group may mimic epileptic seizures (e.g. muscle spasms, gastro-oesophageal reflux, other movement disorders or repetitive behaviours in autism). This group may be undergoing other treatments with potential for interaction with antiepilepsy medication. Children with severe epilepsy (i.e. 'epileptic encephalopathy' in early childhood) have a high prevalence of learning disability and co-morbid conditions, e.g. autism and attention-deficit hyperactivity disorder (ADHD) are common.

Risk factors for learning difficulties

Epilepsy syndromes

Learning outcomes are better in those with idiopathic epilepsy and localization-related epilepsy. However, focal syndromes may be associated with specific deficits in learning. For instance, temporal lobe epilepsy is more likely to be associated with language and memory problems, while in frontal lobe epilepsy there may be disturbance of higher language processes. Specific language deficits have even been shown in idiopathic focal syndromes (e.g. benign rolandic epilepsy with centrotemporal spikes). Symptomatic or cryptogenic generalized epilepsy is associated with a worse outcome (Bulteau et al., 2000). Several severe childhood epilepsy syndromes are strongly associated with learning disability (e.g. West's syndrome, severe myoclonic epilepsy, electrical status epilepticus in slow-wave sleep).

Seizures

Seizure type, timing, frequency and duration are relevant issues. Status epilepticus can cause cognitive impairment. Pre- or post-ictal disturbance of brain processes as well as interictal activity can interfere with learning. Transient cognitive impairment has been associated with interictal epileptiform activity. Nocturnal seizures have a detrimental effect on language function, memory and alertness. Disturbance of sleep stages by nocturnal seizures leads to daytime lethargy and behavioural disturbance. Generalized

---

Introduction to Epilepsy ed. Gonzalo Alarcón and Antonio Valentín. Published by Cambridge University Press.
© Cambridge University Press 2012.

seizures may be associated with attentional difficulties, while focal seizures are associated with focal deficits (e.g. verbal or visuospatial). Early onset of seizures (i.e. during infancy) is thought to disrupt brain development. Age at the time of seizure onset is significantly related to learning difficulties.

Behavioural problems

Clearly, anything that disrupts attention and behaviour can impact on learning and educational performance. Behavioural problems may be inherent, or be related to seizures or antiepilepsy drug treatment or psychosocial issues. Identification and appropriate management of behavioural issues (e.g. by improved seizure control or change of antiepileptic medication) is crucial. On the other hand specific disorders should be identified to ensure appropriate specific management or symptom control (e.g. autism or ADHD). Involvement of child psychiatry and psychology teams should be considered. Psychosocial problems can arise because of overprotection or low expectations of parents and teachers, teasing and bullying from peers, lack of appropriate support in the classroom, low self-esteem or loss of control associated with seizures.

Antiepilepsy medication

There is a complex interrelationship between seizure severity, epilepsy syndrome and medication. Improved seizure control with medication may improve cognitive function. However, side effects from antiepilepsy medication can cause altered cognition (phenobarbitone and phenytoin). Other antiepileptic drugs, particularly at higher serum levels, can cause problems with mental speed and memory. Most antiepileptic drugs can cause drowsiness and attentional difficulties which impact on learning. Topiramate is known to be occasionally associated with cognitive decline and tiagabine may cause non-convulsive status epilepticus. Use of several antiepileptic drugs simultaneously increases the likelihood of drug side effects and polytherapy should be avoided if possible.

Types of learning difficulties and neurophysiological mechanisms

Aldenkamp et al. (2005) has described different 'types' of learning difficulty:

- Memory deficit, which is associated with temporal lobe dysfunction, where there is a specific impairment in short-term memory and memory span.
- Attentional deficit, which causes global academic difficulty, and is associated with generalized seizures and a high frequency of tonic-clonic seizures.
- Speed factor deficit, where there is slowing of information processing especially in performing complex tasks, more likely to cause difficulties with mathematics.
- Problem-solving deficit, 'where there is a disturbance of higher cognitive processing such as concept formation, decision-making and verbal reasoning'.

Several authors describe an 'epilepsy factor' where some cognitive deficits occur regardless of the type of seizure due to reduced alertness and reduced sustained attention.

Epileptiform activity may interfere with our ability to attend to, process and store incoming information (transient cognitive impairment; Aarts et al., 1984). It may disrupt the process of consolidation of learning. Permanent brain damage can affect the brain's ability to adapt to new information, while antiepileptic drugs and sleep disruption by seizure activity disrupt brain function (Binnie et al., 2007).

Management

Optimum treatment of seizures and a holistic approach to management of epilepsy, particularly in childhood, is crucial in order to optimize educational and social outcomes. Benefits of treatment in terms of seizure control should be balanced against drug side effects. Identifying the correct syndrome diagnosis will help to identify the most suitable antiepileptic medication. Underlying co-morbid conditions should be identified and managed. Presence of learning and behavioural issues should be considered at each consultation as these may evolve over time. There should be close links between the medical team and school staff so that important information can be shared. Often the school team may provide important information on seizures and drug side effects. Educational psychologists can help to identify cognitive deficits and advise on strategies in the school setting. A care plan for management of seizures should be implemented in school for staff to follow. NICE guidelines recommend that patients are seen in 'special epilepsy clinics' with access to specialist epilepsy nurses. Specialist nurses have an important role and can facilitate good liaison between school and clinic as well as facilitating training for school staff in administering emergency medication. It is particularly important to identify and investigate patients with inconsistent performance in learning and behaviour, or with deterioration in cognitive functioning so that they can be managed optimally.

References

Aarts JH, Binnie CD, Smit AM, Wilkins AJ. Selective cognitive impairment during focal and generalized epileptiform EEG activity. *Brain* 1984;**107**(Pt 1): 293–308.

Aldenkamp AP, Weber B, Overweg-Plandsoen WC, Reijs R, van Mil S. Educational underachievement in children with epilepsy: a model to predict the effects of epilepsy on educational achievement. *J Child Neurol* 2005;**20** (3):175–80.

Binnie S Channon D Marston CD. Learning disabilities in epilepsy. Neurophsysiological aspects. *Epilepsia* 2007; **31**(s4):s2–8.

Bulteau C, I Jambaque, D Viguier, et al. Epileptic syndromes, cognitive assessment and school placement: a study of 251 children. *Dev Med Child Neurol* 2000;**42**:319–27.

Camfield C, Camfield P, Smith B, Gordon K, Dooley J. Biologic factors as predictors of social outcome of epilepsy in intellectually normal children. A population-based study. *J Pediatr* 1993;**122**:869–73.

Rutter M, Graham P, Yule W. A neuropsychiatric study in childhood. *Clinics in Developmental Medicine*. Philadelphia: Lippincott; 1970.

Sillanpaa M. Epilepsy in children: prevalence, disability, and handicap. *Epilepsia* 1992;**33**:444–9.

Learning objectives

(1) To know the epidemiology of learning and educational issues in children with epilepsy.
(2) To know the risk factors for learning difficulties in patients with epilepsy.
(3) To know the types of learning difficulties and their neurophysiological mechanisms.
(4) To know the principles of management of learning difficulties in patients with epilepsy.

Epilepsy in old age

Gonzalo Alarcón

Seizures in the elderly

In the UK, 25% of people with epilepsy are over 60 years of age. Epilepsy increases above the age of 50, associated with cerebrovascular disease, which is considered by some as the most common cause of epilepsy in all age groups. Epilepsy in the elderly will become a more important problem as the population ages.

The incidence of epilepsy increases with age:

- Incidence in the general population: 69/100 000.
- Incidence among people age 65–69: 87/100 000.
- Incidence among people age 70–80: 147/10 000.

The general principles for diagnosis and management are similar to those for the younger population. Special attention should be paid to the following in the elderly:

- The elderly are often taking multiple medication:
  - Pharmacological interactions between AEDs and other medication can occur.
  - Some common medication, such as antidepressants, might be proconvulsants.
- Lower metabolic rate: more susceptible to dose-related effects. For instance, sodium valproate can induce more pronounced tremor resembling parkinsonian symptoms.
- Low protein levels, particularly when concomitant liver and kidney conditions: free drug levels may be more informative!.
- Impairment of memory is common: simplify medication, use dosette boxes.
- Effects of AEDs on bone metabolism.
- Decreased creatinine clearance.

Impact of seizures in old age

- Typically longer seizures.
- Increased probability of status epilepticus, particularly non-convulsive.
- Increased probability of fractures due to existing osteoporosis and/or falls during seizures. Often followed by decline in independence.

Diagnosis of seizures in old age

- Difficulties in differentiating from other conditions such as: syncope, cerebrovascular disease, cardiac disease, dementia, confusion, hypoglycaemia, vertigo and dizziness.
- Problems in history-taking as many old people live alone and may have a degree of memory impairment.
- To distinguish from syncope, the speed of recovery after seizures can be useful. However, in this age group recovery can be slow.
- Syncope may be associated with incontinence, particularly in old age.
- Nonspecific abnormalities are common in the EEG in old age.

Causes of seizures in old age

- Epilepsy can be associated with asymptomatic imaging evidence of cerebrovascular disease.
- Symptomatic cerebrovascular disease, particularly haemorrhage (more than infarct). Seizures may be the first manifestation of cerebrovascular disease: screening and prevention with aspirin.
- Head injury is the cause of epilepsy in 21% of cases.

Introduction to Epilepsy ed. Gonzalo Alarcón and Antonio Valentín. Published by CAMBRIDGE UNIVERSITY PRESS.
© Cambridge University Press 2012.

- Tumours cause epilepsy in a lower percentage (5–15%).
- Metabolic causes are responsible in 10%: alcoholism, fever, pneumonia.
- Other causes include degenerative disorders (Alzheimer's and other dementias).

Investigation of epilepsy in the elderly

Useful clinical tests include:

- Blood test, including full blood count, erythrocyte sedimentation rate, urea and electrolytes, blood glucose, and γ-glutamyltransferase (marker for recent alcohol consumption).
- Chest X-ray.
- ECG.
- Thyroid function.
- EEG if performed (not indicated if diagnosis and cause of epilepsy is known):
  - Frequent nonspecific interictal abnormalities and slowing can be seen, even in the absence of epilepsy.
  - Supports diagnosis if clear epileptiform discharges are seen.
  - Inconclusive in the absence of clear epileptiform discharges.
  - Crucial for the diagnosis of non-convulsive status epilepticus (NCSE).
- MRI necessary as epilepsy is usually symptomatic.

Frequently asked questions

In most elderly patients, epilepsy in itself:

- does not necessarily imply serious brain damage;
- does not imply dementia;
- can usually be controlled by medication if no progressive disease present.
- medication does not cause brain damage, but can interfere with brain function.

Starting treatment in the elderly

- Lack of studies compared to younger patients.
- Treatment of a single seizure recommended if an organic cause is identified.
- Driving considerations.

Choice of drugs in the elderly

The choice of specific AEDs in an elderly patient should be tailored to each individual case as many drugs have problems in the elderly and drug trials are limited. In general, the doses needed are lower as tolerance to AEDs is lower than for other ages. There are limited trial data regarding specific use of AEDs in the elderly (Leppik et al., 2006), but there are groups that advocate the use of newer AEDs on the grounds of better tolerability. In any case AEDs with no or few interactions with other drugs have an advantage in the treatment of elderly patients. Below are comments regarding a few individual AEDs, although other AEDs may also be used. Note that it is necessary to check potential interactions with concomitant medication.

Carbamazepine

Usually, very useful in younger patients, but generally not well tolerated in older people. It is not a first-line AED in these patients, as it is subject to drug interactions and has the propensity to precipitate heart block in susceptible people If prescribed, an ECG should be recorded, carbamazepine should start on very low doses (50–100 mg) and proceed cautiously.

Phenytoin

It has difficult pharmacokinetics, and it is subject to interactions. Therefore phenytoin should not be considered as a first-line AED in elderly people. Furthermore, the 'therapeutic range' appears to be less tolerated, and lower levels can be aimed for in the first instance, which may well be effective.

Valproate

Relatively easy to use, but drowsiness can be a side effect at moderate to high doses, and it may exacerbate parkinsonian features or tremor. Use low starting doses, increasing only if tolerated.

Levetiracetam

It has the advantage of low interactions with other drugs, but can cause irritability and depression as side effects. Doses used should be lower, as excretion is renal and half-life is likely to be increased in the elderly due to decreased creatinine clearance. Starting doses of 62.5–125 mg/day, increasing slowly depending on tolerance and response.

Lamotrigine

A study has concluded that lamotrigine 'can be regarded as an acceptable choice as initial treatment for elderly patients with newly diagnosed epilepsy' (Brodie et al., 1999). The study compared carbamazepine with lamotrigine, and found a higher incidence of adverse events in carbamazepine, particularly rash. However, this study has been criticized for the choice of carbamazepine formulation and titration. The Veteran's Administration study discussed below also included lamotrigine (Rowan et al., 2005).

Gabapentin

Gabapentin has low interactions. It was included in the Veteran's Association Cooperative Study (Rowan et al., 2005) comparing three treatment groups: gabapentin 1500 mg/day, lamotrigine 150 mg/day and carbamazepine 600 mg/day. The results showed high early terminations (lamotrigine 44.2%, gabapentin 51%, carbamazepine 64.5%) of which the following were due to adverse events: lamotrigine 12.1%, gabapentin 21.6%, carbamazepine 31% ($P = 0.001$) with no significant differences in seizure-free rates. The authors concluded that lamotrigine or gabapentin should be considered as initial therapy for older patients with newly diagnosed seizures.

Important considerations to determine the dose of AEDs in the elderly

- Interactions with concomitant drugs.
- Initial low doses, aiming at low target doses.
- Use free drug fraction of blood levels for treatment monitoring if available, due to the high prevalence of lower protein levels and concomitant disorders.

Complications of epilepsy in old age

- Higher incidence of spontaneous and seizure-induced fractures.
- Status epilepticus after withdrawing sleeping pills (benzodiazepines): often nonconvulsive and difficult to recognize.
- Medication toxicity: poor memory, somnolence, ataxia.
- Complications secondary to drug interactions.

References

Brodie MJ, Overstall PW, Giorgi L. Multicentre, double-blind, randomised comparison between lamotrigine and carbamazepine in elderly patients with newly diagnosed epilepsy. The UK Lamotrigine Elderly Study Group. *Epilepsy Res* 1999;**37**(1):81–7.

Cloyd, JC, Kelly KM, Leppik IE, Perucca E, Ramsay RE (eds). Epilepsy in the elderly. New directions. *Epilepsy Res* 2006;**68**(Suppl 1):S1–83.

Leppik IE, Brodie MJ, Saetre ER, et al. Outcomes research: clinical trials in the elderly. *Epilepsy Res* 2006;**68**(Suppl 1): S71–6. Epub 2006 Jan 18.

Rowan AJ, Ramsay RE, Collins JF, et al. VA Cooperative Study 428 Group. New onset geriatric epilepsy: a randomized study of gabapentin, lamotrigine, and carbamazepine. *Neurology* 2005;**64**(11):1868–73.

Sheorajpanday RV, De Deyn PP. Epileptic fits and epilepsy in the elderly: general reflections, specific issues and therapeutic implications. *Clin Neurol Neurosurg* 2007;**109**(9):727–43.

Learning objectives

(1) To know the epidemiology of seizures in the elderly.
(2) To know the main causes of seizures in old age.
(3) To be aware of the impact of seizures in old age.
(4) To know the general principles for diagnosis and management of seizures and epilepsy in the elderly.
(5) To know the investigations required for the diagnosis and management of epilepsy in the elderly.
(6) To be aware of frequently asked questions when managing epilepsy in the elderly.
(7) To know when to start treatment for epilepsy in the elderly.
(8) To know the criteria for the choice of antiepileptic drugs in the elderly.
(9) To know the principles for adjusting dosage in the elderly.
(10) To know the complications of epilepsy in old age.

Section 6 Epilepsy in specific circumstances

Chapter 102 Epilepsy and learning

Frank M. C. Besag

Prevalence

Epidemiological studies have shown that learning disability (IQ < 70) is common in children with epilepsy. Sillanpää (1992) found that 31.4% of children aged 4–15 years with epilepsy in a region of Finland had an IQ below 70. Learning disability is more common in epilepsy and epilepsy is also more common in people with learning disability. The prevalence of epilepsy increases as the IQ decreases. In addition to global learning disability (mental retardation), specific learning difficulties may also occur. Sillanpää found speech disorders in 27.5% of the children and specific learning disorders in 23.1%.

Relationships between epilepsy and learning disability

The relationship between epilepsy and learning disability falls into three patterns. First, an underlying brain problem may lead both to epilepsy and, independently, to learning disability. For example, a head injury may cause learning disability and may also cause subsequent epilepsy. Second, epilepsy may cause brain damage and consequent learning disability; for example, prolonged status epilepticus may do so. Third, epilepsy can cause learning disability without causing brain damage. To explore this situation further, a distinction must be made between permanent learning disability and 'state-dependent learning disability'. Permanent learning disability is irreversible. Two of the examples already given, namely head injury and prolonged status epilepticus, can cause permanent learning disability. State-dependent learning disability may be defined as learning disability that depends on current reversible factors, for example medication or seizures, which are not necessarily permanent. State-dependent learning disability is potentially reversible and treatable. The first step in managing state-dependent learning disability is to think of the diagnosis. Regrettably, this first step is often not taken, with the result that the state-dependent learning disability goes unrecognized and untreated. Medication as a cause will not be considered in detail.

The way in which the epilepsy itself may affect learning can be broken down into ictal and post-ictal causes.

Frequent absence seizures can affect both cognitive performance and behaviour. Although the classic teaching has been that absence seizures do not affect cognition, the current author's team have shown that spike-wave episodes can occur not only hundreds of times a day but thousands of times a day in some young people. Such frequent discharges can result in withdrawn behaviour, attention problems and fragmented thought processes. The withdrawn behaviour may present with autistic-like traits. It has been suggested, by the current author, that if these frequent discharges/seizures impair social interaction for a prolonged period during a critical developmental stage of childhood, they may result in an ongoing autism-spectrum disorder even when the discharges themselves have resolved or responded successfully to treatment.

Very frequent absence seizures can result in absence non-convulsive status epilepticus. The cognitive and behavioural manifestations of this condition can be remarkably subtle or very dramatic, leading to an almost 'zombie-like' state. Complex partial status epilepticus can also result in reversible cognitive impairment.

Frequent localized discharges can affect learning and behaviour. Treatment with medication or surgery can be of great benefit.

Introduction to Epilepsy ed. Gonzalo Alarcón and Antonio Valentín. Published by Cambridge University Press.
© Cambridge University Press 2012.

Frequent hemispheric discharges can result from a number of different pathologies affecting one hemisphere, including Rasmussen's encephalitis, hemimegalencephaly and a porencephalic cyst. Seizures and epileptiform discharges are often very resistant to medical treatment. The definitive treatment is either anatomical hemispherectomy, involving removal of the pathological cortical hemisphere, or functional hemispherectomy/hemispherotomy, which involves disconnection of the hemisphere. This treatment can abolish both seizures and epileptiform discharges with the result that cognition and behaviour may improve markedly.

Post-ictal state-dependent learning disability includes the effects of frequent daytime seizures, the effects of frequent night-time seizures and electrical status epilepticus of slow-wave sleep (ESES or CSWS).

At first sight, it may appear trivial to include frequent daytime seizures as a cause of state-dependent learning disability because it is so obvious that the post-ictal effect of seizures can be profound. However, if the patient is having several seizures a day and has done so for a prolonged period, both professionals and carers may think of the cognitive impairment as being permanent when it is state-dependent and potentially reversible. If the seizures are better controlled, the individual has the opportunity of recovering from one seizure before having the next, instead of being in the constant state of severe post-ictal state-dependent learning disability. The transformation in terms of cognitive improvement can be dramatic.

Frequent nocturnal seizures can impair daytime performance not only because of direct post-ictal effects but also from a very disturbed sleep pattern. Monitoring carried out by the author's team revealed that two teenage boys each had over 200 seizures in a single night. These were brief tonic seizures which were unobserved and unsuspected by awake night staff but were clearly revealed on split-screen video-EEG monitoring.

Electrical status epilepticus of slow-wave sleep (ESES) or continuous spike-wave during slow-wave sleep (CSWS) is worthy of particular attention. The syndrome of CSWS is described in some detail on the International League Against Epilepsy website (Tassinari *et al.*, 1999). ESES can be associated with the Landau-Kleffner syndrome of acquired epileptic aphasia. After apparently normal early speech progress, the child develops an auditory agnosia and, failing to understand what he or she is saying, also loses expressive speech. This condition is potentially treatable with medication, including sodium valproate, high-dose benzodiazepines or steroids. It can also respond dramatically to the surgical technique of multiple subpial transection, pioneered by Frank Morrell (Morrell *et al.*, 1989). In the past, textbooks have stated that antiepileptic treatment in the Landau-Kleffner syndrome is only effective in treating the seizures and not the loss of speech. This is a highly misleading statement. If the treatment is delayed until permanent speech impairment is established, it will not improve the speech. However, early, effective treatment may result in a dramatic improvement in speech. This is a very striking example of epilepsy-related state-dependent cognitive impairment. It is interesting to note that apparently between one-quarter and one-third of children with the Landau-Kleffner syndrome do not have overt seizures but do have ESES.

ESES does not necessarily affect speech. A patient under the author's care had ESES that affected his visuo-spatial skills profoundly. When the ESES was successfully treated, the boy's visuo-spatial skills improved markedly.

In the child who has lost skills, if this is not the direct result of medication, careful review is necessary. If frequent daytime or nocturnal seizures are not occurring then an EEG is mandatory. If frequent daytime epileptiform discharges are not observed then overnight monitoring should be arranged to check for the possibility of ESES/CSWS. Because early effective treatment can result in dramatic improvement but late treatment may be ineffective, it is of major importance to investigate such individuals promptly.

Parents of children with epilepsy often want to know whether the child is liable to develop permanent loss of learning ability. This is very unlikely unless prolonged seizures occur (see Chapter 76: 'Epilepsy emergency treatment'), if there are very frequent epileptiform discharges in the EEG for long periods of time or if the child has a very rare neurodegenerative condition.

Conclusions

Whatever the cause of the learning disability, appropriate management of the epilepsy with medication and/or surgery should be provided. For those with state-dependent learning disability, such management may improve learning significantly.

References

Besag FMC. Childhood epilepsy in relation to mental handicap and behavioural disorders. *J. Child Psychol Psychiat* 2002;**43**:103–31.

Morrell F, Whisler WW, Bleck TP. Multiple subpial transection: a new approach to the surgical treatment of focal epilepsy. *J Neurosurg* 1989;**70**(2):231–9.

Sillanpää M. Epilepsy in children: prevalence, disability, and handicap. *Epilepsia* 1992;**33**:444–9.

Tassinari CA, Volpi L, Michelucci R. Electrical status epilepticus during slow sleep. ILAE Website: http://www.ilae-epilepsy.org/Visitors/Centre/ctf/electric_stat_slow_sleep.html (accessed 30 May 2010).

Learning objectives

(1) To know the prevalence of learning disability in children with epilepsy.
(2) To be aware of and be able to discuss the relationships between epilepsy and learning disability.
(3) To understand how to diagnose and manage state-dependent learning disability.

Section 6

Epilepsy in specific circumstances

Chapter 103

Epilepsy in chromosomal and related disorders

Elaine Hughes

Epilepsy often arises in association with chromosomal and related disorders. In the majority of cases, the epilepsy does not have specific identifiable features and a variety of seizure types may occur. In a few situations (e.g. Angelman syndrome), the EEG features may suggest the diagnosis. In the main, associated features will prompt the diagnosis rather than the epilepsy, e.g. Down syndrome. Rarely, as in epilepsy associated with ring chromosome 20, there may be no clues prior to seizure onset.

In general, epilepsy is more severe in the presence of ring chromosomes rather than with simple deletions and more severe in cases with duplication/deletion versus simple deletions.

On occasions, the epilepsy arises as a consequence of an underlying genetically determined developmental brain malformation. Such abnormalities associated with underlying chromosomal abnormalities include lissencephaly, a typical example being the lissencephaly associated with 17p13.3 deletion in Miller-Dieker syndrome (MDS). Mutations in the Aristaless Related Homeobox (ARX) have been associated with a range of developmental brain disorders ranging from hydranencephaly, through to agenesis of the corpus callosum. However, different mutations in the ARX gene have been demonstrated to produce other electro-clinical syndromes without abnormalities of brain structure, the first to be identified being X-linked infantile spasms and severe learning difficulties.

Conditions in which epilepsy is almost always a feature include:

- Wolf-Hirschhorn syndrome (4p-);
- Angelman syndrome (deletion 15q11-q13);
- other chromosome 15 anomalies including inversion-duplication 15;
- ring chromosome 20.

Conditions in which epilepsy may be a feature include:

- Down syndrome;
- Rett syndrome;
- fragile X syndrome.

Angelman syndrome (AS)

This may present in the neonatal period with feeding problems. Subsequently delayed motor milestones are a feature alongside severe learning difficulties and lack of speech development. Characteristic facial features are found with fair hair, blue eyes, wide mouth, thin upper lip and prominent jaw. Children are often described as having a happy disposition with bouts of unprovoked or paroxysmal laughter, but these do not represent gelastic seizures.

By age 6, 80% of children develop epileptic seizures. At the onset seizures may be provoked by intercurrent febrile illness, but later multiple seizure types may be found including myoclonic seizures, absences, tonic spasms and myoatonic seizures.

EEG findings are considered characteristic, particularly posterior slow-wave activity, which may be notched or associated with true spikes and this activity is enhanced by eye-closure. In addition there is fast bursting cortical myoclonus. Treatment with piracetam may be helpful for the cortical myoclonus.

The majority of cases of Angelman syndrome are sporadic. The region on chromosome 15 involved in AS shows imprinting (that is, differential expression of genes according to the parent of origin). Most often (in approximately 70%), there is maternally derived de novo deletion of chromosome 15q11–13. In 3–7%, there is paternal uniparental disomy of chromosome 15, so that the child inherits both chromosomes 15 from a single parent, there are no deletions and the

---

Introduction to Epilepsy ed. Gonzalo Alarcón and Antonio Valentín. Published by Cambridge University Press.
© Cambridge University Press 2012.

father is source of both chromosomes 15. Parental chromosomes are normal in both these situations and recurrence risks are low. In a small number of cases, there is an increased risk of recurrence, with UBE-3A mutations, imprinting defects or maternal rearrangements of chromosome 15.

Rett syndrome

This was first described by Dr Andreas Rett in the German literature in 1966 but further delineated and highlighted by Hagberg *et al.* in 1983. The incidence is thought to be between one in 10 000 and one in 23 000 live female births. Girls are often thought to have normal early development but in retrospect they may have been very placid with relative immobility and hypotonia. Regression takes place from around 12–18 months with loss of speech and purposeful hand use, social withdrawal, bouts of unexplained crying and sleep disturbance. An acquired microcephaly is typical but not invariable. Thereafter, periodic marked agitation may occur with alternating hyperventilation and apnoea, bruxism and hand stereotypies, and other autistic features.

Seizures are reported to be common and may be generalized or focal, but it is important to recognize that vacant non-epileptic spells may also be seen and alongside apnoeic episodes may be misinterpreted as seizures. EEGs show bilateral and independent spike-wave complexes, typically central or centrosylvian in location.

Rett syndrome occurs largely in females and is usually sporadic with occasional familial cases. Mutations have been identified in methyl-CpG-binding protein 2 (MECP2) at Xq28. MECP2 mediates transcriptional repression, so regulates other genes. More recently mutations in the same gene have been identified in boys with a severe neonatal onset encephalopathy but also in some males with learning disability.

Down syndrome

Epilepsy is a relatively infrequent feature of Down syndrome, but appears in 1–2% of infants with this condition, typically manifesting as infantile spasms. Interestingly, the EEG features are those of an 'idiopathic' West syndrome, with symmetrical hypsarrhythmia, lack of focus after benzodiazepine suppression and re-emergence of hypsarrhythmia between a cluster of spasms.

Reflex seizures are common and evolution to Lennox-Gastaut syndrome is rare in comparison to other cases of West syndrome – other epilepsy syndromes may occur later and are typically generalized and usually easy to treat. By adulthood rates of epilepsy exceed 12%.

Ring chromosome 20

By contrast, ring chromosome 20 usually presents as severe epilepsy with mild or no dysmorphic features. Children usually have normal early development, with decline in cognitive performance in relation to onset of seizures in early to mid childhood, typically around age 3 to 8 years.

Seizures may manifest as long-lasting states of confusion, which may last minutes to hours, and 'absence status' appears on occasions to be triggered by emotional events. EEGs may show runs of long-lasting bilateral paroxysmal high-voltage slow waves maximal frontally and with occasional spikes. Other seizure types also occur, especially nocturnal partial seizures, and may mimic complex arousals, with EEG showing bursts of frontally dominant, high-voltage fast activity. Epilepsy is characteristically poorly responsive to drug treatment.

Recommended reading

Crespel A, Gelisse P, Bureau M, Genton P. *Atlas of Electroencephalography – The Epilepsies: EEG and Epileptic Syndromes*, vol. 2, pp. 362–79. Paris: John Libbey Eurotext; 2006.

Gobbi G, Genton P, Pini A, Livet M-O. Epilepsies and chromosomal disorders. In Roger J, Bureau M, Dravet C, *et al.* eds. *Epileptic Syndromes in Infancy, Childhood and Adolescence*, pp. 431–56. 3rd edn. London: John Libbey; 2002.

Recommended websites

http://www.angelman.org
http://www.rettuk.org/rettuk-public/rettuk.html

Learning objective

(1) To know the chromosomal abnormalities associated with epilepsy, their clinical manifestations, diagnosis and management of their epilepsy, with particular reference to Angelman syndrome, Rett syndrome, Down syndrome and ring chromosome 20.

Section 6 Epilepsy in specific circumstances

Chapter 104

Epilepsy and cerebral trauma

Charles E. Polkey

There is a wide spectrum of traumatic brain injury and therefore a wide possibility of the factors which favour the occurrence of post-traumatic epilepsy (PTE). Clinical and radiological studies have highlighted these factors. There is a general effect of the severity of the injury. Based on clinical data, Annegers noted that the risk of PTE was 1.5% for mild injury, 2.9% for moderate injury and 17.2% for severe injury (Annegers and Coan, 2000) Other studies have shown that Glasgow Coma Scale (GCS) score at injury, duration of disturbance of consciousness and duration of post-traumatic amnesia have similar significance. It is also known that focal brain injury increases the risk of PTE: data demonstrate that the risk of PTE after penetrating head injury is greater than the overall risk after head injury, which is generally put at 5% (Table 104.1).

MRI findings 2 years after injury were examined for gliomesenchymal scars from focal brain lesions and those with haemosiderin residues either completely or incompletely walled-off. In addition, those patients who had the sequelae of surgical treatment on their scans were noted. It was found that those patients who underwent surgery had 4.38-times higher risk of PTE than those who had not. Also those with haemosiderin incompletely walled-off had a 6.61-times increased risk (Messori et al., 2005). There are other contributing factors, including the region of brain injury: injuries around the central sulcus have a greater incidence of PTE. If injury is complicated by infection but healed in 15 days, the incidence is 36%, rising to 57% if it is healed in more than 60 days and 75% if there is abscess formation. The extent of injury as judged by neurological deficit also affects the incidence, being 47% when there is a persistent monoplegia and 66% if there is a persistent hemiplegia.

The incidence of PTE in children varies from that in adults. They are more prone to have a single seizure

Table 104.1. Incidence of post-traumatic epilepsy

Aetiology	Incidence of PTE
Overall	3–5%
Open head injury	8–9%
Combat head injury	12–24%
Penetrating head injury	34–53%

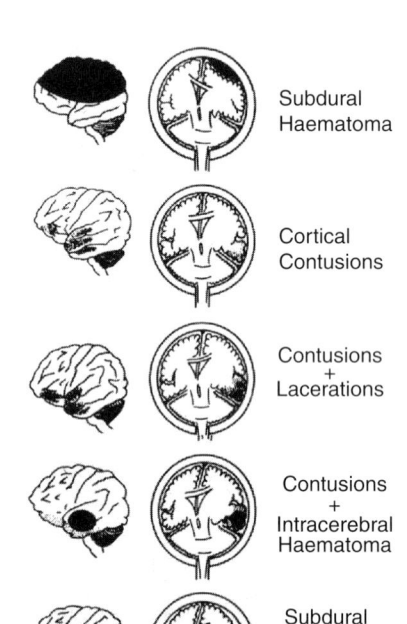

Figure 104.1. Varieties of cortical damage, all of which are potential epileptogenic areas. (Adapted from figures in Indications for surgical treatment, Ch. 33, Hooper R, in *Handbook of Clinical Neurology*, vol. 24., *Injuries of the Brain and Skull*, pt II., pp. 637–667 (1976) Eds. Vinken PJ and Bruyn GW. North Holland Publishing Co, Amsterdam and Oxford, American Elsevier Publishing Co., New York.)

after even a minor injury. In one series of 1785 children the incidence was 8.4%. The risk of PTE in children was increased by a number of factors. Among children aged less than 3 years, 11.3% developed PTE, 30.8% with a GCS of 3–8, 19.3% of

---

Introduction to Epilepsy ed. Gonzalo Alarcón and Antonio Valentín. Published by Cambridge University Press.
© Cambridge University Press 2012.

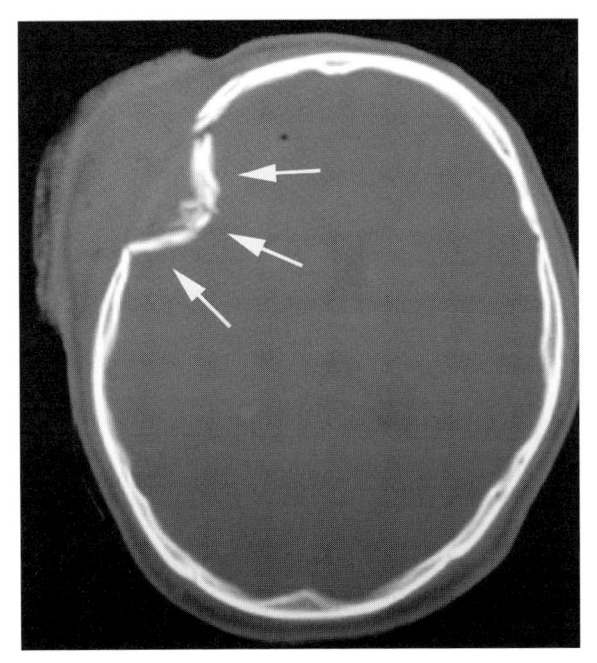

Figure 104.2. CT scan of depressed fracture of the skull. Note how fragments compress the underlying cortex. This is the potential cause of epilepsy and not the fragments themselves. Image from emedicine.medscape.com.

those with a depressed skull fracture, presumed with cortical injury, 13.7% where there was an intraparenchymal haemorrhage and 21.6% of those with cerebral oedema (Ates *et al.*, 2006). Another study showed that children with a normal CT and no neurological signs after a post-traumatic seizure were at low risk of further seizures (Holmes *et al.*, 2004).

Seizures after head injury can be divided into those that occur within the first week, the early seizures, and those that occur thereafter, the late seizures. Early seizures occur in 2–5% of head injuries but are more likely after severe head injury, where the incidence rises to 10–15% in adults and 25–35% in children. Early seizures are followed by late seizures in 25–35% of adults. Although the majority of seizures (80%) occur in the first year after injury, up to 20% may not occur until 4 years after injury.

The management of post-traumatic seizures used to be controversial, but there is now a body of literature that clarifies the situation. The question of prophylaxis was disputed but it is now clear that in cases at risk, early seizures can be prevented with anticonvulsants but this treatment has no effect on late epilepsy (Temkin *et al.*, 1990; Brain Injury Special Interest Group, 1998; Chang and Lowenstein, 2003). It is clear that once the epilepsy is established it should be treated pharmacologically as any other focal epilepsy. A recent review, which is also an excellent source of more detailed information and references, suggests that treatment of early epilepsy may be stopped after weeks or months since seizures seldom recur, but in the case of even a single late seizure, treatment should be continued for at least 2 years (Langendorf *et al.*, 2008). Occasionally there may be grounds for surgical intervention.

Conclusion

(1) Post-traumatic seizures have an overall incidence of 5%.
(2) Severe injury, focal injury or persisting brain damage tends to increase the probability of seizures.
(3) Early seizures, within the first week, remit in up to 50% of cases.
(4) Children have a higher incidence of early seizures with more minor injuries.
(5) Prophylactic treatment may prevent early seizures but not late seizures.
(6) Established seizures should be treated with the usual anticonvulsants.

References

Annegers JF, Coan SP. The risks of epilepsy after traumatic brain injury. *Seizure* 2000;**9**(7):453–7.

Ates O, Ondul S, Onal C, *et al*. Post-traumatic early epilepsy in pediatric age group with emphasis on influential factors. *Childs Nerv Syst* 2006;**22**(3):279–84.

Brain Injury Special Interest Group of the American Academy of Physical Medicine and Rehabilitation. Practice parameter: antiepileptic drug treatment of posttraumatic seizures. *Arch Phys Med Rehabil* 1998;**79**(5):594–7.

Chang BS, Lowenstein DH. Practice parameter: antiepileptic drug prophylaxis in severe traumatic brain injury: report of the Quality Standards Subcommittee of the American Academy of Neurology. *Neurology* 2003;**60**(1):10–16.

Holmes JF, Palchak MJ, Conklin MJ, Kuppermann N. Do children require hospitalization after immediate posttraumatic seizures? *Ann Emerg Med* 2004;**43**(6):706–10.

Langendorf FG, Pedley TA, Temkin NR. Posttraumatic seizures. In Engel JJ Jr, Pedley TA, eds. *Epilepsy:*

A Comprehensive Textbook, pp. 2537–42. 3rd ed. Philadelphia: Lippincott Williams & Wilkins; 2008.

Messori A, Polonara G, Carle F, Gesuita R, Salvolini U. Predicting posttraumatic epilepsy with MRI: prospective longitudinal morphologic study in adults. *Epilepsia* 2005;**46**(9):1472–81.

Temkin NR, Dikmen SS, Wilensky AJ, *et al*. A randomized, double-blind study of phenytoin for the prevention of post-traumatic seizures. *N Engl J Med* 1990;**323**(8):497–502.

Learning objectives

(1) To understand the incidence of epilepsy in relation to different forms of head injury.
(2) To understand the pathological features of traumatic lesions associated with post-traumatic epilepsy.
(3) To understand the difference between early and late epilepsy.
(4) To understand the treatment of established post-traumatic epilepsy.
(5) To understand the use of AEDs in the prophylaxis of epilepsy.

Questions

(1) Describe the relationship between the type of head injury and the incidence of post-traumatic epilepsy.
(2) How does the incidence of post-traumatic epilepsy differ between adults and children?
(3) Outline the usefulness of antiepileptic treatment in the prevention of seizures after head injury.

Section 6 Epilepsy in specific circumstances

Chapter 105

Epilepsy after cerebral tumours, hamartomas and neurosurgery

Charles E. Polkey

Seizures are a common symptom, and frequently the presenting symptom, of intracranial tumours. Tumours can be grouped into malignant tumours (for example, the malignant astrocytoma) and benign tumours (for example, meningiomas). They can also be divided into extra-axial tumours, which occur within the intracranial compartment, and axial tumours, which occur within the brain tissue. Finally, they can be divided into primary tumours, which originate from tissue within the cranial cavity and rarely metastasize, and metastatic tumours from primary tumours outside the cranium such as those arising from the lung or breast. Epilepsy is more likely if tumours occur in susceptible cortex, regardless of their histological type or origin, and the epilepsy is more likely to remit if the tumour is eradicated.

Accurate estimates of the incidence of epilepsy in intracranial tumour are difficult because of the under-reporting of secondary tumours and the scarcity of general population surveys. In the National General Practice Survey, a tumour was the cause of 6% of newly diagnosed epilepsy, 35% of these were primary tumours and 59% secondary tumours. Only 1% of the epilepsy was in patients aged less than 30 years; the maximum incidence was in the 50–59 years group, where it was responsible for 19%, falling in those over 60 years to 11% (Sander *et al.*, 1990). A later survey of an Asian population in Bradford reported tumour in 3.7% of patients with epilepsy. A survey of 222 meningiomas (Figure 105.1) showed that 26.6% presented with epilepsy. Epilepsy was commoner when the lesion was in the supratentorial compartment, especially with convexity tumours and with those with severe peritumoural oedema (Lieu and Howng, 2000). In children, approximately 40% of brain tumours are in the posterior fossa, which should influence the incidence of epilepsy. In a study of

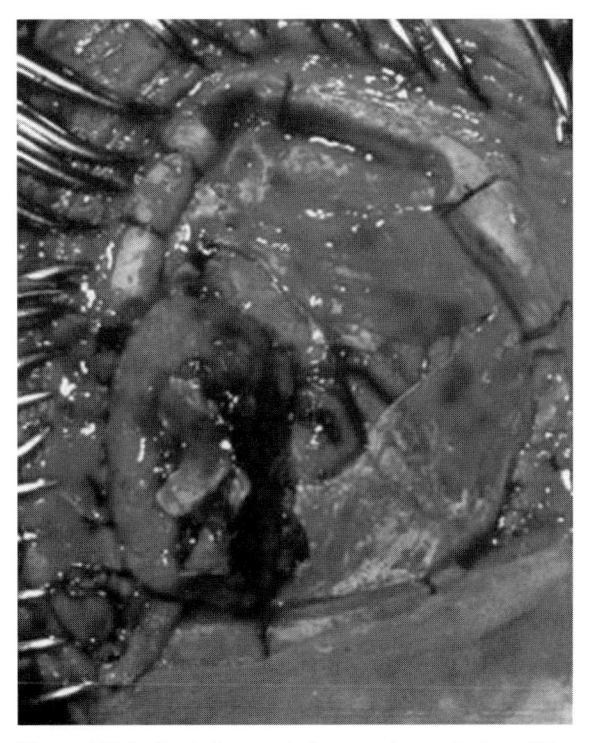

Figure 105.1. Surgical removal of a convexity meningioma. This lesion causes epilepsy by pressure on the underlying cortex. See colour version in plate section.

1046 patients, Kahn *et al.* found 157 children with epilepsy, an incidence of 15%. In these 157 cases the epilepsy was the presenting symptom in 60%. As expected, the proportion of supratentorial tumours was 81%, but in 30 patients (19%) the tumour was in the posterior fossa, and in 12 of these no explanation could be advanced for the epilepsy (Kahn *et al.*, 2006).

Of course, sometimes epilepsy arises as a result of treatment, especially surgical treatment of the tumour. Between 15% and 25% of patients may

---

Introduction to Epilepsy ed. Gonzalo Alarcón and Antonio Valentín. Published by Cambridge University Press.
© Cambridge University Press 2012.

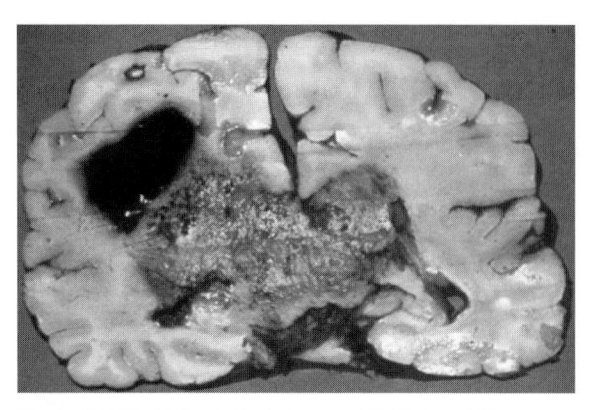

Figure 105.2. Malignant brain tumour (glioblastoma). These lesions cause epilepsy by damaging affected brain structures. See colour version in plate section.

develop epilepsy during treatment of brain tumours. The management of seizures rests on the use of anticonvulsant drugs together with appropriate treatment of the tumour such as surgical resection, radiotherapy and so forth. In both adults and children, seizure control can be established in about 65% of patients by this management. Persistent or breakthrough seizures tend to be associated with incomplete removal or recurrence of the tumour.

A hamartoma is defined as 'a tumour-like mass resulting from the faulty growth or development of normal cells or tissue'. Early papers suggest that lesions of this nature comprise 3% of resected lesions in epilepsy surgery. There is some dispute about the definition, and some believe that hamartomas represent part of a spectrum, which includes lesions with benign glial and neuronal elements. Diehl et al. describe 14 patients with hamartomas operated for drug-resistant epilepsy. They note that the lesions commonly occur in the frontal and temporal lobes, and that 10 of their 14 patients became seizure-free (Diehl et al., 2003). Hamartomas occur in the brainstem, where they give rise to 'non-cortical' seizures which can be relieved by resection of the lesion (Pontes-Neto et al., 2006).

Hypothalamic hamartoma (Figure 105.3; see also Chapter 87: 'Diagnosis and treatment of hypothalamic hamartomas') is a rare condition that can present in infancy with a catastrophic illness of multiple seizure types, developmental delay and behavioural problems. It can also present later in life, with complex partial seizures against a normal background. The best solution for the first group is transcallosal resection of the hamartoma, which has a 53% chance of rendering the patient seizure-free, and a further 30% of a 90% reduction, although with a 12% chance of persisting memory problems (Rosenfeld and Feiz-Erfan, 2007). Other treatments include disconnection, radiosurgery or radiofrequency ablation, which are less effective but less risky.

The relationship between hamartomas and other congenital lesions is complex. A good example of this is tuberose sclerosis where the tubers histologically resemble hamartomas. If the epileptogenic area can be identified then surgery can be helpful in this condition. However, surgical treatment can involve several procedures, including intracranial electrodes and multiple resections in one patient. Jansen et al. in a systematic literature survey involving 177 patients report 57% of patients seizure-free (Jansen et al., 2007). Some advocate the use of AMT (alpha-[11C] methyl-L-trytophan) PET, others magnetic source imaging, as means of identifying the epileptogenic tubers. Teutonico et al. described in detail 42 patients with tuberose sclerosis: in 11 there was good pharmacological control, in 10 presurgical assessments ruled out surgery and in another 11 surgical resections were carried out. Finally there was a group of 10 patients with *forme fruste*, which was defined as patients with only brain manifestations of the condition. Seizure control was much better in the *forme fruste* cases where eight of 10 became seizure-free compared with three of the 11 from the other surgical group. Factors which suggest a more severe form of the condition, including early seizure onset, multiple tubers, bilateral EEG changes and early abnormal EEG background, were associated with a poor surgical outcome (Teutonico et al., 2008).

The incidence of epilepsy after neurosurgical intervention is complex. Many patients have pre-existing epilepsy, the incidence will vary with the site and nature of the intervention, and the use of prophylactic anticonvulsants makes the true incidence difficult to estimate. For simple interventions such as a burr hole and cerebral penetration for biopsy, access for ventricular drainage and so forth the risk is probably around 1%. For more complex procedures such as craniotomy it is greater. Foy, many years ago, estimated it as a cumulative incidence of 17% over 5 years. A more recent paediatric study puts the incidence at 12% (Kombogiorgas et al., 2006). A purer model of the effects of craniotomy is provided by the incidence of epilepsy after subarachnoid haemorrhage

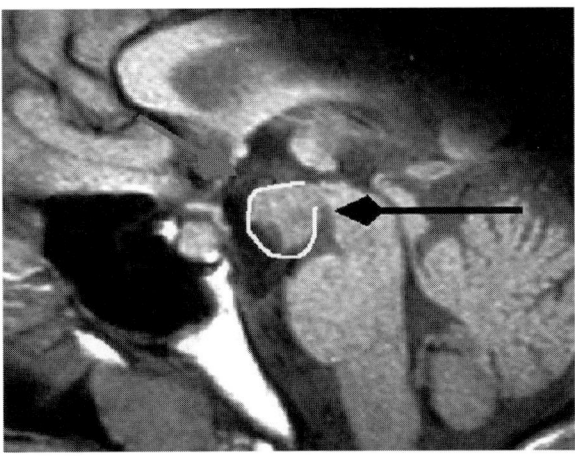

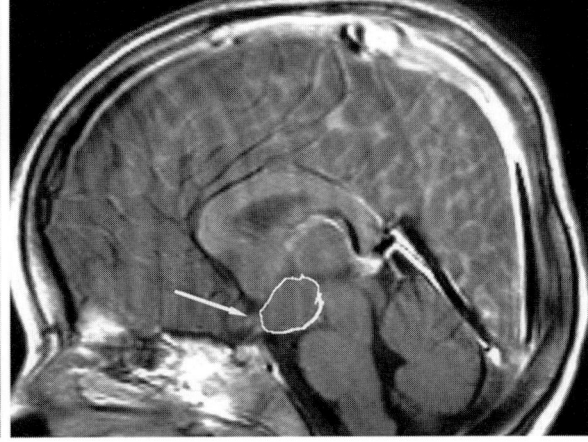

Figure 105.3. Hypothalamic hamartoma shown on sagittal MRI. Pedunculated (left) and sessile (right) varieties outlined and arrowed.

from aneurysm. Here the incidence is around 5–7% more common in patients with a poor initial state and poor outcome (Olafsson *et al.*, 2000; Buczacki *et al.*, 2004). It has been clearly shown that there are fewer seizures after endovascular occlusion of aneurysms, at around 3% (Byrne *et al.*, 2003). There is an extensive literature on prophylaxis in these patients, but the conclusion is that it is appropriate for early seizures but not for long-term prevention.

Conclusions

(1) Seizures are common in patients with all kinds of intracranial tumours and can be controlled in approximately 65% of patients.
(2) Hamartomas are rare lesions in which epilepsy may feature and can be relieved in a number of cases by appropriate treatment.
(3) Seizures occur after 1–17% of neurosurgical treatments, depending upon the underlying condition and the surgery involved.
(4) In all these circumstances, prophylaxis will prevent early but not late seizures. Once seizures are established the usual pharmacological management for focal epilepsy is appropriate.

References

Buczacki SJ, Kirkpatrick PJ, Seeley HM, Hutchinson PJ. Late epilepsy following open surgery for aneurysmal subarachnoid haemorrhage. *J Neurol Neurosurg Psychiatry* 2004;**75**(11):1620–2.

Byrne JV, Boardman P, Ioannidis I, Adcock J, Traill Z. Seizures after aneurysmal subarachnoid hemorrhage treated with coil embolization. *Neurosurgery* 2003;**52**(3):545–52.

Diehl B, Prayson R, Najm I, Ruggieri P. Hamartomas and epilepsy: clinical and imaging characteristics. *Seizure* 2003;**12**(5):307–11.

Jansen FE, Van Huffelen AC, Algra A, van Nieuwenhuizen O. Epilepsy surgery in tuberous sclerosis: a systematic review. *Epilepsia* 2007;**48**(8):1477–84.

Khan RB, Boop FA, Onar A, Sanford RA. Seizures in children with low-grade tumors: outcome after tumor resection and risk factors for uncontrolled seizures. *J Neurosurg* 2006;**104**(6 Suppl):377–82.

Kombogiorgas D, Jatavallabhula NS, Sgouros S, *et al*. Risk factors for developing epilepsy after craniotomy in children. *Childs Nerv Syst* 2006;**22**(11):1441–5.

Lieu AS, Howng SL. Intracranial meningiomas and epilepsy: incidence, prognosis and influencing factors. *Epilepsy Res* 2000;**38**(1):45–52.

Olafsson E, Gudmundsson G, Hauser WA. Risk of epilepsy in long-term survivors of surgery for aneurysmal subarachnoid hemorrhage: a population-based study in Iceland. *Epilepsia* 2000;**41**(9):1201–5.

Pontes-Neto OM, Wichert-Ana L, Terra-Bustamante VC, *et al*. Pontine activation during focal status epilepticus secondary to hamartoma of the floor of the fourth ventricle. *Epilepsy Res* 2006;**68**(3):265–7.

Rosenfeld JV, Feiz-Erfan I. Hypothalamic hamartoma treatment: surgical resection with the transcallosal approach. *Semin Pediatr Neurol* 2007;**14**(2):88–98.

Sander JW, Hart YM, Johnson AL, Shorvon SD. National General Practice Study of Epilepsy: newly diagnosed epileptic seizures in a general population. *Lancet* 1990;**336**(8726):1267–71.

Teutonico F, Mai R, Devinsky O, *et al.* Epilepsy surgery in tuberous sclerosis complex: early predictive elements and outcome. *Childs Nerv Syst* 2008;**24**(12):1437–45.

Learning objectives
(1) To understand the origins and nature of intracranial tumours.
(2) To understand how they might make the patient ill (present) and why they may give rise to epilepsy.
(3) To know the incidence of epilepsy in patients with intracranial tumours both independent of, and in relation to, treatment of these tumours.
(4) To understand the pharmacological treatment of epilepsy caused by intracranial tumours.
(5) To understand the particular nature of the hypothalamic hamartoma.
(6) To understand the problems in the management of hypothalamic hamartoma.

Questions
(1) Describe the principal kinds of intracranial tumours and outline in brief their treatment.
(2) Describe and explain the incidence of epilepsy in patients with intracranial tumours.
(3) Describe the use of prophylactic antiepileptic drugs in general neurosurgical practice.
(4) Describe the hypothalamic hamartoma and its usual presentation.

Section 6　Epilepsy in specific circumstances

Chapter 106

Epilepsy and cerebrovascular disease

R. Shane Delamont

Cerebrovascular disease (CVD) is defined as a pathological process affecting the blood vessels supplying or removing blood from the brain. This process may lead to damage of the brain substance and it is this process that provides the substrate for epilepsy.

Factors in relationship between CVD and epilepsy

The incidence of epilepsy and unprovoked seizures describes a shallow U-shaped curve from birth to senescence and much of this is due to the effects of CVD. The incidence falls from 80/100 000 persons per year in the first year of life to 20/100 000 in young adulthood from 30–50 years, rising to >130/100 000 beyond the age of 75 years. Much of the shape of this curve is due to the contribution of CVD, particularly as the population ages.

Types of CVD

The underlying mechanisms that lead to CVD are amongst the most diverse in internal medicine and teach us a great deal about some of the major causes of morbidity and mortality in modern society. The mechanisms causing brain damage consist of two basic processes with either too little blood supplied (ischaemic) or too much blood present, usually outside the vascular space (haemorrhagic). Both, the mechanisms and the location of the damage, are important in causing epilepsy.

Ischaemia is associated with acute neuronal death, loss of integrity and release of excitotoxins that may act, at least in part, on glutamate receptors. This is followed by inflammation and secondary gliosis and disruption of normal neuronal circuits with the risk of focal epileptogenesis.

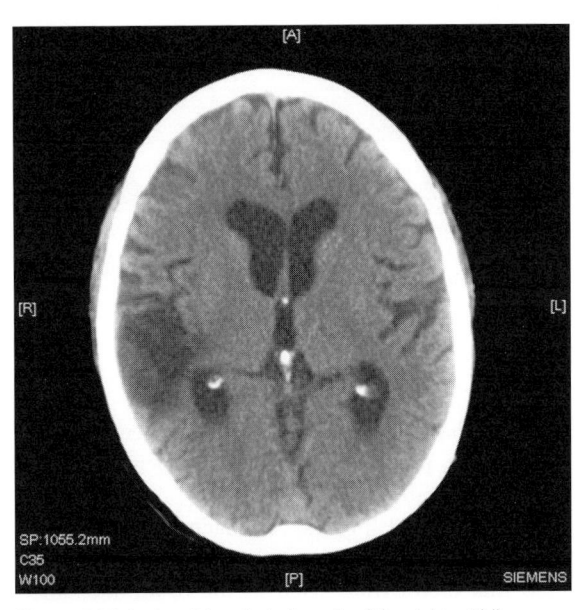

Figure 106.1. An old stroke in branch of the right middle cerebral artery.

Mechanisms for ischaemia

Occlusion of medium-sized arteries, arterioles and draining veins cause ischaemia. There are different causes depending on age, genetic make-up and exposure to lifelong risk factors. The process of occlusion of a vessel may come about as a result of disease affecting the wall of the vessel (e.g. atherosclerosis, inflammation), the lumen of the vessel (e.g. embolic occlusion) or an abnormality in the constituents of the lumen (e.g. hypercoaguable state, Fabry's disease).

Mechanisms for haemorrhage

Haemorrhage acts via similar mechanisms to ischaemia, but has the added effects of blood degradation

---

Introduction to Epilepsy ed. Gonzalo Alarcón and Antonio Valentín. Published by Cambridge University Press.
© Cambridge University Press 2012.

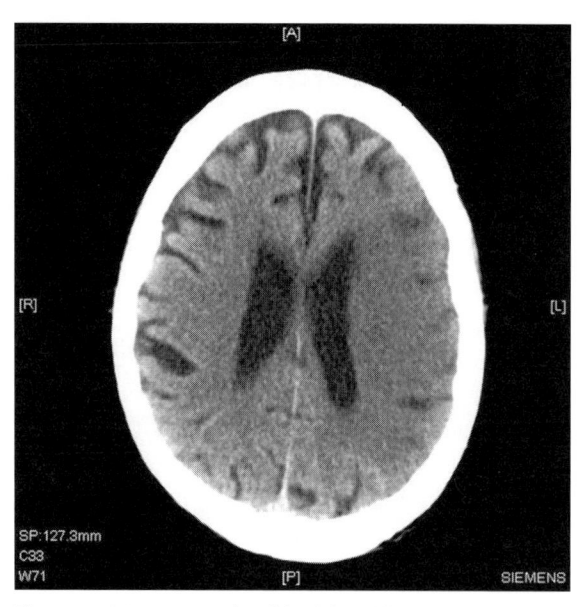

Figure 106.2. Acute stroke of the left middle cerebral artery.

products that are in themselves epileptogenic. Consequently, the presence of blood is associated with a higher risk of developing epilepsy.

The essential process in haemorrhage is the breakdown in the integrity of blood vessel walls such that blood finds itself in the brain substance. When blood enters the brain at arterial pressures, a substantial amount makes egress, disrupting brain architecture, causing acute neuronal concussion, loss of brain perfusion pressure, a mass lesion, secondary inflammation, vasospasm with further ischaemia, and iron deposition with excitatory damage. Age, genetic make-up and exposure to certain risk factors particularly hypertension are important markers.

Epidemiology of CVD

Within Western countries, the incidence of stroke disease is reducing, but because of the ageing population, the total burden for society is increasing. The mortality rate of stroke increases with ageing but more so for men than women. The underlying causes vary between populations. For example, haemorrhagic stroke is more commonly seen in East Asians than in Europeans.

Risk factors for stroke

The major risk factors for CVD in the >65 year age group are: age, family history, smoking, hypertension, cardiac disease, elevated cholesterol, diabetes mellitus. These factors are still relevant for younger populations but other factors need consideration, such as presence of a patent cardiac foramen ovale, using a high-dose oral contraceptive.

Relationship between CVD and epilepsy

Because CVD may not be associated with a clinical stroke event, it can be difficult to correlate epilepsy to specific stroke events. However, using clinical stroke events as a starter, Bladin has shown late epilepsy rates of 8.6% and 10.6% after ischaemic and haemorrhagic strokes respectively. The presence of cortical strokes, haemorrhagic transformation of ischaemic strokes and severe disability (implying extensive stroke disease) have all been associated with higher rates of epilepsy. Recent studies suggest that the presence of embolic strokes is not associated with higher rates of epilepsy.

There is a lower rate of epilepsy in patients with lacunar CVD, initially at 2.6%, but studies suggest a progressive increase in the risk of epilepsy with time, reaching 7.6% at 5 years. As expected, the rate of epilepsy is greater following cerebral haemorrhage: initially 4.6–17%, rising further to 50% of survivors at 5 years post event.

Types of seizures

Eighty per cent of the seizures have a simple partial component and may progress to complex partial or secondary generalized tonic seizures. Status epilepticus, often presenting as complex partial dreamy states, is reported in up to 17% of presentations.

Role of the EEG

The EEG may show changes following a stroke depending on the location and extent of the stroke. If extensive, slowing of background rhythms may be seen acutely down to delta range but with time there is often an improvement into the theta range. The presence of periodic lateralized epileptic discharges (commonly called PLEDs) acutely is a marker for early seizures. In a patient with post-stroke epilepsy, the interictal EEG may be remarkably bland, with few epileptiform discharges seen. Ictal EEG changes usually show slowing of background rhythms whereas a focal spike onset with rhythmic transformation is rarely seen.

Treatment strategies

Treatment should be tailored for the individual patient and should be targeted at the seizures and the underlying CVD. Standard AEDs are usually more effective at controlling seizures than for those with more classic epilepsy. Because many patients are older and may have concomitant medical illnesses, pharmacokinetics and drug interactions are very important for choosing the appropriate drug.

At the same time preventing ongoing damage to brain tissue by addressing risk factors is important in all patients with CVD irrespective of whether they have epilepsy or not.

Prognosis

Using stroke functional outcome measures, the presence of epilepsy has not been shown to reduce the long-term outcome in patients with CVD. However, further work is needed to address the question of functional outcomes using epilepsy measures.

Recommended reading

Ropper AH, Brown RH (eds). *Adam's & Victor's Principles of Neurology*, pp. 684–740. 8th edn. New York: McGraw Hill; 2005.

Learning objectives

(1) To know the epidemiological factors affecting the relationship between cerebrovascular disease and epilepsy.
(2) To know the types of cerebrovascular disease.
(3) To know the mechanisms for ischaemia and haemorrhage in cerebrovascular disease.
(4) To know the epidemiology of cerebrovascular disease and epilepsy:
   - risk factors for stroke
   - relationship between cerebrovascular disease and epilepsy.
(5) To know the types of seizures seen in cerebrovascular disease.
(6) To know the role of the EEG for the diagnosis of epilepsy due to cerebrovascular disease.
(7) To know the treatment strategies for epilepsy due to cerebrovascular disease.
(8) To be aware of the prognosis of epilepsy due to cerebrovascular disease.

Section 6 Epilepsy in specific circumstances

Chapter 107: Abnormalities of neuronal migration

R. Arunachalam

Malformations of cortical development (MCD) are uncommon, but, with ever-improving neuroimaging techniques, are being recognized as an important cause of intractable epilepsy. The classification of MCD is centred on three processes in the development of the brain, which are neuronal proliferation, neuronal migration and cortical organization. Focal cortical dysplasia and tuberous sclerosis are two well-known examples of abnormal proliferation, which can present with refractory focal epilepsy. Polymicrogyria and microdysgenesis are well-described abnormalities of cortical organization. In this chapter, we will be restricting the discussion to disorders of neuronal migration.

During embryonic development, cortical neurons proliferate from the ventricular epithelium or the striatal precursors and migrate considerable distances to reach their destination on a scaffold of glial cells. This migration peaks at 11–15 weeks of gestation and most of the neurons reach the cortex by 24 weeks. The hexalaminar architecture of the cortex is laid down in reverse order and this is followed by cortical organization. This sequence is a rather complex process, which involves the interaction of many different molecules coded for by specific genes. It is therefore not surprising that most of these disorders of development are genetically determined.

The group of disorders due to abnormal neuronal migration can be subclassified into three major categories, namely lissencephaly/band heterotopia spectrum, cobblestone complex and grey matter heterotopia. We will consider each of these in turn.

Lissencephaly/band heterotopia

Lissencephaly in Greek means 'smooth brain'. This was once thought to be a rare condition associated with early death. However, with the advent of MRI, many patients are now known to survive into adulthood and present with epilepsy and mental retardation. The surface of the brain is smooth from lack of or severely reduced gyration. The cortex is thickened and lacks the normal six layers. Deletions or point mutations of two genes, *LIS1* on chromosome 17 and *DCX* (doublecortin) on chromosome Xq, account for most cases of lissencephaly. Heterozygous females with DCX mutations develop a less severe abnormality, wherein the gyral formation is normal but there is abnormal band of grey matter in the subcortical white matter. This is referred to as subcortical band heterotopia, better known as 'double cortex'. Epilepsy is often refractory to drug therapy and surgical treatment is largely unsuccessful due to the extensive nature of the malformation. Genetic counselling has an important role in management.

Cobblestone complex

Previously known as type 2 lissencephaly, cobblestone complex occurs as a consequence of overmigration of neurons beyond the basement membrane (through defects in glia limitans) into the leptomeninges, resulting in an irregular pebbled cortical surface. Multiple brain regions can also be involved with cystic changes in the white matter, ventriculomegaly, brainstem and cerebellar hypoplasia. Cobblestone complex often occurs as part of multiple congenital malformations and in particular is associated with abnormalities of the muscle and eye. Walker-Warburg syndrome, Fukuyama congenital muscular dystrophy and muscle-eye-brain disease are well-described entities and occur as a result of single gene abnormalities. Epilepsy is often present, but in general is not quite as frequent or as severe as in those with lissencephaly.

Introduction to Epilepsy ed. Gonzalo Alarcón and Antonio Valentín. Published by Cambridge University Press.
© Cambridge University Press 2012.

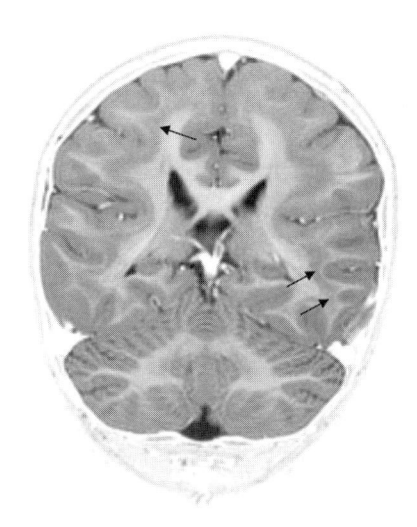

Figure 107.1. Typical findings on MRI of 'double cortex'. The arrows point to the white matter between the two layers of cortex.

Grey matter heterotopia

Heterotopion (plural: heterotopia) is the term used to describe large 'ectopic' accumulations of neurons next to the ventricles (subependymal/periventricular), in the cerebral white matter (subcortical) or rarely in the subpial space (marginal). Subependymal and subcortical heterotopia are well described and have distinct clinico-radiological features and genetics.

The best-studied entity and the most common is the subependymal variety, better known as periventricular nodular heterotopia (PNH). On MRI these are seen as round, ovoid nodules that are isointense with the overlying cortex. They are distinguished from subependymal nodules of tuberous sclerosis by their shape and lack of enhancement with contrast. They usually result from complete failure of migration of neurons from the ventricular epithelium, but can also be due to over-production of neurons. PNH is often found in isolation but can be associated with other CNS malformations. Anatomically they can be unilateral small, unilateral large or bilateral large. Genetically they can be subdivided into X-linked and non-X-linked. The X-linked variety occurs almost exclusively in women as the affected male siblings do not generally survive. It is caused by mutation in the *FLNA* gene on chromosome Xq28. The gene encodes for filamin A, a protein that is essential for neuronal migration. Thanks to lyonization (a process by which one of the two copies of the X-chromosome present in female mammals is inactivated), some neurons migrate normally, while others carrying the mutant gene fail to migrate. The nodules are almost always bilateral and diffuse and the affected women have an 80% chance of developing epilepsy, with the first seizure typically occurring in the second decade of life. Depth electrode studies have shown that these nodules can produce epileptiform discharges. The seizures tend to be focal and have mesial temporal, neocortical temporal or parieto-occipital semiology. Many of these patients have secondary mesial temporal sclerosis. Isolated temporal lobectomy in such individuals is associated with poor outcome. More recent studies have reported better outcome where, in carefully selected patients, the temporal lobes were resected along with the abnormal cortex.

Recommended reading

Andrade DM. Genetic basis in epilepsies caused by malformations of cortical development and in those with structurally normal brain. *Hum Genet* 2009;**126**(1):173–93.

Barkovich AJ, Kuzniecky RI, Jackson GD, Guerrini R, Dobyns WB. A developmental and genetic classification for malformations of cortical development. *Neurology* 2005;**65**(12):1873–87.

Sisodiya SM. Malformations of cortical development: burdens and insights from important causes of human epilepsy. *Lancet Neurol* 2004;**3**(1):29–38.

Learning objectives

(1) To become familiar with the three key processes in the development of the cortex, upon which classification of malformation of cortical development is based.
(2) To become familiar with the three major categories of abnormalities of neuronal migration.
(3) To be aware that patients can present in adulthood with intractable focal epilepsies.
(4) To understand that some can develop secondary mesial temporal sclerosis and surgery is helpful in only carefully selected cases.

Section 6: Epilepsy in specific circumstances

Chapter 108: Malformations of cortical development

Charles E. Polkey

This is a diverse group of conditions mostly related to abnormalities in the development of cortex. Neocortical development consists of a series of overlapping processes:

- proliferation of neuronal and glial cells in the ventricular and subventricular region at four to six weeks;
- radial migration to form layers between seven and 16 weeks;
- terminal differentiation, programmed cell death, synaptic elimination and finally cortical remodelling.

The various identifiable phenotypes can be classified using the first abnormal event as detailed by Kuzniecky and Jackson (2008). The principal conditions considered here will be cortical dysplasia, hemimegalencephaly and heterotopias. Lissencephaly and schizencephaly are of less surgical interest. Their relative frequency typically is (Montenegro et al., 2002):

- focal cortical dysplasia, 21%;
- heterotopias and agyria-pachgyria, 25%;
- polymicrogyria or schizencephaly 47%.

Cortical dysplasia is unilateral in 36% of patients, bilateral and localized in 20% and diffuse in 44%.

Cortical dysplasia (CD) has certain histological features, which were classified by Palmini and are summarized in Box 108.1 (Palmini and Gloor, 1992).

These histological features correlate with the appearances of the lesions on MRI. Type I can be invisible on MRI, whereas type II is invariably visible, and a high intensity on FLAIR imaging is often associated with balloon cells. Independent of its radiological appearances, cortical dysplasia has an electrophysiological signature, which was also described by Palmini.

Box 108.1. Histological characteristics of cortical dysplasia

- Microdysgenesis – abandoned
- Type I
  - IA: isolated architectural abnormalties
  - IB: isolated architectural abnormalities ± giant/immature neurons
- Type II (Taylor's focal cortical dysplasia)
  - IIA: Architectural abnormalities + dysmorphic neurons
  - IIB: Architectural abnormalities + balloon cells

They described the electrographic counterpart of this high degree of epileptogenicity, manifested by continuous or frequent rhythmic epileptogenic discharges recorded directly from CD lesions during intraoperative electrocorticography (ECoG). These ictal or continuous epileptogenic discharges (I/CEDs) assumed one of the following three patterns: (A) repetitive electrographic seizures, (B) repetitive bursting discharges or (C) continuous or quasicontinuous rhythmic spiking (Figure 88.3). They found one or more of these patterns in 23 of 34 patients (67%) with intractable partial epilepsy associated with CD lesions and in only one of 40 patients (2.5%) with intractable partial epilepsy associated with other types of structural lesions. I/CEDs were usually spatially restricted, thus contrasting with the more widespread interictal ECoG epileptiform activity, and tended to co-localize with the magnetic resonance imaging-defined lesion (Palmini et al., 1995). The electrophysiological characteristics seen on SEEG can be used meaningfully to guide resections (Chassoux et al., 2000; Ferrier et al., 2001).

Introduction to Epilepsy ed. Gonzalo Alarcón and Antonio Valentín. Published by Cambridge University Press.
© Cambridge University Press 2012.

Normal   Type I   Type IIA   Type IIB

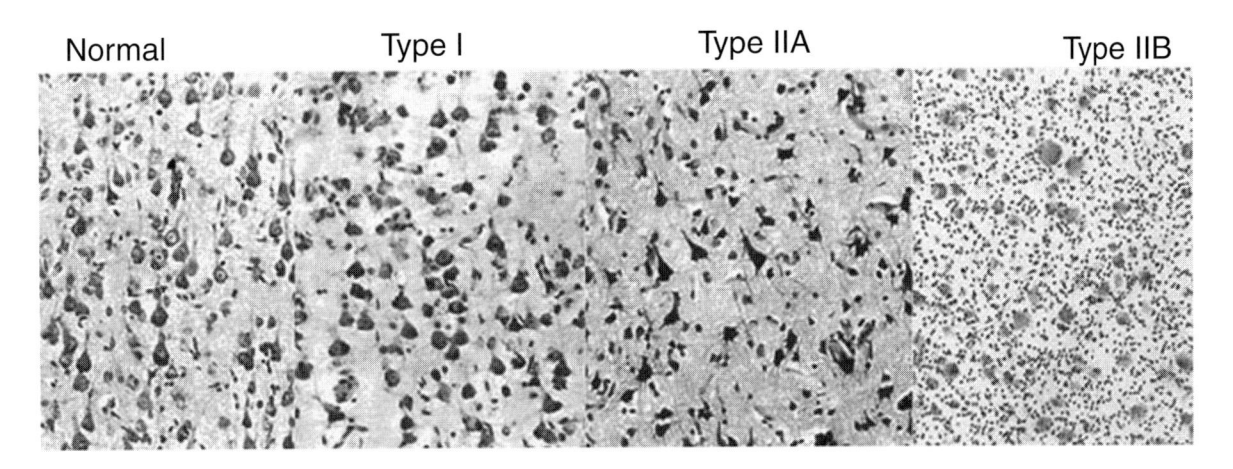

Type I - Architectural abnormalities +/− giant or immature neurons

Type IIA - Architectural abnormalities + dysmorphic neurons

Type IIB - Architectural abnormalities + balloon cells

Figure 108.1. Pathological groups of cortical dysplasia.

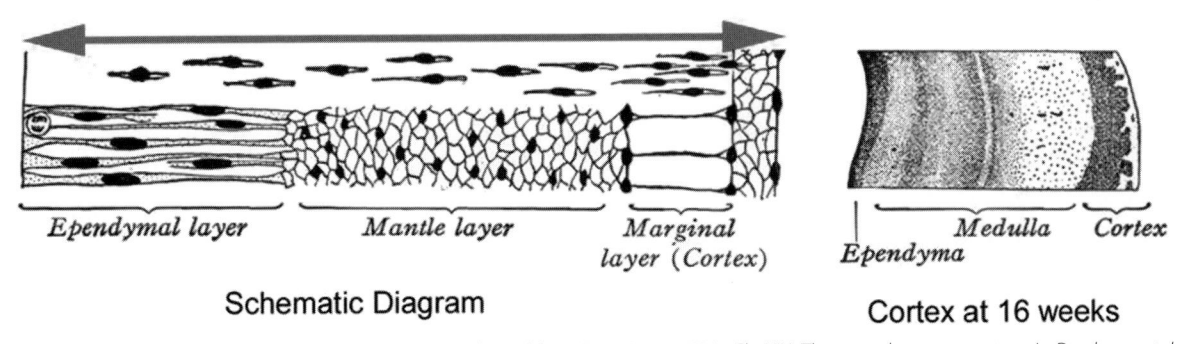

Ependymal layer   *Mantle layer*   *Marginal layer (Cortex)*   *Ependyma*   *Medulla*   *Cortex*

Schematic Diagram   Cortex at 16 weeks

Figure 108.2. Mechanism of cortical development. (adapted from Fig. 431, p. 455 in Ch. XIX, The central nervous system. In *Developmental Anatomy*, Arey LB. 5th edn. WB Saunders Company, Philadelphia and London, 1946.)

The Paediatric Commission of the ILAE, surveying 543 patients treated in 20 surgical centres worldwide, noted that CD was the causative lesion in 42%. In 422 cases operated at the Maudsley hospital the pathology was CD in 9.4%.

The seizure semiology in CD is diverse, but because the majority of the surgical candidates have discrete lesions, the commonest type is appropriately localized focal seizures. However, CD can be the underlying cause of infantile spasms. Presurgical investigation follows the same protocol as for other causes. In a study of 24 MRI negative patients 42% had CD (Chapman et al., 2005). The location of these lesions varies. In 128 cases described by Chung et al., 42.2% were temporal, 37.5% frontal and 20.3% were in other locations (Chung et al., 2005). This last group present difficulties because they are often close to, or within, eloquent cortex. Complex investigations including fMRI and intracranial EEG recordings, may be necessary to justify resection. Other problems may arise. For example, small areas of cortical dysplasia may co-exist with certain tumours such as the DNET, and in the temporal lobe there may be dual pathology. This latter is estimated at between 15% and

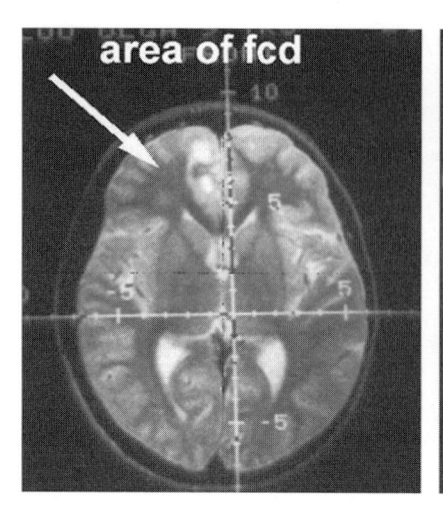

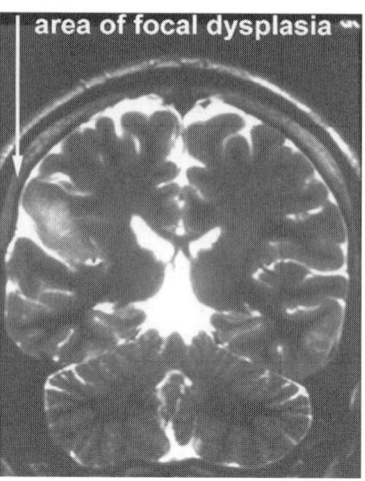

Figure 108.3. Two areas of focal cortical dysplasia on MRI.

87%. Fauser and Schulze-Bonhage, investigating 12 patients with dual pathology in the temporal lobe, showed that in some patients the seizure onset was from the amygdalo-hippocampal complex, whereas in others seizures arose from the CD, and in some patients from both (Fauser and Schulze-Bonhage, 2006). Because of such issues, resection of CD may not always result in seizure freedom.

The possible surgical interventions in cortical dysplasia are resection, multiple subpial transection (MST) and vagus nerve stimulation. The outcome from resection is good but depends on the underlying histology, the extent of the lesion and the location of the lesion, especially in relation to eloquent cortex. In general, type II lesions, corresponding to the original Taylor's focal cortical dysplasia, are easier to image and resect whereas type I lesions tend to be associated with lobar atrophy or hypoplasia, and in the temporal lobe with mesial temporal sclerosis. The patients described by Chung are representative, where 46% of 128 patients were in Engel group I but 40.9% were in Engel groups 3 and 4. There were transient complications in 10% (Chung et al., 2005). A long-term follow-up of 38 children in Alberta seen for at least 10 years showed that 32% remained seizure-free compared with 72% of patients with benign tumours (Hamiwka et al., 2005). A group of smaller series from the literature between 2000 and 2007 showed 64% to 90% being seizure-free. The possible use of MST in this condition is not clear. Some groups describe good results, but in our experience it is of limited or no value.

There are no specific data about the use of vagus nerve stimulation in this condition.

Hemimegalencephaly is a gross cortical malformation, which may be bilateral although then it is usually more marked in one hemisphere. It causes early and severe epilepsy and early operation is recommended. Because of the dangers of major surgery in small infants, the use of hemispherotomy techniques, which minimize operative risk, has improved the outcome in these patients. Generally the outcome in these patients is worse than in hemispherotomy for other major hemisphere disorders. Delalande, reporting his results for hemispherotomy in 83 patients, including 30 with cortical malformations, notes an overall seizure-free rate of 77%, which is reduced to 60% in these patients. Furthermore the mortality and morbidity in these patients is greater than in the remainder of the group. This is partly attributable to the younger age of the group but also reflects the increased difficulty of surgery in this malformation (Delalande et al., 2007). Similar outcomes are reported by others.

Battaglia et al. examined the location of periventricular nodular heterotopia (PNH) in 54 patients, and 27 of them were either unilateral or unilateral with cortical involvement. Interictal and ictal abnormalities were always related to the location of the PNH (Battaglia et al., 2006). Meroni et al. describe 24 patients with heterotopia in the resected specimen. In 14 patients, the lesion had been visible on MRI and was associated with CD in 13. In this group, 78% were seizure-free. The remaining 10 patients had small nodules, not visible on MRI, all associated with gross temporal lobe pathology, and 90% were seizure-free (Meroni et al., 2009). It seems therefore that heterotopic areas may contribute significantly to epilepsy and can be removed.

Conclusions

(1) Malformations of cortical development are complex and arise from a variety of causes, some of which occur early in fetal development.
(2) They may not be visible on MRI scans.
(3) Depending upon the nature and location they may respond well to resective surgery.
(4) Hemimegalencephaly is a gross abnormality, which often presents in the neonatal period with severe epilepsy and developmental delay. In these patients, the quality of life can be improved by some form of hemispherotomy.
(5) Nodular heterotopia, under some circumstances, can respond well to surgery.

References

Battaglia G, Chiapparini L, Franceschetti S, et al. Periventricular nodular heterotopia: classification, epileptic history, and genesis of epileptic discharges. *Epilepsia* 2006;**47**(1):86–97.

Chapman K, Wyllie E, Najm I, et al. Seizure outcome after epilepsy surgery in patients with normal preoperative MRI. *J Neurol Neurosurg Psychiatry* 2005;**76**(5):710–3.

Chassoux F, Devaux B, Landre E, et al. Stereoelectroencephalography in focal cortical dysplasia: a 3D approach to delineating the dysplastic cortex. *Brain* 2000;**123**(Pt 8):1733–51.

Chung CK, Lee SK, Kim KJ. Surgical outcome of epilepsy caused by cortical dysplasia. *Epilepsia* 2005;**46**(Suppl 1): 25–9.

Delalande O, Bulteau C, Dellatolas G, et al. Vertical parasagittal hemispherotomy: surgical procedures and clinical long-term outcomes in a population of 83 children. *Neurosurgery* 2007;**60**(2 Suppl 1):ONS19–32.

Fauser S, Schulze-Bonhage A. Epileptogenicity of cortical dysplasia in temporal lobe dual pathology: an electrophysiological study with invasive recordings. *Brain* 2006;**129**(Pt 1):82–95.

Ferrier CH, Alarcón G, Engelsman J, et al. Relevance of residual histologic and electrocorticographic abnormalities for surgical outcome in frontal lobe epilepsy. *Epilepsia* 2001;**42**:363–71.

Hamiwka L, Jayakar P, Resnick T, et al. Surgery for epilepsy due to cortical malformations: ten-year follow-up. *Epilepsia* 2005;**46**(4):556–60.

Kuznieky RI, Jackson GD. Malformations of cortical development. In Engel JJ Jr, Pedley TA, eds. *Epilepsy: A Comprehensive Textbook*, pp. 2575–88. 2nd ed. Philadelphia: Lippincott Williams & Wilkins; 2008.

Meroni A, Galli C, Bramerio M, et al. Nodular heterotopia: a neuropathological study of 24 patients undergoing surgery for drug-resistant epilepsy. *Epilepsia* 2009;**50**:116–24. Epub 2008 Jul 14.

Montenegro MA, Guerreiro MM, Lopes-Cendes I, Guerreiro CA, Cendes F. Interrelationship of genetics and prenatal injury in the genesis of malformations of cortical development. *Arch Neurol* 2002;**59**(7):1147–53.

Palmini A, Gloor P. The localizing value of auras in partial seizures: a prospective and retrospective study. *Neurology* 1992;**42**(4):801–8.

Palmini A, Gambardella A, Andermann F, et al. Intrinsic epileptogenicity of human dysplastic cortex as suggested by corticography and surgical results. *Ann Neurol* 1995;**4**:476–87.

Learning objectives

(1) To understand the developmental origins of cortical malformations.
(2) To learn about the incidence and distribution of cortical malformations.
(3) To understand the histological, radiological and electrophysiological features of cortical malformations.
(4) To learn about the lesion of hemimegalencephaly.
(5) To understand the surgical management of cortical malformations.

Questions

(1) Describe the developmental origin and histological characteristics of neuronal migration defect.
(2) Discuss the place of electrophysiological investigation in the diagnosis and management of cortical neuronal migration defect.
(3) Describe the factors which are in favour of a good outcome from resection of a cortical malformation.

Rasmussen's disease and epilepsia partialis continua

Charles E. Polkey

Chronic (Rasmussen's) encephalitis

Rasmussen's encephalitis is 'a relentlessly progressive disorder of childhood associated with hemispheric atrophy, severe intractable focal epilepsy, intellectual decline and hemiparesis' (Dubeau *et al.*, 2008). First described from Montreal in 1958 by Theodore Rasmussen, it was called an encephalitis because of the histological appearances (Rasmussen *et al.*, 1958) (Figure 109.1). Typically, it begins in childhood, the median age of onset is 5 years, and in 50% of cases it is preceded by an inflammatory illness. Initially there may be complex partial seizures (28%), or tonic-clonic seizures (33%), or focal motor seizures (28%), but the patient soon shows focal motor seizures. It may also begin with unilateral dystonia. Between 20% and 56% show periods of focal motor status (epilepsia partialis continuans), which can require treatment in an intensive care unit. Bien *et al.* in a European Consensus Statement identify three stages (Bien *et al.*, 2005):

(1) A prodromal stage, with a median duration of 7.1 months, has low seizure frequency and a mild hemiparesis.

(2) An acute stage, with a median duration of 8 months, has increased frequency and severity of seizures and neurological deterioration.

(3) A residual stage with a stable neurological deficit and less frequent seizures.

Patients do not all progress through these stages and some proven cases have arrested with a stable state without a complete hemiplegia or intellectual deterioration. In addition with the passage of time it has become clear that there is a minority of cases with adult onset, or bilateral disease or disease in non-epileptogenic areas such as the brainstem. Andermann *et al.* have recently described children, collected from a number of centres, with an aggressive, bilateral, juvenile form of the disease (Andermann *et al.*, 2006).

There are no absolute radiological features of the condition (Figures 109.2 and 109.3). On CT atrophy is seen and up to one-third of patients may show unilateral atrophy of the head of the caudate nucleus. In addition, in the early stages on MRI there may be multiple hyperintense areas especially in the insular and peri-insular regions. The neurophysiological

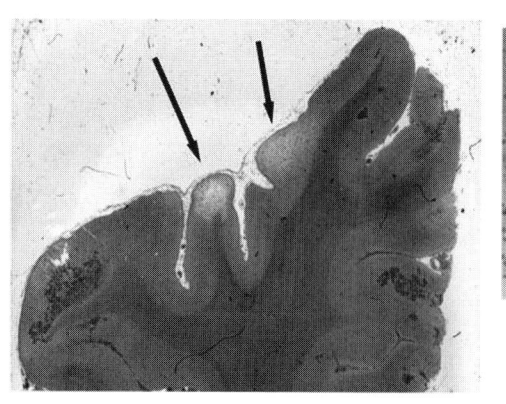

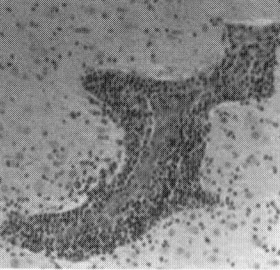

Figure 109.1. Pathological changes in Rasmussen's disease. Left, brain slice showing ischaemic lesions (arrows). Right, photomicrograph showing accumulation of inflammatory cells around a blood vessel. See colour version in plate section.

Introduction to Epilepsy ed. Gonzalo Alarcón and Antonio Valentín. Published by Cambridge University Press.
© Cambridge University Press 2012.

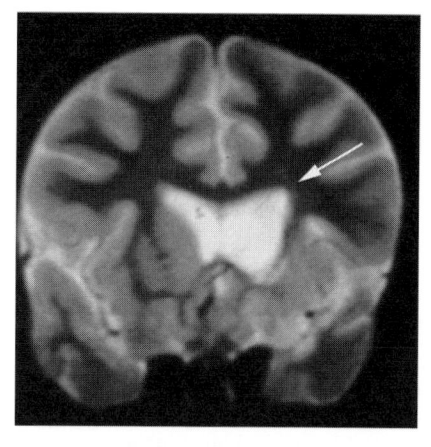

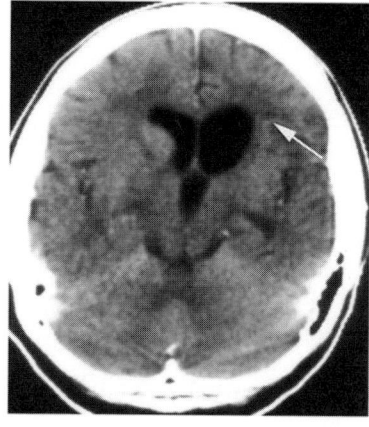

Figure 109.2. MRI in Rasmussen's disease. Note atrophy of the basal ganglia indicated by the arrow.

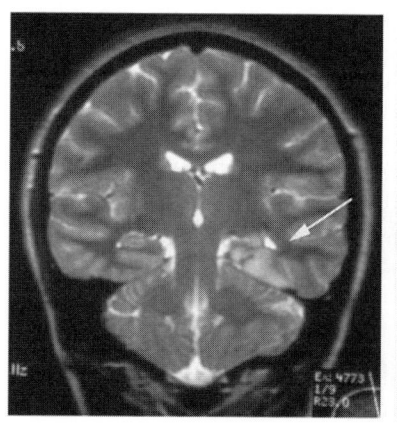

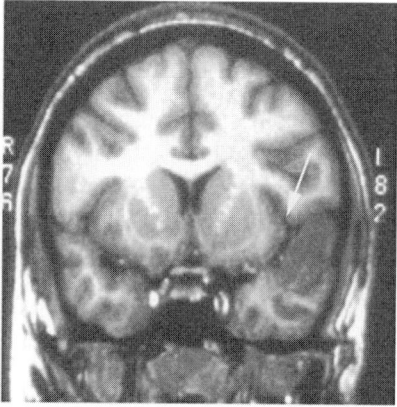

Figure 109.3. MRI in atypical case of Rasmussen's disease. The arrows indicate the abnormal left temporal lobe.

findings depend upon the stage of the disease, there is asymmetry of background activity, and there may be unilateral focal slow activity. There are multiple independent epileptic foci, usually unilateral but they may be bilateral but asymmetric in one-third of cases. The differential diagnosis is very complex but detailed by Bien et al. (2005).

The aetiology of this rare condition is still obscure. The histological changes are those of chronic inflammation. In 1996 an auto-immune mechanism was proposed when Rogers et al. described Rasmussen-type features in rabbits who had become sensitized to the GluR3 protein (Rogers et al., 1994). Although this particular hypothesis did not prove to be robust, the underlying idea of a vicious circle of an auto-immune reaction within the CNS seems to fit the majority of the features of the disease. It does not explain the unilaterality seen in most cases. It has been proposed that this results from the epileptic activity within the hemisphere. Recent investigations have implicated T-cell lymphocytes in this process and this is a more robust finding than the GluR3 antigens (Bien et al., 2002).

Once a diagnosis has been made, often by exclusion, management can be quite complex since both surgical and medical options are available. A suitable schema has been suggested by Bien et al. (2005). The most effective surgery is some form of hemispherectomy or hemispherotomy in suitable candidates. These are usually patients in the acute phase with severe intractable epilepsy, including epilepsia partialis continuans and a severe hemiplegia. The neurophysiological and functional brain imaging results may suggest bilateral disease but often these functional tests probably reflect bilateral epileptogenesis. There may be the addition of a hemianopia but this is usually acceptable. The intellectual consequences are more debatable as surgery is often performed after hemispheric specialization is well advanced and, especially in the dominant hemisphere, there may be considerable deterioration, but all of our patients have regained social speech. The results of hemispherectomy are good, up to 80% of patients are seizure-free and a follow-up of five patients from Alabama over 13 to 26 years show the results to be robust (Tubbs *et al.*, 2005; Delalande *et al.*, 2007). Lesser surgical procedures such as local resection, callosotomy and multiple subpial transection are much less effective. Although they may improve seizure control and quality of life, they never produce seizure freedom and many patients go on to hemispherectomy.

The medical options depend upon theories of the cause of this condition. These measures include antiviral drugs such as gancyclovir, steroids, immunoglobulins and plasma exchange. Reports of antiviral use are few and this treatment has been more or less abandoned. Steroids have been shown to have a short-term effect, as has plasma exchange. Immunoglobulins have been used by a number of groups. All of these options have been used separately or in combination for varying lengths of time and they have all had some effect in some cases but none has been permanently or reliably effective. With theories of a T-cell-mediated process, more recently tacrolimus therapy has been used. Tacrolimus, an immunosuppressive which acts on T cells, in an open study reduced motor deterioration and hemispheric atrophy as judged from radiology, but had no effect on seizure frequency (Bien *et al.*, 2004).

Conclusions

(1) Chronic encephalitis is a rare but devastating disease.
(2) It is not clear whether it has a single cause.
(3) Medical treatments are very inefficient.
(4) If justified, hemispherectomy or hemispherotomy, are very effective.
(5) In the dominant hemisphere there may be considerable cognitive penalties.

References

Andermann F, Farrell K. Early onset Rasmussen's syndrome: a malignant, often bilateral form of the disorder. *Epilepsy Res* 2006;**70**(Suppl 1):S259–62.

Bien CG, Bauer J, Deckwerth TL, *et al*. Destruction of neurons by cytotoxic T cells: a new pathogenic mechanism in Rasmussen's encephalitis. *Ann Neurol* 2002;**51**(3):311–8.

Bien CG, Gleissner U, Sassen R, *et al*. An open study of tacrolimus therapy in Rasmussen encephalitis. *Neurology* 2004;**62**(11):2106–9.

Bien CG, Granata T, Antozzi C, *et al*. Pathogenesis, diagnosis and treatment of Rasmussen encephalitis: a European consensus statement. *Brain* 2005;**128**(Pt 3): 454–71.

Delalande O, Bulteau C, Dellatolas G, *et al*. Vertical parasagittal hemispherotomy: surgical procedures and clinical long-term outcomes in a population of 83 children. *Neurosurgery* 2007;**60**(2 Suppl 1):ONS19–32.

Dubeau F, Andermann F, Wiendl H, Bar-Or A. Rasmussen's encephalitis (chronic focal encephalitis). In Engel JJ Jr, Pedley TA, eds. *Epilepsy: A Comprehensive Textbook*, pp. 2439–53. 2nd ed. Philadelphia: Lippincott Williams & Wilkins; 2008.

Rasmussen T, Obozewski J, Lloyd-Smith D. Focal seizures due to chronic localised encephalitis. *Neurology* 1958;**8**:435–45.

Rogers SW, Andrews PI, Gahring LC, *et al*. Autoantibodies to glutamate receptor GluR3 in Rasmussen's encephalitis. *Science* 1994;**265**(5172):648–51.

Tubbs RS, Nimjee SM, Oakes WJ. Long-term follow-up in children with functional hemispherectomy for Rasmussen's encephalitis. *Childs Nerv Syst* 2005; **21**(6):461–5.

Learning objectives

(1) To understand the aetiology of Rasmussen's disease.
(2) To understand the various clinical scenarios presented by Rasmussen's disease.
(3) To understand the diagnostic criteria involved in the identification of Rasmussen's disease
(4) To describe the management of Rasmussen's disease
(5) To understand the medical and surgical options available to manage Rasmussen's disease

Questions

(1) Discuss the aetiology of Rasmussen's disease.
(2) Describe the usual clinical course of Rasmussen's disease and discuss how this affects management.
(3) Describe and discuss the diagnostic criteria for Rasmussen's disease.
(4) Compare and contrast the surgical and medical treatment of Rasmussen's disease.

Behavioural treatment of epilepsy

Peter Fenwick

In 1881, Sir William Gowers said 'Of all the immediate causes of epilepsy, the most potent are psychical – fright, excitement, anxiety'. He added 'To these were ascribed more than one-third in which a definite cause was given'. This important point, that mental states can lead to the occurrence of seizures, is often forgotten. Its importance is that it points the way to the modification of the frequency of epileptic seizures by behavioural means. The standard medical model suggests that epilepsy is due to genetic causes or brain damage, that fits have physiological causes that are best treated with drugs. The behavioural model stresses that there is a close link between seizures and ongoing brain activity, particularly in the damaged area of brain from which seizures are arising. Seizures are linked to behaviour, so non-drug behavioural treatment is possible. Behaviour therapy recognizes patients as individuals, and that seizures arise as an interaction of the patient with himself, his family, friends and surroundings. Behavioural treatment depends on seeing how patient's seizures are related to his behaviour, lifestyle and relationships. Seizure control may be achieved by modifying these aspects of his life, and teaching him individual behavioural strategies that may help to control his seizures.

The theory behind behaviour therapy is that in the focal epilepsies ongoing abnormal activity is present at the seizure focus. When a seizure occurs, normal cells are recruited into the abnormal discharging, and a wave of abnormal activity spreads out from the focus. The factors that may cause this spread are those which activate surrounding neurons. Thus in the motor cortex movements may lead to the precipitation of seizures, in the parietal areas shapes and sensations, in the visual cortex flashing lights, in the temporal lobes emotional and psychical events.

Animal evidence suggests that seizures may be conditioned using classic conditioning methods in cats, but only in damaged brains. Dogs susceptible to genetic seizures may have seizures when they become excited.

A number of studies have looked at the relationship between seizures and behavioural strategies. In the Maudsley series, 69% of patients said that tension caused their seizures, depression in 67%, tiredness in 49% and anger in 45%. Ten per cent had seizures during sexual intercourse and only 7% had seizures when they were happy. In a study from Sweden, 83% of patients had seizures related to physical activity, 78% to negative stress and 64% to panic. Another study with adolescents showed that the most seizure-provoking situation was to work around home. School was considerably less seizure-provoking, but relaxing by the fire seemed to be the least seizure-provoking state. Some patients can generate their own seizures: 23% in the Maudsley study, 16% in Swedish children and 69% in Swedish adults. The commonest seizure triggers were imitation of seizure onset, thinking of seizure onset and hyperventilation.

Inhibition of seizures in the Maudsley series was shown by 53% of patients using a number of methods, and in Sweden by 89% of patients using positive statements, and by 77% by stimulation of a sensory area.

The main engine of behaviour treatment is detailed seizure analysis using ABC charts, that is, studying:

- **Antecedents**, what happens before a seizure,
- **Behaviour**, what happens during the attack, and
- **Consequences**, what happens after the seizure.

For example, a schoolboy who had seizures in class was taken to the sick room, given warm milk and

---

Introduction to Epilepsy ed. Gonzalo Alarcón and Antonio Valentín. Published by Cambridge University Press.
© Cambridge University Press 2012.

spent the day playing with Lego. Behavioural treatment was to accept that he had a seizure, put him at the back of the class while he recovered, and then let him continue with his work. Seizures in school then faded away to zero.

Countermeasures are also defined by the use of ABC charts. A countermeasure is a technique practised by the patient either in seizure-prone situations or at the beginning of a seizure. Most patients have strategies that they use to reduce either seizure occurrence or seizure spread. These strategies are identified by the ABC charts and the patient is taught how to use them on a routine basis. Hitting a limb that is beginning to tingle at the onset of a seizure, clapping hands, standing up, using smelling salts, may all stop seizures developing. Restriction of movement at seizure onset is a potent anticonvulsant.

An associated behavioural method is that of biofeedback. The first biofeedback method to be used was the augmentation by biofeedback of the sensorimotor rhythm (mu rhythm). It was initially found that in cats given convulsant drugs, enhancement of this rhythm produced an anticonvulsant effect. This was then used in patients, a small proportion of whom became seizure-free. Later, abnormal brain rhythms were fed back in the form of a computer game to the patient and they were asked voluntarily to reduce the amount of abnormal activity. A further method is to feed back positive EEG waves measured on the scalp (CPV), which correlate with cortical inhibition and seizure reduction. The patient is taught in the EEG department how to produce this rhythm, and then practises this at home. Biofeedback of the galvanic skin response can also be used.

Behavioural treatment gives the patient an understanding of themselves, shows them the relationship between seizures and life's difficulties, helps the relationship between peers, and fosters independence and better life adjustment. It is important to remind the patient that both happiness and relaxation are powerful anticonvulsants.

Recommended reading

Dahl J, Brorson L.O, Melin L. Effects of a broad-spectrum behavioural medicine treatment programme on children with refractory epileptic seizures: an 8 year follow-up. *Epilepsia* 1992;**33**(1):98–102.

Fenwick P. Self-generation of seizures by an action of mind. *Adv Neurol* 1998;**75**:87–92.

Lundgren T, Dahl J, Yardi N, Melin L. Acceptance and commitment therapy and yoga for drug refractory epilepsy: a randomised controlled trial. *Epilepsy Behav* 2008;**13**(1):102–8.

Matsuoka H, Takahashi T, Sasaki M, *et al.* Neuropsychological EEG activation in patients with epilepsy. *Brain* 2000;**123**(Pt 2):318–30.

Matsuoka H, Nakamura M. The role of cognitive-motor function in precipitation and inhibition of epileptic seizures. *Epilepsia* 2005;**46**:(Suppl 1):17–20.

Nagai Y, Goldstein L, Fenwick P, *et al.* Clinical efficacy of galvanic skin response via biofeedback training in reducing seizures in adult epilepsy: a preliminary randomised controlled study. *Epilepsy Behav* 2004;5(2): 216–23.

Learning objective

(1) To know the mechanisms of action, objectives, indications, methods and efficacy of the behavioural treatment of epilepsy.

Section 7 Psychiatric, social and legal aspects

Chapter 111
Affective disorders and epilepsy

Nozomi Akanuma

Introduction

Affective (mood) disorders encompass different types of conditions in which a disturbance of affect/mood is the central feature. The altered mood is usually accompanied by symptoms involving thought, perception, biological functioning and behaviour.

A manic episode exhibits elevated mood, accompanied by an increase in the quantity and speed of physical and mental activities, a decreased need for sleep, social dysinhibition and self-important ideas.

A depressive episode is formed with persistent depressed mood (>2 weeks) along with loss of interest and enjoyment, and decreased activities. They are often accompanied by reduced self-esteem and confidence, ideas of guilt, ideas of self-harm, disturbed sleep and diminished appetite.

There are three main entities of mood disorders. Recurrent depressive disorder (or unipolar depression) is an illness with recurrent depressive episodes separated by periods without significant mood disturbance. Bipolar mood disorder (formerly known as manic-depression) is characterized by alternation from depressive mood to mania, and intervals without mood symptoms. An episode of elation may be mild mania (hypomania). Persistent mood disorder is composed of cyclothymia (mood swings between depressive and elated episodes) and dysthymia (chronic depressive mood). Each episode of these two conditions is not as severe as either depressive or manic episodes. However, their course is chronic without a period of remission.

Treatments for mood disorders include medication (antidepressants, mood stabilizers or antipsychotics), and psychological and behavioural therapies. Electroconvulsive therapy can be used for severe depressive and manic episodes when other treatments are deemed unsuitable or have failed.

Mood disorders, particularly depression, are the most common mental health problem in the general population, with a higher prevalence in women. Mood disorders can be a component of psychiatric or physical diseases (co-morbidity). These often lead to decreased social and occupational functioning and reduced quality of life.

Depression in epilepsy
Ictal depression

Depressive mood is a common ictal change of mood/affect in simple partial seizures (SPS) or in SPS followed by complex partial seizure (CPS) and/or secondarily generalized tonic-clonic seizure (sGTCS). Its duration varies. The mood change could outlast the actual ictus. It is most commonly observed in temporal lobe epilepsy.

Peri-ictal depression

In pre-ictal depression, depressed mood or irritability occurs hours to days before a seizure. Mood symptoms preceding a seizure could be perceived as premonitory symptoms, usually before sGTCS in partial epilepsies.

In post-ictal depression, mood changes occur after the seizure. This is more common after a CPS than after other seizure types and in patients with poorly controlled seizures.

Treatment of ictal and peri-ictal depression

Since depressive mood is closely associated with seizures, optimizing seizure control is often effective to lessen or diminish mood symptoms. The use of fast-acting benzodiazepines has been found effective.

Introduction to Epilepsy ed. Gonzalo Alarcón and Antonio Valentín. Published by Cambridge University Press.
© Cambridge University Press 2012.

Interictal depression

Interictal depression is the most common psychiatric disturbance in epilepsy, with a prevalence of 6–70%, which is higher than in the general population. Co-morbid depression is associated with an increased risk of suicide in epilepsy.

While the clinical presentation of interictal depression meets the standard criteria for recurrent depressive disorders, it more commonly includes 'dysthymia-like' symptoms, which are pleomorphic and tend to persist chronically, with recurrent short periods of symptom freedom or euphoric moods.

Interictal depression could affect people with epilepsy across all age groups, including children, both genders, and different types of epilepsies. The following are reported risk factors are shown in Box 111.1.

Box 111.1. Risk factors for interictal depression in epilepsy

- General factors
  - Men (equivalent prevalence in men and women)
  - Family history of mood disorders
  - Brain pathology (e.g. head injury, cerebrovascular accident, space-occupying lesion)
  - Lower intelligence
- Epilepsy-related factors
  - CPSs, focal epilepsies
  - Limbic/temporal or frontal foci
  - Left-sided focus
  - Poor seizure control
- Iatrogenic factors
  - Antiepileptic drugs (AEDs): phenobarbital, primidone, viagabatorine, tiagabine, topiramate (note that all AEDs have the potential to cause depression)
  - Polypharmacy
  - Epilepsy surgery (mainly temporal resection; note that preoperative depression is not a contraindication of epileptic surgery)
- Psychosocial factors
  - Stigma
  - Health locus of control
  - Adjustment to epilepsy
  - Parental overprotection
  - Deterioration of quality of life

Treatment of interictal depression

Optimizing treatment with AEDs is crucial. If it does not resolve the symptoms, similar approaches to depression in the general population can be taken. Antidepressants are a safe option when used with caution (see below). Electroconvulsive therapy is not contraindicated in epilepsy.

Use of antidepressants in epilepsy

Antidepressants are known to decrease the seizure threshold to a varying degree, potentially inducing seizures. Few data are available on antidepressant-induced seizures in people with epilepsy who already are on AEDs. In the general population, the proconvulsive effect of antidepressants is reported to be 0.1–4.0% per year, while the annual incidence of a first seizure is 0.086%. Risks of seizure induction are due to drug-related factors (types, doses and titration rate of antidepressants, and drug interactions) as well as individual-related factors (e.g. neurological, psychiatric or intellectual co-morbidity).

Since both classes of drugs share several cytochrome P450 enzymes, the serum levels of drugs may change, depending on the enzymes involved (either inducer or inhibitor). When antidepressants are administered with AEDs, serum monitoring of AEDs and adjustment of the dosage may be required.

For more details on the use of antidepressants in epilepsy, see Chapter 119 ('Use of psychotropics in people with epilepsy').

Bipolar mood disorder in epilepsy

Bipolar mood disorders are not common in epilepsy, but reportedly more prevalent than in the general population. There is some evidence that interictal manic episodes are more common in patients with fronto-temporal epileptic foci.

For treatment, with bipolar symptoms related to seizures (ictal or peri-ictal), optimizing seizure control is essential. The same approaches to treatment as in non-epileptic patients should be taken, with care for drug interactions and epilepsy-related and psychosocial issues. Many AEDs are used as mood stabilizers (e.g. carbamazepine, sodium valproate, lamotrigine). However, it is not known whether treating epilepsy with these AEDs could have any effect on the development of bipolar symptoms.

Recommended reading

Barry JJ, Lembke A, Huynh N. Affective disorders in epilepsy. In Ettinger AB, Kanner AM, eds. *Psychiatric Issues in Epilepsy: A Practical Guide to Diagnosis and Treatment*, pp. 45–71. Philadelphia: Lippincott Williams and Wilkins; 2001.

Gelder M, Mayou R, Cowen P (eds). Mood disorders. In *Shorter Oxford Textbook of Psychiatry*, pp. 269–325. 4th edn. Oxford: Oxford University Press. 2001.

Lambert MV, Robertson MM. Depression in epilepsy: etiology, phenomenology, and treatment. *Epilepsia* 1999;**40**(Suppl 10):S21–47.

Pisani F, Oteri G, Costa C, Di Raimondo G, Di Perri R. Effects of psychotropic drugs on seizure threshold. *Drug Safety* 2002;**25**:91–110.

World Health Organization. *The ICD-10 Classification of Mental and Behavioural Disorders: Clinical Descriptions and Diagnostic Guidelines*. Geneva: World Health Organization; 1992.

Learning objectives

(1) To be acquainted with the basic classification of psychiatric conditions.
(2) To know the different types of depression and bipolar mood disorder seen in patients with epilepsy, their prevalence, mechanisms, risk factors and treatment.

Section 7: Psychiatric, social and legal aspects

Chapter 112: Anxiety disorders and epilepsy

John Moriarty

Anxiety is probably experienced to some degree by all patients with epilepsy. It is of course a normal phenomenon and so, in considering the clinical problem of anxiety in patients with epilepsy, we need to ensure we and our patients are clear what we mean by the term. We need to be able to recognize when anxiety may be pathological, how it relates to the associated epilepsy, and what treatments or interventions may be of help.

Most of us can recognize anxiety as a subjective sense of fear, worrying or nervousness. This may be normal and appropriate or it may be maladaptive, i.e. not appropriate in the circumstances. It may be thought of as state or trait anxiety. State anxiety is a temporary change of level of anxiety for an individual, often related to real or perceived threat in the external environment. Trait anxiety refers to the fact that the characterological or baseline anxiety experienced by different individuals varies. That is to say, some of us are 'worriers' by nature.

Symptoms of anxiety can be divided into somatic symptoms and psychic symptoms. The former include breathlessness, palpitations, nausea, dizziness, dry mouth, urinary frequency, tremor, sweating and abdominal churning. Psychic symptoms include a feeling of dread, irritability, a sense of panic, poor concentration, insomnia and restlessness.

A detailed account of the biology of anxiety is beyond the scope of this book. It is useful to know, however, that the structures implicated in the biology of anxiety include the amygdala and related limbic structures. Consequently, it is perhaps not surprising that the relationship between epilepsy and anxiety is complex and includes common biological substrates. Seizures and panic attacks can sometimes be difficult to tell apart. Both are unexpected discrete paroxysmal events which can include a sense of fear, of things being unreal or of déjà vu. The EEG in panic disorder does not show epileptic discharges, although nonspecific changes can be seen (Stein and Uhde, 1989). Factors pointing to episodes being ictal include very brief (less than a minute) duration, automatisms or confusion (Vazquez and Devinsky, 2003).

Psychiatric disorders characterized by anxiety are listed in Table 112.1. An example of what a person

Table 112.1. Psychiatric disorders characterized by anxiety with examples of what a person suffering from each might say was worrying him/her

Disorder	Nature of worrying
Panic disorder	'I get a sudden feeling of dread and am worried this may happen again'
Agoraphobia (with or without panic disorder)	'Well, I need to have someone with me – then I'm OK. I can't get on the tube'
Specific phobia	'I feel sick at even the thought of an injection. I won't have any more blood tests'
Social phobia	'I am not too bad one-to-one or if I have had a drink. Otherwise I just can't. I know I am going to make a fool of myself'
Obsessive-compulsive disorder	'I'm worried in case I might have forgotten to take my tablets, then I might have a seizure and die.'
Generalized anxiety disorder	'I'm worried about lots of things, my health, my family, my finances, especially losing my job'

Introduction to Epilepsy ed. Gonzalo Alarcón and Antonio Valentín. Published by CAMBRIDGE UNIVERSITY PRESS.
© CAMBRIDGE UNIVERSITY PRESS 2012.

suffering from each of these disorders might say was worrying them is given alongside. There are formal diagnostic criteria for each of these disorders but they are all characterized by a particular type or circumstance of worrying.

Anxiety disorders may affect up to one in every two patients with epilepsy (Jones *et al.*, 2005). Concerns expressed by patients relate to a wide range of issues including driving, employment, injury, memory, stigma, medication and hospital costs (Gilliam *et al.*, 1997). In addition, the medications used in the treatment of epilepsy can sometimes cause mood or anxiety symptoms while some antiepileptic drugs are anxiolytic (Ketter *et al.*, 1999).

Treatment options for patients with anxiety disorders in epilepsy include medication, including selective serotonin reuptake inhibitors (SSRIs) and buspirone. Benzodiazepines may be very effective, but the risk of addiction is considerable so they should be used with caution. Pregabalin is effective in the shorter term for anxiety, but its role in longer-term management has yet to be established (Rickels *et al.*, 2005). The most important treatment options for patients with anxiety are probably non-pharmacological.

The most influential psychological theories of anxiety have been those derived from behavioural science and especially the concepts of classic and operant conditioning. Classic conditioning refers to the fact that subjects who are exposed to a stimulus which elicits an unconditioned response (for example, a dog salivating in response to the sight of food) can be conditioned to elicit the same response in association with a conditioned stimulus (a bell). Operant conditioning refers to the fact that behaviours can increase or decrease in reaction to reward or punishment systems (e.g. a rat pressing a lever to elicit food). These animal experiments have led through theoretical and practical extrapolations to the current thinking underlying behavioural interventions for anxiety. Non-drug treatment options for anxiety include psycho-education, relaxation techniques and more formal therapies such as cognitive behavioural therapy. The latter will include identifying and challenging reinforcing behaviours, such as too much reassurance, or safety and avoidant behaviours which contribute to an escalating cycle of anxiety.

Although these techniques are primarily useful in reducing anxiety associated with epilepsy, there is evidence that, for at least some patients, these techniques may also be useful in helping patients achieve better control of seizures themselves (Goldstein, 1997).

References

Gilliam F, Kuzniecky R, Faught E, *et al.* Patient-validated content of epilepsy-specific quality-of-life measurement. *Epilepsia* 1997;**38**(2):233–6.

Goldstein LH. Effectiveness of psychological interventions for people with poorly controlled epilepsy. *J Neurol Neurosurg Psychiatry* 1997;**63**:137–42.

Jones JE, Hermann BP, Barry JJ, *et al.* Clinical assessment of axis I psychiatric morbidity in chronic epilepsy: a multicenter investigation. *J Neuropsych Clin Neurosci* 2005;**17**:172–9.

Ketter TA, Post RM, Theodore WH. Positive and negative psychiatric effects of antiepileptic drugs in patients with seizure disorders. *Neurology* 1999;**53**(5 Suppl 2):S53–67.

Rickels K, Pollack MH, Feltner DE, *et al.* Pregabalin for treatment of generalised anxiety disorder. *Arch Gen Psychiatry* 2005;**62**:1022–30.

Stein MB, Uhde TW. Infrequent occurrence of EEG abnormalities in panic disorder. *Am J Psychiatry* 1989;**146**(4):517–20.

Vazquez B, Devinsky O. Epilepsy and anxiety. *Epilepsy Behav* 2003;**4**(S4):S20–25.

Learning objectives

(1) To be aware of the psychiatric conditions characterized by anxiety, with examples of what a person suffering from each might say was worrying him/her.
(2) To know the different types of anxiety seen in patients with epilepsy, their prevalence, mechanisms, risk factors and treatment.

Section 7 Psychiatric, social and legal aspects

Chapter 113

Personality and epilepsy

Peter Fenwick

There is a long history of a relationship between epilepsy and personality characteristics. Aretaeus, in the second century AD, described people with epilepsy as 'languid, spiritless, stupid, unsociable, slow to learn from the torpidity of the understanding and the senses'. By 1857 a more unitary view of the epilepsy personality was described by Morel, who suggested that mental illness was due to a progressive degenerative strain running from generation to generation and showing itself as a moral defect, weakness of character, mental deficiency and epilepsy. This view of mental illness and its linking with epilepsy was supported by Bleuler, Kreplin and Maudsley. Lombroso, an Italian criminologist, in 1876 wrote that a criminal could be identified from birth; he could be defined as a specific physical type with low-slung ears, special facial features, physical degeneration and epilepsy. This erroneous notion of a relationship between epilepsy and psychiatric illness, genetic degeneration and criminality is still held to some extent by the general public today.

By the 1890s the treatment of epilepsy was with bromide and patients with epilepsy were placed in institutions. Their personality at that time was described as violent, aggressive, slow and stupid, with inevitable degeneration. Some of these features were related to endemic bromide toxicity, whereas others were due to recurrent head injury arising from poorly controlled seizures. The modern era began in the 1930s with the introduction of phenobarbitone and much better control of epileptic seizures. The development of the EEG to diagnose epilepsy and the recognition, in the early 1950s, of a specific temporal lobe focus affecting the Papez circuit, now known as the limbic system, led to a clearer understanding of types of epilepsy and consequently the behaviour related to different seizure patterns. The 1960s modern drugs produced better epilepsy control and Lennox (1960) suggested that the personality of patients with epilepsy was normal unless they suffered from brain damage in specific brain systems.

A number of population surveys, starting in the early 1960s, reported a relationship between epilepsy and various personality characteristics. However, these early surveys had variable definitions of epilepsy. Some included people who only had febrile convulsions, while others included only those who were on anticonvulsants. Yet others looked at general practitioner records. It is accepted that the criteria for epilepsy such as anticonvulsant use will lead to higher rates of epilepsy in the population being studied, as 25% of that sample may not actually have epilepsy. Further difficulties were that surveys of general practices, for example the Pond and Bidwell survey of 1960, did not include patients with epilepsy who were in mental hospitals. Pond and Bidwell also pointed out that psychiatric illness and personality difficulties were likely to be over-represented in hospital-based surveys, as often a condition for referral to hospital was not the epilepsy, but rather associated mental illness or personality disorders. For example, in a survey from Warsaw, 1% of those with epilepsy in the community had been admitted to a mental hospital, while 11% of those with epilepsy who had attended medical clinics had been admitted to a mental hospital. The presence of psychiatric morbidity thus varies with the population studied. The Isle of Wight survey gave a figure of 28.6% in uncomplicated epilepsy (4-times higher than in controls) and over 50% in patients with brain damage, while the Medical Research Council longitudinal survey gave a figure of 35% of patients whose epilepsy was graded as complicated. So, an overall prevalence rate of psychiatric morbidity in these populations of a third to a half is likely.

Introduction to Epilepsy ed. Gonzalo Alarcón and Antonio Valentín. Published by Cambridge University Press.
© Cambridge University Press 2012.

Personality difficulties are thus linked to the degree of brain damage, the extent and site of the lesion, the medication being taken, family factors and overall social factors. Studies from the Isle of Wight suggested that if there is no brain damage and the groups are properly matched, then intellectual functioning in populations with epilepsy is normally distributed.

Personality difficulties have been related to a number of specific and nonspecific factors. People with temporal lobe lesions have an increased rate of morbidity but part of this is because they require more drugs, and are also likely to have more seizures. Children with temporal lobe epilepsy, particularly children with left temporal lesions and particularly boys, tend to be more socially isolated and inattentive. Drug toxic effects such as slowness, inattentiveness, irritability and argumentativeness are all chronic long-term effects which are aggravated by polypharmacy. Having a child with epilepsy increases stresses within the family and leads to long-term difficulties for the child. Broken family relationships are more common in such families (one-fifth of mothers have a nervous breakdown and there are higher rates of divorce). In some families, children with epilepsy are over-protected and their activities restricted, leading to chronically dependent personalities. In the 1970s, a new theory was put forward by Bear and Fedio (1977), which argued for an increase in connection between sub-cortical limbic structures and cortical structures due to epileptic spikes (kindling). They argued that this led to a hyper-connection syndrome and suggested that this caused personality differences in those patients who had either right or left temporal lobe spikes. Unfortunately subsequent studies revealed that the personality characteristics which had been attributed to the hyper-connection syndrome were found particularly in patients with epilepsy and high rates of psychiatric morbidity and thus were likely to be related to mental health pathology rather than to their proposed mechanism. The current view is that the traits found by Bear and Fedio are possibly related to deep bilateral or diffuse cerebral pathology, and thus are closely linked to the brain damage rather than to the epilepsy.

Sexual activity is reduced in men with epilepsy, who have a decreased libido and reduced frequency of marriage. This is likely to be due to reduced testosterone due to low follicular stimulating hormone and luteinizing hormone secreted by the pituitary. The cause of this hyposexuality is thought to be both developmental and due to social factors and to anticonvulsant medication. The situation for women is different. Marriage rates are near normal, possibly because women traditionally play a more passive role in initiating and pursuing stable sexual relationships.

References and recommended reading

Bear DM, Fedio P. Quantitative analysis of interictal behaviour in temporal lobe epilepsy. *Arch Neurol* 1977;**34**(8):454–67.

Cornaggia CM, Begbi M, Provenzi M, Beghi E. Correlation between cognition and behaviour in epilepsy. *Epilepsia* 2006;**47**(Suppl 2):34–9.

Lennox W. *Epilepsy and Related Disorders*. London: Churchill; 1960.

Pond D, Bidwell B. A survey of epilepsy in 14 general practices. II Social and psychological aspects. *Epilepsia* 1960;**1**:285–99.

Rutter M., Tizzard J, Yule W, *et al*. Research report: Isle of Wight studies, 1964–74. *Psychol Med* 1976;**6**(2):313–32.

Scott D, Moffat A, Matthews IA, Ettlinger G. The effect of the epileptic discharges on learning and memory in patients. *Epilepsia* 1967;**8**:188–94.

Swinkel WA, van Emde Boas W, Kuyk J, van Dyck R, Spinhoven P. Interictal depression, anxiety, personality traits, and psychological dissociation in patients with temporal lobe epilepsy (TLE) and extra-TLE. *Epilepsia* 2006;**47**(12):2092–103.

Trimble M, Freeman A. An investigation of religiosity and the Gastaut-Geschwind syndrome in patients with temporal lobe epilepsy. *Epilepsy Behav* 2006;**9**(3):407–14. Epub 2006 Aug 17.

Learning objective

(1) To be aware of and be able to discuss the literature findings regarding personality features found in patients with epilepsy and their causes.

Section 7 Psychiatric, social and legal aspects

Chapter 114

The psychoses of epilepsy

Brian Toone

The 'psychoses of epilepsy' is a term used to denote a group of abnormal mental states associated with epilepsy. Most arise on an organic basis. The term 'psychoses' is something of a misnomer as some of the conditions (e.g. minor status) might better be described as acute confusional states. They fall into two groups: the peri-ictal states and the chronic interictal psychoses (CIIP). The former are brief, spontaneously self-limiting conditions, but liable to recur. They may occur immediately before, in conjunction with, or following seizures and, as such, are clearly in some way a direct consequence of that same activity. The CIIP, particularly the schizophrenia-like psychoses of epilepsy (SLPE), are remitting and relapsing chronic psychoses that are associated with epilepsy but largely run their own course independently of the frequency of seizure activity. Bipolar illness is uncommonly associated with epilepsy.

Pre-ictal states

Although they have received little attention they are not uncommon, occurring in up to 10% of cases of epilepsy. Typically, in the hours or days immediately preceding a seizure, the subject becomes increasingly irritable and lacking in concentration. Symptoms increase until the seizure occurs, after which the mental state returns to normal. It is tempting to speculate that aberrant discharge activity is responsible for the abnormal mental state.

Minor status

Two forms of minor status may result in confusional states. Absence (or petit mal) epilepsy occurs most commonly in children and status may occur in 2.6% of absence sufferers. It presents with an alteration of consciousness that may vary from mere inattention to stupor. It may last for hours or days. Once suspected, the diagnosis is readily confirmed by EEG findings, usually of rhythmic three cycles per second spike and wave. Partial complex status occurs more usually in adults but is very rare. The presentation is varied and may be characterized by confusion and hallucinosis punctuated by motor automatisms. The EEG may be characterized by continuous or intermittent fronto-temporal discharges. Both forms of minor status may be terminated by benzodiazepines.

Other diagnostic terms require clarification. A period of post-ictal drowsiness and confusion commonly follows major seizures, particularly in subjects with extensive brain damage. The EEG dominant rhythm is slowing or low amplitude, sometimes with periods of virtually flat EEG. Twilight states and epileptic fugue states are rather out-moded terms. The former refers to a state of excitement and confusion with hallucinosis. These are usually post-ictal psychoses (see below). The latter refers to brief periods of semi-purposeful behaviour and amnesia that occasionally follows seizure activity, particularly when it arises from temporal lobe foci. It is to be distinguished from episodes of longer duration that are usually dissociative.

Forced normalization is said to occur when, during the successful treatment of seizure activity, psychotic symptoms and behaviour emerge whereas at the same time the EEG becomes more normal. This was first described in association with temporal lobe epilepsy, later with absence seizures and the use of ethosuximide. Alternating psychoses is a term used to describe alternating episodes of psychosis and epilepsy. Psychotic episodes may also be precipitated by some AEDs (e.g. vigabatrin in a dose-dependent manner, and less frequently by topiramate).

Introduction to Epilepsy ed. Gonzalo Alarcón and Antonio Valentín. Published by Cambridge University Press.
© Cambridge University Press 2012.

The two psychoses that occur most commonly in association with epilepsy are the post-ictal psychoses (PIP) and the CIIP, also known as the SLPE. The PIP is an acute psychotic episode that develops abruptly following exacerbations of seizures, particularly of complex partial seizures with or without secondary generalization (Logsdail and Toone, 1988). Typically seizure activity subsides and the subject appears to have completely recovered. After a period of normality that may last hours or days (referred to as the lucid interval), psychotic features emerge characterized by a pleomorphic clinical picture with either excitability or withdrawal, hallucinosis and delusions, particularly of a paranoid content, and confusion. This may last for days up to a couple of weeks and resolve spontaneously. Medication may not be needed but patients are not infrequently violent and may need to be sedated. The EEG may show increased focal discharge activity and functional imaging may demonstrate hyperperfusion suggesting an active process. Post-ictal psychoses occur in less than 5% of epilepsy but are liable to recur. Repeated episodes may gradually evolve into a CIIP picture.

The CIIP, which in many respects resembles schizophrenia, may be seen in individuals with epilepsy. Epilepsy and schizophrenia are both common disorders and it was once thought that the CIIP might arise as a chance association. However, recent epidemiological studies have shown that the two conditions occur 2–3-times more frequently than expected while a clinic-based case control study reported schizophrenia to occur 10-times more commonly in patients with epilepsy compared with those with migraine. CIIP develops on average 15 years after the onset of epilepsy. It is more likely to occur in patients with partial epilepsy, particularly if the focus is in the mesial temporal or frontal lobes. Whether or not there is an increased risk of psychotic illness in the relatives in patients with CIIP has not yet been fully determined: a genetic contribution to risk cannot therefore be entirely disregarded. Neuropathological examination has not been particularly helpful in understanding causation, but there does appear to be a particular association with an uncommon tumour, a ganglioglioma that develops in fetal or early life. When compared with schizophrenia as it manifests itself in a non-epileptic population, CIIP is virtually indistinguishable. There is, however, some suggestion that it is a more benign form of schizophrenia, lacking some of the more negative features (e.g. poverty of thinking and poor self-care) and has a better prognosis. Temporal lobe resection for the treatment of epilepsy does not alter the course of CIIP. Indeed, CIIP can develop following a successful resection of the epileptic focus.

Conclusion

In conclusion, PIP and CIIP are the two principal forms of psychosis associated with epilepsy. They are relatively more common in individuals with partial seizures arising from the mesial fronto-temporal region. Repeated episodes of PIP may eventually evolve into CIIP.

Reference

Logsdail SJ, Toone BK. Post-ictal psychoses: a clinical and phenomenological description. *Brit J Psychiat* 1988;**152**:246–52.

Learning objective

(1) To know the prevalence, clinical features and differential diagnosis of the different types of psychoses that can be seen in patients with epilepsy.

Section 7 Psychiatric, social and legal aspects

Chapter 115: Epilepsy and aggression

Peter Fenwick

Patients with epilepsy are commonly thought to be aggressive. A survey in Australia showed that over 60% of the general population believed this to be true. However, matched control groups do not support this view, and with continuing education this perception is slowly changing.

Although aggression is not a general characteristic of epilepsy, it can occur, either in the prodrome, during the ictus, or post-ictally. It can also occur interictally.

During the prodrome many patients are irritable and dysphoric, which may lead to aggressive behaviour. However, it is unlikely that the aggression will be violent and it usually consists of an intensification of continuing interpersonal conflicts.

Ictal aggression is rare, but it does occur. Aggressive acts during a fit are unprovoked and out of character. Although they may seem to be highly coordinated they occur in a confused mental state and are inappropriate to the situation. The behaviour may be the first clinical manifestation of the seizure, and may develop as the seizure progresses. This behaviour is almost always associated with complex partial seizures, although there may be later secondary generalization. Witnesses report that the patient was confused and had glazed eyes. Usually the attack consists of pushing and shoving, though there are reports in the literature of vicious directed violence. The attack has no specific trigger but seems to arise out of the blue and terminates as the seizure progresses. Afterwards the patient is confused and will have little or no memory of the episode. Ictal aggression is less likely to be seen in hospital than in the community, where social tensions are more common. Studies of ictal aggression in hospital will thus underrate its frequency.

Directed ictal aggression occurs when seizure discharges involve the limbic system bilaterally. In patients with implanted electrodes aggressive behaviour has been reported when seizure discharges invade the amygdala.

Post-ictal aggression is very common and takes many forms. It usually occurs either during a post-ictal automatism or during a post-ictal confusional state and sometimes these two mental states overlap. Patients returning to consciousness after a generalized seizure are confused. They make clumsy movements and with a further return of consciousness stand up and walk around in a confused state. They may become resentful if people interfere with them and, in this confusional state, push them away or strike them. Attempts to restrain them only make matters worse and they may become more aggressive and strike out more strongly. Holding patients down after a seizure often results in an aggressive response, whereas giving them space leads to a reduction in their aggressive behaviour.

Post-ictal automatisms usually follow complex partial seizures and during this phase violent behaviour may occur. The patient will be confused and may lash out if approached, especially if restrained. Significant violence in this state is rare but sometimes occurs in units which specialize in patients with severe epilepsy and behaviour disorder. Occasionally patients may be very aggressive and destroy furniture and seriously injure their family if the appropriate avoidance action is not taken. As the confusional state wanes, and automatisms become more complex, the patients' behaviour merges into normality and significant aggression is less likely. During the confusional state after a generalized seizure, the EEG is dominated by delta activity. Automatisms and aggressive activity

---

Introduction to Epilepsy ed. Gonzalo Alarcón and Antonio Valentín. Published by Cambridge University Press.
© Cambridge University Press 2012.

occurring during this time are psychoparetic. This means that there is a dysfunction of the normal psychic mechanisms maintaining consciousness and normal behaviour.

Post-ictal psychosis usually arises after a flurry of complex partial seizures or secondarily generalized seizures, and usually has a confusional element. The majority of schizophreniform post-ictal psychoses have a marked paranoid element. Two to three days after the seizure, the patient becomes intensely paranoid, suspicious and may auditorily hallucinate. Occasionally they may act out their paranoid state by acting impulsively, usually in fear of their lives, jumping through windows ignoring the height of the building, or, less frequently, attacking other people on the ward. Because of these risks, a post-ictal psychosis should always be nursed in hospital.

Interictal aggression is not a unitary syndrome and may be the result of a patient's underlying personality, anxiety, family background and circumstances. Mungus (1983), by means of cluster analysis, showed that in only two of five clusters of aggressive neuropsychiatric out-patients was the aggression related to epilepsy. A study at the Maudsley showed that violent individuals tend to come from violent families and show a long history of violent behaviour since childhood, and are most frequently men under the age of 40 with a large number of soft neurological signs and abnormal EEGs. They are frequently cognitively impaired and show a high proportion of left-handers. They may also have poor attention span and occasionally focal cognitive deficits. They tend to come from the lower socio-economic groups where there are higher levels of perinatal mortality, infections and trauma. When these factors are taken into account, many of the associations of aggression and violence with epilepsy become weaker.

References and recommended reading

Brower M Price B. Epilepsy and violence: when is the brain to blame? *Epilepsy Behav* 2000;**1**(3):145–9.

Fenwick P. Episodic dyscontrol. In Engel J, Pedley T, eds. *Epilepsy, a Comprehensive Textbook,* Ch. 266. Philadelphia: Lippincott-Raven; 1997.

Marsh L, Kraus G. Aggression and violence in patients with epilepsy. *Epilepsy Behav* 2003;**1**(3):160–8.

Mungus D. An empirical analysis of specific syndromes of violent behaviour. *J Nerv Mental Dis* 1983;**171**:354–61.

Learning objective

(1) To know the prevalence, causes, clinical features and differential diagnosis of the different types of aggression episodes that can be seen in patients with epilepsy.

Section 7 Psychiatric, social and legal aspects

Chapter 116: Epilepsy in childhood: effects on behaviour and mental health

Sarah H. Bernard

Introduction

Children with epilepsy are more likely to have behavioural or mental health problems. They are also more likely to have developmental disabilities.

When assessing behavioural problems in children with epilepsy, it is important to understand the underlying nature and cause of the epilepsy. In addition, early treatment of epilepsy is important in order to reduce the risks of behavioural problems and intellectual difficulties.

The causes of childhood epilepsy involve detailed paediatric/neurological investigation.

Behavioural disorders

Behavioural disorders occurring in association with childhood epilepsy are multi-factorial. There are many causes of behavioural problems which are associated with childhood epilepsy including:

- the epilepsy itself;
- the treatment of the epilepsy;
- the reactions to the epilepsy;
- associated brain damage;
- coincidental causes.

There are also many causes of developmental disabilities, which increase the likelihood of behavioural difficulties. Some are common to the underlying cause of the epilepsy, whilst others are discrete. These include:

- chromosomal disorder or genetic defect (e.g. Retts syndrome, Down syndrome);
- structural abnormality of the brain;
- metabolic disorder;
- injury and trauma;
- infection (e.g. encephalitis).

Causes of behavioural problems
The epilepsy itself

- The type of epilepsy: temporal lobe epilepsy is more likely to result in behavioural disturbances than idiopathic generalized epilepsy.
- Brain dysfunction.
- Pre-ictal (e.g. aura which alters emotional state).
- Peri-ictal disturbances (e.g. temporal lobe epilepsy producing automatisms).
- Interictal disturbances (e.g. increased risk of psychotic phenomena).
- Focal discharges.
- Generalized discharges.

The treatment of the epilepsy

- Side effects of medication: phenytoin and phenobarbitone are associated with behavioural problems. Vigabatrin can alter mood. Lamotrigine can improve behavioural disturbances and some anticonvulsants act as mood stabilizers (sodium valproate, carbamazepine).

The reactions to the epilepsy

- Stigma.
- Responses of parents.
- Responses of teachers.
- Response of child.
- Effects of chronic illness.
- Frequent hospitalizations.

The social stigma associated with epilepsy influences psychosocial development and increases the risk of behavioural/mental health problems. In addition, the burden of stress on the family can affect parent–child

---

Introduction to Epilepsy ed. Gonzalo Alarcón and Antonio Valentín. Published by Cambridge University Press.
© Cambridge University Press 2012.

relationships, which, in turn, may relate to behavioural disturbance.

At school the child might be isolated from peers, teased and bullied. Other children (and their parents) might be fearful of the child. The child might experience long absences from school as a result of the epilepsy. Teachers' expectations might differ from those for a child without epilepsy, and the child might be excluded from certain activities which are deemed to pose a risk.

All these factors impact on the child's overall behaviour and should be considered as part of a comprehensive assessment.

Associated brain damage

- Hypoxia
- Injury

Coincidental causes

- All causes of childhood behavioural problems.
- Abuse/neglect.

The child with epilepsy is not protected from all the other factors which normally influence childhood behaviour and mental health.

Assessment

- Full history: parents, teachers, carers, child.
- Interview child.
- Observe child: home, school, structured setting.
- Information from paediatrician/neurologist.
- Functional assessment.
- Speech and language assessment.
- Psychometry.
- Physical investigations in collaboration with paediatrician/neurologist.

In order to manage behavioural or mental health problems in children with epilepsy, it is essential that a comprehensive assessment is undertaken. Such an assessment will involve a number of disciplines and agencies.

The nature of the behavioural disturbance should be considered, as well as any precipitants. Informant and direct observations are essential as is an assessment of the child's intellectual level and the functions served by the behaviour.

Assessments will, in part, take place in the setting the child experiences problems (school, home or respite care settings which the child accesses).

Physical investigations should be offered, if indicated, in collaboration with the child's paediatrician and neurologist.

Management

- Control of epilepsy: medication/other.
- Medication for childhood psychiatric disorder/behaviour.
- Behavioural programme.
- Appropriate education.
- Respite.

It is important that children with epilepsy are able to access specialist epilepsy services. Such services should include psychological assessment and interventions for the child and their family. There should also be a clear means of accessing specialist child psychiatric provision (CAMHS), which will be required by a proportion of children with epilepsy.

The plan of management of behavioural/mental health problems should be agreed with the family, healthcare professionals and the school. This plan, and the implementation of behavioural programmes, must be consistent.

Behavioural difficulties should be considered as part of the regular review offered to children with epilepsy.

Behavioural interventions are more likely to succeed if commenced early rather than when behavioural problems have become ingrained.

If medication is indicated it is important that the family are aware of the indications for its use and any possible side effects which might be experienced. The medication should be monitored by trained professionals such as a school nurse, epilepsy nurse or a community mental health worker.

The child requires appropriate educational provision in an environment that understands and can manage epilepsy. Any developmental delay should be addressed and education planned accordingly.

Families who have a child with a chronic illness such as epilepsy experience significant stress. Respite care should be forthcoming and adapted to the needs of the child and their family.

Recommended reading

Besag FMC. Childhood epilepsy in relation to mental handicap and behavioural disorders. *J Child Psychol Psychiat* 2002;43(1):103–31.

Learning objectives

(1) To know the behavioural disorders associated with epilepsy and their causes.
(2) To know the investigations required to assess behavioural disorders in epilepsy, and their interpretation.
(3) To understand the management of behavioural disorders in epilepsy.

Section 7 Psychiatric, social and legal aspects

Chapter 117 Psychogenic non-epileptic (dissociative) seizures: psychiatric aspects

John D. C. Mellers

The investigation and neurological assessment of psychogenic, non-epileptic seizures is covered in Chapter 56 ('Psychogenic non-epileptic seizures: diagnostic approach'). The current chapter covers clinical and psychiatric aspects of the disorder.

What are dissociative seizures?

Dissociative seizures (DS) are psychologically mediated episodes of altered awareness and/or behaviour that may mimic any type of epilepsy. After syncope, they are the most common cause of diagnostic error in epilepsy and up to one in five referrals to specialist epilepsy clinics will be found to have DS. The term DS is preferred to older terms such as pseudoseizures, hysterical seizures, non-epileptic attacks which are pejorative or lack any widely agreed definition.

DS are regarded, by definition (in ICD 10), as being involuntary or unconscious. This concept is, however, difficult for some clinicians to accept and is probably impossible to prove. For those who doubt the unconscious nature of these episodes, three characteristics of these patients are worth considering:

- the majority of patients are compliant with their antiepileptic drugs, often for many years and sometimes to the point of toxicity;
- when they are admitted for telemetry the majority have a seizure in a setting which they must surely recognize is intensively monitored;
- the seizure is usually a poor imitation of epilepsy.

None of these points is by any means conclusive but if deception is involved, it is of a kind that is difficult to understand. Most experienced clinicians agree that the majority of patients with these seizures are not deliberately fabricating their symptoms.

Occasionally, however, patients are encountered who one strongly suspects are 'putting on' their seizures. In this situation, a diagnosis of factitious disorder (Munchausen's syndrome) is appropriate when the patient's motivation appears to be some psychological gratification derived from adopting the sick role. The term malingering, which is not actually a medical diagnosis, should be reserved for patients who seem to be feigning illness for some obvious practical advantage (e.g. compensation, to avoid a criminal conviction or military service, etc.).

The term dissociation means a psychologically mediated altered state of awareness and/or control over neurological functioning. Normal examples of dissociation, such as 'domestic deafness', illustrate how our awareness of our surroundings can be changed unconsciously (and psychologically) and provide useful examples for discussing DS with patients and their families.

Clinical features of dissociative seizures

The prevalence of DS has been estimated as between 2 and 33 per 100 000. Around three-quarters of patients are female. Seizures typically begin in the late teens or early twenties, but there is a wide range. There is usually a delay of 3 or 4 years before the correct diagnosis is made. Probably no more than 15 or 20% of patients with DS also have epilepsy.

Clinical semiology

No single semiological feature can be relied upon to distinguish DS from epileptic seizures. The most helpful features, as well as some common misconceptions, are listed in Table 117.1. Epileptic seizures are brief, highly stereotyped, paroxysmal alterations in

---

Introduction to Epilepsy ed. Gonzalo Alarcón and Antonio Valentín. Published by Cambridge University Press.
© Cambridge University Press 2012.

Table 117.1. Comparative semiology of dissociative and epileptic seizures

	Dissociative seizures	Epileptic seizures
Duration over 2 minutes	Common	Rare
Recall for a period of unresponsiveness	Common	Very rare
Motor features		
Gradual onset	Common	Rare
Eyes closed	Common	Rare
Thrashing, violent movements	Common	Rare
Side to side head movement	Common	Rare
Pelvic thrusting	Occasional	Rare
Opisthotonus, 'arc de cercle'	Occasional	Very rare
Fluctuating course	Common	Very rare
Automatisms	Rare	Common
Weeping	Occasional	Very rare
Incontinence[a]	Occasional	Common
Injury[a]		
Biting inside of mouth	Occasional	Common
Severe tongue-biting	Very rare	Common
Stereotyped attacks[a]	Common	Common

[a] Three features that are commonly misinterpreted as evidence for epilepsy have been included. Otherwise the table lists clinical features that are useful in distinguishing DS from ES. Figures for frequency of these features are approximate: common > 30%; occasional = 10–30%; rare < 10%; very rare < 5%.

neurological function that conform to a number of now well-described syndromes. Broadly speaking, it is any variation from these clinical pictures – an atypical sequence of events – that will raise the suspicion of DS.

Ictal observation/examination

An opportunity to observe a seizure may provide invaluable information. If the patient's eyes are shut (an important observation in itself, suggesting DS) the examiner should attempt to open them, noting any resistance. If the eyes can be held open easily, evidence of visual fixation may be sought by holding a small mirror in front of the patient, looking for evidence of convergent gaze and fixation on the reflection. This procedure will also often stop the seizure.

Psychiatric co-morbidity

Depression, anxiety, personality disorder and post-traumatic disorder have been reported in patients with DS, but prevalence rates have varied considerably. Many predisposing, triggering and maintaining factors for DS have been described. A disturbed family environment and abuse are common, as is a history of bullying. Many patients have a history of previous medically unexplained symptoms, suggesting a tendency to express emotional distress with physical symptoms (somatization). Sometimes DS occur as a reaction to acute emotional distress but usually no triggers are apparent to the patient. Many patients and their carers will report confusing and sometimes distressing 'confrontations' with medical and paramedical services which only serve to heighten their anxiety, frustration and anger. Carers often become overprotective and inadvertently perpetuate symptoms. If the diagnosis goes unrecognized for years, patients and their families adapt to a life of disability which may be very difficult to change.

Management

An early diagnosis (within a year of onset) and the way in which the diagnosis is conveyed to the patient are probably the two most important factors determining outcome. Points that might be covered in discussing the diagnosis with a patient are outlined in Table 117.2.

There have been no controlled treatment trials in DS. Pharmacotherapy is appropriate for the relatively small proportion of patients with significant psychiatric co-morbidity. For the majority, however, some form of psychological treatment is recommended. Involvement of carers is important in view of the role the patient's social environment may play in perpetuating the disorder. Cognitive behavioural therapy, a well-established treatment for many psychiatric disorders, can be adapted for patients with DS and preliminary evidence suggests that it is effective. AED withdrawal in patients with no epileptic seizures should be gradual and may in itself be therapeutic.

Table 117.2. Presenting the diagnosis of dissociative seizures

The discussion should cover:

1. Explanation of the diagnosis
   - Reasons for concluding they don't have epilepsy
   - What they do have (describe dissociation)
2. Reassurance
   - They are not suspected of 'putting on' the attacks
   - The disorder is very common
3. Causes of the disorder
   - Triggering 'stresses' may not be immediately apparent
   - Relevance of aetiological factors in their case
   - Maintaining factors
4. Treatment
   - DS may improve simply following correct diagnosis
   - Caution that AED withdrawal should be gradual
   - Describe psychological treatments

Long-term, approximately two-thirds of patients will continue to suffer ongoing DS 3 or more years after diagnosis, with more than half remaining dependent on social security. Psychiatric treatment has been associated with a positive outcome in some studies, but not all. A poor prognosis is predicted by a long delay in diagnosis and the presence of severe psychiatric co-morbidity.

Recommended reading

Mellers JDC. The diagnosis and management of dissociative seizures (2007). www.e-epilepsy.org.uk/pages/articles/pdfs/Chapter20Mellers.pdf.

Reuber M. Psychogenic nonepileptic seizures: answers and questions. *Epilepsy Behav* 2008;**12**:622–35.

Learning objectives

(1) To understand the concept and definition of non-epileptic (dissociative) seizures.
(2) To know the clinical features of dissociative seizures and how to distinguish them from those of epilepsy.
(3) To know the psychiatric co-morbidity associated with dissociative seizures.
(4) To know what to discuss when confronted with the diagnosis of dissociative seizures.
(5) To understand the principles of the management of dissociative seizures.

Section 7: Psychiatric, social and legal aspects

Chapter 118: Psychiatric effects of surgical treatment for epilepsy

Richard P. Selway

It is natural that there should be concerns that brain surgery for epilepsy may have effects beyond that on the seizures. It is, however, difficult to study the psychiatric effects of epilepsy surgery due to pre-existing issues, drug adjustments, social impact and changing effects over time.

Patients considered for epilepsy surgery often suffer considerable psychiatric co-morbidity. Anxiety and depression are the commonest diagnoses in this group, constituting, depending on diagnostic criteria, up to half. Severe epilepsy is also associated with more florid psychosis. Disturbance can be interictal or directly associated with the seizures, with abnormal ictal behaviour. Post-ictal psychosis may occur following seizures and can constitute a major cause of morbidity in some.

Psychiatric disturbance in epilepsy may have multiple causes. The brain may be structurally abnormal and this may result in both conditions. Similarly seizures, and the drugs used to treat them, result in changes in brain chemistry which could produce secondary psychiatric problems. Perhaps most importantly, epilepsy produces social disadvantage and stigma that may predispose to psychiatric illness.

Overall, if one compares the incidence of psychiatric disease in preoperative and postoperative surgery patients, the figures are strikingly similar. There does appear to be a short-term increase in depression rates following temporal lobe resections. However, this condition is of varying time-course and often settles within the first year. Depression is often associated with major life events (e.g. bereavement, moving house, changing job) and surgery is obviously such an occasion. Another explanation may be the unmet expectations of surgery. Patients often assume that life will be much improved by abolishing the seizures, but may find that much of the social disadvantage remains. For example, older adults undergoing surgery after long-standing severe epilepsy may not find their job prospects improve significantly. There is also some evidence that the risk of depression in epilepsy correlates with hippocampal volume. Those with temporal lobe epilepsy often have small total hippocampal volume and this obviously is further reduced if one hippocampus is removed at surgery, perhaps explaining the postoperative increase in depression rates.

Much morbidity from epilepsy comes not from the seizures themselves, but from the risk that a seizure might occur. Social exclusion and anxiety result from this risk, even if seizures are quite rare. Unfortunately, following surgery, the chance of seizure freedom is not 100%, and patients may experience similar levels of such risk perception even if no actual seizures occur. Surprisingly there is little evidence that even post-ictal psychosis is improved by successful surgery.

In summary, patients considered for surgery have a high level of psychiatric morbidity. Apart from a short-term increase in depression following an operation, surgery seems to have little effect on this co-existing pathology.

Learning objective

(1) To know the psychiatric effects of surgical treatment for epilepsy and their frequency according to surgical procedure.

Introduction to Epilepsy ed. Gonzalo Alarcón and Antonio Valentín. Published by Cambridge University Press.
© Cambridge University Press 2012.

Section 7 Psychiatric, social and legal aspects

Chapter 119

Use of psychotropics in people with epilepsy

Nozomi Akanuma

People with epilepsy have increased risk of developing psychiatric disorders compared with the general population (Gaitatzis et al., 2004). Co-morbid psychiatric disorders in epilepsy have a negative impact on the quality of life, and the use of psychotropic drugs is often necessary and beneficial. Appropriate psychotropic treatment may not only improve the mental state, but also positively influence seizure frequency and severity (Pisani et al., 2002).

Antipsychotics are drugs that are used to treat schizophrenia and other psychotic disorders. They can also be used for mania, severe depression or anxiety. The older generation of antipsychotics are called 'typical' antipsychotics, which block post-synaptic D_2 receptors. The antipsychotic in the second generation are known as 'atypical' antipsychotics, which block serotonin $5HT_2$ receptors as well as D_2 receptors.

Antidepressants are drugs that alleviate symptoms of moderate to severe depression. They are also used to treat anxiety disorders. They increase the overall level of monoamines at synapses by decreasing either re-uptake or breakdown.

Mood stabilizers are drugs that are used in the treatment of mania, prophylaxis of bipolar disorders and augmentation of antidepressants. They include lithium and some anticonvulsive drugs, such as carbamazepine, valproate and lamotrigine. Table 119.1 summarizes psychotropic drugs.

Special considerations for use of psychotropic drugs in epilepsy
Effects on seizure threshold

Some antipsychotic and antidepressants are recognized as having a propensity to lower the seizure threshold, a concern that may lead to under-treatment of co-morbid psychiatric conditions in people with epilepsy. The incidence of seizures associated with psychotropics varies from 0.1% up to 30% (Pisani et al., 2002), the higher values usually reported from cases with drug overdoses. Recent analysis of clinical trial data shows that the incident of seizures at therapeutic doses of commonly used psychotropics lies between 0 and 0.5% with an exception of a subset of psychotropics (Forsgren et al., 2005) (see below). These rates should be interpreted with caution in comparison to those for newly onset seizures/epilepsy. For reference, the annual incidence of first seizures in the general population is estimated at 0.073–0.086%, the prevalence of active epilepsy in adults under the age of 65 is 0.6%, and its annual incidence is 0.03% (Forsgren et al., 2005).

Various predisposing factors contribute to drug-induced seizures and these factors may be either drug- or individual-related. Proconvulsant effects are well known for some psychotropic drugs (Pisani et al., 2002; Forsgren et al., 2005; Montgomery, 2005; Taylor et al., 2009). The risk of seizures with tricyclic antidepressants at effective therapeutic doses is relatively high (0.4–2%). The risk with SSRIs is considered low at therapeutic levels (up to 0.4%) without clear difference between drugs. The association of clozapine with increased risk of seizures risk at therapeutic serum levels is well established. Chlorpromazine and zotepine are also known to have pro convulsive effects. Among the newer atypical psychotropics, olanzapine and quetiapine appear to mediate higher seizure incidence. For the remaining typical and atypical antipsychotics, their 'Summary of Produce Characteristics' state generic precautions for use in people with a history of seizures or other conditions that potentially lower seizure threshold.

Depot preparations (slow release of the active drug given as an intramuscular injection) are currently available for seven antipsychotics, two of which

---

Introduction to Epilepsy ed. Gonzalo Alarcón and Antonio Valentín. Published by Cambridge University Press.
© Cambridge University Press 2012.

Section 7: Psychiatric, social and legal aspects

Table 119.1. Psychotropic drugs

Type	Class	Examples
Antipsychotics	Typical	Haloperidol Chlorpromazine Trifluoperazine
	Atypical	Risperidone Olanzapine Quetiapine Amisulpride Aripiprazole Zotepine Clozapine
Antidepressants	Selective serotonin reuptake inhibitors (SSRIs)	Fluoxetine Sertraline Paroxetine Fluvoxamine Citalopram Escitalopram
	Serotonin-norepinephrine reuptake inhibitors (SNRIs)	Venlafaxine Duloxetine
	Noradrenaline and specific serotoninergic antidepressants (NASSAs)	Mirtazapine
	Noradrenaline reuptake inhibitors (NARIs)	Reboxetine
	Tricyclic antidepressants (TCAs)	Amitriptyline Clomipramine Imipramine Lofepramine Dosulepin
	Monoamine oxidase inhibitors (MAOIs)	Phenelzine Tranylcypromine
	Reversible inhibitors of monoamine oxidase A (RIMAs)	Moclobemide
	Tetracyclic antidepressants (TeCAs)	Trazodone
Mood stabilizers	Anticonvulsants	Carbamazepine Valproate Lamotrigine
	Other	Lithium

are atypical (Risperidone microspheres and Olanzapine pamoate). Although none of them are known to be highly epileptogenic, depot antipsychotics should be used with extreme caution in people with epilepsy, as the pharmacokinetics of depots are complex and withdrawing the drug may be difficult once seizures occur (Taylor et al., 2009).

Seizures associated with psychotropics are in principle dose-related adverse events. Conditions leading to high plasma level of psychotropics or metabolites, such as drug overdoses, rapid titration or concurrent use of drugs that inhibit metabolism, are likely to increase the risk.

Individual susceptibility to seizures should also be taken into account:
- history of previous seizures and/or abnormal EEG findings prior to starting psychotropics;
- presence of brain damage and head injury, learning disability, alcohol/substance abuse and withdrawal, or dementia;
- family history of a seizure disorder;
- reduced renal/hepatic capacity for eliminating drugs.

Reported seizure incidence in the placebo arms of clinical trials for antidepressants and antipsychotics was greater (7–19-times) in patients with psychotic disorders, depression and obsessive-compulsive disorder than the reported rates of unprovoked seizures in the general population, suggesting that psychiatric disorders themselves are associated with increased risk for seizures (Alper et al., 2007).

Pharmacokinetic interactions

Pharmacokinetic interactions between AEDs and psychotropics are common and usually involve changes in the activity of cytochromes P450 (CYPs) (Spina and Perucca, 2002). As a consequence of CYP inhibition or induction with concurrently administered drugs, plasma concentrations of the drug of interest could be increased or lowered, potentially resulting in adverse events or reduced efficacy. Monitoring of serum levels of AEDs and psychotropics (where possible) is useful and dosage adjustment may be required.

Enzyme-inducing AEDs, such as carbamazepine and phenytoin, may decrease the plasma concentrations of tricyclic antidepressants and many antipsychotics. In contrast, newer AEDs appear to have a lower potential for interactions with psychotropic drugs.

Some SSRIs, such as fluoxetine, paroxetine, sertraline and citalopram, are believed to inhibit CYP enzymes, increasing plasma levels of carbamazepine and phenytoin.

General rules to use psychotropics in people with epilepsy

There are few systematic studies on the effectiveness of psychotropics in people with epilepsy (Farooq and Sherin, 2008). While being cautious with the issues mentioned above, pharmacological treatment should be considered for psychiatric conditions in people with epilepsy whenever clinically indicated. Treatment will be commenced at low doses, titrated slowly to an optimized level and continued for a recommended period for both acute treatment and subsequent maintenance and prophylaxis. Other medication known to reduce seizure threshold should be avoided if possible.

References

Alper K, Schwartz KA, Kolts RL, Khan A. Seizure incidence in psychopharmacological clinical trials: an analysis of Food and Drug Administration (FDA) summary basis of approval reports. *Biol Psychiatry* 2007;**62**:345–54.

Farooq S, Sherin A. Interventions for psychotic symptoms concomitant with epilepsy. *Cochrane Database Syst Rev.* 2008;(**4**):CD006118.

Forsgren L, Beghi E, Oun A, Sillanpaa M. The epidemiology of epilepsy in Europe – a systematic review. *Eur J Neurol* 2005;**12**:245–53.

Gaitatzis A, Trimble MR, Sander JW. The psychiatric comorbidity of epilepsy. *Acta Neurol Scand* 2004; **10**:207–20.

Montgomery SA. Antidepressants and seizures: emphasis on newer agents and clinical implications. *Int J Clin Pract* 2005;**59**:1435–40.

Pisani F, Oteri G, Costa C, Di Raimondo G, Di Perri R. Effects of psychotropic drugs on seizure threshold. *Drug Safety* 2002;**25**:91–110.

Spina E, Perucca E. Clinical significance of pharmacokinetic interactions between antiepileptic and psychotropic drugs. *Epilepsia* 2002;**45**(Suppl 2):7–44.

Taylor D, Paton C, Kapur S (eds). Depression and psychosis in epilepsy. In *The Maudsley Prescribing Guidelines*, pp. 335–8. 10th edn. London: Informa Healthcare; 2009.

Learning objectives

(1) To know the definition, indications and examples of antipsychotics, antidepressants and mood stabilizers.
(2) To know the effects of psychotropic drugs on seizure threshold, and risk of seizures associated with their use at therapeutic doses.
(3) To know the factors increasing the risk of having seizures in patients taking antipsychotics.
(4) To be aware of the main pharmacological interactions between psychotropic agents and other drugs, particularly with reference to antiepileptic drugs.
(5) To know the guidelines on the use of psychotropic drugs in patients with epilepsy.

Section 7 Psychiatric, social and legal aspects

Chapter 120

Time-limited psychodynamic counselling for people with epilepsy

Shiri Spector

Psychodynamic counselling is one of many 'talking therapies' aimed at helping people explore and reflect on aspects of their life at present, and make links to past events and early personal experiences. The focus in counselling for people with epilepsy is an understanding of the relationship between seizures and other aspects of life, both past and present, and between the person's psychological and physical experiences (Cregeen, 1993).

At the basis of my approach to epilepsy counselling is the understanding that epilepsy is a neurological condition. However, the loss of control over body or mind and the unpredictability of seizures can have a significant emotional and psychological impact. In my work, the aim of counselling is not to alleviate seizures but to help patients who experience psychological difficulties to explore the place of epilepsy and seizures in the dynamics of their relationships, their life and their internal world. I consider Steenbarger's (1992) suggestion that time-limited therapy is particularly appropriate when there is a history of successful interpersonal functioning, a specific issue with a recent onset and a person who is motivated and with self-awareness of his/her distress.

This chapter aims to describe some themes and issues which arise in counselling for patients with epilepsy, and help other professionals think more systematically about the various emotional struggles that patients are faced with.

The timing of the onset of epilepsy is often a significant issue. For example, adolescence is a time when young people are considering their own identity, sexuality and independence. Epilepsy can disrupt this process. Parental over-protectiveness and social restrictions are common reactions to epilepsy, and often result in subsequent lower levels of confidence and self-esteem in adolescents (and later adults) with epilepsy. Onset of epilepsy in later life often involves loss. The loss of independence, physical well-being, self-confidence and self-reliance can be as acute and tangible as the loss of a driving licence or a job. As with any loss, mourning and depression are common possible reactions.

Another common issue is one of privacy and secrecy. For many people with epilepsy there seems to be a confusion regarding whether they are not discussing their epilepsy because it is a private matter, or hiding it because it is a bad secret. Such confusion often perpetuates a deep sense of shame and guilt which can be understood and resolved in therapy.

Many people with epilepsy find the physical experience of seizures difficult to share or to describe. Many patients have asked me if I had epilepsy, and expressed their doubts regarding my ability to understand what it's like to have epilepsy if I do not experience it myself. Counselling can be important in helping people learn to talk about their epilepsy, but also acknowledge and tolerate the loneliness of not being able to share the experience in full.

Epilepsy may also evoke high levels of anxiety. Everyday fear of physical injury or embarrassment is often compounded with fear of madness and fear of death. Many patients in therapy initially link their anxiety entirely to their epilepsy. Epilepsy thus tends to become the focus around which the patient builds his/her story. In a paradoxical way, the aim of counselling for people with epilepsy is, in many cases, to steer the person away from thinking about his/her epilepsy, and to try to explore events and themes that may have preceded the onset of seizures. Some brief examples of this follow.

- Peter, a young man in his 20s, came to counselling following serious anger-management issues at work. He is the youngest of nine and one of twins.

Introduction to Epilepsy ed. Gonzalo Alarcón and Antonio Valentín. Published by Cambridge University Press.
© Cambridge University Press 2012.

He was born with congenital problems that made him look odd and developed epilepsy. In therapy he realized that he sometimes used his seizures to get sympathy, to perpetuate injustice and to bully others.
- Ruth is a scientist in her 30s, an only child, born very premature to older parents. She was marked as precious and fragile, and thus had to incorporate into her identity a sense of being physically strong and whole. She was feeling increasingly depressed and vulnerable because of her recent onset of epilepsy and in therapy worked to understand this and find a way to redefine herself.
- Simon, a businessman, father of two, 45 years old and recently diagnosed with epilepsy, was struggling with extreme feelings of inadequacy and anxiety. As a child he had disapproving and critical parents, and realized he developed his own punitive and harsh 'internal parent'. In the counselling sessions we linked his anxiety about his epilepsy to his long-standing anxieties about feeling damaged and worthless.

Conclusion

Being a neurological condition, epilepsy is treated predominantly within the domain of the medical profession, with a focus on seizure type and frequency, drug dosage and side effects. Counselling for people with epilepsy can help with a variety of issues such as the psychological struggle of adjusting to a chronic illness, family adjustment problems, social prejudice and stigma, and issues relating to sexuality, childbearing and parenthood. Psychodynamic counselling allows the exploration of the conscious and unconscious meanings of seizures and the way in which these, rather than the seizures themselves, may be resolved.

Recommended reading

Cregeen S. Making sense: Brain trauma, epileptic seizures and personal meaning. *Psychodynam Psychother* 1996; **10**(1):33–44.

Freud S. *Dostoevsky and Parricide*. Standard edn 21, 1928.

Greenson RR. On genuine epilepsy. *Psychoanal Q* 1944;**13**:139–59.

Miller L. Psychotherapy of epilepsy: seizure control and psychosocial adjustment. *J Cognitive Rehab* 1994; **12**(1):14–30.

References

Cregeen S. Epileptic seizures and infantile states: Some thoughts from psychodynamic therapy. *Seizure* 1993; **2**(4):291–4.

Steenbarger BN. Towards science-practice integration in brief counselling and therapy. *Couns Psychol*, 1992; **20**:403–50.

Learning objective

(1) To know the principles, objectives, indications and efficacy of psychodynamic counselling for people with epilepsy.

Section 7: Psychiatric, social and legal aspects

Chapter 121: Evaluation of quality of life in epilepsy

Jennifer Nightingale

Health-related quality of life (HRQOL) is a concept that has caused much debate and for which there are varying interpretations and definitions available. Shipper defines HRQOL as 'the functional impact of an illness and its consequential therapy upon the patient, as perceived by the patient'.

The social and psychological impact of seizures has been well known for centuries but the study of QOL in epilepsy has only occurred in recent history. Prior to the 1980s, epilepsy management was mainly concerned with seizure control and did not take into account how patients felt or their ability to carry out daily activities. Since then, a number of HRQOL tools have been developed, allowing clinicians a more holistic view of treatment and management. This chapter will outline the broad concepts and scales used to measure HRQOL in epilepsy.

There are four main HRQOL measures:

- generic
- disease-specific
- global and
- cost utility.

The most commonly used measures in epilepsy are generic and disease-specific.

Generic

These are broad measures, which are useful when comparing other patient populations such as comparison with other chronic conditions. Many of the difficulties identified by people with epilepsy mirror those of other chronic conditions, particularly asthma and diabetes, allowing useful comparisons. The generic nature of the models does not allow one to study or detect subtle aspects of those with epilepsy, such as the impact of stigma. Two of the most commonly used generic models are the Rand 36-Item Health Survey and the Nottingham Health profile. Often a generic model is used in tandem with a disease-specific component. Generic studies can be useful in the context of health policy.

Disease-specific

These are more sensitive tools often only able to address a narrow range of issues. This also means it can be difficult to relate data from one tool to another. Epilepsy is complex and has specific areas of study interest, for example, the psychological impacts, such as fear of seizures, stigma and socio-economic limitations which are not addressed in generic scales. Again the vast majority of scales developed in epilepsy use a generic core with disease-specific items. Several authors have reported that disease-specific measures or epilepsy-targeted measures are generally more responsive

Although authors place varying importance upon differing aspects of epilepsy, the majority are in agreement that the following domains are essential when studying HRQOL in epilepsy:

(1) Physical health: identifying the effect that an illness and its treatment have on the patient's ability to carry out daily tasks.
(2) Pyschological health: the emotional impact of the illness (e.g. mood, self-esteem and perception of well-being).
(3) Social health: the interaction of the person with others (e.g. social activities and relationships).
(4) Economic: impact of the illness/treatment on socio-economic status (e.g. ability to gain employment).

Introduction to Epilepsy ed. Gonzalo Alarcón and Antonio Valentín. Published by Cambridge University Press.
© Cambridge University Press 2012.

The design of any study or tool will be dependent on the research question but the following outcome measures of HRQOL tools in epilepsy may include:
- Physical:
  - increased morbidity
  - increased mortality-SUDEP
  - increased risk of suicide
  - adverse effects of AED
- Social:
  - social isolation
  - marriage rates
  - interaction with peers
- Epilepsy-specific:
  - seizure type
  - age of onset
  - seizure duration
  - seizure severity
  - impact of AED
  - underlying aetiology
  - seizure frequency

Physical and psychological impact of seizures and treatment and their impact on QOL

The diagnosis of epilepsy, seizures themselves, and the impact of treatment can have a profound affect on patients' QOL.

Psychological impact of the diagnosis and seizures

The psychological impact of epilepsy is far-reaching. Social stigma and limitations related to employment, social and leisure activities could result in poor quality of life. People report increased rates of social isolation and experience difficulty developing and maintaining relationships. This increased social withdrawal and potential hypo-sexuality can often result in lower levels of marriage and children in comparison with the normal population.

Often economic productivity is affected, resulting in a reduced earning potential. This in turn increases dependency and can result in low self-esteem and depression. A large number of patients will report anxiety or depressive symptoms, which may be related to drug therapy, the diagnosis itself or ongoing seizures. It is thought depression is grossly underdiagnosed in the epilepsy population.

Seizure type and severity

People with a diagnosis of epilepsy who are well controlled on drug therapy obtained the most favourable QOL scores, which were similar to the general population. Those who experience multiple seizure types and frequent seizures have the poorest outcome. All studies to date report ongoing seizures as the clearest indicator to reflect the worst QOL outcome. The earlier the development of epilepsy, the worse the QOL scores, but some recent studies in the elderly suggest late development of epilepsy can have a very negative impact on this group's quality of life. Age of the person at the onset of epilepsy is a less significant indicator than seizure frequency.

Antiepileptic drug therapy

AEDs can have physical, psychotropic and cognitive effects on patients. Effects can be reversible or irreversible.

The commonest reversible side effects include cerebella-vestibular effects, general malaise, occulomotor effects, tremor and fatigue. Often small adjustments in dosage can resolve these but, if left unaddressed, they can have a significant impact on a person's ability to carry out daily tasks. Physical adverse side effects of certain drugs such as weight gain, acne, hirsutism and facial coarsening in rare cases can cause low self-esteem. Patients commonly complain of neuropsychological and behavioural effects of drugs such as cognitive slowing, impaired attention and vigilance, impaired psychomotor speed and memory deficits, particularly in short-term memory. Aggression, irritability and even psychotic episodes have been reported as a side effect of certain AEDs, which can have a marked impact on a person's QOL. Data range from 10% to 70% of patients experiencing adverse effects from AEDs. The most common adverse effect reported is drowsiness.

Irreversible adverse effects include teratogenic effects of AED, both physical fetal malformations such as cardiac defects and possibly intellectual developmental difficulties of offspring. Long-term treatment of enzyme-inducing drugs has been reported to increase the risk of osteoporosis, particularly in women.

Measuring QOL in children and adolescents

Although one can broadly apply the basic principles above to children and adolescents, the models are not transferable due to differing outcome measures such as:

- social life
- school life
- leisure activities
- physical appearance.

Age and development is a complex area to study, particularly in those under 11 years of age. The impact of parents can be difficult to assess and is often reflected in the child's outcomes, e.g. dependence or low self-esteem of the child may be a result of over-protection and not allowing the child to do normal activities for their age. In addition, many children experience seizure worry and anxiety about the burden they place on siblings and their parents. Some researchers attempt to address the differences between adult and child perception by having both child and parental questionnaires.

Restrictions related to driving and employment choice are particularly important to the adolescent group and the effect on self-esteem and relationships (dating). Over-protection and underachievement are common, and age of onset does seem to have an impact: the earlier the diagnosis the poorer the outcome.

Cultural and ethnic considerations

The vast majority of studies have been performed in northern Europe or the USA, although recent studies in China, Russia, Iran and Estonia continue to confirm that seizure frequency and severity are the most important factors. Cultural and ethnic considerations are often lacking in HRQOL studies. Differing cultural and religious beliefs can have an impact on QOL. For example, in certain parts of Africa people may be outcast from society due to a misconception that they are possessed. Nevertheless, transferring tools from one country to another is complicated due to translation and requirement for retesting.

Applications of HRQOL scales in epilepsy

There are three main uses:

- clinical drug trials
- interventions and epilepsy surgery
- clinical practice and monitoring treatment.

Clinical drug trials

The ongoing development of new-generation drugs is mainly targeted at those with continuing seizures requiring add-on therapies. A common end point assessing drug efficacy is a 50% reduction in seizure frequency. There remains debate regarding the validity of this measure. Some authors have suggested at least a 75% seizure reduction as a minimum acceptable end point, as well as the percentage of subjects attaining seizure freedom. It is debatable how meaningful a reduction of 50% is to patients. Using a QOL score in the assessment of new drugs may allow clinicians a greater understanding regarding the impact of drug adverse side effects.

Interventions and epilepsy surgery

Specific tools have been designed to assess the HRQOL outcome of patients who undergo epilepsy surgery. Studies suggest significantly improved QOL after surgery in those who become seizure-free, which is not entirely surprising considering seizure freedom is the most significant indicator for a positive QOL outcome. The most undesirable outcomes were found in those who failed surgery (i.e. continued to experience seizures) and also experienced memory decline as a result of surgery.

Clinical practice and monitoring treatment

Although very useful in a clinical research setting, these scales can be time-consuming and difficult to interpret. Individual patients seem to have differing abilities to cope with ongoing seizures and drug treatment. What is intolerable to one patient may be acceptable to another. Trying to cover the full scope of HRQOL in a single consultation is impossible. That said, enhanced knowledge and regard for the patients' perception of their seizures and treatment, including psychosocial challenges, can improve our patients well-being. Thus these tools should be and continue to be used to assist our clinical practice.

Practical advice: improving people's quality of life

Key areas to address:

- reducing seizure frequency

- minimizing side effects
- reducing stigma.

To achieve this:
- access to specialist diagnosis and treatment
- improved monitoring
- education of patient and wider community
- support and counselling services.

Ultimately, for people with epilepsy to have good quality of life requires seizure freedom, minimal or no side effects and a society which accepts epilepsy, and does not stigmatize the condition.

The most commonly used HRQOL tools in epilepsy

Quality Of life In Epilepsy Instruments (QOLIE 31, QOLIE 89 & QOLIE 10)

Cammer and colleagues developed these scales with the assistance of the non-profit organization Rand. The QOLIE 89 was the original survey developed to assess all aspects of QOL affecting adults with epilepsy containing 17 multi-item measures. The QOLIE 31 is the short-form version and consists of 31 questions about health and daily activites. The QOL10 is a brief survey containing only 10 questions about health and well-being

Epilepsy Surgery Inventory-55 (ESI-55)

This was developed by Vickery and colleagues and uses a generic core with the addition of 19 mainly epilepsy-specific items. The scale assesses HRQOL of post epilepsy surgery patients.

Liverpool Quality Battery

Jacoby and colleagues developed this scale initially to assess psychosocial outcomes after a decision to withdraw or not to withdraw AED. This group have further developed the scale to include physical functioning, e.g. seizure frequency and severity, activities of daily living, social functioning, life fulfilment, stigma, impact of epilepsy, Hospital Anxiety and Depression Scale, self-esteem and mastery components.

Repertory Grid Assessments

This was designed by Kendrick and Trimble, who performed extensive interviews aimed at assessment of a person's abilities and expectations. Patients were asked to identify specific issues that affected their well-being such as physical functioning, cognition, emotion, social functioning, financial and employment status. A repertory grid technique was used.

References and recommended reading

Baker GA, Spector S, McGrath Y, Soteriou H. Impact of epilepsy in adolescence: A UK controlled study. *Epilepsy Behav* 2005;**6**:556–62.

Devinsky O., Baker G, Cramer J. Quality measures of assessment. In Engel J, Pedley T, eds. *Epilepsy, a Comprehensive Textbook*, pp. 1107–13. Philadelphia: Lippincott-Raven; 1997.

Jacoby A, Johnson A, Chadwick DW, on behalf of the Medical Research Council Antiepileptic Drug Withdrawal Group. Psychosocial outcomes of antiepileptic drug discontinuation. *Epilepsia* 1992;**33**:1123–31.

Kendrick AM, Trimble MR. Repertory grid in the assessment of quality of life in patients with epilepsy: the quality of life assessment schedule. In Trimble MR, Dodson WE, eds. *Epilepsy and Quality of Life*, pp. 151–64. New York: Raven; 1994.

Langfitt JT, Westerveld M, Hamberger TS, *et al.* Worsening of quality of life after surgery: effect of seizures and memory decline. *Neurology* 2007;**68**(23):1988–94.

Shipper H, Clinch J, Powell V. Definitions and conceptual issues. In Spilker B, ed. *Quality of Life Assessments in Clinical Trials*, pp. 11–24. New York: Raven; 1990.

Smith D, Baker G, Davies G, Dewey M, Chadwick DW. Outcomes of add-on treatment with lamotrigine in partial epilepsy. *Epilepsia* 1993;**34**:312–22.

Vickery BG, Hays RD, Rausch R, *et al.* Quality of life of epilepsy surgery patients as compared to outpatients with hypertension, diabetes, heart disease and/or depressive symptoms. *Epilepsia* 1994;**35**:597–607.

Wiebe S, Matijevic S, Eliasziw M, Derry PA. Clinically important change in quality of life in epilepsy. *J Neurol Neurosurg Psychiatry* 2002;**73**:116–20.

Learning objectives

(1) To be aware of the relevance of evaluating quality of life in epilepsy.
(2) To know the main health-related quality of life measures and domains on which to apply these measures.

Section 7: Psychiatric, social and legal aspects

(3) To know the physical and psychological impact of seizures and their treatment, and their impact on quality of life:
- psychological impact of the diagnosis and seizures
- impact of seizure type and severity
- impact of antiepileptic drug therapy.

(4) To be aware of the challenges of measuring quality of life in children and adolescents.

(5) To be aware of and be able to discuss cultural and ethnic considerations in measuring quality of life.

(6) To know the main uses of health-related quality of life scales in epilepsy.

(7) To be aware of practical advice to improve people's quality of life in epilepsy.

(8) To know the most commonly used health-related quality of life tools in epilepsy.

Section 7 Psychiatric, social and legal aspects

Chapter 122 Cultural aspects of epilepsy: stigma, prejudice, self-image

Jennifer Nightingale

The term stigma is thought to arise from *stigmata*, which were the symbols used by the Greeks to mark slaves and other less desirable people. Stigma can be defined as an undesirable or discrediting attribute. Any trait that is deemed as deviant or different from the general population results in sanctions and rules against that person. In modern terms stigma could be defined as a characteristic that results in some degree of negative discrimination.

Attitudes towards those who experience seizures historically have been negative. Despite Hippocrates' description of epilepsy as a disease of natural cause around 400 BC, historical texts right up to the nineteenth century associate epilepsy with negative attributes or behaviours. Some of the common themes wrongly associated with seizures and epilepsy are:

- demonic possession
- criminal behaviour
- insanity
- immoral behaviour.

Stigma can be categorized into three domains:

- internalized stigma
- interpersonal stigma
- institutional stigma.

Internalized stigma

This occurs when stigma is felt within the person with the condition, and reflects their feelings and thoughts about being different. Internalized stigma affects self-image and is thought to be strongly associated with the individual's own perception of epilepsy. Many people report feelings of embarrassment, shame and fear when diagnosed with epilepsy. A diagnosis instils feelings of helplessness, loss of control and anxiety. It is very upsetting and embarrassing for patients to experience seizures in public. A small number of people can even go on to develop agoraphobia or social phobia, so it is essential the psychological impact of the diagnosis is always addressed. It is normal that a short period of adjustment to the diagnosis is required, and patients may experience feelings similar to bereavement such as shock, denial, anger, bargaining, depression and acceptance.

Interpersonal stigma

This area of stigma is related to interactions with others, both within and external to the family, and in these interactions the person with the illness is treated differently or negatively. There is little doubt that in the past there has been significant discrimination and stigma against those with epilepsy. Modern studies, however, have highlighted the importance of the person's perception of stigma, identifying that some people with epilepsy experience 'perceived stigma' or 'felt stigma'. Perceived/felt stigma is the feeling that a person is being stigmatized without a definite example of true discrimination/stigma. Authors such as Scambler have found that patients with epilepsy almost always reported they were stigmatized but when asked to give specific examples of prejudice acting against them personally, few were able to. It is thought that people are 'expecting' a negative reaction and seem to develop a self-fulfilling prophecy. Studies though have reported negative attitudes of both families affected by epilepsy and the wider community. Clinicians must be aware that stigma against those with epilepsy continues to exist in modern society.

Below are some of the probable causes for social/interpersonal stigma:

Introduction to Epilepsy ed. Gonzalo Alarcón and Antonio Valentín. Published by Cambridge University Press.
© Cambridge University Press 2012.

- Impact of previous perceptions, e.g. parental beliefs/religious beliefs.
- Public fear of seizures: educating the public (e.g. talks at schools; employers, etc.) can go some way to address this.
- Social exclusion/isolation: this can potentially occur from a young age at school. Educating staff and pupils will help minimize this.
- Fear of developing and maintaining relationships: marriage rates are lower, especially in men with a diagnosis of epilepsy. Disclosure of the diagnosis is often described as a difficult issue for patients.

Institutional stigma

Legal discrimination against people with epilepsy in the past has included limitations on marriage, immigration, employment and even fertility. Legislation continues to restrict patients' choices regarding driving and certain types of employment. This institutional discrimination has an impact on societies' perception of those with epilepsy, often continuing the myth that people with epilepsy are different in some 'essential' way from the normal population.

Identifying and managing the impact of stigma can influence a person's quality of life and psychological well-being.

Real stigma

- Consider cause of stigma
- Educate family, friends and colleagues
- Provide written information
- Provide supportive letters for employment, schooling etc.
- Consider social ramifications of treatment, e.g. cognitive effects of AED
- Ensure patient and family are aware of support groups and voluntary organizations related to epilepsy
- Ensure patient and family are aware of legal aspects, e.g. Disability Discrimination Act

Perceived stigma

- Listen to and validate the person's concerns
- Explore their beliefs and feelings about the diagnosis
- Ensure patient is well informed about epilepsy/seizures
- Encourage independence
- Encourage social activities
- Consider local counselling or referral to psychologist

In order to address the impact of stigma, not only must we counsel and support our patients through perceived and real stigma but also we must address society's attitudes. Only by constant education of the public and local and government lobbying can we change the public perception of epilepsy.

References

Jacoby A. Stigma, epilepsy and quality of life. *Epilepsy Behav* 2002;**3**(6S2):10–20.

Scambler G, Hopkins A. Being epileptic: coming to terms with stigma. *Social Health Illness* 1986;**8**:26–43.

Learning objectives

(1) To be able to define the concept of stigma and its varieties (internalized, interpersonal and institutional, real, perceived).
(2) To be aware of the causes of stigma.
(3) To know and be able to discuss the consequences of stigma.
(4) To be able to discuss how to prevent and manage stigma.

Section 7 Psychiatric, social and legal aspects

Chapter 123 Epilepsy, marriage and the family

Jennifer Nightingale

Epilepsy and marriage

The vast majority of people with epilepsy develop and maintain healthy relationships, although it is well documented that experiencing seizures and a diagnosis of epilepsy have an impact on marriage. The majority of studies suggest marriage rates are lower in those with a diagnosis of epilepsy. Furthermore, the results of virtually every study suggest marriage rates are particularly low for men.

Factors that affect marriage rates:

- age of onset
- severity of epilepsy
- social isolation
- social stigma
- employment status
- fear that offspring will develop epilepsy.

A significant difference occurs between marriage rates for men and women. There remains debate but it is felt the disparity may be based on the socio-economic status of men with epilepsy. Cultural and religious beliefs can also affect the ability to marry. In some cultures, epilepsy continues to have a very negative status, thus affecting a person's chance to marry, which may even lead to concealment of the diagnosis.

Impact of epilepsy on relationships and marriage

A new or existing diagnosis of epilepsy can have a major impact on a person's day-to-day life. One's perception of 'self' can be altered negatively, which impacts on interactions with friends, family and partners. Also ongoing seizures may alter socio-economic status, cause dependence and ultimately have a negative effect on quality of life.

Anxiety concerning pregnancy and parenting is common. Some people with epilepsy wrongly believe that there is a high chance of their offspring developing epilepsy and in some cases this fear may prevent people from marrying. In fact there is usually less than a 10% risk.

The dynamics of relationships can also be affected, such as fear of a spouse's reaction, overprotection of a partner or dependency developing. The psychological impact of the diagnosis, the effect of seizures and the side effects of AEDs may also result in sexual difficulties in a relationship.

Sexuality and epilepsy

There remains controversy about the impact of epilepsy on sexual function. Historically, seizures were thought to be a symptom of 'hyper-sexuality' but later in the 1950s studies suggested hypo-sexuality as a symptom of epilepsy. Hypo-sexuality is thought to affect both men and women. Women experience low libido, with disorders of arousal and desire. Men experience erectile dysfunction and also disorders of both arousal and desire. Epilepsy seems to cause a higher incidence of sexual dysfunction than other neurological conditions. There are multiple factors, including both physiological and psychological.

The cause of sexual dysfunction in epilepsy is primarily physiological. Up to a third of men report poor penile tumescence, anorgasmia and erectile difficulties. Over a third of women experience dyspareunia, vaginismus and lack of vaginal lubrication, with no abnormality in desire or arousal. Hormone

---

Introduction to Epilepsy ed. Gonzalo Alarcón and Antonio Valentín. Published by Cambridge University Press.
© Cambridge University Press 2012.

imbalance has been identified in both genders, i.e. low testosterone in men and low levels of both oestrogen and testosterone in women.

The psychological effect of epilepsy and seizures cannot be underestimated. Poor self-esteem, anxiety and depression are common in patients with epilepsy and can result in sexual difficulties.

Fertility

It is well documented that both men and women with a diagnosis of epilepsy are less likely to produce offspring than the normal population. Although more recent studies have found no significant difference, past studies have reported fertility rates decreased by up to two-thirds. Women with temporal lobe epilepsy have increased rates of anovulatory cycles, irregularities in length of cycles, polycystic ovaries and sexual dysfunction. Men experience imbalances occurring in pituitary gonadal hormones and enzyme-inducing drugs can lower testosterone levels. Reductions in seminal fluid volume and total sperm count have also been reported.

Practical advice

- Consider testing hormone levels
- Refer to sexual dysfunction clinic
- Appropriate treatment for erectile difficulties
- Refer to gynaecology/endocrinology if appropriate
- Provide counselling for marriage/relationship

Recommended reading

Dansky LV, Andermann E, Andermann F. Marriage and fertility in epileptic patients. *Epilepsia* 1980; **21**:261–71.

Gastaut H, Collomb H. Etude du compotement sexuel chez le epileptques psychomoteurs. *Ann Med Psychol* 1954;**112**:657–96.

Jensen P, Jensen SB, Sørenson PS, *et al.* Sexual dysfunction in male and female patients with epilepsy: a study of 86 outpatients. *Arch Sexual Behav* 1990;**19**:1–14.

Morrell MJ. Sexuality in epilepsy. In Engel J, Pedley T, eds. *Epilepsy, a Comprehensive Textbook*, pp. 2021–6. Philadelphia: Lippincott-Raven; 1997.

Yerby MS, Koepsell T, Daling J. Pregnancy complications and outcomes in a cohort of women with epilepsy. *Epilepsia* 1985;**26**:631–5.

Epilepsy and the family

The onset of seizures and diagnosis of epilepsy can have a profound effect on the person with epilepsy and their family. The impact of the diagnosis will differ depending on not only the family involved, but also whether the child or parent has epilepsy, and their role within that family. Many variables impact on the effect of the diagnosis including:

- the age of the individual developing seizures;
- frequency and severity of the seizure disorder;
- socio-economic impact;
- social and educational impact.

If a child develops epilepsy

A new diagnosis for any parent is very frightening. The parent and child may experience some or all of the following:

- over protection of the child
- parental expectations may be altered: lower expectations can occur
- restriction on activities, e.g. swimming
- social stigma: bullying or social isolation
- grief at 'loss of the perfect child'
- feeling of vulnerability, guilt, sadness, shame and anger
- anxiety and depression
- low self-esteem
- loss of control
- change in educational or employment status due to seizures or side effects of medication.

Children are reported to have fear and anxiety about the time and place of seizures. This is particularly associated with the risk that seizures may result in bullying or name-calling. Children can also experience anxiety about how their seizures affect their parents and siblings. A major outcome of the diagnosis is loss of control. This often results in psychological difficulties ranging from mild anxiety to depression.

Parents may feel a mixture of emotions including shock, guilt and anxiety, often resulting in overprotection. Expectations may be lowered and restrictions increased. Siblings may feel sidelined with the parental focus being on the child with epilepsy. This may cause resentment. In some rare cases, the parents may even introduce the concept of stigma to the child. Over protection is common and denies children normal life experiences for their age.

An area of current interest is the effect of epilepsy on the teenager or young adult. This is a challenging time for all young people and there are particularly difficult adjustments for those who have a diagnosis of epilepsy. A recent study by Baker *et al.* (2005) reported low self-esteem, anxiety and depression.

School performance

The cognitive impact of seizures, side effects of AEDs and underlying cause of the epilepsy may prevent optimal achievement. Ongoing seizures and adverse side effects of AEDs may affect school attendance. Teachers' attitudes are generally positive but there is often misinformation and lack of education about epilepsy.

If the parent has a diagnosis of epilepsy

Special attention should be paid to when the person develops epilepsy. Adults who have lived with the condition throughout their lives and go on to have families generally adjust incredibly well. A new diagnosis, though, in adulthood can have a catastrophic effect on some families. Typical issues include:

- employment: possible loss of employment due to seizures, e.g. construction, taxi drivers;
- loss of driving: it can affect ability to drive children to and from school or drive to work;
- single-parent families: child can become a carer;
- psychological impact on the child: child can become anxious or worried about parent;
- restrictions on activities/holidays.

Past studies have suggested that families with a parent with epilepsy experience increased anxiety and stress affecting both parents and children. More recent studies can find no significant difference between families with epilepsy and control groups. In practice, it largely depends on the individual and the family's attitude towards epilepsy. Severity and frequency of seizures also play a role in the family's ability to adjust. Frequent debilitating seizures can have a dramatic psychosocial impact.

Practical advice

All studies researching the impact of epilepsy on the family are unanimous in their agreement about improving education. Individual counselling for the adult or child is essential. Family therapy can be valuable to assist families adjusting to the diagnosis in complex cases.

Where possible refer all patients to a specialist nurse for advice and education.

Ensure families are aware of local support organizations.

Ensure families have access to written literature on all aspects of epilepsy.

Also education for the wider community such as employers, schools and community groups will help reduce the negative impact of the diagnosis on the family.

References and recommended reading

Baker G, Spector S, McGrath Y, Soteriou H. Impact of epilepsy in adolescence: a UK controlled study. *Epilepsy Behav* 2005;**6**:556–62.

Hoare P, Kerley S. Psychosocial adjustment of children with chronic epilepsy and their families. *Dev Med Child Neurol* 1991;**33**:201–15.

Learning objectives

(1) To know and be able to discuss the impact of epilepsy on marriage and on the family.
   - If the parent has epilepsy, its impact on marriage and relationship, on sexuality and on fertility.
   - If the child has epilepsy, on the child's life limitations, activities and school performance.

(2) To be able to discuss and provide practical advice.

Section 7 Psychiatric, social and legal aspects

Chapter 124

Epilepsy and employment

Rona Eade, Sally Gomersall and Stella Pearson

Epilepsy and employment: a historical context

In the late nineteenth century the greatest social difficulty for adults with epilepsy was finding employment. Without a job they were unable to rent lodgings and therefore were often confined to workhouses or asylums.

The National Society for the Employment of Epileptics (NSEE) was launched in 1892 by a group of London philanthropists and physicians. The aim of the Society was to establish a 'colony' for people with epilepsy who were capable of work but couldn't find employment due to their condition and the prevailing social attitudes of the time. It was believed that the fresh Buckinghamshire air and hard labour was beneficial to the 'health and well-being' of the individuals with epilepsy; perhaps more so than drugs and doctors.

Initially, only people of 'reasonable behaviour and mental ability' were admitted to the colony. They either worked six days a week on the land or did domestic work in the home. Later on the men undertook other work such as carpentry, plumbing, painting and bricklaying. A home for women was set up some years later. These women spent the first part of each week washing hundreds of items; then from Wednesday to Saturday they did the ironing. In later years they would also help with fruit-picking and haymaking in the summer.

In the second half of the twentieth century there was a wider choice of antiepileptic drugs, yet securing and retaining work was still difficult for people with seizures. People with epilepsy were twice as likely as people without epilepsy to be at risk of unemployment.

A National Society for Epilepsy 'epilepsy and employment' survey, in 2007, found that:

- 40% of individuals felt they had been treated unfairly by their employer;
- 25% felt that they lost their job because of their epilepsy;
- nearly 75% said their career had been affected by epilepsy;
- nearly 40% felt they had been unsuccessful at interviews because they mentioned their epilepsy.

Epilepsy and employment: what are the issues now?

Nearly all jobs are open to people with epilepsy. As employment can be a vital part of people's lives and identity, it is an important issue for many individuals with epilepsy. While the Equality Act 2010 in the UK protects people from unfair treatment, many people with epilepsy feel that they are, and have been, treated unfairly because of their epilepsy.

Overview of barriers to, and concerns about, employment

Some issues around employment are related to an individual's real or perceived barriers to employment. These may include:

- previous experiences such as rejection by a employer, or being dismissed after disclosing epilepsy or having a seizure;
- having low self-confidence, low self-esteem and lowered expectations (feeling 'not good enough'); and
- having frequent or severe seizures, and needing time off work to recover, or for medical appointments.

Introduction to Epilepsy ed. Gonzalo Alarcón and Antonio Valentín. Published by CAMBRIDGE UNIVERSITY PRESS.
© CAMBRIDGE UNIVERSITY PRESS 2012.

In addition, some issues arise out of the employer's concerns. These may include:

- Will people with epilepsy have lower levels of productivity?
- Will people with epilepsy take more time off work than other employees?
- Will employing a person with epilepsy increase my insurance premiums and claims?
- What are the risks around health and safety at work for people with epilepsy?
- What impact will someone having a seizure have on other employees, clients and the public?

Employers may have little understanding about epilepsy as a condition, or its effect on individuals. They may also have misconceptions about the condition.

The Equality Act 2010

The Equality Act 2010 brings together and strengthens previous legislation to protect people against discrimination because of a 'protected characteristic'. One of the protected characteristics is disability. The Equality Act 'makes it unlawful to discriminate against, harass or victimise a person at work or in employment services' (Equality Act 2010).

The Equality Act 2010 and employment

The Equality Act 2010 applies to all employers (except the armed services, who are exempt), regardless of how many employees they have. It applies from the point of an individual applying for a job, during interview and selection, and throughout employment, and to people with pre-existing disabilities and those who develop a disability while employed.

> An employer discriminates against a disabled person if:
> (a) because of a protected characteristic such as disability, he treats him less favourably than he treats or would treat others, and
> (b) he cannot show that the treatment in question is a proportionate means of achieving a legitimate aim.
>
> Equality Act 2010.

> **Key learning points**
> - The Equality Act 2010 applies in all areas of employment, and to all employers except the armed services.
> - Discriminating against people because of their disability is against the law under the Equality Act 2010.
> - Discrimination happens when someone is treated in a way that is:
>   - different and less favourable than others;
>   - puts the person at a disadvantage compared to others;
>   - without justification; and
>   - without any reasonable adjustments being made.

'Equal' versus 'the same'

Treating someone with a disability equally to someone without a disability is different from treating him/her in exactly the same way. Equality refers to the outcome, such as equal rights, equal access to services or equal opportunities. Discrimination can also happen if an employer treats all employees exactly the same, regardless of their disability, and this results in someone being disadvantaged because of their disability.

> **Key learning point**
> Equality means treating a person with a disability in a way that enables them to have the same, or equal, access, rights or skills as a person without a disability.

Justifiable reasons

While the Equality Act 2010 does not mean that people with epilepsy can be turned down for a job just because of their disability, neither does it mean that every person with a disability can do any job because they have a disability. In some cases there may be a 'justifiable' reason why someone cannot do a job.

The Health and Safety at Work Act (HSWA) can work in harmony with the Equality Act 2010. However, in some situations, employing a person with epilepsy could put them, or others, at risk. If there are no reasonable adjustments that would reduce the risk, under Health and Safety regulations someone may be refused a job. The Equality Act 2010 cannot be used to enforce changes that would break the HSWA.

Reasonable adjustments

Employers are expected to make reasonable adjustments if an individual's disability puts them at a disadvantage compared to someone without a disability. For example, this may be due to a physical feature of the workplace or the working conditions. Making reasonable adjustments means making adjustments so that people with disabilities have the same access, rights and opportunities as people without disabilities.

If an employer fails to make reasonable adjustments for someone with a disability, and this results in the employee being at an unfair disadvantage, this is discrimination.

> (1) Where:
> (a) a provision, criterion or practice applied by or on behalf of an employer, or
> (b) any physical feature of premises occupied by the employer, places the disabled person concerned at a substantial disadvantage in comparison with persons who are not disabled,
> (c) a disabled person would, but for the provision of an auxiliary aid, be put at a substantial disadvantage in relation to a relevant matter in comparison with persons who are not disabled.
>
> It is the duty of the employer to take such steps as it is reasonable to have to take to avoid the disadvantage, or to provide the auxiliary aid. Where the first or third requirement relates to the provision of information, the steps which it is reasonable for the employer to have to take include steps for ensuring that the information is provided in an accessible format.
> Duty to make reasonable adjustments, Equality Act 2010.

Reasonable adjustments could include:
- making adjustments to premises;
- allocating some of the disabled person's duties to another person;
- altering his working hours;
- allowing him to be absent during working hours for rehabilitation, assessment or treatment;
- acquiring or modifying equipment; or
- providing a reader or interpreter.

Except where the Act states otherwise, it would never be reasonable for an employer to pass on any costs of implementing reasonable adjustments to an individual disabled person.

Appropriate reasonable adjustments will depend on the individual employee, their disability, and what would help them to have the same 'rights' as other employees in the same job. So adjustments need to be individualized.

Whether an adjustment is reasonable or not depends on several things:
- how much the adjustment would help;
- how practical it is for the employer to make the adjustment;
- the costs (including financial cost) of making the adjustment, and how this would affect the activities of the organization or company;
- the amount of resources the employer has, including finances; and
- any available assistance for the employer in making the adjustments.

The Equality Act 2010 and epilepsy

Epilepsy is a disability and individuals are protected from unfair treatment, under the Equality Act 2010. This is true even if their seizures are controlled with medication. Each person with epilepsy will have their own needs and abilities, and their epilepsy may affect them differently from how epilepsy affects someone else. However, not every person with epilepsy will feel that they have a disability, as is often the case for people who no longer have seizures.

> A person has a disability for the purposes of this Act if he has a physical or mental impairment which has a substantial and long-term adverse effect on his ability to carry out normal day-to-day activities.
> The Equality Act 2010.

What can employers do to help?

Epilepsy varies from one person to another, so when considering employment and epilepsy it is important to look at each case individually. Making assumptions about someone's epilepsy and how it might affect their work is more likely to result in discrimination than talking through these issues with them, identifying any genuine problems, and looking for ways to resolve them. Consider the following issues.

- The nature of the person's epilepsy.

Knowing about the person's epilepsy, such as whether they have seizures or not, what happens during the seizures, whether they get any warning before and how they need to recover afterwards, can help ensure that employers consider the situation from the individual's point of view, and may help reassure the individual.

- The nature of the work.

Thinking about whether the job involves using equipment or technology, working at heights or near water, working alone, or being responsible for the welfare of others, can help identify any risks and reasonable adjustments to make.

- What is it about their epilepsy that might cause problems in the workplace?

Looking at specific issues, such as individuals who work at heights losing consciousness during seizures, or people who need an ambulance to be called during a seizure, or working alone, can help to identify possible specific risks to individuals.

- How can any potential problems be overcome?

By looking at the issues above, reasonable adjustments to make employment safer can be identified. Adjustments could include adjusting someone's working hours to avoid disrupted sleep patterns if their seizures are affected by being tired, or ensuring the individual does not work alone if they are likely to have seizures and need assistance. A formal risk assessment, including Occupational Health personnel, may help identify the risks, solutions and adjustments.

> **Key learning points**
> - Epilepsy is an individual and variable condition: how it affects one person can be different from how it affects someone else.
> - When looking at employment issues, the situation has to be looked at from the point of view of the individual, their epilepsy and the nature of the work.
> - In some cases it is necessary to carry out a formal risk assessment of the situation before decisions can be made.

Disclosing a disability

A person with a disability is not obliged to disclose their disability: someone with a disability can apply for a job without telling the potential employer about their disability.

Each individual with epilepsy needs to decide whether to disclose their condition to an employer or potential employer.

There are several reasons why it is helpful for an individual to disclose their epilepsy:

- so that employers and colleagues know how to best help them if they have a seizure;
- so that employers make reasonable adjustments to ensure that they are not put at a disadvantage because of their epilepsy; and
- so that employers fulfil their obligations under the Health and Safety at Work Act.

When an individual discloses their epilepsy, they may:

- mention it in a covering letter;
- include a letter from their GP or neurologist, with information about their epilepsy;
- discuss it at their interview, if relevant to the job; or
- only mention it after a job offer is made.

Individuals need to be aware that giving false information on an application form or health questionnaire can be grounds for a job offer being withdrawn.

Employers' obligations

If an employer is aware of an individual's disability, they are required to make reasonable adjustments for that individual. However, if the employer is not aware, or they cannot be expected to know about it, they cannot be held responsible for failing to make reasonable adjustments, or meeting health and safety requirements, for that person.

> (3) [the employer] is not subject to a duty to make reasonable adjustments if [the employer] does not know, and could not reasonably be expected to know:
> (a) in the case of an applicant or potential applicant, that an interested disabled person is or may be an applicant for the employment;
> (b) in any other case, that an interested disabled person has a disability and is likely to be placed at the disadvantage referred to in the first, second or third requirement.
>
> Work: reasonable adjustments, Part 3: Limitations on the duty, Equality Act 2010.

References and useful organizations

The Equality Act 2010 is printed by The Stationery Office. Available from The National Archives at www.legislation.gov.uk.

Directgov has information on public services, including employment, the Equality Act 2010, Health and Safety at Work and disabilities. www.direct.gov.uk.

The Health and Safety Executive can provide information on health and safety and the Health and Safety at Work Act. Infoline 0845 345 0055, www.hse.gov.uk (at October 2011).

The Equality and Human Rights Commission is an independent public body, bringing together the Commission for Racial Equality (CRE), Disability Rights Commission (DRC) and Equal Opportunities Commission (EOC), to reduce discrimination and promote equality. Helplines: England: 0845 604 6610, Scotland: 0845 604 5510, Wales: 0845 604 8810.

Learning objectives

(1) To be able to outline the historical evolution of concepts related to epilepsy and employment.
(2) To be able to discuss the most important present issues on epilepsy and employment.
(3) To know the barriers to, and concerns about, employment in patients with epilepsy.
(4) To be familiar with and be able to discuss the Equality Act 2010, and its relevance for employment of people with epilepsy.
(5) To be aware of the appropriate treatment, adjustments and obligations of employers to people with epilepsy.
(6) To know what employers can do to help.
(7) To know the principles of the UK law on disclosing a disability to employers.

Section 7 Psychiatric, social and legal aspects

Chapter 125 Drivers' and pilots' licences

Peter Fenwick

In the UK there are very strict regulations governing medical fitness to drive. Nobody in the UK can drive without a driving licence. In order to obtain a licence the Department of Vehicle and Licensing Authority (DVLA) in Swansea requires the completion of an application form. On this form the applicant is required to state whether or not they have a diagnosis of epilepsy, if so, whether the epilepsy is well controlled with or without medication, and whether or not they have had any seizure (even a single seizure) no matter how mild or minor. If the answer to any of these questions is yes, then the DVLA will first of all contact the applicant's general practitioner for a medical report, and in the more complex cases will ask the applicant's medical consultant for a report.

Ordinary (Group 1) driving licences

This group consists of light vehicles (private cars, mopeds, motorcycles, invalid carriages and all vehicles up to 3.5 tons). Provided a satisfactory medical report is received, and it can be shown that the applicant has had no epileptic seizures while awake, with or without medication, for a period of 12 months from the date of the last seizure then a licence can be issued. A licence can also be issued if it can be established that for 3 years or more seizures have occurred only during sleep. If these conditions are satisfied, a 3-year licence will normally be issued. Should the applicant remain seizure-free for 7 years, with or without medication, and provided the applicant has no other disqualifying medical condition such as a cardiac or neurological condition, a driving licence valid till the age of 70 years will be issued to the applicant.

For Group 1 the consequences of the occurrence of seizures or blackouts to the licence holder are as follows:

- Newly diagnosed epilepsy: driving ban until 1 year after last seizure.
- Recurrent blackouts of uncertain cause: driving ban for 1 year after last blackout.
- Single blackout of uncertain cause but with epileptic features: driving ban for 1 year.
- Blackout of uncertain cause with no epileptic features: driving ban for 6 months.
- Single provoked seizure: the driving ban is discretionary although DVLA must be informed and sometimes a 6-month ban after the seizure is enforced, provided the cause has been removed, and unless alcohol or drugs are involved.
- Single provoked seizure related to alcohol or drugs: driving ban until 1 year after the last seizure. A medical report, urine and blood tests may be required before a licence is issued. It should be demonstrated that the applicant is alcohol- and drug-free before restoration of the licence.

Group 2 – Heavy goods vehicles or public service vehicle licences: HGV/PSV

For heavy goods vehicles over 7.5 tons and passenger-carrying vehicles with nine seats or more, the rules are more stringent. The application form will again contain questions about epilepsy and will be initially sent to the applicant's general practitioner. The applicant must have had no epileptic seizure in the previous 10 years, must not have taken any antiepileptic drug treatment during the 10-year period, and, most importantly, must not have any continuing liability to epileptic seizures. If the applicant satisfies these regulations, then before a licence is granted they must pass a medical examination with a medical consultant nominated by the DVLA. These consultants are

---

Introduction to Epilepsy ed. Gonzalo Alarcón and Antonio Valentín. Published by Cambridge University Press.
© Cambridge University Press 2012.

usually specialists in medical fitness to drive. The licence cannot be issued before the age of 21 and usually lasts until age 45. It is then issued every 5 years till 65 and thereafter issued annually.

Withdrawal of antiepileptic drugs in a person who is seizure-free

There is no DVLA regulation but the DVLA advise no driving until 6 months after completion of drug withdrawal. There is an overall 40% increased risk of a seizure during the first year.

Informing the police or DVLA that a patient is driving

Every driver has a duty to inform the DVLA as soon as they are aware that they have any medical condition that will affect their driving. So after the occurrence of a single seizure or the diagnosis of epilepsy, the patient must inform Swansea.

The doctor owes a duty of confidentiality to the patient. This duty may be enforced by the General Medical Council. However, the General Medical Council states that the doctor may breach confidentiality in the public interest (for example, a patient or person at risk of causing serious harm or death).

The doctor has a duty to inform the patient after the occurrence of a seizure that they are not to drive and that they are to inform Swansea. If the patient then drives, the doctor should challenge the patient and tell them that the DVLA will be informed. Only in exceptional circumstances should the doctor inform the DVLA without first warning the patient. If the doctor becomes aware that the patient is driving without a licence, they should inform the police.

Only breach confidentiality in good faith and after careful thought.

Drivers may appeal within 21 days of being banned, but, in my view, Swansea are always very careful and this is seldom if ever successful.

Finally, those who are medically disqualified from driving are entitled to apply for a concessionary travel card from their local passenger transport executive.

Pilots' licences

Any seizure or abnormal EEG activity is likely to carry a lifetime ban.

For information and advice contact Drivers Medical Group, Swansea SA99 1TU 0870 600 0301 www.dvla.gov.uk.

Learning objectives

(1) To know the limitations and their timescale of people with epileptic seizures to obtain group 1 and group 2 driving licences in the UK.
(2) To know the DVLA position about antiepileptic drug withdrawal.
(3) To know regulations and obligations about informing the police and DVLA.
(4) To know regulations about pilots' licences.

Section 7 Psychiatric, social and legal aspects

Chapter 126: Treatment with limited pharmacopoeia

Dominic C. Heaney

Introduction

The treatment options available to people with epilepsy have expanded significantly during the second half of the twentieth century. Entering the twenty-first century, physicians have potential access to more than 20 antiepileptic drugs to treat a variety of different seizure disorders.

Nevertheless, up to 80% of people with epilepsy live in the developing world. They may live with economic scarcity, which results in a series of barriers that prevent them from receiving treatments, which could benefit them. This 'treatment gap' is defined by the International League Against Epilepsy as 'the difference between the number of people with active epilepsy and the number whose seizures are being appropriately treated in a given population at a given point in time, expressed as a percentage'. The treatment gap is estimated to be as high as 90% in some regions of the world.

Even where resources exist to diagnose and treat epilepsy, people with epilepsy may be limited to the drugs that are available and affordable in their countries: these drugs are typically those 'off-patent' and whose manufacture can be achieved worldwide. Nevertheless, the use of these 'older' drugs is evidence-based, and can benefit individuals who would otherwise suffer the morbidity and mortality of uncontrolled epilepsy.

What limits drug choices?

Resource-poor countries may be unable to prioritize programmes and health services which allow epilepsy to be understood, diagnosed and appropriately treated. Similarly, the infrastructure that allows provision of good-quality medicines and a consistent supply to those who need them may not exist. Even when antiepileptic drugs are available, they may be offered at prices that cannot be afforded by individuals with epilepsy – or similarly, prescribed by doctors whom people cannot afford to consult.

A further complication is that even when established antiepileptic drugs are available, they may be used irrationally. For example, a study in India demonstrated that 95% of referrals from primary and secondary care facilities to a tertiary care centre were receiving inadequate doses of antiepileptic drugs (AEDs). Many patients were using combinations of inadequate doses of AED – typically phenytoin (PHT) and phenobarbital (PB) but also the more expensive treatments valproate (VPA) and carbamazepine (CBZ).

What drugs are available?

A recent World Health Organization survey performed across a wide range of countries in every region of the world demonstrated that four established treatments for epilepsy were widely available. CBZ, PB, and PHT were included in over 93% of the responding countries 'essential lists': 86.7% also included VPA. However, there were also significant variations observed, with developing countries less likely to include CBZ (82.6%), PHT (68.2%) and VPA (62.5%).

This survey also considered the cost of treatment. Furthermore, median costs of the daily defined dose (DDD) of the first-line AEDs in international dollars also demonstrated significant variation. While the median cost of PB is 0.14 International dollars, it is three times more for PHT, 11 times for CBZ and 16 times for VPA (prices presented in international dollars as at 2000). Compared with the average GDP per capita, without government or health insurance system support, the prices of newer AEDs are beyond the reach of a significant proportion of the population of people with epilepsy.

Introduction to Epilepsy ed. Gonzalo Alarcón and Antonio Valentín. Published by Cambridge University Press.
© Cambridge University Press 2012.

The role of phenobarbital in the twenty-first century

Thus for a significant proportion of people with epilepsy in the world, the only AEDs available for treatment are PB and PHT – both drugs which were initially introduced into clinical practice in the early twentieth century.

As described, PB monotherapy offers significant benefits in terms of its affordability, even in comparison with PHT. It has a broad spectrum of efficacy in a range of epilepsy syndromes. Furthermore, its use in the developing world can be considered as evidence-based, as a number of clinical trials have been published to support its use.

For example, a study in rural India has shown that its efficacy is comparable with phenytoin. Further studies in Mali, Ecuador and Kenya have shown that there was no significant difference between PB and CBZ in either efficacy or safety.

It is often stated that PB may have a negative impact on cognition and behaviour. Certainly, 'head-to-head' comparisons between PB and newer agents have shown an adverse side-effect profile at higher doses. Nevertheless, this observation must be weighed against the consequences of uncontrolled epilepsy for individuals who cannot afford or access other treatments, with the evidence based on trials performed in the developing world. A series of separate trials in Tanzania, Mali, India and more recently China suggest that PB may be both effective and well tolerated. A study from Bangladesh has shown that PB is not associated with excess behavioural side effects when compared with CBZ.

Thus, the efficacy and safety of PB is clear, and its risk of producing cognitive side effects may be to some extent over-stated, particularly when it is considered that the majority of patients may respond well to lower dosages, which may in many patients be perfectly adequate to control epilepsy long term.

Recommended reading

Banu SH, Jahan M, Koli UK, *et al.* Side effects of phenobarbital and carbamazepine in childhood epilepsy: Randomised controlled trial. *BMJ* 2007; **334**:1207–10.

Feksi AT, Kaamugisha J, Gatiti S, Sander JW, Shorvon SD. A comprehensive community epilepsy programme: the Nakuru project. *Epilepsy Res* 1991;**8**:252–9.

Feksi AT, Kaamugisha J, Sander JW, Gatiti S, Shorvon SD. A comprehensive primary health care antiepileptic drug treatment programme in rural and semi urban Kenya. *Lancet* 1991;**337**:406–9.

Jilek-Aall L, Rwiza HT. Prognosis of epilepsy in a rural African community: a 30-year follow-up of 164 patients in an outpatient clinic in rural Tanzania. *Epilepsia* 1992;**33**:645–50.

Kale R, Perucca E. Revisiting phenobarbital for epilepsy. *BMJ* 2004;**329**:1199–200.

Mani KS, Rangan G, Srinivas HV, Srindharan VS, Subbakrishna DK. Epilepsy control with phenobarbital or phenytoin in rural south India: the Yelandur study. *Lancet* 2001;**357**:1316–20.

Nimaga K, Desplats D, Doumbo O, Farnarier G. Treatment with phenobarbital and monitoring of epileptic patients in rural Mali. *Bull World Health Org* 2002;**80**:532–7.

Pal DK, Das T, Chaudhary G, Johnson AC, Neville BG. Randomized controlled trial to assess acceptability of phenobarbital for childhood epilepsy in rural India. *Lancet* 1998;**351**:19–23.

Placencia M, Sander JW, Shorvon SD, *et al.* Antiepileptic drug treatment in a community health care setting in northern Ecuador: A prospective 12 month assessment. *Epilepsy Res* 1993;**14**:252–9.

Scott RA, Lhatoo SD, Sander WA. The treatment of epilepsy in developing countries: Where do we go from here? *Bull World Health Org* 2001;**79**:344–51.

Wang WZ, Wu JZ, Ma GY, *et al.* Efficacy assessment of phenobarbital in epilepsy: a large community-based intervention trial in rural China. *Lancet Neurol* 2006;**5**:46–52.

World Health Organization. *Atlas. Epilepsy Care in the World 2005.* Geneva: WHO; 2005.

Learning objectives

To understand the following issues:

(1) Resource-poor countries carry an enormous burden of epilepsy.

(2) A substantial proportion of patients in resource-poor countries never receive appropriate treatment.

(3) This treatment gap can be minimized by educating primary care physicians on how to diagnose epilepsy and administer phenobarbital treatment.

(4) Epilepsy care programmes cannot be separated from their local socio-cultural, political and economic contexts.

Section 7 Psychiatric, social and legal aspects

Chapter 127: The role of primary care in the management of epilepsy

Greg Rogers

Background

The UK NHS provision of health care in primary care

In the UK, health care is provided free at the point of delivery for every UK citizen and for everyone who is visiting the UK from a country which holds a reciprocal agreement between our countries for health care. Central to this for UK citizens is the possession of an NHS unique identifying number, which enables health care and health checks. The backbone to this care is the network of family general practitioners (GPs) who hold the medical records of everyone registered with them and to whom all NHS healthcare activity is reported and then stored in the patient's medical records.

The importance of this is that there is continuity of care, which for epilepsy is vital, and also it allows the setting up of medical audit, which has the potential to identify, from disease registers, everyone with epilepsy. As will be described later, people with epilepsy are annually invited for an epilepsy check.

Primary care is often the first point of access to care for someone who develops epilepsy, and the role has been strengthened by the recent Transient Loss of Consciousness (TLoC) guidelines which advise GPs to identify and then refer to specialist neurological care anyone who reports the following (http://guidance.nice.org.uk/CG109):

- Suspected epilepsy

Refer people who present with one or more of the following features (that is, features that are strongly suggestive of epileptic seizures) for an assessment by a specialist in epilepsy; the person should be seen by the specialist within 2 weeks (see 'The epilepsies: the diagnosis and management of the epilepsies in adults and children in primary and secondary care': NICE clinical guideline 20).

- A bitten tongue
- Head-turning to one side during TLoC
- No memory of abnormal behaviour that was witnessed before, during or after TLoC by someone else
- Unusual posturing
- Prolonged limb-jerking (note that brief seizure-like activity can often occur during uncomplicated faints)
- Confusion following the event
- Prodromal déjà vu, or jamais vu (see glossary, appendix C)
- Consider that the episode may not be related to epilepsy if any of the following features are present:
  - prodromal symptoms that on other occasions have been abolished by sitting or lying down
  - sweating before the episode
  - prolonged standing that appeared to precipitate the TLoC
  - pallor during the episode
- Do not routinely use EEG in the investigation of TLoC (see 'The epilepsies: the diagnosis and management of the epilepsies in adults and children in primary and secondary care': NICE clinical guideline 20)

Primary care not only has a role in picking up newly presenting cases of epilepsy, but it also has the potential to proactively manage epilepsy using audit of the computerized GP records. This is inherently different from secondary and tertiary care, whose remit is establishing a diagnosis of epilepsy or reviewing

Introduction to Epilepsy ed. Gonzalo Alarcón and Antonio Valentín. Published by Cambridge University Press.
© Cambridge University Press 2012.

people sent to them by primary care or the emergency services who are seeking help with their epilepsy care. The routine medical review of people with epilepsy in primary care was less than satisfactory and help was largely based on an opportunistic basis. This changed with the advent of the NHS Qualities and Outcomes Framework (QOF) in April 2004. For the first time, people with epilepsy were included in a list of long-term conditions, which were proactively reviewed by primary care on a voluntary basis but with financial incentives for the GP surgeries to take part. This facilitated everybody within this group being formally invited to receive a clinical review annually for their epilepsy care (http://www.qof.ic.nhs.uk/).

Through this scheme, GPs are incentivized to:

- produce a register of patients aged 18 and over receiving drug treatment for epilepsy (1 point);
- determine the percentage of patients age 18 and over on drug treatment for epilepsy who have a record of seizure frequency in the previous 15 months (4 points);
- determine the percentage of patients age 18 and over on drug treatment for epilepsy who have a record of medication review involving the patient and/or carer in the previous 15 months (4 points);
- determine the percentage of patients age 18 and over on drug treatment for epilepsy who have been seizure-free for the last 12 months recorded in the previous 15 months (6 points)

There are flaws in this scheme; for example, there is natural reporter bias to do well and indeed many GPs may not be conversant with the subtlety of auras and complex partial seizures. Also practices can 'exception report' on people who are on maximum tolerated dose of medication and still suffering from ongoing seizures or who are non-compliant with medication or attending for the QOF review. The major impact on epilepsy care, however, has been that people with epilepsy are asked how they view their epilepsy care. It marked a historic step forward in bringing epilepsy out of the shadows and since then new epilepsy services have been developed that are more sensitive to the needs of people with epilepsy.

The inclusion of seizure freedom is very important here as we know that for many decades the mortality and morbidity from epilepsy has remained depressingly constant. This is despite the arrival of new antiepilepsy drugs, increased numbers of neurologists and greater knowledge of the aetiology and investigation for epilepsy. At the centre of this lies the problem that while community studies reveal seizure freedom to be around 50%, specialist centres are generally able to achieve in excess of 80% seizure freedom. Hence, there is around a 30% treatment gap. If this group could be identified, the potential to reduce mortality and inherently morbidity from epilepsy presents itself (Rogers, 2002).

The potential of primary care to resolve this issue is still not fully addressed through QOF, in part due to exception reporting, but with the advent of primary care commissioning another way of identifying the group who are at risk due to their suffering ongoing seizures has presented itself. Epilepsy features as being one of the long-term conditions which is heavily represented in acute admission data for A&E departments and indeed even higher in hospital readmission data (http://www.nelm.nhs.uk/en/NeLM-Area/News/2008---November/07/Further-analysis-of-data-on-emergency-readmission-rates-in-England/) Table 127.1.

Schemes to address the needs of those who attend or re-attend are increasingly important, and those who default from care are over-represented in this group. Service redesign to bring care closer to home for this group is being developed at many centres across the UK with intermediate-care epilepsy clinics. These clinics have been developed in partnership with epilepsy clinic users, are designed to be more acceptable to people with epilepsy and are aimed at making epilepsy care more acceptable to those who would otherwise default from formal follow-up. Clinics held in the community are in theory as easy to attend for many as going to the supermarket, and help in clinic surroundings with which patients are familiar and hopefully feel more at ease. One such scheme operates in East Kent.

The East Kent scheme offers a new point of referral for people with epilepsy to a network of GPs with special interest in epilepsy (GPwSI in epilepsy). The route is usually via early discharge from outpatient neurology clinics, freeing space for new cases, or by direct referral from their GP colleagues for people requiring optimization or ongoing active input. The scheme was developed with the collaboration of patients and primary and secondary care.

Through a network of seven GPwSI in epilepsy, referrals are made from both GPs and neurologists for patients who have a current diagnosis of epilepsy and require advice (e.g. epilepsy and pregnancy) or

Chapter 127: The role of primary care in the management of epilepsy

Table 127.1 Original admission health resource groups with most emergency readmissions, adults aged 16–74, 2003–2004 and 2006–2007

HRG code	HRG description	Number of original (index) admissions 2003/4	Number of original (index) admissions 2006/7	Number of emergency readmissions 2003/4	Number of emergency readmissions 2006/7	Emergency readmission rate (%) 2003/4	Emergency readmission rate (%) 2006/7
E36	Chest pain <70 w/o cc	109 741	144 088	9389	11 871	8.6	8.2
F47	General abdominal disorders	88 242	106 722	8080	11 366	9.2	10.7
S16	Poisoning, toxic, environmental and unspecified effects	63 176	83 637	6721	10 720	10.6	12.8
D40	Chronic obstructive pulmonary disease or bronchitis w/o cc	37 783	34 421	7747	7 540	20.5	21.9
F46	General abdominal disorders >69 or w cc	28 553	40 048	3750	6 041	13.1	15.1
E23	Ischaemic heart disease without intervention <70 w/o cc	40 566	33 580	5359	4 288	13.2	12.8
E35	Chest pain >69 or w cc	22 591	30 466	2753	3 719	12.2	12.2
D39	Chronic obstructive pulmonary disease or bronchitis w cc	11 621	14 147	2687	3 600	23.1	25.5
E30	Arrhythmia or conduction disorders <70 w/o cc	32 448	36 917	2963	3 587	9.1	9.7
H42	Sprains, strains, or minor open wounds <70 w/o cc	23 914	38 169	1639	3 491	6.9	9.2
S19	Complications of procedures	22 148	25 852	2688	3 461	12.1	13.4
A30	Epilepsy <70 w/o cc	23 168	26 614	2602	3 370	11.2	12.7
D41	Unspecified acute lower respiratory infection	24 774	26 476	2599	2 926	10.5	11.1
E12	Acute myocardial infarction w/o cc	29 364	24 145	3730	2 921	12.7	12.1
D22	Asthma w/o cc	27 328	27 328	2748	2 773	10.1	10.2

From: http://www.nelm.nhs.uk/en/NeLM-Area/News/2008---November/07/Further-analysis-of-data-on-emergency-readmission-rates-in-England/.

optimization of treatment. GPs also refer people who have suffered a recent seizure or have needed to attend A&E following a seizure. Three local hospitals also discharge newly diagnosed or still unstable patients for further follow-up. The change in the model of care saw networks of GPwSI in epilepsy and epilepsy nurses working in collaboration with the local neurology service, the specialist nurses working mainly with the unstable or new cases of epilepsy and the GPwSI clinicians working in the long-term care of the cohort with epilepsy with high capacity and lower-impact care. In this way, the aim is for all people with epilepsy to potentially be able to access specialist care at the appropriate level of expertise.

Although this has only been running for a few years in Thanet, one of the deprived wards in East Kent, the local consortium has seen an early trend of reduced numbers admitted to their local hospital for epilepsy over the past 24 months. Also the number of neurology outpatient referrals for new patients in the same area has reduced by 20% over the past 3 years, comparing the first 18-month and second 18-month periods. The scheme is warmly received by patients.

In summary, primary care has the potential to identify through audit everyone with a diagnosis of epilepsy and identify problems relating to epilepsy care proactively. On identifying a need which cannot be met by the GP's knowledge and expertise alone a system of intermediate care is being developed which aims to work seamlessly between primary and secondary care and has been identified by Parliament as the direction of travel for epilepsy care in the future (Hansard, 2007). There is also great potential for specially trained pharmacists to become more involved in the active management of long-term conditions such as epilepsy, offering even greater potential in bringing care closer to home for people with epilepsy.

References

Hansard; 17 July 2007; column 42WH.

Rogers G. The future of epilepsy care in general practice . . . A role for the GPWsi? *Brit J Gen Pract* 2002; 52(483):872–3.

The Quality and Outcomes Framework (QOF) is a voluntary annual reward and incentive programme for all GP surgeries in England, detailing practice achievement results. It is not about performance management but resourcing and then rewarding good practice. http://www.qof.ic.nhs.uk/.

Transient loss of consciousness in adults and young people. August 2010. http://guidance.nice.org.uk/CG109.

Learning objectives

(1) Understand the structure of the NHS primary care team and use of personal health audit.
(2) Appreciate the role that primary and indeed intermediate care have in the treatment of epilepsy.
(3) Be further reminded of the importance of striving to obtain seizure freedom.
(4) Have a clearer grasp of how a population with epilepsy require proactive care rather than dispensing health care reactively.

Questions

(1) What roles does IT play in health care in general practice?
(2) How does being registered and having medical records with a family GP allow proactive treatment for epilepsy?
(3) Discuss who should look after the routine care of the 0.9% of the population with epilepsy.
(4) Will doubling the number of epilepsy centres reduce the mortality of people with epilepsy by 50%? If not, why not?
(5) If a person with epilepsy is not taking their medication very often who is likely to be the first health-care professional to notice it and what can they do with the information? Does it matter?

Section 7 Psychiatric, social and legal aspects

Chapter 128

Residential care and special centres for epilepsy

Frank M. C. Besag

History

Attempts to explore the myth that epilepsy was the result of visitation by evil spirits dates back to the time of Hippocrates. However, prejudice about epilepsy and those who have this condition has persisted. An establishment that appears to have had a more caring approach was founded at the end of the fifteenth century by the monks at the Priory of St Valentine at Rufach in Alsace. This was a 'hospice for epileptics'. The Bishop of Wurzburg started a home for people with epilepsy in 1773. It is interesting to note that, much later, in 1815, Esquirol apparently suggested that special provision should be made for people with epilepsy because a healthy individual seeing an epileptic seizure might develop the condition. In 1860, the National Hospital for the Paralysed and Epileptic was founded in Queen Square, London. Particularly influential was the German epilepsy centre in Bielefeld, established in 1867. In 1872 this was taken over by the Pastor Friedrich von Bodelschwingh and it subsequently became the famous Bethel centre, which inspired similar centres in the UK. Other centres were established in Meer en Bosch in Heemstede (Holland) and in the Filadelfia colony in Dianalund (Denmark). In the UK, the Chalfont Centre in Buckinghamshire opened in 1894 and the centre at Lingfield (Surrey), which has undergone many name changes but is now known as the National Centre for Young People with Epilepsy (NCYPE), was founded in 1898. The David Lewis Centre in Cheshire was founded in 1904. There are currently active centres throughout Europe, including Norway, France, Holland, Germany and the UK.

Concept and role

The concept of the residential epilepsy centre has changed dramatically over the years. In the past, the epilepsy centre was, perhaps, analogous to the leper colony. It was a place where those who had the condition could be segregated from the general public – out of sight and out of mind. Such attitudes are unacceptable in current society. Against this background, one might ask: do residential epilepsy centres still have a role?

There are at least five current roles for residential epilepsy centres:

Longer-term placement for those with severe epilepsy, particularly with a high risk of status epilepticus

Severe epilepsy would usually be managed in the community. However, if there is a risk of frequent injury requiring medical attention or if there is a high risk of status epilepticus that does not respond promptly to out-of-hospital treatment, then the medical risks of managing the individual in the community might be unacceptably high. Prolonged seizures can cause permanent brain damage (see Chapter 76: 'Epilepsy emergency treatment'). Although the availability of treatment that can be administered by carers, namely rectal diazepam and, more recently, buccal midazolam, implies that even those at risk of status epilepticus can usually be managed in the community, for those who do not respond reliably to such treatments the only safe way of managing this situation might be long-term placement at the residential epilepsy centre. If a review of the regular antiepileptic medication reduces the risk of status epilepticus, however, the need for the placement should also be reviewed.

A situation that may be difficult to measure in the community is the occurrence of frequent drop

---

Introduction to Epilepsy ed. Gonzalo Alarcón and Antonio Valentín. Published by Cambridge University Press.
© Cambridge University Press 2012.

attacks that are liable to lead to injury. Although atonic seizures are notorious in this regard, other seizure types leading to falls may also carry a high risk of injury, for example tonic seizures and massive myoclonic jerks. Even though protective helmets are often provided for those who have frequent drop attacks liable to result in injury, helmets are not always effective and their value has been questioned.

Severe co-morbidity that is difficult to manage

Learning disability and psychiatric disorders occur at a higher rate in people with epilepsy. The prevalence of psychiatric disorder is particularly high in those who have both epilepsy and learning disability. An individual who has a schizophreniform psychosis, a mood disorder or seriously aggressive behaviour may be very difficult to manage in the community and residential placement might be necessary.

Short-term assessment to clarify diagnostic uncertainty

Most modern residential centres offer prolonged video-EEG monitoring facilities, together with observation by trained expert staff who are experienced in diagnosing unusual seizure types. A short-term assessment period at a residential centre, typically lasting from a few days to a few weeks, may resolve diagnostic uncertainty and allow appropriate management of the epilepsy to be implemented. Sometimes the presumptive diagnosis of epilepsy proves to be incorrect, allowing antiepileptic medication to be withdrawn.

Short-to-medium-term management of complex antiepileptic medication changes

In some cases, admission to a residential epilepsy centre can greatly facilitate medication changes. Such placement can be particularly useful if antiepileptic drug reductions that are liable to lead to withdrawal seizures are being considered. Such drugs typically include barbiturates and benzodiazepines. Other situations in which medication review might require close supervision would include those in which suspected adverse reactions to antiepileptic drugs, including skin rash, have previously occurred. Some adverse reactions to antiepileptic drugs can be potentially life-threatening.

Drug interactions, either between antiepileptic drugs or with essential medication to treat other conditions, can be complicated to manage, requiring close supervision of the type that can be provided at the epilepsy centre.

Presurgical assessment

The assessment of candidates for neurosurgery to treat epilepsy may require prolonged video-telemetry. Although such investigations can be carried out in a hospital setting, they are often better performed in a residential centre that is specially set up for such procedures. Sometimes withdrawal of antiepileptic drugs is undertaken to allow an adequate number of seizures to be captured. The associated risk can usually be managed well in a specialist epilepsy centre.

The future of residential epilepsy centres

The trend over recent years has been for epilepsy centres to be firmly established as academic centres of excellence that not only provide first-class investigation, diagnostic facilities and treatment, but also act as the nucleus for ground-breaking research. It is anticipated that this trend will become even more firmly established. High-quality research will continue to be carried out at such centres. Innovative treatments will be pioneered in settings where close specialist supervision can be provided. Multidisciplinary management of complex cases, including those with psychiatric or other co-morbidity, can be offered in such centres but would be difficult to emulate elsewhere. The emphasis will be on short-term diagnosis, assessment and treatment. This will include both antiepileptic drug reviews and presurgical assessment. The provision of high-quality diagnostic, treatment and rehabilitation services at the residential epilepsy centres should imply that the proportion of people requiring longer-term placement will become smaller. The majority of those who previously required long-term placement at a residential epilepsy centre will be effectively managed in the community, but residential epilepsy centres are likely to continue to have a valuable role in providing highly specialist facilities for those whose needs cannot be met adequately in the community.

Reference

Besag FMC, Brown SW. Residential epilepsy centers: United Kingdom. In Engel J Jr, Pedley TA, Aicardi J, eds. *Epilepsy: A Comprehensive Textbook*, pp. 2947–9. 2nd edn. Philadelphia: Lippincott-Raven; 2008.

Learning objectives

(1) To have an overview of the history of residential care and special centres for epilepsy.
(2) To know the present role of residential care and special centres for epilepsy.
(3) To be able to discuss the future of residential care and special centres for epilepsy.

Section 7 Psychiatric, social and legal aspects

Chapter 129 Main UK charities supporting epilepsy

Shiri Spector

In 1892 a group of philanthropists and medical men from London launched the National Society for the Employment of Epileptics (NSEE) and established a 'colony' where people with epilepsy of 'reasonable behaviour and mental ability' could live and work.

We have come a long way from the days when people with epilepsy were confined to workhouses or asylums because they could not find employment or accommodation and, alongside the medical and scientific advances in the understanding and treatment of epilepsy, significant and important leaps were made in educating the public and supporting those with epilepsy and their families.

This chapter briefly explores what is available to the public (patients, professionals and carers) in terms of education and support. These are the national organizations only. A comprehensive list of local organizations and services is found on both the Epilepsy Action website and the JEC website (see below).

National Society for Epilepsy (NSE)

'The National Society for Epilepsy's mission is to enhance the quality of life of people affected by epilepsy, by promoting research, education and public awareness and by delivering specialist medical care and support services.

'We strive to raise awareness to combat ignorance, misunderstanding and the stigma attached to epilepsy. We support everyone with epilepsy by providing up to date information on all aspects of living with the condition. We provide face to face support, help and information, as well as running a dedicated helpline and a nationwide Epilepsy Information Network (EIN).'
  www.epilepsysociety.org.uk
  Helpline: 01494 610 400
  NSE switchboard: 01494 601 300

Epilepsy Action (until 2002: British Epilepsy Association – BEA)

'Since May 2002 BEA has worked under the name Epilepsy Action. However, its aims are still the same as those in 1950, namely to improve the quality of life for people with epilepsy. As well as campaigning to improve epilepsy services and raise awareness of the condition, Epilepsy Action offers assistance to people in a number of ways, including a national network of branches, accredited volunteers, regular regional conferences, an Epilepsy Helpline and website.'
  www.epilepsy.org.uk
  Main office: 0113 210 8800
  Epilepsy Helpline: freephone 0808 800 5050

Epilepsy Bereaved (EB)

'Epilepsy Bereaved is committed to preventing Sudden Unexpected Death in Epilepsy and other epilepsy death through research, awareness and influencing changes. EB provides a contact line enabling people to get initial support and information. Core to the work of the charity is providing information and support to bereaved families, friends and carers who have lost a loved one through epilepsy. EB provides support individually and the opportunity to meet each other in regional peer support groups.'
  www.sudep.org
  Bereavement support line: 01235 772 852

Joint Epilepsy Council (JEC)

'The Joint Epilepsy Council of the U.K. and Ireland (JEC) is an umbrella organization which exists to represent the united voice of the voluntary sector and presents evidence based views on the need to

---

Introduction to Epilepsy ed. Gonzalo Alarcón and Antonio Valentín. Published by Cambridge University Press.
© Cambridge University Press 2012.

improve services for people with epilepsy, their families, and carers in the UK and Ireland.

'The JEC provides a way for 24 epilepsy organizations, operating in England, Wales, Scotland, Northern Ireland and the Republic of Ireland, to work collaboratively in a focussed, professional and effective manner, facilitating the sharing of information, expertise and skills, promoting good practice, maximizing resources and identifying unmet needs. We work to unite the efforts of member organizations to reduce stigma, challenge discrimination and disadvantage and improve the quality of life for people with epilepsy.'

www.jointepilepsycouncil.org.uk
General Secretary: 01943 871852

Learning objective

(1) To be aware of the objectives of the four main UK charities supporting epilepsy.

Section 7 Psychiatric, social and legal aspects

Chapter 130: Public education and resources

Stephen Brown

Epilepsy voluntary organizations, in addition to providing services and information for people with epilepsy and sponsoring research, are also typically concerned with campaigning on two main fronts. First, there is a general aim to reduce epilepsy-related stigma and increase awareness of epilepsy among the general public in everyday life. Second, there is a desire to influence legislators and public policy decision-makers to provide a social framework in which people with epilepsy are not disadvantaged by ignorance in school, in the workplace or in public settings such as public transport, and have satisfactory access to the optimum level of healthcare.

To whom is the campaigning addressed, and who are the public?

This process of public education includes campaigning by charities or other voluntary groups with an interest in epilepsy. In this context, the target audience will include people living with epilepsy themselves as well as their families, carers and friends. Professional groups other than politicians that may be targeted include not only health professionals, but also educationalists and employers. Recently several studies have examined public attitudes in a variety of countries and cultural settings. It seems that higher levels of education generally are associated with more positive attitudes towards epilepsy (Njamnshi et al., 2009; Neni et al., 2010), and that specific community-based programmes aimed at reducing stigma and educating the public can have a positive impact (Wang et al., 2009). Cultural attitudes prevalent in the developing world may be mirrored in first-generation immigrant populations in developed countries (Rhodes et al. 2008), and programmes aimed at raising awareness in European settings need to take this mixture into account.

What needs to be addressed in the educational message?

Surveys of public attitudes, even in developed countries, reveal shortfalls in knowledge that have a negative impact on the way people with epilepsy are perceived. For example Bagic et al. (2009) found 15% of respondents would object if their child played with a child with epilepsy. A primary task therefore is to correct misconceptions and myths about epilepsy such as that it is contagious or a sign of insanity. Some more subtle misconceptions may be held by employers regarding the risk of accidents in the workplace or the amount of sick leave a person might take, and in one recent UK study 21% of employers surveyed thought that employing people with epilepsy would be a major issue and 16% considered there were no jobs in their company suitable for a person with epilepsy (Jacoby et al., 2005). Obviously there are opportunities here for reducing fear in those whose value base is diminished by a small knowledge base, and providing practical information such as first aid for seizures and giving the general public, including employers, more appropriate expectations about people with epilepsy. This extends to the school situation, where children with epilepsy are at risk of underachieving (Aldenkamp et al., 2005) and may have specific learning needs of which their teachers may be unaware (Dunn et al., 2010).

How may the message be delivered?

Once the target audience is identified, it is essential that successful communicators of the message are identified as well. Ideally these will be led by people with epilepsy, and their families and friends. In most cases competent and motivated professionals may also

---

Introduction to Epilepsy ed. Gonzalo Alarcón and Antonio Valentín. Published by Cambridge University Press.
© Cambridge University Press 2012.

play a vital role. The context in which campaigning, lobbying or public education takes place is crucial to the choice of method or approach, so an appropriately facilitating environment needs to be identified. An example of a facilitating environment in the UK is the Parliamentary All Party Group on Epilepsy, which consists of legislators from both Houses of Parliament who have an interest in the subject (sometimes personal but typically stimulated by approaches from constituents). The UK epilepsy voluntary sector played a major part in lobbying for the group to form originally in the 1990s, and it is generally thought to achieve positive outcomes; e.g. in 2007 the group published a report on the human and economic cost of epilepsy in England (Wasted Money, Wasted Lives, 2007).

For a number of years the various UK epilepsy organizations agreed a joint theme for campaigning during National Epilepsy Week (the third week in May), though recently there has been increasing additional emphasis on round-the-year activity. The strength of a united voluntary sector was able to lead to government-sponsored but charitable-sector-produced publications such as the National Statement of Good Practice (Frost et al., 2002), and a coalition of clinicians and the voluntary sector was responsible for securing, carrying out and publishing the government-sponsored National Sentinel Clinical Audit of Epilepsy-Related Death (Hanna et al., 2002), which has had a significant impact on priority-setting for epilepsy service provision in the UK, and achieved considerable international recognition.

As far as epilepsy is concerned, it has been necessary to maintain campaigning pressure or else ground which is gained may be lost as other priorities compete or key personnel responsible for implementing policy move on. Following a sustained campaign combining professionals and the voluntary sector, the Department of Health in England produced an Executive Letter stating certain expectations about the quality of epilepsy services that should be provided in the NHS (EL (95)120). Although this was an end result of a campaign, it was also an opportunity to set up the next piece of work, and so the British Epilepsy Association surveyed NHS commissioners regarding their plans for epilepsy services in the context of the Executive Letter (Brown and Lee, 1998), and then delivered a series of seminars about epilepsy to a selection of NHS managers and clinicians around the country who were responsible for such services. A follow-up nationwide survey one year later revealed that areas where the seminar had occurred did indeed advance in their commissioning intentions, but in areas where there had been no seminars the commissioning approach to epilepsy had deteriorated (Brown et al., 1999).

Essential components for success therefore seem to include strong locally based advocacy as well as national initiatives. This advocacy can arise from the active involvement of people with epilepsy, their friends and family and committed clinicians, and the process must involve engagement with legislators. It must also be a long-term and continuous process.

References and recommended reading

Aldenkamp AP, Weber B, Overweg-Plandsoen WCG, Reijs R, van Mil S. Educational underachievement in children with epilepsy: a model to predict the effects of epilepsy on educational achievement. *J Child Neurol* 2005;**20**:175–80.

Bagic A, Bagic D, Zivkovic I. First population study of the general public awareness and perception of epilepsy in Bosnia and Herzegovina. *Epilepsy Behav* 2009;**14**(1): 154–61.

Brown SW, Lee P. Developments in UK provision for people with epilepsy: the impact of NHS Executive Letter 95/120. *Seizure* 1998;**7**:185–7.

Brown SW, Lee P, Buchan S, Jenkins A. Further developments in UK provision for people with epilepsy: where is the commitment to quality? *Seizure* 1999;**8**:128–31.

Dunn DW, Johnson CS, Perkins SM, et al. Academic problems in children with seizures: relationships with neuropsychological functioning and family variables during the 3 years after onset. *Epilepsy Behav* 2010;**19**:455–61.

EL(95)120 *A Positive Approach to Epilepsy*. NHS Executive Letter EL (95)120. Leeds: NHS Executive Headquarters; 1996.

Frost S, Crawford P, Mera S, Chappell B. *National Statement of Good Practice for the Treatment and Care of People who have Epilepsy*. Leeds: Joint Epilepsy Council; 2002.

Hanna NJ, Black M, Sander JWS, et al. *The National Sentinel Clinical Audit of Epilepsy-Related Death: Epilepsy – death in the shadows*. London: The Stationery Office; 2002.

Jacoby A, Gorry J, Baker GA. Employers' attitudes to employment of people with epilepsy: still the same old story? *Epilepsia* 2005;**46**:1978–87.

Neni SW, Latif AZ, Wong SY, Lua PL. Awareness, knowledge and attitudes towards epilepsy among rural populations in East Coast Peninsular Malaysia: a preliminary exploration. *Seizure* 2010;**19**(5):280–90.

Njamnshi AK, Angwafor SA, Tabah EN, Jallon P, Muna WF. General public knowledge, attitudes, and practices with respect to epilepsy in the Batibo Health District, Cameroon. *Epilepsy Behav* 2009;**14**(1):83–8.

Rhodes PJ, Small NA, Ismail H, Wright JP. 'What really annoys me is people take it like it's a disability': epilepsy, disability and identity among people of Pakistani origin living in the UK. *Ethnicity Health* 2008;**13**:1–21.

Wang W, Zhao D, Wu J, *et al*. Changes in knowledge, attitude, and practice of people with epilepsy and their families after an intervention in rural China. *Epilepsy Behav* 2009;**16**(1):76–9.

Wasted Money, Wasted Lives: the Human and Economic Cost of Epilepsy in England. Report by the All Party Parliamentary Group on Epilepsy. Leeds: Joint Epilepsy Council; 2007.

Learning objectives

To know the following about epilepsy voluntary organizations:

(1) Their main objectives.
(2) To whom is their campaigning addressed, and who are the public?
(3) What needs to be addressed in their educational message?
(4) How may the message be delivered?

Section 7 — Psychiatric, social and legal aspects

Chapter 131

Organizations and support services for people with epilepsy

Stephen Brown

The epilepsy voluntary (charitable) sector in the UK may be classified in at least three ways; by mandate, function, and locus of action.

Mandate

Most epilepsy organizations can trace their mandate in one of three ways:

Consumer-led

Some epilepsy organizations take steps to involve people with epilepsy in the determination of policy and consider themselves directed in this way. This may mean trustees or non-executive directors are elected by the membership, which in turn consists mainly of people with epilepsy and their families. These consumer-led groups will therefore tend to have their policy and priorities directed by people with epilepsy. An example of this is Epilepsy Action (formerly known as the British Epilepsy Association).

Professional-led

There are also groups whose members and leaders are professionals, especially clinicians, with particular interest in epilepsy. An example is the International League Against Epilepsy UK Chapter, but this category would also include various epilepsy interest groups that meet in different parts of the country. These are included here because they play an important part in the delivery of care and organization of services at national and local levels, as well as maintaining clinical standards.

Patronage

Many charitable organizations, often originally established with a specific financial endowment, continue to be governed by boards of trustees that effectively appoint their own members, usually from the same social class as the founders. These tend to be providers of care services, such as the David Lewis Centre.

Function

An organization may fulfil more than one function. Some examples are given here but the list, especially of those charities involved in various activities, is not exhaustive.

Care provider

Although statutory agencies such as the NHS are tasked with supplying assessment and treatment services, and local government has responsibility for special education, a number of epilepsy charities interact with this system to provide clinical, educational and social care services, such as those found in the David Lewis Centre, the National Centre for Young People with Epilepsy and the National Society for Epilepsy.

Information, support and training

Some organizations supply dedicated telephone helplines. Some help set up local support groups for people with epilepsy, or their carers, and some provide training for carers, including professional training (e.g. Epilepsy Action, National Society for Epilepsy).

Fundraising for research, and awarding research grants

At the present time in the UK there is one major charity exclusively concerned with research, and that is Epilepsy Research UK. Some of the other charities also consider research sponsorship to be part of their portfolio of activity, including the National Society for Epilepsy, Epilepsy Action and Epilepsy Bereaved.

Introduction to Epilepsy ed. Gonzalo Alarcón and Antonio Valentín. Published by CAMBRIDGE UNIVERSITY PRESS.
© CAMBRIDGE UNIVERSITY PRESS 2012.

Seeking to influence

Most of the larger charities and organizations regard representing the case for epilepsy services to legislators and to relevant media in order to shape public policy and attitudes in a positive way as an important part of their activity.

Locus of action

Finally, some charities are active in the whole nation and regard themselves as having a national role, e.g. Epilepsy Action, Epilepsy Bereaved or Epilepsy Scotland, while others confine their activities to a smaller geographical region, e.g. Mersey Region Epilepsy Association.

With such a multiplicity of organizations involved in such a spread of activities, it is perhaps not surprising that attempts have been made to produce some coordination of approach. Most of the epilepsy voluntary sector in the UK is currently contained within the membership of the Joint Epilepsy Council of the UK and Ireland, an umbrella body with a membership of 24 organizations. Some aspects of the current legislative environment in the UK will now be discussed.

Disability legislation in the UK

The 1995 Disability Discrimination Act defined disability as 'physical or mental impairment which has a substantial and long-term adverse effect on the ability to carry out normal day-to-day activities' with an interesting addition that 'where an impairment is being treated or corrected the impairment is considered as having the effect it would have without the measures in question'. It afforded civil rights protection to individuals with disabilities similar to those granted to women and minorities and made it illegal for employers to discriminate on the basis of disability. Subsequently the Act has been repealed and its provisions are now included in the newer 2010 Equality Act, which requires equal treatment in access to employment as well as private and public services, regardless of the protected characteristics of age, disability, gender reassignment, marriage and civil partnership, race, religion or belief, sex, and sexual orientation. The new Act also abolished the Disability Rights Commission and established instead a new Equality and Human Rights Commission to take on a wider brief.

Disabling aspects of epilepsy

The greatest impact on quality of life is generally taken to be whether seizures are well controlled as well as the presence of any additional disabilities. Hoare (1993) drew attention to three areas of particular relevance in children; epilepsy and its treatment, effects on personal development and the effect on the rest of family. A diagnosis of epilepsy has been reported as resulting in twice the expected unemployment rate, worse if there is active epilepsy and increased more so if there are added neurological or psychiatric problems. There was a risk that a person with epilepsy was less likely to leave school with qualifications or undergo subsequent training (Elwes *et al.*, 1991).

Cooper (1995) described some of the barriers in a survey of employers' attitudes. Employers are not always aware of the problems people with epilepsy face, there was a lack of monitoring of recruitment or promotion so that equal opportunities policies, even if present, were not being applied, and line managers were often left to make decisions about recruitment with no awareness training. Jacoby *et al.* (2005) found little had changed in 10 years. Furthermore, the effect on family, marriage, financial and moral consequences goes beyond traditional concern with stigma in at least some societies (Kleinman *et al.*, 1995). Coping skills seem to be related to being different or not being able to do things (Devlieger *et al.*, 1994). Particular problems might arise where epilepsy or its treatment has a negative effect on mobility, continence, coordination or the ability to perceive the risk of physical danger. Yet on the other hand, some researchers have described a more positive picture in first-hand studies of families' views (Laybourn and Hill 1994) and Collings (1990) found that people's perceptions of themselves and of their epilepsy were the variables most strongly related to overall well-being, although some seizure variables, including seizure frequency and being in full-time employment, also seemed of some importance.

Politicizing disability

The 1996 Disability Discrimination Act was passed after intense lobbying from the voluntary sector, and the epilepsy organizations played a part in this. However, the Charity Commission for England and Wales, which regulates the governance of charities, subsequently issued guidance reminding these organizations that overt political campaigning would in future have a negative bearing on their charitable status (CC9, CC9a) and since then the organizations have had to adopt a somewhat different approach.

Final thoughts

Much of the recent expansion in epilepsy services has been fuelled by the voluntary sector, e.g. the Sapphire project, which set up many new epilepsy specialist nurse posts and was led by the British Epilepsy Association. It is probably still too early to assess the impact of disability rights legislation and the new Equality and Human Rights Commission. Current changes in NHS reorganization provide opportunities for the voluntary sector to influence the standard of care locally, and there remains an obligation to consult service users. However, the challenge is to ensure that local campaigners have adequate resources, including training and information, and that actions are coordinated. The long-term effects of devolved government in Scotland, Wales and Northern Ireland are also still to be assessed, but these seem to be part of a trend to seeking more locally based solutions. The epilepsy charities are well placed to take advantage of this.

References

CC9 – Political Activities and Campaigning by Charities. London: Charity Commission; 1996.

CC9a – Political Activities and Campaigning by Local Community Charities. London: Charity Commission; 1996.

Collings JA. Epilepsy and well-being. *Soc Sci Med* 1990;**31**: 65–170.

Cooper M. Epilepsy and employment – employers' attitudes. *Seizure* 1995;4(3):193–9.

Devlieger P, Piachaud J, Leung P, George N. Coping with epilepsy in Zimbabwe and the Midwest, USA. *Int J Rehabil Res* 1994;17:251–64.

Elwes RD, Marshall J, Beattie A, Newman PK. Epilepsy and employment. A community based survey in an area of high unemployment. *J Neurol Neurosurg Psychiatry* 1991; 4(3):200–3.

Hoare P. The quality of life of children with chronic epilepsy and their families. *Seizure* 1993;2(4):269–75.

Jacoby A, Gorry J, Baker GA. Employers' attitudes to employment of people with epilepsy: still the same old story? *Epilepsia* 2005;46:1978–87.

Kleinman A, Wang WZ, Li SC, *et al*. The social course of epilepsy: Chronic illness as social experience in interior China. *Soc Sci Med* 1995;**40**:1319–30.

Laybourn A, Hill M. Children with epilepsy and their families: needs and services. *Child Care Health Dev* 1994;20:1–14.

Learning objectives

(1) To be aware of the classification of the epilepsy voluntary (charitable) sector in the UK: by mandate, function and locus of action.
(2) To know the rights of people with epilepsy according to the Disability Legislation in the UK.
(3) To know the disabling aspects of epilepsy in addition to the seizures themselves.
(4) To be aware of the risks of politicizing disability.

Section 7 Psychiatric, social and legal aspects

Chapter 132

Can a joined-up primary–secondary care approach help people with epilepsy?

Leone Ridsdale

Introduction

The aim in this chapter is to describe disabilities in epilepsy and provoke interest and debate about applying a joined-up primary–secondary care approach, which draws on the model of rehabilitation. Epilepsy is not usually conceptualized as requiring rehabilitation. Most adults with epilepsy experience paroxysmal loss of consciousness and between attacks they have no signs of weakness, rigidity or incoordination. Disability is likely to be cognitive, psychological and social, so hidden. This chapter highlights the cognitive and psychosocial challenges experienced by people with epilepsy, and identifies limitations in current service patterns, using as an example the United Kingdom (UK). It proposes that health-care systems, in this case the National Health Service (NHS), adopt a rehabilitative approach designed to increase patients' capacity to participate in the community, and reduce distress (and inequality) throughout life (Wade and de Jong, 2000). This can be achieved more efficiently by developing skills and partnerships between hospital-based specialist services and general practice.

There are about 48 million adults (Statistics Government UK, 2008) in the UK. The prevalence of adults treated for epilepsy in general practice is about 288 000 (0.6%) (Ridsdale *et al.*, 1996a). There are about 575 full-time adult neurologists, so every neurologist has about 500 adults with epilepsy who they could see for long-term follow-up. The incidence of epilepsy used to be highest in children. The onset of epilepsy is now higher in older adults, with cerebrovascular disease being the commonest cause of epilepsy (15%) (Sander *et al.*, 1990). Sudden death is three times commoner in epilepsy, it affects about 800 people with epilepsy per year (Majeed *et al.*, 2000). It is more likely to affect working-age people, particularly young men; it frequently occurs in a context in which there has been loss of continuity and communication about care; mortality had not declined in recent years.

New-onset epilepsy

The role of the general practitioner (GP) in epilepsy involves problem definition first, differentiating between syncope and epilepsy, and asking a witness to be available at a specialist appointment. When the diagnosis is suspected, the GP needs also to give advice on risk management, including the positioning of an unconscious person, and not driving. Although important, this advice is frequently not given. The National Institute for Health and Clinical Excellence Guidelines (NICE, 2004) recommend that patients with suspected epilepsy see a doctor with specialist training. Assuming a ratio of 2:1 patients referred with suggestive symptoms for every one diagnosed, specialists (mostly neurologists) may see on average 100 new referrals for suspected epilepsy per year. Rehabilitation after diagnosis is arguably the weakest link in epilepsy care (Ridsdale *et al.*, 2003).

A factor likely to be important for patient self-management of epilepsy in the long term is the individual's own knowledge and understanding of their condition. In people with newly diagnosed epilepsy our research group found the median score for knowledge of epilepsy was 43/55 on a knowledge questionnaire (range of 12 to 51) (Ridsdale *et al.*, 2000). Not having general educational qualifications (GCSE's) predicted lower knowledge of epilepsy (one-third of the general population has no qualifications). Compared to those in the highest knowledge of epilepsy quartile at baseline, those who were in the lowest

Introduction to Epilepsy ed. Gonzalo Alarcón and Antonio Valentín. Published by Cambridge University Press.
© Cambridge University Press 2012.

quartile had scores 12 points lower on the knowledge scale (36 versus 48) (Ridsdale et al., 2000). This is likely to be important.

Ideally, an epilepsy specialist nurse or other keyworker will start rehabilitation by offering advice and support after diagnosis. We randomized new patients with epilepsy after seeing a neurologist to see nurse specialists or to have usual medical care. The nurses acted as key workers and referrals were made when indicated, to social services, psychology, neurology, occupational therapy, an employment officer, or the learning disability team. After a nurse-led input, the mean knowledge score was 5 points higher in the intervention group (43 versus 37) for the group (Ridsdale et al., 2000) in the lowest quartile of knowledge of epilepsy compared to the control group. Whatever their baseline scores were, patients who were offered nurse-led input were significantly more likely to report they had received enough information to manage different aspects of life, and were significantly more satisfied with this input.

Long-term epilepsy

After patients have been diagnosed, some are difficult to stabilize. Sometimes this is a straightforward biomedical challenge, requiring a trial of different medications. However, the management of epilepsy by doctor and patient involves coping with psycho-social challenges. The diagnosis of epilepsy is a loss or blow to the patient's self-perception. The range of reactions include denial, anxiety, anger, guilt, bargaining, depression as well as acceptance. Psychological responses to the diagnostic label may limit individuals' ability to take in new knowledge. In responding to new information about a long-term condition, patients can be described as information avoiders, weavers and seekers (Pinder, 1990). Providers of education and support must negotiate and adapt as individuals with epilepsy go through stages of emotional adjustment, and when they change their social roles throughout life. Medical staff who work in hospitals are less well situated to see the social and family context.

After diagnosis, most patients are transferred back to their GP, with a recommended drug regime. In the past, GPs expressed lack of confidence and competence in providing epilepsy care (Thapar et al., 1998). This does not correspond with patients' preferences. Our research group found 50% of patients prefer GP care, 20% prefer shared GP and specialist care, 10% prefer specialist care, and 20% have no preference (Ridsdale et al., 1996a). Epilepsy became the first neurological condition for which doctors in primary care are paid specifically to do routine monitoring, through the Quality and Outcome Framework (The Information Centre, 2008). With this, GPs must gradually increase their competence and confidence. Traditionally, neurologists have been less available or involved in GP education and advice in the district than diabetes or asthma specialists. This may change as the number of neurologists in the UK has tripled over the last 15 years. There is evidence emerging that GPs with additional training and with Special Interest (GPwSI) in neurology can provide education to other GPs, as well as contributing to service planning (Ridsdale et al., 2008; Rogers, 2008).

Ideally, those with long-term epilepsy should get services that match their illness severity at different points in their lives. Attacks vary in type, frequency and severity. Research in one region found those with an epilepsy attack in prior 6 months were more likely to see a specialist (Ridsdale et al., 1996a). This was reassuring, but a national study found no association (Hart and Shorvon, 1995). If specialists hold on to some patients regardless of illness severity, specialists become less accessible to new referrals for diagnosis, and to patients with long-term epilepsy, who have difficulty managing at a later point in their lives. GPwSI and nurse specialists may have a useful role in helping patients who are newly diagnosed to transfer away from specialist care, and manage their condition in the community (Rogers, 2008).

GPwSI and nurse specialists can additionally help patients with long-term epilepsy, when they have life changes, for example planned pregnancy, loss of epilepsy control, or conversely no attacks, with questions about whether an individual can come off medication. There is evidence about the characteristics of patient groups who are more likely to have no recurrence following planned medication withdrawal (Medical Research Council, 1991; Kwan and Sander, 2004). A false perception that epilepsy is a permanent diagnosis, held by some professionals and patients, may mean that patients do not benefit from this evidence.

The experience (not just the diagnosis) of epilepsy has psychological and social impact. Depression is the consequences of life events and difficulties without sufficient support in terms of close, intimate confiding relationships. Using questionnaires to estimate the likelihood of being 'a case', we found age affected the reaction to epilepsy; older people with epilepsy were more depressed, whilst younger people felt more stigmatized (Ridsdale et al., 1996b). Depression, anxiety and stigma is increased if there has been an increased frequency of epilepsy attacks (Ridsdale et al., 1996b; Kimiskidis et al., 2007). People with poorly controlled epilepsy are not vocal in their demands. It is important to enquire about these psychological symptoms in ongoing assessments for rehabilitation to take place. Untreated psychological symptoms create a vicious circle. If psychological distress following epilepsy attacks, it is likely further to impair individuals' ability to manage their epilepsy.

In a study of people with long-term epilepsy (average 23 years), we found people had similar median knowledge scores (42.5) as those with newly diagnosed epilepsy (Ridsdale et al., 1999). We found people with chronic epilepsy, with no general educational qualifications (General Certificate of Secondary Education, GCSEs) have less knowledge of epilepsy compared to those with GSCEs or higher qualifications (39 vs 43). Lower epilepsy knowledge scores were found in older people compared to younger people, (37 vs 43), those who left school earlier rather than later (40 vs 43) and those not belonging to self-help groups versus those belonging (42 vs 45). Multiple regression showed these have independent effects. The additive consequences of social disadvantage on knowledge of epilepsy are considerable (Ridsdale et al., 1999). An understanding of this is important to rehabilitation.

A bio-psycho-social team approach is a core attribute of general practice. It is also the hallmark of rehabilitation. This approach is required to manage people with epilepsy. Being emotionally stuck prevents patients from taking in the information that they need to self-manage a long-term condition effectively. Patients need to be offered information intermittently when they can use it. A structured format allows different members of the team to know what has been discussed, and to discuss new issues that could not be covered or were not relevant at one point, at another time. In interviews we found that younger people with epilepsy were more affected by the consequences on driving, jobs and managing their families' lives. Older people tended to see epilepsy as just another problem to cope with, but often needed to add new drugs to an already complicated regime (Ridsdale et al., 2003).

Linking primary and specialist services to tackle inequalities

The addition of neurology to training for General Practice (Education Unit, 2008) and financial remuneration for epilepsy monitoring for GPs provided by the Quality and Outcomes Framework (QOF) (The Information Centre, 2008) marks a watershed. It heralds acceptance of responsibility for neurological problems in UK primary care. At present the number of criteria and points achievable for epilepsy care are small. An incremental approach is sensible if GPs and their practice nurses are to build up their capacity through education and experience, just as they did previously with diabetes and asthma. In the long run patients with epilepsy need ongoing rehabilitation with personalized care plans including information about diagnosis, investigation, prognosis, medications, efficacy, side effects, adherence, drug interactions, free prescriptions, epilepsy triggers, lack of sleep, alcohol, drugs and stress, first aid management, women's issues if applicable, safety in the home, driving, stigma, anxiety and depression, and support organizations. This approach is supported by self-groups, and will merit more QOF points.

There is some way to go, particularly in tackling inequalities. Ashworth et al. (2007) have pointed out that the collection of points which result in payments through the QOF is lower in socially deprived areas. When epilepsy care is measured specifically, there is worrying variation in control. For example in two inner London boroughs, Lambeth and Southwark, the organizing Primary Care Trusts include a population served by two Foundation Trusts with expertise in epileptology and epilepsy surgery; but they are also deprived areas. Whilst current national Quality and Outcomes Framework (QOF) data suggest 40% of people with epilepsy have had an attack in the prior year (Ashworth M, personal communication, 3 Feb 2008), 50% of people with epilepsy in these two boroughs have had an attack in the prior year. Shohet et al. (2007) showed that poor epilepsy control measured by the QOF is strongly associated with higher levels of emergency epilepsy-related hospitalization. About 6:1 of hospital admissions for epilepsy are for emergency and not planned (Majeed et al., 2000). Rehabilitation for those identified through QOF could therefore improve lives, and reduce cost.

Teams working together across primary and hospital sectors can hopefully show the extent to which poor epilepsy control in socially deprived areas is remediable. Doctors are often cynical about government policy initiatives; some have benefits. Arguably the plan to provide access for diagnosis and management to everyone in the NHS within 18 weeks will be one. In at least one area, GPs, GPwSI, neurologists and managers are planning for common neurological conditions at regular meetings, producing integrated pathways for common disorders and in making recommendations for care in the area.

There is scope for research too. Interventions for epilepsy need development and evaluation in order to reduce inequalities, unnecessary hospital attendance, and sudden unexplained death. If joined up policy-making can be supported by resources, training and evaluation, epilepsy may cease to be Cinderella condition.

References

Ashworth M, Seed P, Armstrong D, Durbaba S, Jones R. The relationship between social deprivation and the quality of primary care: a national survey using indicators from the UK Quality and Outcomes Framework. *Br J Gen Pract* 2007;**57**(539):441–8.

Education Unit. RCGP. 2008. Available from: http://www.rcgp.prg.uk/default.aspx?page=4020.

Hart YM, Shorvon SD. The nature of epilepsy in the general-population.2. Medical-care. *Epilepsy Res* 1995; **21**(1):51–8.

Kimiskidis VK, Triantafyllou NI, Kararizou E, *et al*. Depression and anxiety in epilepsy: the association with demographic and seizure-related variables. *Ann Gen Psychiatry* 2007;**6**(28):1744–859.

Kwan P, Sander JW. The natural history of epilepsy: an epidemiological view. *J Neurol Neurosurg Psychiatry* 2004;**75**(10):1376–81.

Majeed A, Bardsley M, Morgan D, O'Sullivan C, Bindman AB. Cross sectional study of primary care groups in London: association of measures of socioeconomic and health status with hospital admission rates. *Brit Med Jl* 2000;**321**(7268):1057–60.

Medical Research Council Antiepileptic Drug Withdrawal Study Group. Randomized study of antiepileptic drug withdrawal in patients in remission. *Lancet* 1991;**337** (8751):1175–80.

National Institute for Health and Clinical Excellence. Epilepsy in adults and children: *NICE guideline*. Available from: http://www.nice.org.uk/nicemedia/pdf/2004_043_Launch_of_epilepsy_guidelines.pdf. 27-10-2004.

Pinder CM. *The Management of Chronic Disease: Patient and Doctor Perspectives on Parkinson's Disease*. Basingstoke: MacMillan Press; 1990.

Ridsdale L, Robins D, Fitzgerald A, Jeffery S, McGee L. Epilepsy monitoring and advice recorded: general practitioners' views, current practice and patients' preferences. *Br J Gen Pract* 1996a;**46**(402):11–14.

Ridsdale L, Robins D, Fitzgerald A, Jeffery S, McGee L. Epilepsy in general practice: patients' psychological symptoms and their perception of stigma. *Br J Gen Pract* 1996b;**46**(407):365–6.

Ridsdale L, Kwan I, Cryer C. The effect of a special nurse on patients' knowledge of epilepsy and their emotional state. *Br J Gen Pract* 1999;**49**(441):285–9.

Ridsdale L, Kwan I, Cryer C, Epilepsy Care EG. Newly diagnosed epilepsy: can nurse specialists help? A randomized controlled trial. *Epilepsia* 2000; **41**(8):1014–19.

Ridsdale L, Kwan I, Morgan M. How can a nurse intervention help people with newly diagnosed epilepsy? A qualitative study of patients' views. *Seizure* 2003; **12**(2):69–73.

Ridsdale L, Doherty J, McCrone, Seed P. A new GP with special interest headache service: observational study. *Br J Gen Pract* 2008;**58**(552):478–83.

Rogers G. This house believes that only general practitioners with a specialist interest in epilepsy should be treating the condition. *Pract Neurol* 2008; **8**:138–40.

Sander JWAS, Hart YM, Shorvon SD, Johnson JL. National General Practice Study of Epilepsy: newly diagnosed epileptic seizures in a general population. *Lancet* 1990;**336**:1267–71.

Shohet C, Yelloly J, Bingham P, Lyratzopolous G. The association between the quality of epilepsy management in primary care, general practice population deprivation status and epilepsy-related emergency hospitalisations. *Seizure* 2007;**6**(4):351–5.

Statistics Government UK. 2008. Available from: www.statistics.gov.uk/census2001/profiles/commentaries/people.asp.

Thapar AK, Stott NCH, Richens A, Kerr M. Attitudes of GPs to the care of people with epilepsy. *Fam Pract* 1998;**15**(5):437–42.

The Information Centre. *The Quality and Outcome Framework. 2008*. Available from: www.ic.nhs.uk/services/qof.

Wade D, de Jong B. Recent advances in rehabilitation. *Brit Med J* 2000;**320**(7246):1385–8

Learning objective

(1) To be able to discuss the role of primary and secondary care in the management of newly diagnosed and chronic epilepsy and the advantages of their joint management.

Section 7 Psychiatric, social and legal aspects

Chapter 133: Support groups and their role in care in the community

Jane Juler

Support groups can be run by health professionals for their patients, or, more usually, by a mixture of sufferers, carers and others with an interest in the subject. Whatever the detailed make-up, support groups depend on volunteers and the extent of their activities will depend on the resources available.

Typically a group's activities will include some of the following:

(1) Support for sufferers (and families, friends and carers)
- Someone to talk to: many newly diagnosed patients find it a great relief to be able to talk to people who know about the condition and aren't bothered by it. The need for this has been reducing as facilities to chat online have developed.
- A source of information: though, again, to a large degree, the internet is taking over in this area.
- Helpful hints: including ideas for improving compliance, e.g. talking to consultant about changing times for taking AEDs if the current ones make things difficult (partying teenagers may not find last thing before bed the best time to remember to take their medication).
- Social events (where fits don't matter)!: some people find that the worry that they will have a fit when they go out, will precipitate one. Such people can attend support group meetings, knowing that it doesn't matter if they do have a fit (and then they rarely do).

(2) Educating the local community: the public at large, teachers, employers.

(3) Fundraising: for group needs (e.g. hall hire or advertisement costs) and for wider needs (e.g. national activities).

(4) Advertisement: most of the above activities are ineffective if no-one knows the group is there.

This list is, of course, not exhaustive and specialized skills by volunteers can widen it.

Support for sufferers, families, friends and carers

Many newly diagnosed patients are feeling shocked, bewildered and frightened. Often, they don't know much about epilepsy except that it sounds terrible, they've been told they can't drive, and they may have had very strange experiences (e.g. jamais vu, indescribable sensations). Meeting people who are familiar with epilepsy, may have shared their experiences (or at least have known of others who have shared them) and are not bothered by it can be a tremendous relief.

Spouses, partners, parents, relatives and friends can be frightened by seizures, especially by tonic-clonic seizures. They usually want to know what they can do to help. In particular, parents of children with epilepsy can be very distressed, and wanting information about epilepsy, as well as the chance to compare notes with other parents, and ideas for what they can do to help. Where parents perceive their children as suffering side effects of medication, and the clinicians seem uninterested, they can become frantic. Support groups can explain how keeping good records and reporting precisely on observed side effects can help in such circumstances.

When a sufferer has a partner who is frightened by seizures and there are children, the partner can be desperate to protect the children from being present during seizures, putting tremendous strains on the relationship.

Introduction to Epilepsy ed. Gonzalo Alarcón and Antonio Valentín. Published by CAMBRIDGE UNIVERSITY PRESS.
© CAMBRIDGE UNIVERSITY PRESS 2012.

Resisting overprotectiveness is another situation where it can be helpful to talk things over with others faced with similar temptations.

Support groups can help the epileptologists, too!

Support groups can provide information at leisure, in a relaxed atmosphere, so that it can be taken in better. At the lowest level, this can spare the medical staff some time spent in passing on general information about epilepsy.

Most people want to know what they can do to help themselves or their child/partner/parent/friend. Support groups can encourage all involved to keep good records of what is happening, so improving the quality of information available to the medical staff at the same time as reducing feelings of helplessness. This again can save time being wasted.

Improving the quality of information provided by the sufferer and associates will often help to resolve matters when they are not happy with the quality of medical care. It not only saves time, it saves aggro too!

Support groups can pass on tips for improving compliance – and again, can explain the need at leisure, so it's more likely to be taken in. Few, if any, doctors let their patients know that pharmacists have discretion to supply small quantities of vital medications in an emergency without a prescription – so that if the patient suddenly finds themselves caught without their AEDs, they can talk to a chemist. The chemist will have to check their story, preferably but not necessarily contacting the patient's GP or regular pharmacist in the process.

They can also explain that there are other advantages in having a regular pharmacist, and of making sure that this pharmacist is aware that their AEDs have been prescribed for epilepsy. AEDs are prescribed for other conditions where variability of supply formulation is unlikely to be a problem. If the chemist knows AEDs are for epilepsy they will usually try to keep the precise formulation unchanged.

General comments

No one will use a support group if they don't know it is there. If you know of a local group do help make it known.

Support groups do need help too. Remember they depend on volunteers and their activities will reflect the resources available.

Whilst there are good leaflets available (from BEA, NSE, etc.), most groups welcome talks from health professionals as part of their programme of events.

However, it is as well for prospective speakers to be aware that bad experiences of mismanagement by the medical profession have embittered some people and left a deep distrust of doctors. Such people are not likely to be deeply involved with running a support group but may come to meetings to air their grievances.

Learning objectives

(1) To be able to discuss the role of support groups to support sufferers from epilepsy and their relatives, friends and carers.
(2) To be aware of the advantages in the cooperation between support groups and the specialists.

Section 7: Psychiatric, social and legal aspects

Chapter 134: The International League Against Epilepsy (ILAE) and the International Bureau for Epilepsy (IBE)

Edward H. Reynolds

Foundation and history

The International League Against Epilepsy (ILAE) was founded in 1909 in Budapest by a group of European neurologists, psychiatrists and physicians attending the 16th International Medical Congress. In the same year, the journal *Epilepsia* was launched as the official publication of the ILAE. After a promising start with meetings in Europe every year, including London in 1913 at the time of the 17th International Medical Congress, the progress of the ILAE was interrupted by World War I and its aftermath.

The ILAE was revived and reconstituted at Lingfield, Surrey, UK, in 1935 during the second International Neurological Congress in London dedicated to the centenary of the birth of Hughlings Jackson (1835–1911). After a further pause for World War II, the ILAE grew steadily such that it now has 100 affiliated country 'chapters' in every continent, i.e. in over half the countries of the world. In July 2009, the ILAE celebrated its centenary with a special anniversary Congress jointly with the International Bureau for Epilepsy (IBE), again in Budapest. The ILAE and *Epilepsia* are the oldest neurological sub-speciality organization and journal in the world (Shorvon et al., 2009).

Objectives

The objectives of ILAE have changed very little since its inception. As a non-profit charitable non-government organization (NGO) the objectives are to:

(1) Advance and disseminate throughout the world knowledge concerning the epilepsies.
(2) Encourage research concerning the epilepsies.
(3) Promote prevention, diagnosis, treatment, advocacy and care for all persons suffering from these disorders.
(4) Improve education and training in the field of the epilepsies.

The main methods for promoting these objectives have been to:

(1) Encourage the establishment of national societies (chapters) with the same objectives, and of which there are now 100 such chapters.
(2) Establish effective cooperation with other worldwide organizations active in medical science, public health and social care, e.g. neurology, psychiatry, the World Health Organization (WHO) etc.
(3) Promote publications about epilepsy, especially *Epilepsia*, and organize international congresses or symposia.
(4) Appoint special commissions for the study of specific issues relating to epilepsy and to make recommendations.

The ILAE now holds international congresses every two years, jointly with IBE, as well as several regional congresses separate from IBE in the intervening year. The best-known commission of the ILAE has been that on classification and terminology. The recommendations of that commission for classification of seizures (1981) and of the epilepsies and epileptic syndromes (1989) have been widely adopted throughout the world (see Shorvon et al., 2009). Other important commissions have included those on developing countries, education, epidemiology and economics, all of which are relevant to the ILAE/IBE/WHO Global Campaign against Epilepsy (see below). Other commissions deal specifically with, for example, antiepileptic drugs, genetics, neurobiology, neurosurgery, paediatrics etc, the reports of which may appear in *Epilepsia* or in one of its supplements.

Introduction to Epilepsy ed. Gonzalo Alarcón and Antonio Valentín. Published by Cambridge University Press.
© Cambridge University Press 2012.

Chapter 134: The International League Against Epilepsy (ILAE) and the International Bureau for Epilepsy (IBE)

With the international growth of ILAE in the last two decades, regional commissions of ILAE, based mainly on WHO regions, have been set up to coordinate regional cooperation in political, educational and research activity.

The International Bureau for Epilepsy (IBE)

From the beginning ILAE's objectives included a strong commitment to the social care and rehabilitation of people with epilepsy. However, there was often a tension between those officers or members interested in either medical or social aspects. At the ILAE Congress in Rome in 1961 this led to the proposal to establish an International Bureau for Epilepsy which would enable lay organizations to participate in the work of the ILAE, especially in relation to such social dimensions as education, employment, legislation, stigma, transport and mobility. At first this was a social arm of the ILAE, but by 1966 it became an independent organization with its own constitution (Shorvon et al., 2009).

The objectives of IBE are to:

(1) Identify the needs of people with epilepsy and their families.
(2) Provide information and support to them.
(3) Promote public awareness and education about epilepsy.
(4) Improve social services, care and quality of life for people with epilepsy.

From the beginning, IBE, which evolved out of ILAE, has worked closely with the ILAE through interlocking executive committees, i.e. the president, secretary general and treasurer of each organization serve also on the executive of the other organization. Full joint executive committee meetings are also held on matters of common interest. Each organization holds parallel democratic international elections of officers for simultaneous four-year terms. The most obvious manifestations of this cooperation have been the joint international congresses every two years. However, like the ILAE the IBE holds independent Regional Congresses in the intermediate year. The IBE also establishes its own commissions, for example, on employment, social care etc, but occasionally joint commissions of ILAE and IBE have been established, for example, on developing countries or driving licences. A more recent major collaborative effort has been that of the ILAE/IBE/WHO Global Campaign against Epilepsy.

In the UK the League has a single British chapter, which holds a scientific meeting at least once a year. The Bureau has two UK chapters, i.e. Epilepsy Action covering England, Wales and Northern Ireland, and Epilepsy Action Scotland, which is independent.

The ILAE/IBE/WHO Global Campaign against Epilepsy

Epilepsy is a unique global problem that affects all ages, races, social classes and countries. Eighty-five per cent of at least 50 million people with active epilepsy are in developing countries, where as many as 6–98% receive no adequate treatment (Jallon, 1997).

The ILAE and IBE are now global in scale and structure and both are NGOs affiliated to WHO. As President of ILAE in the mid-1990s, I proposed a global partnership and campaign by the League (professional), the Bureau (patients and public) and the WHO (political) to bring epilepsy 'out of the shadows' and to address the 'treatment gap' described above (Reynolds, 2001). The campaign was launched at WHO headquarters, Geneva, in 1997 with the following specific objectives:

(1) To increase public and professional awareness of epilepsy as a universal treatable brain disorder.
(2) To promote public and professional education about epilepsy.
(3) To change attitudes, dispel myths and raise epilepsy on to a new plane of acceptability in the public domain.
(4) To identify the needs of people with epilepsy on a national, regional and global basis.
(5) To encourage governments and departments of health to develop their own national campaigns to improve prevention, diagnosis, treatment, care, services and public attitudes.

The Campaign has inter-related global, regional and national components. During Phase 1 (1997–2001) which concentrated on the first three objectives, the WHO raised the priority of the Campaign to its highest level, making epilepsy the first neurological disorder to be accorded this status. Regional conferences and declarations on the needs of people with epilepsy were held in Europe, Africa, Latin America, North America and Asia and Oceania. A White Paper on Epilepsy was presented to the European Parliament. All of this culminated in the launch of the second phase of the Campaign in 2001 with the emphasis on objectives 4 and 5 (Reynolds, 2002). This has included specific regional demonstration projects in several developing countries, notably China, to estimate prevalence, to promote awareness-raising and training, and to develop models of treatment (Wang et al., 2006). As of 2008, 103 countries or chapters have initiated projects under the umbrella of the Campaign. The campaign secretariat has also undertaken a major review of epilepsy services available throughout the world (Atlas, 2005).

References

Atlas: Epilepsy Care in the World. Geneva: World Health Organization; 2005.

Jallon P. Epilepsy in developing countries. ILAE workshop report. *Epilepsia* 1997;**38**:1143–51.

Reynolds EH. ILAE/IBE/WHO Global Campaign 'Out of the Shadows': Global and regional developments. *Epilepsia* 2001;**42**:1094–100.

Reynolds EH (ed.). Epilepsy in the world: launch of the second phase of the ILAE/IBE/WHO Global Campaign Against Epilepsy. *Epilepsia* 2002;43 (Suppl 6).

Shorvon S. Weiss G, Avanzini G, et al. *International League against Epilepsy 1909-2009: A Centenary History.* Chichester: Wiley-Blackwell; 2009.

Wang WZ, Wu JZ, Ma GY, et al. Efficacy assessment of phenobarbital in epilepsy: a large community-based intervention trial in rural China. *Lancet Neurol* 2006;5:46–52.

Learning objective

(1) To know the historical development of the International League Against Epilepsy and of the International Bureau for Epilepsy, their objectives, activities and achievements.

Section 7 Psychiatric, social and legal aspects

Chapter 135

Health economics and epilepsy

Dominic C. Heaney

Introduction

Health economics is a branch of economics concerned with issues related to scarcity in the allocation of health and health care. Its methods can be used to inform a range of situations that arise in the treatment of epilepsy.

For example, simple and important questions such as 'How much do we spend on epilepsy?', 'Could we do what we do more cheaply?' or 'How can we measure the financial impact of epilepsy?' can all be approached using health economic methods.

At its most complex, health economics requires a sophisticated understanding of mathematics, statistics and choice theory. Nevertheless, the basic principles of health economic analysis are simple to understand, and can be applied by identifying which resources are 'used' (i.e. resource-use) and what they cost ('unit costs'). The product of resources used and unit costs can be compared between health-care interventions (for example, comparing different drugs, surgery vs non-surgery or even nurse specialists vs generic health-care workers).

Resource use

One of the first steps when investigating the health economic impact of a condition or its treatment has been to consider its impact in the widest sense. There has traditionally been great focus on the cost of anti-epileptic drugs (AEDs). This narrow perspective is important particularly when: (i) the large number of people with epilepsy is considered (for example up to 400 000 in the UK may suffer the condition); and (ii) the observation that a significant, less well-defined, proportion of these will require regular treatment for many years. Thus AEDs are important because it represents a 'mid-cost', 'high-volume' pharmaceutical burden.

But any individual with epilepsy will state that their condition and its treatments has effects on a wide range of other 'resources' – ranging from a need to attend doctors' appointments to discrimination in the workplace. Health economists classify these by considering their relation to medical care.

Direct costs are those resources used in relation to delivery of medical care. They can be 'medical' (such as hospitalization, health-care professional wages, medication, laboratory tests and investigations) or 'non-medical' (including social services, transport and communication costs).

Indirect costs are borne outside the context of medical treatment. Work (and absence from work) is commonly regarded as the primary indirect cost – indeed the term 'productivity' cost is often used synonymously. Depending on the context, it may also be appropriate to consider the effect of epilepsy and its treatments on education and leisure time. For example, studies of the cost-effectiveness of paediatric surgery should include consideration of the impact on education.

There is some controversy surrounding the term 'indirect costs' as it is used elsewhere (for example, in accountancy) with a different meaning. However defined, these costs can be very significant in epilepsy. They include unemployment, absenteeism, reduced productivity, premature mortality, under-employment, indirect costs imposed on carers, and schooldays or university days missed – all of which have been shown in numerous studies to be over-represented among people with poorly controlled epilepsy.

It may also be appropriate to consider 'intangible' costs, which include the financial impact of reduced quality of life, pain and suffering arising from epilepsy. They are described as 'intangible' as their value is difficult to define without using contingent

---

Introduction to Epilepsy ed. Gonzalo Alarcón and Antonio Valentín. Published by Cambridge University Press.
© Cambridge University Press 2012.

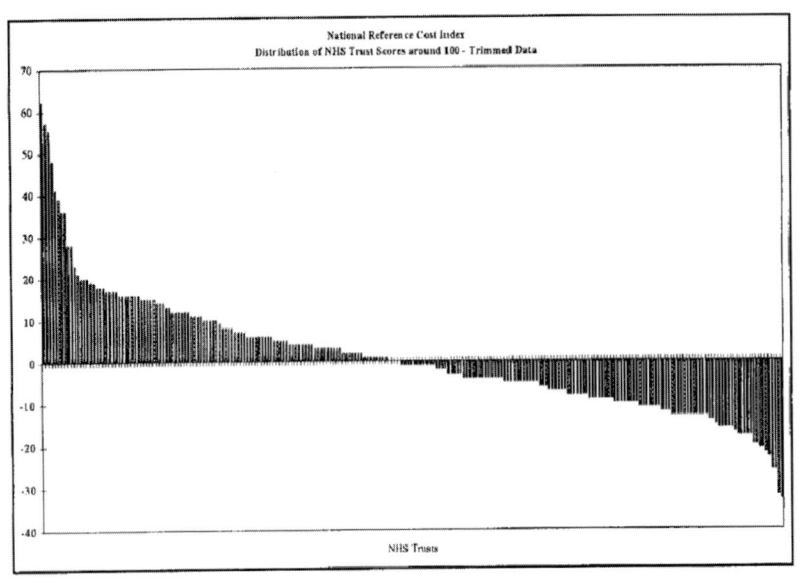

Section 7: Psychiatric, social and legal aspects

Figure 135.1. Example of how unit cost for a surgical procedure varies across NHS hospitals (data from NHS Reference Costs 2005)

valuation (CV) techniques. In their most commonly used form, CV methods involve asking individuals to choose between hypothetical scenarios – with their choices implying how they value various aspects of their condition. For example, patients may be offered a hypothetical operation that might offer them a small chance of 'ridding' them of epilepsy permanently – but with a risk of mortality or injury. Their choices in these scenarios may give some information about how that individual 'values' a cure for their condition. Although interesting insights into epilepsy may be gained through these methods, their applicability and validity of the estimates they generate is contested.

Unit costs

A health economic study must consider the value of resources (direct, indirect and intangible) relevant to a particular economic question. The value of each unit is considered in financial terms and described as the 'unit cost'. In most cases, the focus is on direct medical costs and productivity losses as these are likely to represent the majority of all costs incurred.

There are several issues that should be considered when using unit costs.

First, the economic perspective of a study should be considered. This concept dictates that only costs or benefits directly relevant to the viewpoint of a study should be considered. In an extreme case, if an economic study is being considered from the narrow perspective of a pharmacy or hospital (perhaps trying to reduce their drug budget) it would be inappropriate to include the impact of treatments on employment since even if an unemployed patient is rendered seizure-free and returns to work full-time, the benefits of this outcome will not be seen by the pharmacy. Similar issues arise when considering health insurance plans where there are high patient co-payment for pharmaceuticals or, alternatively, where a patient is responsible for social care costs.

Second, a researcher must consider whether to use the unit costs of an individual organization or institution – or instead use national rates. This is significant because unit costs for individual procedures or items can vary significantly between hospitals (Figure 135.1). Therefore, the results of a cost-study of an inner-city teaching hospital may be very different to that in a rural clinic setting, where many overheads may be significantly lower. Furthermore, within-institution prices do not reflect true cost – for example, there may be inter-departmental cross-subsidization, or inadequate pricing information. In most cases, the researcher will consider both institution-specific costs and national tariffs.

Sources of information about unit costs

Once the economic perspective has been defined and a decision made about which type of costs to use, the researcher can obtain appropriate unit costs.

Direct medical and non-medical unit costs are usually easy to obtain. In many countries, published databases contain details of a wide range of health-care costs including drug prices, admission costs and hospital staff salaries. In the UK, the Department of Health produces reference costs for a very wide range of reference costs and tariffs.

Indirect/productivity employment costs can be considered in terms of average wage rates, or more specifically for people with epilepsy. This is significant, because people with epilepsy are more likely to be unemployed – or through discrimination employed in the workforce in positions below their potential abilities.

The most commonly used method by which indirect/productivity costs are valued is the 'human capital' method. Very simply stated this method is:

Indirect/productivity cost = Number of days work missed × Value of work

'Intangible' costs are included in studies that attempt to measure quality-of-life impact of epilepsy and its treatments – but typically as part of the numerator (rather than the denominator) in cost-effectiveness studies.

Different types of economic study

Budget impact and cost-of-illness study

The most straightforward form of economic evaluation is a cost-of-illness study. These studies are a simple account of all the relevant costs associated with a condition.

These studies can provide a useful assessment of the 'headline' impact of a condition, which is easily communicated in a non-medical setting. For example, studies of the cost of epilepsy in the UK in the 1990s allowed statements such as 'epilepsy costs the UK £2 billion' (Cockerell et al., 1994) to be made based on published evidence. Whereas these facts allowed those who may have been unfamiliar with the prevalence and impact of epilepsy to consider it in comparison with national health-care budgets, cost-of-illness studies clearly do not allow any evaluation of whether increased (or decreased) spending on different aspects of epilepsy treatment or education might produce better outcomes.

Cost-effectiveness study

Cost-effectiveness studies are more complex and allow comparison between different treatment interventions. The impact of a treatment on resources used is calculated and a ratio between this cost and the clinical benefit is derived.

In its simplest form, the clinical benefit is the same for each treatment (e.g. seizure freedom) and the study is described as a 'cost-minimization study'. Different health gain outcomes (or even quality-of-life outcomes) may be compared in cost-effectiveness or cost-utility studies. For two outcomes, A and B, the incremental cost-effectiveness ratio (ICR) is calculated as follows:

ICR = (cost A − cost B)/(health gain A − health gain B)

Cost-effectiveness studies have been performed to consider a variety of economic questions in epilepsy treatment. Typically, the cost-effectiveness of AEDs has been considered, for example considering the use of different antiepileptic drugs in newly diagnosed epilepsy, but there have also been cost-effectiveness studies of a range of other issues including the use of generic versus branded treatments, and epilepsy surgery.

Sensitivity analysis

One unifying feature of economic analysis of epilepsy has been the significant amount of 'uncertainty' incorporated in studies. Cost-effectiveness studies of antiepileptic drugs have typically extrapolated clinical data from trials that were originally performed primarily to establish safety and effectiveness for licensing reasons. Resource use and unit costs therefore have been simply estimated from these clinical trials, and consequently the potential for error is great. Even when resource use and unit cost data are collected during clinical trials, the validity of extrapolating these data to an every-day, 'naturalistic' setting is another source of uncertainty.

This uncertainty is recognized by health economists and the requirement to use economic models and estimates (rather than primary data) is well known. Standard statistical analysis can account for natural variation in populations and sampling variation, but economic sensitivity analysis can handle uncertainty arising where no patient-level data on resources costs and health outcomes are directly available.

At its most simple, sensitivity analysis will involve exploration about whether changes in assumptions about, for example, certain unit costs, will alter the conclusions reached in the study as a whole. A change in a single basic assumption can be tested (univariate sensitivity analysis) or a more complex effects from changing a number of assumptions (multivariate sensitivity analysis). Random scenarios may be generated in probabilistic sensitivity analysis – although clearly the models for generating these scenarios rely on additional assumptions about the statistical distribution of the variable being tested.

Conclusions

Epilepsy is a common and chronic condition – often requiring lifelong treatment. Its economic impact is great, and questions about the benefit of different interventions to treat people with this condition can be answered in part by health economic methods. Fundamental to any health economic analysis is an understanding of how a condition impacts on a range of resources – defined as direct, indirect and intangible costs. The uncertainty that arises from economic models can be accounted for, in part, by sensitivity analysis.

References

Cockerell OC, Hart YM, Sander JWAS, Shorvon SD. The cost of epilepsy: an estimation based on the results of two population based studies. *Epilepsy Res* 1994;**18**:249–60.

Drummond MF, Sculpher MJ, Torrance GW, O'Brien BJ, Stoddart G. *Methods for the Economic Evaluation of Health Care Programmes*. Oxford: Oxford University Press; 2005.

Heaney DC, Begley CE. Health economic evaluation of epilepsy treatment: a review of the literature. *Epilepsia* 2002;**43**(Suppl 4):10–17.

http://www.dh.gov.uk/en/Publicationsandstatistics/Publications/PublicationsPolicyAndGuidance/DH_123459.

Learning objectives

To understand the following issues:

(1) That health economics offer a method by which questions about allocation of scarce resources can be applied to epilepsy and its treatment.
(2) That fundamental to any health economic analysis is an understanding of how a condition impacts on a range of resources – defined as direct, indirect and intangible costs.
(3) That cost of illness studies have limited use in determining which treatment or treatment programme should be adopted – but cost-effectiveness analysis allows comparison between treatment options.

Section 7 Psychiatric, social and legal aspects

Chapter 136 Epilepsy, crime and legal responsibility

Peter Fenwick

Under English law, everyone who has reached the age of discretion is deemed responsible for their acts. This is enshrined in the principle *'Actus non facit reum nisi mens sit rea'* (The deed does not make a man guilty unless his mind is guilty). In Court it has to be shown that there is an 'actus rea', that is, by whose hand the crime was committed, and then secondly, the principle of 'mens rea' is applied. Mens rea includes the concept that the person knew what they were doing and that it was wrong. There are several defences against a mens rea:

(1) Provocation. This is now a technical defence but it is essentially that the person was so provoked by the person with whom they were arguing that any reasonable man would have responded as they did.
(2) Self defence, which is self-explanatory.
(3) Duress, which is again self-explanatory.
(4) That the mind was innocent, i.e. the person did not know the difference between right and wrong. This is seldom used now as there are a number of statutes in the Mental Health Act 1983 and other Acts which cover lack of mental capacity.
(5) The mind was insane at the time of the crime
(6) The mind was absent at the time of the crime.

These last two (an absent mind or an insane mind) are applied to patients with epilepsy who commit a crime.

In the case of insanity, the rules were laid down by the House of Lords in the 1850s, following, in 1843, the case of Daniel McNaughton, who tried to kill the Prime Minister, Sir Robert Peel, against whom he had an imaginary grudge. By mistake, he shot his secretary, Mr. Drummond. A hue and cry followed and McNaughton was found not guilty but insane by the Court. This created a furore: Queen Victoria was incensed and forced the law to be changed to 'guilty but insane', which led to the McNaughton rules formulated by the House of Lords. These rules state that it has to be proved that: 'At the time of committing the act, the party accused was labouring under such a defect of reason from disease of the mind as not to know the nature and quality of the act he was doing, or if he did know it, that he did not know he was doing what was wrong.'

The legal definition of an absent mind, or automatism, is given by Viscount Kilmuir: 'The state of a person who, though capable of action, is not conscious of what he is doing ... it means unconscious, involuntary action, because the mind does not go with what is being done.'

The medical definition of automatism

A state of clouding of consciousness which occurs during or immediately after a seizure, during which the individual retains control of posture, muscle tone, and performs simple or complex movements without being aware of what is happening.

These two definitions are very similar, but the lawyers divide automatism into two classes, sane automatism, or *automatism simpliciter*, which leads to an absolute acquittal, and insane automatism, which leads to the judge deciding according to the facts of the case on the disposal of the defendant.

Insane automatism is due to an internal factor, as it is recognized in law that states internal to the individual are likely to recur. In the case of Bratty, Lord Denning said that those acts which are likely to recur and have resulted in violence are the type of acts for which the defendant needs to be sent to hospital and for which there should not be a direct acquittal. This ruling has meant that brain damage, sleepwalking, epilepsy and many psychiatric states that depend on an inherent cause are classified as insanity.

Introduction to Epilepsy ed. Gonzalo Alarcón and Antonio Valentín. Published by CAMBRIDGE UNIVERSITY PRESS.
© CAMBRIDGE UNIVERSITY PRESS 2012.

Sane automatism is defined as those states leading to an absence of mind which results from an external factor. This could be an injection of insulin, as in the case of Quick, or a blow to the head such as might occur in a rugby match, or even the confused state after an anaesthetic. Clearly included in this group would be the reflex reaction to a bee sting.

In 1991, the Criminal Procedure and Insanity Act allowed the judge freedom to decide on the sentence and disposal of a defendant who had carried out an act automatically due to an internal factor. He would be able to free the individual or send him to a secure mental hospital with, if he had killed, a restriction order. Thus patients with epilepsy who commit a criminal offence during a seizure and who enter a plea of insane automatism, as they must do if they say they had no control over their actions, face the double jeopardy of the stigmata of being declared insane and being sent to hospital. For example, a patient with a temporal lobe automatism picking up a lampshade, putting it on her head and walking out of a shop is guilty of shoplifting and if prosecuted her defence would be insanity. This seems unreasonable. The key case is that of R. v. Sullivan 1982, who in a seizure pushed an 80-year-old woman to the ground. She struck her head in falling and later developed a thrombosis and died. He was charged with murder and at that time had the option of pleading not guilty due to insanity and going to Broadmoor for life or pleading guilty to murder. He was persuaded to plead guilty to manslaughter and the judge put him on probation. This led to an examination of the law by the House of Lords. The Lords confirmed that epilepsy arose from an internal factor and epileptic defendants would have to plead insanity. They recognized that it was unfair that patients with epilepsy who committed crimes in a seizure should be labelled insane, but said it was up to Parliament to change the law. This, so far, has not been done.

References and recommended reading

Bratty v. Attorney General for Northern Ireland (1961) Northern Ireland Law Reports 78–110.

R. v. Quick 1973 Queens Bench 910.

R. v. Sulllivan 1983 House of Lords Weekly Law Reports, July 8th.

Fenwick P. Epilepsy, automatism and the English law. *Med Law* 1997;**16**(2):349–58.

Learning objective

(1) To know and be able to discuss the responsibilities of criminal actions carried out by patients during epileptic seizures.

Section 7 Psychiatric, social and legal aspects

Chapter 137: The law and its consequences for people with epilepsy

Peter Fenwick

The Disability Discrimination Act

Patients with epilepsy have been stigmatized over many years, as have many other disadvantaged groups. The legislation concerning disability and the unfair treatment of the disabled was brought up to date in 1995 by the Disability Discrimination Act. This Act can be found in full on the following website: http://www.hmso.gov.uk/acts/acts1995/1995050.htm.

It is important to note that nothing in this part of the Act applies to an employer who has fewer than 20 employees.

The aim of the Act is to make certain that those with a disability are not discriminated against. The Act states: (1) Subject to the provisions of schedule 1, a person has a disability for the purposes of this Act if he has a physical or mental impairment which has a substantial and long-term adverse effect on his ability to carry out normal day-to-day activities. (2) In this Act 'disabled person' means a person who has a disability. It is clear from this definition that some patients with epilepsy will have either a physical or a mental impairment, or both, which has a substantial long-term adverse effect on their ability to carry out day-to-day activities and thus people with epilepsy fall within the benefits detailed in the Act. The meaning of 'a substantial adverse effect' and the meaning of 'long-term' are both discussed within the Act.

In Part II, Employment, there is a section headed Discrimination by Employers. 4(1) 'It is unlawful for an employer to discriminate against a disabled person. a) in the arrangements which he makes for the purpose of determining to whom he should offer employment b) in terms on which he offers that person employment; or c) by refusing to offer or deliberately not offering him employment.'

The Act goes on to note: (2) 'It is unlawful for an employer to discriminate against a disabled person whom he employs – a) in terms of the employment which he affords him b) in the opportunities which he affords him for promotion, a transfer, training or receiving any other benefit; c) by refusing to afford him, or deliberately not affording him, any such opportunity; or d) by dismissing him or subjecting him to any other detriment.'

The section goes on to define the meaning of discrimination.

5–(1) '. . . An employer discriminates a disabled person if a) for a reason which relates to the disabled person's disability, he treats him less favourably than he treats or would treat others to whom that reason does not or would not apply; and b) he cannot show that the treatment in question is justified.'

6–(1) There is a duty on the employer to make adjustments for the disabled, so that a) any arrangements made by or on behalf of an employer, or b) any physical features of premises occupied by the employer face the disabled person concerned at a substantial disadvantage in comparison with persons who are not disabled. It is the duty of the employer to take such steps . . . in order to prevent the arrangements or features having that effect. (3) There are 12 steps mentioned in the act which the employer may have to take in relation to a disabled person, including (a) making adjustments to the premises, (b) allocating some of the disabled person's duties to another person, (d) altering his working hours, (e) assigning him to a different place of work, (f) allowing him to be absent during working hours for rehabilitation, assessment or treatment, (g) giving him or arranging for him to be given training, (j) modifying procedures for testing or assessment, (l) providing supervision.

Introduction to Epilepsy ed. Gonzalo Alarcón and Antonio Valentín. Published by Cambridge University Press.
© Cambridge University Press 2012.

There are enforcement procedures for this Act and Section 8 deals with this aspect and notes: (1) (a) 'A complaint by any person that another person (a) has discriminated against him in a way which is unlawful under the Act . . . . may be presented to an industrial tribunal . . ..'

Section 11 is important as it deals specifically with advertisements, particularly those 'suggesting that employers will discriminate against disabled persons'.

The Health and Safety at Work Act

Since 1974 the Health and Safety at Work Act has required employers to be concerned about and take care of the health and safety of their employees. The Act, in conjunction with the new Disability Discrimination Act of 1995, already discussed, places an additional responsibility on employers concerning the health and safety of their workers. The 1974 Act states that the employer has a duty to 'ensure so far as is reasonably practical the health, safety and welfare at work of all employees.' This means that they have to carry out a risk assessment of all workers' activities, including the additional risks to certain groups of workers such as disabled people. The employer of someone with epilepsy must carry out a risk assessment. There are several requirements. The assessment must: focus on the person as an individual; not make assumptions; consider the facts; consider the essential elements of their job; identify the duration and frequency of any hazardous situations; if necessary get individual specific medical advice. The two following are important. The assessment must consult the employee in question about how reasonable adjustments can be made and look at any reasonable adjustments to reduce the risk.

Finally, if there is still an unacceptable risk even with adjustments, either to the employee with epilepsy or to others, then the employer has to make a decision about whether to dismiss them. However, before dismissal the employer should consider redeploying the employee to a job they can do.

References

DRC website (www.drc-gb.org/knowyourrights/employment.asp)

Health and Safety Executive: Tel: 08701 545 500

Website www.hse.gov.uk

Health and Safety pamphlet 3 contains much of the advice on health and safety given above.

Learning objective

(1) To know the consequences of the Disability Discrimination Act and the Health and Safety at Work Act for people suffering with epilepsy in the UK.

Section 7 Psychiatric, social and legal aspects

Chapter 138: Epilepsy and lifestyle issues

Frank M. C. Besag

Lifestyle issues might be viewed as a relatively unimportant topic for professionals managing people with epilepsy. Surely the important issue is to control the seizures. However, seizure freedom at any cost is not acceptable: a seizure-free patient in coma from excessive antiepileptic medication would not be considered a successful therapeutic outcome. A balance has to be struck between seizure control, on one hand, and an acceptable quality of life, on the other. A significant factor in enhancing quality of life is establishing a good therapeutic relationship between the professional and the patient/family. Most professionals would wish to be open, honest, knowledgeable, humane, sensitive and available for discussion.

Independence, risks and death

With regard to risk-taking, how much direct guidance should be given? A father in my epilepsy outpatient clinic demanded, in relation to his 14-year-old son with epilepsy: 'We want you to tell Jimmy if he can ride his bicycle'. How should you respond in this situation? Some professional decisions are straightforward. In an emergency, the doctor might need to act immediately. In some circumstances, it would be inappropriate for a doctor to offer an opinion at all, because the decision concerns a life situation choice, not a medical matter. Many of the decisions facing people with epilepsy lie somewhere between these two extremes. Some professionals simply make the decision for the family. Does this imply that, whenever the family needs to make a decision about the epilepsy that might involve some risk, they have to consult the doctor? Some might view this as a failing to enable the family to make decisions for themselves. With regard to Jimmy and his bicycle, it would be highly appropriate for the professional to explore the possible risks and benefits of bicycle-riding in the individual case but is it appropriate for the professional to make the decision? If Jimmy did not have epilepsy or any other relevant medical condition, would the doctor be asked to make this decision? No. The medical condition has a major influence on the decision-making process, in this particular case, but perhaps it is still up to the family to weigh the factors carefully and then make their own final decision. If pressed, I am prepared to say: 'If he were my child, I think my decision would be ....' However, I always add: '– but he is not my son and the final decision must be yours'. This approach does not always apply. If someone with the uncontrolled epilepsy asks: 'Can I drive a car?' the answer is: 'No, it is against the law'. If someone with absence seizures asks if the doctor will support their application for a motorcycle licence the answer should be 'No', because this would involve an unacceptable risk.

Families sometimes make statements that appear to be sensible but are not. For example: 'If there was any risk involved, I couldn't possibly let him do it'. If that was the criterion used, then no parent would allow their child to go to university or to drive or, for that matter, to ride a bicycle. The issue is not whether there is a risk involved; so many situations in life involve some risk. The issue is whether it is an unreasonable risk. However, this needs to be balanced by the question: 'Is this an unreasonable limitation?'

Some specific risk situations for epilepsy should be discussed. For swimming, someone competent and confident must provide one-to-one supervision of the person with epilepsy while they are in the water. With regard to taking baths, the risk is very high and supervision must be recommended very strongly. The exact nature of supervision will depend on the seizure type and on other factors.

Introduction to Epilepsy ed. Gonzalo Alarcón and Antonio Valentín. Published by Cambridge University Press.
© Cambridge University Press 2012.

Death

Should professionals discuss the risk of sudden unexplained death in epilepsy (SUDEP) at an early stage? Does this raise unnecessary anxieties? Providing accurate information can actually decrease rather than increase anxiety. A careful decision needs to be made for each family. Some families might not be ready for this information if, for example, they have been overwhelmed by the recent diagnosis of epilepsy.

Sex, drugs and rock & roll

Sex

Self-image is often of major importance, especially in teenagers with epilepsy. Imagine a teenage girl with epilepsy who is wearing her favourite dress but is terrified of having a seizure and being incontinent. This is hardly likely to increase her self-confidence or improve her self-image. A teenage boy wants to talk to a girl but is terrified of having a seizure at the moment when he wants to appear at his best. What can professionals do to assist? Some find it helpful to remind the teenager who has recently developed epilepsy that they still remain the same person. Peer-group support from other teenagers may prove to be very valuable.

Enzyme-inducing antiepileptic drugs can affect the efficacy of the oral contraceptive. Clear and accurate information should be provided (see Chapter 97: 'Management of epilepsy in women').

Antiepileptic medication can also be associated with major malformations in the offspring of women with epilepsy. However, in most cases the risk is relatively small (less than 5%) if monotherapy is used (Morrow *et al.*, 2006). The risk appears to be related to dose; the lower the dose, the lower the risk. Sodium valproate is the antiepileptic drug that has been particularly associated with major malformations but, again, the effect is dose-related. Polytherapy, especially with sodium valproate, should be avoided if possible. Sodium valproate can also be associated with decreased verbal IQ in the offspring but so can having frequent tonic-clonic seizures during pregnancy (Adab *et al.*, 2004).

Genetic counselling may be appropriate. The risk, in most cases, is relatively small if only one parent has epilepsy. There are certain exceptions. For example, tuberous sclerosis is a dominant condition that is frequently associated with epilepsy. Genetic counselling if either parent has this condition would be totally appropriate.

Drugs

If a teenager presents with unexplained seizures, cocaine-induced seizures should be considered in the differential diagnosis. Alcohol itself probably does not usually induce seizures but withdrawal seizures may occur after alcohol intake. Alcohol is also an enzyme-inducing substance and will decrease the blood levels of some antiepileptic drugs.

Rock & roll

Some types of epilepsy, notably juvenile myoclonic epilepsy, are strongly associated with sleep-deprivation seizures. If a person with juvenile myoclonic epilepsy wants to attend an all-night party, for example, they should be warned of the possible risks of loss of seizure control. However, the final decision should be theirs. They should be encouraged to have someone confident and competent in the management of seizures with them the day after undertaking any activity that involves disruption of the sleep pattern and/or sleep deprivation.

There is probably much unnecessary restriction around discotheque lights. Photosensitivity is relatively infrequent in people with epilepsy (less than 5%, overall), although it is frequent in people with JME (30–60%). If the individual is not photosensitive then there should be no risk from the lights. If the lights comply with regulations, the flash frequency will usually be too low to precipitate seizures even in the relatively small percentage of people with epilepsy who are photosensitive. However, discotheque lights that contravene the regulations and could precipitate seizures in photosensitive subjects are readily available through the internet.

Conclusions

Life is for living. The role of the professional is neither to overemphasize nor to ignore the issues but to provide accurate, understandable information and to be available for discussion so that individuals can be encouraged to make responsible decisions for themselves.

References

Adab N, Kini U, Vinten J, *et al.*, The longer term outcome of children born to mothers with epilepsy. *J Neurol Neurosurg Psychiatry* 2004;75(11):1575–83.

Morrow J, Russell A, Guthrie E, *et al.*, Malformation risks of antiepileptic drugs in pregnancy: a prospective study from the UK Epilepsy and Pregnancy Register. *J Neurol Neurosurg Psychiatry* 2006;77(2):193–8.

Learning objectives

(1) To be able to provide accurate information regarding the risks associated with epilepsy and its treatment that may affect lifestyle issues.

(2) To be able to discuss risk affecting lifestyle issues in a way that empowers individuals and families to make responsible decisions for themselves.

Section 7 Psychiatric, social and legal aspects

Chapter 139: Bereavement, SUDEP and Epilepsy Bereaved

Maureen Lahiff and Jane Hanna

There are at least three seizure-related deaths every day in the UK, but many people, mistakenly, think that seizures are benign. Sudden unexpected death in epilepsy (SUDEP) accounts for just over half of these deaths, with young people most affected. When SUDEP occurs families and carers often experience bewilderment, isolation and prolonged distress because they do not realize that a seizure can be fatal; the death usually occurs during sleep and is wholly unexpected.

> Epilepsy Bereaved exists to prevent unnecessary deaths from SUDEP (Sudden Unexpected Death in Epilepsy) and other epilepsy deaths.

Epilepsy Bereaved began with a campaign by five women: Catherine Brookes, Jane Hanna, Sheila Pring, Sue Kelk and Jennifer Preston. Jennifer's son William died in 1988 (aged 22); Jane's partner and Sheila's son Alan died in 1990 (aged 27); Catherine's son Matthew died in 1991 (aged 21) and Sue's daughter Natalie died in 1992 (aged 22). In the early 1990s the subject of SUDEP was not being addressed except by a handful of clinicians and talking about SUDEP even at educational conferences was sometimes viewed as a taboo. It was the partnership between these dedicated clinicians and Epilepsy Bereaved that made the campaign not only possible, but also highly successful. The group used the tactics developed many years before by the campaign to abolish slavery to stimulate debate and change – organizing a group, involving politicians, allies and opinion formers; producing literature and giving talks!

In 1995, Epilepsy Bereaved was founded as a charity. In 1996, Epilepsy Bereaved, with the support of an educational grant from The Wellcome Trust, convened a workshop of international epilepsy experts and epilepsy organizations to address sudden death and epilepsy. The workshop produced a series of published papers on SUDEP (Nashef and Brown, 1997) addressing issues of definition, mechanisms, risk factors, information and prevention, and acted as a catalyst for research.

Further campaigning led to funding for a national investigation into epilepsy deaths and in 1998 Epilepsy Bereaved became the first voluntary-sector organization to lead a national clinical audit. The NICE 'Epilepsy – death in the shadows' report (Hanna et al., 2002) was the first national and international report to address the preventability of SUDEP deaths, establishing in 2002 that 42% of epilepsy deaths in the UK are potentially avoidable.

Since founding in 1995, there has been a seismic shift in thinking and practice on SUDEP in the UK. The context of overwhelming lack of recognition and interest in SUDEP during the early 1990s has changed to a situation today where SUDEP potential prevention strategies are recognized in NICE national clinical guidelines.

National Guidelines on the Epilepsies 2004 state that the risk of SUDEP can be best managed if a person's seizures are being controlled and people with epilepsy and their carers are alert to the risks of night-time seizures. Tailored information on the individual's risk of SUDEP should be part of the counselling checklist for people with epilepsy and their families and/or carers, taking account of the small but definite risk of SUDEP.

NICE also recommends that when SUDEP occurs, health professionals should offer information on SUDEP support services.

Epilepsy Bereaved works today to support and enable people affected by SUDEP and other epilepsy deaths, to educate about ways to minimize risk and to promote research dedicated to prevention of unnecessary deaths.

Support and enablement

Our contact line responds to about 100 newly bereaved people during the year and just under 800 bereaved people continue to seek regular information and access to the services of the charity.

Research commissioned by Epilepsy Bereaved from the College of Health with bereaved relatives revealed the emotional impact on the family, ranging from shock and devastation, to guilt, anger, difficulty accepting the death and loneliness. Among relatives of SUDEP victims, these grief reactions can be traumatic because of the added dimensions of being unexpected, as the family may not have been told of any risk. Further, with sudden deaths, the bereaved are thrust into an unfamiliar world of investigation into the death.

Everyone's reaction is different, as is their way of grieving. However, to begin with people generally want information and answers to their questions: What is SUDEP? Why did they not know that a seizure could be fatal? How could this happen? Could they have saved their loved one? etc. They may also want information regarding the post mortem or inquest. The charity can listen, provide information and explain the process, since people who ring us can often feel too daunted and upset to ask questions from the authorities.

Calls to our contact line or emails to the charity from bereaved relatives are responded to initially by our support and liaison manager.

For some people, it is very important to talk about what has happened and the effect on them. They want, and need, to express the strong emotions they are feeling, particularly to someone who had not been involved in any way prior to the death. Where appropriate, a person will choose to speak with a family support befriended who are at least 2 years beyond their own experience of bereavement and are trained in listening and befriending skills. The charity runs two national weekend events during the year and the charity is developing more informal regional meetings. This gives our members a chance to meet face-to-face with others who have had similar experiences. Every three years Epilepsy Bereaved holds an inclusive memorial service. This is another occasion for meeting together for remembrance of our loved ones, celebration of their lives and recognition of their deaths.

After receiving information some bereaved people want to grieve by doing rather than talking, so we believe in developing the charity's work to mirror the needs of those in contact with us. The charity produces two magazines a year, which include their writings, poems and other contributions. People can also be supported by the charity's education and awareness manager to get involved with a range of opportunities such as fundraising, running an information table or joining our speakers team.

Raising awareness and informing of ways to reduce risks

One in four of the people we support become active in the work of the charity. This enables the charity to inform and educate a larger audience. Surveys of people affected by SUDEP who choose to get involved indicate that people find being active in the work of the charity a positive way to channel their grief.

Prevention of deaths

The charity continues to be uniquely placed to champion research on SUDEP because of the number of deaths reported to the charity each year and our dedicated focus on targeting our research funds on projects that can easily translate into prevention measures that can be put into practice to prevent deaths.

The charity is currently working with King's College Hospital and King's College London on a SUDEP research initiative including a monitor of deaths reported to the charity.

References

Hanna NJ, Black M, Sander JWS, *et al. The National Sentinel Clinical Audit of Epilepsy-Related Death: Epilepsy-death in the shadows.* London: The Stationery Office; 2002.

Nashef L, Brown SW (eds). Epilepsy and sudden death. *Epilepsia* 1997;**38**(Suppl 11).

Learning objective

(1) To know the objectives, activities and achievements of Epilepsy Bereaved, and the support that can be provided to patients with epilepsy and their families.

Index

ABC (antecedents/behaviour/
  consequences) 513–14
absence epilepsy/seizures
  animal studies 51
  atypical **153**. *See also* Lennox-
    Gastaut syndrome
  classification 112
  epileptogenesis in vivo 61
  hyperventilation 123
  juvenile 131–2, 135–6
  and learning disability/behaviour 489
  management 406–7
  psychiatric disorders 291, 522
  typical 160, **164**
  video-EEG monitoring 284
  See also childhood absence epilepsy
absolute refractory period 26
accidental deaths 341
acquired epileptic aphasia (Landau
  Kleffner syndrome) 131–2, 140,
  333–4, 339
acquired mechanisms of
  epileptogenesis 53
action potentials 25–6, **27**, **96**
activation clinic, King's College
  Hospital, London 315–16
activation maps 266
active controls 372
active movement 24
acute electrocorticography **445**, 447–50
acute experimental models, 47–9
acute symptomatic seizures 53, 189,
  190, 299
acute viral encephalitis, EEG
  applications 213–16
acutely isolated neurons 31
adaptation action potentials 26
ADD (Antiepileptic Drug
  Development) program 367–8
adjustments, employment 550
adolescent syndromes. *See* childhood/
  adolescent epilepsy
AEDs (antiepileptic drugs) 46–7,
  330–1, 403–4
  behavioural/mental health effects
    403–4, 413–14, 526
  blood tests 300
  BOLD effect 244
  childhood epilepsy 135, 479–81

clinical neuropsychological
  evaluation 410
compliance 577
dose selection 369, 488
economics 581–2
elderly patients 487–8
GABA-mediated inhibitory
  transmission 354–6
glutamatergic neurotransmission 355
health-related quality of life 539
iatrogenic damage 66
idiopathic generalized epilepsies 166
interactions. *See* pharmacological
  interactions
interictal EEG 119–20
learning disability 484
mechanism of action **354**, 357
migraine 293
monotherapy/polytherapy 372, 392,
  393, 394–5
myoclonus 140, 154, 184, 188
neonatal seizures 145, **148**
neurochemistry 353–7
neuropsychological effects 413–14
pharmokinetics 358–9, **360**, 366
preclinical trials 367–8, 373
residential care/specialist
  centres 562
screening 46–7
side-effects 279, **354**, 357, 539.
  See also behavioural effects
  of AEDs
toxicity 300, **375**, 376, 392–3
voltage-gated ion channels 353–5
withdrawal 401–2
See also clinical trials; therapeutic
  drug monitoring; treatment gaps
AEDs, new 367, 380–2, 384
  behavioural effects 404–5
  neuropsychological effects 414
  selected features of specific drugs
    382–3, 396–400
  under development 396–400
AEDs, traditional 374–8, 379
  behavioural/mental health effects
    403–4, 413–14
  neuropsychological effects 413–14
  principles of drug treatment 374–5
  toxicity 375, 376

aetiology of epilepsy. *See* causes
affective disorders 515–17.
  See also anxiety; depression
after-hyperpolarization 26
age-effects 329, 414. *See also* elderly
  patients
aggression, and epilepsy 524–5
agonist/antagonist pharmacology 19
alcohol use 330–1, 339, 590
algorithms, tractography 261
allosteric modulation, GABA system
  355
Alpers disease (progressive neuronal
  degeneration of childhood with
  liver disease) 187
alpha brain waves 81
alternating psychoses 522
Alzheimer's disease 183, 213, 330–1
ambulatory EEG 281
amobarbital procedure 61
AMPA receptors 40–1, 53–4, 356
amygdalo-hippocampectomy **431–2**
amytal test (Wada test) 61,
  415–16, 423
anatomy
  CNS 8–15, 16
  hippocampus 10, 37–9
Angelman syndrome 44, 181, 492–3
animal models 58, 464–5, 513.
  See also experimental models;
  laboratory studies
anoxia 97, **98**, 213–14, 283
anterior temporal lobectomy 431, **432**
antidepressant medication 516,
  533, **534**
antidromic stimulation 33
antipsychotic medication 533, **534**
anxiety 513, 518–19
  clinical evaluation 411
  families of epilepsy sufferers 546
  marriage 545–6
  and surgery 532
  treatment 536–7.
  See also behavioural treatment
apnoea 289
artefacts, EEG 82–4
artificial membrane-channel
  preparations 31
aspiration 341

594

Index

assessment. See investigations
association analysis 348–9
association areas, lesion studies 11–12
asterixis 181
atonic seizures 111
attention, neuropsychological evaluation **411**
attention deficit hyperactivity disorder 291
A-type potassium channels 28–9
atypical absence seizures 153.
   See also Lennox-Gastaut syndrome
atypical benign partial epilepsy 154–5
audiogenic epilepsy 464–5
auditory evoked potentials 220, 459
auditory stimuli, reflex epilepsy 459
auras 110, 277, 290–1, 293, 421
autoimmune disease 302–3
automatisms 110, 112, 282–3, 524–5, 585–6
autonomic failure 286
autonomic symptoms 109
autoregulatory systems 285
autosomal dominant cortical reflex myoclonus 176, 181
axons 17

bacterial meningitis 330–1
Baltic myoclonus epilepsy 74
band heterotopia 504
barbiturates 376
Batten disease 220, **221**
beamformer algorithms 270, 274
behavioural disorders, childhood epilepsy 526–8
   differential diagnosis 297
   and learning disability 484
behavioural effects of AEDs 403–5
   new AEDs 404–5
   older/established drugs 403–4, 413–14
behavioural treatment 513–14
benign childhood epilepsy with centrotemporal spikes (BECTS) 131–3, **134**
   EEG 200, 208–10
benign childhood epilepsy with occipital spasms. See Panayiotopoulos syndrome
benign epilepsy 158, 164.
   See also idiopathic focal epilepsies
benign familial (idiopathic) neonatal convulsions 333–4
benign myoclonic epilepsy of infancy 161, 200, 204–7
benign paroxysmal vertigo 298
benzodiazepines 378, 408–9
bereavement. See Epilepsy Bereaved

beta brain waves 81
bilateral independent temporal interictal discharges 428
biochemical abnormalities 283, 300, 306–7, 337
biochemistry of neurotransmission 40–5
biofeedback 514. See also behavioural treatment
biological matrixes, therapeutic drug monitoring 361
bio-psycho-social approaches 574
bipolar mood disorder 515–16
birth hazards 337
bizarre behaviours 288–9, 534
blinding, clinical trials 369
blood tests 300
BOLD (blood oxygenation-level dependent effect) 244, 266
brain activity, fMRI 245
brain damage
   childhood epilepsy 527
   EEG phenomenology 97, **98**
   perinatal 70
   prevention 407–8, 409
   secondary changes 64–6
brain diseases, EEG applications 213–16
brain slices 31, **47**, 50, 55–7, 52
brain stem death 214–16
brain stimulation 436, 439, 442, **443**.
   See also single pulse electrical stimulation; vagus nerve stimulation
brain tumours. See tumours
breath-holding in children 297
brief seizures, management 407
British Epilepsy Association 564
brivaracetam 396
buccal midazolam 378, 409
budget impact studies 583

calcium ion channels 28, 48, 54, 353–4
calcium IT oscillating currents **50**, 55
callosotomy, preoperative assessment 420
candidate genes 348
carbamazepine 135, **375**, 377
   benign epilepsy of childhood with centrotemporal spikes 132
   elderly patients 487
   late-onset occipital epilepsy 134
   pharmacological interactions 386–7, **388**
   therapeutic drug monitoring 362, **363**
   treatment gaps 556
cardiac arrhythmia 103–5
cardiology assessment 299

cardiovascular syndromes simulating epilepsy 285–6
care approaches. See joined-up primary-secondary care approach; primary care; specialist centres
carers, community support groups 576–7
carotid amobarbital test (Wada test) 61, 415–16, 423
case scenarios, paediatric epilepsy **307**, 308, 312
case-control studies 330
catamenial seizures 476–7
caudate stimulation 442
causes
   of death in epilepsy 341–2
   of epilepsy 330
cell electrophysiology 22–9, 30
cell membranes. See membranes
cellular level epileptogenesis in vitro 54–5, 62
central nervous system (CNS), functional anatomy 8–15, 16
centrencephalic hypothesis 60–1
cerebellar atrophy 66
cerebral cortex 8–12
cerebral hemispheres 8–10, **13**.
   See also lateralization
cerebral malformations, 67–70
cerebral perfusion 285
cerebral trauma. See head injury
cerebral tumours. See tumours
cerebrovascular disease 330–1, 501–3
   EEG 97–8, 502–3
chain reactions, excitatory neurotransmission 48
charities supporting epilepsy 564–5.
   See also organizations/support services
childhood absence epilepsy (CAE) 131–2 135, **136**, 161, **165**
   case scenarios
   EEG 200, 204–7
childhood/adolescent epilepsy 131–2, 304, 307, 482, 540, 141
   AEDs 479–81
   behavioural/mental health effects 527
   case scenarios **307**, 308, 312
   classification 131
   cognitive decline 306–7
   differential diagnosis 296–8, 339
   EEG reporting sessions 318–19, 326, 327
   epidemiology 337–9
   health-related quality of life 540
   management 478–82

595

Index

childhood/adolescent epilepsy (cont.)
  neuroimaging 305–6
  neurophysiology/EEG 304–5
  non-genetic risk factors 331
  other investigations 306–7
  surgery 438–9, 440
  syndromes 131–2
  See also learning disability
chromosomal epilepsies 351, 492–3.
    See also genetics; lissencephaly;
    ring chromosome
chronic encephalitis. See Rasmussen's
    encephalitis
chronic epilepsy 6, 49–50
  experimental models 49–51
  neuroimaging indications 238
  secondary changes 64–6
chronic interictal psychoses 522–3
chronic progressive epilepsia partialis
    continua of childhood
    (Kojewnikow syndrome) 131,
    134–5, 333–4
chronically cultured neurons 31
classical conditioning
classification 107, **115–16**, 117–18,
    300–1
  childhood/adolescent epilepsy
      131, 338
  EEG manifestations 113
  evolution of 113–14
  focal seizures 107–11
  generalized seizures 107, 111–13
  international classifications 107
  multi-axial **307–8**,
  myoclonus, epileptic 183
  neonatal seizures 142–3, **145**
  neuroimaging guidelines 237
  newly diagnosed/chronic epilepsy,
      300–1
  other classifications 118
  practical examples 116
  psychogenic non-epileptic
      seizures 313
  relevance 117
  status epilepticus 468–9
  terminology 107–8
  video-EEG monitoring 283
  See also diagnosis
clinical trials, AEDs 292, 369–73
  health-related quality of life
      measures 540
  status epilepticus 472
clonic convulsions/seizures 111, 282–3
CLV (continuous low-voltage inactive
    EEG) 195–6
cobblestone complex 504
Cochrane reviews, new AEDs 381
Coffin Lowry syndrome 465

cognitive behavioural therapy
  See also behavioural treatment
cognitive decline, investigations
    302–3, 306–7
cognitive impairment, effects
    of AEDs 403
cohort studies 330
commissures, posterior/anterior 8
community support groups 576–7,
    593
co-morbidity 530, 562
comparative genomic hybridization
    (CGH) **306**
complex partial seizures 110, 406–7
compliance, medication 577
conditioning, classical/operant
confidentiality, patient 551, 554
continuous low-voltage inactive EEG
    (CLV) 195–6
continuous spike-wave during
    slow-wave sleep (CSWS) 131,
    140–1, 490
contraception 474, 590
controls, clinical trials 369, 372
convulsions, clonic 282–3
convulsive movements 108
convulsive seizures, management 406
cornu ammonis 38
corpus callosum 8, 12, 67–8, 74, 418
cortical action-reflex myoclonus 183
cortical dysplasia 67–8, 506–8
cortical resection 75
cortical stimulation 442
corticobasal degeneration 183
corticoreticular epilepsies model 61
cost of illness studies 583
cost-effectiveness studies 583
counselling, psychodynamic 536–7
Creutzfeldt–Jakob disease (CJD) **101**,
    213, **214**
criminal responsibility 585–6.
    See also Disability Discrimination
    Act; Health and Safety at Work
    Act
cross-over studies, clinical trials 370
CT (computerized tomography) 224,
    226–36. See also neuroimaging
cumulative incidence of epilepsy 330
current clamp recordings 33
cyanosis 282–3
cyclothymia 515

Davy, Sir Humphrey 3
death. See mortality; sudden
    unexpected death
declarative memory 262–3
definitions of epilepsy 6–7, 114,
    329, 332

delayed rectifier potassium channels
    28–9
delta brain waves 82
dementia 213, **214**
dendrites 17
dentato-rubro-pallido-luysian atrophy
    (DRPLA) 186
depersonalization 292
depression 330–1, 513, 515–16, 545–6
  definition 515
  joined-up care approach 573–4
  neuropsychological evaluation 411
  risk factors 516
  surgery effects 434, 532
  treatment 515, 516.
    See also behavioural treatment
depth electrodes 424
developing world, treatment gap
    555–6,
developmental regression 310
diagnosis 6–7
  elderly patients 486
  electro-clinical 6–7
  ictal EEG 128
  molecular/genetic techniques 36
  neonatal seizures 143–7
  residential care/specialist
      centres 562
  video-EEG monitoring 281–2,
      282–3
  See also classification; differential
    diagnosis; investigations
dialeptic seizures 108
diazepam 378, 408
dietary measures 138, 154, 456–7
differential diagnosis 298
  audiogenic epilepsy 465
  behavioural/psychiatric
      disorders 297
  childhood epilepsy 296–8, 339
  ictal EEG 128
  movement disorders 294–5
  neurological disorders 297–8
  other possible conditions 296
  psychiatric disorders simulating
      epilepsy 290
  syncope 296–7
  West syndrome/infantile
      spasms 151
  See also specific conditions
diffuse neocortical atrophy 66
diffusion tensor imaging (DTI)
    259–65
dipolar source localization 269–70
dipole electroencephalography 79
direct costs 581
Disability Discrimination Act (1995)
    549–51, 570, 587–8

Index

disabling aspects of epilepsy, organizations/support services 570
dissociative seizures 313, 317, 529–31
   clinical semiology 529, **530**
   definitions/terminology/classification 313, 529
   diagnosis 297, 313, 315–16, 531
   investigations 313–16
   psychiatric co-morbidity 530
   video-EEG monitoring 282–3
distributed source localization 270–1
DNA diagnosis 36. *See also* genetics
Doose syndrome (myoclonic-astatic epilepsy) 131, 138–40, 154, 200
   EEG 208–9
dormant cell hypothesis 58
double cortex **505**
Down syndrome 181, 493
Dravet syndrome. *See* severe myoclonic epilepsy of infancy
driving 335–6, 341, 540, 553–4
   AED withdrawal 401, 554
   elderly patients 487
   joined-up approach 572
   parents with epilepsy 547
drop attacks 111
drowning 341
drug use 590. *See also* AEDs; antidepressant medication; antipsychotic medication; mood stabilizers; psychotropic drugs
DTI (diffusion tensor imaging) 259–65
DWI (diffusion-weighted imaging) 260
dysembryoplastic neuroepithelial tumour (DNT) 73
dysthymia 515

early (neonatal) myoclonic encephalopathy 152, 197–8
early infantile epileptic encephalopathy (Ohtahara syndrome) 152, 197
early myoclonic encephalopathy 184
early-onset benign occipital epilepsy. *See* Panayiotopoulos syndrome
East Kent scheme, primary care 558–9
ECG (REVEAL) 286
economics, health 581–4
ECT (electro-convulsive therapy) 330–1
education. *See* learning disability; public education
EEG (electroencephalography) 76, 80
   case reporting sessions 318–19, 326–7

continuous low-voltage inactive 195–6
definitions 191
history 3
indications 301
interpretation 77–**8**
intracranial 34
montages 78
recording methodology 76–7
recording/reviewing principles **76**, 77–8
source reconstruction 266
techniques 191
terminology 79
types 305
See also ictal EEG; interictal EEG
EEG - normal phenomenology 81, 95
   artefacts 82–4
   children/neonates 191–4, 198–200
   normal background 81–3, **84**
   normal transients/benign variants 83–93
   state/age effects 95–4
EEG - pathological phenomenology, 96–7, 106
   atypical benign partial epilepsy 154–5
   brain diseases 213–16
   cardiac arrhythmia 103–5
   cerebrovascular disorders 97–8, 502–3
   childhood absence epilepsy 135–6
   children/neonates 194–6, 200, 212
   continuous spike-waves during slow-wave sleep 141
   Creutzfeldt–Jakob disease 100, **101**
   Dravet syndrome 157
   early epileptic encephalopathies with suppression-burst EEG 152
   early (neonatal) myoclonic encephalopathy 197–8
   early infantile epileptic encephalopathy 197
   encephalitis 99–102
   encephalopathies, infancy/early childhood 200–6
   hepatic encephalography 101–2, **103**
   hypoxic brain damage 97, **98**
   idiopathic focal epilepsies 208–11
   idiopathic generalized epilepsies **164**, 166, 204–10
   juvenile absence epilepsy 136
   juvenile myoclonic epilepsy 137
   Landau Kleffner syndrome 140
   late-onset occipital epilepsy 134
   Lennox-Gastaut syndrome 138, 154
   management applications 304–5
   myoclonic-astatic epilepsy 139, 154

   neonatal seizures 197–9
   newly diagnosed/chronic epilepsy 300–1
   occipital lobe epilepsies 161, 177–9
   Panayiotopoulos syndrome 133, 160
   preoperative assessment 428
   rolandic epilepsy 158–9, **160**
   status epilepticus 102–5
   temporal lobe epilepsy 170–1
   tumours 97
   typical absence seizures 160, **164**
   West syndrome/infantile spasms 151, **338**
EEG-correlated fMRI 266–8, 301–2
elastic Van Gieson 35
elderly patients 486–8
electrical extracellular stimulation 33
electrical source imaging 269, **271**.
   See also source localization
electrical status epilepticus of slow-wave sleep 490
electrocorticography, acute **445**, 447–50
electrodes, intracranial EEG 424–5
electrographic seizures 52
electromagnetic theories, history 2–3
electron microscopy 36
electrophysiology of cells 22–9, 30
electroretinography 217–22
emergency treatment 339, 409, **559**.
   See also management
emotions, physiology 13–14
employment 552
encephalitis 99–102, 330–1
encephalopathy 184, 213–14
   early childhood 153–5
   first year of life 150–2
   infancy/early childhood 200–6
epidemiology of epilepsy 329–31
   cerebrovascular disease 502
   childhood epilepsy 337, **338**, 339
   learning disability 483
   non-genetic risk factors 331
   status epilepticus 468
epidural peg electrodes 424–5
epilepsia partialis continua 176, 181, 333–4. *See also* Rasmussen's encephalitis
Epilepsy Action 564
Epilepsy Bereaved 564, 592–3.
   See also sudden unexpected death
Epilepsy Surgery Inventory 541
epilepsy with continuous spike and wave during slow-wave sleep 333–4
epilepsy with generalized tonic-clonic seizures 165, 333–4

Index

epilepsy with myoclonic absences 165–6, 184
epileptic seizures, definitions 6
epileptiform discharges 119–22
epileptogenesis in vitro 52, 57
  cellular level 50, 54–5, 56, 62
    mechanisms 53
    molecular level 53–4
    network level (brain slices) 55–7
    reactive (induced) seizures 53
    stages 53
epileptogenesis in vivo 58, 59, 60–2, 63, 60
epileptogenic lesions 67
equality/inequality 549, 574–5
Equality Act (2010) 570
equilibrium potentials 23–4
eslicarbazepine acetate 362, 387
ethnic considerations, health-related quality of life 540
ethosuximide 362, 387
evoked potentials 217–23
  role in epilepsy 219–21
examination. *See* history-taking; physical examination
excitability, cell 24–5
excitation (resonance) 240
excitatory neurotransmission, 40–2
  chain reactions 48
  epileptogenesis 53–4
  experimental models 47
excitatory postsynaptic potentials 25
excitement 513
exclusion criteria, clinical trials 369
executive functioning, neuropsychological evaluation 411
exercise 513. *See also* behavioural treatment
experimental models 32, 46–51. *See also* epileptogenesis in vitro; laboratory studies
eyelid myoclonia with absences (Jeavons' syndrome) 112, 140, 165, 166
eyewitnesses 276, 290–1, 296–8

factitious disorder (Munchausen's syndrome) 529
families of epilepsy sufferers 521, 546–7
  community support groups 576–7
  practical advice 547
FDG tracers 252–3, 301–2
febrile convulsions 156–7, 330–1
  epidemiology 338
  and febrile seizures 156
  generalized epilepsy with febrile seizures plus 157

neuropathology 71–2
severe myoclonic epilepsy of infancy 157
felbamate 362, 382, 405
females with epilepsy 474–7, 493
fertility 546
fetal damage 70, 539
fimbria 8
fissures 8
fixation-off sensitive epilepsy 462–3
FLAIR (fluid-attenuated inversion-recovery) imaging 301
flumazenil tracers 252–3
fluorofelbamate 397
fMRI (functional MRI) 244–7, 301–2, 426
  EEG-correlated 266–8, 301–2
focal cortical dysplasia 68–70
focal epilepsy
  acute models 47–9
  chronic models 49–50
  ILAE classification 131
  mechanisms 59, 60, 60
  terminology 115, 132
  Wyler's hypothesis 58
  See also frontal lobe epilepsy; idiopathic focal epilepsies
focal onset seizures, AEDs 480
focal seizures, electroclinical classification 107–8
  autonomic symptoms 109
  classification by site of origin 111
  gelastic seizures 110
  hemiclonic seizures 111
  with impaired consciousness 110
  myoclonias 111
  with preserved consciousness 109–10
  psychic symptoms 109–10
  sensory symptoms 109
  terminology 108
focus localization 269–72, 283–4, 417–18, 421, 427
foramen ovale electrodes 424
forced normalization 522
forward problem 269
frontal association cortex, lesion studies 11–12
frontal lobe epilepsy 174–6
frontal lobe seizures, classification 111
frontal lobe surgery 450
fugue states 522
functional anatomy. *See* anatomy
functional imaging 306. *See also* fMRI
functional localization, history 2
functional neurosurgery 74, 418
functional surgery 436
fundraising, research 569

GABA (γ-amino butyric acid) system 20, 42–5
  AEDs, neurochemistry 354–6
  B receptors 44
  epileptogenesis at molecular level 54
  epileptogenesis in vivo 62
  GABA-transaminase 44
  genetic defects 44
  phasic/tonic inhibition 44
  A receptors 42–4, 47
  surround/recurrent inhibition 44–5
  transporters 42
gabapentin 362, 382, 387, 404, 488
GABA-transaminase 44
gamma knife irradiation 436, 445
ganaxolone 397
ganglioglioma 73
Gastaut type late-onset occipital epilepsy 131–4
Gaucher disease 187
gelastic seizures 110, 444
gelegenheitsanfälle (acute symptomatic seizures) 189, 190, 299
gender and epilepsy 329, 521. *See also* women with epilepsy
general anaesthesia 447–9
generalized epilepsies 183. *See also* idiopathic generalized epilepsies
generalized epilepsy with febrile seizures plus (GEFS +) 44, 157
generalized seizures 60–2, 107, 111–13, 132, 480
generalized tonic-clonic seizures 163, 165
Genetically Epilepsy Prone Rat (GEPR) 50–1
genetics 330–1
  basic principles 345–6
  diagnosis 36
  epilepsy classification 115
  GABA receptors 44
  investigations 306
  mechanisms of epileptogenesis 53
  methodology 347–9
  neuropathology 75
  progress 350–2
  ring chromosome 20, 310–11, 492–3
Global Campaign against Epilepsy 579–80
glutamate 40–2
glutamate metabotropic receptors 42, 357
glutamatergic neurotransmission 255, 355
Goldman constant field flux 24
gradients, ion 23
grey matter 8, 20, 505

Index

guidelines 305–6
  childhood epilepsy 480, 481
  management of epilepsy 478
  new AEDs 381
  psychotropic drugs 535
guilt 536
gyri 8
gyrus dentatus 38

haemorrhage mechanisms 501–2
half-life, AEDs 359
hamartomas, hypothalamic 444–6, 500
  and epilepsy 498, **499**
happiness 513. *See also* behavioural treatment
head injury 494–5, 496
  chronic epileptic brain damage 66
  and learning disability/epilepsy 489
  neuropathology 72
  risk factors for seizures 332
Health and Safety at Work Act 549, 588
health economics 581–4
health-related quality of life (HRQOL) 538–42, 570
hemiclonic seizures 111
hemimegalencephaly 67–8
hemispherectomy/hemispherotomy 75, 420, 432–3
hemispheres, cerebral 8–10, **13**. *See also* lateralization
hepatic encephalography 101–2, **103**, 213–14
herpes simplex encephalitis 99, **100**, 213–16
hippocampus
  anatomy/connections 10, 37–9
  chronic epileptic brain damage, 65–6
  epileptogenesis in vitro 56–7
  histochemistry 35, **65**–**7**, **69**, **74**
historical contexts 1–2, 5
  employment 548
  ILAE 578–9
  personality 520
  psychiatry of epilepsy 3–4
  residential care/specialist centres 561
  social disorders 4
  temporal lobe epilepsy 168
  vascular/electromagnetic theories 2–3
history-taking 6, 276–8, 280
  cardiovascular syndromes simulating epilepsy 285
  childhood epilepsy 338
  preoperative assessment 421
Hughlings Jackson, J. 2–3, 168, 578

Human Genome Project 346
Huntington's disease 183
hydantoins 376
hydrogen nuclei 240, **241**
hyper-connection syndrome 521
hyperekplexia 294–5, 465
hyperkinetic seizures 174
hypermotor seizures 108, 174
hyperpolarization 24, **25**
hyperpolarizing inward rectification 29
hypersynchrony, hippocampal 56
hypertension 330–1
hyperventilation 77, 123, **125**
hypnic jerks 289
hypocalcaemia 283
hypoglycaemia 283, 339
hypothalamic hamartomas. *See* hamartomas, hypothalamic
hypoxic brain damage 97, **98**, 213–14, 283
hypsarrhythmia **338**, 150–1

iatrogenic damage, AEDs 66
ictal EEG 124–30, **134**, 175
  benign epilepsy of childhood with centrotemporal spikes 132, **133**–**4**
  frontal lobe epilepsy 175
  infantile spasms/West syndrome 200–3
  preoperative assessment 423
  temporal lobe epilepsy 170–1
idiopathic childhood occipital epilepsy of Gastaut 200
idiopathic focal epilepsies 116, 158–62
  EEG 208–11
  prognosis 333–4
idiopathic generalized epilepsies 116, 163–7
  EEG 204–10
  myoclonus, epileptic 183–4
  prognosis 333–4
idiopathic (primary) epilepsy
  acute models 48–9
  chronic models 50–1
  history 2
  ILAE classification 131
idiopathic photosensitive occipital epilepsy 131, 134, 463
ILAE (International League Against Epilepsy)
  global campaign against epilepsy 579–80
  history 578–9
  neuroimaging guidelines 237
  See also classification
immunohistochemistry 35–6

in vitro experimental models 31–3, 47. *See also* epileptogenesis in vitro
in vivo experimental techniques/models 34, 47
incidence of epilepsy 329–30
inclusion criteria, clinical trials 369
independence, lifestyle 589
independent component analysis 270
indirect brain stimulation 436
indirect costs 581
individualized therapeutic concentrations 361–2
individual variations, reactions to AEDs 358
inequality/equality 549, 574–5
infantile spasms 150–2
  case scenarios 309
  EEG 200–3
  epidemiology **338**
  prognosis 333–4
infants, epidemiology of epilepsy 337
infection, CNS 213–16
information sources, unit costs 582–3
inhibitory neurons 20
inhibitory neurotransmission 42–5
  epileptogenesis 54
  experimental models 47
inhibitory postsynaptic potentials 25
insula 8, 111
intangible costs 581
intelligence 411, 521
intensive monitoring. *See* video-EEG monitoring
intention-to-treat analyses 369
interictal EEG 52–124, **125**, 130
  frontal lobe epilepsy 175
  infantile spasms/West syndrome 200–3
  preoperative assessment 422–3
  temporal lobe epilepsy 170–1
International Bureau for Epilepsy 579–80
international classifications 3, 107
International League Against Epilepsy. *See* ILAE
interneurons 20
interventions. *See* management interventions
intracellular electrodes 32
intracranial EEG recordings 34, 423–5
  complications 426
  indications 425–6
  interpretation 426–7
intractable epilepsy, new AEDs 381
intraoperative (acute) electrocorticography **445**, 447–50
inverse problem 269

599

Index

inversion recovery sequences 301
investigations, adult epilepsy 299, **300-1**, 303
   neuropsychological evaluation 410-12
   psychogenic non-epileptic seizures 313-16
   single seizures 336
inward-rectifying potassium channels 28-9
ion channels 22
ionic currents 273
irreversible side effects, AEDs 539
ischaemia mechanisms 501
isolated brain laboratory studies 31-2

Janz syndrome. *See* juvenile myoclonic epilepsy
Jeavons' syndrome 112, 140, **165**, 166
jerks (generalized myoclonic seizures) 112
joined-up primary-secondary care approach 572-5
Joint Epilepsy Council 564-5
juvenile absence epilepsy 131-2, 135-6, 164, **165**, 200
juvenile Gaucher disease 187
juvenile myoclonic epilepsy (Janz syndrome) 131-2, 136-8, 161, **164-5**
   EEG 200, 208-10
   genetic defects 44
   lifestyle 590
JZP-4 397

kainate receptors 41, 356
ketogenic diet 138, 154, 456-7
kindling, experimental models 49, **50**
King's College Hospital, London 315-16, 452-4
knowledge/understanding of epilepsy 572-4, 577, 593. *See also* public education
Kojewnikow syndrome (chronic progressive epilepsia partialis continua of childhood) 131, 134-5, 333-4

L calcium channels 28
laboratory studies 31-6
   photosensitivity 461-2
   See also experimental models; neuropathology
lacosamide 364, 382, 387
Lafora body disease 73, 185
laminar necrosis 64
lamotrigine 364, 377-8, 383, 389, 404, 488

Landau-Kleffner syndrome (acquired epileptic aphasia) 131-2, 140, 333-4, 339
language disturbances
   clinical neuropsychological evaluation **411**
   functional anatomy 12-13
   lateralization 12-14, **246**, 261-2
   location, fMRI **246**
   terminology 108
   Wada test 415
late infantile neuronal ceroid lipofuscinosis 187
late-onset occipital epilepsy (Gastaut type) 131-4
lateral temporal lobe epilepsy 170
lateralization, cerebral hemispheres
   functional MRI **246**
   language function 12-14, 261-2, 415
   memory function 415-16
   preoperative assessment 421
laughing (gelastic) seizures 110, 444
law 585-6. *See also* Disability Discrimination Act; Health and Safety at Work Act
layers of cortex 20
lead toxicity 213-14
learning disability 483-5, 489-91
legal responsibility 585-6. *See also* Disability Discrimination Act; Health and Safety at Work Act
legislation, UK 570
Lennox-Gastaut syndrome 131-2, 138, **139**, 153-4, 493
   EEG 200, 204-6
   prognosis 333-4
lesionectomy 431-2
lesions
   classification 114
   epileptogenic 67
   experimental studies 11-12, 34
   stereotactic 74
   See also neuropathology of epilepsy
Leskell Gamma Knife 436, 445
levetiracetam 364, 383, 389, 404, 487
lifestyle 589-90
   AEDs withdrawal 401-2
   avoiding accidental deaths 341
   and prognosis 335-6
ligand-gated ion channels 353-7
limbic system 10, 13-14
linkage analysis 347-8
lissencephaly 67-8, 504
Liverpool Quality Battery 541
local drug application 34
localization, source 269-72, 283-4, 417-18, 421, 427

long-term epilepsy, joined-up primary-secondary care approach 573-4
long-term extension studies, AEDs 370
long-term placements, residential care/specialist centres 561-2
low-dose controls, AEDs 372

macrocephaly 67-8
magnetic resonance imaging. *See* MRI
magnetic source imaging 269. *See also* source localization
magnetoencephalography 273-5, 301-2
malformations of cortical development 506-9
   PET **255**
   See also neurones migration abnormalities
malignant migrating partial seizures in infancy 200, **205**, 518
malingering 529
management interventions 409
   anxiety
   behavioural 513-14, 527-8
   catamenial seizures 477
   cerebrovascular disease 503
   childhood epilepsy 337, 478-82
   depression 515-16
   dissociative seizures 530-1
   emergency treatment 409
   hamartomas, hypothalamic 444
   health-related quality of life measures 539-40
   learning disability 484-5
   photosensitivity 463
   and prognosis 333
   seizures 406-7
   single seizures 336
   status epilepticus 471-2
   See also AEDs; emergency treatment; ketogenic diet; surgery; treatment gaps
manic episodes, definitions 515
marriage 545-6
maximal electroshock model 367
measures, health-related quality of life 540-1
medial/mesial temporal lobe epilepsy 169
medical history-taking. *See* history-taking; physical examination
medication. *See* AEDs; antidepressant medication; antipsychotic medication; mood stabilizers; psychotropic drugs
MEG (magnetoencephalography) 273-5, 301-2

Index

megalencephaly 67–8
membranes, neuronal 17, **28**
  electrophysiology 22, 27–9
  laboratory studies 31
  potentials 22
  receptors 19
  resting behaviour 22–3
memory function
  clinical evaluation 411
  fMRI 246–7
  parahippocampal gyrus 262–3
  surgical outcomes 434
  Wada test 415–16
Mendel, Gregor 345
Mendelian epilepsies 347–8, 350, **351**
meningitis, bacterial 330–1
mercury toxicity 213–14
mesial temporal epilepsy 434
mesial temporal memory function 246–7
mesial temporal sclerosis 168
  chronic epileptic brain damage 65–6
  surgical techniques **431**
meta-analyses, new AEDs 381
metabolic abnormalities 283, 300, 306–7, 337
metabolic interactions, AEDs 385–6, 388–7
microcephaly 67–8
microdialysis 34
midazolam 378, 409
migraine and epilepsy 293–5
migration abnormalities, neuronal 504–5
mild malformation of cortical development 68
minimum norm solution 270
misdiagnosis, psychogenic non-epileptic seizures 313.
  See also differential diagnosis
mitochondrial myopathy with ragged red fibres 74, 187
molecular genetics. See genetics
molecular level epileptogenesis in vitro 53–4
molecular techniques of diagnosis 36
monitoring. See video-EEG monitoring
monotherapy/polytherapy 372, 392, **393**, 394–5
montages, electroencephalography 78
mood stabilizers 533, **534**
mood state
  clinical evaluation 411
  neuropsychological effects of AEDs 414

mortality in epilepsy 340–3.
  See also Epilepsy Bereaved; sudden unexpected death
mossy fibres 39
motor cortex 9, 10–11, 246
motor skills, clinical neuropsychological evaluation **411**
mouth-to-mouth resuscitation 408
movement artefacts, fMRI 245
movement disorders 289, 294–5
MR-compatible EEG recording systems 267
MRI (magnetic resonance imaging) 224, **225–6**, 240
  image formation 241–2
  management of childhood epilepsy 305–6
  negatives 256
  newly diagnosed/chronic epilepsy 300–1
  preoperative assessment 421–2
  structural imaging 226–36, **227–36**
  temporal lobe epilepsy 170
  volumetric 242
  See also DTI; functional MRI; neuroimaging; NMR
MRS (magnetic resonance spectroscopy) 240, 242–3
multi-axial classification **308**
multiple sclerosis 294, 330–1
multiple sleep latency test 288
multiple subpial transactions (MST) 418, 436
Munchausen's syndrome 529
muscarine-sensitive potassium currents 28–9
musicogenic epilepsy 464–5
myoclonic-astatic epilepsy. See Doose syndrome
myoclonus, epileptic 181–4
  absence seizures 112, 131, 140, 165–6
  focal seizures 111
  generalized myoclonic seizures 112
  idiopathic generalized epilepsies 160, 183–4
  management 407
  negative 112, 181
  neuropathology 73–4
  progressive 183, 185–6, 188
  variations **113**, 116

N calcium channels 28
narcolepsy 283, 288–9, 465
nasal midazolam 378, 409
National Epilepsy Week 567

National Institute for Health and Clinical Excellence, neuroimaging guidelines 237
National Sentinel Clinical Audit of Epilepsy-related Death 567
National Society for Epilepsy (NSE) 564
natural history of epilepsy 333
negative myoclonus 112, 181
neonatal convulsions, prognosis 333–4
neonatal myoclonic encephalopathy 152, 197–8
neonatal seizures 142–6, **147–8**, 149
  EEG 197–9
Nernst equation 24
network level brain slices 55–7
neurocardiogenic syncope 286
neurochemistry, AEDs 353–7
neurochemistry/receptor pharmacology 17–21
neurodegenerative conditions presenting with epilepsy **307**
neuroimaging 224, **225–6**
  indications 237–9
  management role 305–6
  preoperative assessment 421–2
  See also CT; DTI; MEG; MRI; MRS; PET; SPECT
neurological disease 297–9
neuromodulators 21
neuronal body 17
neuronal ceroid lipofuscinoses 220, **221**
neurones
  anatomy, 17–20
  inhibitory 20
  laboratory studies 31
  layers of cortex 20
  migration abnormalities 504–5
  neurochemistry/receptor pharmacology 19–20
  thalamic 55
neuropathology of epilepsy 35, 64, 75
  chronic epileptic brain damage 64–6
  electron microscopy 36
  febrile convulsions 71–2
  genetics 75
  histochemistry 35, **69**, 74
  immunohistochemistry 35–6
  molecular/genetic techniques 36
  myoclonic epilepsy 73–4
  neurosurgery 58, 75
  Rasmussen's encephalitis 71–2
  secondary neuropathological changes 64–7
  status epilepticus 64
  surgical specimens, handling 35
  symptomatic epilepsy 67–71
  trauma **66**, 72
  tumours 72–3

601

Index

neurophysiology of epilepsy 304–5, 484
neuropsychiatric/neuropsychological assessment 410–12, 421–2, 427
neuropsychological effects of AEDs 413–14
neurosurgery. *See* surgery
neurotransmission 40–5
new-onset epilepsy
    joined-up primary–secondary care approach 572–3
    new AEDs 381
NHS 558. *See also* primary care
NICE guidelines 305–6, 381, 478, 481
NMDA receptors 40–1, 53–4, 356–7
NMR (nuclear magnetic resonance) 240, 243
    basic principles 240–2
    volumetric MRI (VMRI) 242
    See also MRI; MRS
non-cerebral transients 82–4
non-epilepsy seizures 339
non-epileptic attack disorder 297
non-linear source localization 269–70
non-Mendelian epilepsies 348–51
novel designs, clinical trials 372
NREM (non-rapid eye movement) sleep 287–9
nuclear spin 240
nuclei, cerebral 8

occipital lobe epilepsies **159**, 163, 177–80
    and migraine 294
occipital lobe seizures 111
ohmic currents 273
Ohtahara syndrome 152, 197
old age 486–8
olfactory stimuli, reflex epilepsy 459
operant conditioning
operculum 8
opiate neurotransmission 253–4
optical recording 33
organizations/support services 569–71
    disability 570–1
    employment 552
    See also charities
orthodromic stimulation 33
orthostatic control, disorders of 296
oscillating currents, thalamic relay neurons 50, 54–5
osteoporosis 539
over-determined source localization 269–70
oxcarbazepine
    behavioural effects 404
    pharmacological interactions 389
    selected features 383
    therapeutic drug monitoring 364

P calcium channels 28
pachygyria 67–8
paediatrics. *See* childhood/adolescent epilepsy syndromes
Panayiotopoulos syndrome (early-onset benign occipital epilepsy) 131–3, **159**, 160, 309–10
    EEG 209–11
panic disorder 290–1
parahippocampal gyrus 262–3
paraldehyde, rectal 378, 408–9
parallel-group studies, clinical trials 370
parents with epilepsy 547
parietal association cortex lesion studies 11–12
parietal lobe epilepsy, 177–80
parietal seizures, classification 111
Parliamentary All Party Group on Epilepsy 567
paroxysmal abnormalities
    ataxia/tremor 294
    interictal EEG 119–22
    photoparoxysmal responses 122–3
paroxysmal depolarizing shift **28**, 29, 52, 55, **56**
paroxysmal kinesigenic choreoathetosis 294
paroxysmal non-kinesigenic choreoathetosis 294
partial epilepsy 47–9
partial seizures 107, 110, 522
passive movement 24
patch clamps 32
pattern electroretinography 219
pattern sensitive epilepsy 462
Penfield homunculus 11
per protocol (PP) analyses 369
perforant path 39
perforated patch clamps 32
perinatal brain damage 70
periventricular nodular heterotopia
persistent mood disorder, definitions 515
personality, and epilepsy 520–1
PET (positron emission tomography) 252, **253**–5, 256, 258
    management of childhood epilepsy 306
    preoperative assessment 422
petit mal seizures. *See* absence seizures
pharmacological interactions, AEDs 385, 390–1
    between different AEDs 386–90
    factors affecting significance 388–7
    mechanisms 385
    pharmacodynamic interactions 386

pharmacokinetic interactions 385–6, 535, 385
    specific drugs 386–90
pharmacology, receptor 17–21
pharmokinetics, AEDs 358–9, **360**, 366
    interactions 385–6, 535
phases, AED clinical trials 370–2
phasic inhibition, GABA receptors 44
phenobarbitone 364, 376, **388**, 389, 556
phenytoin 376
    elderly patients 487
    pharmacological interactions **388**, 389
    therapeutic drug monitoring 364
    treatment gap, developing world 556
photic stimulation 77
photoparoxysmal responses, interictal EEG 122–3
photosensitivity 461–3
    differential diagnosis 339
    lifestyle 590
    occipital epilepsy 131, 134, 463
physical abnormalities, association with epilepsy 278–9
physical examination, 278–80. *See also* history-taking
pilots' licences 554
politicizing disability 570–1
polymicrogyria 67–8
polytherapy//monotherapy 372, 392, **393**, 394–5
positional cloning 347
positron emission tomography. *See* PET
postanoxic encephalopathy 183
post-ictal phenomena
    aggression 524–5
    automatisms 524–5
    drowsiness 522
    psychosis 523, 525
postsynaptic potentials 24–5
potassium channels 28–9, 54, 354
potassium IH oscillating currents 50, 55
precession, NMR 240
precipitants, epilepsy 284, 459–61
preclinical trials, AEDs 367–8, 373
precocious puberty 444
pregabalin 364, 383, 389
pre-ictal states 110, 277, 515, 522
prejudice 543–4
preoperative assessment 430
    admission criteria 420
    contraindications for surgery 419
    DTI 263–4
    functional mapping 426

history-taking/physical examination 421
ictal EEG 423
indications for surgery/timing 419
interictal EEG 422–3
intracranial EEG 423–5
intracranial EEG complications 426
intracranial EEG indications 425–6
intracranial EEG interpretation 426–7
methods 420–1
misconceptions 427–8
neuroimaging 421–2
neuropsychiatric assessment 421
neuropsychology 422, 427
phased evaluation 427–9
residential care/specialist centres 562
seizure semiology 421
Wada test 423
prevalence
epilepsy 330
learning disability 489
prevention, sudden unexpected death in epileptics 593
primary care, role 557–60.
  See also joined-up primary–secondary care approach
primary motor cortex 9, 10–11, 246
primary parasomnias 298
primidone 365, 389
privacy, patient 536.
  See also confidentiality
prodromal symptoms 110, 277, 515, 522
prognosis, newly diagnosed/chronic epilepsy 332–4
investigations/management 336
after a single seizure 332, 335–6
specific syndromes 333–4
progressive myoclonus 183, 185–6, 188
progressive neuronal degeneration of childhood with liver disease (Alpers disease) 187
prolactin levels 282, **315–16**
proportional mortality 340
prospective cohort studies 330
protein binding, AEDs 361, 385
provoked (acute symptomatic) seizures 189, 190, 299
pseudo-seizures 297
psychiatric disorders associated with epilepsy 290, 292
  anxiety **518**
  co-morbidity 530
  differential diagnosis 290, 297
  effects of surgery 434, 532

history 3–4
other disorders 291–2
panic disorder 290–1
  See also psychoses
psychic symptoms 109–10
psychodynamic counselling 536–7
psychogenic non-epileptic seizures.
  See dissociative seizures
psychological impact of diagnosis/seizures, health-related quality of life 539
psychomotor seizures 110
psychoses of epilepsy 291, 522–3
  effects of AEDs 403, 404
  surgical outcomes 434, 532
psycho-social history of patient 278
psychotherapy, time-limited 536–7
psychotropic drugs 533–5
  See also mood state
puberty, precocious 444
public education 566–7, 568.
  See also knowledge/understanding of epilepsy
Purkinje cells 66
pyramidal cells 20, 48

Q calcium channels 28
Qualities and Outcomes Framework (QOF) 558, 574
quality of life 538–42, 570
Quality Of Life In Epilepsy Instruments (QOLIE) 541

race, and epilepsy 329
radial electrical currents 76
radiosurgery, stereotactic 436
Ramsay Hunt syndrome 74
randomization, clinical trials, AEDs 369
randomized clinical trials. *See* clinical trials
Rasmussen's encephalitis 134–5, 510–12
  neuropathology of epilepsy 71–2
  prognosis 333–4
reactive (induced) seizures 53, 189, 190, 299
reading epilepsy 466, **467**
reasonable adjustments, employment 550
receptor pharmacology 17–21
rectal benzodiazepine administration 378, 408–9
recurrent depressive disorder, definition 515.
  See also depression
recurrent inhibition, GABA system 44–5
reference ranges, AEDs 361–2, 366

reflex epilepsy 6, 459–60.
  See also audiogenic epilepsy; photosensitivity
reflex seizures 112–13
rehabilitation 410. *See also* joined-up primary–secondary care approach
relationships, and epilepsy 545.
  See also families of epilepsy sufferers; marriage
relative refractory period 26
relaxation, NMR 240–2
relaxation techniques
REM (rapid eye movement) sleep 287–8, 289
remission, spontaneous 333
renal excretion 386
Repertory Grid Assessments 541
research fundraising 569
resective neurosurgery 74, 417–18, 434–6, 444–5
residential care/specialist centres 561–3
resonance, NMR 240
resource use economics 581–2
respiratory syncope 297
responsibility, legal 585–6.
  See also Disability Discrimination Act; Health and Safety at Work Act
reticular reflex myoclonus 184
retigabine 397–8
retrospective cohort studies 330
Rett syndrome 493
rhythmic myoclonus 181
right-hand grip rule 273
ring chromosome 20, 310–11, 492–3
risk factors
  cerebrovascular disease 502
  depression in epilepsy 516
  epidemiology 330–1
  learning disability 483–4
  surgery 418
risk-taking lifestyles 589
rodent models 465. *See also* animal models
rolandic epilepsy 158–9, **160**, 294
rolandic fissure 8
rotarod test 367
rufinamide 383, 389–90

safinamide 385
sample size, clinical trials 369
sampling time, therapeutic drug monitoring 360–1
scales, health-related quality of life 540–1
schizencephaly 67–8

schizophrenia-like psychoses of
    epilepsy 291, 522–3.
    See also psychoses
school performance 547.
    See also learning disability
sclerosis, tuberous 70
secondarily generalized seizures
    50, 110
secondary parasomnias 298
seizure onset, terminology 108
seletracetam 398
self-image 543–6, 590
sensitivity analysis, health
    economics 508
sensory evoked potentials 221–2
sensory symptoms, focal seizures 109
septum nuclei 8
septum pellucidum 8
serotenergic neurotransmission 254
severe myoclonic epilepsy of infancy
    (Dravet syndrome) 157
    differential diagnosis 339
    EEG 200, 201–4
    prognosis 333–4
sexual functioning 513, 521, 545–6,
    590. See also behavioural
    treatment
shame 536
sharp electrode technique 32
sharp waves, EEG 96
short-term assessment, residential
    care/specialist centres 562
sialidosis 186
    side effects, AEDs **354**, 357, 401,
    539. See also behavioural effects
    of AEDs
signal aperture magnetometry **274**
simple partial seizures 109–10, 407
single-cell extracellular recordings 34
single-channel patch clamps 32
single-pulse electrical stimulation
    450, 452–4, 455
situation related seizures 53,
    189–90, 299
sleep deprivation 590
sleep disorders 283, 287–9
    differential diagnosis 298
    and learning disability 490
sleep physiology **15**
slice cultures 31, **47**, 50, 52, 55–7
social disorder, epilepsy as 4
sodium amytal test 61
sodium channels 27–8, 54, 157, 353–4
sodium valproate 137–8, 377
sodium–potassium currents 29
sodium–potassium pump 24
somatization 530
somatosensory cortex 9–11

somatosensory stimuli, reflex
    epilepsy 459
source localization 269–72, 283–4,
    417–18, 421, 427
South East Thames Paediatric Epilepsy
    Interest Group 480
space-occupying lesions 214
spasms 111–12
specialist centres 561–3
SPECT (single positron emission
    computed tomography) 248,
    250–1
    ictal **249**
    interictal 248
    investigations, adult epilepsy 301–2
    investigations, childhood
        epilepsy 306
    preoperative assessment 422
speech. See language
spikes. See action potentials
spike-related BOLD maps 267
spike-wave complexes 97
spontaneous remission 333
spontaneous seizures 53
SQUIDs (superconductive quantum
    interference devices) 273
staining techniques, histochemistry
    35, **65–7, 69**, 74
standardized mortality ratio 340
staring symptoms 110, 112
startle epilepsy 464
state-dependent learning disability 489
statistical thresholds, fMRI 245
status epilepticus 468–70, 473
    accidental deaths 341
    convulsive 472–3
    diagnosis/management 471–3
    EEG 102–5
    emergencies 339, 407–8
    experimental models 49, **50**
    and learning disability 489
    management 407
    non-convulsive 473
    randomized clinical trials 472
    secondary neuropathological
        changes 64
    treatment principles 471–2
stereotactic
    lesions 74
    radiosurgery 436
    thermocoagulation 445
stigma 526–7, 543–4. See also public
    education
stimuli, epilepsy 284, 459–61
stiripentol 390
stress 513
stroke. See cerebrovascular disease
structural imaging 226–36, **227–36**,
    301, 305–6

study designs
    clinical trials 370
    epidemiological 330
    functional MRI 245
    health economics 583
sub-acute sclerosing panencephalitis
    102, 213–16
subcortical structures 9, 15
subcutaneous pentylenetetrazol
    model 367
subdural electrodes 424–5
subpial resection 74
substance misuse 330–1
subthalamic nucleus stimulation 442
subtle seizures 308–10
sudden unexpected death in epileptics
    66–7, 341–2, 590, 592–3.
    See also Epilepsy Bereaved;
    mortality in epilepsy
suicides 341
sulci 8
superior longitudinal fasciculus 261–2
support groups 576–7, 593.
    See also organizations/support
    services
surgery 418, 434–7, 500, 417
    case scenarios, paediatric epilepsy
        308–9
    and epilepsy 498–9
    functional 418, 436
    neuropathology 58, **75**
    neuropsychological evaluation 410
    outcomes 434–6, 438–9
    paediatric 438–40
    psychiatric effects 532
    resective 417–18, 434–6
    specimen handling 35
    techniques **431–2**, 433
    temporal lobe epilepsy 172
    See also intraoperative
        electrocorticography;
        preoperative assessment
surround inhibition 20–1, 44–5
sylvian fissures 8
symptomatic focal epilepsy 116,
    333–4. See also frontal lobe
    epilepsy
symptomatic generalized epilepsy **116**,
    333–4
symptomatic (secondary) epilepsy
    history 2
    ILAE classification 131
    myoclonus, epileptic 183
    neuropathology 67–71
symptomatic seizures, acute 53, 189,
    190, 299
synaptic anatomy/physiology, 18–19
synaptic function 62

Index

synchronization, epileptogenesis in vitro 56
syncope
  cardiology assessment 299
  and cardiovascular syndromes 285–6
  differential diagnosis 296–7
  EEG 214
  neurocardiogenic 286
  treatment of 286

T calcium channels 28
T2000 398–9
talampanel 399
Task Force of the ILAE 118
teamwork. See joined-up primary–secondary care approach
telemetry 281, 284, 313–14, **315–16**
temporal lobe epilepsy 168, **171**, 173
  DTI 261–2
  memory impairment 262–3
temporal lobe seizures 110–11, **169**
temporal lobe surgery 74, 449–50
tension, nervous 513
teratogenic effects, AEDs 539
terminal remission, definition 332
tetanus toxin 49, **50**
thalamic
  clock theory 62
  hypothesis 62
  neurones **55**
  relay neurons 54–5
  stimulation 442, **443**
therapeutic drug monitoring 359–62, 363, 366
  specific drugs 362–6
therapeutic ranges, AEDs 361–2, 366
theta brain waves 81
thresholds, seizure 533–5
tiagabine 365, 383, 390, 404
tilt-table testing 286
time-limited psychotherapy 536–7
time trends, epidemiology of epilepsy 330
tiredness 513. See also behavioural treatment
tonabersat 399
tonic-clonic seizures 110–11

tonic inhibition, GABA receptors 44
tonic seizures 111, 407
topiramate 365, 383, 390, 404
toxic poisons, EEG applications 213–14
toxicity, AEDs 300, 375–6, 392–3
tractography 260, 261. See also DTI
trauma. See head injury
treatment. See management interventions
treatment gaps
  developing world 555
  NHS 558
triggers, epilepsy 284, 459–61
tuberous sclerosis 67–8, 70, 181
Tullio's phenomenon 465
tumours 330–1, 500
  case scenarios, paediatric 308–9
  EEG 97
  and epilepsy, 497–9
  neuropathology 72–3
  PET 256
twilight states 522
2-deoxy-D-glucose 396–7
typical absence seizures 160, **164**

UK
  disability legislation 570
  primary care 557–60. See also joined-up primary–secondary care approach
under-determined source localization 270–1
unilateral seizures, history 2
unit costs 582–3
unusual behaviours 534, 288–9
Unverricht-Lundborg disease 74, 185
uraemia 213–14

vagus nerve stimulation 436, 439, 441
valproic acid 365, **388**, 390, 487
valrocemide 399–400
variations, inter-individual 358
vascular malformations 70–1
vascular theories, history of epilepsy 2–3
vasculo-degenerative dementia 213
vestibular stimuli, reflex epilepsy 459

video games, photosensitivity 462
video-EEG monitoring (video-telemetry) 281, 284, 313–14, **315–16**
vigabatrin 135, 220–1, 365–6, 383, 390, 404
visual evoked cortical potentials 217–21
visual field defects 263–4
visual stimuli 459, 462–3. See also photosensitivity
visuospatial abilities, clinical neuropsychological evaluation 411
VMRI (volumetric MRI) 242
voltage clamp recordings 33
voltage-gated ion channels 22, 47–8, 353–7. See also calcium ion channels; potassium channels; sodium channels
voltage-gated K^+ currents 47–8
voltage-sensitive sodium channels 54
volumetric acquisition 301
volumetric MRI 242

Wada test 61, 415–16, 423
warning symptoms 110, 277, 515, 522
water safety 589
websites
  Epilepsy Action 564
  Epilepsy Bereaved 564
  Joint Epilepsy Council 564–5
  National Society for Epilepsy 564
  new AEDs 382
  pilots' licences 554
  relevant organizations 552
Wernicke's area 10
West syndrome 150–2, 200–3, 333–4
white matter 8, 20, 259
whole-cell patch clamps 32
withdrawal, AED 401–2
witnesses 276, 290, 291, 296–8
women with epilepsy 474–7, 493. See also gender
World Health Organization 3, 579–80

YKP3089 400

zonisamide 366, 383, 390, 404